£2oo

COMPLICATIONS OF UROLOGIC SURGERY

Prevention and Management

FOURTH EDITION

Samir S. Taneja, MD
The James M. Neissa and Janet Riha Neissa Associate Professor of Urologic Oncology
Director
Division of Urologic Oncology
Department of Urology and New York University Cancer Institute
New York University Langone Medical Center
New York, New York

SAUNDERS

ELSEVIER

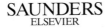

SAUNDERS
ELSEVIER

1600 John F. Kennedy Boulevard
Suite 1800
Philadelphia, PA 19103-2899

COMPLICATIONS OF UROLOGIC SURGERY   ISBN: 978-1-4160-4572-4

Library of Congress Cataloging-in-Publication Data

Complications of urologic surgery: prevention and management / editor, Samir S. Taneja.—4th ed.
     p. ; cm.
  Revised edition of Complications of urologic surgery / edited by Samir S. Taneja, Robert B. Smith and Richard M. Ehrlich. 2001.
  Includes bibliographical references and index.
  ISBN 978-1-4160-4572-4 (alk. paper)
  1. Genitourinary organs–Surgery–Complications. I. Taneja, Samir S.
  [DNLM: 1. Urologic Surgical Procedures, Male. 2. Postoperative Complications–prevention & control. 3. Urinary Tract–surgery. WJ 168 C737 2010]
  RD571.C65 2010
  617.4'601–dc22

                                       2009018387

Acquisitions Editor: Stefanie Jewell-Thomas
Associate Developmental Editor: Martha Limbach
Publishing Services Manager: Tina Rebane
Senior Project Manager: Amy L. Cannon
Design Director: Steven Stave

Printed in China

Last digit is the print number: 9 8 7 6 5 4 3 2 1

Working together to grow
libraries in developing countries

www.elsevier.com | www.bookaid.org | www.sabre.org

ELSEVIER   BOOK AID International   Sabre Foundation

This book is dedicated to the memory of my dear friend and colleague, John P. Stein. When he passed last year, John left a void in the community of urologic oncology, particularly among those of us in the generation of his contemporaries. John's optimism and energy for life charismatically drew us to him. The fact that so many were deeply affected by his passing coupled with his uncanny ability to make each of us feel special and important reflects his impact.

John left an eternal legacy through his unending pursuit of perfection and excellence in the care of patients. Despite his tremendous academic accomplishments, his zeal for scientific inquiry, and his global outreach as an educator, John always placed the care and outcome of his patients first. No matter how good the outcome, he always felt it could and would be made better through his efforts. In this regard, John will always live on as an example to all of us and stands as a wonderful symbol of the spirit of this text.

On a personal level, I would like to offer thanks for the love and support given to me by my own family, Uttama, Sorab, and Sabina. The family of every surgeon makes sacrifices through time lost and hours waiting. Without them, the time lost in our work would have little meaning. Through my wife Uttama's guiding hand, I find life's balance and meaning, and through the eyes of my children, Sorab and Sabina, I find its promise and discovery. I thank all three of them for the sacrifices they made in the preparation of this text.

SST

PREFACE

Regardless of the number of years in practice or cases performed, the prevention and management of surgical complications remain primary challenges for any operating surgeon. Although directly impacted by surgical technique, patient selection, and underlying disease processes, some complications inevitably arise even in the perfect candidate receiving the perfect operation. Despite this, the surgeon must continue throughout his or her career to make every effort to reduce the possibility of complication through careful patient selection, methodical preoperative patient optimization, and careful attention to technique.

First and foremost, complications take a tremendous emotional and physical toll on our patients, and surgeons must remember this when confronted with a complication. For the patient, the process of surgery is one in which control is given completely to the surgeon. The uncertainty of outcome, the loss of control, and the fear of mortality are tremendously stressful for the patient even in the setting of an uncomplicated surgery. When complications arise, these stresses are magnified and patients and their families are often confused, depressed, or angry. Careful, calm, and comprehensive communication are essential to enable them to understand the nature of the complication, its probable causes, and the planned management. Discussing potential outcomes, concerns going forward, and specific benchmarks for improvement can allow the patient a structured process to mentally cope with the situation. Patients with complications often fear the surgeon will abandon them, and reassurance can go a long way toward maintaining a good relationship.

Physical concerns in the setting of complications relate to the patient's ability to tolerate the stresses and the relative risk of prolonged hospitalization. In patients with pre-existing comorbid conditions, careful attention to management of underlying disease processes, particularly those influencing recovery, will help in avoiding secondary complications. Maintaining nutrition, preventing infection, and carefully monitoring fluids and electrolytes are fundamental surgical principles that directly affect recovery from most intra-abdomenal and intrathoracic surgeries but that can be forgotten in the heat of a stressful complication. Although not all patients recover from complications, the surgeon's primary goal must be to ensure that the patient's odds of recovery are optimized by optimizing his or her condition.

The balance between action and inaction is a difficult one for surgeons. An underlying desire to make a complication go away often leads to the decision to act quickly through intervention or reoperation. Although sometimes indicated, quick decisions to intervene often result in worsening of the problem or development of secondary complications. At the time of complication, careful diagnostic evaluation to fully understand its nature and extent are critically important before any action is taken. Although stressful for both the patient and surgeon, sometimes waiting it out is the best course of action.

It is the intent of this fourth edition of *Complications of Urologic Surgery: Prevention and Management* to provide both general and specific guidelines for surgeons in the management of most common, and many uncommon, urologic surgery complications. The response to the third edition of the book has been uniformly positive with many commenting on its tremendous utility in preparing for both a urologic career and day to day practice. Using this helpful feedback I have structured the book's fourth edition. Over the 10 years since I began constructing the third edition, urologic surgery has changed dramatically. The rapid growth and adoption of minimally invasive techniques and surgical technologies have altered the way we perform most common procedures and, in doing so, have changed the way we train urologists in residency. As a direct result, urologists less frequently perform open surgery and conventional transurethral procedures. Understanding complications of these procedures is perhaps of *greater* importance now because contemporary urologists have less experience with these procedures.

As such, in this fourth edition I have tried to balance the content between contemporary and classic techniques by including more chapters that specifically focus on minimally invasive procedures, laparoscopic surgery, and robotic surgery. Open surgical techniques remain a focus of the book with inclusion of additional chapters on specific procedures such as partial nephrectomy, orthotopic neobladder, and transurethral bladder tumor resection. Classic chapters from the third edition such as transurethral resection of the prostate and perineal prostatectomy have been re-printed as little could be added to the work of the previous authors.

It is my sincere hope that the additional chapters, along with the online case studies and multiple-choice questions, offer expanded utility for the book and a continued positive response among readers in the decade to come.

Samir S. Taneja MD
June 2009

LIST OF CONTRIBUTORS

William J. Aronson, MD
Clinical Professor, Department of Urology, David
  Geffen School of Medicine, University of California–
  Los Angeles, Los Angeles, California
  Complications of Ureteral Surgery

Dean G. Assimos, MD
Professor of Surgical Sciences, Department of Urology,
  Wake Forest University School of Medicine,
  Winston-Salem, North Carolina
  Complications of Extracorporeal Shock Wave Lithotripsy

Katie N. Ballert, MD
Fellow, Department of Urology, New York University
  School of Medicine, New York, New York
  Complications of Surgery for Male Incontinence

Gaurav Bandi, MD
Assistant Professor, Department of Urology, Jefferson
  Medical College, Thomas Jefferson University,
  Philadelphia, Pennsylvania
  Complications of Lasers in Urologic Surgery

Lionel L. Bañez, MD
Assistant Professor of Surgery, Division of Urological
  Surgery and The Duke Prostate Center, Department
  of Surgery, Duke University Medical Center,
  Durham, North Carolina
  Impact of Host Factors and Comorbid Conditions

Yagil Barazani, MD
Resident, Department of Urology, Beth Israel Medical
  Center, New York, New York
  Complications of Pediatric Laparoscopy

Laurence S. Baskin, MD
Professor and Chief, Pediatric Urology, University of
  California–San Francisco Children's Hospital, San
  Francisco, California
  Complications of Surgery for Disorders of Sex Development

Aaron P. Bayne, MD
Pediatric Urology Fellow, Scott Department of
  Urology, Baylor College of Medicine; Urology
  Service, Texas Children's Hospital, Houston, Texas
  *Complications of Adrenal Surgery; Complications of Hypospadias
  Repair*

Nelson E. Bennett, MD
Director, Sexual Medicine and Surgery, Institute of
  Urology, Lahey Clinic Medical Center, Burlington;
  Assistant Professor of Urology, Department of
  Urology, Tufts School of Medicine, Boston,
  Massachusetts
  *Complications of Surgery for Erectile Dysfunction and Peyronie's
  Disease*

David A. Berger, MD
Fellow in Urologic Oncology, Division of Urologic
  Surgery, Washington University School of Medicine,
  St. Louis, Missouri
  Complications of Radiation Therapy for Urologic Cancer

Bernard H. Bochner, MD
Attending Surgeon, Department of Surgery, Urology
  Service, Memorial Sloan-Kettering Cancer Center,
  New York, New York
  Complications of Lymphadenectomy

Donald R. Bodner, MD
Professor and Interim Chair, Department of Urology,
  Case Western Reserve University School of
  Medicine, Cleveland, Ohio
  Complications of Renal Stone Surgery

Stephan A. Boorjian, MD
Fellow in Urologic Oncology, Department of Urology,
  Mayo Clinic, Rochester, Minnesota
  Complications of the Incision and Patient Positioning

Steven B. Brandes, MD
Professor of Urologic Surgery, Division of Urologic
  Surgery, Washington University School of Medicine,
  St. Louis, Missouri
  Complications of Radiation Therapy for Urologic Cancer

Maurizio Buscarini, MD
Resident, Department of Urology, University of
  Southern California, Norris Comprehensive Cancer
  Center, Los Angeles, California
  Complications of Radical Cystectomy

Jeffrey A. Cadeddu, MD
Ralph C. Smith, MD, Distinguished Chair in
  Minimally Invasive Urologic Surgery; Professor,
  Department of Urology, University of Texas
  Southwestern Medical Center at Dallas, Dallas, Texas
  Complications of Renal Tissue Ablation

David Canes, MD
Assistant Professor of Urology, Tufts University
Medical School, Boston, Massachusetts
Complications of Renovascular Surgery

Bruce I. Carlin, MD
Former Assistant Professor of Urology, Washington
University School of Medicine, St. Louis, Missouri
Complications of Renal Stone Surgery

Sachiko T. Cochran, MD
Professor Emeritus, Division of Abdominal Imaging
and Cross Sectional Interventional Radiology, David
Geffen School of Medicine, University of California–
Los Angeles, Los Angeles, California
Complications of Therapeutic Radiologic Procedures

Tasha Cooke, MBBS, DM(Urol)
Urologist, The Cornwall Regional Hospital, St. James,
Jamaica
Pharmacologic Complications

Michael S. Cookson, MD
Professor, Department of Urologic Surgery, Vanderbilt
University Medical Center, Nashville, Tennessee
Complications of Orthotopic Neobladder

John M. Corman, MD
Medical Director, Virginia Mason Cancer Institute,
Virginia Mason Medical Center; Associate Clinical
Professor of Urology, University of Washington
School of Medicine, Seattle, Washington
Complications of Interstitial Seed Implantation

Rahul A. Desai, MD
Surgeon, Urology, The Polyclinic, Seattle, Washington
Complications of Extracorporeal Shock Wave Lithotripsy

Matthew D. Dunn, MD
Assistant Professor of Urology, Department of
Urology, Keck School of Medicine, University of
Southern California, Los Angeles, California
Complications of Continent Cutaneous Diversion

Jack S. Elder, MD
Clinical Professor of Urology, Case Western Reserve
School of Medicine, Cleveland, Ohio; Chief,
Department of Urology, Henry Ford Hospital;
Associate Director, Vattikuti Urology Institute,
Detroit, Michigan
Complications of Surgery for Posterior Urethral Valves

William J. Ellis, MD
Professor, Department of Urology, University of
Washington, Seattle, Washington
Complications of Simple Prostatectomy

Christopher P. Evans, MD
Professor and Chairman, Department of Urology,
University of California–Davis, Sacramento,
California
Complications of Nephrectomy

David Fenig, MD
Associate Director, Male Fertility and Sexuality,
Chesapeake Urology Associates, Baltimore, Maryland
*Complications of Surgery of the Testicle, Vas, Epididymis, and
Scrotum*

Neil E. Fleshner, FRCSC, MD, MPH
Chief of Urology, Princess Margaret Hospital,
University Health Network; Associate Professor,
University of Toronto, Toronto, Ontario, Canada
Complications of Hormonal Treatment for Prostate Cancer

Stephen J. Freedland, MD
Associate Professor of Urology and Pathology, Division
of Urological Surgery and The Duke Prostate Center,
Department of Surgery, Duke University Medical
Center, Durham, North Carolina
Impact of Host Factors and Comorbid Conditions

Andrew L. Freedman, MD
Director, Pediatric Urology, Minimally Invasive
Urology Institute, Cedars-Sinai Medical Center,
Los Angeles, California
Special Considerations in the Pediatric Patient

Rodrigo Frota, MD
Fellow, Glickman Urological Institute, Cleveland
Clinic, Cleveland, Ohio
Management of Vascular Complications

Gerhard J. Fuchs, MD
Medallion Chair in Minimally Invasive Urology;
Director, Minimally Invasive Urology Institute;
Vice Chairman, Department of Surgery, Cedars-Sinai
Medical Center, Los Angeles, California
Complications of Ureteroscopic Surgery

John P. Gearhart, MD
Professor and Chief of Pediatric Urology, Brady
Urological Institute, Johns Hopkins Medical
Institutions, Baltimore, Maryland
Complications of Exstrophy and Epispadias Repair

Joel Gelman, MD
Associate Clinical Professor, Department of Urology,
University of California, Irvine Medical Center,
Orange, California
Complications of Urethral Reconstruction

Scott M. Gilbert, MD, MS
Assistant Professor, Urologic Oncology, Department of
Urology, University of Florida College of Medicine,
Gainesville, Florida
*Complications Following Laparoscopic Robot-Assisted Radical
Prostatectomy*

David A. Ginsberg, MD
Associate Professor of Urology, Department of
Urology, Keck School of Medicine, University of
Southern California, Los Angeles; Chief of Urology,
Rancho Los Amigos National Rehabilitation Center,
Downey, California
Complications of Bladder Augmentation

Guilherme Godoy, MD
Fellow in Urologic Oncology, Bruce and Cynthia
Sherman Fellowship in Urologic Oncology, Division
of Urologic Oncology, Department of Urology, New
York University Langone Medical Center, New York,
New York
*Complications of Partial Nephrectomy; Complications of Radical
Retropubic Prostatectomy; Complications of Conduit Urinary
Diversion*

Sam D. Graham Jr, MD
Retired Professor and Chairman, Department of
Urology, Emory University, Atlanta, Georgia
Complications of Radical Perineal Prostatectomy

H. Albin Gritsch, MD
Surgical Director, Renal Transplantation, Kidney and
Kidney-Pancreas Transplantation Program,
Department of Surgery, University of California–Los
Angeles Medical Center; Associate Professor of
Urology, David Geffen School of Medicine,
University of California–Los Angeles, Los Angeles,
California
Complications of Renal Transplantation

Gregory R. Hanson, MD
Surgeon, Metro Urology, Maple Grove, Minnesota
Complications of Interstitial Seed Implantation

David J. Hernandez, MD
Assistant Professor, Division of Urology, University of
South Florida College of Medicine, Tampa, Florida
Complications of Exstrophy and Epispadias Repair

Oscar Joe Hines, MD
Professor of Surgery, Department of Surgery, David
Geffen School of Medicine, University of
California–Los Angeles, Los Angeles, California
Management of Bowel Complications

Susie N. Hong, MD
Cardiology Fellow, Division of Cardiology,
Department of Medicine, New York University
Medical Center, New York, New York
Cardiac Complications of Urologic Surgery

R. Alex Hsi, MD
Section Head, Radiation Oncology, Virginia Mason
Medical Center, Seattle, Washington; Adjunct
Assistant Professor, University of Pennsylvania
School of Medicine, Philadelphia, Pennsylvania
Complications of Interstitial Seed Implantation

George J. Huang, MD
Clinical Instructor, Department of Urology, Keck
School of Medicine, University of Southern
California, Los Angeles, California
Long-term Outcomes of Radical Prostatectomy

William C. Huang, MD
Assistant Professor, Department of Urology, New York
University, New York, New York
Pulmonary Complications of Urologic Surgery

Elias S. Hyams, MD
Resident Physician, Department of Urology, New York
University School of Medicine, New York, New York
*Complications of Minimally Invasive Reconstruction of the Upper
Urinary Tract*

Brian H. Irwin, MD
Assistant Professor of Surgery, Division of Urology,
University of Vermont College of Medicine,
Burlington, Vermont
Complications of Robotic Surgery

Niels-Erik B. Jacobsen, MD, FRCSC
Fellow, Urologic Oncology, Department of Urology,
Indiana University, Indianapolis, Indiana
Metabolic Complications of Urologic Surgery

Sudheer K. Jain, MD
Assistant Professor of Clinical Anesthesiology, New
York University Medical Center, New York, New
York
Anesthetic Complications in Urologic Surgery

Eric A. Jones, MD
Assistant Professor, Scott Department of Urology,
Baylor College of Medicine; Urology Service, Texas
Children's Hospital, Houston, Texas
Complications of Hypospadias Repair

Jamie A. Kanofsky, MD
Resident in Urology, Department of Urology, New
York University Langone Medical Center, New York,
New York
Complications of Conduit Urinary Diversion

Eric L. Kau, MD
Fellow in Endourology, Minimally Invasive Urology
Institute, Cedars-Sinai Medical Center, Los Angeles,
California
Complications of Ureteroscopic Surgery

Jeremy Kaufman, MD
Resident, Department of Urology, New York University
Langone Medical Center, New York, New York
Hematologic Complications

Melissa R. Kaufman, MD, PhD
Assistant Professor, Department of Urologic Surgery,
Vanderbilt University Medical Center, Nashville,
Tennessee
Complications of Orthotopic Neobladder

Adam S. Kibel, MD
Professor of Urologic Surgery, Division of Urologic Surgery, Washington University School of Medicine, Alvin J. Siteman Cancer Center, St. Louis, Missouri
Complications of Radiation Therapy for Urologic Cancer

Simon P. Kim, MD, MPH
Resident, Division of Urologic Health Services Research, Department of Urology, University of Michigan Medical Center, Ann Arbor, Michigan
Assessing Quality of Care in Urologic Surgery

Michael O. Koch, MD
Professor and Chairman, Department of Urology, Indiana University, Indianapolis, Indiana
Metabolic Complications of Urologic Surgery

Venkatesh Krishnamurthi, MD
Director, Kidney/Pancreas Transplant Program, Glickman Urological Institute, Cleveland Clinic, Cleveland, Ohio
Management of Vascular Complications

William Lea, MD
Resident, Department of Surgery, Indiana University School of Medicine, Indianapolis, Indiana
Management of Urinary Fistulas

Richard Lee, MD
Urology Resident, Weill Medical College of Cornell University, New York, New York
Complications of Minimally Invasive Procedures for Benign Prostatic Hyperplasia

Bradley C. Leibovich, MD
Associate Professor, Department of Urology, Mayo Clinic, Rochester, Minnesota
Complications of the Incision and Patient Positioning

Steven E. Lerman, MD
Associate Professor of Urology, Department of Urology, David Geffen School of Medicine, University of California–Los Angeles, Los Angeles, California
Complications of Pediatric Laparoscopy

John A. Libertino, MD
Chairman, Institute of Urology, Lahey Clinic, Burlington; Professor of Urology, Tufts University Medical School, Boston, Massachusetts
Complications of Renovascular Surgery

Daniel W. Lin, MD
Associate Professor and Director of Urologic Oncology, Department of Urology, University of Washington/ Seattle Cancer Care Alliance; Attending Physician, Veterans Administration Puget Sound Health Care System, Seattle, Washington
Toxicities of Chemotherapy for Genitourinary Malignancies

Michael Lipkin, MD
Resident, Department of Urology, New York University Langone Medical Center, New York, New York
Complications of Percutaneous Renal Surgery

Surena F. Matin, MD
Associate Professor, University of Texas M. D. Anderson Cancer Center, Houston, Texas
Special Considerations in Laparoscopy

Jeff M. Michalski, MD
Professor of Radiation Oncology, Division of Radiation Oncology, Washington University School of Medicine, Alvin J. Siteman Cancer Center, St. Louis, Missouri
Complications of Radiation Therapy for Urologic Cancer

Kiarash Michel, MD
Urologist, Cedars-Sinai Medical Center, Los Angeles, California
Complications of Transurethral Resection of the Prostate

Rosalia Misseri, MD
Assistant Professor, Pediatric Urology, James Whitcomb Riley Hospital for Children, Indiana University School of Medicine, Indianapolis, Indiana
Complications of Ureteral Reimplantation, Antireflux Surgery, and Megaureter Repair

Bruce Montgomery, MD
Associate Professor, Department of Medicine, University of Washington/Seattle Cancer Care Alliance; Attending Physician, Veterans Administration Puget Sound Health Care System, Seattle, Washington
Toxicities of Chemotherapy for Genitourinary Malignancies

Patrick W. Mufarrij, MD
Chief Resident, Department of Urology, New York University, New York, New York
Pulmonary Complications of Urologic Surgery

John P. Mulhall, MD
Director, Male Sexual and Reproductive Medicine Program, Urology Service, Department of Surgery, Memorial Sloan-Kettering Cancer Center, New York, New York
Complications of Surgery for Erectile Dysfunction and Peyronie's Disease

Stephen Y. Nakada, MD
Professor and Chairman, Division of Urology, Department of Surgery, University of Wisconsin School of Medicine and Public Health, Madison, Wisconsin
Complications of Lasers in Urologic Surgery

Mischel G. Neill, BHB, MBChB, FRACS
Consultant Urologist, North Shore Hospital, Auckland, New Zealand
Complications of Hormonal Treatment for Prostate Cancer

Eric C. Nelson, MD
Clinical Research Fellow, Department of Urology, University of California–Davis, Sacramento, California
Complications of Nephrectomy

Christopher S. Ng, MD
Attending, Minimally Invasive Urology Institute, Cedars-Sinai Medical Center, Los Angeles, California
Complications of Ureteroscopic Surgery

Alan M. Nieder, MD
Associate Professor, Division of Urology, Columbia University, Mount Sinai Medical Center, Miami Beach, Florida
Pharmacologic Complications

Victor W. Nitti, MD
Professor and Vice Chairman, Department of Urology, New York University School of Medicine, New York, New York
Complications of Surgery for Male Incontinence

Rebecca L. O'Malley, MD
Resident in Urology, Division of Urologic Oncology, Department of Urology, New York University Langone Medical Center, New York, New York
Complications of Partial Nephrectomy

Priya Padmanabhan, MD, MPH
Instructor, Department of Urologic Surgery, Vanderbilt University School of Medicine, Nashville, Tennessee
Management of Urinary Fistulas

Michael Paik, MD
Urologist, Private Practice, Northwest Community Hospital, Arlington Heights, Illinois
Complications of Renal Stone Surgery

Ganesh S. Palapattu, MD
Assistant Professor of Urology, Pathology, and Oncology, University of Rochester School of Medicine, Rochester, New York
Complications of Transurethral Resection of Bladder Tumors

Erik Pasin, MD
Resident, Department of Urology, University of Southern California, Norris Comprehensive Cancer Center, Los Angeles, California
Complications of Radical Cystectomy

David F. Penson, MD, MPH
Professor of Urology, Vanderbilt University, Nashville, Tennessee
Long-term Outcomes of Radical Prostatectomy

Phuong M. Pham, MD
Surgical Resident, Department of Surgery, David Geffen School of Medicine, University of California–Los Angeles, Los Angeles, California
Management of Bowel Complications

Lee Ponsky, MD
Assistant Professor, Case Western Reserve University, Cleveland, Ohio
Special Considerations in Laparoscopy

Steven S. Raman, MD
Associate Professor of Radiology, Division of Abdominal Imaging and Cross Sectional Interventional Radiology, David Geffen School of Medicine, University of California–Los Angeles; Director, Abdominal Imaging Fellowship, Radiological Sciences, University of California–Los Angeles, Los Angeles, California
Complications of Therapeutic Radiologic Procedures

Martin I. Resnick, MD†
Former Chair, Department of Urology, Case Western Reserve University School of Medicine, Cleveland, Ohio
Complications of Renal Stone Surgery

Polina Reyblat, MD
Urology Resident, Department of Urology, Keck School of Medicine, University of Southern California, Los Angeles, California
Complications of Bladder Augmentation

Richard C. Rink, MD
Professor and Chief, Pediatric Urology, James Whitcomb Riley Hospital for Children, Indiana University School of Medicine, Indianapolis, Indiana
Complications of Ureteral Reimplantation, Antireflux Surgery, and Megaureter Repair

Eric S. Rovner, MD
Professor of Urology, Department of Urology, Medical University of South Carolina, Charleston, South Carolina
Complications of Female Incontinence Surgery

Rajiv Saini, MD
Clinical Assistant Professor of Urology, Weill Medical College of Cornell University, New York; Attending Urologist, Voiding Dysfunction, Brookdale University Hospital and Medical Center, Brooklyn, New York
Complications of Minimally Invasive Procedures for Benign Prostatic Hyperplasia

Harriette Scarpero, MD
Associate Professor, Department of Urologic Surgery, Vanderbilt University School of Medicine, Nashville, Tennessee
Management of Urinary Fistulas

†Deceased

Arthur Schwartzbard, MD
Director, Non-Invasive Cardiology Lab, Manhattan Campus, New York Harbor Healthcare System; Director, Clinical Lipid Research, New York University Center for Prevention of Cardiovascular Disease; Assistant Professor of Medicine, New York University School of Medicine, New York, New York
Cardiac Complications of Urologic Surgery

Ojas Shah, MD
Assistant Professor of Urology and Director of Endourology and Stone Disease, Department of Urology, New York University Langone Medical Center, New York, New York
Hematologic Complications; Complications of Percutaneous Renal Surgery

Ellen Shapiro, MD
Professor of Urology, Director of Pediatric Urology, Department of Urology, New York University School of Medicine, New York, New York
Complications of Surgery for Posterior Urethral Valves

Katsuto Shinohara, MD
Professor, Department of Urology, University of California–San Francisco, San Francisco, California
Complications of Cryosurgical Ablation of Prostate

Eric A. Singer, MD, MA
Chief Resident in Urology, University of Rochester School of Medicine, Rochester, New York
Complications of Transurethral Resection of Bladder Tumors

Jennifer S. Singer, MD
Assistant Professor, Pediatric Urology and Renal Transplantation, Department of Urology, David Geffen School of Medicine, University of California–Los Angeles, Los Angeles, California
Special Considerations in the Pediatric Patient

Eila C. Skinner, MD
Professor of Clinical Urology, Department of Urology, Keck School of Medicine, University of Southern California, Los Angeles, California
Complications of Continent Cutaneous Diversion

Robert B. Smith, MD
Professor of Urology, David Geffen School of Medicine, University of California–Los Angeles, Los Angeles, California
Complications of Transurethral Resection of the Prostate

Mitchell H. Sokoloff, MD
Professor of Surgery and Chief, Section of Urology, University of Arizona College of Medicine, Tucson, Arizona
Complications of Transurethral Resection of the Prostate; Complications of Adrenal Surgery

Elizabeth A. Soll, PhD
Research Associate, Division of Urologic Health Services Research, Department of Urology, University of Michigan Medical Center, Ann Arbor, Michigan
Assessing Quality of Care in Urologic Surgery

John P. Stein, MD†
Professor, Department of Urology, University of Southern California, Norris Comprehensive Cancer Center, Los Angeles, California
Complications of Radical Cystectomy

Michael D. Stifelman, MD
Director of Robotic Surgery and Minimally Invasive Urology, Department of Urology, New York University School of Medicine, New York, New York
Complications of Minimally Invasive Reconstruction of the Upper Urinary Tract

Samir S. Taneja, MD
The James M. Neissa and Janet Riha Neissa Associate Professor of Urologic Oncology; Director, Division of Urologic Oncology, Department of Urology and New York University Cancer Institute, New York University Langone Medical Center, New York, New York
Hematologic Complications; Complications of Intravesical Therapy; Complications of Partial Nephrectomy; Complications of Radical Retropubic Prostatectomy; Complications of Conduit Urinary Diversion

Basir Tareen, MD
Fellow in Urologic Oncology, Bruce and Cynthia Sherman Fellowship in Urologic Oncology, Division of Urologic Oncology, Department of Urology, New York University Langone Medical Center, New York, New York
Hematologic Complications; Complications of Intravesical Therapy; Complications of Radical Retropubic Prostatectomy

Alexis E. Te, MD
Associate Professor of Urology and Director, Brady Prostate Center, Weill Medical College of Cornell University, New York, New York
Complications of Minimally Invasive Procedures for Benign Prostatic Hyperplasia

Matthew K. Tollefson, MD
Fellow in Urologic Oncology, Department of Urology, Mayo Clinic, Rochester, Minnesota
Complications of the Incision and Patient Positioning

Burak Turna, MD
Fellow, Glickman Urological Institute, Cleveland Clinic, Cleveland, Ohio
Management of Vascular Complications

---

†Deceased

George T. Vaida, MD
Assistant Professor of Clinical Anesthesiology; Medical Director and Anesthesia Director, Minimally Invasive Urology Unit, New York University Medical Center, New York, New York
Anesthetic Complications in Urologic Surgery

Jeffrey L. Veale, MD
Assistant Professor, Department of Urology, David Geffen School of Medicine, University of California–Los Angeles, Los Angeles, California
Complications of Renal Transplantation

Joseph R. Wagner, MD
Director of Robotic Surgery, Connecticut Surgical Group/Hartford Hospital, Hartford, Connecticut
Complications of Robotic Surgery

John T. Wei, MD, MS
Associate Professor, Division of Urologic Health Services Research, Department of Urology, University of Michigan Medical Center, Ann Arbor, Michigan
Assessing Quality of Care in Urologic Surgery

Alon Z. Weizer, MD
Assistant Professor, Department of Urology, University of Michigan, Ann Arbor, Michigan
Complications of Laparoscopic Renal Surgery

Philip Werthman, MD
Director, Center for Male Reproductive Medicine, Los Angeles, California
Complications of Surgery of the Testicle, Vas, Epididymis, and Scrotum

Jason M. Wilson, MD
Associate Professor, Division of Urology, Department of Surgery, University of New Mexico, Albuquerque, New Mexico
Complications of Surgery for Disorders of Sex Development

J. Stuart Wolf Jr, MD
David A. Bloom Professor of Urology, Department of Urology, University of Michigan, Ann Arbor, Michigan
Complications of Laparoscopic Renal Surgery

David P. Wood, MD
Professor of Urology, Division of Urologic Oncology, Department of Urology, University of Michigan, Ann Arbor, Michigan
Complications Following Laparoscopic Robot-Assisted Radical Prostatectomy

Jonathan L. Wright, MD, MS
Assistant Professor, Department of Urology, University of Washington, Seattle, Washington
Complications of Simple Prostatectomy

Ofer Yossepowitch, MD
Attending Surgeon, Department of Urology, Rabin Medical Center, Petah-Tikva, Israel
Complications of Lymphadenectomy

Ilia S. Zeltser, MD
Instructor, Department of Urology, University of Texas Southwestern Medical Center at Dallas, Dallas, Texas
Complications of Renal Tissue Ablation

CONTENTS

NONUROLOGIC COMPLICATIONS OF UROLOGIC SURGERY

Chapter 1

IMPACT OF HOST FACTORS AND COMORBID CONDITIONS

Lionel L. Bañez MD

Assistant Professor of Surgery, Division of Urological Surgery and The Duke Prostate Center, Department of Surgery, Duke University Medical Center, Durham, North Carolina

Stephen J. Freedland MD

Associate Professor of Urology and Pathology, Division of Urological Surgery and The Duke Prostate Center, Department of Surgery, Duke University Medical Center, Durham, North Carolina

Every urologist would prefer that any patient who has a consultation for a urologic disease would be solely afflicted with the disease for which he or she seeks medical attention, that every surgical patient would be healthy enough to tolerate the proposed surgical intervention to treat the condition, and that complications would occur with only miniscule probability. Unfortunately, this situation is far removed from reality and certainly is becoming less common in current clinical practice in which medical histories, physical examinations, preoperative laboratory examinations, and imaging scans are likely to reveal coexisting medical problems in the urologic patient.

In the present era, with life expectancy ever increasing, the prevalence of comorbid conditions such as obesity, heart disease, and diabetes, which affect urologic diseases and their clinical outcome following management, has congruently reached alarming proportions in the general population. Whether driven by improved medical science, rapid technologic advancement, or an effect of natural selection, men and women are living longer (**Fig. 1-1**). The medical community recognizes special considerations for elderly patients, and most of these considerations are brought about by medical conditions that are diagnosed in later life and progress with advancing age. In urologic disease entities such as erectile dysfunction in men, pelvic floor disorders in women, and urologic malignant diseases such as prostate and bladder cancer, the predisposition and clinical effects related to advanced age have direct biologic implications for the urologic condition. Moreover, because most of these disease entities are diagnosed in the more mature stages of life, the probability of preexisting medical conditions in these patients at the time of consultation is significantly high.

Notwithstanding the effect of age on comorbid medical conditions in the urologic patient, the past decades have also seen a dramatic rise in the prevalence of disease entities closely linked to harmful lifestyle choices such as smoking and alcohol consumption, unhealthy diets, lack of exercise and physical activity, and intravenous narcotic abuse. These lifestyle choices adversely affect patients of all ages who may seek urologic consultation and who may present with detrimental comorbidities such as childhood obesity, juvenile diabetes, chronic obstructive pulmonary disease, liver disease, and human immunodeficiency virus/acquired immunodeficiency syndrome (HIV/AIDS).

Although biologic links to known urologic diseases may be less apparent, the overall outcome and incidence of complications following surgical intervention are directly affected by coexisting health problems. Indeed, assessing the urologic patient for preexisting comorbidities is of critical importance because host factors play an important role in postoperative complications. Awareness of comorbidities allows the urologist to institute the proper measures to control preexisting diseases to optimize the overall health status of the individual patient, maximize the likelihood of a good outcome, and minimize the risk of a complication. The urologist also can assess the need for ancillary examinations for a more comprehensive evaluation of comorbid conditions more accurately and can determine the need for intraoperative monitoring and specialized intensive postsurgical care. More importantly, comprehensive knowledge of all concurrent illnesses in the urologic patient aids the urologist in the deciding whether surgical intervention is the optimal treatment option or whether conservative management may be the only viable therapeutic alternative.

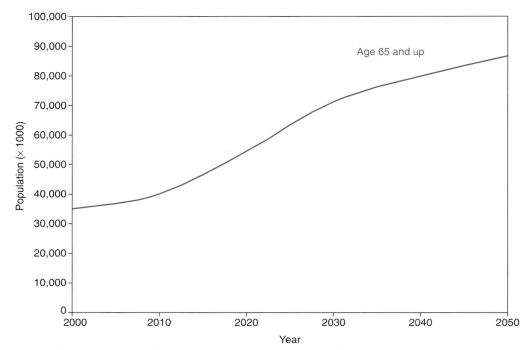

Figure 1-1 Projected population of the United States for adults ≥65 years old (2000-2050). *Based on data from the United States Census Bureau (http://www.census.gov/ipc/www/usinterimproj/)*

To serve as an introduction to the succeeding chapters in this section, we tackle host factors that significantly affect the occurrence of nonurologic complications following urologic surgery. We provide an overview of comorbidities in the urologic patient and highlight current prevalent disease entities that influence outcome following definitive surgical management. Comorbidities to which whole chapters are devoted, such as those pertaining to cardiovascular, pulmonary, hematologic, and anesthetic complications, are discussed only briefly here, to leave room for a more detailed discussion of topics of special interest such as obesity that are of major interest in the field of contemporary urology. We also provide insight into clinical tools such as useful comorbidity indices and scoring systems that aim to quantify the severity of comorbidities and predict post-treatment morbidity and mortality.

OBESITY

The importance of nutritional status to surgical outcomes and the deleterious effects of obesity are of significant interest in the field of urology. Interest has centered on obesity for two main reasons: (1) the prevalence of obesity has been growing at epidemic proportions worldwide, particularly within the United States[1]; and (2) scientific evidence suggests a relationship between obesity and multiple urologic conditions including urologic malignant diseases, benign prostatic hyperplasia (BPH), incontinence, erectile dysfunction, and stone disease, to name a few.[2]

Most of the leading causes of death in the United States are linked to obesity, including heart disease, cancer, stroke, chronic respiratory disease, and diabetes. Viewed as a growing national health crisis, obesity has surpassed tobacco smoking as the leading cause of preventable death; obesity not only results in a potentially avoidable toll in human lives but also incurs a substantial cost in health expenditure for the country.[3] Affecting nearly a third of all adults in the United States, obesity is further associated with various comorbidities, such as hypertension, hypercholesterolemia, sleep apnea, cholecystolithiasis, osteoarthritis, and depression, that may aggravate the overall health status of the overweight or obese patient and may contribute to the occurrence of surgical complications. Childhood obesity is also on the rise and would have undesirable consequences for children and adolescents undergoing pediatric urologic procedures.[4]

Obesity is defined as an excess accumulation of adipose tissue in the body; however, functionally, *overweight* and *obese* are labels used to denote ranges of weight that are in excess of what is generally considered healthy for the given height of a person. Because of its simplicity, body mass index (BMI) is a widely accepted method to assess for obesity. BMI is calculated by dividing the weight (in kilograms) of an individual by the height (in meters) squared.[5] **Figure 1-2** illustrates the standard weight status categories associated with BMI range for adults. Although other anthropometric measurements such as skinfold thickness and midarm circumference may be used for more accurate estimation

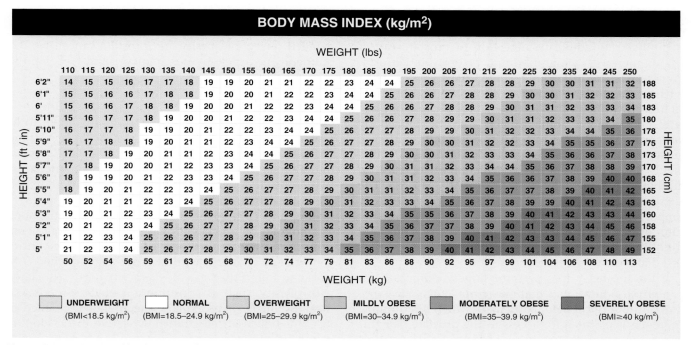

Figure 1-2 Estimates of body mass index using measured height and weight.

of body fat, these measurements are not routinely recorded in clinical practice and are of limited availability for retrospective studies.[5]

Fat distribution may also be an important determinant of obesity because individuals with high BMI who have upper body fat distribution (android) have been shown to be at greater risk for comorbidities such as cardiovascular disease, cerebrovascular disease, and hypertension compared with men and women who have lower body fat distribution (gynecoid).[6] Newer studies found better accuracy in gauging obesity with the use of waist circumference and waist-to-hip ratios; however, these parameters are more cumbersome to measure compared with BMI.[7] *Central obesity* correlates with visceral fat accumulation in the abdomen and is diagnosed when the waist-to-hip ratio exceeds 1.0 in men and 0.9 in women. This condition is in contrast to *peripheral obesity,* in which fat accumulation occurs subcutaneously in the gluteofemoral region. However, the distinction is clinically important because central obesity imparts a significantly higher risk of insulin resistance and type 2 diabetes, blood lipid disorders, hypertension, and heart disease compared with peripheral obesity.[8]

The medical consequences of obesity result in part from increased secretion of pathogenic macromolecules from enlarged adipose cells. Increased release of fatty acids from fat cells that are consequently stored in the liver or muscle results in an insulin-resistant state that is commonly seen in obesity. Diabetes ensues as the mounting insulin resistance overwhelms the secretory response of the pancreas.[9] Bioactive cytokines, particu-

larly interleukin-6, released from adipocytes promote the proinflammatory state that is characteristic of obesity. Secretion of prothrombin activator inhibitor-1 from adipose cells coupled with impaired endothelial function plays a key role in the hypercoagulable state of obesity and ultimately increases the risk of cardiovascular disease, stroke, and hypertension in obesity. This prothrombotic state is further aggravated directly by increased estrogen levels and is complicated indirectly by decreased antiangiogenic cytokines such as adiponectin.[10] The overall effect of these multiple pathologic consequences of increased fat stores ominously leads to a risk of shortened life expectancy.[11]

Obesity and Urologic Malignant Diseases

Investigations since the late 1980s have sparked keen interest in the link between obesity and urologic cancer, especially for prostate adenocarcinoma and kidney cancer.[12] Investigators have hypothesized that diet and obesity affect the underlying biologic mechanisms that ultimately lead to carcinogenesis including promotion of angiogenesis and mitogenesis, increased cellular proliferation, impairment of immune response, increased exposure to oxidative damage by free radicals, and promotion of a proinflammatory state.[13] Obesity can directly influence surgical outcome as a result of these proposed biologic linkages with urologic malignant diseases.

Prostate Cancer

Because obese men with prostate cancer have lower serum prostate-specific antigen (PSA) levels relative to men of normal weight,[14,15] and because physical assessment of the prostate through digital rectal examination is hindered by adiposity, detection of prostate cancer among men with a high BMI may be delayed. Performing a transrectal ultrasound–guided biopsy to establish a tissue diagnosis of prostate cancer can also be more technically difficult in obese men, and because of prostatic enlargement, some cancers may be missed by undersampling.[14] After histopathologic confirmation of prostate cancer, the patient may opt for surgical treatment, but urologists may be reluctant to operate on morbidly obese patients for several reasons. The anesthetic risks pertaining to adequacy of ventilatory support and difficulty in fluid monitoring[16] are further complicated by the increased incidence of comorbid conditions such as hypertension, heart disease, stroke, and diabetes.[9]

If the urologist does perform surgery, adiposity can be a physical hindrance that may curtail adequate exposure of the surgical field, particularly when a retropubic approach is planned for access to the prostate. For this reason, some urologists have advocated that perineal prostatectomy should be favored over the retropubic approach for treatment of obese men with prostate cancer. However, a study by Fitzsimons and associates[17] suggested that both surgical approaches have comparable outcomes in terms of estimated blood loss and operative time for obese patients. Indeed, performing a watertight vesicourethral anastomosis may be relatively more difficult in morbidly obese men undergoing radical retropubic prostatectomy. This situation led to innovative techniques such as the novel Vest suture, developed by Kamerer and colleagues,[18] which is aimed at alleviating the difficulties surrounding surgical treatment of prostate cancer in obese men. However, to date, solid data to substantiate our anecdotal experience regarding the technical difficulties in performing radical prostatectomy in obese men are limited.

Beyond technical issues, obesity may also influence the oncologic outcome among men undergoing radical prostatectomy. First, earlier studies found an increased incidence of positive surgical margins and capsular incision among men with higher BMIs.[19,20] Similarly, men with higher BMIs present with higher-grade tumors and more advance pathologic stages.[21] On postsurgical follow-up, men with an elevated BMI (≥ 30 kg/m^2) are at significantly increased risk of biochemical recurrence relative to men with a lower BMI, as denoted by an elevated postoperative PSA test result (>0.2 ng/mL or two values at 0.2 ng/mL).[19,22,23] More ominously, increased body weight was found to be associated with an increased risk of death from prostate cancer in a large, prospectively studied population.[24] Thus, obesity may well exert a biologic effect on prostate cancer that promotes aggressiveness and disease progression. However, in terms of health-related quality of life after radical prostatectomy, prospective studies have so far failed to demonstrate large differences between mildly obese men and men of normal weight.[25-27] For a more detailed review of obesity and prostate cancer, we recommend the article by Buschemeyer and Freedland in *European Urology*.[28]

Kidney Cancer

Obesity, particularly in women, has been shown to be associated with renal cell carcinoma (RCC).[24,29] A high BMI was found to be a strong risk factor for RCC; several underlying mechanisms were suspected, including higher insulin and estrogen levels, hypertension, hypercholesterolemia, and impaired host immune response.[30] Boeing and colleagues[31] examined determinants such as smoking, diet, occupational hazards, beverage consumption, medications, and obesity in a case-control cohort of 277 patients with RCC and 286 matched controls and found that specific dietary patterns associated with obesity, such as consumption of fatty foods and meat products, may explain the higher incidence of RCC in industrialized countries relative to developing countries.[31] Indeed, in a large retrospective study involving 363,992 men, investigators from the National Institutes of Health found that obese men, especially those with a history of tobacco use and elevated systolic blood pressures, have an increased long-term risk for RCC.[32]

As in prostate cancer, open surgical procedures for RCC can be technically difficult in patients with severe adiposity. Thus, wide interest exists in prescribing laparoscopic procedures for obese patients because these less invasive approaches have been found to be safe and effective for these subsets of patients.[33,34] However, a study of 210 patients who were treated with laparoscopic surgery for RCC revealed that BMI was a significant risk factor for major postoperative complications.[35] The investigators further reported that with every unit increase in BMI, the risk of a major complication increased by 14%. Finally, with regard to clinical outcome and cancer-specific mortality, overweight and obese patients have higher risk of death from kidney cancer relative to patients of normal weight.[24]

Bladder Cancer

Compared with prostate and renal cancer, published reports of relationships between bladder cancer and obesity are scarce. In 1994, an epidemiologic study of 514 patients with bladder cancer found that beyond the well-known link with smoking, obesity was also a significant risk factor for bladder cancer.[36] However, a large prospective study of nearly 1 million people found no link between BMI and bladder cancer mortality.[24] With regard to diet, reports on the association between high fat intake and bladder cancer have been conflicting.[37,38]

With respect to surgical outcome for radical cystectomy, abundant reports show not only that obesity contributes to the technical challenge of the operation but also that higher BMI increases the risk of perioperative complications. In a retrospective analysis of 304 consecutive patients who underwent radical cystectomy and urinary diversion for bladder cancer, increased BMI was independently associated with higher estimated blood loss.[39] This finding was later confirmed in a cohort of 498 patients; the investigators further concluded that, along with greater blood loss, an increased BMI was also independently associated with prolonged operative time and increased rate of complications.[40]

Obesity and Benign Urologic Conditions

Several nonmalignant urologic conditions are also unfavorably affected by an increased BMI and morbid obesity.

Benign Prostatic Hyperplasia and Lower Urinary Tract Symptoms

Obesity is a known risk factor for lower urinary tract symptoms (LUTS) and BPH. Indeed, a large-scale, cross-sectional study from the Prostate Study Group of the Austrian Society for Urology found a link between BPH and obesity.[41] The relationship between obesity and LUTS was further confirmed in a report from Johns Hopkins University in Baltimore on 2797 men from the Third National Health and Nutrition Examination Survey.[42] In another confirmatory study, BPH was found to be associated with increased serum insulin levels and abdominal obesity as opposed to BMI itself.[43] The biologic link between obesity and BPH likely has its origin in the association of obesity with hyperinsulinemia and the status of insulin as a direct prostate growth factor.[44]

Erectile Dysfunction

Obesity, particularly central obesity, is a known predictor of erectile dysfunction in men.[45] Both atherosclerosis and diabetes mellitus, which are associated with obesity, play significant roles in the development of erectile dysfunction. Although the underlying cause for erectile dysfunction is thought to be multifactorial, investigators have suggested that obesity increases the risk of erectile dysfunction of vascular origin as a result of the development of chronic vascular disease.[46] Obesity is also known to increase the risk of diabetes. The microvascular complications characteristic of diabetes exert deleterious effects on erectile tissue similar to the pathologic features of diabetic nephropathy, retinopathy, and gastroparesis.[47] Furthermore, weight loss is the only known lifestyle intervention that can improve erectile dysfunction.[48]

Stress Urinary Incontinence

Pelvic floor weakness leading to stress urinary incontinence (SUI) in women is aggravated by increased intra-abdominal pressure and is closely associated with truncal obesity.[49] A report examined the association of bladder function with smoking, food consumption, and obesity in 6424 women with SUI and found a strong relationship between SUI and obesity.[50] These findings were confirmed in a questionnaire-based study conducted in Norway involving 27,936 women.[51] The proposed underlying mechanism for the association between high BMI and incontinence is that a high BMI leads to increased intravesical pressures and thus lowers the differential between the detrusor pressure and leak point pressure such that incontinence is more likely to occur.[52] With regard to the perioperative effect of obesity in surgical treatment of SUI, a study involving 250 women who underwent retropubic anti-incontinence procedures revealed that operative time was significantly longer for obese women; however, blood loss and major perioperative complications were similar across BMI groups.[53]

Urolithiasis

Urinary stone formation has been linked to obesity, as illustrated by a report on 527 calcium oxalate stone formers wherein an increased BMI was strongly associated with an elevated risk of stone formation for both men and women.[54] However, a retrospective study of 5492 stone formers revealed that the association between obesity and stone formation was significant only in women.[55] In a study conducted at Duke University in North Carolina, the major metabolic abnormalities found in obese stone formers that were possible contributors to recurrent stone formation were hypocitraturia, gouty diathesis, and hyperuricosuria.[56] An inverse association between pH and body weight suggests that production of excessively acidic urine promotes urate nephrolithiasis in obese stone formers.[57]

With respect to urologic procedures to treat stone disease, obesity adversely affects outcome following extracorporeal shock wave lithotripsy (ESWL). In a report examining clinical and radiologic variables associated with poor outcome after ESWL, along with obesity, pelvic ureteral stones, stones >10 mm, and obstruction were independent predictors of unsuccessful outcome.[58] Thus, because of the probability of treatment failure, obese patients may be better served by endourologic procedures than by ESWL.

MALNUTRITION

At the opposite end of the nutritional spectrum from overnutrition and obesity is malnutrition. With regard to the surgical patient, malnutrition has been associated with an increased incidence of nosocomial infection, poor wound healing, an increased length of hospital stay, multiorgan dysfunction, and mortality.[59] Various scientific investigations have demonstrated that deterioration of nutritional status has an invariably deleterious effect on surgical outcome. As early as 1932, Cuthbertson[60] reported the association of impaired wound healing with negative nitrogen balance in trauma patients. A more recent prospective study conducted in a cohort of patients who did not have cancer used four clinical parameters to predict perioperative morbidity:

1. Percentage of ideal body weight
2. Preoperative percentage of weight loss
3. Arm muscle circumference
4. Serum albumin

Results of the study revealed that patients with at least one abnormal clinical parameter had a significant increase in the incidence of major complications and in length of hospital stay relative to patients with normal preoperative parameters.[61] Not only has malnutrition per se been implicated in surgical complications, but also certain types of nutrient deficiency, protein malnutrition in particular, may lead to more severe postoperative problems. Relative to protein-calorie malnutrition, which is characterized by a lack of both proteins and carbohydrates, severe protein malnutrition leads to low serum albumin concentration, edema, and a high prevalence of acute infections.[62] Thus, it is evident that nutritional status is a key clinical parameter demanding thorough evaluation in the surgical patient to prevent nutrition-related complications.

NUTRITIONAL STATUS ASSESSMENT

Traditionally, clinicians relied on anthropometric measurements, which they compared with tables providing ideal weight-for-height estimates to evaluate the nutritional status of patients.[63] Clinicians also determined body mass composition determinants such as lean body mass based on limb skinfold or circumference measurements and used these variables as indicators for adequacy of nutrition. However, problems pertaining to the precision of anthropometric measurements, the wide intraobserver and interobserver variations, and the lack of reliable reference standards have challenged the validity of these methods in ascertaining nutritional health of the surgical patient.[59] These issues surrounding the traditional methods of screening for malnutrition led to an interest in studying serum markers for more accurate determination of preoperative nutritional competence.

Serum albumin is by far the most commonly used biochemical parameter to assess for nutritional status in the surgical patient. The National Veterans Affairs Surgical Risk Study involved a very large prospective observational investigation of 54,215 patients and found that preoperative serum albumin level was a highly reliable predictor of 30-day operative mortality and morbidity after major noncardiac surgery.[64] To validate this finding in urologic surgery, McLaughlin and colleagues[65] performed a similar analysis on 643 patients who under-

went major urologic operations, compared preoperative and intraoperative factors, and sought to identify risk factors associated with complications after urologic surgery. Their study revealed that serum albumin was one of the five most significant preoperative determinants associated with 30-day morbidity (along with histories of congestive heart failure, diabetes with end-organ damage, angioplasty, and quadriplegia). Specifically, low serum albumin levels ($\leq$35 g/L) conferred 2.5 times greater risk of incurring a postoperative morbidity in patients undergoing urologic operative procedures.

Although serum albumin is emerging as a robust clinical marker of nutritional status with clear advantage over anthropometrics, controversies remain especially with regard to the reliability of the serum marker in more elderly patients.[66] Other visceral protein biomarkers of interest to both physicians and nutritionists include prealbumin and retinol-binding protein,[67] which are fairly well maintained in the geriatric population compared with albumin. However, the use of these soluble proteins to gauge nutritional insufficiency can be limited by fluid shifts, increased vascular permeability, and altered hepatic protein metabolism in response to stress. Technologic advances such as total body nitrogen measurement, dual radiographic absorptiometry, and bioelectrical impedance may circumvent these limitations[68] and become the future standards of care. Until these newer modalities are fully tested and validated in a true patient population, serum albumin determination will remain a simple and readily available applicable test for nutritional assessment in the urologic patient.

INFECTION AND UROSEPSIS

Although community-acquired urinary tract infections (UTIs) are very common and are considered relatively easy to treat, complicated UTIs such as those acquired in the hospital setting are a legitimate cause for concern in urology. The term *complicated UTI* connotes infections brought about by a functional or anatomic abnormality in the urinary tract, but it may also be used to indicate an infection that occurs in a patient with altered defense mechanisms.[69] When an infection previously localized to the urinary tract enters the bloodstream and causes a systemic infection, urosepsis ensues.

Judicious use of prophylactic antibiotics in surgical procedures has served to minimize the incidence of these preventable yet potentially lethal complications in urologic practice.[70] However, the rising incidence of antimicrobial resistance, especially of gram-positive pathogens such as methicillin-resistant *Staphylococcus aureus* (MRSA) and vancomycin-resistant enterococci (VRE), can lead to treatment failure and life-threatening sepsis.[71] Moreover, the increasing numbers of patients who are immunocompromised either by an underlying disease (e.g., HIV/AIDS) or through concurrent medical therapy (e.g., steroids, anticancer chemotherapy)[72] also lead to greater infection risk. These risk factors are particularly relevant when surgery entails instrumentation and manipulation of the urinary tract. Given that certain host factors predispose the urologic patient to complicated infection, it is necessary to determine the need for antimicrobial prophylaxis preoperatively and to prevent the occurrence of systemic septicemia.

Both demographic factors and medical conditions play a role in susceptibility to complicated UTI. Advanced age in a patient should alert the urologist to the possible presence of UTI. The prevalence of UTI increases with age and reaches approximately 3.6% in men ≥70 years old and 7% in women ≥50 years old.[73] As previously discussed, nutritional imbalances leading to obesity and malnutrition could impair cellular immunity and thereby predispose patients to UTI. Preexisting local or systemic infections intuitively are associated with complicated UTI.

Recent antimicrobial use has been linked to complicated UTI, possibly through two mechanisms: (1) antibiotic therapy fails, and the initial infection, either systemic or local, progresses to complicated UTI or frank urosepsis; or (2) antibiotics used to eliminate competing pathogens promote the growth of resistant strains and lead to infection with a more virulent strain.[74] Diabetes mellitus not only increases the incidence of UTI in adults but also contributes to a complicated course despite antibiotic prophylaxis and treatment. This situation is the result of defects in the secretion of urinary cytokines and increased adherence of microorganisms to the uroepithelial cells in diabetic patients.[75]

Not surprisingly, many urologic and medical renal conditions are associated with an increased incidence of complicated UTIs and urosepsis. One of the most consistent contributors to complicated UTI is obstruction of the urinary tract.[76] This underlying mechanism encompasses the following: intrinsic disorders of the kidney, renal pelvis, and ureters (e.g., congenital anomalies including vesicoureteral reflux, renal or ureteral calculi, neoplasms, strictures); extrinsic abnormalities of the upper urinary tract (e.g., aberrant vessels, retroperitoneal hematomas or fibrosis, nonurologic neoplasms); and disorders of the bladder and bladder neck (e.g., BPH, prostate and bladder cancer, cystolithiasis, bladder neck contracture) and urethra (e.g., valves, strictures). Functional impairment of the bladder, as seen in spastic or atonic neurogenic bladder, may have the same consequences as conditions causing physical obstruction.[77] Renal diseases, whether unilateral, bilateral, or segmental, may also complicate UTI and include conditions such as azotemia, polycystic kidney disease, and papillary necrosis, as well as nephropathies brought about by abuse of analgesics such as nonsteroidal anti-inflammatory drugs.[78]

Immunosuppressed urologic patients present a unique problem with regard to susceptibility to compli-cated UTI. Whether impairment of immunologic response was brought about iatrogenically (e.g., patients with cancer who are undergoing chemotherapy, transplant recipients receiving steroids) or is the result of a disease process (e.g., HIV/AIDS, persistent neutropenia or granulocytopenia),[72] avid use of broad-spectrum antibiotics not only for common infections but also for opportunistic organisms should be considered by the urologist for an optimal clinical outcome. Finally, urologic instrumentation leads to an increased probability of introducing microorganisms into an otherwise sterile urinary tract and thus predisposes patients to infections. The same principle applies to urologic procedures in which foreign bodies are purposefully left in the human body (e.g., ureteral stents, penile prostheses).[79] Although intended to elicit only a minimal inflammatory response, any foreign body can serve as a nidus of infection and must be removed promptly when it is determined to be the source of infection or when its presence in the body contributes to a complicated UTI.

QUANTIFYING COMORBIDITY

In medicine, *comorbidity* is defined as the effect of all other pathologic conditions an individual patient may have other than the primary disease of interest. The very nature of comorbidities, as secondary or lesser diseases of interest, has led to some indifference among practicing clinicians and research investigators regarding the significance of these illnesses in treatment decision making and survival outcomes. Because of the significant correlation between advanced age and increased prevalence of preexisting comorbidities at the time of surgery, physicians have traditionally used age as a surrogate for the effects of concurrent medical conditions, especially in elderly urologic patients.[80] Although no one can discount the value of age in treatment decisions,[80] the use of age as a strict criterion that may deny appropriate curative therapy to healthy older patients is unacceptable and may even have litigious consequences.

The impact of comorbidities is substantial in the field of urology, particularly in urologic oncology. An analysis of 34,294 newly diagnosed cases of cancer in patients from the Netherlands Eindhoven cancer registry showed that, aside from lung cancer (58%) and stomach cancer (53%), the crude prevalence of comorbidities was highest in malignant diseases of the kidney (54%), bladder (53%), and prostate (51%).[81] In terms of prognosis, Post and colleagues[82] acknowledged that comorbidity was the most important prognostic factor for 3-year survival in a population-based study of 1337 patients with localized prostate cancer. In a series of 1023 consecutive radical nephrectomies and nephron-sparing surgical procedures for RCC in Dresden, Germany, comorbidities were closely associated with overall morbidity and mortality.[83] With regard to treatment-related side effects, both peripheral vascular disease and diabetes have been shown to be significant risk factors for development of impotence following external beam radiation for prostate cancer as well as for gastrointestinal and genitourinary toxicities.[84] Thus, comorbidities can affect almost all aspects of urologic disease but most importantly the incidence of posttreatment morbidity and all-cause death.

Up until the late 1980s, the effects of comorbidities were largely unquantifiable and subjective. As a result, certain beliefs and attitudes in clinical practice were based mostly on anecdotal data rather than on appropriate evidence-based information. This need for methods to quantify the effects of comorbidities adequately led to the development of comorbidity scoring systems, which are gaining utility for both research and clinical purposes.

The most extensively studied and most commonly used comorbidity scoring scheme in medicine is the *Charlson Index score*.[85] Dr. Mary E. Charlson, a clinical epidemiologist and methodologist who was interested in improving clinical outcome in both medical and surgical patients, first published the index in 1987 at Cornell University in Ithaca, New York. The Charlson Index is a list of 19 pathologic conditions (Table 1-1). Based on the proportional hazards regression model that Charlson constructed from clinical data, each condition is an assigned a weight from 1 to 6. The Charlson

TABLE 1-1	Weighted Index of Comorbidity [Defined by the Charlson Index]
Assigned Weights for Diseases	**Conditions**
1	Myocardial infarct
	Congestive heart failure
	Peripheral vascular disease
	Cerebrovascular disease
	Dementia
	Chronic pulmonary disease
	Connective tissue disease
	Ulcer disease
	Mild liver disease
	Diabetes
2	Hemiplegia
	Moderate or severe renal disease
	Diabetes with end organ damage
	Any tumor
	Leukemia
	Lymphoma
3	Moderate or severe liver disease
6	Metastatic solid tumor
	AIDS

Assigned weights for each condition that a patient has. The total equals the score. Example: chronic pulmonary (1) and lymphoma (2) = total score (3).
From Charlson ME, Pompei P, Ales K, MacKenzie CR. A new method of classifying prognostic comorbidity in longitudinal studies: development and validation. *J Chronic Dis.* 1987;40:373-383.

Index score is the sum of the weights for all concurrent diseases aside from the primary disease of interest. Thus, for example, in men with prostate cancer, although cancer is generally assigned a score of 2, in this case, men are assigned no points for prostate cancer because it is the primary index disease. In a cohort of 685 patients with breast cancer in the original study, the Charlson Index score showed a strong association of a 2.3-fold increase in the 10-year risk of mortality per 1-point increment in the comorbidity level.

The Charlson Index score provides a simple means to quantify the effect of comorbid illnesses, incorporate the severity of a particular disease (diabetes without complications versus diabetes with end-organ damage), and account for the aggregate effect of multiple concurrent disease processes on clinical outcome, most often mortality. In prostate cancer research, the Charlson Index score has been avidly evaluated as a predictor of both cause-specific mortality and all-cause mortality. Albertsen and colleagues[86] showed that the Charlson Index score provided significant predictive information on cancer-specific and all-cause survival independent of age, Gleason score, or clinical stage in a cohort of 451 patients with Jewett-Whitmore stage A1-B prostate cancer treated with hormonal ablation. In 2002, a competing risk analysis of 751 men who were undergoing radical prostatectomy for clinically localized prostate cancer at the Mayo Clinic in Rochester, Minnesota showed that whereas the Gleason score emerged as the only significant predictor of prostate cancer–specific mortality, both the Charlson Index score and the Gleason score were predictive of overall mortality.[87] Comparable results were reported by other groups who performed similar analyses using Charlson Index scores in prostate cancer out`come studies.[82,88,89]

The clinical utility of the Charlson Index score extends to other urologic diseases as well. With regard to bladder cancer, the Charlson Index score was evaluated in predicting adverse pathologic characteristics, cancer-specific death, and overall survival following radical cystectomy.[90] Logistic regression revealed that the Charlson Index score was independently associated with an increased risk of extravesical disease. Cox regression models further revealed that the index was significantly associated with decreased cancer-specific survival. In 302 men undergoing transurethral resection of the prostate (TURP) or simple prostatectomy for BPH, the Charlson Index score correlated with 5-year mortality.[91] Thus, even for nononcologic urologic operations, comorbidity indices have demonstrated power for predicting mortality following surgery.

Aside from being scientifically validated for use in urologic surgery, the Charlson Index has other notable advantages in urologic practice and clinical research. Administrative database codes known as *International Classification of Diseases codes, ninth revision with or without clinical modification (ICD-9/ICD-9CM)* and implemented by almost all hospitals in the United States can be used to calculate the Charlson Index score for a particular patient.[92] Ideally, meticulous chart review for each individual patient should be done to ensure a completely accurate Charlson Index score because the ICD-9 codes may not be up to date for that particular patient. However, studies have shown that the predictive properties of indices computed using either ICD-9 codes alone or detailed chart review are comparable.[93]

The Dartmouth-Manitoba version was the first adaptation of the Charlson Index score to use ICD-9 diagnoses.[94] Other adaptations published by Deyo and associates,[95] D'Hoore and colleagues,[96] and Ghali and associates[97] further simplified the translations from ICD-9 to Charlson Index score while maintaining validity and relevance for prediction of clinical end points such as 1-year mortality, in-hospital mortality, or postoperative death. Limitations to the Charlson Index score, as previously alluded to, include coding errors (particularly when relying on ICD-9 codes), incomplete medical histories, and determination of whether a diagnosis is a comorbidity at hospital admission or a complication arising during the hospital stay.[98] Furthermore, because of the lack of definitive comorbidity studies for all urologic diseases, the correlations of the comorbidity index to outcome may vary among disease entities and surgical procedures.

Other indices of comorbidity are available but have not been as broadly used as the Charlson Index. Three prime examples are the Index of Co-Existent Disease (ICED),[99] the Kaplan-Feinstein Index (KFI),[100] and the Cumulative Illness Rating Scale (CIRS).[101] Similar to the Charlson Index, the ICED, KFI, and CIRS are designed to measure the impact of concurrent diseases on prognosis. Because of the lack of definitive head-to-head comparisons of the various methods of comorbidity assessments, no clear-cut evidence exists to establish the advantage of one scale over the other.[102] In fact, in a study in which Charlson Index scores were shown to be predictive of 5-year mortality following TURP for BPH, similar analysis using the KFI and ICED demonstrated comparable predictive power.[91]

Although the Charlson Index is the most widely used, its role as a robust prognostic indicator for many disease entities remains unclear. Given the upswing in interest in this field, we anticipate that future validation of this and other indices will be forthcoming.

CONCLUSION

It is the ultimate goal of every urologist to provide the best possible care for the urologic patient. The projected surge in life expectancy in this new millennium translates into an analogous increase in urologic patients who will potentially present with various comorbid diseases. These patients will require thorough evaluation including addressing of associated comorbidities to obtain an excellent outcome. The impact of host factors and comorbidities cannot be taken lightly because more and more scientific evidence points to associations of these pretreatment parameters with a heightened risk for undesirable posttreatment complications. In particular, obesity, which is associated with other significant comorbidities and has been found to affect both the urologic disease process and consequent complications, must be investigated comprehensively. Furthermore, adequate assessment of nutritional status to ensure sufficient nutritional support in the surgical patient is also warranted.

Patients with host factors that predispose them to infections may require prophylactic antibiotic coverage and must be closely monitored to anticipate the need for further antimicrobial treatment to prevent urosepsis. Finally, various comorbidity scoring systems are being investigated for their clinical value and may further provide urologists and other clinicians with more accurate predictive models for assessing the risk of complications among patients with urologic diseases. As subsequent chapters in this book delve into more organ-specific, urologic disease–specific, or procedure-specific complications, we encourage the readers to make every effort in taking a broad, encompassing approach when evaluating urologic patients by diligently considering the effects of comorbid conditions in each individual person.

KEY POINTS

1. With increasing life expectancy in the general population, the prevalence of comorbid conditions such as obesity, heart disease, and diabetes has increased to alarming proportions.
2. Awareness of comorbidities allows the urologist to institute the proper measures to control preexisting diseases to optimize the overall health status of the individual patient, maximize the likelihood of a good outcome, and minimize the risk of a complication.
3. Obesity can directly influence surgical outcome because of certain proposed biologic linkages with urologic malignant diseases.
4. Nutritional status is a key clinical parameter demanding thorough evaluation in the surgical patient to prevent nutrition-related complications.
5. Given that certain host factors predispose the urologic patient to complicated infection, it is necessary to determine the need for antimicrobial prophylaxis preoperatively and to prevent the occurrence of systemic septicemia.

REFERENCES

Please see www.expertconsult.com

Chapter 2

PULMONARY COMPLICATIONS OF UROLOGIC SURGERY

Patrick W. Mufarrij MD
Chief Resident, Department of Urology, New York University, New York, New York

William C. Huang MD
Assistant Professor, Department of Urology, New York University, New York, New York

Some say we can get along on only 20 percent of our lung capacity, but that dragging sort of existence is a poor substitute for the vitality we enjoy when the twin bellows of our lungs are taking in great drafts of oxygen.

—Gene Tunney
World heavyweight boxing champion, 1926 to 1928

Indeed, the lungs are the essential respiratory organ of air-breathing vertebrates and sustain the fire of life by absorbing oxygen into the body and excreting carbon dioxide into the atmosphere. For surgical patients, safe airway management and the maintenance of optimal perioperative pulmonary function are instrumental to a successful recovery. Unfortunately, pulmonary complications do occur on multiple levels and at varying rates of clinical urgency. Although these complications have a wide range of causes, all affect either oxygenation or ventilation of the patient.

Postoperative pulmonary complications are a major cause of morbidity and mortality, and they result in prolonged hospital stays and increased health care costs. The risks of such complications depend on the susceptibility of the patient and on the type of procedure undertaken. Although definitions and analytical methods vary throughout the literature, the incidence of postoperative pulmonary complications, ranging from clinically significant atelectasis to respiratory failure, following abdominal or pelvic surgery has been reported to be between 20% and 30%.[1-4] We define *respiratory complication* as any pulmonary abnormality that produces identifiable disease or dysfunction that is clinically significant and impairs a patient's clinical course.[5]

PREOPERATIVE PULMONARY ASSESSMENT AND POSTOPERATIVE PULMONARY REHABILITATION

Patients who are at risk for developing pulmonary complications need to be identified preoperatively so that special measures can be undertaken in the perioperative period either to avoid or to mitigate these potential setbacks. As outlined by Smetana and coworkers,[5] definite risk factors for developing postoperative pulmonary complications are as follows:

1. Chronic obstructive pulmonary disease (COPD)
2. Active tobacco smoking history
3. Cessation of smoking <8 weeks preoperatively
4. American Society of Anesthesiologists class >2
5. Serum albumin concentration <3 g/dL
6. Blood urea nitrogen level >30 mg/dL
7. Surgical procedures lasting >3 hours

Smoking tobacco is a well-known risk factor for postoperative pulmonary complications that increases the relative risk of these events among smokers as compared with nonsmokers by an odds ratio of 1.4 to 4.3.[2,3] In their prospective study of 200 patients undergoing coronary artery bypass surgery, Warner and associates[6] demonstrated that patients who had stopped smoking ≥8 weeks preoperatively had a significantly lower risk of pulmonary complications than did patients who were active smokers (14.5% versus 33%). Moreover, patients who had stopped smoking for >6 months had pulmonary complication rates similar to those patients who had never smoked (11.1% versus 11.9%). Surprisingly, patients who had quit smoking <8 weeks preoperatively experienced more untoward pulmonary events than did active smokers (57% versus 33%).

The most important patient-related risk factor for developing a postoperative pulmonary complication is

COPD.[7] Patients with severe COPD are up to six times more likely to have such a complication than are patients who do not have this disease. The subset of patients with COPD must be medically optimized before elective surgical procedures by the use of bronchodilators, physical therapy, antibiotics, smoking cessation (if they are active smokers), and corticosteroids in selected cases.[8]

The evaluation of preoperative pulmonary risk begins with a detailed history and physical examination to identify factors that prompt a thorough pulmonary evaluation such as exercise intolerance, tobacco smoking, chronic cough, sputum production, previous pulmonary surgery, previous chemotherapy (see later), dyspnea at rest or on exertion, wheezing, rales, cyanosis, or weakness or debilitation. Chest radiographs should be obtained in all patients with any of the foregoing risk factors for developing postoperative pulmonary complications. Smetana and colleagues[9] published evidence-based guidelines for preoperative pulmonary function testing. According to this review, preoperative spirometry should be obtained in patients with COPD or asthma and in patients with unexplained dyspnea or exercise intolerance.

Postoperative pulmonary rehabilitation is as important as is the preoperative evaluation of each surgical patient. For any patient receiving anesthesia, and especially for patients undergoing urologic surgical procedures involving an incision that breaches muscles used during respiration, pulmonary rehabilitation is critical in preventing complications and in fostering the recuperation of normal respiratory status. Deep breathing exercises, incentive spirometry, coughing, sputum clearance, and early ambulation are all part of postoperative pulmonary rehabilitation.

In a prospective, randomized, controlled trial, Morran and coworkers[10] concluded that routine prophylactic postoperative chest physical therapy significantly decreased the incidence of chest infection in patients who underwent open cholecystectomy (7% versus 19%). More recently, however, these notions were called into question. Pasquina and colleagues[11] performed a systematic review of published randomized trials investigating prophylactic respiratory physical therapy and pulmonary outcomes after abdominal surgical procedures. Of the 13 trials that included a "no-intervention" control arm (and thus could produce meaningful conclusions), 9 studies failed to report significant differences. Pasquina's group concluded that because of the paucity of trials that reported significant benefit, the routine use of prophylactic pulmonary physical therapy following abdominal surgery remains unproven and requires further study.[11] Nonetheless, we still employ a rigorous postoperative respiratory rehabilitation program, especially in patients with pulmonary risk factors or in patients undergoing surgical procedures lasting >3 hours.

ATELECTASIS AND RESPIRATORY INFECTION

Atelectasis is the reversible collapse of alveoli in dependent lung areas. Studies suggest that atelectasis could also represent alveoli that are filled with fluid and foam.[12] Ninety percent of anesthetized patients develop atelectasis, a complication believed to result from surfactant inhibition, gas resorption, or lung compression.[13] Atelectasis occurs with both intravenous (IV) and inhalational anesthesia regimens, regardless of whether the patient is breathing spontaneously or is mechanically ventilated. Surgical patients are also predisposed to atelectasis because of the rapid, shallow breathing pattern and the inhibiting effect of analgesia on spontaneous sighing that is commonly seen in the postoperative setting.[14] Although increased age was once thought to be a risk factor, it has not been shown to increase the propensity for development of atelectasis.[15]

Atelectasis is associated with the development of several pathophysiologic respiratory effects, including decreased compliance, impairment of oxygenation, increased pulmonary vascular resistance, and development of lung injury.[16] Impairment of gas exchange, often the most obvious effect of atelectasis, leads to worsened arterial oxygenation in the absence of supplemental oxygen. The consequences of impaired oxygenation are frequently insignificant in a healthy lung, but they may necessitate the application of higher inspired oxygen concentration in a diseased lung.

The diagnosis of atelectasis is usually suspected when the alterations in lung physiology consistent with this entity (described earlier) occur in a likely setting, such as the postoperative period. Clinical findings such as dyspnea, tachypnea, or hypoxemia usually confirm this suspicion, but imaging with chest radiography or computed tomography (CT) often reliably confirms the diagnosis.[17] Reversing or preventing atelectasis is possible in many patients in the postoperative period and is of proven benefit in preventing pulmonary complications.[18] The most clinically important techniques or devices are those that encourage patients to inspire deeply and thus to produce a large and sustained increase in transpulmonary pressure to distend the lung and to reexpand collapsed lungs. Although some controversy exists regarding the routine use of prophylactic pulmonary physical therapy following abdominal surgical procedures, we strongly encourage the practice.

Postoperative pulmonary infections have an incidence in the literature widely ranging from 2.8% to 50% depending on the type of anesthesia, type of surgery, and patient risk factors.[19] Infectious respiratory complications are not surprisingly more common in patients with risk factors such as COPD, altered lung defenses, and active smoking. Postoperative pneumonia delays recovery from the surgical procedure, and the resulting impairment of tissue oxygenation can delay wound healing. Rodgers and coworkers[20] reported that patients who developed postoperative pneumonia had a 10% mortality rate, which was substantially higher when systemic sepsis ensued. Another large study of patients undergoing major noncardiac surgical procedures found that 1.5% developed postoperative pneumonia, and this cohort of patients had a 10-fold higher 30-day mortality rate did than patients who did not develop this complication.[21]

The two types of pneumonia most frequently encountered in the postoperative patient are aspiration and nosocomial. *Aspiration pneumonia* occurs after abnormal entry of fluid, particulate matter, or gastrointestinal secretions into the respiratory tract and can result in pulmonary complications by way of chemical pneumonitis, bacterial infection, or mechanical obstruction.[22] Pneumonia resulting from aspiration is caused primarily by anaerobic bacteria that comprise the normal flora of the patient. Treatment of aspiration pneumonia involves antibiotics, supportive care, and removal of any aspirated material that is obstructing the respiratory tree.

Nosocomial pneumonia is acquired in the hospital and manifests ≥48 hours after admission; the definition of this condition excludes any infection present or incubating at the time of hospital admission.[23] Unlike aspiration pneumonias, nosocomial infections of the lung are frequently polymicrobial and result from highly virulent bacteria, with gram-negative bacilli the predominant organism in 60% of cases.[23]

Treatment entails supportive care and empirical antibiotic coverage, with specific attention paid to frequent pathogens of a particular institution, such as methicillin-resistant *Staphylococcus aureus*, *Pseudomonas aeruginosa*, or *Acinetobacter baumannii*.[24] *Ventilator-associated pneumonia*, a specific subset of nosocomial pneumonia, is bacterial pneumonia in patients with acute respiratory failure who have been intubated for >48 hours.[23] Treatment of ventilator-associated pneumonia is similar to that for nosocomial pneumonia. Mortality rates of ≤40% have been reported for ventilator-associated pneumonia, and grave complications such as acute respiratory distress syndrome (ARDS) can develop.[24]

ARDS, a severe lung disease characterized by inflammation of the lung parenchyma that leads to impaired gas exchange with concomitant systemic release of inflammatory mediators, causes inflammation and hypoxemia, and frequently results in multisystem organ failure.[25] Essentially, the pathophysiology of ARDS involves massive capillary leak resulting from excessive inflammatory response in the host's lung tissue. Treatment of ARDS involves mechanical ventilation, treatment of underlying causes, supportive care, and antibiotic coverage if indicated.

PULMONARY EMBOLISM

Pulmonary embolism (PE) has historically been reported in ≤10% of patients following urologic surgical procedures, and with deep vein thrombosis (DVT) has been observed in ≤30% of patients who do not receive prophylaxis.[26] One prospective observational study suggested a marked decrease in the incidence of PE, largely because of the institution of routine DVT prophylaxis, such as early ambulation, use of graduated compression stockings, and intermittent pneumatic compression.[27] In this study, urologic patients, 40% of whom underwent open surgical procedures, had an overall PE rate of 0.87%. At our institution, we routinely use nonpharmacologic methods of thromboprophylaxis, such as compression stockings or pneumatic compression devices placed before induction of general anesthesia and then in the early postoperative period, particularly if the patient is not ambulatory. The 3-month mortality of PE has been reported to be 15%, despite current aggressive treatment guidelines.[28] The use of anticoagulation treatment for venous thromboembolism (VTE), the clinical entity that comprises both DVT and PE, must be weighed against the risk of bleeding, especially in the postsurgical patient.

The statistically significant risk factors for postoperative DVT include the following[29]:

1. Increased age
2. Obesity
3. Previous history of VTE
4. Varicose veins
5. Oral contraceptive therapy
6. Malignant disease
7. General anesthesia
8. Orthopedic surgery
9. Factor V Leiden gene mutation (a thrombophilia)

Regional and spinal anesthetic regimens have been associated with a decreased risk of PE when compared with general anesthesia, purportedly as a result of the vasodilation of the lower extremities afforded by sympathetic blockade.[30] This finding is of particular interest because many endoscopic urologic procedures can be performed with spinal anesthesia.

The most common symptoms of PE, according to two large prospective studies, are dyspnea (73%), pleuritic chest pain (63%), and cough (37%).[31,32] More than 97% of patients with confirmed PE complain of at least one of these symptoms.[31] Clinical decision models have been created to help in the diagnosis of PE.[33,34] According to one such model developed by Kruip and coworkers,[33] patients are stratified according to a points system. Patients who are considered "unlikely" to have PE should undergo D-dimer serum testing; if test results are negative, the diagnosis of PE is excluded.[33] All other patients considered "likely" to have PE and patients with an abnormal serum D-dimer test results should undergo spiral CT of the chest. The spiral chest CT scan is the prevailing imaging modality used in the diagnosis of PE because it is readily available and safe. It cannot, however, be used in patients with renal insufficiency or an allergy to contrast dye. In these patients, a ventilation-perfusion scan is preferred, but many clinicians would rather treat patients with suspected PE empirically rather than rely on the poor sensitivity (41%) and specificity (10%) of this scan.[31] A negative result on the spiral CT scan of the chest excludes the diagnosis of PE, whereas patients with positive scan results proceed to appropriate therapy.[35]

Anticoagulation therapy is the treatment of PE in patients without signs of cardiogenic shock or right ventricular dysfunction. Patients with evidence of right-sided cardiac dysfunction (submassive PE) or with signs of shock (massive PE) may also benefit from more aggressive therapies, such as fibrinolysis or embolectomy.[36] The addition of thrombolytic therapy causes faster clot lysis than does heparin therapy alone, but the 12% incidence of major hemorrhage requires careful patient selection.[36,37]

The decision to use thrombolytic therapy should be made in consultation with a cardiologist. Inpatient anticoagulation therapy is initiated with IV heparin, which accelerates the actions of antithrombin III, helps to prevent the formation of additional clots, and promotes fibrinolysis of the existing clot. Therapeutic partial thromboplastin times (PTT) while patients are receiving IV heparin should be reached within 24 hours of treatment initiation; failure to do so has been associated with higher rates of further embolic episodes.[38] Patients receiving heparin should have daily hemograms to monitor for the rare development of heparin-induced thrombocytopenia, which necessitates immediate cessation of heparin therapy and possible initiation of alternative forms of anticoagulation.

Absolute contraindications to heparin therapy are active bleeding, severe bleeding diathesis, a platelet count $\leq$20,000/mm^3, neurosurgical or ocular surgical procedures performed within the past 10 days, or intracranial bleeding within the past 10 days.[39] The placement of an inferior vena cava filter is indicated in patients with a contraindication to anticoagulation therapy or with recurrent VTE despite maximal medical anticoagulation therapy. Warfarin sodium, an oral vitamin K antagonist, remains the mainstay of outpatient anticoagulation therapy, although patients can also be maintained on subcutaneous injections of heparin or low-molecular-weight heparin.

The seventh American College of Chest Physicians Conference on Antithrombotic and Thrombolytic Therapy made recommendations for the use of antithrombotic and thrombolytic therapy in urologic patients.[40] For patients undergoing transurethral, lapa-roscopic, or low-risk procedures, early and persistent mobilization is recommended. Recommendations for patients undergoing major open urologic procedures include intermittent pneumatic compression, use of graduated compression stockings, and early ambulation. These recommendations in combination with the identification of VTE risk factors offer reasonable guidelines for urologic thromboprophylaxis.

PULMONARY COMPLICATIONS OF OPEN AND LAPAROSCOPIC UROLOGIC SURGERY

Given the anatomic proximity of the kidneys and adrenal glands to the costodiaphragmatic pleural spaces, inadvertent violation of the thoracic cavity during open or laparoscopic surgical procedures is possible. Pleural entry during surgical procedures of the flank can result from the intimate association between the pleura and lower ribs: the pleura extends down to the 11th rib in the posterior axillary line and to just below the 12th rib in the area of the vertebral column. Riehle and Lavengood[41] observed that pleural violation usually occurs while the surgeon attempts to separate the pleura and diaphragm during dissection within the intercostal space or because of failure to mobilize the diaphragm sufficiently before retractor placement. Entry into the pleural space is sometimes expected during a flank incision, especially if a rib resection is necessary. Investigators have also reported cases of a kidney tumor invading the diaphragm and necessitating resection of that tissue with subsequent repair.[42]

Open flank surgical procedures for nephrectomy are associated with a risk of pleural injury in >23% of cases, and pneumothorax is a known complication of this surgical approach.[43] In reports by Shaffer and associates[44] and by Stephenson and colleagues,[45] pneumothorax incidence after open nephrectomy ranged from 1% to 10%; 1% of patients undergoing open nephrectomy required postoperative chest tube placement. Most pleural injuries during flank surgical procedures are recognized intraoperatively, and 99% of pneumothoraces are found in patients who sustained an intraoperative injury.[46] Modifications of the traditional flank incision, such as the *supra-11th mini-flank incision,* help to prevent pleural injury during open surgical procedures of the kidney.[47]

Pleurotomies recognized intraoperatively during open flank surgical procedures can usually be repaired without difficulty or sequelae.[48] Adequate mobilization of the diaphragm is usually paramount to facilitate these closures. A 12-Fr rubber catheter is initially placed through the defect and into the pleural cavity, and the pleura is closed with absorbable or nonabsorbable suture in a running pattern. Next, the lung is expanded with positive pressure ventilation; this maneuver forces out the remaining air within the pleural cavity through the end of the catheter, which has been submerged in a container of fluid. The catheter is removed when air ceases to bubble out of its submersed tip. At the same time the catheter is removed from the pleural space, the running suture is tied while the lung remains expanded.

Compared with open flank surgical procedures, diaphragmatic injury during laparoscopic nephrectomy or adrenalectomy is rare, with a reported incidence as low as 0.6%.[49,50] Unlike its open counterpart, laparoscopic urologic surgical procedures are performed during insufflation of the peritoneum or retroperitoneum with carbon dioxide. This gas can seep into the pleural space through small diaphragmatic injuries and can cause sudden collapse of the ipsilateral lung. The resulting pneumothorax can be catastrophic if it is not recognized quickly. The diaphragm may also begin to billow into the surgical field, the so-called *floppy diaphragm sign* of pleural injury.[51] These injuries can also result from endoscopic instruments, such as retractors, that are not in view of the laparoscope, and recognition of the problem may be delayed until the patient begins to show signs of decompensation. Because laparoscopic diaphragmatic injuries may not be as obvious as in open surgical procedures, they manifest more commonly as emergencies.

As in open surgical procedures, suspected diaphragmatic tears during laparoscopy should be repaired primarily, if possible. Depending on the severity of the injury and the clinical status of the anesthetized patient, these repairs can be performed either immediately or after the specimen has been removed. Delaying repair until after specimen extraction may provide better visualization of the injury; however, unstable patients require immediate attention to this complication. In a review of 1765 laparoscopic renal procedures, Del Pizzo and colleagues[50] noted that diaphragmatic injury was able to be addressed at the end of the case when the patient remained hemodynamically stable without acute respiratory decompensation.[50] If repair can be delayed, then it is advised to decrease the pneumoperitoneum to 10 mm Hg to limit the extent of any present pneumothorax, to facilitate patient ventilation, and to allow for tension-free anastomosis.[52]

In repairing large diaphragmatic injuries, the laparoscope can be used to inspect the pleural cavity for any direct pulmonary injuries. Laparoscopic suturing devices or needle drivers are used to close the injury with interrupted figure-of-eight nonabsorbable sutures.[50] Before complete closure of the injury, the laparoscopic suction device is inserted through the rent into the pleural cavity to evacuate any residual air, while a large inspiratory breath is given to the patient by the anesthesiologist. Then the final stitch is secured as the suction device is removed from the pleural cavity. For smaller diaphragmatic insults, such as cautery burns, simply oversewing the area of injury usually suffices, as in open surgical procedures.[50]

Other techniques have been described for repair of diaphragmatic injuries during laparoscopy. These include the use of nonabsorbable sutures with pledgets for tenuous closures, polyglactin mesh stapled over the defect or gelatin thrombin matrix for small defects, and placement of allogenic material, such as polytetrafluoroethylene (PTFE), for large defects.[52-55] Insertion of a chest tube is generally unnecessary unless there is pleural bleeding, injury to the visceral pleura, or failure of the foregoing techniques.[50] If a thoracostomy tube is indicated, it can be placed under vision by passing the laparoscope through the diaphragmatic opening before inserting the chest tube. Postoperatively, patient hemodynamic or respiratory decompensation would certainly justify thoracic surgical consultation and chest tube insertion.

Historically, it had been the standard of care to obtain a chest radiograph after every open flank surgical procedure regardless of the index of suspicion for pleural injury. Latchemsetty and colleagues[46] concluded that postoperative chest radiographs are not routinely needed after open nephrectomy unless they are clinically indicated by, for example, one of the following:

1. Central line placement
2. Intraoperative diaphragmatic injury
3. Respiratory distress
4. Abnormal physical examination findings

Similarly, investigators have noted that postoperative chest radiographs are not useful in patients who undergo uncomplicated laparoscopic surgical procedures.[56]

PULMONARY COMPLICATIONS OF PERCUTANEOUS NEPHROLITHOTOMY

Percutaneous nephrolithotomy (PCNL) is generally a safe treatment option. Most of the complications and injuries to surrounding organs develop from the initial puncture. Total complication rates, including insignificant bleeding and fever, are reported to be as high as 83%.[57,58] The rates of significant bleeding requiring transfusion and of sepsis are 5% to 18% and 1% to 4.7%, respectively.[59] Regarding pleural injuries, complication rates have been reported to range from 2.3% to 23%, depending on the definition of injury.[58-60]

Anatomically, the lower border of the pleural reflection crosses the 10th rib in the midaxillary line and crosses the 12th rib posteriorly at the lateral border of sacrospinal muscle.[61] The posterior portion of the diaphragm arises from the tips of the 10th to 12th ribs and from the lateral and medial arcuate ligaments. Meanwhile, the 11th and 12th ribs cross the upper pole of the kidney. Thus, all supracostal nephrostomy tracts traverse the diaphragm, and in many cases also the pleural space, but the lung may be avoided.[62]

Not surprisingly, the rates of thoracic complications are higher with the supracostal approach for PCNL.[60,63] Subcostal punctures are associated with fewer complications, but under certain circumstances, such as scoliosis, high kidney position, staghorn calculi, upper calyx stone, stone in proximal ureter or pelvis, or duplicated collecting systems, the optimal access route is through a supracostal approach to the upper pole of the kidney.[64] Decreased pulmonary complications have been reported under C-arm fluoroscopic guidance, a technique that also helps to prevent injury to the spleen, liver, bowl, and renal hilum.[65] In addition, punctures should be performed after maximal exhalation, when the lungs are smallest. Hopper and Yakes[66] observed that at end expiration, the likelihood of violating the pleura with supracostal access was 29% on the right and 14% on the left. Nonetheless, a 16-fold greater risk of pleural injury is reported when the puncture is made above the 11th rib as compared with supra-12th rib access.[60] Thus, many urologists avoid supra-11th rib access if possible.

The use of an adequately sized working sheath during supracostal PCNL seals the pleural opening and prevents pneumothorax and hydrothorax while allowing for stone removal and irrigation.[60] During PCNL, maintaining low pressure within the irrigation system minimizes the chances of fluid and air entering the pleural space through the pleural opening from a supracostal approach. Postprocedurally, the drainage catheter should be large enough to tamponade the tract.[65]

Intrathoracic complications, most of which are hydropneumothoraces, following supracostal access for PCNL occur at rates between 3.1% and 12.5%.[60,67] Many urologists routinely obtain postoperative upright chest radiographs to evaluate for these possible injuries. Ogan and coworkers[68] prospectively noted that intraoperative chest fluoroscopic examination during PCNL is sufficient to detect clinically significant hydropneumothoraces and recommended that routine immediate, postoperative chest radiographs are not necessary unless postoperative clinical symptoms become suspicious. These investigators found that both fluoroscopic examinations and upright chest radiographs yielded high false-negative rates when compared with chest CT scans; however, most missed fluid collections were clinically insignificant. Pleural fluid that becomes clinically significant most likely accumulates later in the postoperative period, at which time the development of symptoms or signs warrants imaging and possible intervention.[68]

Golijanin and coworkers[63] reported a 3.5% incidence of thoracostomy tube placement in 115 patients who underwent supracostal PCNL. The incidence of pulmonary complications that necessitate surgical intervention after a supra-12th rib approach ranges from 3% to 23%.[65,68] To avoid painful chest tube placement postoperatively by a thoracic surgeon, Ogan and Pearle[69] described inserting an 8- to 10-Fr loop nephrostomy tube intraoperatively using real-time fluoroscopic guidance into the pleural space of patients who had developed significant hydropneumothorax following supracostal PCNL. These investigators detected significant hydropneumothoraces using intraoperative fluoroscopy and believed that an advantage of this procedure is maintained drainage in cases requiring second-look flexible nephroscopy, which could introduce additional fluid and air into the pleural space. Traditional thoracostomy tube placement is recommended when significant drainage, blood, or parenchymal injury to the lung is detected.

A rare pulmonary complication of PCNL is *nephropleural fistula*. Lallas and colleagues[70] retrospectively reported rates of nephropleural fistulas following supracostal PCNL as 2.3% (2 of 87 cases) in supra-12th rib access and 6.3% (2 of 32 cases) in supra-11th rib access. These fistulas were managed with decompression of the collecting system with ureteral stent, endourologic treatment of any obstruction resulting from residual stone fragments, and decompression of the pleural space with a thoracostomy tube. Refractory cases of intra-thoracic fluid accumulation may require decortication with pleural sclerosis via a thoracic surgical procedure. This group also suggested obtaining antegrade nephrostograms before removing the nephrostomy tube in patients to aid in the diagnosis of this uncommon fistula; however, the cost-effectiveness of this practice is admittedly unknown. To reduce the probability of this relatively rare complication further, Lingeman and associates[71] suggested removing all tubes from the upper pole access site and placing a nephrostomy tube in a remote lower pole location. This method, however, requires an additional puncture and trauma to the kidney and therefore may not be worth the risk reduction of an already infrequent complication.

PATIENTS WITH PRIOR BLEOMYCIN CHEMOTHERAPY

Fortunately for patients with testicular cancer, chemotherapy offers durable responses in almost all patients including those with widely disseminated disease. The current standard of treatment for patients with metastatic germ cell tumors is the following regimen:

1. Bleomycin, an antibiotic with antineoplastic activity
2. Etoposide, a DNA topoisomerase inhibitor
3. Cisplatin, an alkylating agent

This multidrug chemotherapeutic regimen is commonly referred to as BEP. Although patients with good-risk disease can avoid treatment with bleomycin,[72] many patients including those with poor-risk or intermediate-risk disease are subjected to bleomycin.

Urologists should be well aware of potential complications associated with administration of bleomycin. Bleomycin-related toxicities include interstitial pneumonitis (bleomycin-induced pneumonitis [BIP]), which can result in pulmonary fibrosis (2%-40%).[73] In a few patients, this complication may eventually result in death.[74] Toxicity is believed to be related to multiple factors including cumulative bleomycin dose, increasing age, thoracic radiation, poor renal function, exposure to high inspired oxygen concentrations, and a history of smoking.[75] BIP typically begins gradually and manifests in the first few months of therapy but may develop even 6 months following discontinuation of therapy. Initial symptoms of BIP include nonproductive cough, dyspnea with exertion, and fever. Symptoms may progress to dyspnea at rest and cyanosis.[75] Because of similarities in symptoms, a diagnosis of infectious pneumonitis is excluded before the drug is discontinued.

Patients undergoing surgical procedures such as retroperitoneal lymph node dissection after BEP therapy should have a thorough preoperative evaluation. This assessment should include pulmonary function testing because pulmonary fibrosis may result in significant perioperative complications. In a retrospective study of patients undergoing retroperitoneal lymph node dissection after chemotherapy, Baniel and associates[76] identified pulmonary complications as the largest contributors to severe postoperative complications. The conclusion from this study was that conservative fluid administration and limited inspired oxygen concentrations minimized pulmonary complications in patients with bleomycin exposure.[76] Subsequent studies confirmed the importance of meticulous fluid management, although they raised questions regarding the significance of high inspired oxygen concentrations.[77]

KEY POINTS

1. Patients who are at risk for developing pulmonary complications need to be identified preoperatively so that special measures can be undertaken in the perioperative period either to avoid or to mitigate complications.
2. For any patient receiving anesthesia, and especially for those undergoing urologic surgical procedures involving an incision that breaches muscles used during respiration, pulmonary rehabilitation is critical in preventing complications and in fostering the recuperation of normal respiratory status.
3. Surgical patients are also predisposed to atelectasis because of the rapid, shallow breathing pattern and the inhibiting effect of analgesia on spontaneous sighing that is commonly seen in the postoperative setting.
4. Infectious respiratory complications are more common in patients with risk factors such as COPD, altered lung defenses, and active smoking.
5. In preventing PE in patients undergoing transurethral, laparoscopic, or low-risk procedures, early and persistent mobilization is recommended.
6. Recommendations for patients undergoing major open urologic procedures include intermittent pneumatic compression, use of graduated compression stockings, and early ambulation, in addition to VTE prophylaxis when indicated based on risk factors.

REFERENCES

Please see www.expertconsult.com

Chapter 3

CARDIAC COMPLICATIONS OF UROLOGIC SURGERY

Susie N. Hong MD

Cardiology Fellow, Division of Cardiology, Department of Medicine, New York University Medical Center, New York, New York

Arthur Schwartzbard MD

Director, Non-Invasive Cardiology Lab, Manhattan Campus, New York Harbor Healthcare System; Director, Clinical Lipid Research, New York University Center for Prevention of Cardiovascular Disease; Assistant Professor of Medicine, New York University School of Medicine, New York, New York

Cardiac complications can pose significant risks to patients undergoing urologic surgical procedures. Several strategies and guidelines have evolved to help identify patients at greatest risk and therapies have been developed to help modify and minimize cardiac surgical complications. In this chapter, we review the general approach to preoperative assessment as well as perioperative management of cardiovascular disease states that are often encountered.

GENERAL APPROACH TO THE PATIENT

A detailed history and physical examination combined with a baseline electrocardiogram (ECG) can elucidate cardiac disease states, such as coronary artery disease (CAD), congestive heart failure, valvular abnormalities, or arrhythmias. If a cardiac disease state is identified or known, it is important to know the degree, stability, and severity of the condition. Information about previous management and treatment for the condition is helpful in optimizing the patient's preoperative, perioperative, and postoperative course. Additionally, assessments of the patient's baseline functional capacity, comorbid conditions (e.g., diabetes, renal failure), and type of surgical procedure required are important in assessing overall cardiac risk.

PREOPERATIVE CLINICAL EVALUATION

Multiple algorithms have been devised to assess periopverative risk. In this chapter, we review the American College of Cardiology/American Heart Association (ACC/AHA) 2007 guidelines,[1] which incorporate the elements of the Revised Cardiac Risk Index[2] in an algorithm to assess cardiac risk before noncardiac surgical procedures.

American College of Cardiology/ American Heart Association 2007 Guidelines

The ACC/AHA 2007 guidelines on perioperative cardiovascular evaluation for noncardiac surgical procedures concluded that identifying patients with active cardiac conditions, by careful history taking and clinical assessment, is crucial before elective surgical procedures. Terminology such as *cleared for surgery* as a preoperative assessment is not recommended by the ACC/AHA[1] because such statements may not accurately assess a patient's overall cardiac risk during surgery and can possibly be misleading.

The ACC/AHA 2007 guidelines recommend obtaining at least four components from a patient's history and physical examination to assess whether a patient can safely proceed to surgery, the patient's overall cardiac risk, and whether additional testing is needed. Additionally, these variables are needed to navigate the stepwise approach algorithm devised by the 2007 ACC/AHA guidelines. These components are as follows:

1. Clinical risk factors (Box 3-1)
2. Cardiac risk assessment: identification of active cardiac conditions requiring evaluation and treatment (Table 3-1)
3. Functional capacity (Table 3-2)
4. Surgery-specific risk (Table 3-3)

Clinical Risk Factors

The ACC/AHA 2007 guidelines incorporate several elements of the Revised Cardiac Risk Index,[2] one of the most widely used risk indices for preoperative evaluation for noncardiac surgery, into its assessment of clinical risk factors for preoperative assessment before noncardiac surgical procedures (see Box 3-1). Active cardiac disease indicates a major clinical risk. The pres-

BOX 3-1 Clinical Cardiac Risk Factors

- History of ischemic heart disease*
- History of compensated or prior heart failure†
- History of cerebrovascular disease‡
- Diabetes mellitus (insulin treated)
- Renal insufficiency (creatinine >2 mg/dL)

Ischemic heart disease is defined as history of myocardial infarction, history of positive treadmill test result, use of nitroglycerin, chronic stable angina, or electrocardiogram with abnormal Q waves.
†*Congestive heart failure* is defined as history of heart failure, pulmonary edema, paroxysmal nocturnal dyspnea, peripheral edema, bilateral rales, S_3, or radiograph with pulmonary vascular redistribution.
‡*Cerebrovascular disease* (history of transient ischemic attack or stroke).

TABLE 3-1 Active Cardiac Conditions for Which the Patient Should Undergo Evaluation and Treatment Before Noncardiac Surgery (Class I, Level of Evidence: B)

Condition	Examples
Unstable coronary syndromes	Unstable or severe angina* (CCS class III or IV)† Recent MI‡
Decompensated HF (NYHA functional class IV; worsening or new-onset HF) Significant arrhythmias	High-grade atrioventricular block Mobitz II atrioventricular block Third-degree atrioventricular heart block Symptomatic ventricular arrhythmias Supraventricular arrhythmias (including atrial fibrillation) with uncontrolled ventricular rate (HR >100 bpm at rest) Symptomatic bradycardia Newly recognized ventricular tachycardia
Severe valvular disease	Severe aortic stenosis (mean pressure gradient >40 mm Hg, aortic valve area <1.0 cm², or symptomatic) Symptomatic mitral stenosis (progressive dyspnea on exertion, exertional presyncope, or HF)

bpm, beats per minute; CCS, Canadian Cardiovascular Society; HF, heart failure; HR, heart rate; MI, myocardial infarction; NYHA, New York Heart Association.
*According to Campeau L. Grading of angina pectoris [letter]. *Circulation.* 1976;54:522-523.
†May include "stable" angina in patients who are unusually sedentary.
‡The American College of Cardiology National Database Library defines *recent MI* as >7 days but ≤1 month (≤30 days).
From Fleisher LA, Beckman JA, Brown KA, et al. ACC/AHA 2007 guidelines on perioperative cardiovascular evaluation and care for noncardiac surgery: a report of the American College of Cardiology/American Heart Association Task Force on Practice Guidelines (Writing Committee to Revise the 2002 Guidelines on Perioperative Cardiovascular Evaluation for Noncardiac Surgery): developed in collaboration with the American Society of Echocardiography, American Society of Nuclear Cardiology, Heart Rhythm Society, Society of Cardiovascular Anesthesiologists, Society for Cardiovascular Angiography and Interventions, Society for Vascular Medicine and Biology, and Society for Vascular Surgery. *Circulation.* 2007;116(17):e418-e499.

ence of one or more active cardiac conditions (see Table 3-1) mandates intensive management and may result in the delay or cancellation of the operation unless it is an emergency.

The ACC/AHA chose to replace the intermediate-risk category with the clinical risk factors from the index, with the exclusion of the type of surgery, which is incorporated elsewhere in the approach to the patient. Clinical risk factors include the following:

1. History of ischemic heart disease
2. History of compensated or prior heart failure
3. History of cerebrovascular disease
4. Diabetes mellitus
5. Renal insufficiency

Ischemic heart disease is defined as history of myocardial infarction (MI), a history of a positive treadmill test result, use of nitroglycerin, chronic stable angina, or an ECG with abnormal Q waves. *Congestive heart failure* is defined as a history of heart failure, pulmonary edema, paroxysmal nocturnal dyspnea, peripheral edema, bilateral rales, S_3, or a radiograph showing pulmonary vascular redistribution cerebrovascular disease (history of transient ischemic attack or stroke). *Diabetes mellitus* is defined as preoperative insulin treatment for diabetes mellitus, and *renal insufficiency* is defined as a preoperative creatinine concentration of >2 mg/dL. Increasing numbers of risk factors correlate with increased risk. Although no adequate clinical trials on which to base firm recommendations have been conducted, it appears reasonable to wait 4 to 6 weeks after MI to perform elective surgical procedures.[1]

Cardiac Risk Assessment

Identifying the highest-risk patient is critical to avoid serious complications and adverse outcomes in elective noncardiac surgery. History taking should attempt to identify serious cardiac conditions such as unstable coronary syndromes, prior angina, recent or past MI, decompensated heart failure, significant arrhythmias, and severe valvular disease (see Table 3-1). The presence of one or more of these conditions mandates intensive management and may result in delay or cancellation of a surgical procedure unless it is an emergency.

Exercise Capacity

The assessment of functional capacity provides important prognostic information, since patients with good functional status have a lower risk of complications. Functional status can be expressed in metabolic equivalents (MET). Perioperative cardiac and long-term risks are increased in patients unable to meet a 4-MET demand during most normal daily activities. Various activity scales provide the clinician with a set of questions to determine a patient's functional capacity. See Table 3-2 for a functional status assessment and estimated energy requirements for various activities.

Confounding factors in assessing functional capacity include a history of arthritis or peripheral vascular disease. If ambulation cannot be assessed because of these limitations, a careful history of other METs (e.g., household chores not involving walking, upper extremity activities) can be helpful in evaluating a patient's functional capacity.

Surgery-specific Risk

Urologic procedures are generally considered intermediate-risk procedures. However, the timing of surgery (emergency versus elective) can alter the patient's risk significantly. Additionally, urologic procedures involving large volume shifts, as well as procedures in elderly patients, can increase cardiac risk. Cardiac risk stratification is listed in Table 3-3. Intermediate-risk procedures are generally associated with a 1% to 5% cardiac risk. Care should be taken in optimizing a patient preoperatively and perioperatively to minimize risk and to maximize medical therapy based on overall cardiac risk.

In emergency surgery, which generally is associated with substantial risk, risk indices do not necessarily apply because these indices are derived mostly from elective procedures,. However, these algorithms can assist in providing an estimate of the patient's minimal risk. Further testing and interventions are likely not very beneficial given that patients are usually better off proceeding directly to surgery. In general, emergency surgical procedures should be assumed to be high risk, and much care should be taken in optimizing the medical management of these patients. If a patient has a known cardiac condition, medical therapy should be targeted to the specific disease state to optimize medical care and to minimize complications (see "Management of Specific Preoperative Cardiac Conditions").

Urgent surgery (need for a procedure during the same admission but able to be delayed a few days without significant patient compromise) is another category that likely increases cardiac risk.[3] With urgent surgery, initial risk estimates should be made preoperatively. However, additional testing and subsequent therapies are often limited, except for identifying and stabilizing patients with unstable cardiac disease.

Overall Risk Assessment

A stepwise approach generalizing cardiac risk assessment can be seen in **Figure 3-1**, which combines the

TABLE 3-2	Estimated Energy Requirements for Various Activities		
	Can you ...		**Can you ...**
1 MET	Take care of yourself?	4 METs	Climb a flight of stairs or walk up a hill?
	Eat, dress, or use the toilet?		Walk on level ground at 4 mph (6.4 kph)?
	Walk indoors around the house?		Run a short distance?
	Walk a block or 2 on level ground at 2-3 mph (3.2-4.8 kph)?		Do heavy work around the house such as scrubbing floors or lifting or moving heavy furniture?
4 METs	Do light work around the house like dusting or washing dishes?		Participate in moderate recreational activities like golfing, bowling, dancing, playing doubles tennis, or throwing a baseball or football?
		>10 METs	Participate in strenuous sports like swimming, singles tennis, football, basketball, or skiing?

kph, kilometers per hour; MET, metabolic equivalent; mph, miles per hour.

Modified from Hlatky MA, Boineau RE, Higgenbotham MB, et al. A brief self-administered questionnaire to determine functional capacity (the Duke Activity Status Index). *Am J Cardiol.* 1989;64:651-654.

TABLE 3-3	Cardiac Risk* Stratification for Noncardiac Surgical Procedures	
Risk Stratification		**Procedure Examples**
Vascular (reported cardiac risk often >5%)		Aortic and other major vascular surgery Peripheral vascular surgery
Intermediate (reported cardiac risk generally 1%-5%)		Intraperitoneal and intrathoracic surgery Carotid endarterectomy Head and neck surgery Orthopedic surgery Prostate surgery
Low[†] (reported cardiac risk generally <1%)		Endoscopic procedures Superficial procedure Cataract surgery Breast surgery Ambulatory surgery

*Combines incidence of cardiac death and nonfatal myocardial infarction.

†These procedures do not generally require further preoperative cardiac testing.

From Fleisher LA, Beckman JA, Brown KA, et al. ACC/AHA 2007 guidelines on perioperative cardiovascular evaluation and care for noncardiac surgery: a report of the American College of Cardiology/American Heart Association Task Force on Practice Guidelines (Writing Committee to Revise the 2002 Guidelines on Perioperative Cardiovascular Evaluation for Noncardiac Surgery): developed in collaboration with the American Society of Echocardiography, American Society of Nuclear Cardiology, Heart Rhythm Society, Society of Cardiovascular Anesthesiologists, Society for Cardiovascular Angiography and Interventions, Society for Vascular Medicine and Biology, and Society for Vascular Surgery. *Circulation.* 2007;116(17):e418-e499.

four elements in risk assessment into a preoperative algorithm for noncardiac surgery. **Figure 3-1** is broken down into five steps that aid in deciding which patients would benefit from further evaluation of CAD and which patients are at greatest risk for cardiac complications perioperatively.

In general, emergency surgical procedures do not allow for preoperative cardiac evaluation because it may delay the patient from a potentially lifesaving procedure. Such patients should be medically optimized perioperatively and postoperatively. For patients whose cardiac risk assessment may require that their surgical

procedure be delayed, formal consultation with a cardiologist is recommended.

PREOPERATIVE TESTING

Resting Electrocardiogram

A preoperative 12-lead resting ECG is recommended in the following patients:

1. Patients with at least one clinical risk factor (see Box 3-1) who are undergoing vascular (high-risk) surgical procedures (see Table 3-3)

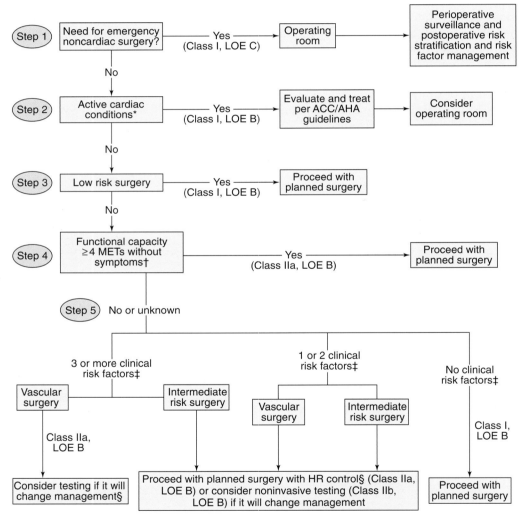

Figure 3-1 Cardiac evaluation and care algorithm for noncardiac surgery based on active clinical conditions, known cardiovascular disease, or cardiac risk factors for patients ≥50 years old. *See Table 3-1 for active clinical conditions. †See Table 3-2 for estimated metabolic equivalent (MET) level. ‡Clinical risk factors include ischemic heart disease, compensated or prior heart failure, diabetes mellitus, renal insufficiency, and cerebrovascular disease. §Consider perioperative β-blockade for populations in which this has been shown to reduce cardiac morbidity and mortality. ACC/AHA, American College of Cardiology/American Heart Association; HR, heart rate; LOE, level of evidence. (From Fleisher LA, Beckman JA, Brown KA, et al. ACC/AHA 2007 guidelines on perioperative cardiovascular evaluation and care for noncardiac surgery: a report of the American College of Cardiology/American Heart Association Task Force on Practice Guidelines [Writing Committee to Revise the 2002 Guidelines on Perioperative Cardiovascular Evaluation for Noncardiac Surgery]: developed in collaboration with the American Society of Echocardiography, American Society of Nuclear Cardiology, Heart Rhythm Society, Society of Cardiovascular Anesthesiologists, Society for Cardiovascular Angiography and Interventions, Society for Vascular Medicine and Biology, and Society for Vascular Surgery. *Circulation.* 2007;116[17]:e418-e499.)

2. Patients with known CAD, peripheral arterial disease, or cerebrovascular disease who are undergoing inter-mediate-risk surgical procedures

A preoperative ECG is generally not recommended as a routine test in asymptomatic patients undergoing low-risk procedures. Q waves or significant ST-segment deviation (elevations or depression) are often associated with an increased incidence of cardiac complications and should be further evaluated.

Stress Testing

Routine screening for cardiac disease of asymptomatic men or women is generally not recommended for pre-operative evaluation for noncardiac surgery. Stress testing is a good way of evaluating CAD in patients with an intermediate pretest probability of CAD and assess-ing a patient's functional capacity, if exercise stress testing is used. Poor functional capacity in patients with chronic CAD or those convalescing after an acute cardiac event is associated with an increased risk of subsequent cardiac morbidity and mortality.[4] The

ACC/AHA provides a prognostic gradient of ischemic responses during an ECG-monitored exercise test in Table 3-4, as developed for a general population of patients with suspected or proven CAD. However, much thought should be taken into account in using informa-tion obtained by noninvasive stress testing, because this information can lead to further unnecessary testing (both noninvasive and invasive), complications of such testing, and possible delay of surgical procedures.

PREOPERATIVE AND PERIOPERATIVE MEDICAL THERAPY

Physiologic factors associated with surgery predispose patients to myocardial ischemia, which is more pro-nounced in patients with underlying CAD. These factors include volume shifts and blood loss, enhanced myo-cardial oxygen demand from elevations in heart rate and blood pressure secondary to stress from surgery, and an increase in postoperative platelet reactivity. Optimizing medical therapy alone with close cardiac monitoring is often a reasonable strategy for patients undergoing urologic procedures.

TABLE 3-4	Prognostic Gradient of Ischemic Responses During an ECG-Monitored Exercise Test in Patients With Suspected or Proven CAD
Risk Level	**Ischemic Response Gradient**
High	Ischemia induced by low-level exercise* (<4 METs or heart rate <100 bpm or <70% of age-predicted heart rate) manifested by one or more of the following: Horizontal or downsloping ST-segment depression >0.1 mV ST-segment elevation >0.1 mV in noninfarct lead 5 or more abnormal leads Persistent ischemic response >3 minutes after exertion Typical angina Exercise-induced decrease in systolic blood pressure by 10 mm Hg
Intermediate	Ischemia induced by moderate-level exercise (4-6 METs or heart rate 100-130 bpm [70%-85% of age-predicted heart rate]) manifested by one or more of the following: Horizontal or downsloping ST-segment depression >0.1 mV Persistent ischemic response >1-3 minutes after exertion 3-4 abnormal leads
Low	No ischemia or ischemia induced at high-level exercise (>7 METs or heart rate >130 bpm [>85% of age-predicted heart rate]) manifested by: Horizontal or downsloping ST-segment depression >0.1 mV 1 or 2 abnormal leads
Inadequate Test	Inability to reach adequate target workload or heart rate response for age without an ischemic response; for patients undergoing noncardiac surgery, the inability to exercise to at least the intermediate-risk level without ischemia should be considered an inadequate test

bpm, beats per min; CAD, coronary artery disease; MET, metabolic equivalent.
*Workload and heart rate estimates for risk severity require adjustment for patient age. Maximum target heart rates for 40- and 80-year-old subjects taking no cardioactive medication are 180 and 140 bpm, respectively.
From Fleisher LA, Beckman JA, Brown KA, et al. ACC/AHA 2007 guidelines on perioperative cardiovascular evaluation and care for noncardiac surgery: a report of the American College of Cardiology/American Heart Association Task Force on Practice Guidelines (Writing Committee to Revise the 2002 Guidelines on Perioperative Cardiovascular Evaluation for Noncardiac Surgery): developed in collaboration with the American Society of Echocardiography, American Society of Nuclear Cardiology, Heart Rhythm Society, Society of Cardiovascular Anesthesiologists, Society for Cardiovascular Angiography and Interventions, Society for Vascular Medicine and Biology, and Society for Vascular Surgery. *Circulation.* 2007;116(17):e418-e499.

β-Blockers

β-Blockers may be beneficial in higher-risk patients who are undergoing major noncardiac surgery.[5] However, a 2006 ACC/AHA guideline update on perioperative β-blocker therapy noted major limitations in the published literature regarding this issue.[6] More recently, a large randomized controlled trial of patients undergoing noncardiac surgery with risk factors found that although β-blockade decreases the risk of MI, it may increase the risk of stroke and overall mortality.[7]

As a result of newer evidence and questionable benefit of perioperative β-blocker treatment for noncardiac surgery, we recommend the following:

1. β-Blockers should be continued in patients undergoing surgery who are already receiving β-blockers to treat angina, symptomatic arrhythmias, hypertension, or other ACC/AHA class I guideline indications.
2. β-Blockers are probably recommended for patients in whom preoperative assessment for high-risk surgery (e.g., vascular surgery) identifies high cardiac risk owing to the findings of ischemia on preoperative testing.

We do not recommend using β-blockers in patients at low to intermediate risk who are not already being treated with a β-blocker. However, β-blockers should not be withdrawn before noncardiac surgical procedures from patients already receiving β-blocker therapy for other indications.

Statins

Among patients who are undergoing major vascular surgery or those with known CAD, we recommend continuing statin therapy in patients already being treated and, in previously untreated patients, initiating statin therapy before elective vascular surgical procedures. Among patients not previously treated with statins who are undergoing urgent or emergency major vascular surgical procedures, we suggest initiating statin therapy in the perioperative period and, if possible, preoperatively. Over the long term, we recommend that statin therapy be titrated to recommended goals.

MANAGEMENT OF SPECIFIC PREOPERATIVE CARDIAC CONDITIONS

Hypertension

Known hypertension, particularly stage 3 hypertension (systolic blood pressure ≥180 mm Hg and diastolic blood pressure ≥110 mm Hg) should be controlled preoperatively. In most cases, an effective medical regimen can be achieved over several days to weeks of preoperative outpatient treatment.

If surgery is more urgent, rapid-acting agents can be administered that allow effective blood pressure control in a matter of minutes or hours. β-Blockers are particularly effective agents and may reduce perioperative complications in high-risk patients. Most important, continuation of preoperative antihypertensive treatment through the perioperative period is critical, and a patient's medical antihypertensive regimen must be ascertained before the procedure. Because of potential heart rate or blood pressure rebound, particular care should be taken to avoid withdrawal of β-blockers and clonidine.

Ischemic Heart Disease

Evaluation for Coronary Artery Disease

One of the most important historical assessments of patients with known CAD is to determine whether the patient is experiencing angina. If the patient is asymptomatic and receiving an effective cardiac regimen, medical optimization without further testing for CAD is generally recommended. However, if a patient experiences symptoms, great care should be taken in determining whether the angina is stable or unstable.

Patients with *chronic stable angina* (chest pain worsened by exercise and relieved by rest or sublingual nitrogen) should be managed with optimal medical therapy before surgical procedures. Preoperative noninvasive or invasive cardiac testing is generally not recommended.

Unstable angina (chest pain that occurs at rest or sleep and is unrelieved by rest or sublingual nitroglycerin) should be evaluated further before surgical procedures. If a patient is experiencing symptoms of unstable angina or an MI, medical optimization, a baseline ECG, and referral to a cardiologist for further testing or cardiac catheterization are highly recommended. Cardiac revascularization may delay the patient's surgical procedure, especially if percutaneous intervention (PCI) with stenting is performed. Given evidence regarding the limited value of coronary revascularization before noncardiac surgical procedures,[8] the indication for preoperative testing is limited to patients with active cardiac disease and groups in whom coronary revascularization may be beneficial independent of noncardiac surgical procedures.

Noninvasive Testing Exercise ECG testing is the preferred stress test given the importance of exercise tolerance as a predictor of outcome. Exercise ECG testing is usually performed with perfusion imaging or echocardiography because imaging can better identify high-risk features that would warrant referral for angiography. For patients who cannot exercise, adenosine/dipyridamole stress testing and dobutamine echocardiography are other options for noninvasive cardiac testing to assess CAD.

We recommend the following patients for noninvasive testing:

1. Patients with active cardiac conditions (see Table 3-1) in whom noncardiac surgical procedures are planned; these patients should be evaluated and treated by a cardiologist preoperatively
2. Patients with three or more clinical risk factors and poor functional capacity (<4 METs) who require vascular surgical procedures, if it will change management

Preoperative Percutaneous Interventions

Preoperative PCI should be limited to patients with active unstable CAD who would possibly benefit from emergency or urgent revascularization.[9,10] In patients with acute coronary syndrome in whom a noncardiac surgical procedure is imminent, despite an increased risk in the peri-MI period, a strategy of balloon angioplasty or bare metal stent (BMS) use should be considered. However, patients with asymptomatic ischemia or stable angina do not appear to be candidates for prophylactic preoperative coronary revascularization unless cardiac catheterization reveals high-risk surgical anatomy, including left main artery or triple-vessel CAD.

Management of Patients With Coronary Stents

Perioperative coronary artery stent thrombosis is a potentially catastrophic surgical complication. Coronary stents, especially recently placed stents, can be a challenge for the patient, anesthesiologist, and surgeon, especially when the patient is receiving dual antiplatelet therapy. Noncardiac surgical procedures appear to increase the risk of thrombosis to recently placed stents, likely because of several factors including lack of endothelium of a recently placed stent, a proinflammatory state during surgery, and discontinuation of dual antiplatelet therapy perioperatively.

One of the important ways to manage a patient with known coronary stents is to determine how recently the stent was placed, in which coronary artery it was placed, and what type of stent was placed (BMS versus drug-eluting stent [DES]). It is important to hold a preoperative discussion with the cardiology, anesthesia, and urology departments regarding optimal management, especially if a patient had a recent PCI. In such patients, if possible, urologic surgery should occur in a center with interventional cardiology capability so any complication that may occur can be immediately evaluated and treated with PCI.

Bare Metal Stents It is recommended that patients with BMSs delay noncardiac surgical procedures for ≥2 weeks and ideally 6 weeks after implantation for allow for partial endothelialization.[1] The earlier the surgical procedure after stenting (<6 weeks), the higher the risk for in-stent thrombosis.[11-15] After 6 weeks of BMS placement, the patient can be maintained on aspirin therapy, which should be continued during and after the surgical procedure.

Drug-Eluting Stents DESs were designed to reduce neointimal formation and therefore result in lower restenosis rates. Sirolimus and paclitaxel, the two currently used medicated coatings on DES, delay endothelialization and healing. DESs may also induce hypersensitivity to the drug or polymer used and lead to an increased risk of thrombosis.[16,17] Thrombosis of DES may occur late and has been reported up to 1.5 years after implantation, particularly in the context of discontinuation of antiplatelet agents before noncardiac surgical procedures.[18,19] Because few data are available regarding long-term outcomes regarding DESs, the optimal delay of noncardiac surgical procedures is unknown. However, current recommendations suggest that is it likely to be >12 months.

Recommendations Regarding Preoperative Aspirin and Clopidogrel Use

If preoperative PCI is considered, any potential benefit must be balanced against the requirements for a full course of aggressive antiplatelet therapy with aspirin and clopidogrel. Premature discontinuation of antiplatelet therapy carries a substantial risk of stent thrombosis, MI, and death, a risk that may be exacerbated by surgery. A science advisory by multiple medical and surgical societies was published in 2007 regarding the withholding of antiplatelet therapy with aspirin and clopidogrel given the data concerning complications associated with DESs.[20] This advisory stresses the importance of 12 months of dual antiplatelet therapy after placement of a DES and education of the patient and health care providers about hazards of premature antiplatelet therapy discontinuation. Additionally, it recommends postponing elective surgical procedures for 1 year, and if operations cannot be deferred, considering the continuation of aspirin during the perioperative period in high-risk patients with DESs.

Patients who undergo PCI with BMSs within 6 weeks, and particularly within 2 weeks, of major noncardiac surgical procedures have an increased risk of death or MI, a finding usually reflecting stent thrombosis, which may be associated with withholding or reducing antiplatelet therapy to minimize bleeding.[11] This risk continues for a much longer period in patients with DESs, probably because of delayed neointimal coverage. In contrast, the thrombotic risk is low with angioplasty alone, although this approach is associated with substantially higher rates of restenosis and target vessel revascularization. In general, it is recommended that dual antiplatelet therapy (aspirin and clopidogrel) be continued, whenever possible, during and after surgical procedures, especially in patients with DESs.[20]

In patients in which clopidogrel must be discontinued preoperatively, the following strategy is recommended[8]:

1. Continue low-dose aspirin (81 mg/day) during and after the surgical procedure.
2. Hold clopidogrel 5 to 7 days preoperatively but "bridge" the patient to surgery using a short-acting antiplatelet agent with a glycoprotein IIb/IIIa inhibitor or an antithrombin (e.g., heparin) in the interim.
3. Restart clopidogrel as soon as possible postoperatively.

Heart Failure

Heart failure has been identified in several studies in association with a poorer outcome of noncardiac surgical procedures.[21-23] For patients with known heart failure, it is important to identify the cause of their cardiac disease because management and prognosis may differ depending on the disease process (e.g., ischemic, hypertensive, hypertrophic cardiomyopathy). *Hypertrophic obstructive cardiomyopathy* poses special problems. Reduction of blood volume, decreased systemic vascular resistance, and increased venous capacitance may reduce left ventricular volume and thereby potentially increase outflow obstruction, with potentially malignant results. If a patient is known to have hypertrophic obstructive cardiomyopathy, a cardiologist should be consulted before noncardiac surgical procedures for optimal medical management in the preoperative, perioperative, and postoperative periods.

Regardless of origin, a baseline transthoracic echocardiogram to evaluate left ventricular function is recommended preoperatively for patients with known heart failure. Fluid status, assessed clinically, is critical regarding preoperative management, and a baseline preoperative weight measurement is essential. Strict intake and outputs should be recorded during and after the surgical procedure.

The use of pulmonary artery catheters should be reserved for patients with tenuous fluid status with potential large volume shifts perioperatively, in which the ability to assess volume overload cannot be ascertained on physical examination. Additionally, a pulmonary artery catheter is useful if the patient is critically ill and findings may be confounded by a septic picture.

Therapy

All efforts regarding optimizing medical management for heart failure as recommended by the ACC/AHA guidelines (e.g., β-blockers, angiotensin-converting enzyme [ACE] inhibitors, diuretics)[24] should be made preoperatively to minimize complications that may occur in the perioperative and postoperative periods. Preoperative consultation with the patient's internist or cardiologist regarding dose titration of the heart failure regimen is recommended.

Valvular Heart Disease

Indications for evaluation and treatment of valvular heart disease are the same as those in the non-preoperative setting.[25] A baseline transthoracic echocardiogram is recommended preoperatively for patients with known valvular abnormalities or a cardiac murmur not previously evaluated. If a patient is found or known to have a moderate to severe valvular abnormality, consultation with a cardiologist is recommended preoperatively for evaluation for need for repair or replacement as well as optimal medical management before and during the surgical procedure.

Severe Stenotic Lesions (Aortic Stenosis and Mitral Stenosis)

Symptomatic severe stenotic lesions are associated with risk of perioperative heart failure or shock and may require percutaneous valvulotomy or valve replacement before noncardiac surgical procedures to lower cardiac risk. Severe aortic stenosis poses the greatest risk for noncardiac surgery.[25] When aortic stenosis is symptomatic, elective noncardiac surgical procedures should generally be postponed or canceled. Such patients require aortic valve replacement before elective but necessary noncardiac surgical procedures. When aortic stenosis is severe but asymptomatic, noncardiac surgical procedures should be postponed or canceled if the valve has not been evaluated within the year. Conversely, in patients with severe aortic stenosis who refuse cardiac surgery or are otherwise not candidates for aortic valve replacement, noncardiac surgical procedures can be performed with a mortality risk of approximately 10%.[26] If a patient is not a candidate for valve replacement because of serious comorbid conditions, percutaneous balloon aortic valvuloplasty may be considered, with careful consultation with a referring cardiologist and interventional cardiologist.

Significant mitral stenosis increases the risk of heart failure; however, preoperative surgical correction of mitral valve disease is not indicated before a noncardiac surgical procedure unless the valvular condition should be corrected to prolong survival and to prevent complications that are unrelated to the proposed noncardiac surgical procedure.[1] When stenosis is severe, the patient may benefit from balloon mitral valvuloplasty or open surgical repair before high-risk surgical procedures are performed.[27]

Severe Regurgitant Lesions (Aortic Insufficiency and Mitral Insufficiency)

Symptomatic regurgitant valve disease is usually better tolerated perioperatively and may be stabilized preoperatively with intensive medical therapy and monitoring. Regurgitant valve disease can then be treated definitively with valve repair or replacement after a noncardiac surgical procedure. Medical therapy and monitoring are appropriate when a significant delay before noncardiac surgical procedures may not have severe consequences. Exceptions may include severe valvular regurgitation with reduced left ventricular function, in which overall hemodynamic reserve is so limited that destabilization during perioperative stresses is likely. Patients who have severe symptomatic mitral regurgitation or aortic insufficiency should be considered for further evaluation, and a cardiologist should be consulted for optimal preoperative management.

Cardiac Arrhythmias and Conduction Defects

The stress of surgery or large fluid shifts seen in certain urologic procedures (e.g., retroperitoneal dissections) can trigger many types of cardiac arrhythmias (atrial or ventricular). The presence of an arrhythmia or cardiac conduction disturbance should provoke a careful evaluation for underlying cardiopulmonary disease, drug toxicity, or metabolic abnormality. Therapy should be initiated for symptomatic or hemodynamically significant arrhythmias, first to reverse an underlying cause and then to treat the arrhythmia. Indications for antiarrhythmic therapy and cardiac pacing are identical to those in the nonoperative setting. Frequent ventricular premature beats or asymptomatic nonsustained ventricular tachycardia have not been associated with an increased risk of nonfatal MI or cardiac death in the perioperative period, and therefore aggressive monitoring or treatment in the perioperative period generally is not necessary.

In the setting of any hemodynamically unstable arrhythmia, acute cardiopulmonary life support (ACLS) protocol should be instituted with the goal of patient stabilization. Once the patient is stabilized or if the patient is already stable, a general approach to a patient with an arrhythmia should include determining whether the arrhythmia has an atrial or a ventricular origin.

Atrial Arrhythmias

Sinus Tachycardia The most common atrial arrhythmia is *sinus tachycardia*. In most cases, treatment of the underlying cause of sinus tachycardia (e.g., blood transfusion, infection control, pain relief) should be the therapy of choice.

Atrial Fibrillation *Atrial fibrillation* is another very common atrial arrhythmia found postoperatively. It is important to know whether the patient has underlying atrial fibrillation (chronic versus paroxysmal) or whether this is a first-time event because as anticoagulation with heparin or warfarin to prevent future cerebrovascular events must be addressed. An underlying transthoracic echocardiogram and consultation with a cardiologist

are recommended to assess any structural cardiac abnormalities and future management. Rate control with atrioventricular (AV) nodal blocking agents (e.g., β-blockers) in the preoperative, perioperative, and postoperative periods is highly recommended. Additionally, postoperatively, patients often experience an increase in catecholamine levels (e.g., blood loss, infection, pain) that can make rate control challenging. In such cases, treating underlying causes is also recommended because AV nodal blocking agents are often vasodilators, a property that can make blood pressure management difficult with increasing dose titration.

Amiodarone is a common rate-controlling AV nodal blocking agent that is often used in patients with postoperative atrial fibrillation. In the setting of a hemodynamically unstable patient, this may be a first-line medication if electrical cardioversion is not readily available. However, one must take the risk of chemical cardioversion with amiodarone, a risk that can present a problem in patients with known chronic atrial fibrillation who may have a preexisting atrial thrombus. Intravenous amiodarone can be associated with hypotension, proarrhythmia, and liver toxicity.[28] Additionally, amiodarone carries a risk of multiorgan toxicity, especially with long-term use. Its use in young patients should be carefully considered. In general, β-blockade, calcium channel blockers, or digoxin should be considered before use of amiodarone in a young patient with a structurally normal heart.

Other Atrial Tachycardias *Supraventricular tachycardias,* including atrial flutter, AV nodal reentrant tachycardias, AV reentrant tachycardias, and atrial tachycardias can be extremely difficult to manage medically. Such atrial arrhythmias should be evaluated by a cardiologist and potentially referred to an electrophysiologist for electrophysiologic study and consideration for percutaneous ablation therapy.

Ventricular Arrhythmias

Ventricular Premature Contractions *Ventricular premature contractions* are usually not associated with increased mortality, but a patient who is found to have frequent ventricular premature contractions should be evaluated by transthoracic echocardiography for any structural abnormalities. Additionally, the patient's electrolytes should be checked and corrected because metabolic derangements can predispose a patient to significant arrhythmias.

Nonsustained Ventricular Tachycardia *Nonsustained ventricular tachycardia* can be a harbinger for ventricular tachycardia or ventricular fibrillation and should be evaluated. A baseline transthoracic echocardiogram, ECG, and electrolyte panel should be the initial first steps. Nonsustained ventricular tachycardia in the setting of cardiomyopathy may warrant evaluation for an implantable cardioverter-defibrillator (ICD), and consultation with a cardiologist is recommended. Medical management with β-blockade is recommended, as is treatment of any underlying any structural heart disease.

Ventricular Tachycardia and Ventricular Fibrillation All hemodynamically unstable ventricular arrhythmias *(ventricular tachycardia/ventricular fibrillation)* should be managed according to ACLS protocol guidelines, which include electrocardioversion or amiodarone. A cardiologist should be consulted for an evaluation of precipitation causes (e.g., ischemia, electrolyte abnormalities, medications) and to see whether an implantable defibrillator is warranted for secondary prevention.

Pacemakers and Implantable Cardioverter-defibrillator

Patients with a pacemaker or an ICD require management perioperatively if an electrocautery device is to be used intraoperatively because the electrocautery unit may interfere with the pacemaker's or ICD's sensing capabilities and subsequent energy delivery. The pacemaker or ICD can be managed by the anesthesia or cardiology department. It is imperative that the type and manufacturer of the device be identified to assist the consultant who may need to perform programming. In general, ICD devices should be programmed off immediately preoperatively and then on again postoperatively, with defibrillator pads placed on the patient intraoperatively as backup. Pacemakers, pending their use, may need to have their sensing turned off with default pacing.

CONCLUSION

For many patients undergoing noncardiac surgical procedures, a preoperative evaluation is wonderful opportunity to receive appropriate cardiac assessment in the short and long term. Because the field of medicine is dynamic, with constant updating of guidelines and novel therapies for specific disease processes, it is important that all involved share data and optimize patients' outcomes as well as modifying CAD risk factors. In general, the use of both noninvasive and invasive preoperative tests should be limited to those circumstances in which the results of such tests will clearly affect patient management. Ultimately, successful outcomes of urologic surgery with minimal cardiac complications require careful preoperative evaluation and good communication among the patient and team of specialists.

KEY POINTS

1. A detailed history and physical examination may elucidate cardiac disease states and avoid unnecessary cardiac testing prior to elective surgery.
2. Active cardiac conditions (e.g., unstable coronary syndromes, decompensated heart failure, and severe valvular disease) should be further evaluated prior to elective surgery.
3. Patients with a history of recent stenting of the coronary arteries must be evaluated by a cardiologist to determine whether discontinuation of anti-platelet therapy (aspirin and/or clopidogrel) is safe prior to urologic surgery. If discontinuation of anti-platelet therapy is not safe, surgery may need to be delayed or performed with patient on anti-platelet therapy.
4. Patients with pacemakers or ICDs undergoing surgery with an electrocautery device should be managed by anesthesia or cardiology intraoperatively. The type and manufacturer of the device should be identified to assist the consultant for programming.

REFERENCES

Please see www.expertconsult.com

Chapter 4

HEMATOLOGIC COMPLICATIONS

Basir Tareen MD
Fellow in Urologic Oncology, Bruce and Cynthia Sherman Fellowship in Urologic Oncology, Division of Urologic Oncology, Department of Urology, New York University Langone Medical Center, New York, New York

Jeremy Kaufman MD
Resident, Department of Urology, New York University Langone Medical Center, New York, New York

Ojas Shah MD
Assistant Professor of Urology and Director of Endourology and Stone Disease, Department of Urology, New York University Langone Medical Center, New York, New York

Samir S. Taneja MD
The James M. Neissa and Janet Riha Neissa Associate Professor of Urologic Oncology; Director, Division of Urologic Oncology, Department of Urology and New York University Cancer Institute, New York University Langone Medical Center, New York, New York

The nature of urologic surgery mandates that the practicing urologist have a comprehensive understanding of the normal physiology of the hematologic system as well as of potential abnormalities. Early identification and evaluation of hypercoagulable or coagulopathic patients are essential, to limit possible complications that may arise from either of these disease states. In this chapter, we outline a comprehensive approach to the hematologic evaluation of the urologic patient including the preoperative and intraoperative management of coagulopathies, the identification and management of the hypercoagulable state, and the management of deep venous thrombosis (DVT).

PREOPERATIVE EVALUATION

When evaluating patients for potential hematologic complications before any urologic surgical procedure, the most important first steps are thorough history taking and physical examination. The clinician taking the patient's history should pay specific attention to the following: any personal or family history of known bleeding disorder; a history of prolonged bleeding after trauma, surgery, or a dental procedure; a history of liver disease, malabsorption, or malnutrition; recent use of anticoagulants (aspirin, clopidogrel, warfarin, and

heparin). Physical findings suggestive of coagulopathy include petechiae, ecchymoses, hematomas, purpura, and the stigmata of acquired disease, such as liver failure or uremia.

Bleeding symptoms in the patient or in a member of the patient's family should prompt a laboratory evaluation. In addition, routine laboratory screening tests are often performed in asymptomatic patients, including complete blood count, platelet count, prothrombin time (PT), and activated partial thromboplastin time (APTT). The PT measures the activity of the extrinsic clotting system, and the APTT measures the intrinsic clotting system (**Fig. 4-1**). Measurement of the bleeding time is used to identify patients with possible platelet function defects. Further laboratory evaluation is unnecessary unless history, physical examination, or routine laboratory tests reveal an abnormality.

In obtaining preoperative screening PT, APTT, and platelet counts, surgeons attempt to identify asymptomatic patients at increased risk for intraoperative or postoperative hemorrhage. The evaluation of symptomatic patients is not considered screening. Most patients experiencing significant perioperative bleeding, however, would not be identified by preoperative screening measures because most such bleeding episodes are the result of surgical technique rather than of

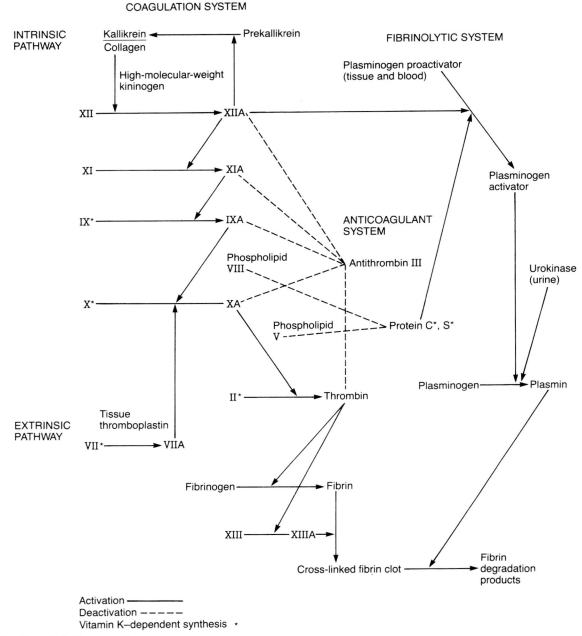

Figure 4-1 Normal clotting cascade.

intrinsic coagulopathy. The risk of preexisting coagulopathy, in the absence of historical symptoms and signs of bleeding, is extremely low.

Some studies evaluated the cost effectiveness of baseline preoperative screening,[1-4] and collectively, these studies recommended that preoperative screening for coagulopathy is unnecessary and should not be performed in the absence of clinical findings suggestive of an increased bleeding risk. Preoperative testing should always be performed in all patients in whom adequate clinical assessment is not possible. The elimination of routine screening based on these criteria would reduce the total number of preoperative tests of coagulation by approximately 50%.[2] These data do not support the use

of routine preoperative screening coagulation tests in asymptomatic patients,[2,4] but despite these recommendations we continue to obtain routine PT, PTT, and platelet counts on all patients undergoing major extirpative or reconstructive procedures in which significant blood loss is possible.

ABNORMALITIES OF BLOOD COMPONENTS

Red Blood Cells

Anemia detected in routine preoperative screening should be evaluated with regard to its functional significance and origin. Typically, a preferred preoperative hemoglobin level is >10 g/dL. Although lower intraoperative hemoglobin levels can generally be tolerated by most patients, these values are associated with an increased risk of morbidity and mortality. Additionally, anemia may reflect a previously unsuspected coexisting disease process that could have a significant effect on the perioperative course. Because anemia can be a primary disorder or can occur secondary to other systemic processes, a careful history and physical examination are essential and can provide extensive information about the underlying cause.[5]

Initial diagnostic studies should include reticulocyte count, mean corpuscular volume (MCV), examination of the peripheral blood smear, and a fecal occult blood test.[5] Many urologic conditions can be associated with anemia, including malignant disease and chronic renal failure. Iron deficiency anemia has been associated with states of renal cell carcinoma. Direct involvement of the bone marrow by cancer may result in myelofibrosis and subsequent anemia, most often seen in metastatic prostate cancer.[6] Radiation therapy can lead to bone marrow suppression or vitamin B_{12} deficiency secondary to radiation ileitis.[7] Many chemotherapeutic agents can cause myelosuppression. Commonly used antibiotics in urology, such as nitrofurantoin, sulfa compounds, and quinolones, can produce hemolytic anemia in patients with glucose-6-phosphate dehydrogenase deficiency. Hemolytic anemia has also been reported in association with renal cell carcinoma and seminoma.[8,9] Finally hematuria itself can cause anemia if it is chronic or severe.

Understanding the cause of the anemia can dictate the appropriate perioperative course of action to minimize operative morbidity. For patients with a correctable underlying cause of anemia who are judged to be at risk for functional compromise, therapy consists of transfusion. In patients who are undergoing surgical procedures that are deemed elective, it is advisable to proceed after correcting the underlying cause of anemia preoperatively and thereby avoiding transfusion. In certain conditions, recombinant erythropoietin can be used to elevate the hemoglobin level, and this agent is often used in the preoperative period. Preoperative transfusions should ideally be performed 24 hours in advance to allow regeneration of 2,3-diphosphoglycerate, which shifts the oxygen dissociation curve to increase oxygen availability to the tissues. Transfusions incur a potential risk of morbidity, including hemolytic reactions, allergic reactions, and transmission of viral diseases (Table 4-1).[11]

Elevation of the hematocrit level significantly higher than normal (erythrocytosis) increases blood viscosity and decreases oxygen transport. A significant increase in surgical morbidity and mortality occurs, particularly related to thromboembolic complications. This increase in red blood cell (RBC) mass can be primary, as in polycythemia vera, or secondary. Common causes of secondary erythrocytosis are hypoxic states or paraneoplastic syndromes (as seen in renal cell carcinoma and Wilms'

TABLE 4-1	Complications of Transfusions Per Unit Transfused	
Complications	**Frequency**
Immune	
Acute hemolysis	1/12,000
Delayed hemolysis	1/1500
Febrile nonhemolytic	1-4/100
Allergic cutaneous	1-4/100
Anaphylactic	1/150,000
Alloimmunization (RBC)	1/100
Alloimmunization (HLA)	1/10
Nonimmune	
Hepatitis C	1/103,000
Hepatitis B	1/200,000
HIV-1	1/490,000
HIV-2	None reported
Malaria	1/4,000,000
Bacterial sepsis	Rare
Hypothermia	Rare

HIV, human immunodeficiency virus; HLA, human leukocyte antigen; RBC, red blood cell.
Adapted from Dzieczkowski JS, Anderson KC. Transfusion biology and therapy. In: Fauci AS, Braunwald E, Isselbacher KJ, et al, eds. *Harrison's Principles on Internal Medicine,* 14th ed. New York: McGraw-Hill; 1998:718-724.

tumor) likely resulting in increased production of erythropoietin. Patients with polycythemia vera should undergo preoperative phlebotomy to lower hematocrit levels to <45% to reduce the risk of thromboembolic complications. In patients with secondary erythrocytosis, the hematocrit should be lowered to <50%.[12]

Platelets

Although a normal platelet count can vary greatly among patients, a platelet count >50,000 is usually adequate for surgical hemostasis. Thrombocytopenia results from decreased production of platelets (radiation, primary marrow disorders, alcohol, drugs), increased peripheral destruction (autoimmune disease, disseminated intravascular coagulation [DIC], sepsis, drugs), sequestration (splenomegaly), or extracorporeal platelet loss (exsanguination). Initial therapy should consist of treating a possible underlying cause, but if this cannot be done than the next step is platelet transfusion. One unit of platelets can be expected to raise the platelet count by 5000 to 10,000.

Primary thrombocytosis, as in myeloproliferative diseases, can increase the risk for thrombotic or hemorrhagic complications. Qualitative platelet disorders are identified by an increased bleeding time despite a normal platelet count. The most common type is *von Willebrand's disease,* which results from the absence of von Willebrand factor (vWF). Inherited intrinsic defects of platelet function are rare.[13] Treatment is with desmopressin (DDAVP), platelet transfusion, or both. Acquired intrinsic platelet dysfunction occurs with the use of aspirin, clopidogrel, and nonsteroidal anti-inflammatory drugs (NSAIDs). Because the platelet life span is approximately 7 to 10 days, platelet function typically resumes 7 to 10 days after the last dose of these medication types.[14,15] Platelet dysfunction can also occur in patients with liver disease, uremia, and hypothyroidism. For acquired defects, treatment is directed at the underlying cause.

von Willebrand's Disease

von Willebrand's disease results from the deficiency of vWF, which is required for adequate platelet function. The disease is transmitted as an autosomal dominant or recessive trait. Characteristically, factor VIII levels are reduced, and factor VIII–related antigen (vWF) levels are also low. This situation leads to prolonged bleeding time. Moreover, ristocetin-dependent platelet aggregation is absent in 70% of these patients. Although spontaneous bleeding may be mild, serious gastrointestinal bleeding can occur. Treatment is preferably with cryoprecipitate and DDAVP. Direct factor VIII transfusions do not work because they generally contain very little vWF.[13]

Factors VIII and IX

Factor VIII and IX deficiencies are extremely rare inherited disorders. The underlying pathophysiology behind both diseases is based on the insufficient generation of thrombin by factor IXa/VIIIa complex. Both deficiencies are typically inherited as a recessive X-linked trait. *Hemophilia A, or factor VIII deficiency,* occurs in 1 in 5000 male births.[18] The APTT is prolonged, whereas PT, fibrinogen level, and platelet count are normal. In severe deficiency, spontaneous bleeding may occur, whereas patients with moderate disease may have traumatic bleeding. The diagnosis is established by a reduction of factor VIII activity. Whereas patients with minor bleeding can generally be treated with factor levels that are 25% to 30% of normal, surgical patients generally require target levels that reach 75% to 100% of normal activity. Many different factor VIII preparations can be given, but the half-life of factor VIII is 8 to 12 hours and administration must be on a steady-state basis. Most patients require 2 to 3 weeks of postoperative hematologic support to allow sufficient wound healing and scar formation.[16]

Factor IX deficiency (Christmas disease) resembles hemophilia A, but it occurs in 1 in 30,000 male births.[18] Replacement therapy with factor IX, as in hemophilia A, is recommended.

Rare Inherited Factor Deficiencies

Other factor deficiencies are much less common, and not all are associated with coagulopathies. The presentation and management of these disorders are outlined in Table 4-2. In general, these patients may present with ecchymosis, hematoma, or delayed traumatic bleeding.

TABLE 4-2	Laboratory Findings and Treatment of Factor Deficiencies				
Deficient Factor	**PT**	**APTT**	**TT**	**Bleeding Time**	**Replacement Factor**
I	↑	↑	↑	↑, N	FFP, cryoprecipitate
II	↑	↑	N	N	FFP, factor IX concentrate
III*					
IV*					
V	↑	↑	N	N	FFP
VII	↑	N	N	N	FFP, factor IX concentrate
VIII	N	↑	N	N	cryoprecipitate, factor VIII concentrate
IX	N	↑	N	N	FFP, factor IX concentrate
X	↑	↑	N	N	FFP, factor IX concentrate
XI	N	↑	N	N	FFP
XII	N	↑	N	N	
XIII	N	N	N	N	FFP
vWF	N	↑	N	↑	FFP, cryoprecipitate

*Deficiency affecting coagulation is unknown.
APTT, activated partial thromboplastin time; FFP, fresh frozen plasma; N, normal time; PT, prothrombin time; TT, thrombin time; vWF, von Willebrand factor; ↑, prolongation.
Adapted from Wilner ML, Rosove MH. Hematologic complications. In: Smith RB, Ehrlich RE, eds. *Complications of Urologic Surgery: Prevention and Management,* 2nd ed. Philadelphia: WB Saunders; 1990:441-452.

Factor II deficiency, hypothrombinemia, is a very rare autosomal recessive disorder with prolonged PT and variably prolonged APTT. Maintenance of >15% of normal levels should be adequate for surgery and can be achieved with fresh frozen plasma (FFP). *Factor V deficiency* is also a very rare disorder in which the PT and APTT are prolonged. Approximately 25% of normal activity is maintained for surgery. *Factor VII deficiency* is uncommon and is inherited as an autosomal gene with intermediate penetrance. The PT is prolonged and the APTT is normal. Replacement is achieved by transfusing plasma or factor VII replacement.

Inherited factor X deficiency is autosomal recessive. Maintenance of levels >40% of normal may be achieved with plasma transfusion in preparation for surgery. *Factor XI deficiency* is uncommon as well and is inherited in an autosomal dominant fashion. A higher frequency of this deficiency is noted in the Ashkenazi Jewish population. These patients may not have bleeding histories but often present with epistaxis. Severe bleeding may occur with trauma or major surgery. Patients can successfully undergo urologic surgical procedures with adequate FFP therapy.

Factor XII deficiency is not usually associated with bleeding manifestations, although the APTT is prolonged. Therapy is not needed for this deficiency. Factor XIII stabilizes fibrin into a covalent network, and in *factor XIII deficiency* coagulation studies are normal except fibrin stability. Abnormal clot solubility and specific factor XIII assay establish the diagnosis, and transfusion of FFP is sufficient for hemostasis.[17] *Fibrinogen deficiency, or dysfibrinogenemia,* is uncommon and FFP or cryoprecipitate may be given to maintain a level adequate for normal hemostasis.

DISORDERS OF INCREASED BLEEDING

Coagulation and bleeding abnormalities are among the major problems encountered in the surgical or critically ill patient. Although most of these patients have no intrinsic abnormalities of hemostasis, either their underlying disease or the therapy of the disease may produce clinically significant bleeding problems. The urologist must be able to recognize these abnormalities quickly and address them before clinically significant problems arise. Failure to do so may result in a significant increase in morbidity and mortality in the acutely ill patient or the surgical patient. In this section, we discuss the major critical disorders that may lead to increased bleeding.

Renal Failure

Renal disease can be associated with functional defects in RBCs, platelets, leukocytes, and coagulation factors. Significant bleeding conditions can occur in the uremic patient, most commonly the result of impaired platelet function. Investigations of the hemorrhagic tendency associated with uremia have mostly been performed in patients with chronic renal failure, and whether these findings can be extrapolated to acute renal failure is unclear.[19]

Uremic bleeding is multifactorial in origin and is mainly the result of impaired platelet–vessel wall interaction. Increased prostacyclin and nitric oxide production by the endothelium, abnormalities in vWF, and several biochemical and functional abnormalities of uremic platelets have also been described.[20] The finding that acquired platelet dysfunction is at least partially corrected by hemodialysis suggests that accumulation of uremic toxins in the blood may contribute to the observed effects. Despite the hemorrhagic tendency, activation of coagulation has been demonstrated in uremic patients and is more prominent in those who are treated with hemodialysis. The safest treatment to relieve uremic bleeding is administration of DDAVP, but its effect is often short-lived. High-dose intravenous (IV) conjugated estrogens can significantly improve the bleeding time and have a longer duration of action.[21-24]

Disseminated Intravascular Coagulation

DIC is an acquired coagulopathy and is the most commonly entertained diagnosis in a bleeding, critically ill patient. Of all acute causes of coagulopathy, it is potentially the most life-threatening. DIC is not a single entity, but rather a clinicopathologic syndrome that is the end product of a variety of underlying disorders, most commonly bacterial sepsis and malignant disease in the urologic patient.[25-28]

Central to the pathogenesis of DIC is the unregulated and excessive generation of thrombin.[26] Normally, the cumulative effect of clot production, clot dissolution (fibrinolysis), and inhibition of clot activation is to produce the steady-state equilibrium of hemostasis. In DIC, however, excess thrombin is generated, resulting in the inappropriate activation of fibrinolysis and the shifting of the steady state to excessive clot dissolution. A secondary result is that fibrin thrombi are formed in the microvasculature, and platelets and RBCs are trapped and consumed. As the cycle continues, platelets, fibrinogen, and other clotting factors are consumed beyond the body's ability to compensate, and excessive bleeding ensues. It should be clear from this description that DIC is initially a thrombotic process with secondary hemorrhage occurring only when platelets and clotting factors are sufficiently consumed and depleted. Approximately 10% of patients with DIC present with only thrombotic manifestations.[28]

Patients in whom DIC is suspected generally present with diffuse bleeding from several sites, petechiae or ecchymoses, hypoxemia, hypotension, or oliguria. In acute DIC, laboratory evaluation demonstrates variable degrees of thrombocytopenia, hypofibrinogenemia, and prolongation of PT and APTT. Assays for fibrin split products (FSPs), fibrin degradation products (FDPs), or the D-dimer fragment of fibrin are generally markedly elevated. The D-dimer assay is theoretically more specific for DIC because this fragment is produced by the action of plasmin on polymerized fibrin.[32] Patients with malignant disease often have chronic, compensated DIC in which bleeding is minimal in the steady state, and these patients often present with normal PT/PTT, platelet, and fibrinogen test results. Patients in this subset demonstrate an elevation of FDPs, FSPs, or D-dimer. These patients are also at increased risk for significant bleeding following anything that may activate their clotting system, such as relatively minor surgical procedures.[28-30]

The diagnosis of DIC relies heavily on laboratory results, but one must also consider the clinical picture. Of all the laboratory findings, thrombocytopenia, hypofibrinogenemia, and D-dimer fragments appear to be the most sensitive in making a laboratory diagnosis.[28,29,32] In addition to the coagulation abnormalities, microangiopathic hemolytic anemia is present with fragmented RBCs (schistocytes) on the peripheral blood smear.[28]

The primary management strategy in patients with DIC consists of aggressive basic support measures and prompt treatment of the underlying process causing the DIC.[25,28,33] When this is not possible, when treatment of the underlying disease accentuates the DIC, or when the DIC is progressing despite appropriate treatment of the underlying process, the general approach is to support the patient's hemostatic system with the transfusion of FFP, cryoprecipitate, or platelets.[28] The idea that this approach will add to the consumption coagulopathy has never been clinically proven. If hemorrhage is excessive, replacement with packed RBCs is advised. When the underlying process is not immediately controllable, or when intensive blood replacement therapy does not improve clinical parameters, heparin infusion may be beneficial.[34]

Primary Fibrinogenolysis

Primary fibrinogenolysis is the condition in which the fibrinolytic pathway is activated independent of the activation of coagulation. This process results in the pathologic degradation of fibrinogen and fibrin by plasmin. Urologic conditions associated with abnormal activation of fibrinolysis are metastatic malignant disease (primarily prostate cancer) and infections.[35] In patients with metastatic carcinoma, the tumor cells are presumed to release a substance that directly activates fibrinolysis.[27]

Patients do not typically present with gross bleeding but are at significant risk for hemorrhage resulting from hypofibrinogenemia. Marked thrombocytopenia should raise the suspicion of the development of DIC. The major laboratory discriminant between primary fibrinogenolysis and DIC is the absence of an elevated level of D-dimer. Once active bleeding develops, it is very difficult to distinguish the two entities because fibrin is generated through the action of thrombin and lysis of fibrin produces D-dimers.[27]

Unlike in DIC, the treatment of choice of primary fibrinogenolysis is the use of antifibrinolytic agents, such as ε-aminocaproic acid or tranexamic acid.[27,35,36] Transfusion support with cryoprecipitate may also be given for severe hypofibrinogenemia. If DIC has developed, the use of antifibrinolytic agents in the absence of systemic anticoagulation (heparin) is contraindicated because of the risk of increased microvascular thrombosis. The best approach in individuals with primary hyperfibrinogenolysis secondary to malignant disease is often aggressive treatment of the underlying malignant condition. Caution should be used in balancing chemotherapy-related bone marrow suppression with bleeding complications resulting from fibrinogenolysis.

Vitamin K–related Disorders

Liver disease and *vitamin K deficiency* are common causes of abnormal coagulation tests and clinical coagulopathies. The pathophysiology of these disorders is the decreased production of vitamin K–dependent clotting factors (factors II, VII, IX, X) and of proteins C and S. Of all these changes, a decrease in factor VII is the most common because of its short half-life (6-10 hours). The liver is the major source of all coagulation proteins except factor VIII and vWF. Liver disorders may also produce abnormalities in fibrinolysis.[37,38] Primary vitamin K deficiency is extremely rare in healthy people. A wide variety of animal and plant sources can provide sufficient vitamin K, and the bacterial flora in the intestine is able to synthesize a significant portion of the required dietary vitamin K. Vitamin K is fat soluble, and therefore adequate bile salt circulation is necessary for absorption.

Vitamin K deficiencies can result from a wide range of conditions. These include, but are not limited to, the following:

1. Newborns, owing to poor transfer of vitamin K by the placenta and lack of vitamin K synthesis in the initially sterile intestine
2. Severe malnutrition or total parenteral nutrition
3. Extrahepatic biliary obstruction
4. Intestinal malabsorption syndromes
5. Broad-spectrum antibiotic use

The liver also synthesizes factor V, which plays a critical role in fibrin generation. Significant impairment of hepatic synthetic function may result in the decreased production of any of these clotting factors despite normal vitamin K status.

Patients with liver disease or vitamin K deficiency initially have isolated prolongation of the PT resulting from a depletion of factor VII without any signs of clinically significant bleeding. In more severe deficiencies, the PTT can also be elevated because of depletion of factors II, IX, and X. A marked reduction in fibrinogen solely on the basis of decreased synthesis is an ominous sign and suggests very severe liver disease. Patients with long-standing liver disease develop portal hypertension, which may result in splenic pooling of platelets. A valuable assessment of liver synthetic function is the measurement of albumin or cholesterol.

In a patient with vitamin K deficiency and no evidence of active bleeding, observation with repletion of vitamin K is indicated. Vitamin K may be administered orally, subcutaneously, intramuscularly, or intravenously. Of these routes of administration, the safest and most reliable is subcutaneous injection as long as the patient's cutaneous perfusion is adequate. However, this route may take 12 to 36 hours for PT correction. Studies have assessed the risk of anaphylactic reaction when vitamin K is given intravenously, and although the actual number of reports is low, prudent administration is recommended.[39] The response to vitamin K may be poor in the presence of liver disease. Patients who fail to respond to vitamin K, who demonstrate increasing abnormalities of PT or PTT, or who are to undergo an invasive procedure may be treated with FFP infusions. Given the short half-life of factor VII, aggressive support with FFP every 6 hours in the perioperative period is generally necessary to produce sustained correction in clotting.[40]

Massive Transfusion Syndrome

Massive transfusion syndrome results from replacement of total blood volume in <24 hours without the concomitant transfusion of platelets and FFP, as can often be seen in trauma.[41] This situation leads to dilutional coagulopathy because stored RBCs contain no viable platelets and may be deficient in clotting factors, which can give a clinical and laboratory picture resembling DIC.[41] This diagnosis should be suspected in any patient who presents with bleeding, prolonged PT and PTT, and thrombocytopenia after receiving >5 U of blood. The key element in making the diagnosis is the transfusion history.

Treatment of this disorder is replacement of clotting factors by FFP and of platelets with platelet transfusions. However, the best treatment is avoiding the situation, and this can be achieved by transfusion of 1 U of FFP and platelets for every 5 U of packed RBCs transfused. In individuals with continued or excessive blood loss, empirical treatment with FFP or platelets may be advisable. In the absence of uncontrolled or continued bleed-ing, it is acceptable to hold the use of FFP and platelets unless they are clinically indicated for postoperative bleeding.

ANTICOAGULATED PATIENT

Patients receiving chronic anticoagulation therapy who require a urologic procedure represent a challenge to the urologist. Perioperative management of these patients should be aimed at minimizing both surgical and medical risks. To accomplish this goal, the urologist must have an understanding of the indication for anticoagulation therapy, the consequence of withholding the therapy, and the pharmacologic mechanism of action of the particular anticoagulation medication.[42]

The most common indications for chronic anticoagulation include venous thromboembolism (VTE), mechanical prosthetic heart valves, and chronic atrial fibrillation. In addition, the urologist is seeing more and more patients who are managed on antiplatelet therapy following the placement of metallic cardiac stents, particularly drug-eluting stents. Discussion of VTE is addressed later in this chapter. Mechanical prosthetic heart valves require anticoagulation secondary to the risk of thrombotic complications including systemic embolization and occlusive thrombosis. Patients with atrial fibrillation require anticoagulation because of their six times normal increased rate of stroke.[42]

A discussion of commonly used anticoagulation agents should include aspirin (acetylsalicylic acid [ASA]), warfarin, heparin, and now clopidogrel (Plavix). ASA exerts its anticoagulant effect by inhibiting platelet aggregation by inhibiting thromboxane A production. This effect is irreversible and lasts for the life of the platelet, which is approximately 7 to 10 days. Therefore, patients taking ASA who are undergoing an elective procedure should discontinue ASA for approximately 10 days before the procedure. In theory, if the platelet count is normal and 20% of the platelets are ASA free, near-normal hemostasis can be achieved, and it has been suggested that ASA can be discontinued 3 days before the procedure. Typical patients taking ASA include those with coronary artery disease, those with a history of stroke, and some patients with atrial fibrillation. Discontinuing ASA in these patients for a urologic procedure is often of minimal risk, and ASA treatment can be restarted as soon as reasonable after the procedure.

Although the urologist now faces an aging population of patients, many of whom are taking clopidogrel as a result of prior cardiac stent placement, guidelines have yet to be established regarding the safety of cessation of this drug, even for a short time. Most patients who have had a drug-eluting cardiac stent placed are advised to take lifelong antiplatelet therapy. Each case needs to be addressed individually, however, and the risk-to-benefit ratio of stopping the medication must be weighed against the necessary planned procedure. In any event, this decision needs to involve the urologist, the cardiologist, and often a hematologist.

Warfarin exerts its anticoagulant effect by inhibiting vitamin K–dependent procoagulation factors II, VII, IX, and X and anticoagulant proteins C and S. Warfarin's effect usually occurs 2 to 3 days after initiation of therapy because of the prolonged half-life of the different procoagulant factors; factor II has the longest half-life (72 hours). In the past, the PT was used to measure the effect of warfarin, but because of variability in PT measurements the INR (international normalized ratio) is currently used. The therapeutic range for all anticoagulant indications is 2 to 3, except for prosthetic mechanical heart valves for which an INR of 2.5 to 3.5 is recommended. Most procedures can be performed safely when the INR is 1.4 or less. Warfarin is used in patients with prosthetic heart valves, atrial fibrillation, and a history of stroke as well as in preventing recurrent myocardial infarction and death in patients with an acute myocardial infarction.[43] However, the most common indication for warfarin therapy is management of patients with VTE.

The management of patients taking warfarin who require an invasive procedure depends on the procedure, the risk of bleeding, and the risk of thromboembolism once the warfarin is stopped. Patients who are at lower risk such as those with atrial fibrillation can often discontinue the warfarin, allow the INR to correct, and restart therapy when it is clinically safe following the procedure. For those patients at higher risk for a thromboembolic event, including patients with a mechanical prosthetic mitral valve and patients with a mechanical prosthetic valve and atrial fibrillation or left ventricular dysfunction, should discontinue warfarin 3 to 5 days before admission and start heparin therapy once the INR is <2.0. Traditionally patients required hospital admission for continuous infusion of dose-adjusted unfractionated heparin. However, the current trend is toward the use of low-molecular-weight heparin (LMWH), which can generally be administered in the outpatient setting and does not require monitoring.

One consideration is patients with renal failure, in whom LMWH is contraindicated. If emergency surgery is required, then patients receiving warfarin therapy can receive FFP. Vitamin K to reverse the effect of warfarin should be used with caution because it can complicate the reinitiation of warfarin therapy.[44]

Heparin acts by inactivating free thrombin through its interaction with antithrombin III (AT III). The inactivation of thrombin prevents the conversion of fibrinogen to fibrin. Heparin also inactivates factors XA and IXA of the coagulation cascade. Heparin's anticoagulant effect is monitored by APTT. Heparin should be discontinued 3 to 4 hours before a procedure. If reversal is necessary on an emergency basis, protamine can be given.

For patients with a mechanical prosthetic valve who require a minor urologic procedure with a low risk of bleeding, one may perform the procedure safely with an INR in the low therapeutic range (2.5). Patients with nonrheumatic atrial fibrillation without concomitant risk factors for thromboembolism should be managed similarly to patients with an isolated aortic valve (i.e., warfarin should be discontinued 3 to 5 days preoperatively and resumed as soon as possible or ≤3 days). Higher-risk patients should undergo reversal of warfarin with concurrent heparin administration.

Finally, patients with thromboembolic disease that has occurred beyond 3 to 6 months should be managed by discontinuing anticoagulation 3 to 5 days preoperatively and resuming it as soon as possible postoperatively. Patients with a history of a more recent thromboembolic event should be managed with concurrent heparin anticoagulation during the discontinuation of warfarin.[43,44]

MANAGEMENT OF INTRAOPERATIVE BLEEDING

On occasion, the urologist is faced with a patient who has extreme intraoperative coagulopathy. This condition has many possible causes, and it is imperative for the surgeon to identify the appropriate factors. When the operative field is infected, such as in abscess drainage or resection of xanthogranulomatous pyelonephritis, coagulopathy should be a clue to progressive intraoperative sepsis. In individuals with excessive surgical bleeding, dilutional coagulopathy is a likely source. Finally, in patients with known abnormalities of hepatic synthetic function, the bleeding may be a function of the underlying disease state. The immediate management of such patients varies according to the cause of bleeding.

In patients with dilutional coagulopathy or transfusion reaction, empirical replacement of clotting factors with administration of FFP, cryoprecipitate, or platelets may be enough to slow bleeding and allow completion of the surgical procedure. The patient's core temperature should be maintained because hypothermia may worsen the bleeding. Devices such as warming blankets, as well as warm irrigation of the surgical field, may allow rapid improvement in core temperature in such a setting. Obviously, in patients with consumptive coagulopathies, such efforts may be of little help, and in these cases, the surgeon's effort should be focused on prompt completion of the procedure with maximal drainage of the infected cavity, to minimize ongoing bacteremia.

In the absence of visible arterial bleeding, exhaustive efforts to control the bleeding with cautery or ligature are often unsuccessful, and liberal use of packing should be implemented. Extensive efforts to achieve hemostasis only delay the completion of the procedure and, indirectly, worsen the coagulopathy through progressive blood loss and hypothermia. On completion of the procedure, widespread coagulation with devices such as the argon beam coagulator can be useful as long as they do not delay completion of the surgical procedure.

On rare occasions, the procedure must be aborted if the patient is unstable, or packing can be left in place even if the procedure is complete. When this is necessary, packing is generally left in place and the wound is closed in a single layer. The patient is then transported to the intensive care unit for resuscitation and correction of coagulopathy before reoperation and removal of packing, usually 24 to 48 hours later. In cases of extirpative surgical procedures, organ resection should be completed if possible because this allows more prompt resolution of coagulopathy. Reconstruction can then be carried out at time of reexploration. In patients with active infection, drainage or resection of infected tissue is extremely important before the procedure is aborted because ongoing infection will likely perpetuate the coagulopathy. Obviously, acquisition of new infection is a concern in aborted procedures, and the patient should be maintained on broad-spectrum antibiotics while packing materials are in place.

PROBLEMS OF INCREASED COAGULATION

Hypercoagulable State

Patients with a history of recurrent or spontaneous venous thrombosis may have an underlying *familial or acquired hypercoagulable state* (Table 4-3).[45,46] Historically, it was thought that underlying hereditary defects were the source of <10% of such cases.[46] More recently, it was determined that, in fact, >50% of such cases have a specific underlying cause. The coagulation cascade is influenced by certain regulatory factors. Abnormalities of these factors may increase the risk of thrombosis and include deficiencies of AT III, protein C, and protein S. Activated protein C (APC) resistance (factor V Leiden mutation) was discovered to account for the majority of diagnosable coagulation defects (Table 4-4).[47-50] Factor V Leiden occurs with an estimated frequency of 5% in the general population of European ancestry.[51,52]

Physiology

Most coagulation proteins are serine proteases that act sequentially on one another. These proteins are regulated by another series of proteins called *serapins* (serine protease inhibitors). Serapins may be activated under normal homeostatic situations, in stress conditions, or as part of administered therapy. Serapin deficiencies may cause the hypercoagulable state. The best-studied serapin is AT III, a heparin cofactor that allows heparin to inactivate factors II, IX, XI, and XII. A decrease in the concentration of AT III predisposes patients to thrombosis by allowing uncontrolled activity of the majority of coagulation factors. AT III deficiency is responsible

TABLE 4-3	Familial or Acquired Disorders Leading to Hypercoagulable State	
Familial	**Acquired**
Antithrombin III deficiency	Malignant disease
Protein C deficiency	Regulatory protein deficiency (malnutrition/nephrotic syndrome)
Protein S deficiency	Acute-phase reactants (trauma/surgery)
Activated protein C resistance	Antiphospholipid syndrome
Factor V Leiden	Myeloproliferative disorders
Abnormal factor V cofactor activity	Heparin-associated thrombocytopenia
Hypoplasminogenemia	Disseminated intravascular coagulation
Abnormal plasminogen	Oral contraceptives
Plasminogen activator deficiency	Pregnancy/postpartum state
Dysfibrinogenemia	
Factor XII deficiency	
Abnormal platelet reactivity	

TABLE 4-4	Prevalence of Disorders Leading to Hypercoagulation in Patients With Thrombosis	
Disorder	**Prevalence (%)**
Activated protein C resistance	20-50
Protein C deficiency	2-5
Protein S deficiency	2-5
Antithrombin III	2-4
Antiphospholipid syndrome	2-3
Fibrinogen deficiency	1

Adapted from Brigden ML. The hypercoagulable state: who, how, and when to test and treat. *Postgrad Med.* 1997;101:249-252, 254-256, 259-262.

for hypercoagulability in 2% to 4% of studied patients, and it is present in 0.2% to 0.4% of the general population.[53]

In addition to regulation by serapins, the clotting cascade is influenced a complex group of receptors at the endothelial surface termed *thrombomodulins*. These receptors function as anticoagulants because of their ability to neutralize thrombin on the endothelial surface. Once formed, the thrombin-thrombomodulin complex activates a vitamin K–dependent factor called *protein C*, which metabolizes activated factors V and VIII and thus suppresses coagulation. This activation is facilitated by another vitamin K–dependent factor called *protein S,* which also functions to metabolize activated factors V and VIII. Deficiencies in proteins C or S may result in a thrombotic tendency, are observed in 2% to 5% of hypercoagulable patients, and are present in approximately 0.5% of the general population.[45,46,50]

For APC to exert its control on activated factor V, it must first attach itself to and then cleave this factor. A mutation in factor V, called *factor V Leiden,* has been identified that results in the inability of APC to cleave factor V, a condition referred to as *APC resistance.* This abnormality accounts for approximately 90% of cases of APC resistance and has a prevalence of approximately 5% in the general population.[47-50,53,55]

Deficiencies of AT III, protein C, and protein S, as well as APC resistance, are all inherited in an autosomal dominant fashion.[45] Whereas deficiencies of these proteins have an incidence of <1% each, APC resistance is present in 3% to 8% of the population.[45,50] The presence of APC resistance increases the likelihood of a simultaneous additional inherited disorder. In such cases, the risk for thrombosis is dramatically increased compared with the risk in individuals with APC resistance alone.[56-60] Coexisting acquired conditions (see Table 4-1), as well as immobilization, trauma, pregnancy, malignant disease, hormone replacement therapy, and surgery, also significantly add to the risk for thrombosis in individuals with hereditary hypercoagulable states.[45,61]

An acquired condition that has been increasingly recognized as a common cause of thrombosis is the *antiphospholipid syndrome,* which is present in 2% to 3% of the general population. Antiphospholipids predispose patients to both arterial and venous thrombosis.[62] The diagnosis involves the detection of lupus anticoagulant or anticardiolipin antibodies in conjunction with arterial and venous thromboses or thrombocytopenia.[55,63,64] Individuals with lupus anticoagulant may present with an elevation of serum APTT. The mechanism of thrombosis in antiphospholipid syndrome, however, has not been well delineated.

Evaluating the Hypercoagulable Patient

Screening for an underlying coagulation abnormality in cases of venous thrombosis should be performed in the presence of any of the following situations:

1. Family history of thrombosis
2. Thrombosis at an early age (<45 years)
3. Recurrent thrombosis, especially without precipitating factors
4. Recurrent thrombosis despite adequate anticoagulant therapy
5. Thrombosis at an unusual site
6. Elevated APTT (lupus anticoagulant), hematocrit, white blood cells, and platelets
7. Apparent warfarin-induced skin necrosis

Several additional indications suggest the need to test for antiphospholipid antibodies. These indications include a history of recurrent fetal loss, venous or arterial thrombosis associated with thrombocytopenia, and thrombosis associated with neurologic abnormalities such as stroke or transient ischemic attacks. A specific cause of spontaneous venous thrombosis is found in ≤50% of outpatients, but all individuals should be evaluated because of the potentially lethal consequences of an untreated underlying abnormality.[53]

Abnormalities of AT III, protein C, or protein S in screened individuals can manifest with either a normal or deficient level. Individuals with normal levels may have dysfunctional or inactive forms of these proteins, thereby resulting in a clinically deficient state. A comprehensive discussion of specific assays is beyond the scope of this chapter, but for the aforementioned reasons, functional assays are initially more informative than antigenic assays that simply measure the presence or absence of the factor. Ideally, the patient should not be in an active thrombotic state or taking anticoagulants at the time of testing.

Whenever possible, anticoagulant therapy should be discontinued several weeks before testing because warfarin and heparin can interact with the various assays. When concern exists that a patient is still at risk for thrombosis if anticoagulation is discontinued, it is possible to continue anticoagulation while testing for certain hypercoagulable states. Deficiencies in AT III, lupus anticoagulant, and anticardiolipin antibodies, as well as APC resistance (in factor V–deficient plasma), can be detected during warfarin administration. Additionally, protein C or S deficiencies or anticardiolipin antibodies can be tested for while patients are receiving heparin (Table 4-5).[53]

A positive test result should be confirmed before the diagnosis of an inherited deficiency is made. To confirm the diagnosis of the antiphospholipid syndrome, antibodies must be shown to be present on two occasions >3 months apart.

Management

Acute thrombosis with an underlying hypercoagulable condition requires treatment as discussed in the next section, on DVT, but some special considerations should be kept in mind in patients with known hypercoagulable states and an acute thrombotic event. After the initial therapy and the recommended 3 to 6 months of therapy with anticoagulation, the question remains which patients require continued anticoagulation. The number of sites involved, the severity of thrombosis, the presence of recurrent thrombosis, and whether the thrombosis was spontaneous or secondary to a precipitating event should all be taken into consideration. Special attention must be paid to such factors as reproductive status and potential risks for immobilization or trauma.

TABLE 4-5	Effects of Anticoagulants on Functional Assays for Hypercoagulable States	
Functional Assay	**Effect of Anticoagulant**	
	Heparin	**Warfarin**
Antithrombin III	Decrease	No effect
Protein C	No effect	Decrease
Protein S	No effect	Decrease
Activated protein C resistance	False-positive result	Modified assay may avoid interaction
Lupus anticoagulant	Possible false-positive result	Modified assay may avoid interaction
Anticardiolipin antibodies	No effect	No effect

For patients with antiphospholipid syndrome, available studies suggest that lifelong anticoagulant therapy should be considered in the setting of any arterial or venous thrombotic event.[55,63] Conversely, lifetime anticoagulation is recommended only for patients with two or more thromboembolic events following the diagnosis of an inherited deficiency. Finally, in asymptomatic adults with hereditary deficiencies, short-term prophylaxis with heparin (subcutaneous or LMWH) should be considered when the risk of thrombosis is increased, such as during prolonged bed rest, surgery, or trauma.[45,46,53]

Deep Venous Thrombosis and Pulmonary Embolism

Thromboembolic disease, in particular DVT and pulmonary embolus (PE), is a significant cause of morbidity and mortality especially in the surgical patient. DVT accounted for nearly 100,000 hospital visits in 2000, according to the Centers for Medicare and Medicaid Services.[54] Approximately 5 million cases of DVT, 500,000 to 630,000 cases of PE, and 200,000 cases of fatal PE occur annually.[51] DVT incidence rates of 30% and PE incidence rates of 14.1% have been reported in the general surgical population. Although the most extensive work has been done in orthopedic surgery, thromboembolic disease is known to be a major potential complication of urologic surgery, especially pelvic surgery. In a review, Kibel and associates[65] reported a DVT incidence rate of approximately 30%, a PE incidence rate of 10%, and a fatal PE rate of 5% in patients undergoing pelvic surgical procedures without prophylaxis. Investigators have reported that 1% to 5% of patients undergoing major urologic surgical procedures have symptomatic VTE.[66]

The risk factors for venous thrombosis can be thought of in the context of Virchow's triad for the pathophysiology of thrombus formation:

1. Stasis
2. Hypercoagulability
3. Intimal injury

Risk factors include advanced age (>60 years old), obesity, history of previous DVT, prolonged immobility, pregnancy, malignant disease, fracture, estrogen use, major medical conditions leading to venous stasis (congestive heart failure, nephrotic syndrome, sepsis, myocardial infarction, inflammatory bowel disease, erythrocytosis, myeloproliferative disorder), and thrombophilia, which is the tendency to recurrent VTE.[59,67,68] That these risk factors are additive is important. For instance, Wheeler showed that patients with no risk factors had an 11% and 1% rate of DVT and PE, respectively, whereas those patients with one risk factor had a 24% and 4% rate, and finally those with four risk factors had a much higher risk of 100% and 67%, respectively.[69]

Thrombus formation is believed to occur during the surgical procedure.[69,70] Furthermore, investigators have proposed that the likelihood of thrombus formation increases with the duration of anesthesia, especially if it exceeds 1 hour.[71,72] This finding seems to be related to an increase in venous stasis secondary to prolongation of intraoperative muscle relaxation.

Urologic patients, by the nature of the diseases for which they are surgically treated, often have multiple risk factors for thromboembolic disease including advanced age, malignant disease, and prolonged operative time. The incidences of DVT and PE have been examined in various urologic procedures. Historically, Colby in 1948 reported a 6.26% thromboembolic rate and a 2.64% fatal PE rate in patients undergoing open prostate surgical procedures.[61a] The DVT and fatal PE rate for suprapubic prostatectomy has been reported to be 17.39% and 8.69%, respectively. Igel and associates[73] reported similar rates of 1.2% for DVT and 2.7% for PE in a review of postoperative complications after radical retropubic prostatectomy in a series of 692 consecutive patients. In the setting of cystectomy, incidences of 8.1% for DVT, 1.8% to 4.1% for PE, and 2% for fatal PE have been reported.[74,75] Soloway and colleagues[76a] reported a DVT rate of 0.21% in their series of 1364 patients who underwent open radical prostatectomy with only mechanical compression device prophylaxis.

The challenge of diagnosing DVT stems from the nonspecific nature of its clinical presentation. The classic triad of pain, swelling, and erythema can be found in both patients with and without DVT, and the classic Homans sign is found in only 10% of patients with DVT.[69] In view of these findings, objective testing is required to confirm the diagnosis before treatment, particularly because the treatment of thromboembolic disease is not without its own additional complications. Once DVT is suspected, compression ultrasonography of the proximal veins or duplex ultrasonography should be performed. Compression ultrasonography has a sensitivity of >90% for detecting proximal vein thrombosis.[77,78] It is less invasive than the gold standard diagnostic test, contrast venography, and is more accurate than impedance plethysmography.[67] If the initial ultrasound finding is abnormal, then a diagnosis of DVT can be comfortably made. Conversely, when the test result is normal, one cannot completely rule out the possibility of a DVT. Ginsberg, in a review of DVT management, recommended a repeat ultrasound study for those patients with clinically suspected DVT who had normal findings on their initial ultrasound examination.[67]

Because of the difficulty of definitively diagnosing DVT definitively, attempts have been made to develop strategies to accomplish this without the need for repeat testing. One investigated strategy involves measuring plasma D-dimers, often in combination with impedance plethysmography or other assays.[78] More extensive work needs to be conducted in this area before this approach can become standard practice.

The diagnosis of acute PE is also difficult given the wide range of presentation (see Chapter 2).[59,79,80] More recent approaches, such as use of the Wells score, have suggested using a D-dimer test and categorizing patients as having a low, intermediate, or high probability of PE.[81] When the index of suspicious is high, particularly in patients in the postoperative period, a spiral computed tomography (CT) scan is warranted and is considered by most clinicians to be the standard initial diagnostic test.

At present, we often employ spiral chest CT as a first test for PE. If results are negative, then we proceed with pulmonary angiography only if a strong clinical suspicion still exists for PE. A potential shortcoming of both spiral CT and pulmonary angiography is the need for a large bolus of IV or intra-arterial contrast material. In individuals with preexisting renal compromise, a ventilation-perfusion scan is clearly the best first test to consider.

Newer modalities for diagnosis and exclusion of PE have been evaluated. These techniques include ventilation-perfusion single photon emission CT (SPECT), single-detected and multi-detected CT, and magnetic resonance angiography (MRA) with gadolinium enhancement and perfusion magnetic resonance imaging (MRI).[82] Real-time MRI has been suggested for patients in whom contrast studies should be avoided or who have renal failure.[82] MRA may be used more in the future as techniques are improved and more data become available.

Management

The goals of treating thromboembolic disease are to prevent further propagation of the thrombus, to prevent embolization of the thrombus, and in certain situations to promote fibrinolysis. Once the diagnosis is made, then anticoagulation therapy should be instituted unless a contraindication exists. If the patient is hemodynamically unstable or has extensive ileofemoral DVT, thrombolytic therapy may be considered. This therapy usually entails the use of streptokinase (SK), urokinase (UK), or tissue plasminogen activator (tPA). The use of thrombolytic therapy is limited by the associated increased risk in major bleeding, especially in the postoperative patient. The Food and Drug Administration currently recommends two regimens for thrombolytic therapy: (1) IV SK with a bolus of 250,000 U followed by an infusion of 100,000 U/hour for ≤72 hours for the treatment of DVT; and (2) 100 mg IV tPA over 2 hours for the treatment PE.[67,67a] Again, thrombolytic therapy should be reserved for those patients with hemodynamic instability, extensive disease, and low risk of bleeding.

If the patient is not hemodynamically unstable, then heparin therapy should be instituted immediately on confirmation of DVT. Various regimens for the administration of IV unfractionated heparin have been developed, are based on weight or dose titration nomograms.[67] An APTT of 1.5 to 2.5 times the control is recommended. Furthermore, attempts should be made to achieve therapeutic APTT values as rapidly as possible because persistent subtherapeutic values likely increase the risk of DVT recurrence. Heparin therapy is usually maintained for 4 to 7 days.

Warfarin therapy is started 24 hours after heparin therapy and is monitored by INR with a goal of 2.0 to 3.0 times control. The clinician should confirm that the patient has no evidence of major bleeding with a therapeutic APTT before warfarin therapy is instituted. Heparin therapy can be discontinued once therapeutic levels of INR have been achieved for 2 days. The duration of treatment is determined by the risk for future thromboembolic disease. Patients with a first episode of thromboembolic disease and a reversible risk factor such as surgery should be treated for 6 weeks to 3 months (depending on the severity of the episode). As described later, patients with idiopathic thromboembolic disease should be treated for 3 to 6 months. Longer and, in certain instances, indefinite treatment is recommended in patients with a predisposition for recurrent venous thrombus.

Complications of heparin therapy include bleeding, thrombocytopenia with and without thrombosis, osteoporosis, skin necrosis, and less common complications including anaphylaxis, hypoaldosteronism, and alopecia.[59,83] Similar complications are associated with warfarin therapy; bleeding is the most common. Particular attention should be paid to concomitant medications that may interact with warfarin and affect INR, the most prevalent of which are fluoroquinolones, macrolides, and sulfonamides in the treatment of urologic patients.[84,85]

Because of potential complications, alternative anticoagulation regimens have been sought. Several studies have been conducted in the past 2 decades to evaluate LMWH. LMWHs are synthesized from larger unfractionated heparin molecules by enzymatic or chemical depolymerization.[86-89] The advantages of LMWH include superior bioavailability, lower incidence of bleeding, lower incidence of heparin-induced thrombocytopenia, ease of administration and monitoring (subcutaneous once or twice daily), and the availability of outpatient use.[86,87] Several trials comparing LMWH with unfractionated heparin concluded that LMWH significantly reduced recurrence, had a superior relative risk reduction of thromboembolic complications, and incurred a statistically significant reduction in bleeding.[87,90] Although the actual cost of LMWH is 10 to 20 times that of unfractionated heparin, the potential lower complication rates, the reduced need for laboratory and hospital monitoring, and the availability of outpatient treatment may make LMWH a more cost-effective alternative. For these reasons, LMWH is preferable to unfractionated heparin in most settings.[87]

For those patients with a contraindication to anticoagulation therapy, an inferior vena caval filter can be considered. However, no definitive evidence confirms the efficacy of these devices in preventing PE. Surgical intervention (i.e., thrombectomy) has been replaced by thrombolytic therapy. The only definitive indication for surgical thrombectomy is in a patient with chronic thromboembolic pulmonary hypertension or in a patient with a massive PE and a contraindication to thrombolytic therapy.

Because of the significant morbidity and mortality associated with thromboembolic disease, prevention is critical, especially in the surgical patient. Radical pelvic surgery is considered to be a serious risk factor for postoperative DVT; it is associated with a DVT rate of approximately 30% and PE rate of 10% in patients without prophylaxis.[65] With prophylaxis, these rates decrease to 10%, and 1.5% respectively. However, currently no large, randomized prospective studies have examined various methods of prophylaxis in the urologic patient. Chandhoke and colleagues[91] conducted a prospective randomized study comparing warfarin and intermittent pneumatic leg compression as prophylaxis for postoperative DVT in the urologic patient and concluded that low-dose warfarin is as effective as is intermittent pneumatic leg compression. Unfortunately, this study involved only 100 patients.

Based on data in general and orthopedic surgical patients, Clagget and associates[91a] developed a general strategy for prevention based on a patient's risk. For the low-risk patient (<40 years old; undergoing minor surgical procedures), early ambulation is all that is recommended. Patients with moderate risk (>40 years old; undergoing major surgical procedures; no other risk factors) should receive low-dose unfractionated heparin at a dose of 5000 U subcutaneously 2 hours preoperatively and then postoperatively every 8 hours or intermittent pneumatic compression (IPC) stockings during and after surgery. IPC stockings not only increase blood flow but also promote fibrinolysis. Low-dose unfractionated heparin, LMWH, or use of IPC stockings is recommended for high-risk patients (>40 years old; undergoing major surgical procedures; and additional risk factors). High-risk patients with a history of previous VTE, malignant disease, orthopedic surgery, hip fracture, stroke, or spinal cord injury should receive LMWH, oral anticoagulation, IPC stockings, or adjusted-dose heparin given at a dose of 3500 U three times a day beginning 2 days preoperatively to maintain an APTT at the upper limit of normal.

We routinely use IPC stockings in all patients undergoing open pelvic surgery, particularly for malignant disease. Individuals with bulky pelvic malignant tumors should be evaluated preoperatively for the presence of a preexisting DVT before the placement of IPC stockings. IPC stockings are placed before the induction of anesthetic and muscle relaxation and are maintained until the patient is ambulating on a regular basis postoperatively. In patients undergoing flank surgery, the decision to use IPC stockings is based on the anticipated length of the procedure. Given the position of the patient during flank surgery, we generally employ IPC stockings in most patients.

A review of 5900 patients undergoing laparoscopic prostatectomy showed that only 31 developed symptomatic VTE within 90 days of the surgical procedure. The investigators found that prior DVT, current tobacco smoking, larger prostate volume, longer operative time, and longer hospital stay were associated with VTE in univariate analysis. The data did not support the routine use of heparin prophylaxis in this multi-institution study.[92]

A topic of concern is late thromboembolic complications. In the past, it was believed that DVT occurred in the first 3 postoperative days and that prophylaxis was indicated during that period. More recent studies, however, suggested that significant numbers of DVT and PE cases occur after hospital discharge. Huber and associates[93] determined that ≤25% of DVT and 16% of PE occurred after hospital discharge. This finding of late DVT has been noted in urologic patients as well. In a series reviewing postoperative complications in patients undergoing radical retropubic prostatectomy, investigators noted that DVT was diagnosed an average of 12 days postoperatively.[73] Late thromboembolism is thought to result from a prolonged hypercoagulable state that extends beyond the period of prophylaxis. Such prolonged states may be of particular concern in patients at prolonged bed rest or with concurrent malignant disease. Unfortunately, the trend toward minimally invasive surgical procedures and earlier hospital discharge may make addressing this question more difficult.

KEY POINTS

1. Although routine preoperative coagulation defect screening is not shown to be cost effective, we have continued its use in patients at risk of significant bleeding during a planned procedure.

2. Anemia can affect surgical outcomes and should be corrected whenever possible before elective surgical procedures.

3. Individuals undergoing elective surgical procedures should discontinue the use of ASA, clopidogrel, or NSAIDs a full 7 to 10 days preoperatively to allow normalization of platelet function.

4. In patients with drug-eluting coronary stents, or specific indications for anticoagulation, the risk of stopping anticoagulation should be weighed against the risk of intraoperative bleeding, depending on the planned procedure.

5. Patients with an abnormal preoperative PTT value and no history of anticoagulation should undergo careful evaluation for clotting factor deficiency.

6. The distinction between DIC and primary fibrinogenolysis is essential because treatments are distinct and antifibrinolytic therapies are contraindicated in DIC.

7. In patients with certain risk factors for a hypercoagulable state, and in patients at risk for venous thrombosis, evaluation for factor deficiency or lupus anticoagulant is indicated.

8. The risk factors for venous thrombosis can be thought of in the context of Virchow's triad for the pathophysiology of thrombus formation (stasis, hypercoagulability, and intimal injury).

9. VTE prophylaxis recommendations should be risk adjusted.

10. High-risk patients with a history of previous VTE, malignant disease, orthopedic surgery, hip fracture, stroke, or spinal cord injury should receive VTE prophylaxis in the form of LMWH, oral anticoagulation, IPC stockings, or adjusted-dose heparin given at a dose of 3500 U three times a day beginning 2 days preoperatively to maintain an APTT at the upper limit of normal.

REFERENCES

Please see www.expertconsult.com

Chapter 5

METABOLIC COMPLICATIONS OF UROLOGIC SURGERY

Niels-Erik B. Jacobsen MD, FRCSC
Fellow, Urologic Oncology, Department of Urology, Indiana University, Indianapolis, Indiana

Michael O. Koch MD
Professor and Chairman, Department of Urology, Indiana University, Indianapolis, Indiana

Implicit with the medical and surgical management of genitourinary disorders, metabolic complications are commonly encountered in urologic practice. To facilitate the diagnosis, management, and prevention of such complications, the urologist must maintain a firm understanding of the pathophysiology involved. This chapter provides an in-depth discussion of metabolic complications commonly encountered as sequelae of urologic surgery, including transurethral resection (TUR) syndrome, post-obstructive diuresis (POD), and metabolic complications of urinary diversion. Additionally, special consideration is given to the perioperative management of patients with chronic kidney disease (CKD).

PERIOPERATIVE MANAGEMENT OF THE PATIENT WITH CHRONIC KIDNEY DISEASE

CKD affects an estimated 35% of adults over the age of 20 years in the United States.[1,2] It is associated with numerous complications and comorbid conditions that, together, pose a definite morbidity and mortality risk. Fortunately, adverse outcomes from renal insufficiency can be delayed or prevented through appropriate monitoring and early treatment. As such, it is essential that the urologist maintains a basic understanding of the pathophysiology of CKD, particularly as it applies to perioperative management.

Definition of Chronic Kidney Disease

In 2002 the Kidney Disease Outcome Quality Initiative (K/DOQI) Working Group of the National Kidney Foundation defined CKD according to the presence of objective renal damage (e.g., proteinuria >300 mg/day) or a glomerular filtration rate (GFR) below 60 mL/min/1.73 m² for >3 months.[2] GFR, the best measure of overall renal function, represents the product of the number of functioning nephrons and single-nephron GFR. GFR can be estimated using the Cockcroft-Gault equation for creatinine clearance. Normal reference levels of GFR vary with age, gender, and body size. A GFR of 60 mL/min/1.73 m² represents roughly half the normal adult GFR. The K/DOQI definition makes allowance for the normal age-related decline in GFR (~1 mL/min/1.73 m² per year) that occurs after the age of 20 or 30 years.

Irrespective of GFR, all patients with objective evidence of kidney damage are considered to have CKD because they remain at risk for progressive loss of renal function and related complications (Table 5-1). CKD is classified into five stages according to GFR (Table 5-2). Although the cut-off values between stages are arbitrary, the prevalence and severity of complications associated with CKD worsen as GFR declines.

Management of Comorbidities and Complications

The numerous complications and comorbid conditions associated with CKD may negatively impact patient outcome independent of the renal dysfunction itself (see Table 5-1). Each deserves individual consideration and management so as to minimize the potential for adverse events in the perioperative period.

Diabetes mellitus and hypertension represent the first and third leading causes of end-stage renal disease (ESRD), respectively.[3] New-onset or worsening hypertension, secondary to hypervolemia and stimulation of the renin angiotensin system, also represents a common complication of CKD.[4] Strict glycemic control and optimization of blood pressure are obvious goals in the perioperative period. Angiotensin-converting enzyme (ACE) inhibitors and angiotensin-receptor blockers (ARBs) are first-line anti-hypertensive agents used in this setting; their use is based on studies that demonstrate effective blood pressure control and reduced risk of progression to ESRD in both diabetic and non-diabetic CKD patients.[5,6] Diuretics, followed by calcium channel or beta-blocking agents, may be added if blood pressure remains high despite ACE inhibitors or ARBs.[7] Loop diuretics are preferred over thiazides if the GFR is <30 mL/min/1.73 m^2.[8]

Cardiovascular disease is a common complication of CKD. Relative to the general population, the cardiovascular risk is 3-fold higher among patients with mild renal insufficiency and 65-fold higher in patients with ESRD.[9,10] Reasons for this include extraskeletal calcification (e.g., valvular, atherosclerosis) secondary to calcium-phosphorous dysregulation, ventricular hypertrophy secondary to chronic anemia, congestive heart failure (CHF) exacerbated by hypervolemia, as well as hypertension, diabetes, and dyslipidemia.[11] Patients with longstanding CKD or a history of myocardial ischemia warrant preoperative cardiac evaluation, particularly if invasive surgery is planned.

Anemia is common in patients with a GFR <60 mL/min/1.73 m^2.[12] It is typically normochromic normocytic and reflects insufficient production of erythropoietin. Most patients with CKD are symptomatic (e.g., fatigue) at hemoglobin values <11 g/dL. Chronic anemia may promote left ventricular hypertrophy, CHF, and myocardial ischemia if untreated.[11] Supplemental iron and vitamins are usually ineffective and repeated transfusion risks the development of immune sensitization, which may compromise future transplantation. Recombinant erythropoietin is recommended as primary treatment. Maintaining the serum hematocrit at 33% to 36% or hemoglobin at 11 to 12 g/dL has been shown to reduce cardiovascular mortality by 30%.[13,14]

Patients with renal insufficiency may develop a bleeding diathesis late in the course of disease as demonstrated by a prolongation in bleeding time. The primary defect involves an abnormality in von Willebrand factor (vWF)-related platelet aggregation and platelet–vessel wall interaction. Measures to correct this include administration of cryoprecipitate, factor III, or DDAVP (1-deamino-8-D-arginine vasopressin), all of which raise circulating levels of vWF. Correction of anemia with either erythropoietin or red blood cell transfusion also may improve the bleeding profile. These strategies are recommended as both prophylaxis and treatment in uremic patients undergoing major surgery.

Fluid and Electrolyte Considerations

Most patients with CKD are able to maintain fluid and electrolyte homeostasis until the GFR is 15 mL/min/1.73 m^2.[15,16] Homeostasis occurs because an adaptive increase in both single nephron GFR and tubular function causes an increase in the fractional excretion of water and electrolytes. Such adaptation can only maintain homeostasis under the conditions of a normal diet, however. Extreme changes in diet, as may occur perioperatively, often lead to fluid and electrolyte imbalance.

Patients with CKD progressively lose the ability to both conserve and excrete sodium. When the GFR falls below 15 mL/min/1.73 m^2, sodium excretion becomes relatively fixed and the kidneys are no longer able to compensate for changes in sodium intake and nonrenal sodium loss.[17] At a GFR of 5 mL/min/1.73 m^2, the excretion of 120 to 140 mEq of sodium per day allows

TABLE 5-1	Comorbidities and Complications of Chronic Kidney Disease
Comorbidities	**Complications**
Diabetes mellitus (type 1 or 2)	Cardiovascular disease
	Hypertension
Hypertension	Anemia
Cardiovascular disease	Bone disease (renal osteodystrophy)
	Platelet dysfunction
	Malnutrition
	Neuropathy
	Drug toxicity
	Fluid and electrolyte imbalance
	Hypervolemia
	Increased total body sodium
	Hyper- or hypokalemia
	Hypocalcemia
	Hyperphosphatemia
	Metabolic acidosis

TABLE 5-2	K/DOQI Classification of Chronic Kidney Disease		
Stage	**Description**	**GFR (mL/min/1.73 m^2)**	**Estimated Prevalence**
1	Kidney damage with normal GFR	≥90	64.3%
2	Kidney damage with mildly reduced GFR	60-89	31.2%
3	Moderately reduced GFR	30-59	4.3%
4	Severely reduced GFR	15-29	0.2%
5	Renal failure	<15	0.2%

GFR, glomerular filtration rate.
Adapted from Kidney Disease Outcome Quality Initiative. K/DOQI clinical practice guidelines for chronic kidney disease: evaluation, classification, and stratification. *Am J Kidney Dis.* 2002;39(2 Suppl 1):S46.

for a daily sodium intake of 5 to 10 g. Dietary intake below 2 g per day risks sodium depletion, whereas intake above 10 g risks total body sodium excess. Sodium depletion secondary to non-renal loss is not uncommon in the perioperative period. Risk factors for sodium depletion include nasogastric suction, vomiting, diarrhea, and fistula drainage. Perioperative diuretic therapy may worsen the situation by augmenting renal sodium excretion. Patients without risk factors for sodium depletion require 5 to 10 g of sodium per day (diet or intravenous [IV]) to maintain homeostasis, whereas those with established risk factors require additional supplementation. In the setting of severe peripheral (or pulmonary) edema or hypertension, sodium intake should be limited to 2 g per day in order to avoid further fluid overload.

As renal failure progresses, the kidneys also lose the ability to concentrate and dilute urine. The concentration defect results from an impairment in the medullary solute gradient, which often overshadows the dilution defect until renal failure is quite advanced. Typically, water loads are well tolerated until the GFR approaches 15 mL/min/1.73 m^2.[15,16] In conjunction with the inability to regulate sodium excretion, the concentration defect predisposes patients with CKD to dehydration. The solute load generated by the intake of 5 to 10 g of sodium per day results in an obligate urine volume of 1.5 to 2.0 L.[17] Consideration of perioperative fluid replacement must take into account obligate urine output in addition to the customary loss that occurs through hemorrhage, drainage, or insensible routes. Failure to do so may result in severe dehydration and an acute worsening of renal function through inadequate renal perfusion (pre-renal failure). Fluid intake should be maintained at a minimum of 1.5 L per day unless the patient has ESRD, in which case intake should match urine output plus insensible losses.

Hyponatremia is common in patients with severe CKD due to the impaired excretion of free water (i.e., dilution defect). Fluid restriction to less than 1 L per day is generally sufficient.

Hyperkalemia is uncommon in CKD until the GFR falls below 25% of normal. Patients with severe CKD are unable to fully excrete the daily potassium load, thus they are exquisitely sensitive to changes in intake. Exogenous intake of potassium, be it through diet or medications, is the most common cause of hyperkalemia in CKD. As such, potassium restriction is an important component of therapy.

Preoperative Evaluation

Patients with CKD require a careful preoperative determination of overall health. The basic evaluation includes a careful history and physical examination, complete metabolic profile, coagulation times, electrocardiogram, and plain radiograph of the chest. The presence of comorbid or complicating conditions should be determined preoperatively and managed accordingly. A detailed list of prescribed medications should be made because polypharmacy is common. Medications that adversely affect renal function or whose clearance depends on adequate renal function may require substitution or a reduction in dose. Nephrology consultation is advised for both perioperative and long-term care if the GFR is below 30 mL/min/1.73 m^2.

TUR SYNDROME

Etiology

TUR syndrome is a constellation of signs and symptoms caused by the intravascular absorption of hypotonic fluids during endoscopic surgery. It is most commonly reported following transurethral resection of the prostate (TURP), but it may complicate any endoscopic procedure in which hypotonic irrigation is used,[18] including cystoscopy, bladder tumor resection, percutaneous nephrolithotripsy, and transcervical endometrial resection. Intravascular absorption of irrigant occurs primarily through direct infusion into open venous channels; however, reabsorption of extravasated fluid following inadvertent perforation of the prostatic capsule or bladder wall also may occur. This distinction is important because TUR syndrome secondary to direct intravascular absorption presents acutely, whereas TUR syndrome associated with extravasation may be delayed up to 24 hours.[19]

Early reports of TUR syndrome noted reddish discoloration of the serum, progressive oliguria, azotemia, pulmonary edema, and even death following the absorption of large amounts of sterile water during TURP. Non-electrolyte solutions with osmolalities similar to serum (275-290 mOsm/kg H_2O) were introduced when it was recognized that the rapid absorption of water could cause intravascular hemolysis and subsequent renal failure. These solutions included glycine, mannitol, and sorbitol. Although the risk of hemolysis with such solutions is negligible, TUR syndrome remains a concern, albeit less common, because all modern irrigants are hypo-osmolar relative to serum (1.5% glycine = 200 mOsm/kg). The incidence of TUR syndrome among patients undergoing TURP with glycine is 1% to 10%.[18] Mortality ranges from 0.2% to 0.8%.[19]

Mechanism

The mechanism of TUR syndrome is not universally agreed upon. Leading theories include the following[18,20]:

1. Intravascular fluid absorption
2. Hyponatremia

3. Hyperammonemia
4. Hyperglycinemia

Although many consider hyponatremia to be the primary cause of TUR syndrome, multiple factors are likely responsible. This may help to explain the heterogeneous presentation of this syndrome.

It is estimated that 20 mL of irrigation fluid is absorbed per minute of resection during TURP.[50] Rapid or prolonged intravascular absorption causes a transient hypervolemia as demonstrated by an initial rise in central venous pressure (CVP), which plateaus within 15 minutes.[18,22] Hypertension and reflex bradycardia are common early; however, as the syndrome progresses, a hypokinetic hemodynamic phase characterized by hypotension and bradycardia often develops. This hemodynamic shift reflects a decline in both cardiac output and intravascular volume, which begin once irrigation is discontinued.[18,23,24] Factors responsible include natriuresis, osmotic diuresis, intracellular uptake of water, hyponatremia, hypocalcemia, and hypothermia among others.

Hyponatremia results from (1) expansion of the extracellular compartment by the infusion of hypotonic fluid (i.e., dilutional hyponatremia), and (2) increase in the urinary excretion of sodium (i.e., natriuresis). The relative contribution of dilution and natriuresis toward hyponatremia depends on the amount of irrigation absorbed and the timing of serum sodium analysis.[25] Early in the course of absorption, sodium dilution predominates because the majority of fluid remains extracellular. As the osmotic gradient widens, water is progressively drawn into the intracellular space such that hyponatremia reaches nadir when hypotonic irrigation is stopped. Less than 50% of the absorbed fluid remains extracellular 30 minutes after infusion has ended.

Serum sodium is commonly used to quantify extracellular fluid (ECF) volume expansion; however, this suggests that it is only at the completion of surgery that such an estimate is accurate. The degree of hyponatremia is an inaccurate measure of extracellular hydration at all other points in the postoperative period. Cases of irrigant extravasation represent an exception to this rule because hyponatremia in this setting is most pronounced 2 to 4 hours after surgery due to delayed reabsorption. The systemic absorption of glycine stimulates renal sodium excretion.[18] Natriuresis accounts for 20% of the hyponatremia at the conclusion of glycine infusion and 30% to 60% when measured 30 minutes later. Taken together, the extracellular volume contraction, intracellular volume expansion, and natriuresis that occur following the absorption of hypotonic fluids call into question the use of fluid restriction and loop diuretics as treatment for TUR syndrome.

Severe acute hyponatremia (<120 mEq/L), particularly in the context of hypervolemia, is a risk factor for cerebral edema and possible mortality. Early symptoms of cerebral edema include nausea, vomiting, and confusion. Seizures, obtundation, and coma may develop if the hyponatremia is not corrected promptly. Hypertension and bradycardia (i.e., Cushing reflex) also may arise as a consequence of heightened intracranial pressure. Radiologic studies demonstrate that cerebral edema may occur following the absorption of as little as 1 L of hypotonic irrigation.[26] By comparison, irrigation with normal saline causes a greater expansion of the intravascular space, but cerebral edema is uncommon.[18]

The most common irrigant used during TURP today is 1.5% glycine. Independent of volume and electrolyte imbalance, glycine and its metabolites retain properties that directly contribute to TUR syndrome in a dose-dependent manner.[27,28] Glycine is metabolized by the liver into ammonia and glyoxylic acid. A small proportion (10%) is excreted unchanged by the kidneys and promotes an osmotic diuresis and natriuresis.[18] Within the retina and central nervous system, glycine functions as an inhibitory neurotransmitter. Visual disturbance is reported in 10% of patients absorbing more than 500 mL of 1.5% glycine solution.[18,27,28] With continued absorption, this may progress to transient blindness, which generally resolves within 24 hours and requires no specific treatment.[29] Depending on the volume of glycine absorbed, a spectrum of mental status changes may be noted. The spectrum includes confusion, depressed consciousness, and coma. Glycine also impairs cardiac conduction and contractility through the generation of subendocardial hypoxic lesions.[30]

Ammonia represents an intermediate product in the hepatic metabolism of glycine. Normally, ammonia is further metabolized by the liver into urea, which is then excreted by the kidneys. In cases of renal or hepatic insufficiency, however, the metabolism of ammonia is impaired and hyperammonemic encephalopathy may occur. Serum ammonia levels tend to correlate with the incidence and severity of neurologic symptoms.[31] Hyperammonemic encephalopathy secondary to glycine absorption is self-limited and will gradually correct once the infusion is stopped. Only supportive measures need be provided.

Risk Factors

Potential risk factors for the development of TUR syndrome are listed in Box 5-1.[18] Although the extent of resection correlates with the volume of irrigation absorbed and the incidence of TUR syndrome, in turn, the relationship between TUR syndrome and irrigation pressure is not as precise. Two large studies have failed to demonstrate any correlation between bag height and fluid absorption during TURP.[32,33] Smoking has been shown to be an independent predictor of large-scale fluid absorption (>1 L) in patients undergoing TURP.

BOX 5-1	Risk Factors for Transurethral Resection Syndrome During Transurethral Resection of the Prostate

Extensive resection
  >45 g
  >90 min
Open venous sinus
Capsular perforation
High pressure irrigation
  >40 cm H_2O
Intermittent flow resection
Smoking history

Data from Hahn RG. Fluid absorption during endoscopic surgery. *Br J Anaesth.* 2006;96(1):8-20.

TABLE 5-3	Symptoms of Transurethral Resection Syndrome
Cardiovascular	**Neurological**
Bradycardia	Nausea
Hypertension	Vomiting
Hypotension	Restlessness
Shortness of breath	Confusion
Chest pain	Depressed consciousness
	Headache
	Blurred vision
	Blindness

This is thought to reflect an increase in prostatic microvessel density among smokers.[34]

Presentation

The presentation of TUR syndrome is heterogeneous and depends on the volume, rate, route, and type of fluid absorbed. Mild cases usually present 30 to 45 minutes after the completion of surgery and may be overlooked.[18] Symptoms are usually neurologic or cardiovascular in origin (Table 5-3). During the intraoperative and early postoperative period, nausea, vomiting, restlessness, confusion, and visual disturbance are common as are the sensations of facial prickling and warmth. Blindness, seizures, and coma may occur in extreme cases. Although transient hypertension and bradycardia can be seen initially, hypotension secondary to gradual ECF volume contraction is more common and problematic. Pulmonary edema may develop in patients with left ventricular dysfunction. In the event of extravasation, abdominal pain radiating to the shoulder is common.

Evaluation

Suspicion of TUR syndrome intraoperatively warrants prompt termination of the procedure after hemostasis is attained. Serum sodium and osmolality should be measured at the completion of surgery because it is only at this time that they accurately quantify ECF volume expansion. Most patients are not symptomatic until the serum sodium concentration falls <125 mEq/dL.

Supplementary measures of fluid absorption include volumetric fluid balance (volume irrigation – volume recovered = volume absorbed), patient weight, CVP, and ethanol breath measurement; however, these are not in widespread clinical use. In addition to laboratory evaluation, hemodynamic stability and intravascular volume status should be determined. This may involve central venous or pulmonary capillary wedge pressure monitoring in unstable patients.

Management

The treatment of TUR syndrome must address both volume status and hyponatremia. On one hand, hypertension secondary to volume overload is usually transient and will resolve spontaneously as the osmotic diuresis and intracellular transfer of fluid proceed. Cardiovascular collapse, on the other hand, requires urgent treatment. Unstable patients with profound hypotension and bradycardia are treated with atropine, epinephrine, and IV calcium.[35]

Although fluid restriction and loop diuretics were recommended in the past to correct volume overload and hyponatremia, the extracellular volume contraction and natriuresis that occur in the postoperative period question whether such steps are appropriate. Loop diuretics, in particular, would be expected to exacerbate the hyponatremia and hypovolemia.[36] Instead, plasma volume expansion and sodium supplementation should be the goal. This can be achieved using IV normal saline (0.9% NaCl) in patients with mild symptoms and serum sodium >130 mEq/L or hypertonic saline (3% NaCl, 513 mOsm/kg H_2O) in severe cases, particularly if the serum sodium is <120 mEq/L.[18,23] The primary indication for use of loop diuretics is acute symptomatic pulmonary edema that fails to resolve with spontaneous diuresis. No studies support the routine use of diuretics in TUR syndrome; however, the combination of hypertonic saline and furosemide may be appropriate in severe cases (e.g., seizure, obtundation, or coma) wherein rapid correction of hyponatremia is necessary.[37,18] The addition of furosemide (20-40 mg) in this manner accelerates the rise in serum sodium 2-fold over hypertonic saline alone.

Unless the patient is severely symptomatic, correction of hyponatremia should proceed slowly so as to avoid the development of central pontine myelinolysis (CPM). This devastating neurologic complication is usually reported in context of chronic hyponatremia; however, it also may occur following the overly rapid correction of acute hyponatremia. Mildly symptomatic hyponatremia should be corrected at a rate of 1 mEq/L/hr.[2] In contrast, patients with severe neurologic symptoms (e.g., seizures, coma) require rapid correction to a serum

TABLE 5-4	**Management of Acute (<48 Hours) or Symptomatic Hyponatremia**				
Treatment Level	**Indication**	**Sodium Solution**	**Dosage**	**Duration**
1	Asymptomatic plus serum Na >120 mEq/L	0.9% NaCl	Based on Na+ deficit	Until serum Na normal
2	Serum Na <120 mEq/L or symptomatic	3% NaCl	1-2 mL/kg/hr	Until symptoms improve
3	Severe symptoms	3% NaCl	4-5 mL/kg/hr	1-2 hr

Notes
Administer hypertonic saline via central venous catheter.
If furosemide is added, it may double the rate of SNa rise.
Measure SNa q 1-2 hours in early stages.
Regress through levels of treatment as SNa and symptoms improve.

Na, sodium; NaCl, sodium chloride; SNa, serum sodium concentration.
Adapted from Decaux G, Soupart A. Treatment of symptomatic hyponatremia. *Am J Med Sci.* 2003;326(1):25-30.

sodium level of 120 mEq/L over 1 to 2 hours, or until symptoms regress. Beyond this point, correction should proceed slowly (0.5-1 mEq/L/hr). Guidelines for hypertonic saline administration are provided in Table 5-4. Calculation of the sodium deficit may serve to guide replacement. Serum electrolytes (sodium) should be monitored frequently to guide treatment every 1 to 2 hours, initially. Central venous access is necessary for the administration of hypertonic saline because this fluid scleroses peripheral veins.

POST-OBSTRUCTIVE DIURESIS

POD refers to the dramatic urine output that may occur following the relief of bilateral ureteral obstruction (BUO) or obstruction of a solitary kidney. The true incidence of POD is not known; however, it does appear to be an uncommon event. Factors necessary for its development include an accumulation of total body water, sodium, and urea or an impairment of tubular reabsorptive capabilities. Most cases of POD involve chronic urinary obstruction; however, significant changes in glomerular and tubular function are evident within 24 hours of complete ureteral obstruction.[38] Although ipsilateral renal function is compromised in all cases of ureteral obstruction, clinically significant POD is uncommon in patients with a normal contralateral kidney. This reflects the continued maintenance of fluid and electrolyte homeostasis by the contralateral kidney. For the purpose of this review, only the pathophysiology of BUO (or obstruction of a solitary kidney) as it pertains to obstructive uropathy and POD is discussed.

Etiology

Urinary obstruction may be anatomic or functional (e.g., neurogenic bladder) in etiology and intrinsic or extrinsic in location. A multitude of etiologies exist, the most common of which include benign prostatic hyperplasia (BPH) or prostate cancer in males and cervical cancer or pregnancy in females. Although nephrolithiasis is a relatively frequent cause of acute obstruction, most cases of POD involve chronic and progressive urinary obstruction as may occur with bladder outlet obstruction (e.g., BPH) or extrinsic bilateral ureteral obstruction (e.g., cervical cancer).

Pathophysiology of Obstructive Nephropathy

Obstructive nephropathy refers to the functional and pathologic damage sustained by the renal parenchyma during urinary obstruction. The severity and consequences thereof depend on the degree and duration of obstruction as well as the presence or absence of an unobstructed contralateral kidney. Our present understanding of the involved pathophysiology comes mainly from animal models of complete unilateral or bilateral ureteral obstruction for 24 hours or more.

Upon the initiation of complete obstruction, profound changes in renal hemodynamics and glomerular filtration take place. In the case of BUO, such changes follow a biphasic pattern.[38] Within the first 2 hours of obstruction, GFR begins to fall as a consequence of elevated tubular hydraulic pressure (P_T). Beyond this period, P_T continues to rise and, more importantly, renal blood flow (RBF) falls dramatically as a result of intense efferent arteriolar vasoconstriction caused by angiotensin II, thromboxane A_2, and neural input.[39] Intrarenal blood flow is also preferentially directed toward the outer cortex in BUO, leaving many glomeruli nonperfused.

The end result is a profound reduction in single nephron and whole kidney GFR by 24 hours. Animal models report ipsilateral GFR at roughly 25% of normal following 1 week of complete unilateral ureteral obstruction.[40] Glomerular filtration appears to be better maintained in BUO, likely on the basis of elevated levels of atrial natriuretic peptide (ANP).[41] Secreted in response to intravascular volume expansion, ANP improves RBF and GFR through the following means[42,43]:

1. Afferent arteriolar vasodilation
2. Tubulo-glomerular feedback inhibition
3. Renin-angiotensin system (vasoconstrictive) inhibition
4. Glomerular filtration coefficient (Kf) increase

Along with its direct natriuretic properties, the actions of ANP are thought to contribute to the diuresis, natriuresis, and rapid return to maximal renal function observed following the relief of BUO. Persistent obstruction also exerts deleterious effects on renal tubular function, primarily through the down-regulation of important transporter and co-transporter activity along the entire nephron.[44] This impairs the reabsorption of sodium (Na^+), potassium (K^+), hydrogen (H^+), and water which, in turn, dissipates the medullary solute gradient and limits the generation of concentrated urine. Together, glomerular and tubular dysfunction manifest as profound natriuresis and diuresis following the relief of BUO.

Mechanism

POD may involve a water diuresis, a solute diuresis or a combination thereof. In most cases, POD represents an appropriate and self-limited physiologic response to volume and solute overload. On occasion, however, the diuresis may extend inappropriately beyond the euvolemic state, usually as a result of excessive free-water loss caused by collecting duct insensitivity to antidiuretic hormone (i.e., nephrogenic diabetes insipidus). Similar to physiologic POD, this form of diuresis is often self-limited and easily managed. True pathologic POD usually refers to the inappropriate excretion of both water and solute as reflected by a urine osmolality >250 mOsm/kg water (Table 5-5).[45] The inability to concentrate urine in pathologic POD stems from the defective generation and maintenance of a medullary solute gradient. Reasons for this include the following[45]:

1. Decreased reabsorption of sodium chloride in the loop of Henle
2. Decreased reabsorption of urea in the collecting tubule

TABLE 5-5	Diuresis Subtype Based on Urine and Plasma Osmolalities	
Diuresis	**Uosm (mOsm/kg water)**	**Uosm:Posm**
Pure water	<150	<0.9
Solute	≥250	>0.9
Mixed	≥250	<0.9

Posm, plasma osmolality; Uosm, urine osmolality.
Adapted from Gulmi FA, Felsen D, Vaughan ED. Management of post-obstructive diuresis. *AUA Update Series*. 1998;17(23):177-183.

3. Medullary solute washout caused by increased medullary blood flow
4. Increased tubular flow rate and solute concentration in the distal tubule

Presentation

The manner of presentation of urinary obstruction depends on the etiology, the time over which it develops, whether it is unilateral or bilateral, and whether it is complete or partial. In the context of chronic BUO, the signs and symptoms are often non-specific. Although most patients with complete obstruction describe anuria or oliguria, some patients with partial obstruction may report polyuria secondary to impaired renal concentrating ability.

Volume expansion is common and may present as weight gain, peripheral edema, or even shortness of breath if CHF is a complicating factor. Patients with long-standing obstruction may present with uremic symptoms including mental status change, tremor, and gastrointestinal (GI) bleeding. Volume expansion or azotemia in the setting of BUO should raise suspicion for possible diuresis following the relief of obstruction. As such, these patients should be monitored and treated accordingly. In clinical practice, a urine output in excess of 200 mL/hr over 12 consecutive hours constitutes POD.[45] It is important to note, however, that significant derangement in fluid and electrolyte status can take place during the initial 12 hours and, as such, appropriate investigation and treatment should not be delayed.

Evaluation and Management

Upon presenting with BUO, patients should undergo a thorough baseline evaluation including a complete blood count (CBC) and complete metabolic profile. Elevations in serum blood urea nitrogen (BUN) and creatinine may be identified as well as hyperkalemia and metabolic acidosis which require correction. The development of a brisk diuresis (>200 mL/hr) following the relief of obstruction constitutes POD and warrants appropriate monitoring, investigation and treatment.

Most cases represent physiologic POD and, as such, the diuresis is allowed to proceed until the euvolemic state is reached as determined by clinical parameters such as orthostatic vital signs, breath sounds, jugular venous distention, and peripheral edema. During this time, serum electrolytes should be evaluated every 6 to 12 hours because electrolyte imbalance, particularly hypokalemia and hypomagnesemia, may develop.[46]

If the diuresis persists beyond the euvolemic state, a pathologic concentrating defect or salt wasting nephropathy should be suspected. In this case, urinary diagnostic indices are useful to determine the type of diuresis (water versus solute versus mixed) and to guide fluid replacement (see Table 5-5). With excessive free water loss, plasma osmolality will rise while urine osmolality remains inappropriately low (<150 mOsm/kg water).

Most patients with an intact thirst mechanism and free access to water can compensate for this defect. Patients in whom oral replacement is not an option because of mental status, nil per os (NPO) status, or limited access to water require IV supplementation with hypotonic saline solutions (0.45% NaCl).

Most recommendations call for the replacement of half the urine output at 2 hourly intervals so as to not perpetuate the diuresis. However, animal models suggest that maintenance of a volume expanded state may improve ultimate renal recovery.[47] This has led some centers to replace the entire urine output until renal function plateaus. Contraindications to excessive hydration include CHF and hypertensive crisis. Fluid replacement may be withheld in these cases until such time that the heart failure or hypertension resolves with diuresis and appropriate medical management.

Pathologic POD secondary to salt-wasting nephropathy is a rare, yet potentially life-threatening, event. Dehydration and electrolyte imbalance (Na^+, K^+, magnesium [Mg^{2+}]) are common as the persistent natriuresis promotes the loss of water, potassium and magnesium. Urine osmolality ($\geq$250 mOsm/kg water) is often slightly higher than that of plasma. These patients warrant careful hemodynamic monitoring, possibly including CVP, as well as frequent monitoring of both serum and urine electrolytes.

Sodium and volume replacement is accomplished using normal saline (0.9% NaCl) supplemented on occasion with hypertonic saline (3% NaCl) if the sodium deficit is profound. Serum and urine electrolytes serve as a guide in this regard. Volume replacement should match urine output in a 1:1 fashion until vital signs and renal function stabilize. Hypokalemia and hypomagnesemia are common and require correction. Hyperkalemia and acidosis also may occur, particularly in the event of profound dehydration and consequent worsening of renal function.

METABOLIC COMPLICATIONS OF URINARY DIVERSION

Metabolic complications are common to all forms of bowel urinary diversion as a result of continued solute transport by the interposed segment. These include electrolyte and acid-base abnormalities, altered sensorium, drug toxicity, osteomalacia, urinary calculi, and GI malabsorption syndromes. Factors which influence the type and severity of such complications include the following[48]:

1. Segment of bowel used
2. Surface area (length of bowel)
3. Contact time with urine
4. Urine composition (solutes, pH)
5. Renal function

These factors are particularly important with regard to the development of electrolyte and acid-base disturbance, the focus of this discussion.

Gastrointestinal Transport of Water and Electrolytes

A basic understanding of GI transport facilitates the management of potential complications. The primary functions of the GI tract are digestion, absorption of water and nutrients, and excretion of solid waste. Most water and electrolyte transport occurs through the paracellular and transcellular pathways, respectively.[48]

An Na^+/K^+ ATPase located on the baso-lateral membrane drives the transport of water and solute across the intestinal mucosa by generating an electrochemical gradient. This gradient favors the absorption of sodium through luminal Na^+/H^+ exchange or non-coupled Na^+ channels. Variable expression of luminal transport proteins helps to explain differences in the type, incidence, and severity of electrolyte abnormalities amongst the different bowel segments used for urinary reconstruction. For example, the jejunum has very loose intracellular junctions, allowing for the rapid movement of fluid and electrolytes through paracellular pathways. It also lacks an Na^+/H^+ antiporter but has a Cl^-/HCO_3^- antiporter, which allows for movement of bicarbonate and chloride.

Sodium rapidly follows the existing concentration gradient such as that between plasma (140 mEq/L) and urine (20-40 mEq/L). The frequent association of hyponatremia and hypovolemia with jejunal conduits reflects this fact. Chloride absorption is linked to bicarbonate secretion throughout the small bowel and colon.[48] Bicarbonate, generated by intracellular carbonic anhydrase, is secreted in a 1:1 ratio for chloride. In contrast, gastric parietal cells generate bicarbonate for systemic absorption in the process of acid (H^+) secretion in exchange for potassium. The ileum and colon have less permeable intracellular junctions and can exchange both Na^+/H^+ and Cl^-/HCO_3^-.[49-51] For the most part, the intestinal transport of potassium is passive as dictated by the electrochemical gradient and movement of water. The luminal concentration of potassium is an important determinant of net potassium secretion or absorption.[52]

The majority of water transport and a minority of solute transport occurs paracellularly. GI osmotic permeability, as determined by mucosal tight junctions, decreases caudally such that the permeability of proximal small bowel is four to six times that of the distal ileum and colon.[53] The heightened permeability of jejunum to both solute and water explains the frequent

TABLE 5-6	Metabolic Abnormalities of Urinary Diversion		
Segment	Electrolyte Abnormality	Treatment	Prevention
Stomach	Hyperchloremic, hypokalemic metabolic alkalosis	Rehydration with normal saline KCl replacement H_2 receptor antagonists Proton pump inhibitors	H_2 receptor antagonists Proton pump inhibitors
Jejunum	Hyponatremic, hypochloremic, hyperkalemic metabolic acidosis	Rehydration with normal saline Alkalinization (IV/PO) $NaHCO_3$	PO hydration PO NaCl supplementation PO $NaHCO_3$
Ileum or colon	Hyperchloremic metabolic acidosis ± Hypokalemia	Alkalinization (IV/PO) ± KCl replacement	PO $NaHCO_3$, sodium citrate, potassium citrate Chlorpromazine Nicotinic acid

IV, intravenous; KCl, potassium chloride; PO, oral.
Adapted from Tanrikut C, McDougal WS. Acid-base and electrolyte disorders after urinary diversion. *World J Urol.* 2004;22(3):168-171.

association of electrolyte abnormalities with use of this segment.

Stomach

The interposition of gastric mucosa in the urinary tract has been performed more commonly in pediatric patients than in adults. Purported advantages to the use of stomach include the prevention of short gut syndrome, less mucus production, a relative reduction in the risk of electrolyte or acid-base disturbance, recurrent infection, and urolithiasis.[54] The most frequent electrolyte abnormality is a hypochloremic hypokalemic metabolic alkalosis, which occurs as a result of hydrogen, chloride, and potassium secretion and bicarbonate generation/systemic absorption (Table 5-6).[55]

Patients are also at risk for dehydration secondary to the loss of water through the gastric mucosa. Rarely does this metabolic abnormality achieve clinical significance except in cases of severe renal dysfunction or acute dehydration. Although patients with normal renal function are able to minimize the development of alkalosis through an increase in renal bicarbonate excretion, those with renal insufficiency cannot.

Hypergastrinemia also may be important.[55,56] Secreted by gastrin cells in response to distention (among other stimuli), gastrin stimulates proton secretion by parietal cells through activation of the luminal H^+/K^+ ATPase. This mechanism becomes clinically relevant in cases of gastrocystoplasty wherein bladder distention caused by chronic outlet obstruction may stimulate the secretion of gastrin and precipitate this syndrome.

Symptomatic patients may present with lethargy, weakness, altered mental status, seizures, respiratory depression, and cardiac dysrhythmia.[57] Treatment begins with rehydration using IV normal saline (0.9% NaCl) and correction of hypokalemia as outlined in Table 5-6.[55] Long-term supplementation with oral salt or potassium chloride also may be of benefit.[56] Patients

with persistent mild metabolic alkalosis warrant treatment with histamine-2 (H_2) receptor antagonists, which competitively inhibit histamine-mediated gastric acid secretion. Proton pump inhibitors, which directly inhibit the gastric H^+/K^+ ATPase, are useful in cases refractory to H_2 blockade.[48,55]

Jejunum

Of all bowel segments used for urinary reconstruction, electrolyte abnormalities occur most commonly with the use of jejunum.[55] As a result, this segment is only used when ileum or colon are either unavailable or inadvisable. The typical metabolic changes that occur when jejunum is used include hyponatremia, hypochloremia, hyperkalemia, volume contraction, and metabolic acidosis, all of which reflect the propensity of jejunum for sodium and chloride secretion and potassium and hydrogen ion absorption (see Table 5-6).[58] Significant dehydration is common because the osmotic gradient generated by sodium secretion results in the net loss of water. Hypovolemia stimulates the secretion of aldosterone which, in turn, stimulates renal sodium reabsorption and potassium secretion.[59] This produces a urine low in sodium and high in potassium. When exposed to such urine, jejunum loses sodium and absorbs potassium as driven by the electrochemical gradient. This further perpetuates the metabolic disturbance. At least 25% or more of patients may develop metabolic changes, although only 4% are severe if short segments are used.[60-62] The incidence and severity of this syndrome also appears to be less if distal rather than proximal jejunum is used.

In severe cases, patients may present with lethargy, nausea, vomiting, dehydration, and weakness. Treatment involves rehydration with IV normal saline and correction of metabolic acidosis using sodium bicarbonate ($NaHCO_3$). In the acute setting, standard management of hyperkalemia includes the use of insulin or glucose infusion, bicarbonate infusion, and orally or rectally administered potassium-binding resins such as sodium polystyrene sulfonate (Kayexalate). In the normovolemic state, most patients are able to excrete excess potassium if renal function is normal. If this is not the case, thiazide diuretics may be used to augment the renal excretion of potassium in the long-term.[63] Likewise, vigilant oral hydration and sodium chloride supplementation are recommended as prophylactic strategies.

Ileum and Colon

Ileum and colon, the bowel segments used most commonly in urinary diversion, possess similar transport properties. When exposed to urine in which the concentration of potassium and hydrogen is typically higher and the concentration of sodium is lower than intestinal contents, these segments secrete sodium and bicarbonate and absorb hydrogen, chloride, and ammonium.

Ammonia, generated by the kidneys, buffers free urinary hydrogen ions through the formation of ammonium. Ammonium, in turn, competes with sodium for absorption through the intestinal Na^+/H^+ antiporter, whereas bicarbonate is excreted in exchange for chloride absorption.[55,64] The net result is a hyperchloremic metabolic acidosis.[65] It appears that the absorption of ammonium chloride accounts for the majority of the acid load.[64]

Hypokalemia and total-body potassium depletion also may occur. Most commonly, this reflects intracellular potassium depletion secondary to chronic metabolic acidosis in combination with renal potassium wasting and intestinal potassium secretion.[55,66] Hypokalemia is less common with ileal versus colonic diversions because ileum demonstrates a higher capacity for potassium absorption than does colon.[67]

Hyperchloremic metabolic acidosis is not uncommon following urinary reconstruction with ileum or colon (see Table 5-6).[65,68] In most cases, however, the metabolic disturbance is quite mild because of renal and hepatic compensation. Metabolic acidosis is minimized through an increase in acid excretion by the kidneys, whereas the toxic effects of hyperammonemia are avoided through the hepatic metabolism of ammonium to urea.[48] As discussed, the incidence and severity of metabolic disturbance depends on numerous factors including length of bowel segment (surface area), contact time with urine, and renal function. Commensurate with these risk factors, the incidence of hyperchloremic metabolic acidosis is higher with continent diversions (50%) than with conduit diversions (10%-15%) using ileum or colon.[69-70] This highlights the importance of normal renal and hepatic function at baseline in patients considered for continent urinary diversion. Basic requirements for continent diversion include a serum creatinine <2.0 mg/dL and a normal urine protein concentration. Patients with a GFR >35 mL/min and minimal urine protein who are able to generate a urine pH <5.8 following ammonium chloride loading and urine osmolality >600 mOsm/kg following water deprivation also may be suitable candidates.[60] Otherwise, conduit urinary diversion is more appropriate.

Patients with significant hyperchloremic metabolic acidosis may present with fatigue, weight loss, anorexia, and polydipsia. Laboratory studies reveal a significant nonanion gap metabolic acidosis with hyperchloremia and azotemia. It is estimated that up to 10% of patients with conduit diversion and a higher proportion with continent diversion require treatment for chronic acidosis.[60,71] Treatment involves alkalinization and simultaneous potassium replacement. Correction of acidosis without adequate potassium repletion may precipitate or worsen hypokalemia as potassium is driven into the intracellular space. Sodium bicarbonate is used most commonly for alkalinization; however, sodium citrate plus citric acid (Bicitra) and potassium citrate are suitable alternatives. Unless potassium supplementation is contraindicated, potassium citrate may be more appropriate in patients with CHF or renal insufficiency in whom an excessive sodium load may be poorly tolerated. Patients generally require 1 to 2 mEq/kg of alkali supplementation per day to neutralize the acid load.[60]

Specific management considerations in patients with a continent urinary diversion include the establishment of prompt drainage (i.e., indwelling catheter) as well as empiric antibiotic therapy if urinary tract infection (UTI) is suspected. Urinary obstruction perpetuates the transport of water and solute across the bowel segment, whereas systemic infection has been known to precipitate ammoniagenic encephalopathy through bacterial endotoxin-induced hepatic dysfunction.[72]

Altered Sensorium

Among patients with urinary diversion or reconstruction, an altered sensorium may develop secondary to magnesium deficiency, drug toxicity, or ammoniagenic encephalopathy. Hypomagnesemia, although uncommon, reflects GI malabsorption or renal magnesium wasting caused by chronic acidosis.[73] Drug intoxication may develop whenever a particular medication or its active metabolite is excreted unchanged by the kidneys and then absorbed systemically by interposed bowel. This may occur with such drugs as phenytoin or methotrexate among others.[74] Although chemotherapy (including methotrexate) has been found to be equally safe among patients with continent and incontinent diversions, it seems prudent to catheterize continent patients during therapy.[75]

Excreted by the kidneys, ammonium is absorbed by the intestinal segment and transported to the liver via the portal circulation. Ammonium (or ammonia) is metabolized by the liver into urea, which is then excreted by the kidneys. Under normal conditions, hepatic metabolism is able to adapt to the increased delivery of portal ammonia such that systemic levels remain unchanged. In the setting of liver dysfunction, however, serum ammonia may accumulate to toxic proportions.

Ammoniagenic encephalopathy is a rare complication of bowel urinary diversion. Although this syndrome develops most commonly in patients with liver dysfunction, case reports also exist among patients with normal hepatic function.[76] Often, such cases involve systemic bacterial infection or UTI with urea-splitting organisms. Systemic infection may induce transient hepatic dysfunction secondary to the proliferation of bacterial endotoxin.[77] Alternately, urea-splitting bacteria may generate ammonia through the enzymatic action of urease on urea.[55,76] In both cases, the absorbed ammonia load may overwhelm hepatic metabolism and precipitate encephalopathy.

Depending upon the degree of hyperammonemia and the time course over which it develops, symptoms of encephalopathy vary from mild changes in mental state to deep coma. Evaluation includes an assessment of liver function as well as a thorough search for possible systemic or UTI. In patients with continent urinary diversion, obstruction should be ruled out because urinary stasis may augment the absorption of urinary ammonium. Acute management includes prompt urinary drainage by way of Foley catheter and empiric systemic antibiotics tailored toward urea-splitting bacteria.[55] Dietary protein restriction, neomycin (oral), and lactulose (oral or rectal), which reduce the production or absorption of ammonia in the GI tract, also are appropriate.[78]

KEY POINTS

1. Unless the patient is severely symptomatic, correction of hyponatremia should proceed slowly so as to avoid the development of central pontine myelinolysis.

2. The mechanism of TUR syndrome likely involves a combination of hyponatremia, hyperammonemia, and hyperglycinemia. The extracellular volume contraction and natriuresis that take place call into question the customary use of diuretic therapy. Fluid resuscitation, possibly with hypertonic saline (3% NaCl), is more appropriate.

3. Brisk diuresis (>200 mL/hr) following the relief of urinary obstruction constitutes POD. Patients with POD should be monitored and treated to ensure that volume depletion and electrolyte disturbance do not occur. Most often, however, the diuresis is physiologic and will cease spontaneously without significant sequelae.

4. The frequency and severity of metabolic complications following urinary diversion depend on the segment of bowel used, surface area, contact time, urine composition, renal function, and liver function. Metabolic disturbance is most common with the use of jejunum. This segment should only be used if ileum or colon are either unavailable or inadvisable. Complications with continent urinary diversion can be minimized if this form of diversion is limited to patients with a serum creatinine <2.0 mg/dL and a normal urine protein concentration.

REFERENCES

Please see www.expertconsult.com

Chapter 6

ANESTHETIC COMPLICATIONS IN UROLOGIC SURGERY

George T. Vaida MD
Assistant Professor of Clinical Anesthesiology; Medical Director and Anesthesia Director, Minimally Invasive Urology Unit, New York University Medical Center, New York, New York

Sudheer K. Jain MD
Assistant Professor of Clinical Anesthesiology, New York University Medical Center, New York, New York

Urologists gain significantly from understanding different anesthesia techniques, their risks, their benefits, and their complications. Thorough knowledge of the patient's preexisting medical, surgical, and psychological condition is essential to design a judicious surgical and anesthesia plan. Together, the urologist and anesthesiologist can pursue an integrated strategy to produce the safest patient outcome.

This chapter details the choice of anesthetic technique for specific urologic surgeries, and discusses the major types of anesthesia (i.e., general, regional, and nerve blocks) used in urology with their respective risks and complications. Additionally, the chapter includes sections covering postoperative pain management and the special anesthetic management complications of transurethral resection (TUR) syndrome and urologic laparoscopy.

SAFETY OF ANESTHESIA

Anesthesia safety has been steadily improving for the past several decades. Over the past 20 years, incidence of anesthetic mortality, in which anesthesia was the primary cause of death, ranged between 1 in 2500 and 1 in 220,000. This shows a tremendous improvement over anesthetic mortality 30 to 50 years ago, at which time the anesthetic mortality rate was between 1 in 852 and 1 in 14,075.[1] The reasons for this improvement include better intraoperative monitoring, more targeted preoperative testing, improved institutional practices, and more awareness and knowledge of potential surgical and anesthesia complications. Today, anesthetic techniques are safer than they have ever been.

PREOPERATIVE ASSESSMENT

In anesthesia for urological surgery, the best choice of anesthetic technique requires a thorough preoperative evaluation of the patient. This minimally includes a detailed assessment of cardiac risks, pulmonary risks and airway, infectious complication risks, and anticoagulation risks. All this data, along with the American Society of Anesthesiologists (ASA) anesthesia risk classification and an understanding of procedure-specific surgical and anesthetic risks, influence the choice of anesthesia technique.

Preanesthetic Evaluation

A preanesthesia evaluation involves assessment of information from multiple sources, including patient's history and physical examination, previous medical records, and findings from preoperative tests. According to the ASA practice advisory for preanesthesia evaluation,[2] the patient's history and physical condition should dictate what kind of preoperative testing is appropriate, and routine preoperative testing should be avoided. A presurgical testing unit (PST) is very useful in determining what selective preoperative tests should be obtained. Each hospital should have its own experience-based decision-making parameters for the timing, quality, and quantity of the specific preoperative tests required for each given procedure. It is beyond the scope of this chapter to greatly detail all required preoperative testing regimens for urologic surgery.

At a minimum, however, complete blood cell count (CBC), basic metabolic, blood urea nitrogen (BUN)/creatinine, and urinalysis are obtained. If urinalysis is positive, a culture and sensitivity (C&S) test is obtained and patients placed preoperatively on the culture-specific antibiotic in order to sterilize the urinary tract to prevent bacteremia and possibly urosepsis during surgery.

The patient's preexisting cardiac and pulmonary conditions are the two most common risks for anesthetic morbidity and mortality.

Cardiac Risks

The cardiovascular complication of utmost concern is perioperative acute myocardial infarction (MI). Heart failure, arrhythmias, hypertensive crisis and thromboembolism (e.g., pulmonary embolism [PE], stroke) are also major perioperative risks. The initial history and physical examination, along with electrocardiogram (ECG), will identify potentially serious cardiac disorders.

Risk factors for coronary artery disease can be classified as follows[3,4]:

1. *Major risk factors:* Smoking, high blood pressure (BP), high low-density lipoprotein (LDL) cholesterol, low high-density lipoprotein (HDL) cholesterol, advanced age, and diabetes
2. *Predisposing risk factors:* Obesity, physical inactivity, family history, ethnic factors, and psychosocial factors
3. *Conditional risk factors:* high triglycerides, high homocysteine, high lipoproteins, and inflammatory markers such as C-reactive proteins

Clinical predictors for increased risk of perioperative MI, heart failure, and death can be classified into three categories[3]:

1. *Major predictors:* Unstable coronary syndromes such as MI within a week or unstable angina, decompensated heart failure, significant arrhythmias of various kinds, and severe valvular disease
2. *Intermediate predictors:* Stable angina, previous MI, congestive heart failure (CHF), renal insufficiency, diabetes
3. *Minor predictors:* Advanced age, abnormal ECG, atrial fibrillation, low physical functional capacity, history of stroke, uncontrolled hypertension

The type and anatomic location of the proposed surgery greatly affects cardiac risk. High cardiac risk (>5%) surgeries include major emergency operations in the elderly, aortic and major vascular surgeries, and extensive operations with large fluid shifts. Intermediate risk (1%-5%) surgeries include intraperitoneal, intrathoracic, carotid, head and neck, orthopedic, and prostate procedures. Low cardiac risk (<1%) surgeries include endoscopic, superficial biopsy, eye, and breast procedures.[4]

Optimization of the associated cardiac and other comorbidities should be done preoperatively. Perioperative β-blockers are used to prevent perioperative hypertension and atrial fibrillation and are recommended in coronary artery disease, heart failure, insulin-dependent diabetes, and high-risk surgeries.

Pulmonary Risks and Airway

A focused pulmonary history inquires about symptoms such as shortness of breath, cough, productive sputum, and wheezing, and about smoking history. Auscultation of the lungs is mandatory before anesthesia administration. These factors dictate what further tests (e.g., chest radiograph, arterial blood gas, pulmonary function test) need to be performed or if consultation with a pulmonary specialist is necessary. A preoperative pulmonary function test showing diffusion defects <80% of predicted and forced expiratory volume in the first second of expiration (FEV_1) <70% of predicted will identify patients at risk for pulmonary complications.[5]

Of special interest to the anesthesiologist is the patient's airway examination. An ASA closed claims study reveals that most adverse outcomes related to anesthesia involve respiratory problems, most commonly hypoventilation, airway obstruction, and difficult intubation.[6] Additionally, it is important to look for the patient's ability to flex and extend the neck, range of mouth opening, presence or absence of dentition, thyromental distance, presence of a large tongue, body mass index, and neck circumference.

In extreme cases, videoscope or fiberoptic intubation might be required. If that fails, the surgical technique might need to be modified to accommodate regional anesthesia (i.e., no intubation).

Risk of Anticoagulation

Patients taking oral anticoagulant therapy for medical conditions such as chronic atrial fibrillation, recurrent venous thromboembolism, or prosthetic heart valves, and those patients with medical problems predisposing to thromboembolism, are at increased risk for intraoperative bleeding and spinal cord hematomas following spinal or epidural anesthesia.

Ideally, warfarin is discontinued 4 to 5 days preoperatively, allowing the prothrombin time to correct itself (preoperative retesting is mandatory). An international normalized ratio (INR) of <1.4 is required for surgery under general and regional anesthesia. Oral vitamin K (5-10 mg dose) reverses the therapeutic effect of oral anticoagulation within 12 to 48 hours. Fresh frozen plasma can be used for the same purpose in emergency surgery.

Patients at very high risk of thromboembolic events may be hospitalized before surgery and a replacement therapy with heparin initiated. Heparin should be discontinued 3 to 4 hours preoperatively. Where low molecular weight heparin (LMWH) is used as a preoperative regimen, it should be discontinued 12 to 14 hours preoperatively. In high risk patients with chronic or recurring thromboembolism or recent or recurring PE, or in whom bleeding would be catastrophic postoperatively, the preoperative insertion of a vena caval filter (e.g., Greenfield filter) should be entertained.

Platelet inhibitors, such as aspirin (acetylsalicylic acid) and ticlopidine hydrochloride (Ticlid) remain effective for the entire life cycle of the platelets (8 days). They should be discontinued 8 days before surgery, except in patients with recently (<1 year) inserted drug-eluting cardiac stents, in whom early discontinuation of antiplatelet medication can lead to stent thrombosis and is associated with a 20% to 45% chance of death. For these patients, a cardiologist-driven special preoperative "bridging" protocol is recommended.[7,8]

Dipyridamole (Persantine) and pentoxifylline (Trental) are not considered anticoagulants and can be continued before surgery without affecting bleeding.[9]

See "Spinal Hematoma" section for a discussion of the impact of anticoagulant timing on the insertion and removal of the spinal needle and epidural catheter.

Infectious Complications: Antibiotic Prophylaxis in Urology

Urologic diagnostic and therapeutic procedures can often induce severe deep surgical site infections (SSIs), complex urinary tract infections (UTIs), pyelonephritis, and sepsis. This is of great concern to the anesthesiologist because it is known that urosepsis can occur a few minutes after manipulating the infected urinary tract, thus placing the patient in a life-threatening situation. Regional anesthesia should be avoided in contaminated and dirty or infected procedures in order to prevent dissemination of the infection into the patient's nervous system.

Specific antibiotic prophylaxis is required for the patient with mitral valve prolapse or other valvular disorders and any type of preexisting surgical implant (e.g., prosthetic heart valve, coronary stent, metal screws and plates, penile prosthesis, pacemaker, automatic implantable cardioverter defibrillator [AICD] device, cosmetic implant), at least 1 hour preoperatively.

Choice of antibiotics is a hospital-specific matter, based on regional experience (local ecology and infectious disease strategy).

Anesthesia Risk: The American Society of Anesthesiologists Physical Status Classification System

Once all the preoperative information is evaluated, the anesthesiologist assigns an ASA score. The score is intended to create a uniform system of describing the patient's preoperative physical condition. ASA classification is important because studies have demonstrated that with increasing ASA class, there is increased incidence of adverse events and adverse outcomes.[10]

The modern classification system consists of the following six physical status categories:

ASA I: Normal healthy patient
ASA II: Patient with one mild systemic disease
ASA III: Patient with two severe systemic diseases
ASA IV: Patient with several systemic diseases, at least one life threatening
ASA V: Moribund patient who is not expected to survive without the operation

ASA VI: Declared brain-dead patient who will become an organ donor

Choice of Anesthesia Technique in Urologic Surgery

Adult patients requiring anesthesia for renal and genitourinary surgery are often very old, and they may have a host of comorbidities, which pose serious problems before, during, and after surgery and anesthesia. The choice of anesthetic technique depends on a myriad of factors, including patient's preexisting conditions; type, site, and length of surgery to be performed; skill of the urologist and anesthesiologist and their intimate knowledge of potential surgical and anesthetic complications; and predictability and limitations of the surgical and anesthesia procedures. Based on all of these factors, the ultimate decision of anesthesia method needs to be the product of a well-informed discussion between the surgeon and the anesthesiologist.

Patient-Specific Risk Stratification

The modern ASA classification system, in conjunction with the full preoperative workup data of the patient, provides a degree of perioperative risk stratification that is very useful in choosing the optimal anesthetic technique for a given patient undergoing a particular surgery.

ASA I patients who are young, healthy, normal patients with good exercise tolerance and no organic physiologic or psychiatric disturbance may have general anesthesia, regional anesthesia, nerve blocks, or clinical sedation for their procedure. Any obvious difficulty with general anesthesia (e.g., difficult airway, full stomach, allergies to anesthetics, hyperreactive airway) will necessitate modifications in the general anesthesia technique (e.g., fiberoptic intubation, fast sequence induction and endotracheal intubation, avoidance of certain drugs, modification or deepening of induction). General anesthesia will be used in cases in which patient stillness during the procedure is essential, for example brachytherapy, renal and upper ureteral stone lithotripsy, and most laparoscopic and robotic surgeries.

ASA II patients with mild systemic disease who have no functional limitations and have a well-controlled one body system disease (e.g., diabetes, hypertension, smoking without chronic obstructive pulmonary disease [COPD]) can tolerate general anesthesia as well as regional anesthesia or nerve blocks. The one system disease must be stabilized under full medical control. If the patient presents with full stomach or hyperreactive airway, regional anesthesia or nerve blocks might provide extra safety for the patient and ease postoperative recovery.

ASA III patients have severe systemic disease, involving more than one major body system. They are in no immediate danger of death, but they have some functional limitations (e.g., stable angina, CHF, old heart attack, poorly controlled hypertension and diabetes, morbid obesity, chronic renal failure). With the advent of modern monitoring and mandatory use of pulse oximetry and end tidal carbon dioxide monitoring ($ETCO_2$), contemporary general anesthesia has greatly improved. Most recent clinical studies comparing general with regional anesthesia show no substantial difference in outcomes. However, when using general anesthesia in this patient population, utmost care must be exercised in maintaining steady normal vital signs throughout the case (e.g., use etomidate for induction, use cardiovascular support, if needed, and maintain normal blood volume). If there are no contraindications, regional anesthesia or nerve blocks with their pulmonary and cardiovascular sparing effect, along with the prolonged postoperative analgesia they provide, are our favorite modalities for predictable, stable, safe, and comfortable outcomes in this patient group.

ASA IV patients have multiple system disease, where one or more disease may present a constant threat to life. These diseases may be poorly controlled or at their end stage (e.g., unstable angina, symptomatic COPD, symptomatic CHF, hepatorenal failure). Preoperatively, these patients require time and specialist support to maximally control their unstable diseases. Intraoperatively, heavy monitoring (e.g., A-line, central venous pressure [CVP], Swan-Ganz catheter, cardiac output) and pharmacologic cardiovascular and pulmonary support are needed. In this patient group, general anesthesia poses high risk. For urologic procedures, regional anesthesia in skilled hands, using minidoses of local anesthetic, ensures minimum respiratory and cardiovascular risk, as well as less eventful, stable, and comfortable recovery. Importantly, using only minimum sedation with the regional block, the mental status of these sicker, older patients will remain unimpaired throughout the case and during the recovery period.

Procedure-specific Indications

Because most urologic procedures are performed in an anatomic area primarily innervated by thoracolumbar and sacral nerve supply, these procedures are excellent candidates for regional anesthesia and nerve blocks. The great versatility of regional anesthesia relies on the fact that, if skillfully done, it can greatly preserve pulmonary and cardiovascular functions in all patients. This gives maximum benefit to older patients or those with severe comorbidities. Major contraindications for regional anesthesia are patient refusal, skin infection, sepsis, cardiac outflow tract obstruction (aortic stenosis, idiopathic hypertrophic subaortic stenosis [IHSS]), serious previous neurologic deficiencies, anticoagulation, shock, hypotension, or allergies to local anesthetics.

In some urologic procedures patient awareness is an advantage, as in transurethral resection of the prostate (TURP) in which the patient can voice any discomfort and early symptomatology (see "Transurethral Resection Syndrome," later). In other procedures, slight sedation or a total intravenous (IV) anesthesia (TIVA) helps the patient accept the operative surroundings (operating room [OR] noises, uncomfortable positioning) and length of procedure (e.g., long perineal reconstructive procedures done under combined spinal or epidural block, radical prostatectomy under regional block, penile prosthesis insertion, artificial urinary sphincter insertion, complex female incontinence surgery, endourethral procedures, longer procedures done under pudendal or penile block).

TIVA is always used successfully for physical and emotional comfort before pudendal blocks and penile blocks. Patients are unaware of the block and after the procedure, they wake up comfortable and enjoy a prolonged postoperative analgesia. A propofol-based TIVA predictably prevents postoperative nausea and vomiting (PONV) in most patients, including those with a history of PONV. See "Propofol Total Intravenous Anesthesia for Postoperative Nausea and Vomiting," later.

INTRAOPERATIVE ANESTHESIA MANAGEMENT

Anesthesia for urologic surgery includes general anesthesia, regional anesthesia, and specific nerve blocks. Each technique has its own specific complications.

General Anesthesia

Adverse pulmonary events are the cause of most anesthetic complications that occur under general anesthesia. In Caplan's study of the ASA closed claims database, adverse respiratory events accounted for 34% of all adverse events, with death or brain damage occurring in 85% of those patients.[6] Three mechanisms accounted for 75% of these injuries: inadequate ventilation, esophageal intubation, and difficult tracheal intubation.

Less common but equally important mechanisms of adverse respiratory-related events included airway obstruction, bronchospasm, aspiration, airway trauma, and pneumothorax.[11] Proper airway management is essential in avoiding most of these pulmonary event–related anesthetic complications. Other specific complications occurring during general anesthesia administered for urologic procedures also will be mentioned.

Difficult Airway

When the anesthesiologist has difficulty ventilating or intubating the patient, the airway is defined as difficult. The ASA has devised a complex algorithm to help manage the difficult airway. Preoperatively, the most important question is whether or not oxygenation and ventilation can be provided.[12] Using a laryngeal mask airway (LMA), videoscope or fiberoptic intubation can help solve this problem. Alternatively, using regional anesthesia will circumvent these difficulties. In extreme cases, surgical technique might need to be adapted to the modified anesthesia choice.

Bronchospasm and Hyperreactive Airway
Patients with bronchial asthma or with a history of it, COPD, smokers, patients with atopies (e.g., eczema), or those with recent upper respiratory infections (within 4-6 weeks) will present either with a hyperreactive airway or with an overt asthmatic condition. Their usual medications, such as β_2-agonists (e.g., albuterol) and anticholinergics (e.g., ipratropium), should be used preoperatively. Most importantly, an adequate depth of anesthesia should be achieved before manipulating the airway with endotracheal intubation or before patient positioning and any surgical manipulation. The same principle applies when extubating these patients. In this patient population, regional anesthesia techniques are preferable, whenever feasible.

Aspiration
Aspiration pneumonitis due to aspiration of gastrointestinal (GI) contents is associated with a significant degree of morbidity and mortality, especially in patients in ASA class III and above. Many risk factors exist for aspiration, including full stomach, gastroesophageal reflux disease (GERD), hiatal hernia, ileus or bowel obstruction, pregnancy, obesity, diabetes, emergency cases, trauma, gastric motility disorders, inadequate general anesthesia, difficult intubation, enteral tube feeding, sepsis, and severe renal failure.

Aspiration occurs because the protective airway reflexes (e.g., gag, cough) are missing or blunted by anesthesia. For prevention, patients should be nil per os (NPO) 4 to 8 hours before surgery, and a host of pharmacologic agents may be used preoperatively to diminish gastric acidity and/or volume (e.g., antacids; proton pump inhibitors such as omeprazole; and histamine-2 receptor antagonists such as cimetidine, famotidine, and ranitidine; or GI stimulants such as metoclopramide). For patients at risk of aspiration pneumonitis, rapid sequence induction and endotracheal intubation should be used in all general anesthesia cases. Alternatively, aspiration of stomach contents can be avoided entirely by using a regional anesthesia technique.

Laryngeal, Pharyngeal, and Esophageal Trauma
In an ASA closed claims analysis, the larynx was the most common site of injury (33%), followed by the pharynx (19%) and the esophagus (18%).[6] Most airway injuries are of minor significance and are temporary in nature, although some can result in severe sequelae (e.g., mediastinitis) or even death. Whenever a difficult intubation is encountered or if the patient complains of specific symptoms postoperatively, the surgeon and the anesthesiologist should keep a high index of suspicion for airway injury. These injuries may require further

evaluation by an otolaryngologist and further intervention.

Avoiding intubation altogether or using fiberoptic laryngoscopy or LMA will prevent most of these complications. Regional anesthesia is a safe choice.

Airway Obstruction
Airway obstruction occurs with some frequency during anesthesia. Most airway obstructions (89%) occur during general anesthesia, and 70% of these involve the upper airway.[11] Causes of upper airway obstruction may include laryngospasm, foreign body, laryngeal polyps, laryngeal edema, pharyngeal hematoma, kinked endotracheal tube (ETT), and kinked breathing circuits. Tracheobronchial obstruction may occur as well, usually secondary to blood or mucous in the lumen or external compression from a mass (e.g., tumor, mediastinal mass, hematoma). Airway obstruction also may occur during monitored anesthesia care (MAC).

Most cases of airway obstruction can be relieved with proper airway management or placement of an LMA or an ETT. Cautious placement of a nasal trumpet can be invaluable in preventing and relieving airway obstruction, especially in MAC cases. Vigilance is the key in preventing airway obstruction—watching the patient's chest and diaphragmatic movement, looking and feeling for exhaled air, and so on—along with $ETCO_2$ and airway pressure monitoring.

Pneumothorax
Pneumothorax is a relatively rare complication. Most causes for pneumothorax may be divided into two categories: needle-related or airway management related. Most needle-related pneumothorax cases are due to nerve blocks or central venous catheter placement. Airway management related pneumothorax cases involve airway instrumentation (e.g., laryngoscopy, ETT placement, bronchoscopy) and barotrauma (e.g., ventilator).[11]

Specific urologic procedures are associated with a higher incidence of pneumothorax. Procedures performed abutting the diaphragm (e.g., nephrectomy, partial nephrectomy, percutaneous nephrolithotomy [PCNL]) and laparoscopic cases run the risk of puncturing the diaphragm and creating a pneumothorax. Pneumothorax should be suspected when there is an increase in the patient's respiratory rate and peak airway pressure, hypoxemia, hypercarbia, and hemodynamic changes, particularly hypotension and mediastinal shift, as in tension pneumothorax (which is an emergency). Definitive diagnoses can be confirmed with a chest radiograph. Treatment includes needle thoracotomy and chest tube placement along with supportive therapy. Prevention includes avoidance of positive pressure ventilation whenever possible (use manual ventilation instead) and discontinuation of nitrous oxide (N_2O).

Hypothermia

Perioperative hypothermia and shivering are risks for all patients, especially for older and sicker patients. A 0.5°C drop in body core temperature stimulates the hypothalamus, which initiates shivering. Abnormally large muscle masses are involved in this exothermic reaction to reestablish lost body heat. Shivering increases oxygen consumption by 100% to 400%, with potential deleterious effects; in that respect, shivering mimics a grand mal seizure.[13] The cardiovascular system may be affected with bradycardia, atrial fibrillation, ventricular arrhythmias, and even cardiac arrest.[14,15] Patients feel extremely cold and uncomfortable and may experience confusion, delayed awakening, brain infarct, and even brain death.[16] The musculoskeletal system will show slowness, rigidity, and cramps, among other effects. Surgical blood loss will be increased.[17,18]

Several pharmacologic treatments for shivering (e.g., meperidine 25-50 mg IV or chlorpromazine 2-5 mg IV) work within a few minutes, and as soon as shivering stops, patients suddenly feel comfortable and warm.[19] Treatment for hypothermia includes body warming and fluid warming. Fast rewarming is dangerous because it rapidly increases oxygen consumption, on a temporary basis (100%-200%).

Best prevention for hypothermia includes using a fluid warmer (for all IVs), a body warmer (e.g., Bair Hugger) for all cases, warm irrigation fluids, warm ORs, and shorter surgical procedures. Also, epidural or spinal use of narcotics for anesthesia counteract a tendency to shiver.

Tetraplegic and paraplegic patients are at highest risk for prolonged hypothermia. They must be warmed throughout the entire surgery and through postoperative care. They cannot shiver and are vasodilated at all times; therefore, they will take an extremely long time to rewarm postoperatively.

Hyperkalemic Cardiac Arrest

Patients with spinal cord injury (paraplegics and tetraplegics who frequently undergo endourologic procedures) and those who are bedridden long-term run the risk of hyperkalemic cardiac arrest secondary to succinylcholine (SCH) administration used to facilitate intubation. This occurs due to massive extra-junctional proliferation of SCH receptors of the neuromuscular junction in this subset of patients, and also can be secondary to massive burns, brain and peripheral nerve injury, or muscle atrophies or dystrophies.

In these patients, SCH produces intense muscle fasciculations with massive release of intracellular potassium and cardiac arrest. If SCH is not used for these patients or if regional anesthesia is used, these complications will be avoided.

Autonomic Hyperreflexia

Autonomic hyperreflexia is characterized by an uncontrolled sympathetic response secondary to a precipitant, due to loss in descending inhibition from higher centers and due to alterations in connections within the distal spinal cord. Autonomic hyperreflexia usually occurs in patients with spinal cord injuries at the T6 level and above; it occurs in 50% to 70% of this patient population. Signs and symptoms of autonomic hyperreflexia are caused by the vasoconstriction and sympathetic response below the level of the spinal cord lesion and by the compensatory parasympathetic response above the level of the lesion.

Major symptoms include hypertension, headache, sweating, flushing or pallor above the level of the lesion, and bradycardia. Other less common signs include pupillary changes, Horner syndrome, nausea, and anxiety. The most common precipitants of autonomic hyperreflexia involve the urinary tract. Importantly, bladder distention has been shown to account for up to 85% of cases. UTIs, genital stimulation, urologic procedures, and even catheterization can also elicit a response.

When autonomic hyperreflexia is suspected, treatment should begin immediately, before serious complications result, such as intracranial hypertension, seizures, or intracranial hemorrhage. Removal of the stimulus and pharmacologic treatment of the hypertension should be done immediately. A short acting α-blocker (e.g., phentolamine 5-30 mg IV in divided boluses) is generally effective in normalizing BP.

Preventing autonomic hyperreflexia begins by identifying those patients at risk (T6 and above spinal cord lesions) and maintaining a high index of suspicion. For the urologist, measures that reduce the incidence of bladder distention (e.g., anticholinergic, intermittent catheterization) may reduce the incidence of attacks.

For these patients, spinal anesthesia is the anesthesia technique of choice, especially for urologic procedures, because it prevents most cases of autonomic hyperreflexia, avoids the need for general anesthesia, and provides excellent cardiovascular stability.[20] The slight disadvantage of spinal anesthesia is that it may be difficult to reliably determine the level of blockade. General anesthesia also has been used successfully and autonomic hyperreflexia avoided as long as deep anesthesia is maintained. However, these patients have a host of other medical issues associated with their spinal cord injury (e.g., immobility, muscle wasting, respiratory issues, thermoregulation problems), which may increase the risk of general anesthesia. Epidural and MAC (sedation, local anesthetic infiltration) have been reported as less successful in preventing autonomic hyperreflexia when compared with spinal and general anesthesia.

Malignant Hyperthermia

Malignant hyperthermia (MH) is an uncommon pharmacogenetic clinical syndrome of hypermetabolism triggered by specific anesthetic agents. MH is an inherited disorder that occurs in 1 in 10,000 to 1 in 50,000 patients. It occurs as a result of abnormally increased intracellular release of calcium from the sarcoplasmic reticulum. All inhalational anesthetics, except N_2O, can trigger MH. SCH is a very frequent trigger. Safe anesthetic agents include N_2O, barbiturates/IV anesthetics, all narcotics, and all antianxiety medications. MH can begin during administration of anesthetic agents, or it may occur postoperatively.

Testing for susceptible patients, the so-called in vitro caffeine-halothane contracture test, is done on freshly collected muscle biopsy specimens. Newly developed molecular genetic testing, which identifies about 50 mutations as causal for MH, is still in early development. A complete list of testing center locations in North America is available from the Malignant Hyperthermia Association of the United States (MHAUS) at www.mhaus.org.

Predisposing diseases include certain muscle disorders, such as central core disease, Duchenne or Becker muscular dystrophies, specific types of myotonia, and hyper- or hypokalemic paralyses.

Special clinical syndromes have been grouped as masseter muscle rigidity (a sustained contracture of the jaw muscles after SCH administration, which may or may not progress to full MH), sudden unexpected cardiac arrest (especially soon after the use of succinylcholine), and myopathies (muscle rigidity and/or hyperthermia—if hyperkalemia is successfully treated, the outcome may be good). These syndromes may occur alone or in the context of fully developed MH.

To diagnose MH, the most consistent indicator is an unanticipated increase (tripling or quadrupling) of $ETCO_2$ when minute ventilation is normal. Sudden unexpected cardiac arrest may occur, especially in boys and young men (aged 5-15 years), and hyperkalemia should be suspected. Unexpected tachycardia is an early symptom, as are tachypnea and masseter spasm. Respiratory and metabolic acidosis usually indicate advanced or fulminant MH (late clinical development). Body rigidity is a specific sign of MH in patients under general anesthesia. Core body temperature elevation is often a late sign of MH. Postoperative rhabdomyolysis and acute myoglobinuric renal failure are usually later events. There is a 25% MH recrudescence rate in the postoperative period, thus patients should be watched carefully after any initial MH event.[21]

Treatment begins by immediately discontinuing the triggering agent. Hyperventilate with 100% oxygen. Treat with IV 2.5 mg/kg dantrolene sodium (because this solution does not have significant side effects, it should be used for all cases in which MH is suspected). Treat acidosis with bicarbonate; treat hyperkalemia with glucose, insulin, and calcium; treat hyperthermia with cooling (nasogastric lavage, rectal lavage, intraperitoneal lavage, surface cooling—to end point of 38°C). Avoid calcium channel blockers (use other antiarrhythmics). Carefully monitor serum potassium; measure cre-

atine phosphokinase (a good measure of muscle destruction) every six hours until decreased (though in severe MH, high creatine phosphokinase might last for 2 weeks). Follow coagulation profile because disseminated intravascular coagulation may occur.

Prevention begins by identifying patients at risk of MH through positive history or previous testing. Patients with known or suspected MH who need surgery can be safely operated on using a non-triggering anesthesia technique (total avoidance of triggering agents) and a mandatory fresh oxygen (O_2) flushing of the anesthesia circuit for a minimum 20 minutes preoperatively (in order to eliminate any traces of inhalational agents). ASA recommends measuring core body temperature in all anesthesia cases lasting >30 minutes. It is recommended that a full complement of fresh dantrolene ampules and chilled IV fluids, along with full resuscitative medications, be readily available at all times in the OR.

Postoperative Nausea and Vomiting

If untreated, up to 30% of all surgical patients will have PONV after general anesthesia with inhalational anesthetics, whereas high risk patients will have an incidence up to 80%. Patients with an increased incidence of PONV tend to be young children; women; or patients with preoperative pain and anxiety, delayed gastric emptying, and, most importantly, a positive history of motion sickness and PONV. Anesthesia risk factors for PONV include dehydration, general anesthesia with inhalational anesthetics, anesthesia lasting longer than 3 hours, and the use of N_2O, narcotics, sedatives (e.g., ketamine, etomidate), and neostigmine. Urologic factors that increase the likelihood of PONV include laparoscopic surgery, hernia repair, and orchiopexy. Postoperative risks include sudden motion, pain, and early fluid intake.

Various antiemetic medications are used to treat nausea and vomiting. One group of antiemetics works by antagonizing neurotransmitters at various receptor sites (e.g., dopamine, histamine, serotonin, or cholinergic-muscarinic receptors). These include antihistamines (diphenhydramine and promethazine), butyrophenones (droperidol and haloperidol), phenothiazines (chlorpromazine and prochlorperazine), benzamides (metoclopramide) and anticholinergics (scopolamine). Another group works as anti-inflammatories or specific antiserotonin ($5-HT_3$) antagonists (ondansetron, granisetron, and dolasetron). Dexamethasone is a corticosteroid that works through anti-inflammatory and some unknown properties.

Various side effects occur after using antiemetic medications. Their most significant side effect is sedation.

As prophylaxis for PONV, dexamethasone combined with an antiserotonin antagonist proves to be one of the most efficient regimens, if used at induction of general anesthesia. For treatment of PONV, combinations of antiemetics seem to be more efficient (through their additive effect) than single medications. In our experience, however, when everything else fails, one of the best rescue medications is haloperidol 1.25 mg to 2.0 mg used intramuscularly (an IV dose is too short acting), which provides >15 hours of intense antiemetic effect without excessive sedation or any hallucinations.

The most effective way to prevent PONV is to entirely avoid inhalational anesthetics, unnecessary sedatives, and N_2O (which causes a 30% increase in PONV). See "Propofol Total Intravenous Anesthesia for Postoperative Nausea and Vomiting," next.

Propofol Total Intravenous Anesthesia for Postoperative Nausea and Vomiting

TIVA is a modern form of general anesthesia. Propofol TIVA, which uses a propofol drip along with fentanyl, seems to be the most effective general anesthetic technique for preventing PONV. Propofol TIVA proves especially useful in patients at higher risk for PONV (those with a history of motion sickness or previous PONV).

Propofol TIVA general anesthetic can be administered with the patient breathing spontaneously or with the patient muscle relaxed and mechanically ventilated. In either TIVA technique, N_2O, benzodiazepines, or other sedative medications are not needed (bispectral index [BIS] monitor tested), and should be avoided because they tend to produce PONV, unnecessarily delay patients' awakening, and prolong recovery. Propofol TIVA predictably provides a well-anesthetized patient who has no operative recall, is easy to wake up, has satisfactory postoperative analgesia, and has no PONV.

For patients with a history of hypersensitive (hyperreactive) airway such as asthma (even if childhood asthma), smokers, patients with recent upper respiratory infections (within the past 6-8 weeks), chronic bronchitis, or eczema, low concentrations of inhalational agents (e.g. 0.2%-0.4% sevoflurane) should be added (for deeper anesthesia level and bronchodilation) to either of the TIVA regimens listed. The same regimen should be used for an obese patient or any intubated patient. Adding low concentration inhalational agents does not diminish the potent anti-PONV qualities of the propofol/fentanyl TIVA.

Patient Positioning

Urologic surgeries require the patient to be in specific positions (e.g., supine, prone, lithotomy, or lateral position), which can cause inadvertent nerve injury. Most nerve injuries involve the ulnar nerve (28%), brachial plexus (20%), lumbosacral nerve roots (16%), and the spinal cord (13%).[22] Nerve injuries usually occur as a result of compression or stretching of the nerve.

With patients in supine position, the most commonly injured nerve is the ulnar nerve, regardless of whether the patient has both arms tucked at the side or out on armboards. With patients in lithotomy position, sciatic, femoral, and peroneal nerves are at increased risk for injury. In lateral position, the brachial plexus is at increased risk. Meticulous attention must be paid to positioning a patient, ensuring that he or she is not stretched beyond the physiologic range, and padding all pressure points to reduce the incidence of nerve injury.

According to the ASA practice advisory for prevention of perioperative peripheral neuropathies,[23] arm abduction should be limited to 90 degrees in supine patients. Arms also should be positioned to decrease pressure on the postcondylar groove (ulnar nerve) and the spiral groove of the humerus (radial nerve). Neutral forearm position or supination of the arms with proper padding should meet this recommendation.

For lower extremity positioning, excessive stretching of the hamstring muscle group beyond a comfortable range must be avoided (especially in lithotomy position), as this may cause sciatic neuropathy. Prolonged pressure on the peroneal nerve at the fibular head should be avoided by using proper padding (especially in lithotomy position). Neither flexion nor extension of the hip has been shown to increase the risk of femoral neuropathy, although it is advised that excessive flexion or extension be avoided.

Preventing peripheral neuropathies begins in the preoperative phase. Certain patient characteristics have been shown to be associated with perioperative neuropathies, including smoking, diabetes, vascular disease, arthritis, and extremes of body weight and age. Preoperatively, any preexisting neuropathies should be identified during the initial history and physical examination, and the patient's normal comfortable range of motion should be determined. Intraoperatively, patient positioning and padding should be checked periodically. Postoperatively, patients should be watched for early signs of any nerve injury and appropriate steps taken, including obtaining neurologist consultation if necessary.

Regional Anesthesia

A preponderance of outcome data suggests that regional anesthesia improves patient morbidity and mortality,[24] as compared with general anesthesia. Also, regional anesthesia was found to reduce overall mortality by approximately 30%. Regional anesthesia decreased the odds of deep venous thrombosis by 44%, PE by 55%, transfusion by 50%, pneumonia by 39%, respiratory depression by 59%, MI by 33%, and renal failure by 43%, thus greatly reducing overall morbidity as well. The benefits of regional anesthesia include the following[24]:

- Attenuation of the body's stress response perioperatively (preserves cardiovascular function)
- Preservation of respiratory function and decrease in pulmonary complications
- Faster recovery of postoperative GI function
- Decrease in intraoperative blood loss
- Decrease in postoperative hypercoagulability
- Preservation of perioperative immune function
- Superior postoperative analgesia compared to systemic opiates
- Decreased length of stay in the post anesthesia care unit (PACU) due to adequate pain control
- Increase in patient satisfaction

Contraindications for regional anesthesia include patient refusal, cardiac outflow tract obstruction (as in IHSS and aortic stenosis), the anticoagulated patient (when INR >1.4), skin infections, serious previous neurologic deficiencies, hypotension, allergy to local anesthetic, sepsis, and hemorrhagic shock.

Regional anesthesia can be divided into two categories: neuraxial anesthesia (e.g., spinal, epidural, combined spinal/epidural) and peripheral nerve block anesthesia (e.g., pudendal, penile).

Neuraxial anesthesia deposits a local anesthetic within the subarachnoid (spinal) or epidural space. This produces sympathetic block (vasodilation), sensory block (painlessness), and motor block (muscle relaxation), with separate corresponding levels, each producing distinctive physiologic changes.

The sympathetic block results in vasodilation, with an increase in volume of the capacitance vessels, causing a decrease in cardiac preload and secondary hypotension. This undesirable hypotension can be abrupt and severe, directly proportional to the degree of sympathetic denervation, and it must be treated early and aggressively with vasopressors, fluids, and head-down position (thus increasing cardiac preload). The sympathetic denervation may involve the entire lower extremities, the pelvis, or the thoracoabdominal cavity, depending on the height of the sympathetic level achieved. The sympathectomy slowly wears off throughout the surgery and outlasts the sensory block by about 3 hours.

The sensory blockade renders the patient insensitive up to a certain level, which can be manipulated in various ways in order to achieve painlessness for the entire dermatomal distribution of the surgical procedure and for the duration of surgery and recovery.

The motor blockade also can be manipulated at will to produce full muscle relaxation extending from the lower extremities all the way up to the thoracic wall, depending on the type of surgery performed. For surgical anesthesia, solid sensory and motor denervation are needed, whereas for postoperative analgesia, only sensory block is required.

Spinal Anesthesia

Spinal anesthesia is achieved by injecting small amounts of various local anesthetics below L1 spinal level directly into the cerebrospinal fluid (CSF) through a fine needle inserted beyond the arachnoid membrane. A sensory dermatomal level and a three dermatomal segments higher sympathectomy (vasodilation) are obtained. The motor block is about two dermatomal levels lower than the sensory level. Duration of the spinal block depends on the type, dose, and baricity of the local anesthetic used; it also depends on patient positioning. The major side effect of spinal anesthesia is drop in BP, proportionate to the level of sympathectomy (vasodilation). For best treatment of this side effect, see "Further Prevention of Regional Anesthesia Complications," later.

The following important complications may occur with spinal anesthesia.

Postdural Puncture Headache

Postdural puncture headache (PDPH) is a headache that may occur 24 to 48 hours after spinal anesthesia (or inadvertent epidural subarachnoid puncture). It is thought to be due to a continuous leak of CSF through the spinal puncture hole, decompressing the subarachnoid space with secondary stretching of the cranial nerves. PDPH has two specific characteristics: it is frontal and positional. It typically appears as a throbbing frontal headache (of variable intensity). Its main positional characteristic is used as a test. When the patient is lying in bed, he or she may have no headache at all. However, when the patient sits up or walks, a throbbing frontal headache will occur, which disappears when the patient lies down again. In severe cases, even a slight lift of the head from the horizontal position elicits the headache. This positional test differentiates PDPH from sagittal sinus thrombosis, which produces a continuous throbbing headache in any position.

Associated symptoms of PDPH include neck ache or stiff neck (57%), upper back ache (35%), nausea (22%), and visual and auditory disturbances. If untreated, PDPH spontaneously resolves within 1 to 6 weeks, but it is very distressing to patients.

Conservative treatment relies on hydration, caffeine (cerebral vasoconstrictor), sumatriptan succinate (serotonin type 1d receptor agonist, a powerful cerebral vasoconstrictor), and adrenocorticotropic hormone (a controversial treatment, which works through increased CSF production and/or β-endorphin release). Epidural blood patch, an invasive PDPH treatment used only for unrelenting symptomatology, consists of injecting 10 to 15 mL autologous blood into the patient's epidural space. PDPH disappears immediately in 85% of such cases, and recurrence is rare.

Cauda Equina Syndrome/ Transient Neurologic Syndrome

Cauda equina syndrome (CES) is a clinical representation of local anesthetic neurotoxicity. It can present as varying degrees of pain or neurologic deficit limited to the lower extremities, and it can create functional deficiencies (e.g., urinary and fecal incontinence). It may present with transient symptomatology, or it may evolve into permanent neurologic lesions with permanent loss of function. Permanent CES is very rare.

All local anesthetics are potentially neurotoxic in high doses. CES may be caused by maldistribution, high concentration, and/or high and repetitive doses of local anesthetics. See "Local Anesthetic Systemic Toxicity," later.

Transient neurologic syndrome (TNS) is another clinical representation of local anesthetic neurotoxicity. TNS has been described in conjunction with continuous spinal anesthesia, where frequent topoff reinjections of the same local anesthetic cause toxicity. Consequently, continuous spinal anesthesia is rarely performed. TNS also may appear on rare occasions after spinal administration of single doses of lidocaine, mepivacaine, bupivacaine, or any other spinal anesthetic, if used in excessive doses. However, in our experience, following thousands of subarachnoid meperidine blocks, TNS has not occurred. We strongly recommend using meperidine in regular doses of 35 to 50 mg or in minidoses of 20 to 30 mg in all cases. See "Further Prevention of Regional Anesthesia Complications," later.

Epidural Anesthesia

Epidural anesthesia is achieved by injecting local anesthetic into the epidural space, which is located between dura mater and the yellow ligament (ligamentum flavum). Consequently, a sensory dermatomal block is obtained, associated with a 3 to 6 dermatomal segment higher sympathectomy (vasodilation). A motor block is also obtained. In clinical practice, epidural anesthesia can be obtained with a single injection or through an epidural catheter used for reinjection with local anesthetic in order to prolong surgical anesthesia or to provide postoperative pain relief. The major side effect of epidural anesthesia is hypotension, proportionate to the level of sympathectomy (vasodilation). The onset of this hypotension is slower than the hypotension associated with spinal anesthesia. For best prevention or treatment of this side effect, see the use of ephedrine in "Further Prevention of Regional Anesthesia Complications," later.

The following complications may occur with epidural anesthesia:

Inadvertent Subarachnoid Injection

Inadvertent subarachnoid injection is an accidental local anesthetic injection into the subarachnoid space (CSF). This occurs when the epidural needle accidentally penetrates the dura mater and arachnoid membranes and ends up in the subarachnoid space. Epidural anesthesia requires much higher local anesthetic volumes than spinal anesthesia (~1.5 mL per dermatomal segment blocked); if some of this high volume anesthetic ends up in the subarachnoid space, it will create undesirably high levels of subarachnoid block (total spinal). This will cause widespread sympathectomy and vasodilation, with sudden drop in BP and cardiac output, leading to a clinical picture of shock, often rapidly progressing to respiratory and cardiovascular arrest.

As a first measure, the patient is immediately placed in the Trendelenburg position in order to increase preload to the heart. Treatment then is geared toward cardiovascular and respiratory support.

Prevention includes keeping patients awake and conversant, using a subarachnoid test (injecting small fractionate doses of local anesthetic), and slowly raising the dermatomal sensory level of anesthesia with frequent testing (cold or pinprick test).

Inadvertent Intravascular Injection

Inadvertent intravascular injection is unintended injection of a large dose of local anesthetic into a blood vessel within the epidural space. This may occur during a single injection through the epidural needle or following even small fractionate doses of local anesthetic through an epidural catheter. Local anesthetic intravascular toxicity may occur with the following symptoms, usually appearing in a clinically predictable sequence: tinnitus, perioral numbness, dizziness, fainting, drop in BP, bradycardia, seizures, coma, and death.

Treatment is symptomatic. Immediately stop injecting the local anesthetic and, in cases of seizure or cardiovascular collapse, use sedatives and cardiovascular support measures. In case of clinical shock with cardiorespiratory arrest, administer cardiopulmonary resuscitation.

Prevention starts with the correct placement of the epidural catheter. Then the epidural catheter is tested with an IV testing dose using small, non-seizure producing, tracer-laced (e.g., epinephrine) local anesthetics while looking for tachycardia on ECG. It is essential to inject slowly, keeping the patient conversant and asking for the presence of early symptoms of local anesthetic intravascular toxicity (i.e., tinnitus, perioral numbness, dizziness). If these symptoms appear, immediately stop the injection and assume toxicity. The use of benzodiazepines at this point will prevent seizures; however, these drugs will not prevent the cardiovascular collapse secondary to a massive intravascular injection. Use basic monitoring (ECG, BP cuff, pulse oximetry, ETCO$_2$) for the entire epidural and surgical procedure in order to observe any other symptoms of inadvertent intravascular injection (e.g., drop in BP, drop in arterial saturation, bradycardia).

Maintain general awareness of this potential complication throughout the case. Even if the local anesthetic is injected properly (negative IV test), if massive toxic doses accumulate over time, a similar delayed clinical picture may occur. The anesthesiologist must not trespass into the generally acknowledged toxic doses of each specific local anesthetic. See also "Local Anesthetic Systemic Toxicity," later.

Combined Spinal/Epidural Anesthesia

Combined spinal/epidural (CSE) anesthesia blends the advantages of both types of anesthesia. Classically, the spinal anesthesia component, with its early onset and dense block, is used for surgical anesthesia; this might be sufficient for the entire surgery. The epidural catheter, however, may be accessed for additional anesthesia during surgery if, at any time, the spinal anesthesia wears off. The same epidural catheter also can be used for prolonged postoperative analgesia.

Complications can arise from either the spinal or the epidural component of the technique. Prevention of most potential CSE complications is identical to the separate spinal and epidural preventive measures.

Local Anesthetic Systemic Toxicity

Local anesthetic systemic toxicity may occur in two ways: massive reabsorption after tissue injection or secondary to inadvertent intravascular injection. If the quantity (in milligrams) of the local anesthetic injected exceeds certain toxic peak levels, the following symptoms may be produced:

1. *Central nervous system (CNS) excitability/depression:* Tinnitus, perioral numbness, dizziness, confusion, seizures, coma, death
2. *Cardiovascular effect:* Peripheral vasodilation with hypotension, heart block, bradycardia, ventricular tachycardia, asystole, cardiovascular collapse
3. *Respiratory effect:* Respiratory depression due to direct local anesthetic effect and/or secondary to CNS and cardiovascular effects
4. *Methemoglobinemia:* Central cyanosis refractory to supplemental oxygen administration appears at a methemoglobin level >15%. At 50% to 60%, methemoglobinemia may produce confusion, arrhythmias, hemodynamic instability, and seizures, leading to death. Chocolate-colored blood that keeps its color despite exposure to air is diagnostic. Methemoglobinemia can occur after large doses of benzocaine topical administration and absorption (usually used for various endoscopic procedures). Also it may occur when large doses of prilocaine (>600 mg) are admin-

istered. (Prilocaine is no longer available for use as a local anesthetic.)[25]

There are various ways to estimate the toxic dose of a given local anesthetic. Clinically useful and generally acknowledged local anesthetic toxic doses (when used with epinephrine) are tetracaine 1.5 mg/kg, bupivacaine 3 mg/kg, lidocaine 7 mg/kg, mepivacaine 7 mg/kg, procaine 20 mg/kg, and 2-chlorprocaine 20 mg/kg.

There are two general categories of local anesthetics: ester and amide. The ester types are tetracaine, procaine, 2-chlorprocaine, and benzocaine. They are metabolized in the body by the natural esterases, which limit and terminate their inherent toxicity. The amide types—bupivacaine, levobupivacaine, ropivacaine—are metabolized in the liver, a longer process, thus making these local anesthetics available for a longer time, and prolonging the potential toxicity.

Treatment

Treatment depends on the severity of the event. CNS excitability can be treated with sedatives such as benzodiazepines. The respiratory and cardiovascular depressant effects should be addressed by supportive measures. Severe methemoglobinemia is treated by using 1 mg/kg IV methylene blue.

Recently, IV lipid emulsion has been used successfully to bind and quickly remove the highly liposoluble local anesthetics from the intravascular system. There are numerous clinical reports of life-saving rapid reversal of major local anesthetic toxic symptomatology.[26-29]

Prevention

The overall injected quantity (in milligrams) of local anesthetic always must be kept below the toxic dose (see "Local Anesthetic Systemic Toxicity," earlier). Maintain constant vigilance during and after local anesthetic injection. Resuscitative equipment and medications must be available at all times. Monitor patients fully whenever local anesthetics are injected. When infiltrating tissues, constantly move the needle while injecting, and whenever the needle stops, before injecting, apply 90-degree double aspirations to make sure the needle tip is not inadvertently in a blood vessel. Inject small fractionate doses when performing nerve blocks. Whenever possible, add a tracer substance (e.g., epinephrine) to diminish tissue reabsorption of the local anesthetic and also to provide an early sign (tachycardia) of inadvertent intravascular injection of the local anesthetic.

Spinal Hematoma

Bleeding associated with neuraxial blockade is a rare complication, occurring in an estimated 1 in 220,000 for spinal anesthesia and in <1 in 150,000 for epidural anesthesia.[30] Spinal hematoma may occur in patients with known or unknown coagulopathies and in patients who may be anticoagulated for various medical or surgical reasons.

Symptoms include progression of the existing sensory or motor block (68%), bladder or bowel dysfunction (8%), and pain of radicular nature.[31] Whenever spinal hematoma is suspected, a computed tomography (CT) or magnetic resonance imaging (MRI) scan is diagnostic.

If the hematoma is symptomatic, it should be surgically evacuated as soon as possible. If possible, the anticoagulant involved also should be discontinued.

Preventing spinal hematoma requires judicious perioperative planning and good communication among the urologist, anesthesiologist, cardiologist/internist, and pain clinic staff. Nonsteroidal anti-inflammatory drugs (NSAIDs) do not seem to pose a serious risk, either on insertion or removal of the neuraxial needle or catheter.[32]

When subcutaneous unfractionated heparin is used, there are no added significant risks on insertion (needling) or removal; however, it is recommended to wait 1 hour postremoval before resuming anticoagulation.

When IV unfractionated heparin is used, however, hold it 2 to 4 hours before insertion and 1 hour after insertion before resuming anticoagulation; hold it 2 to 4 hours before catheter removal and 1 hour after catheter removal before resuming anticoagulation.

When low molecular weight heparin (LMWH) is used, hold it 10 to 12 hours before insertion, and >2 hours after insertion before resuming anticoagulation; hold it 10 to 12 hours before catheter removal and >2 hours after catheter removal before resuming anticoagulation. The American Society of Regional Anesthesia recommends the removal of indwelling epidural catheters before starting LMWH.

When warfarin is used for thromboprophylaxis, the INR should be allowed to normalize to ≤1.4 preoperatively.[30] For patients with drug-eluting cardiac stents, there is a new specific "bridging" protocol, which recommends that patients continue their antiplatelet medication.[7,8]

Further Prevention of Regional Anesthesia Complications

Meperidine Spinal Anesthesia

In my practice (Vaida), we use regional anesthesia extensively for most urologic procedures. The judicious use of meperidine spinal anesthesia prevents many major and minor anesthetic complications, and provides superior long lasting postoperative pain relief.

We have perfected a technique over the past several decades in which regular doses or minidoses of meperidine have been used without any respiratory depressant effect or otherwise deleterious side effects in thousands of ASA III-IV patients. We have used this regimen with great success in a wide variety of urologic procedures, ranging from cystoscopy to long TURPs, female and male reconstruction for incontinence, radical retropubic prostatectomy, and endourology procedures, including transurethral lithotripsy.

Meperidine has a fast onset and, when used alone, provides a deep sensory and motor block completely resembling plain lidocaine spinal (both drugs used as 50 mg yield a T6 sensory level, which covers ~1.5 hours of surgical anesthesia). Subarachnoid meperidine is the only short-acting narcotic with local anesthetic properties that provides 8 to 12 hours of postoperative analgesia. In the PACU, patients who received meperidine during surgery are completely awake, have a clear sensorium, are recovered fully from the initial motor block, and do not require pain medications.

As a rare side effect, itchiness occurs in <1% of cases. If itchiness becomes intense, treat it with naloxone 40 μg IV, followed by 80 to 100 μg IM for prolonged effect.

Meperidine does not increase the risk of spinal headache (we have observed 0% in our patient population). Meperidine does not produce TNS as do the other local anesthetics. Meperidine does not delay time to void in the recovery room.

Meperidine may be used alone or in combinations. We add minidoses of local anesthetic in order to prolong meperidine anesthesia during longer surgeries. This allows great versatility in matching a spinal anesthesia regimen to the length of a particular surgical procedure, so that the motor blockade will wear off very soon after the conclusion of surgery while still providing very long postoperative analgesia.

Meperidine can provide the spinal component of the CSE technique used in extra long cases in which postoperative pain relief must be maintained for several days.

Combined Intravenous and Intramuscular Ephedrine for Cardiovascular Stability

In order to counteract the potential drop in BP secondary to any spinal anesthesia, we use ephedrine immediately following spinal injection, as 5 mg IV bolus, with simultaneous IM injection of 25 mg to 40 mg (depending on patient's size). The IV dose starts working within a minute, without producing undue tachycardia, and lasts up to 10 minutes. The IM dose becomes effective within 10 minutes and works for 2.5 hours (using the muscle as a depot), with only minor increases in BP or heart rate (<10%), thus ensuring a continuum of BP support.

If given early enough, at the onset of sympathectomy due to the spinal administration, this ephedrine regimen will simply maintain the patient's original heart rate and BP, independent of the hydration status. Thus, a completely stable cardiovascular status is assured for the length of the case. This ephedrine regimen confers great cardiovascular stability to spinal anesthesia, making it an extremely attractive choice for all patients, and especially older and sicker ASA III-IV patients.

NERVE BLOCKS IN UROLOGY

Nerve blocks offer a safe anesthetic approach to a multitude of urologic procedures and a rapid painless recovery for all patients. These blocks prove to be especially safe and useful in old and sick ASA III-IV patients because these blocks eliminate the risks and complications general and regional anesthesia cause while providing a stressless operative and postoperative course (pain free, no PONV, clear postoperative mentation).

Contraindications to these nerve blocks include patient refusal, anticoagulation, allergy to the local anesthetic, and local infection.

Pudendal block and penile block are the nerve blocks most frequently used in hospital-based urologic surgery.

Pudendal Nerve Block

Pudendal nerve block may be used in all superficial male and female perineal surgeries; male and female lower urinary reconstructive procedures; sling procedures for incontinence; rectal and urinary sphincter procedures; and procedures on the penis, clitoris, scrotum, and labia majora. The pudendal nerve block can be used in conjunction with a short spinal anesthesia, general anesthesia, or continuous propofol/fentanyl TIVA.

The pudendal nerve innervates the perineum, the anal and urethral sphincters, the penis, and the clitoris. A number of male and female urologic procedures depend on knowledge of pudendal innervation, including anal and stress incontinence surgeries via suprapubic, perineal, or vaginal approaches, and pudendal canal decompression for pudendal canal syndrome and pudendal artery syndrome (with erectile dysfunction).[33]

The sacral plexus gives off the pudendal nerve by using the S_2, S_3, and S_4 anterior rami. The pudendal nerve roots emerge from the anterior sacral foramen. The pudendal nerve contains autonomic and motor nerve fibers together, making it a mixed nerve.

Out of the pudendal canal, the pudendal nerve gives off three terminal branches: the inferior rectal nerve, the perineal nerve, and the dorsal nerve of penis or dorsal nerve of clitoris.[34]

The inferior rectal nerve supplies the external anal sphincter, the mucus membrane, and the lower half of the perianal skin and the inner anal canal. The perineal nerve gives off deep branches to the muscles of the urogenital triangle and superficial branches to the skin of the lower labia majora and lower scrotum. The dorsal nerve of the penis or clitoris supplies sensory nerve endings to the skin surface of clitoris and penis.

The pudendal nerve runs through three significant anatomical regions: the gluteal region, the pudendal canal, and the perineum. The course of the pudendal nerve in the area of the ischial spine is important because this is where the pudendal nerve block is placed.

There are three approaches to the pudendal nerve block:

1. Transvaginal approach
2. Perineal approach (Aburel method)
3. Direct percutaneous approach (Vaida method)

Transvaginal Approach

This method, often used in obstetrics, provides perineal analgesia during the third stage of delivery, when the presenting part of the newborn is visibly bulging the perineum. It is also useful in urologic surgery.

The block is done with the patient in lithotomy position. Palpate with the left hand (5-6 cm intravaginally) the left ischial spine through the left lateral vaginal wall. Affix the tip of an Iowa Trumpet between the palpating fingers and the tip of the ischial spine. Pass a long injecting needle through the trumpet and through the vaginal wall until it punctures the sacrospinous ligament and advances another 1 cm. Perform two 90-degree safety aspirations and, if there is no blood return, inject 5 to 8 mL local anesthetic.

Repeat the same exact technique on the patient's right side, using the right hand for vaginal examination and the left hand for the aspiration-injection sequence. The sensory block obtained between the anus and clitoris can be ascertained by pinprick testing the skin of this area. Any local anesthetic may be used, such as 3% 2-chloroprocaine (providing a 1-2 hour block), lidocaine 1.5% or 2% (providing a 2-3 hour block), or bupivacaine 0.25% or 0.5% (providing a 4-8 hour block).

Complications Potential problems may include accidental rectal puncture, bleeding (rare), pudendal blood vessel puncture (with local anesthetic systemic toxicity), and infection (rare). Avoid injecting large volumes of local anesthetic because toxicity may occur. See "Local Anesthetic Systemic Toxicity," earlier.

Prevention The 90-degree double safety aspiration before the injection (to ascertain that the needle tip is not in intravascular position) is essential. When the patient is in the lithotomy position, the rectum is located medial and inferior to the ischial spine; therefore, the palpating hand entirely protects the rectum. Do not do any puncture until the Iowa Trumpet is firmly affixed between the palpating fingers and the ischial spine.

Perineal Approach

In the 1960s, Aburel described a percutaneous perineal approach used in female and male urology cases. With the patient in lithotomy position, the block is done midway between the rectum and the base of the penis or vagina on the midperineal line. With the area thoroughly prepared, pass the injecting needle posteriorly and laterally from this point, aiming toward the ischial spines, one at a time. When the ischial spine is contacted, walk the needle off the bone, medioinferiorly, about 1 cm past the sacrospinous ligament. After two 90-degree safety aspirations (ensuring no blood return), deposit 5 to 8 mL local anesthetic.

Complications Complications include accidental rectal puncture, pudendal vascular puncture (local anesthetic systemic toxicity), and infections (rare). Avoid injecting large volumes of local anesthetic because toxicity may occur. See "Local Anesthetic Systemic Toxicity," earlier.

Prevention Rectal puncture is prevented by guiding the needle with simultaneous transrectal palpation of the ischial spine. Inadvertent puncture of blood vessels is prevented by the 90-degree double safety aspirations.

Direct Percutaneous Approach (Vaida Method)

Direct percutaneous approach can be used easily in male or female urology. It is done with the patient in lithotomy position, with the entire perineum and gluteal areas thoroughly prepared with antiseptic solution. A syringe containing 10 to 16 mL local anesthetic is outfitted with a 20-gauge spinal needle. In lithotomy position, the ischial spine can be palpated easily directly through the skin about 3 to 4 cm lateral from the anus. Through a puncture done at this level, insert the needle in a 10-degree posterolateral direction. When the needle tip contacts the ischial spine, walk it off medioinferiorly, through the sacrospinous ligament, for another 1 cm. After two 90-degree aspirations, deposit 5 to 8 mL local anesthetic. Repeat again over the other ischial spine.

Complications The direct percutaneous approach avoids rectal injury, which is most likely in the perineal approach, and inadvertent intravascular injection (the slight angulation keeps the injecting needle in a more medial position away from the pudendal vessels). However, infection is a potential, although rare, complication.

Prevention Double 90-degree safety aspirations are used in order to prevent local anesthetic systemic toxicity. Thorough skin preparation is essential to prevent infections.

Penile Block

Thorough understanding of pudendal nerve anatomy is essential to the penile block. Terminal branches of the pudendal nerve innervate the rectum, the perineum, the scrotum, and the penis.

Perineal Nerve

After emerging from the pudendal canal, the perineal nerve courses downward for 2 to 3 cm and gives rise to two terminal divisions: a lateral scrotal branch and the medial striated urethral branch.[35,36] The scrotal branch unites with the inferior rectal nerve to form the common scrotal branch, which innervates the posterior aspect of scrotum.

Deep Dorsal Nerve of Penis

This is one of the two branches of pudendal nerve leaving the pudendal canal. It courses forward along the inferior pubic ramus, along the end of the ischiorectal fossa, into the deep perineal pouch. The nerve courses forward into the suspensory ligament of the dorsum of penis, sending terminal branches to the entire dorsum.[37] It is noteworthy that very often a well done dorsal penile block spares the anterior lower part of the penis, which is innervated by rami of the perineal branch of the pudendal nerve as well.[38] By contrast, the circumferential block done at the base of the penile shaft is a complete block of the dorsal nerve of penis and the perineal branches of the pudendal nerve, which provide sensory innervation to the midanterior aspect of the penis all the way up to the frenulum.[39]

Indications of Penile Block (Adults Only)

Although circumcision is performed on an estimated one in six newborn males worldwide and about 60% of newborn males in the United States,[40] adult circumcision is much less frequently performed. The usual indications for adult circumcision are social, personal, or medical, including the following: phimosis, paraphimosis, acute paraphimosis (emergency), recurrent infections such as balanitis and posthitis, or preputial neoplasms. General anesthesia, penile block, or a combination of both is used in the majority of these cases.

The penile block is always done before the surgery begins, preferably using long-acting local anesthetics (e.g., 30 mL bupivacaine 0.375% or 0.5% provides 8-15 hours analgesia). Because the penis is an organ with terminal circulation, the local anesthetic used for penile block must never contain epinephrine. See "Penile Ischemia and Necrosis," later. The block is intensely painful; therefore, it should be done under a TIVA using continuous propofol/fentanyl technique, with the patient spontaneously breathing oxygen by mask. This technique may be continued throughout the entire surgical procedure, as a light or medium sedation. See "Propofol Total Intravenous Anesthesia for Postoperative Nausea and Vomiting," earlier.

Penile Block Techniques

There are two accepted penile block techniques that may be used separately or together.

Dorsal Penile Nerve Block   Dorsal penile nerve block[41] is done by injecting 5 to 8 mL local anesthetic through a 27-gauge needle, deep to Buck's fascia, where the two (left and right) dorsal nerves of the penis emerge from under the pubic bone. Inject at the 10-o'clock and 2-o'clock positions at the base of the penis, walking the needle off caudad the pubic bone and popping through Buck's fascia.

A 4% to 6.7% failure rate has been reported using the dorsal block alone.[39] See "Deep Dorsal Nerve of Penis," earlier. To complete the block on the upper ventral side of the penis, a subcutaneous ring block must be done at the base of the frenulum.

Circumferential Block   This is our preferred technique because it provides 100% sensory block to the penis.[41] With the penis pulled up vertically and thoroughly prepped, 15- to 30-mL local anesthetic is injected subcutaneously at the very base of the penile shaft, circumferentially. The injection is done with a 25-gauge needle, continuously moving the needle forward then backward while injecting, raising a contiguous ring around the base of the penis. When close to the dorsal vein of the penis, lift the needle over the vein subcutaneously while constantly advancing and injecting, making sure that no local anesthetic is deposited intravenously. The needle must be kept subcutaneous at all times.

Complications and Prevention

Bleeding and Hematomas   Bleeding and hematomas can be prevented by using a continuous mode of injection with small 25- or 27-gauge needles. When approaching the large dorsal vein of penis, it is possible to skillfully lift the needle and course it subcutaneously above the vein while still injecting. This will avoid inadvertent IV injection of local anesthetic and bleeding or hematoma.

Local Anesthetic Toxicity   Even small amounts of local anesthetic, if directly injected intravenously, may cause toxicity. Additionally, if overly large volumes of local anesthetics are used for the block, they may get absorbed and cause delayed systemic toxicity. It is important to calculate and stay below the tissue toxic dose of the local anesthetic used. See "Local Anesthetic Systemic Toxicity," earlier.

Penile Ischemia and Necrosis   The arterial supply of the penis is through terminal branches of the pudendal artery, which gives rise to the bulbourethral arterial branches. The glans is supplied by the dorsal arteries, which give off circumflex branches perforating the tunica albuginea and supplying the distal end of corpora penis.

Penile ischemia/necrosis is a grave complication, usually caused by accidental use of vasoconstrictors (e.g., epinephrine).[42] All end organs with terminal vasculature are at risk of prolonged ischemia and necrosis (nose, fingers, toes, penis). Many cases of penile necrosis have been described in the pediatric literature; never use epinephrine in this block.

The local anesthetic ropivacaine also seems to be a potent vasoconstrictor. When comparing epidural ropivacaine and bupivacaine using xenon clearance technique, ropivacaine produced large decreases (37%) in epidural blood flow, whereas bupivaine produced an increased epidural blood flow.[43] Ropivacaine's vasoconstrictor property is further substantiated by animal studies.[44] Consequently, ropivacaine should not be used in end organ blocks with terminal arterial supply.

A possible temporary ischemia (presenting as pallor, pain, swelling, necrosis) has been successfully treated with vasodilation provided either by a regional block (caudal, spinal, epidural) or use of prostacyclin (PGI_2), the major prostanoid produced by the blood vessels. PGI_2 relaxes smooth vasculature, inhibits platelet aggregation, and can be administered intravenously or intraarterially.

Infection   Both methods of penile block must be done respecting full sterility precautions. In case of any infection, suspect skin flora.

INTRAOPERATIVE PENILE ERECTION

Intraoperative penile erection is a serious problem that may preclude Foley catheterization or cystoscope insertion and may increase bleeding and injuries to the corpora cavernosa and urethra during penile surgery. The mechanism for intraoperative penile erection is complex and poorly understood. It can be traced to a combination of neuroendocrine, vascular, and psychological factors acting upon the penile erectile organs.

Parasympathetic fibers (nervi erigentes) originating from S_2-S_4 sacral spinal segments innervate the penis. If parasympathetic tone predominates, the arteriolar dilation with subsequent erection of the corpora cavernosa causes erection. High sympathetic nervous tone causes arteriolar vasoconstriction with a subsequent reduction of the blood flow to the corpora cavernosa, causing penile flaccidity. Vasoactive mediators also can affect the tumescence of the penis through a host of mediators like nitric oxide, bradykinin, or vasopressin.

The overall incidence of intraoperative penile erection is 2.5% for all male patients undergoing surgery, affecting those under general and epidural anesthesia evenly. The lowest incidence of 0.3% is encountered in spinal anesthesia.[45]

Clinically, intraoperative penile erection may occur from a multitude of factors. The most frequent are Foley catheterization (in 1% of general anesthesia cases) and penile manipulation (most frequently in patients <50 years of age).

Treatment

Cooling the penis with ethyl chloride spray or anesthetizing with a penile block are frequently effective. Additionally, numerous pharmacologic methods have been used to obtain detumescence. Phenylephrine, a pure α-blocker, injected as 50 to 150 μg intracavernosally, provides detumescence within a few minutes. Vasodilators such as IV nitroprusside and inhaled amyl nitrate act through their relaxing effect upon the corpora cavernosa to produce detumescence. These might be contraindicated in hypotension, regional blocks (sympathectomy) and cases of increased intracranial or intraocular pressure. IV ketamine in doses of 0.5 to 1 mg/kg may be used. Ketamine's dissociative affect upon the limbic nervous system, coupled with its penile relaxing effect (decrease in central parasympathetic outflow), produce detumescence.[45]

Terbutaline 0.2 to 0.5 mg IV, a β$_2$ adrenergic agonist, has been used successfully to terminate erections. It causes direct relaxing effect over the corpora cavernosa smooth muscles. Care must be taken in cardiac patients due to the tachycardia it may cause. Glycopyrrolate 0.2 to 0.3 mg IV, an anticholinergic with reduced chronotropic and CNS effects (better than scopolamine and atropine), works through its acetylcholine blocking effect in the nitric oxide penile erection mechanism.

Most sympathomimetics mentioned as useful penile detumescents in the urologic literature need to be evaluated seriously against their major cardiovascular complications. Epinephrine, norepinephrine, and metaraminol, to name a few, should be avoided if possible due to their intense β$_1$ activity.[45]

Prevention

Initial deepening of general anesthesia and avoiding early penile stimulation are important in preventing intraoperative penile erection. Spinal anesthesia (instead of general) needs to be considered more frequently for urologic procedures. In some elective cases, if prevention or milder treatment methods do not work, cancelling the case might be a better choice than causing inadvertent cardiovascular complications in a very sick ASA III-IV patient.[46]

OBTURATOR REFLEX

Obturator reflex is a problem potentially encountered during transurethral bladder tumor resections (TURBTs). Whenever the tumor resection gets close to the lateral wall of the bladder, the energy of the resectoscope can directly stimulate the obturator nerve through the bladder wall, which initiates a sudden violent pelvic thrust secondary to powerful contraction of the thigh adductor muscles. This may cause the resectoscope to inadvertently perforate the bladder. Obturator nerve block,[47,48] however risky[49] and difficult to perform, seems to be useful in preventing obturator reflex in conjunction with general or regional anesthesia. It was hoped that the use of the newest technologies, such as the new bipolar thermocoagulation devices,[50,51] would diminish the incidence of obturator reflex.

However, the obturator reflex can be totally prevented only if the patient is under general anesthesia, fully muscle relaxed. General anesthesia can be selected at the beginning of the case or initiated at any point later during the case if the tumors to be resected seem to be positioned on the unfavorable lateral wall of the bladder. Awareness of the problem and good communication between the urologist and anesthesiologist are essential to prevent the occurrence of obturator reflex.

POSTOPERATIVE PAIN MANAGEMENT

Most urologic procedures produce significant postoperative pain. Postoperative pain management should be discussed and planned jointly by the urologist and anesthesiologist before the surgery. The choice of anesthesia is crucial in partially or totally preventing postoperative pain. Patients waking up after general anesthesia have full pain, whereas patients after regional anesthesia have somewhat less pain.

The need for heavy pain medication produces its own unnecessary symptomatology, such as PONV, unpleasant sedation, confusion (prolonged in the very old), residual pain, and longer recovery times. Ideally, the anesthesia technique simultaneously provides adequate stress-free anesthesia for the urologic procedure and prolonged postoperative pain relief in the PACU. This is best accomplished through the judicious use of nerve blocks and meperidine spinal anesthesia in association with propofol TIVA. See "Further Prevention of Regional Anesthesia Complications," earlier.

Various pain management techniques can be employed postoperatively:

Narcotics

Major narcotics still are relied upon heavily for immediate postoperative pain management. Morphine has been successfully used in single injectable doses on demand. It produces only moderate pain relief, with deep sedation, confusion, PONV, and histamine release. Morphine is very useful in narcotic addicted patients, alone or in association with other methods of analgesia. See "The Narcotic-addicted Patient," later.

We find that fentanyl 100 to 150 μg (depending on patient's weight), used IM rather than IV (using the patient's large quadriceps muscle as a drug depot) along with 10 mg lidocaine added to alleviate injection discomfort, is a more potent analgesic than morphine and causes less deleterious side effects. Fentanyl used in this fashion causes no significant immediate respiratory depression, less PONV, and no histamine release (tachycardia, hypotension, itchiness) and provides very good pain relief for several hours. Fentanyl proves even more useful in patients with relative or absolute contraindications to other pain medications such as morphine, meperidine, hydromorphone (Dilaudid), or NSAIDs.

Nonsteroidal Anti-inflammatory Drugs

NSAIDs are very useful after shorter, less painful procedures, alone or in conjunction with minor narcotics (Percocet, Tylenol with Codeine, Vicodin) or in the context of multimodal analgesia. Most patients tolerate NSAIDs well for short treatment courses. Patients with known asthma history, allergy to NSAIDs, renal failure, GI problems (e.g., gastritis, ulcer), or coagulopathies should not be given NSAIDs. Acetaminophen (Tylenol) is a viable substitute, alone or in conjunction with narcotics.

Ketorolac tromethamine (Toradol) is safe in single IM doses of 30 to 60 mg and provides excellent 6 to 8 hour analgesia without any sedation. IV Toradol has an extremely short effect, and thus is never useful for significant postoperative pain relief (as per label warning). Toradol also may be used in combination with other medications. We prefer a novel IM combination injection of Toradol 60 mg, plus 100 to 150 µg fentanyl, plus 10 mg lidocaine (prevents fentanyl injection discomfort) for even more potent, long-acting postoperative analgesia, without significant sedation. To accommodate this slightly increased volume, we do a double injection (in two directions) through the same puncture hole in the patient's quadriceps muscle.

Tramadol

Tramadol (Ultram), a centrally acting moderate analgesic, is used in doses of 50 mg or 100 mg PO every 4 to 8 hours, and is safe for patients <75 years old. Tramadol decreases the seizing threshold of patients with seizure disorder and interacts negatively with a host of psychotomimetic drugs (serotoninergic syndrome).[52]

Multimodal Analgesia

Different regimens mixing NSAIDs with minor or major narcotics and local anesthetics/nerve blocks prove to be very efficient, facilitating an early recovery.[53,54] Multimodal analgesia is heavily relied upon in ambulatory surgery.

Morphine Intravenous Patient-controlled Analgesia

When postoperative pain is prolonged, morphine IV–patient-controlled analgesia (IV-PCA) may be used.

Many physicians tend to underdose morphine IV-PCA. In healthy patients, use a continuous rate of 1 to 1.2 mg/hr, a patient demand bolus of 1.3 to 1.5 mg, and a lockout time of 8 to 10 minutes, based on the patient's weight and gender (lower weight patients use the lower doses/longer lockout times). Less frequent or lower doses leave the patient in constant pain. We prefer fentanyl IV-PCA in all cases, except for the narcotic-addicted patient.

Fentanyl Intravenous Patient-controlled Analgesia

Fentanyl IV-PCA provides superior analgesia, with less respiratory depressant effect (shallow breathing, respiratory rate <6/min, CO_2 retention), less CNS depressant effect (somnolence, disorientation), less histamine release (tachycardia, hypotension, itchiness), and less PONV than morphine. Fentanyl IV-PCA is administered at a continuous rate of 10 µg/hr in women, with a patient demand bolus of 30 µg and a lockout time of 8 minutes (in patients weighing 150-170 lb) or 6 minutes (in patients weighing 180-250 lb). Men get the same regimen, except the continuous dose is higher (20 µg/hr). All doses should be decreased by 10 µg for less painful surgeries (e.g., laparoscopies, robotics).

IV-PCAs are mainly maintenance regimens. For them to be successful, the patient must already be comfortable (painless) before the IV-PCA is engaged. Sometimes, several narcotic boluses have to be administered to render the patient comfortable before starting the IV-PCA so that the IV-PCA maintains comfort at that level.

Epidural Patient-controlled Analgesia

Compared to any IV-PCA, epidural PCA has the advantage of better analgesia achieved with diminished sedative effect and even less frequent PONV. Epidural PCA uses various combinations of low concentration local anesthetic mixed with a potent narcotic (fentanyl, sufentanil). We use two distinct regimens: for patients <65 years of age we use bupivacaine 1.25% mixed with fentanyl 5 µg/mL (called *BF-5*); for patients >65 years of age we use bupivacaine 0.625% mixed with fentanyl 2 µg/mL (called *BF-2*). Both regimens are used at a continuous rate of 3 to 5 mL/hr, with a patient demand bolus of 2 to 3 mL, and lockout time of 12 to 15 minutes (depending on the patient's height and/or the dermatomal level of the surgery).

The Sleep Apnea Patient

For safe treatment of the clinically documented sleep apnea patient, use a non-narcotic–based epidural PCA (e.g., bupivacaine 0.1% or 0.125%), administered at a continuous rate of 4 to 5 mL/hr, with a patient demand bolus of 2 to 3 mL and lockout time of 12 to 15 minutes. Most sleep apnea patients tolerate a fentanyl IV-PCA after a regular general anesthesia (using IV narcotics); however, these patients must be observed carefully in the PACU for signs of respiratory depressant effect. If that occurs, a non-narcotic–based epidural PCA is substituted.

The Narcotic-addicted Patient

Fentanyl IV-PCA and fentanyl epidural PCA do not provide satisfactory pain management for the narcotic-addicted patient, even in the best circumstances. These patients crave the pleasing effect of μ-receptor stimulation. This effect can be achieved only by using morphine or Dilaudid. We use morphine IV-PCA or Dilaudid IV-PCA only for the narcotic-addicted patient.

TRANSURETHRAL RESECTION SYNDROME

Transurethral resection (TUR) syndrome is an iatrogenically induced severe condition due to absorption of irrigation fluid (glycine). It may occur during various types of surgery, such as transurethral resection of the prostate (TURP),[19,55,56] PCNL,[57,58] TURBT (mostly if perforation occurs),[59,60] hysteroscopic resections (the female TUR syndrome),[61-64] shoulder arthroscopy,[65] and potentially any endoscopic procedure using large volumes of glycine.

Irrigation fluid is used to ensure even current dispersion during electric loop cutting, to prevent hemolysis if absorbed, and to ensure good distention of the urinary bladder with clear optical visibility for the performance of TURP.

Absorption of this fluid creates a host of adverse effects in the cardiovascular system and CNS, which has been known as TUR syndrome since the 1950s. Numerous studies show an overall incidence of TUR syndrome between 0%[66] and over 10%.[64,67-70]

Special Considerations

Pathophysiology

There are two mechanisms of inadvertent absorption of glycine during surgery: direct intravascular absorption and extravasation.

Direct intravascular absorption occurs after the electric cutting loop opens up blood vessels and large venous sinuses, and the pressure of the overhang irrigant exceeds the mean venous pressure of the patient (8-12 mm Hg). The volume absorbed is a direct function of the length of time the intravesical irrigant pressure exceeds 15 mm Hg.[71,72] Once major fluid absorption begins, it tends to continue, and frequently coincides with decreases in the patient's mean arterial BP.[73]

Extravasation occurs after penetration of the prostatic capsule during TURP, the bladder wall during TURBT[59,60] or cystoscopy,[74] or uterine wall in hysteros-

copy with endometrial resection.[75] It also may occur in PCNL.[57,58] The irrigant fluid fills up the retroprostatic intraperitoneal and retroperitoneal spaces and only needs to exceed the usual intraabdominal pressure of 3 to 4 mm Hg for extravasation and absorption to occur.[76]

Risk Factors

The only documented patient-related risk factor for a large scale fluid absorption during TURP is smoking.[77] Length of procedure is a well known intraoperative risk factor for irrigant absorption.[73] PCNL increases the risk and the volume of irrigant absorption.[58,78] Furthermore, capsular penetration by the urologist, along with depth and extent of the procedure, greatly increase the volume of fluid absorbed.[73,79] Hysteroscopies for fibroid resection present a somewhat higher risk of irrigant absorption because the pressures needed to keep the uterine cavity open are greater than those needed in cystoscopy or TURP.[63,64,80-82] In patients with prostates >45 g, the rate of TUR syndrome increases up to 1.5%.[83]

Glycine: The Irrigant Solution

Glycine 1.5%, first introduced in 1940, is the most frequently used irrigant in the United States. With a distribution half-life of 6 minutes and a dose-dependent terminal half-life between 40 minutes to several hours,[84,85] glycine 1.5% tends to accumulate intracellularly.[86] It has a somewhat restricted penetration into the CNS[87] but, nevertheless, it seems to cause serious CNS symptomatology.[88,89]

The plasma concentration of glycine increases 25-fold after the administration of only 1 L of this irrigant. Glycine's plasma concentrations measured in fatal TUR syndrome cases were 21 to 80 mmol/L.[90,91]

Visual disturbances occur at plasma concentrations of 5 to 8 mmol/L; higher plasma concentrations cause transient blindness.[92] Nausea and vomiting occur at plasma concentrations of >10 mmol/L glycine.[70,93]

Glycine is eliminated through the liver, in the form of ammonia. In the case of glycine overhydration, only 10% of the absorbed dose is eliminated unchanged by the kidneys. This promotes an intense osmotic diuresis, increasing the renal elimination of many other nonessential amino acids as well.[93-95]

Clinical Course and Mechanisms of TUR Syndrome

TUR syndrome can appear at various times: as soon as 15 minutes into the surgery, during the recovery period, or even the next day.

Hemodynamics

A transient hypervolemia follows irrigant absorption. BP and central pressures increase but plateau within 15 minutes.[96] Hypervolemia may be followed by a depressed cardiovascular state, characterized by hypovolemia, low

BP, and low cardiac output.[97,98] These symptoms largely are generated by the osmotic diuresis with a secondary natriuresis and intracellular edema. A persistent, deep (down to 60-70 mm Hg) hypotension and bradycardia are frequently the first clinical signs of severe TUR syndrome.[97] This may be followed later by pulmonary edema marked by severe hyposmolar state[99] and hyponatremia (<100 mmol/L).[100] Associated hypothermia[101] and a release of endotoxins[102] might increase the gravity of the situation. Low serum calcium, sodium, and osmolality may present during TUR syndrome.[103-105]

Mini-TUR syndrome, easy to overlook, is characterized by slightly lowered serum sodium (by up to 10 mmol/L),[62,106] nausea, and moderate sudden hypotension.[107,108] Usually, this presents 1 hour postoperatively, during the recovery period.

Cardiac Function

In humans, absorption of massive volumes of irrigant may cause myocardial depression, bradycardia with slowing of the conduction system, and ST-T segment changes (depression).[91,100,109] This is supported by animal studies, where glycine causes subendocardial hypoxic lesions[98,110,111] and various damage to the myocardial hystoskeleton.[112]

Cerebral Function

Global brain swelling followed by acute cerebral herniation may develop postoperatively.[91,103,113] CT scan is a sensitive test for diagnosing brain edema following the absorption of only 1 L of glycine. Interestingly enough, patients may become comatose even with a negative CT scan (no brain edema), and they may progress toward a metabolic type of encephalopathy in the presence[114-116] or the absence[117] of large levels of serum ammonia, a direct byproduct of glycine metabolism.

Hematologic Function

Absorption of large fluid volumes causes metabolic acidosis (pH 7.10-7.25). Metabolic acidosis develops when massive volumes of fluid are absorbed (15 L).[118] Plasma potassium increases 15% to 25%, secondary to massive tissue cellular uptake of the glycine irrigant.[94]

Even moderate decreases in serum sodium cause muscle weakness, twitching, epileptic seizures and shock (<120 mmol/L).[70] Most irrigant solutions are hyposmolar (200 mOsm/kg); therefore, reduction of the serum osmolality will correspond well to the gravity of the symptoms listed.[70]

Renal Function

Moderate amounts of irrigant absorption induce an intense osmotic diuresis that will result in great losses of total body sodium. Larger absorption causes renal swelling with secondary anuria.[110] In cases of massive extravasation, anuria and hypotension coexist due to renal tubular necrosis (hypoxic).[108,119]

Respiratory Function

Respiratory depression is thought to be secondary to brain edema, pulmonary edema, or various cardiovascular causes leading to poor myocardial performance, low flow state, and hypoxia.[99,100,103]

Extravasation

Diffuse abdominal pain, radiating to the shoulder, is a common indicator of extravasation.[73,120] Intense hyponatremia ensues, as the tissues slowly lose sodium to the absorbed fluid. This is followed by hypotension, bradycardia, and hypovolemia.[57,59,73,121] Sometimes the symptoms of extravasation might be delayed up to 24 hours after the surgery, due to the slow development of these changes.[74]

Special Warning About Glycine and Other Irrigants

In spite of its widespread usage, glycine proves to be a poor performer, as documented by a large series of objective studies. Glycine is an inhibitory neurotransmitter, which occasionally causes transient blindness, usually resolving within 24 hours. Glycine absorption and the presence of glycine byproducts (ammonia, glycolic acid, glyoxylic acid, glutamic acid)[114] share a parallel time course with clinical symptoms (confusion).[93,122] In response to glycine absorption, massive amounts of vasopressin are released.[88] In animal studies, general survival rate is poor with glycine 1.5%. Glycine 1.5% irrigant has been implicated in the most severe cases of TUR syndrome, mostly when severe neurologic symptoms occur.[56]

Normal saline solution primarily is used with bipolar thermocoagulation. If massively absorbed, it causes lip numbness, dyspnea, progressive edema of the limbs with generalized swelling, and mental changes. It may produce hyperchloremic acidosis[123] and pulmonary edema.

Sterile water must never be used as an irrigant solution, based on extensive experiments in animals and humans.

Symptoms of Transurethral Resection Syndrome

Knowing and rating the symptoms of TUR syndrome quickly determines the onset and gravity of the complication. Verbal feedback from the patient is just as important as careful monitoring during the TURP, thus most anesthesiologists prefer regional anesthesia (spinal, epidural, or a CSE anesthesia technique), which allows intraoperative communication with the patient.

Early Symptoms

Early symptoms include numbness, pins and needles or burning sensation of the face and neck, restlessness, headache, and transient chest pain. A patient saying "I don't feel good" is slightly more common than nausea and vomiting.[56] Chest pain occurs in 5% of the patients who absorb >1 L of irrigant[114] but becomes a more frequent symptom when the overall blood loss is minimal. Frequently occurring symptoms are bradycardia and hypotension.[56]

Late Symptoms

Late symptoms tend to develop toward the end of surgery or, more commonly, postoperatively: as more irrigant fluid is absorbed, the predominant symptoms are nausea, hypotension, vomiting, and low urinary output, occurring in that order.[107,124]

Other

Severe TUR syndrome is rare, but it has been described. In a review of 29 severe cases of glycine absorption, 92% had neurologic signs, 54% had cardiovascular symptoms, 42% had various visual disturbances, 25% had GI signs, and 21% had renal failure. Of the patients in this review, 25% died.[103]

Depressed mental status appears in 4% to 5% of patients who absorbed >1 L fluid. Visual disturbances are reported by 10% of patients who absorb >500 mL of glycine.

Extravasation frequently presents as hypotension associated with GI disturbances and reduced urinary output.[59] Large volumes of irrigant absorbed (>1-2 L) coincide with spatial confusion,[70] progressing to obtunded consciousness,[113,57] seizures,[89] and coma.[103,116,125]

Prevention and Treatment

Measuring Fluid Absorption

Measuring fluid absorption during TURP is useful in early prevention of TUR syndrome. Volumetric fluid calculation (the difference between in-out fluids) and the use of a tracer substance (ethanol)[72,94,126-129] are reliable methods. Measuring intraoperative increases in BP, decreases in serum sodium or potassium level, decreases in body temperature, or changes in CVP are all unreliable methods.

Surgical Methods

Varying or altering surgical approach to TURP can help prevent TUR syndrome. One of the most important methods is to reduce the surgical resection time; <1 hour resection is deemed optimal.[19,99] Lowering the fluid bag, although it might seem important intuitively, proves to be ineffective.[130,131] Several modern techniques show promise. Powerful lasers produce less bleeding and less irrigant absorption. Bipolar thermocoagulation produces less bleeding and less absorption and, because it uses normal saline, it completely eliminates glycine toxicity.[132]

Anesthesia Methods

The anesthesiologist has a major role in recognizing and treating TUR syndrome. General anesthesia should be used rarely because it eliminates one of the most important early diagnostic tools: communication with the patient. Regional anesthesia (spinal, epidural, or CSE) is preferred for TURP. Despite the fact that it does not reduce irrigant absorption per se, regional anesthesia provides a powerful vasodilation effect through its inherent sympathectomy, which greatly increases the capacity of the vascular bed. Moreover, patients stay awake, and they can voice their very early symptoms (e.g., "I don't feel well," chest pain, shortness of breath, visual problems, and nausea and vomiting). Thus, any gross change in mental status can be assessed early.

For spinal anesthesia, we use meperidine, which provides a convenient surgical analgesia for 1.5 to 2 hours during the procedure and an 8- to 12-hour postoperative analgesia, enables clear postoperative mental status, and has a very high patient satisfaction. We also use prophylactic ephedrine (IV and IM) to maintain steady BP throughout the entire surgery. This obviates the need for heavy hydration (diminishing patient's overall fluid load). This inexpensive low-tech method ensures predictably good results in all patients, especially old and ASA III-IV patients. See "Further Prevention of Regional Anesthesia Complications," earlier. However, the reduced hydration method does not prevent the occurrence of TUR syndrome due to glycine absorption. Only complete elimination of glycine as an irrigant will achieve that.

Epidural anesthesia is used primarily when difficulty with spinal anesthesia occurs, or when it is thought that prolonged postoperative analgesia will be required after the TURP. CSE anesthesia has its own advantages. When long procedures are envisioned, the combination of meperidine spinal with epidural backup will provide great surgical anesthesia and prolonged postoperative analgesia.

Myth and Reality

A variety of popular myths about TUR syndrome are not supported by objective clinical data:

Myth 1: TUR syndrome always appears early during the TURP procedure. In reality, TUR syndromes start at the end and mostly hours after the end of the procedure. Rarely does a massive syndrome develop during surgery of <1 hour. Severe symptoms develop several hours after TURP. In cases of massive extravasation, symptoms develop slowly over the next 24 hours; therefore, constant, prolonged vigilance is important.

Myth 2: Hyponatremia is an early symptom of TUR syndrome, heavily relied upon for early diagnosis. In reality, severe hyponatremia occurs as a very late symptom, mostly secondary to a delayed osmotic diuresis following glycine absorption. Severe hyponatremia is implicated in the most severe manifestations of the

TUR syndrome: seizures, cardiomyopathy, skeletal myopathy. Mild hyponatremia is incidental to the mini-TUR syndrome—overhydration, obtunded CNS, confusion, twitching, hypertension—and usually appears 1 hour after surgery.

Myth 3: Glycine is a relatively safe irrigant, comparable to mannitol-sorbitol or normal saline. In reality, glycine 1.5% proves to be worse than any other irrigant, as supported in the majority of animal and human studies. It has been implicated in most fatal cases of TUR syndrome.

Myth 4: Monopolar loop surgery is comparable to lasers or bipolar thermocoagulation. In reality, monopolar loop surgery provides fast, deep, and efficient cutting, but it is known to leave bleeders in its wake and has been implicated in most of the severe TUR syndromes to date.

Myth 5: General anesthesia is acceptable for TURP in old and sick patients. In reality, regional anesthesia with an awake or lightly sedated patient is the safest way to operate. Direct observation of the patient's sensorium alerts the team to early symptoms of TUR syndrome. General anesthesia is used only when there are absolute contraindications to regional anesthesia.

Myth 6: A small, short TURP is safe under general anesthesia. In reality, all TURPs are big invasive procedures, however short (small gland) they might appear at the outset. Regional anesthetic, along with adequate monitoring of the patient's sensorium and cardiovascular status, should be used whenever possible.

Myth 7: IV hypertonic saline is dangerous to use in treatment of TUR syndrome. In reality, fear of rapid sodium replenishment, causing an acute demyelinating syndrome (pontine myelinolysis), placed hypertonic saline on the "do not use" list in many institutions. However, in severe cases of hyponatremia (<120 mmol/L), the patient's sodium level should be brought up to 120 mmol/L using hypertonic saline. After that, slow replacement over several days should be done with normal saline. In mild cases, simple replacement with normal saline is adequate. Hypertonic saline is not known to induce pulmonary edema.[133] If judiciously used (1 mmol/L/hr),[134] it will diminish cellular swelling, reduce brain edema, increase diuresis, and expand plasma volume, thus improving BP, tissue oxygenation, and glomerular filtration rate (GFR). In very severe cases (<100-120 mmol/L), a delay in sodium administration will lead to permanent neurologic damage or death.[70,134]

Myth 8: Furosemide (Lasix) is important in therapy for all forms of TUR syndrome. In reality, Lasix is important only in early treatment of the mini-TUR syndrome in order to facilitate the quick removal of excess irrigant. Later on, sodium replacement becomes more important because by then the patient will intensely diurese due to the osmotic load of glycine. Lasix should be used only in the oliguric patient, after hypertonic saline has been used and the patient is hemodynamically stable, or in patients with acute pulmonary edema.

Myth 9: Fluid restriction must be used early in the treatment of TUR syndrome. In reality, fluid restriction might work initially on a small scale, if mini-TUR syndrome occurs. However, in a patient with severe hypovolemia and compromised hemodynamics (low BP, low cardiac output), intravascular volume should be restored under the guidance of heavy cardiovascular monitoring (CVP, Swan-Ganz catheter, cardiac output measurements). Hypertonic saline should be slowly administered (raising sodium to 120 mmol/L).[134] Vasopressors, chronotropes, inotropes, and calcium should be used, if necessary, to support the cardiovascular system. Patients should be closely followed for several days in an intensive care unit setting.

Myth 10: One can never perform TURP on the anticoagulated or coagulopathic patient. In reality, recent surgical technologies for TURP, such as high powered laser surgery and bipolar thermocoagulation, provide easier hemostasis. Relatively good results have been obtained without excessive bleeding or death in patients on continued warfarin (Coumadin) and even heparin use.[135-142]

UROLOGIC LAPAROSCOPY

Today, a wide array of urologic surgeries are performed laparoscopically or via robotic-assisted laparoscopy. Similar anesthesia considerations and techniques apply to most of these procedures.

Pathophysiologic Effects of Laparoscopy Under General Anesthesia

Several processes constantly interplay during laparoscopy: the pressure effect of the insufflated CO_2, a neurohormonal effect, a cardiovascular effect, absorption of the CO_2, positioning of the patient, and other systemic effects.

Mechanical Effects of Carbon Dioxide Insufflation

Increasing intraabdominal pressure (IAP) with CO_2 insufflation compresses the venous system in the abdomen and causes a transient increase in venous return, followed by a drop in cardiac preload. The result is a drop in cardiac output up to 48%.[143] There is also a clinically significant reduction in functional residual capacity (FRC) of the lungs. Remarkably, in an animal model of CO_2 insufflation, a pressure of 12 mm Hg exerted a minimal effect on hemodynamic function.[144] This has useful potential implications for the laparoscopic surgeon.

Neurohormonal Effects

Increase in IAP and hypercapnia cause a release of vasopressin and catecholamines. The renin-angiotensin-aldosterone axis becomes activated. A parallel time course profile between these changes and the changes in BP, systemic vascular resistance (SVR), and cardiac index (CI) suggests a cause-effect relationship.[145]

Cardiovascular Effects

Alterations in cardiovascular performance are well described in the literature. The interaction of several factors, including neurohormonal release,[145] intravascular volume,[146] cardiorespiratory status,[147] and positioning[148] affect cardiovascular changes during pneumoperitoneum.

Hemodynamic changes occur in phases. A study by Joris and associates[149] using CI measurements is very evocative of the serial changes that occur. Induction of anesthesia in Trendelenburg position and then placing the patient into a steep reverse Trendelenburg (rT) position greatly decreases CI (35% to 40%). With CO_2 insufflation, CI further drops to 50% of preoperative awake values. The filling pressures of the heart (CVP, pulmonary capillary wedge pressure) also are reduced by induction of anesthesia and rT positioning; they tend to recover soon after the CO_2 insufflation starts. SVR increases markedly at the beginning of insufflation, to recover later (within 10-15 minutes) during establishment of the pneumoperitoneum. The mean arterial BP increases during insufflation and stays high, even as CI recovers to previous values. The recovery of CI and decrease in SVR occur simultaneously.[149]

In patients with mild heart disease, or in ASA III or ASA IV patients with severe systemic disease, the direction of changes in CI, SVR, and mean arterial BP is the same as in healthy patients, except that the initial decrease in CI and increase in SVR are more pronounced. Also, there is a significant increase in oxygen demand, as expressed by great increases in left ventricular stroke work index.[150-152] Interestingly, if CO_2 insufflation is done in the supine position, there is a lesser initial decline in CI.

All these changes revert to normal upon release of the CO_2.

Temperature Effects

Body core temperature drops significantly during surgery with continuous CO_2 insufflation.[147] This change is more pronounced in older patients and may continue, despite patient warming, throughout the procedure.

Respiratory Effects: Mechanical

Changes in pulmonary function during CO_2 insufflation include reduction in lung volumes, decrease in pulmonary compliance, increase in peak airway pressures, and reduction in FRC.[153-155] Insufflation of CO_2 at 15 mm Hg lowers an already decreased FRC (due to induction of general anesthesia and positioning), exacerbating the ventilation/perfusion ($\dot{V}/\dot{Q}$) mismatch.[156] Hypoxia may be the result. Positive pressure ventilation will recover some of the FRC, reducing the chance for hypoxia.[157] The greatest reduction in FRC is seen in obese patients, thus creating a significant $\dot{V}/\dot{Q}$ mismatch during pneumoperitoneum.[158] The existence of intrapulmonary shunting in COPD patients places them at extra risk of hypoxia during laparoscopic surgery.

Respiratory Effects: Carbon Dioxide Absorption

CO_2 is used in laparoscopy because it is not flammable (permitting the use of electrocautery), is highly diffusible, and can be eliminated rapidly through the lungs by slight increases in minute ventilation, which comes in handy when accidental gas embolism occurs. CO_2 absorption is greater during extraperitoneal than during intraperitoneal procedures.[159,160]

Elimination of CO_2 is biphasic; early rapid elimination occurs at the beginning of insufflation and is followed by a slower elimination later on. This biphasic mode is maintained at lower as well as at higher inflating pressures.[159] Intentional hypercarbia increases plasma catecholamines and cardiac output, and it decreases SVR directly through the vasodilating effect of CO_2 and indirectly by stimulating the sympathetic nervous system. N_2O administered during CO_2 insufflation tends to exaggerate the cardiovascular depressive effects of CO_2.

Elimination of CO_2 is not problematic in healthy patients, but in sicker ASA III or ASA IV patients, the minute ventilation requirements and peak airway pressures are higher during laparoscopy.[161] In some ASA III and ASA IV patients, ETCO2 may not be a true reflection of their arterial partial pressure of CO_2 (PaCO2). In these patients, refractory hypercapnia might occur during laparoscopy. Preoperatively, a pulmonary function test showing diffusion defects <80% of predicted and FEV_1 <70% of predicted identify patients at risk.[5]

Specific Circulatory Changes

Regional blood flow changes during laparoscopy have been carefully studied. These circulatory effects alter organ perfusion in specific ways, and pose problems when operating on ASA III and IV patients.

Cerebral Blood Flow Cerebral blood flow and intracranial pressure (ICP) increase significantly during CO_2 insufflation, regardless of the level of PaCO2.[162] There is a linear increase in ICP with increasing IAP. The Trendelenburg position further increases ICP to 150% of initial.[163]

Splanchnic Blood Flow Changes in splanchnic blood flow are mediated through a direct increase in IAP and through mesenteric vasculature compression.[164] The effect of low IAP (7 mm Hg) on splanchnic perfusion is negligible. Higher IAP (14 mm Hg) decreases portal and hepatic blood flow and decreases intestinal mucosal pH.[165]

Increased IAP through CO_2 insufflation stimulates the release of antidiuretic hormone (ADH), with subsequent vasoconstriction of the splanchnic bed. Splanchnic ischemia is a serious risk factor for sepsis and multi-organ system failure, which can outlast CO_2 deflation by as much as 18 hours.[166]

Hepatic Blood Flow Hepatoportal blood flow varies in direct proportion to changes in IAP. At low IAP (7 mm Hg), the portal blood flow is reduced 37%. At higher IAP (14 mm Hg), portal blood flow is reduced 53%.[167] The reverse Trendelenburg position significantly reduces the hepatoportal flow.[168]

Renal Blood Flow CO_2 insufflation reduces flows in the renal cortex and medulla. There is a transient reduction in GFR, creatinine clearance, and urinary output.[169,170] Urine output and creatinine clearance tend to decrease at higher IAP (14-15 mm Hg). Any method that diminishes IAP, such as retraction[171] or abdominal wall lifting,[172] promotes stable renal hemodynamics during laparoscopy. Humoral factors such as renin[173] and ADH are released by increased IAP and cause vasoconstriction with decreased urine output and urea excretion (GFR unchanged).[174]

Pathophysiologic Effects of Laparoscopy in Awake Patients (Under Regional or Local Anesthesia)

Respiratory Changes

The previously described respiratory changes in patients under general anesthesia are less evident in patients under regional anesthesia. In a study of a small series of awake patients done under epidural anesthesia, no significant changes of the respiratory parameters were observed in Trendelenburg position. By contrast, on insufflation, expired volume per unit time ($\dot{V}E$) increased significantly (from 9.1 to 11.8 L/min), and respiratory rate increased (from 16.9 to 23.1 breaths/min) while venous CO_2 remained unchanged along with $PaCO_2$.[175] Under epidural anesthesia, respiratory mechanisms remain intact; patients can adjust their minute ventilation during CO_2 insufflation in order to normalize their ETCO_2. These results suggest that epidural anesthesia may be a safe alternative to general anesthesia because it is not associated with ventilatory depression.

Cardiovascular Changes

Hemodynamic changes during regional anesthesia are different from general anesthesia. The Trendelenburg position and CO_2 insufflation have little effect on heart rate and mean arterial pressure.[175] However, they affect the sensory level of the hyperbaric spinal anesthesia, which ends up significantly higher than expected, thus magnifying the normal cardiovascular impact of the spinal block (sympathectomy leading to low mean arterial pressure). To counteract this, smaller doses (minidoses) of local anesthetic in combination with potentiating narcotic minidoses are recommended.[176]

Operative Management

Patient Monitoring

It is well accepted practice to use general monitoring such as electrocardiogram, SaO_2, ETCO_2, BP, and temperature during laparoscopy in healthy and slightly obese patients.[177] There might be larger differences between ETCO_2 and $PaCO_2$ in patients with serious pulmonary disease or the morbidly obese; therefore, an arterial line is advisable for serial blood sampling, for SaO_2 determinations, and for tighter BP monitoring. Unchecked increases in CO_2 might cause arousal in patients under general anesthesia because of the intense catecholamine release secondary to hypercarbia. The use of a BIS monitor helps with anesthesia depth assessment.[178]

General Anesthesia

The majority of urologic laparoscopies, both diagnostic and therapeutic, are done under general anesthesia in the United States. Propofol TIVA is also a good choice, with specific benefits for patients with a past history of PONV. See "Propofol Total Intravenous Anesthesia for Postoperative Nausea and Vomiting," earlier.

Choice of Airway Endotracheal intubation is used for most patients. This ensures an airway protected against gastroesophageal reflux and enables the anesthesiologist to effectively change the mechanical ventilation (minute ventilation) in response to the increases in ETCO_2 during insufflation.

LMA also has been used extensively in laparoscopic surgeries.[179] The fear of inadvertent gastroesophageal reflux has not been substantiated in studies done with clinical monitoring[179] and continuous esophageal pH monitoring.[180] General anesthesia can be performed safely using a correctly placed LMA Supreme (LMA North America, San Diego, California).

During pneumoperitoneum, satisfactory ETCO_2 (34-35 mm Hg) is obtained by only a 15% to 25% increase in minute ventilation. In patients with COPD, it is safer to increase the respiratory rate rather than the tidal volume because of the risk of tension pneumothorax caused by the rupture of alveolar bullae.[181,182]

When the patient is breathing spontaneously through an LMA or a mask under regional block, if inappropriately high levels of ETCO_2 are reached or are difficult to prevent (as in patients who are morbidly obese or who have severe pulmonary disease), the surgery should be stopped, the abdomen deflated, and the patient intubated for the conclusion of the surgery. High ASA status (III or IV) coupled with preoperative low vital capacity volumes and low forced expiratory volumes are good predictors of intraoperative hypercapnia and acidosis in laparoscopic procedures.[5]

Nitrous Oxide N_2O is the second most diffusible gas in the body after CO_2. In conjunction with insufflated CO_2, N_2O readily overdistends most closed cavities such as the bowel, colon, and bladder and increases the resident gas volumes by 100% to 200%. N_2O exaggerates the deleterious cardiovascular effects of CO_2. It also is associated with increased rates (30%) of PONV. Because of these negative characteristics, N_2O must never be used in conjunction with laparoscopic surgery.

Regional Anesthesia

Regional anesthesia (spinal, epidural, or combined spinal/epidural) is used in laparoscopic surgery as an alternative anesthesia choice in patients with severe cardiopulmonary disorders, which contraindicate general anesthesia. Other advantages of regional anesthesia include decreased or lack of postoperative pain, decreased PONV, more rapid recovery with shorter PACU stay, fewer hemodynamic changes,[182] fewer respiratory changes,[183] and the availability of an epidural catheter for postoperative analgesia.[184] A disadvantage of regional anesthesia for laparoscopy is that it often requires the surgeon to work with a lower IAP (9-12 mm Hg). Additional disadvantages include the requirement of a cooperative patient and gentler surgical technique. Oversedation can cause hypoxia.[185]

Epidural Anesthesia Epidural anesthesia is considered safe and practical in short procedures and in outpatient laparoscopic surgery. It does not inhibit respiratory function, thus patients can increase their minute ventilation easily to compensate for the increase in $PaCO_2$ and $ETCO_2$ remains unchanged.[175] The epidural technique has been used successfully for patients with advanced COPD.[175,183,184] Epidural anesthesia also has been used successfully in gasless laparoscopic procedures, providing cardiovascular and respiratory safety similar to general anesthesia.[186]

Spinal Anesthesia In this age of short outpatient laparoscopic surgery, spinal anesthesia is used increasingly to provide fast onset, deep, and reliable blocks with easily controllable length of action. The classic hyperbaric spinal technique should be replaced by minidose spinals because of the propensity for cephalad spread of the sensory level during the increased IAP and Trendelenburg position.[176,187] Ideally, minidoses of local anesthetic, potentiated by the addition of minidoses of narcotics, are used.[188] Even more effectively, minidoses of meperidine (30-40 mg) also provide long-lasting postoperative pain relief.

Local Anesthesia However controversial, local anesthesia is used for ultra-short diagnostic laparoscopies and is adequate for special microlaparoscopic procedures done in non-obese patients.[182,189-194] In all these cases, preemptive port site local anesthetic infiltration greatly diminishes postoperative pain.

Peripheral Nerve Blocks Several nerve block techniques have been described in conjunction with laparoscopic surgery, including rectus sheath block,[195] inguinal block,[195] and paravertebral block.[196] These blocks prove to be useful adjuncts to general anesthesia or TIVA, and they provide effective postoperative pain relief in various types of laparoscopic surgery. They result in reduced PONV and increased patient satisfaction.

Intraoperative Complications

A variety of surgical complications can occur that affect anesthesia management for laparoscopic procedures. Major vascular injuries may appear from the moment the trocar is inserted[197-199]; therefore, large bore IV lines need to be inserted at the beginning of each case and the patient crossmatched for blood preoperatively.

Subcutaneous Emphysema

Following CO_2 insufflation, an inadvertent SC emphysema might occur, with a reported incidence of 0.4% to 2%.[200,201] It may be limited to the abdominal wall, or it may dissect all the way around the chest wall, neck, head, and thighs, creating a lot of easily palpable SC crepitus. On some occasions, increased $ETCO_2$ and respiratory acidosis have been described.[202] Careful deep insertion of the needle, maintaining the inflating pressures at <15 mm Hg, and visualization of the intraperitoneal position prevent this complication.[203]

Pneumopericardium, Pneumomediastinum, and Pneumothorax

Complex rare cases of pneumothorax associated with pneumopericardium, pneumomediastinum, and periocular emphysema have been described. High inflating pressures probably contribute to the occurrence of these complications.[204,205] Signs of cardiac tamponade may occur, including arrhythmias, muffled heart sounds, jugular vein distention (JVD), drop in BP and cardiac output, and superior vena cava syndrome, which manifests as a "blue cape" cyanosis and swelling of the head and neck (due to the impingement upon the venous return to the right heart). Decreasing the inflating pressures to <15 mm Hg or completely releasing the CO_2 from the abdominal cavity is sufficient to halt and reverse these complications.[206]

Pneumothorax leading to tension pneumothorax, a rare but potentially life-threatening complication, has been described in both intraperitoneal[207] and extraperitoneal[208] laparoscopy. CO_2 can enter the thoracic cavity through the natural esophageal or aortic hiatus, or it might dissect through a congenitally open pleuroperitoneal hiatus.[209,210] A sudden large accumulation of CO_2 in the pleural cavity or an accidental rupture of lung bullae may cause tension pneumothorax. Sudden increase in airway pressure, drop in BP, hypoxia-hypercapnia, cardiovascular collapse, and silent lung alert of such a complication. An immediate chest radiograph is diagnostic. In emergencies, when cardiovascular collapse is imminent, the best method is to stop surgery and immediately deflate the abdomen. Careful manual ventilation soon promotes CO_2 reabsorption, re-expands the affected lung, and restores normal cardiovascular function. In extreme cases, an emergency thoracocentesis releases the CO_2, allowing manual re-expansion of the lung. Maintaining inflating pressures at <15 mm Hg might prevent such occurrences.

Carbon Dioxide Gas Embolism

CO_2 gas embolism during laparoscopic surgery can be non-fatal[211] or fatal.[212] Gas embolism can occur following accidental puncture of veins or a very vascular organ (e.g., liver). Hypoxia, arrhythmias, cyanosis, precordial "mill wheel" murmur, and sudden drop in $ETCO_2$ and $PaCO_2$ (due to the reduction in pulmonary venous return) may be followed by cardiovascular collapse. Gas embolism may occur at any time during CO_2 insufflation. In the presence of a patent right to left communication (e.g., patent atrial septal defect, patent foramen ovale), coronary and cerebral CO_2 embolism may result.[213]

Subclinical forms of CO_2 embolism occur somewhat frequently and may be detected using transesophageal echocardiography (TEE).[214]

Careful surgery done by an experienced surgeon, a high suspicion index by the anesthesiologist, the use of a precordial stethoscope, a large bore central line, and TEE used in high-risk patients with advanced multisystem disease help in early detection and treatment of gas embolism.

Advantage of Low Pressure and Normobaric Gasless Laparoscopy

An alternative to high pressure (13-15 mm Hg) laparoscopy, the low pressure technique (9-12 mm Hg) has been used successfully in various surgeries. It is a good choice in difficult sick patients with advanced cardiopulmonary disease and in patients who are pregnant. An abdominal lift device was described and used in the early 1990s.[215] This method, however difficult to use, creates a very low IAP of 1 to 4 mm Hg through insufflation of only 2 to 5 L of CO_2. Very minimal respiratory and cardiovascular changes occur, rendering the procedure safer in patients with multisystem disease.[216] A second generation of anterior abdominal retractor (described in 1993) is a totally gasless method, which creates enough space, through a 15-cm elevation of the abdominal wall, to perform surgery with minimal disturbance to the cardiopulmonary or urinary systems.[217,218]

KEY POINTS

1. Urologic diagnostic and therapeutic procedures can often induce SSIs, UTIs, and sepsis; most procedures need to be covered with prophylactic antibiotics. If there is an active infection or any infectious source (e.g., Foley catheter) preoperatively, it should be diagnosed (urinalysis, C&S) and specifically treated before surgery. Choice of antibiotics is hospital-specific and the most active antibiotics reserved for therapy.

2. The ASA classification system is a useful tool for perioperative risk stratification in conjunction with a specific surgery. Choice of anesthesia must be tailored to the specific patient (e.g., age, comorbidities), the specific procedure (e.g., potential complications, surgical site, length and difficulty of surgery, patient positioning), and the skills of both the anesthesiologist and the surgeon. Deciding which anesthesia technique to use is a complex byproduct of thorough preoperative assessment and good communication between anesthesiologist and urologist.

3. Adverse pulmonary events are the cause of most anesthetic complications under general anesthesia. Inadequate ventilation, esophageal intubation, and difficult tracheal intubation are responsible for most of these injuries. Less common but equally important mechanisms of adverse respiratory-related events include airway obstruction, bronchospasm, aspiration, airway trauma, and pneumothorax. Proper airway management is essential in order to avoid most of these complications.

4. In the right hands, when there are no contraindications, regional anesthesia (spinal, epidural, CSE) is a good choice for most urologic surgeries. It ensures good surgical analgesia; fast, alert, comfortable recovery; and excellent postoperative pain relief (8-12 hours) when meperidine spinal anesthesia is used.

5. Complications of regional anesthesia include hypotension, PDPH, CES/TNS, total spinal through inadvertent subarachnoid injection, and systemic local anesthetic toxicity through inadvertent intravascular injection. Although these complications are rare, awareness of them must be maintained and proper patient monitoring and safeguards used.

6. Two of the most common debilitating conditions in the recovery room are pain and PONV, and both conditions are largely preventable. The use of regional anesthesia, nerve blocks, and meperidine spinal anesthesia can prevent or minimize pain while providing stress-free anesthesia. PONV largely can be prevented by avoiding inhalational anesthetics, N_2O, and unnecessary intraoperative sedatives. Using antiemetics early, along with propofol TIVA, further reduces the incidence and severity of PONV.

7. Pudendal and penile nerve blocks are minimally invasive and easy to perform. They are good primary or adjuvant methods for surgical analgesia and postoperative pain relief. These blocks are especially safe and useful in the old and sick ASA III/IV patients because these blocks eliminate the risks and complications caused by general and regional anesthesia while providing a stressless operative and postoperative course (pain-free, no PONV, clear postoperative mentation).

8. The urologist and anesthesiologist must discuss and plan postoperative pain management before surgery. The ideal anesthesia technique simultaneously provides adequate stress-free anesthesia for the urologic procedure and prolonged postoperative pain relief in the PACU. Currently, this ideal is best accomplished through the judicious use of nerve blocks and meperidine spinal anesthesia in association with propofol TIVA.

9. TUR syndrome is a complex dangerous condition that may occur in any type of surgery using glycine as irrigant solution. TUR syndrome may occur during surgery, but most develop postoperatively, especially the severe forms. The most important risk factors are surgery >1 hour and use of glycine.

10. A wide array of urology cases are being performed laparoscopically. Intimate knowledge of CO_2 insufflation pathophysiology is essential. Intraoperative complications such as SC emphysema, pneumopericardium, pneumomediastinum, pneumothorax, and CO_2 gas embolism must be understood, anticipated, and avoided. Although general anesthesia is used for most laparoscopies, regional anesthesia is feasible and greatly underutilized in the United States.

REFERENCES

Please see www.expertconsult.com

Section II

COMPLICATIONS OF MEDICAL THERAPIES

Chapter 7

PHARMACOLOGIC COMPLICATIONS

Tasha Cooke MBBS, DM(Urol)
Urologist, The Cornwall Regional Hospital, St. James, Jamaica

Alan M. Nieder MD
Associate Professor, Division of Urology, Columbia University, Mount Sinai Medical Center, Miami Beach, Florida

The objective of this chapter is to review drug reactions that are likely to be encountered by the practicing urologist. Urinary retention, impotence, infertility, hematuria, and priapism are genitourinary adverse effects of drugs prescribed by all physicians. Drugs that cause these specific genitourinary disorders are presented. This chapter also highlights the adverse drug reactions of pharmacologic agents commonly prescribed for urologic diseases. We have limited our review to drugs used to treat benign prostatic hyperplasia (BPH), prostate cancer, erectile dysfunction, overactive bladder (OAB), renal calculi, and metastatic renal cell carcinoma.

UROLOGIC COMPLICATIONS OF DRUG THERAPY

Infertility

Many pharmacologic agents have been found to decrease male fertility. Some inherent difficulties in evaluating fertility are that many patients do not take these medications their entire life, they take them at an early age, and they may never attempt to father children. Furthermore, the standard in defining fertility is obviously the fathering of children. Many of the reports and reviews that implicate specific agents in the inhibition or damage of spermatogenesis are based on either experimental animal models or isolated case reports. Although the effects of drugs on male fertility can be evaluated by experimental models, the data are not 100% extrapolatable. Moreover, for many patients with infertility that is suspected to be caused by pharmaceutical preparations, pretreatment fertility parameters are frequently unknown; these patients may have neither fathered children nor been given a semen analysis. Although studies have demonstrated the relative reliability of semen analyses in assessing fertility, the results again are not perfect markers for the ultimate product: conception of a child.[1] Therefore, demonstrating a precise cause-and-effect relationship among infertile patients who have taken various medications is extremely difficult, if not impossible.

Antibiotics are a large class of medications that have been shown clinically and experimentally to affect male fertility adversely. Schlegel and colleagues[2] published a comprehensive review of antibiotics that had previously been found to decrease fertility in both animal and human studies. The antibiotics listed included nitrofurans, macrolides (erythromycins), aminoglycosides, tetracyclines, sulfa drugs, and penicillins. The mechanisms by which these drugs negatively influence fertility are often multiple and affect more than one aspect of spermatogenesis. Timmermans[3] investigated the effects of antibiotics on rat spermatogenesis. He found that gentamicin, nitrofurantoin, penicillin, and other drugs altered germ cell mitotic and meiotic divisions so that metaphase never occurred. Furthermore, testis biopsies from men receiving gentamicin before prostate surgery were found to also show an arrest of spermatogenesis with an increased number of primary spermatocytes.

Sulfasalazine, a drug widely prescribed for the treatment of inflammatory bowel disease, has been associated with decreased male fertility. The mechanism is not clear; however, the effects have been noted to be reversible.[4] In one report, four patients taking sulfasalazine had oligospermia and infertility. Findings on semen analyses rapidly improved in all patients when the medication was withdrawn, and the partners of three of the four patients became pregnant. Furthermore, restarting sulfasalazine treatment resulted in findings of rapid deterioration on semen analyses in two of the men.[5] Mesalazine, an analogue of sulfasalazine also used for the treatment of inflammatory bowel disease, has not been found to alter spermatogenesis as significantly. After substituting mesalazine for sulfasalazine in nine patients, improvements in sperm count, motility, and morphology were noted in all patients.[6]

Cimetidine, a histamine receptor type II (H₂) antagonist and an extremely popular antiulcer medication, has been shown to interfere with endocrine function and the binding of androgens to their receptors. In a study of seven men, investigators noted a 43% reduction in sperm count following cimetidine administration. Furthermore, a statistically significant decrease in the level of luteinizing hormone (LH) response to LH-releasing factor occurred.[7] Because of cimetidine's antiandrogenic properties, the drug has also been implicated as a cause of erectile dysfunction.[8]

Chemotherapeutic agents that have had great success in treating both urologic and nonurologic malignant diseases also have a toxic effect on testicular function and male fertility. The question of long-term fertility in patients with cancer is significant, especially for those patients treated as children and young adults in whom the potential for parenthood may be lost forever unless pretreatment semen preservation is undertaken. Testis cancer is a malignant disease in which the treatment and the disease directly affect fertility. Because this is a disease of younger men, many patients have not yet fathered children at the time of diagnosis or treatment. Importantly, many studies have demonstrated a primary abnormality in spermatogenesis in men with testicular tumors before any chemotherapeutic treatments are administered.[9,10]

Some patients definitely demonstrate long-term semen abnormalities following treatment for testis tumors. In a study by Stephenson and colleagues,[11] who evaluated the reproductive capacity of 30 patients with germ cell tumors following treatment with cisplatin, etoposide, and bleomycin, significant decreases were observed in semen analyses. Of the 30 patients, 13 (43%) developed oligospermia, and only a single patient had >50% normal spermatozoa. Nevertheless, 8 of these 30 patients eventually fathered children. Different chemotherapeutic agents affect the testis with different degrees of severity; nitrogen mustard, vincristine, prednisolone, mechlorethamine, cyclophosphamide, chlorambucil, and procarbazine produce severe effects on testis function. Investigators have reported that <20% of the patients receiving these drugs will ever recover spermatogenesis.[12] Doxorubicin has also been shown to affect fertility. Drasga and coworkers reported that of 25 patients who had received chemotherapy for testis tumors, the 8 (32%) whose partners had successful pregnancies had not received doxorubicin.[10]

Reports in the literature on whether normal spermatogenesis returns following the administration of chemotherapeutic agents have been conflicting. Buchanan and colleagues[13] demonstrated that the recovery of testicular function was not significantly dependent on the interval of treatment or the total dose of cyclophosphamide received. These investigators found that a return of spermatogenesis occurred in 38% of patients within 15 to 49 months after completing treatment. However, other investigators found that total chemotherapeutic dose does determine whether fertility will be adversely affected. Richter and coworkers[14] observed that the degree of testicular damage in men with lymphoma was related to the total dose of chlorambucil administered. As the dose of chlorambucil approached 400 mg, severe oligospermia occurred. Testis biopsies in these men demonstrated only Sertoli cells and peritubular fibrosis. Another group of investigators similarly found that irreversible damage to fertility is likely to occur at cumulative doses of cisplatin >400 mg/m^2.[15]

Finally, immunosuppressive agents have been found to decrease androgen levels. Rajfer and colleagues[16] measured testosterone and LH levels in male rats after oral administration of cyclosporine. These investigators found a statistically significant decrease in testosterone and LH levels, a finding suggesting that cyclosporine has an inhibitory effect on the hypothalamic-pituitary axis.

Hematuria

Both microscopic hematuria and gross hematuria should typically warrant quick referrals to the urologist. A complete drug history is a critical component of the urologic workup because many common prescription and nonprescription medications can cause hematuria. Hemostasis is maintained by both platelets and the coagulation factors that ultimately produce thrombin and fibrin. Aspirin directly affects platelet function and prolongs the bleeding time. This effect is the result of the irreversible acetylation of platelet cyclooxygenase and the consequent reduced formation of thromboxane A_2, an inducer of platelet aggregation and a potent vasoconstrictor. Because platelets lack nuclei and cannot synthesize new proteins, the action of aspirin on platelet cyclooxygenase is permanent and lasts the life of the platelet (7-10 days).[17] A single dose of 650 mg of aspirin (two tablets) approximately doubles the mean bleeding time for a period of 4 to 7 days.

Hematuria may also result from the administration of nonsteroidal anti-inflammatory drugs (NSAIDs) other than aspirin; these NSAIDs similarly prolong bleeding time by inhibiting platelet cyclooxygenase. Unlike with aspirin, however, the effect is reversible and thus shorter lasting. Kraus and colleagues[18] reported that >50% of those patients with idiopathic hematuria after a negative urologic workup had been receiving either aspirin or other NSAIDs. Thienopyridine derivatives (ticlopidine and clopidogrel) have been used as effective antiplatelet agents for years. Clopidogrel blocks the activation of platelets by adenosine phosphate by selectively and irreversibly inhibiting the binding of this agonist to its receptor on platelets. The drug thereby affects the adenosine diphosphate–dependent activation of the glycoprotein IIb/IIIa (GpIIb/IIIa) complex, the major receptor for fibrinogen present on the platelet surface. In a review of randomized clinical trials of low-dose aspirin (75-325 mg/day) or clopidogrel administered for cardiovascular prophylaxis, low-dose aspirin increased the risk of major bleeding by 70%, but the absolute increase was modest. Compared with clopidogrel, aspirin increases the risk of gastrointestinal bleeding but not other bleeding.[19]

In one study, a cause for microscopic and gross hematuria was not identified in 24 of 116 (21%) patients undergoing complete urologic workups.[18] However, 54% of these patients with so-called idiopathic hematuria were receiving either aspirin or other NSAIDs on a regular basis. Other agents commonly used for anticoagulation include warfarin and heparin, both of which affect specific coagulation factors. Bleeding following heparin therapy tends to be dose related; however, other factors increase the incidence of bleeding, such as female gender, severe illness, and concurrent treatment with aspirin.[20] Some studies have demonstrated that patients >70 years of age had a four-fold increased risk of bleeding compared with patients <50 years of age.[21] In a pilot study addressing the safety of combination low-dose aspirin and warfarin therapy, microscopic hematuria was the most common (20%) adverse effect; however, it was unrelated to the international normalized ratio (INR).[22]

Hematuria should always be addressed with a thorough workup, whether or not the patient has received anticoagulants. In a small series of patients, 82% of those with hematuria during anticoagulant therapy were subsequently found to have urologic disease such as urethral strictures, calculi, and carcinoma of the prostate and bladder.[23] In a similar retrospective review, significant urologic findings were found in 59% consecutive patients in whom gross or microscopic hematuria developed while they were receiving heparin or warfarin anticoagulation therapy.[24] The explanation for the increased risk of hematuria in association with anticoagulation is that neoplastic and inflammatory tissues are more prone to bleed than is normal tissue.

Urinary Retention

The activity of the lower urinary tract is precisely controlled by the autonomic nervous system. The autonomic nervous system has two discrete components: the sympathetic nervous system (originating in the thoracolumbar nerves) and the parasympathetic nervous system (originating in the sacral nerves). The postganglionic sympathetic receptors are adrenergic, responding to norepinephrine, whereas the postganglionic parasympathetic receptors are muscarinic, responding to acetylcholine. *Micturition* involves the simultaneous coordinated contraction of the bladder detrusor muscle, which is controlled by parasympathetic (cholinergic) nerves, and the relaxation of the bladder neck and sphincter, which are controlled by sympathetic (α-adrenergic) nerves. Theoretically, urinary retention

should be precipitated by inhibiting muscarinic receptors and stimulating β-adrenergic receptors in the bladder (inhibition of detrusor contraction) and by stimulating α-adrenergic receptors in the sphincter (increased bladder outlet resistance).

Clinically, urinary retention occurs following the administration of muscarinic receptor antagonists such as propantheline bromide and adrenergic agonists such as phenylephrine. Drugs that have relatively potent anticholinergic properties, such as phenothiazines, tricyclic antidepressants, and antispasmodics, may also promote urinary retention. Although the bladder contains a significant number of β-adrenergic receptors, isoproterenol and other β-adrenergic agonists do not appear to induce urinary retention in human beings.

Men with BPH appear to be more susceptible to the development of urinary retention following the administration of anticholinergic and α-adrenergic drugs. α-Adrenergic agonists may promote urinary retention in men with BPH by increasing the tension of the smooth muscle cells in both the bladder neck and prostatic adenoma. In the Health Professionals Follow-up Study, certain antihypertensive medications, specifically calcium channel and β-blockers, were found to increase the risk of acute urinary retention in men.[25]

Whereas older antihistamines were prone to induce urinary retention, newer more selective antihistamines that do not cross the blood-brain barrier tend to have fewer anticholinergic effects. Terfenadine, one of the first selective H_1 receptor antagonists developed (and no longer available in the United States), was associated with approximately the same incidence of retention as was placebo.[26] However, sporadic reports of urinary retention did occur.[27] Reports of urinary retention related to other selective antihistamines, such as astemizole, also exist.[28]

Erectile Dysfunction

The mechanism by which penile erections occur is a complex series of pharmacologic reactions, and many commonly prescribed medications alter the ability to obtain and maintain erections. This section describes some of the more commonly cited classes of agents that cause erectile dysfunction.

Anticholinergics

Atropine sulfate, benztropine, diphenhydramine (Benadryl), and propantheline bromide are commonly prescribed drugs with anticholinergic properties. Anticholinergic drugs presumably cause erectile dysfunction by inhibiting preganglionic cholinergic receptors.

Antidepressants

The pharmacology of tricyclic antidepressant drugs such as amitriptyline, doxepin, nortriptyline, and imipramine is complex because these drugs interfere with the reuptake of norepinephrine at nerve terminals. These drugs also bind to acetylcholine receptors with variable affinities. Penile blood flow may be diminished secondary to the preganglionic cholinergic blockade or α-adrenergic potentiation resulting from the inhibition of norepinephrine reuptake. Newer non–tricyclic antidepressant medications also significantly cause male sexual dysfunction. In a retrospective review, 23 of 56 patients receiving selective serotonin reuptake inhibitors (SSRIs)—fluoxetine, paroxetine, and sertraline—complained of sexual dysfunction.[29] Lithium, a drug used to treat manic depression, has also been implicated in erectile dysfunction.[30]

Antihypertensives

Antihypertensive medications may interfere with erections by pharmacologically altering the perfusion pressure of the corpora cavernosa. Antihypertensive agents may also act on central and peripheral neural pathways that influence erections. Many antihypertensive medications have been reported to cause erectile dysfunction in men.[31] Diuretics have been reported to induce erectile dysfunction, although the mechanism is poorly understood.

Chang and colleagues[32] published a prospective, randomized, placebo-controlled trial comparing thiazides with placebo. Thiazides were found to cause statistically significant decreases in libido, difficulty in gaining and maintaining an erection, and difficulty with ejaculation. Spironolactone, another diuretic known to induce erectile dysfunction, is a steroid analogue that competitively inhibits the binding of aldosterone to its receptor.[33] The drug produces low serum testosterone levels, increased testosterone clearance, and elevated levels of estradiol and LH. This endocrine dysfunction may cause the erectile dysfunction.

β-Adrenergic antagonists are another group of antihypertensive medications that cause erectile dysfunction, presumably by decreasing blood flow to the corpora. The Veterans Administration Cooperative Study on Antihypertensive Agents reported the development of erectile dysfunction in 7% of patients treated with propranolol alone.[34]

Centrally acting antihypertensives also induce erectile dysfunction. Methyldopa reduces hypertension by antagonizing adrenergic receptors on peripheral smooth muscle and by stimulating α-adrenergic receptors in the brain. The incidence of erectile dysfunction secondary to methyldopa reported in the literature ranges between 3% and 50%.[35,36] Clonidine is a selective α$_2$-adrenergic antagonist that presumably reduces blood pressure through central receptors. Clonidine has been associated with erectile dysfunction in 10% to 20% of male patients.

In a prospective trial comparing erectile responses to papaverine injections in men taking antihypertensive medications, Muller and colleagues[37] found that patients taking antihypertensive medication demonstrated a worse arterial response to papaverine than did those not taking medication. Furthermore, the best response to papaverine injections was found in men taking a combination of β-adrenergic antagonists and vasodilators as opposed to men taking thiazides either alone or in combination.

Antipsychotics

Phenothiazines such as chlorpromazine (Thorazine) and thioridazine (Mellaril) cause erectile dysfunction secondary to peripheral anticholinergic and antiadrenergic effects. Kotin and coworkers[38] reported that 44% of patients treated with thioridazine specifically reported erectile dysfunction, whereas 60% of all patients treated suffered from sexual dysfunction. Sexual function has been shown to be affected by the central monoamine neurotransmitters serotonin and dopamine. The dopaminergic blocking properties of the phenothiazines and the butyrophenones may alter sexual behavior, presumably by depleting central monoamine neurotransmitters. Most cases of erectile dysfunction occur shortly after initiation of the drug, often within 24 hours. Nevertheless, the erectile dysfunction usually improves fairly quickly after the antipsychotic drug is withdrawn.[39]

Narcotics

Morphine, meperidine, and codeine cause erectile dysfunction, presumably by depressing central nervous system (CNS) activity.

Antiandrogens

Drugs with antiandrogenic properties may impair erectile function, libido, and fertility.

Priapism

Priapism, a prolonged, painful erection of the penis, has multiple causes, including medications. Iatrogenic priapism has become a well-recognized complication of the treatment of erectile dysfunction; this specific cause is discussed in the section "Erectile Dysfunction Medications." Pohl and colleagues[40] evaluated a series of patients presenting with priapism and found 38 different causes. Trazodone, a triazolopyridine-derived oral antidepressant, is the drug most commonly associated with the development of priapism.[41] Even low-dose trazodone therapy (50 mg) administered for a short duration (10 days) has been reported to induce priapism.[42] Investigators have suggested that the mechanism of trazodone-induced priapism is through its α-adrenergic blocking activity.[43] Trazodone has also been reported to induce priapism of the clitoris in women.[44]

Other psychopharmacologic agents that induce priapism include clozapine (Clozaril),[45,46] thioridazine,[47] chlorpromazine,[48] and other neuroleptic agents.[49] In addition to the psychopharmacologic agents, antihypertensive medications have also been recognized to induce priapism. The most often cited agent is prazosin, an α-adrenergic antagonist.[50-52] Other antihypertensive agents that induce priapism include guanethidine and hydralazine.[53] Hydralazine induces priapism by its direct relaxation of vascular smooth muscle. The development of an erection requires relaxation of the cavernosal and sinusoidal smooth muscle. Nitric oxide is the primary mediator of cavernosal smooth muscle. Cavernosal smooth muscle relaxation is mediated by α-adrenergic agonists. α-Adrenergic antagonists are therefore one class of agents that have *not* been associated with erectile dysfunction. In fact, α-adrenergic antagonists have been reported to promote erections.[54]

In addition to prescription medications, illicit drugs, such as intranasal cocaine, have the potential to cause priapism.[55] Moreover, the use of intraurethral cocaine,[56] topical application of cocaine to the glans penis,[57] and the use of cocaine in its solid form, crack,[58] have all been reported to cause priapism. Finally, investigators have reported that the combination of trazodone and cocaine may cause an additive risk for priapism.[59]

COMPLICATIONS OF UROLOGIC DRUG THERAPY

Medications for Benign Prostatic Hyperplasia

Since the late 1980s, the management of clinical BPH has evolved considerably secondary to the widespread acceptance of medical therapy. Furthermore, the treatment of clinical BPH, which was once the strict domain of urologists, is now being managed by both urologists and nonurologists alike. Medical therapy for the treatment of clinical BPH has replaced transurethral resection of the prostate in many men without absolute indications for intervention primarily because patients are willing to minimize adverse events at the expense of efficacy. Importantly, although α-blockers and 5α-reductase (5AR) inhibitors have recognized adverse events, they are almost always reversible and are not life-threatening.

Terazosin (Hytrin), doxazosin (Cardura), tamsulosin (Flomax), and alfuzosin (Uroxatral) are the α_1-blockers approved by the U.S. Food and Drug Administration (FDA) for the treatment of BPH. Terazosin and doxazosin are long-acting α_1-blockers that show no selectivity for the α_1 subtypes. Tamsulosin and alfuzosin are newer agents that show some selectivity for the a_{1a} versus a_{1b} subtype. The a_{1a} subtype mediates prostate smooth muscle contraction. Terazosin is the most extensively studied and widely used α_1-blocker. The incidence of terazosin-related adverse events reported in the literature depends on the duration of the study and the daily dose. The most common adverse events are asthenia, dizziness, and postural symptoms.

Lepor and colleagues performed a multicenter, randomized, double-blind placebo-controlled study in 1229 U.S. veterans and compared the safety and efficacy of terazosin, finasteride, a combination of both, and placebo in the treatment of clinical BPH.[60] In this study, the investigators noted a significant increase in dizziness and postural hypotension in men treated with terazosin. The treatment-related rates of dizziness, asthenia, postural hypotension, and syncope were 19%, 6%, 6%, and 1%, respectively. Lowe[61] reported that the terazosin-mediated incidence of dizziness at 1 mg, 2 mg, 5 mg, and 10 mg was 1.4%, 1.6%, 3.6%, and 7.4%, respectively, based on six randomized placebo-controlled trials. A bedtime dose has been suggested to minimize the incidence and severity of these adverse events.

The incidence of adverse effects with doxazosin is comparable to that of terazosin, based on a comparison of nonconcurrent studies. Terazosin and doxazosin are also widely used antihypertensive agents. Both terazosin and doxazosin lower blood pressure in those patients who are hypertensive at baseline. Therefore, these a_1-blockers should be considered for the concomitant treatment of BPH and high blood pressure. Owing to the effect on blood pressure, terazosin and doxazosin are dose titrated to avoid the "first-dose" phenomenon.

Tamsulosin and alfuzosin exhibit some selectivity for the a_{1a} compared with the a_{1b} subtype; tamsulosin has less effect on blood pressure in both normotensive and hypertensive patients relative to terazosin or doxazosin. It is unclear whether this diminished effect on blood pressure is the result of the modest subtype selectivity or the slow-release formulation. Thus, no dose titration is required to achieve a clinical effect, and the drug may be prescribed without a change in the patient's hypertensive medications. Relative to terazosin and doxazosin, tamsulosin at equivalent doses appears to cause less asthenia and dizziness; however, the incidence of rhinitis and retrograde ejaculation is greater.

Lepor[62,63] reported the results of a phase III multicenter, double-blind, placebo-controlled trial comparing once-daily dosing of either 0.4 mg or 0.8 mg of tamsulosin compared with placebo in patients with BPH. The reported incidence of dizziness was 10%, 11%, and 5% for the three arms of the trial, respectively. The incidence of abnormal ejaculation was 18%, 6%, and 0%, respectively. In a Brazilian 12-week, randomized, double-blind study comparing controlled release doxazosin and tamsulosin, the proportion of satisfied patients was observed earlier in the doxazosin cohort.[64] However, at week 12 the risk of ejaculatory dysfunction was higher in the tamsulosin-treated group.

The efficacy and safety of a once-daily formulation of alfuzosin in a pooled analysis of three parallel, randomized, double-blind, placebo-controlled 3-month studies of patients with lower urinary tract symptoms consistent with clinical BPH were determined by Roehrborn and colleagues.[65] Patients were randomized to receive alfuzosin or placebo for 12 weeks. Dizziness, the most frequently reported adverse event, was greater in the alfuzosin cohort compared with the placebo cohort, 6.1% versus 2.9%, respectively. However, no significant changes in blood pressure were noted with alfuzosin compared with placebo, including in elderly and hypertensive patients. Furthermore, sexual adverse events were rare in the alfuzosin cohorts (<1%).

Other reported rare adverse effects of α-blockers are polyarthralgia[66] and sinus bradycardia.[67] Stress urinary incontinence in women has also been reported to be caused by α-adrenergic antagonist therapy.[68-70] The mechanism for the stress urinary incontinence is α_1-adrenergic blockade of the smooth muscle of proximal urethra and bladder neck. Intraoperative floppy iris syndrome has been reported with the use of α_{1a}-adrenergic blockade.[71]

Two 5AR inhibitors, finasteride and dutasteride, have been approved for the treatment of BPH. 5AR is the enzyme responsible for the conversion of testosterone to dihydrotestosterone. Dutasteride and finasteride are 5AR competitive inhibitors; finasteride inhibits type 1 and dutasteride inhibits both type 1 and type 2. In a large, noninterventional observational cohort of 14,772 patients, the reported treatment-related incidence of ejaculatory dysfunction, loss of libido, and gynecomastia was 2.1%, 1%, and 0.4%, respectively.[72] Another adverse effect related to the use of finasteride is severe myopathy.[73]

One study randomized 4325 men to 0.5 mg dutasteride or placebo.[74] At 24 months, the serum dihydrotestosterone concentration was reduced from baseline by a mean of 90.2%, and the total prostate and transition zone volumes were reduced by a mean of 25.7% and 20.4%, respectively. The adverse events most commonly seen included impotence (1.7%), reduced libido (0.6%), ejaculation disorders (1.3%), and gynecomastia (0.5%). In a review of clinical trials comparing finasteride and dutasteride, no significant clinical difference in the adverse event profiles of dutasteride and finasteride was found.[75]

Erectile Dysfunction Medications

First reported by Virag in 1982,[76] the use of intracavernosal papaverine injections for the management of erectile dysfunction revolutionized the treatment options for patients with this disorder. In 1983, Brindley[77] described intracavernosal injections of phentolamine and used himself as an initial subject, and in 1985, Zorgniotti and Lefleur[78] introduced the papaverine-phentolamine combination. Currently, the most common regimens are prostaglandin E_1 (PGE_1) and a combination of phentolamine, papaverine, and PGE_1 (Trimix). Although many men find the use of intracavernosal injections extremely satisfying, this therapy has potential risks. Patients need to be carefully selected for this treatment: they need to be motivated, responsible, and compliant.

Priapism has been reported to occur in ≤7% of men receiving injection therapy.[79] The patient predisposed to develop priapism is, however, somewhat predictable. Lomas and Jarow[80] demonstrated that younger men and men with neurologic disease were at increased risk for papaverine-induced priapism. In addition, men with coronary artery disease had a decreased risk. Moreover, those men who had previously had an episode of priapism had a greater likelihood of a repeat episode. Kava[81] reviewed the adverse effects of different injection therapies (Table 7-1).

Systemic effects related to injection therapy include orthostatic hypotension and dizziness. PGE_1 tends to produce fewer systemic effects than do other medications because it is rapidly metabolized; however, PGE_1 more often causes local burning on injection.[82] Although the risk of penile fibrosis and scarring increases with long-term use, papaverine induces an area of severe fibrosis with degeneration and atrophy of the smooth muscles with a complete loss of normal architecture.

TABLE 7-1	Complications of Intracavernous Injection Therapy in Several Contemporary Series			
	Casabe et al (1998)	Kunelius and Lukkarinen (1999)	Baniel et al (2000)	Linet et al (1996)
Patients studied, N	189	69	625	683
Agent	Trimix	PGE_1	Progressive*	PGE_1
Penile ecchymoses, n (%)	40 (20.9)	7 (10.1)	31 (4.9)	57 (8)
Corporeal fibrosis, n (%)	10 (5.3)	4 (5.8)	19 (3)	15 (2)
Prolonged erection, n (%)	7 (3.7)	3 (4.3)	19 (3)	40 (6)
Urethral bleeding, n (%)	2 (1.1)	0	0	0
Penile pain, n (%)	0	5 (7.2)	106 (16.9)	343 (50)

*Several combinations, including (1) papaverine/phentolamine, (2) PGE_1, (3) Trimix, and (4) Quadramix were used in a progressive manner.
PGE_1, prostaglandin E_1; Trimix, phentolamine, papaverine, and PGE_1; Quadramix, Trimix plus atropine.
From Kava BR. Advances in the management of post–radical prostatectomy erectile function: treatment strategies when PDE-5 inhibitiors don't work. *Rev Urol.* 2005;7(Suppl 2):S39-S50.

Other rare adverse effects related to the use of intra-cavernosal injection therapy can be diminished with good patient teaching and compliance. One case report noted intracorporeal needle breakage requiring surgical extraction.[83] In addition, single case reports have described fatal pulmonary embolism secondary to pria-pism and thrombosis of the entire corpus cavernosum, extending to the penile, pudendal, and internal iliac veins. This patient had multiple sclerosis and within 30 minutes had injected two doses of 6.25 mg papaverine and 0.2 mg phentolamine.[84]

Alprostadil is an intraurethral agent marketed as MUSE (medicated urethral system for erection). The medication has fewer adverse effects compared with intracorporeal injections. Padma-Nathan and cowork-ers[85] conducted a double-blind, placebo-controlled study of 1511 men that assessed the efficacy of MUSE. After the effective dose was determined (125, 250, 500, or 1000 µg), the 996 patients who found the drug effec-tive and could tolerate it were randomized either to active treatment or placebo pellets to be used for 3 months at home. Penile pain occurred in 32.7% of patients treated with alprostadil versus only 3.3% of those treated with placebo. Pain was reportedly usually mild and rarely caused patients to discontinue treat-ment. Hypotension occurred in 3% of patients during the first dose-ranging stage of the trial, and dizziness occurred in 2% during home use. No men experienced penile fibrosis, priapism, or urethral strictures; however, the study was limited to 3 months.

The three oral agents for the treatment of erectile dysfunction are sildenafil (Viagra), tadalafil (Cialis), and vardenafil (Levitra). They all work by inhibiting cyclic guanosine monophosphate phosphodiesterase. The most often reported adverse effects are headache, dys-pepsia, and mild pelvic musculoskeletal pain.[86] Although the drug is well tolerated by most men, important safety issues have been raised by both physicians and the general media, owing to the drug's extreme popularity. An absolute contraindication to sildenafil is the use of nitrates, which in combination can cause hypotension. Although spontaneous reports of death among men using sildenafil exist, reporting of spontaneous events has limitations. Clinical trials have not shown any increase in myocardial infarction rates in age-matched populations of men.[87]

A comparison of the side effects of all the three oral agents is given in Table 7-2. Moore and associates[88] reviewed 50 randomized trials evaluating the phospho-diesterase type 5 inhibitors. Reported rates of with-drawal for sildenafil, tadalafil, and vardenafil were 8%, 13%, and 20%, respectively. All three drugs were well tolerated; headache, the most commonly reported event, occurred in 13% to 17% of patients. Serious adverse events were recorded more frequently in tadala-fil and vardenafil trials rather than in sildenafil trials, a finding possibly reflecting the newness of the studies. Overall, sildenafil offered better efficacy and lower rates of adverse events.

Overactive Bladder Medications

As previously discussed in the section on urinary reten-tion, the bladder detrusor muscle is controlled by parasympathetic cholinergic input. For this reason, anticholinergic drugs should be considered first-line agents for patients with detrusor instability.[89] The FDA-approved drugs for the treatment of OAB include oxy-butynin chloride, tolterodine, trospium chloride, propantheline bromide, solifenacin, and darifenacin.

Oxybutynin chloride (Ditropan) was the initial anti-cholinergic drug available in the United States for the treatment of neurogenic bladder. Oxybutynin has both an anticholinergic effect and a local anesthetic effect on the bladder.[89] Oxybutynin decreases urgency, frequency, and urge incontinence. However, the anticholinergic side effects can be severe, and many patients discon-tinue using the drug. These side effects include dry mouth, constipation, dizziness, tachycardia, palpita-tions, and blurred vision. Furthermore, all antimusca-rinic agents are relatively contraindicated in patients with narrow-angle glaucoma because these drugs can cause an increase in intraocular pressure. Oxybutynin has been released in a once-daily, long-acting formula-

TABLE 7-2	Common Adverse Events of All Three Phosphodiesterase Type 5 Inhibitors (Higher Recommended Doses)					
	Placebo	Sildenafil (100 mg)	Placebo	Tadalafil (20 mg)	Placebo	Vardenafil (20 mg)
Headache (%)	6	19	6	21	6	16
Flushing (%)	2	14	2	5	1	12
Dyspepsia (%)	2	9	2	17	1	4
Rhinitis (%)	2	5	4	5	4	10
Abnormal vision (%)	1	6			0	<2
Back pain (%)			5	9		
Myalgia (%)			2	7		

From Hatzimouratidis K, Hatzichristou DG. A comparative review of the options for treatment of erectile dysfunction: which treatment for which patient? *Drugs.* 2005;65(12):1621-1650.

tion (Ditropan XL). In a multicenter, randomized, double-blind study comparing two formulations, both groups of patients had similar reductions in urge and total incontinence episodes.[90] However, the incidence of dry mouth of any severity was reported by 68% and 87% of the controlled and immediate-release groups, respectively, and moderate or severe dry mouth occurred in 25% and 46%, respectively.

Thuroff and colleagues[91] conducted a randomized, double-blind, placebo-controlled, multicenter trial comparing oxybutynin, propantheline, and placebo. Mean improvement of voiding symptoms was significantly higher with oxybutynin than with propantheline; however, the percentage of patients reporting adverse effects—most commonly dry mouth—with oxybutynin (63%) was greater that in patients given propantheline (44%).

Appell[92] evaluated four randomized, multicenter trials comparing tolterodine, oxybutynin, and placebo. Adverse effects in patients treated with placebo, 1 mg tolterodine twice daily, 2 mg tolterodine twice daily, and oxybutynin were reported in 78%, 74%, 75%, and 93% of patients, respectively. The OBJECT (Overactive Bladder: Judging Effective Control and Treatment) trial compared oxybutynin extended-release (ER) with tolterodine immediate-release (IR) formulations.[93] Adverse effects, including dry mouth and CNS effects, occurred with similar frequencies in both groups, and both drugs were equally well tolerated, resulting in similar discontinuation rates.

The OPERA trial (Overactive Bladder: Performance of Extended-Release Agents) compared tolterodine ER with oxybutynin ER.[94] Dry mouth, although mild, was significantly more common with oxybutynin. Other adverse effects, including CNS effects, had similar frequencies.

Oxytrol is a transdermal formulation of oxybutynin. The transdermal application is designed to bypass the first-pass effect seen with the oral preparation and thus decreases systemic side effects. In a double-blind study, patients were randomized to 12 weeks of treatment of twice-weekly transdermal oxybutynin, daily tolterodine ER, or placebo.[95] The most common adverse event for the transdermal medication was localized application site pruritus (14% versus 4% placebo), yet overall systemic side effects were low, with dry mouth seen in only 4%.

Trospium chloride (Sanctura) is a novel quaternary ammonium derivative of nortropan that is a competitive inhibitor of acetylcholine at muscarinic receptors. Because the drug does not cross the blood-brain barrier, CNS and cognitive performance adverse effects such as dizziness should be minimal.[96] In a placebo-controlled, randomized, double-blind, multicenter study comparing trospium chloride with placebo, trospium chloride significantly improved bladder function.[97] The most frequently seen adverse effect was dry mouth.

Solifenacin (Vesicare) is a selective M_3 muscarinic receptor antagonist. One study compared solifenacin 2.5 mg, 5 mg, 10 mg, or 20 mg once daily with tolterodine 2 mg twice daily. Solifenacin had no serious treatment-related adverse events. The incidence of dry mouth was 14% for solifenacin 5 mg and 10 mg, 2.6% for placebo, and 24% for tolterodine.[98] Similar to solifenacin, darifenacin (Enablex) is a muscarinic receptor antagonist with enhanced specificity for the M_3 receptor subtype. Another study evaluated darifenacin and placebo in a pooled analysis of three phase III studies.[99] The overall incidence of adverse effects was 54% with darifenacin 7.5 mg and 65.6% with darifenacin 15 mg versus 48.7% with placebo. The most common adverse effects were dry mouth and constipation, and most of these effects were mild to moderate.

Intravesical administration of traditional drugs has been tried as an alternative to conventional oral administration for the unstable bladder. This route of instillation offers the possibility to obtain a high concentration of drug at the target organ and thus avoid systemic side effects. In motivated patients or patients who cannot tolerate oral anticholinergic agents, intravesical instillation should be considered as a nonsurgical option. These agents all have varying degrees of success; however, oxybutynin may be tolerated much better intravesically, may reach plasma levels comparable to those with oral administration, and may cause less dry mouth.

Intravesical delivery of two newer agents, capsaicin and resiniferatoxin, shows promise. Capsaicin is derived from capsicum peppers; it is a vanillyl amide and interacts with vanilloid receptors within the urinary bladder. Resiniferatoxin, derived from the cactus relative *Euphorbia resinifera,* shares a vanilloid configuration with capsaicin and is an analogue with much higher potency.[100] Kuo[101] evaluated the effectiveness and tolerability of multiple intravesical instillations of resiniferatoxin in patients with detrusor overactivity. The results were excellent or improved in nearly 50% of patients. However, side effects, often related to the required multiple injections, included decreased voiding efficiency, hematuria, and urinary tract infections.

Botulinum toxin A (BTX-A) is one of the most potent biologic neurotoxins, produced by the gram-positive bacterium *Clostridium botulinum.* It selectively blocks the release of acetylcholine from nerve endings and has therefore been used by some urologists as second-line treatment for neurogenic detrusor overactivity.[102] A single-center, prospective, nonrandomized study evaluated the safety, tolerability, and efficacy of a single dose of 300 U of BTX-A injected intravesically in 15 women with detrusor overactivity. All patients voided spontaneously; no episodes of urinary retention occurred, and no major adverse events were reported. Overall improvement lasted ≤24 weeks.

The main advantages of BTX-A are its efficacy, safety, lack of adverse effects, and temporary action. The temporary action of BTX-A necessitates repeated injections, and as a result some investigators were concerned about the development of antibodies and hence the long-term efficacy of treatment. The development of antibodies to BTX protein and clinical resistance to treatment with BTX-A was reported with the original BTX formulation. However, the current BTX introduced in 1997 has a much lower antigenic potential, and immunoresistance to treatment is rare and has not been reported in any studies of lower urinary tract disorders.[103] Although intravesical instillations of BTX-A have been relatively safe, the known side effects of BTX can obviously be severe: nausea, vomiting, dry mouth, dysphagia, weakness of the respiratory muscles, and paresis.[104]

Desmopressin is used in children with nocturnal enuresis and has shown some promise in the treatment of OAB in adults. Desmopressin is a synthetic analogue of vasopressin and thus acts as an antidiuretic. Although desmopressin at bedtime does not "cure" OAB, it can effectively decrease urine output for approximately 6 hours. Desmopressin administration does have risks: fluid overload and hyponatremia may result from concurrent excessive fluid intake. Severe hyponatremia may induce seizures and coma. Patients with electrolyte or fluid balance abnormalities, such as patients with congestive heart failure and cystic fibrosis, should be monitored carefully or should not be given this medication at all.[105] Nevertheless, the medication has been demonstrated to be safe even in elderly patients.[106]

Imipramine HCl (Tofranil) is a tricyclic antidepressant useful for increasing urine storage by decreasing detrusor contractility and by increasing outlet resistance. However, the exact mechanism of action of this drug remains a matter of debate. Besides anticholinergic side effects, patients may also complain of centrally mediated side effects such as weakness, fatigue, and sedation. The medication also has a depressant effect on the myocardium and thus must he used with caution in patients with preexisting cardiovascular disease. The drug is contraindicated in patients using monoamine oxidase inhibitors.

Alkalinizing Agents

Nephrolithiasis is a common condition affecting nearly 5% of U.S. men and women during their lifetimes. Depending on the type of stone, medications may be given to decrease stone formation or to aid in the breakdown and excretion of the material causing the stone. Agents may include such medications as diuretics, phosphate solutions, allopurinol, antibiotics (for struvite stones), and medications that alkalinize the urine. Alkaline citrate has been used to promote the excretion of urinary citrate.[107]

For uric acid stones, the use of potassium citrate (30-60 mEq/day) promotes urinary alkalinization with a consequent dissolution of excreted uric acid and reduction of urinary uric acid supersaturation.[108] Potassium is the preferred citrate preparation because the sodium salt can increase urinary calcium excretion. Potassium citrate therapy may be limited by gastrointestinal intolerance, particularly in older patients and patients with dyspepsia. One formulation of magnesium and potassium citrate may minimize this side effect.[109] Sodium bicarbonate has been used for many years and has the advantage of being inexpensive and generally well tolerated. The usual dose is 650 mg three times daily. Adverse effects of sodium bicarbonate include increased sodium and fluid load, which can be detrimental in patients with congestive heart failure, liver cirrhosis, and hypertension. Additionally, the sodium load may promote calcium oxalate stone formation by increasing urinary excretion of calcium and sodium.

Uric acid dissolution by oral alkalinization is generally effective, with a reported success rate of 80%. If oral alkalinization is ineffective, intravenous alkalization with one sixth molar sodium lactate is faster and more effective.[110] In a study conducted to test the efficacy of potassium-magnesium citrate in preventing recurrent calcium oxalate calculi formation, potassium-magnesium citrate did not cause frequent or troublesome diarrhea, and when this treatment is given for up to 3 years it reduces the risk of stone recurrence by 85%.[111]

KEY POINTS

1. Demonstrating a precise cause-and-effect relationship of pharmacologic agents among infertile patients is extremely difficult, if not impossible.
2. A complete drug history is a critical component of the urologic evaluation of hematuria because many common prescription and nonprescription medications can be the cause.
3. Urinary retention occurs following the administration of muscarinic receptor antagonists or drugs that have relatively potent anticholinergic properties.
4. α-Adrenergic agonists may promote urinary retention in men with BPH by increasing the tension of the smooth muscle cells in both the bladder neck and prostatic adenoma.
5. Erectile dysfunction can be the result of multiple drug therapies, and a careful medication history is essential in evaluation.
6. Drug therapy for erectile dysfunction may result in priapism, as can the commonly cited antidepressant, trazodone.
7. Because of the tremendous potential for side effects with drugs commonly employed in the management of urologic disease, knowledge of potential outcomes is critical for the practicing urologist.

REFERENCES

Please see www.expertconsult.com

Chapter 8

COMPLICATIONS OF INTRAVESICAL THERAPY

Basir Tareen MD
Fellow in Urologic Oncology, Bruce and Cynthia Sherman Fellowship in Urologic Oncology, Division of Urologic Oncology, Department of Urology, New York University Langone Medical Center, New York, New York

Samir S. Taneja MD
The James M. Neissa and Janet Riha Neissa Associate Professor of Urologic Oncology; Director, Division of Urologic Oncology, Department of Urology and New York University Cancer Institute, New York University Langone Medical Center, New York, New York

More than 75% of newly diagnosed bladder cancer represents early-stage urothelial carcinoma (stage Ta, stage T1, or carcinoma in situ [CIS]).[1] Numerous intravesical agents may be used in the management of these cancers, and as such specific knowledge of the toxicity of these agents is imperative for the practicing urologist.

INTRAVESICAL IMMUNOTHERAPY

Bacille Calmette-Guérin

Bacille Calmette-Guérin (BCG) is used for patients with stage T1 tumors, CIS, or stage Ta tumors of high grade. Originally introduced for this indication by Morales and colleagues in 1976,[2] BCG is now accepted as the most efficacious of the intravesical agents.[3,4] Although numerous studies have proven the benefit of BCG in delaying disease recurrence, its benefit in terms of disease progression has been more difficult to demonstrate in clinical trials.[5-7]

BCG's mechanism of action involves creating an inflammatory reaction in the bladder by means of live attenuated *Mycobacterium*.[8-11] For this reason, the rate of local side and systemic side effects is high. The primary cytokines released following intravesical BCG administration are interferon-γ (IFN-γ) and interleukin 2 (IL-2); therefore, many of the systemic side effects noted with BCG are similar to those seen with the systemic administration of cytokines.[12,13] The primary cytokine-related side effects of BCG often do not occur until the third or fourth instillation, a finding suggesting cumulative cytokine release with increasing exposure to the antigen.

Traditionally, BCG was given in six weekly instillations, although numerous more recent studies showed a significant benefit from maintenance therapy as opposed to induction therapy alone.[14-16] The largest of these studies was the Southwest Oncology Group (SWOG) trial, which examined patients with recurrent Ta, T1, and CIS and randomized 550 patients to receive either induction alone or induction and maintenance using 3-week treatments given at 3, 6, 12, 18, 30, and 36 months. Median time to disease recurrence was 35.7 months in the no maintenance group and was 60 months in the maintenance group. At 5 years, the recurrence-free rate was 41% and 60%, respectively.[13] Maintenance therapy, however, was not well tolerated; only 16% of the 243 patients completed all eight scheduled maintenance courses over 3 years.

Low-dose BCG was proposed as a means of decreasing toxicity and improving tolerance.[17] The largest randomized trial compared 500 patients using a BCG dose of either 27 or 81 mg and found no statistically significant difference in results for recurrence and progression in the two groups.[17] The investigators reported significant reduction in toxicity in the low-dose group. Patients with urothelial cancer that is refractory to BCG therapy also have been treated with low-dose BCG in combination with IFN therapy, with similar results.[18,19]

Numerous strains of BCG are widely used: TICE, Connaught, RIVM, Armand Frappier, Pasteur, and Tokyo. In a large meta-analysis, Lamm and colleagues[20] found no difference among the different strains in terms of clinical efficacy or side effects.

Overview of Complications

Although BCG is generally well tolerated, every urologist should be familiar with the expected minor and unexpected other adverse effects. Soloway and associates[21] reviewed 234 patients referred from community urologists and found significant numbers of patients treated for Ta G1 disease, a pathologic stage or grade in which one must seriously consider the side effects of BCG to outweigh the small benefit in treatment of typically indolent disease.

TABLE 8-1 Frequency of Bacille Calmette-Guérin Complications

Study (year)	No. Patients	Induction Dose	Maintenance Dose	Irritative Voiding Symptoms	Fever	Sepsis	Death
Pagano et al (1991)	126	75 mg Pasteur, 6 wk	Monthly × 1 yr, every 4 mo × 1 yr	30%	17%	0	0
Lamm et al[25] (1992)	2602	50 mg, 6 wk		95%	3%	0.40%	0
Witjes et al[22] (1993)	140	5×10^8 CFU/50 mL, 6 wk TICE	3 and 6 mo, give 6 weekly treatments if recurs	30%	2%	0.71%	0
Martinez-Pineiro et al (1990)	252	81 mg/50 mL, Connaught, 6 wk	Weekly × 6 wk, 6 more instillations fortnightly	71%	2%	0	0
	248	27 mg/50 mL Connaught, 6 wk		62%			
Vegt et al[23] (1997)	290	50 mg, 6 wk	3 weekly at 3, 6, 12, 18, 24, 30, 36 mo	53%	11%	0	0
Bassi et al (1999)	126	Pasteur 75 mg	Monthly/1 yr, every 4 mo/1 yr	27%	17%	0	0
Steinberg et al (2001)	2602			90%	75% (2.9%)	10.4%	7
Laurenti et al (2002)	41	TICE 5×10^8 CFU/50 mL	Weekly × 6, monthly × 11, every 3 mo × 4, every 6 mo × 6	Dysuria 25/41, hematuria 15/41	1% (2.9%)	0	0
Lorenz et al (2002)	102	TICE 5×10^8 CFU/50 mL × 6 weeks	3 weekly instillations at 3, 6, 2, 18, 30, and 36 mo	84%	13% (13%)	?	0

A distinction should be made between expected side effects and true complications of BCG therapy (Table 8-1). Local and systemic toxicities can be divided into immune-mediated or infection-mediated complications. Local toxicities are generally treatable and unavoidable symptoms. Some degree of local toxicity is experienced by virtually all patients, although the reported incidence in contemporary series ranged from 27% to 90% depending on sample size, dose and regimen, and definition of local toxicity.[20,22,23] Although many investigators believe that a strong correlation exists between BCG toxicity and efficacy, this link has never been proven in clinical trials.[24]

Systemic complications are uncommon, and >95% of patients will tolerate the treatment well. In a review of 2400 cases, Lamm and colleagues[25] found that fever >103°F was the most severe adverse event (2.9%). Other systemic complications include granulomatous changes, sepsis, pneumonitis, hepatitis, arthralgias, and cutaneous manifestations. Although major adverse reactions are unusual, it is important that the urologist recognize, diagnose, and treat these conditions early. When these complications are diagnosed and treated appropriately, virtually all patients recover from them with no long-term sequelae.

In an attempt to reduce side effects and improve tolerability, isoniazid (INH) has been tested as a prophy-lactic adjunctive treatment with BCG. A study by Vegt and associates[26] did not show any reduction in local or systemic reactions when INH was used prophylactically. In addition to not providing any protection against reactions to BCG, INH was associated with a significantly higher risk of developing abnormal hepatic transaminase levels.[26] More recently, ofloxacin was given in a randomized, blind, multicenter trial to 115 patients undergoing BCG treatment. Prophylactic ofloxacin was found to decrease the incidence of moderate to severe adverse events, which many investigators believe cause patients to discontinue treatment. No negative effect on efficacy was reported in the ofloxacin-treated group.[27]

Specific Complications

We generally categorize the side effects of BCG as local, inflammatory, or infectious. Management and prevention of these side effects depend on the timing of BCG administration and the early recognition of symptoms.

Local Toxicity The most commonly seen local toxicity of BCG is cystitis-like irritative voiding symptoms, reported in ≤90% of patients.[28,29] Severe symptoms typically occur after the third instillation when lymphokine release causes the maximal inflammatory response. Consideration should always be given to secondary bacterial infection, and a negative urine culture should be obtained before further BCG administration.

Treatment should include local analgesics such as phenazopyridine and antimuscarinics if severe bladder overactivity is noted. Dose reduction may be considered on follow-up administration, but unless the problem is severe, doses should not be withheld on the basis of local irritative symptoms alone. Most local symptoms subside within 2 to 3 days of administration, but in severe cases, symptoms can persist for several weeks after completion of therapy.

Gross hematuria occurs in 1% to 34% of patients receiving BCG.[29,30] It is usually self-limiting and most commonly occurs after the second or third dose. Urine culture should be obtained. If hematuria does not resolve after 2 to 3 weeks of observation, repeat cystoscopy is indicated to exclude the possibility of recurrent tumor.

Inflammatory Toxicity Flulike symptoms, such as low-grade fever <38.5°C, often accompany the irritative voiding symptoms. Malaise, myalgia, and low-grade fever typically last 24 to 48 hours. Treatment with acetaminophen and nonsteroidal anti-inflammatory drugs (NSAIDs) is typically successful. In some cases, we have used prophylactic acetaminophen administered at the time of BCG instillation. If symptoms are severe or if no resolution is noted after 48 hours, consideration should be given to antituberculin therapy until symptoms resolve.[29]

Infectious Toxicity High fever (>102°F-103°F) or shaking chills suggests fever resulting from systemic absorption and warrants empiric treatment with antituberculosis therapy. Failure to treat or delay in diagnosis can result in a progression to sepsis and mortality.

In patients who develop BCG sepsis, therapy must be immediate and aggressive. Sepsis typically occurs in <4% of patients.[29] More than 10 deaths have been attributed to BCG sepsis, and the rate is estimated to be 1 death for every 12,500 patients treated with intravesical BCG. The classic presentation is a patient with history of traumatic catheterization who presents with fever, chills, hypotension, and mental confusion. Respiratory failure, jaundice, leukopenia, and disseminated intravascular coagulopathy can occur. Results of culture are typically negative for mycobacteria, and treatment must be started based on clinical suspicion.

Treatment is with INH, rifampin, and prednisone.[29] Lamm proposed that BCG sepsis is, in part, the result of a delayed-type hypersensitivity reaction, and for this reason the administration of 40 mg prednisolone may improve survival.[30] Ethambutol is added if the patient does not respond to the foregoing regimen. Whereas prednisone may be discontinued after the resolution of symptoms, rifampin and INH are continued for ≥6 months. The use of cycloserine has been proposed by some investigators for systemic BCG absorption.

Although the use of this agent has shown a survival advantage in mice, it appears to be ineffective against currently used BCG strains.[31,32]

Prevention of Systemic Absorption Numerous factors may contribute to the risk of systemic absorption. Most commonly, traumatic catheterization, a nonhealing resection site, and unrecognized urinary tract infection (UTI) are the leading suspects. During catheterization of a patient for BCG instillations, any difficulty or trauma should raise concern. At least seven reported deaths have resulted from systemic BCG infection after traumatic catheterization.[29] At the time of instillation, atraumatic catheterization is essential. If traumatic catheterization does occur, BCG therapy should be withheld. A history of significant urethral stricture may be a contraindication to BCG therapy. In these patients, the stricture disease should be treated definitively before to intravesical therapy is begun. On rare occasions, a patient can be treated with a catheter in place. Following catheterization, the BCG is instilled and the catheter is left capped for 2 to 3 hours, depending on the patient's bladder capacity. Caution must be exercised to ensure that the patient does not have poor compliance or detrusor instability, which may result in high intravesical pressure and systemic absorption. Such individuals may not be appropriate candidates for BCG therapy if they also have poor bladder capacity. BCG should not be administered in the setting of known muscle invasive or necrotic bladder cancer.

BCG instillation should be performed by gravity, not by pressurized instillation. Generally, a syringe with piston removed can be attached to the catheter and used as a reservoir for gravity-driven instillation.

Following tumor resection, most investigators recommend withholding BCG for a minimum of 7 days. We have found an interval of 2 to 3 weeks from administration with resolution of hematuria is usually sufficient to allow healing without affecting therapeutic outcome. In patients with a large resection bed, flexible cystoscopy can be used to ensure healing before BCG instillation. Gross hematuria or significant microscopic hematuria should have resolved before instillation. Periodic urine culture is useful to identify UTI. Symptoms alone may not be helpful for identification of UTI because most patients experience some irritative voiding symptoms.

Granulomatous Complications Granulomatous prostatitis is reported to occur in 1% to 27% of patients receiving BCG therapy, depending to some degree on the treatment regimen.[29,30] The true incidence of this complication is likely much higher and was found to be as high as 40% among patients undergoing biopsy in one study.[33] Granulomatous prostatitis is usually discovered incidentally on digital rectal examination in patients with or without an elevated prostate-specific antigen (PSA) level. In the small percentage of patients who are symptomatic

(6%), Lamm and associates[34] noted that these patients usually present with acute prostatitis or urinary retention. Biopsy is needed to rule out cancer, and once the diagnosis is made, asymptomatic patients can be observed. Treatment of symptomatic disease is with 300 mg INH and 600 mg rifampin for 3 to 6 months.[34]

It is wise to obtain a PSA level before BCG therapy. This test should be performed at a time distant from lower tract instrumentation. If test results are normal, PSA need not be measured until 1 year following BCG instillation. In individuals undergoing maintenance therapy, we determine the PSA level immediately before the 12-month maintenance dose. Given the frequent instrumentation, rises in PSA level are difficult to interpret. One may give a course of INH for 2 to 3 months to assess the cause of PSA elevation. If the BCG treatment was given in the remote past, the urologist should proceed directly to biopsy.

More infrequently, granulomatous epididymo-orchitis or even granulomatous balanoposthitis can occur.[35] Patients with granulomatous epididymo-orchitis generally present with local induration and pain. Local symptoms may be accompanied by fever or leukocytosis. Treatment is with INH and rifampin for 3 to 6 months. A diagnosis of bacterial infection should be excluded. Some cases may proceed to abscess formation requiring orchiectomy for definitive treatment.

Granulomatous hepatitis and pneumonitis represent systemic infection and occur in <1% of patients treated with BCG.[29] Patients typically present with general malaise, shortness of breath, and fever >101°F. One death has been reported from granulomatous hepatitis and BCG sepsis.[36] A full fever workup that includes elevated liver enzymes and a chest radiograph are needed to delineate the diagnosis. Liver biopsy is required to confirm the presence of granulomatous hepatitis. Hospitalization, fluid resuscitation, and acetaminophen are essential. INH and rifampin are given for 3 months with ethambutol added for severely ill patients. The incidence of hypersensitivity reaction from BCG is unclear, but investigators have reported that some granulomatous reactions result from an immune rather than an infectious process.[37-39] Although no controlled studies have been conducted of steroid therapy in BCG-infected patients, preliminary data reveal that prednisolone (40 mg/day) may be added in unremitting conditions, as in the case of BCG sepsis.[40-42]

Granulomatous reactions also occur in the bladder.[42,43] Contracted bladder occurs in <1% of patients, but patients receiving maintenance therapy may be at higher risk, and some investigators have advocated use of prophylactic INH to decrease likelihood of this complication. Treatment of contracted bladder consists of hydrodistention and withholding of BCG. If conservative measures fail, cystectomy may be required.[44] Ureteral obstruction may occur secondary to edema or inflammation of the orifice and is reported in <0.3% of patients. CIS and vesicoureteral reflux are probably predisposing factors.[45]

Granulomatous reactions of the bone marrow also may occur. Organisms are usually not found on bone marrow aspirates. The presence of cytopenia should arouse suspicion of bone marrow involvement. Treatment is with symptomatic support and cessation of BCG therapy.

Arthralgic Complications Arthralgia and arthritis are some of the rare severe complications associated with BCG therapy. Joint involvement occurs in approximately 0.5% of cases.[29] Arthritis usually occurs ≤2 weeks after the last instillation, whereas arthralgias can appear within a few days of instillation and become more severe with further instillations.[46] The symptoms usually resolve with NSAID treatment, cessation of BCG therapy, and in some cases steroids. Arthritis may occur within the complex of Reiter syndrome.[47]

Rare Complications Penile edema and meatal ulceration have been reported with and without lymph node enlargement.[48] A 3-month course of INH and rifampin therapy should be given. Cutaneous complications of BCG therapy are rare, but penile edema and meatal ulceration suggest the possibility of local spillage.[49] Other rare reported complications include nephrogenic adenoma, immune complex glomerulonephritis, choroiditis, cardiac toxicity, suppurative lymphadenitis, mycotic aneurysm, aortoduodenal fistula, lupus vulgaris, and musculoskeletal lesions.[49]

Continuing Therapy and Maintenance

Patients experiencing mild local and systemic inflammation side effects can be safely continued on an unmodified dose of BCG. In individuals experiencing severe local side effects or systemic toxicity lasting >48 hours, we recommend holding the dose until symptoms have resolved and then resuming treatment with a lower dose of BCG (1/3, 1/6, 1/12, or 1/100 dilution) to reduce the severity of symptoms.[29,50] In general, prophylactic use of INH is not indicated unless the clinician suspects systemic absorption of the organism.

In patients with high fever or severe local symptoms, once the symptoms resolve, the clinician should rule out obvious reasons for systemic absorption such as traumatic catheterization, bladder wall ulceration, or timing in relation to transurethral resection. BCG therapy may then be resumed, but it is advisable to use prophylactic INH, typically at the standard dose of 300 mg for 2 days before instillation and 1 day after instillation. Individuals who have experienced severe systemic illness or sepsis should not receive further BCG therapy.

Numerous studies have shown that long-term maintenance therapy is associated with a poor rate of compliance, ranging from 16% to 65.5%.[18,51-53] In comparison with nonmaintenance regimens, patients undergoing maintenance therapy clearly have a greater incidence of side effects, and compliance seems directly related to the duration and total number of instillations.[51] The high rate of adverse events necessitates a dose reduction in most patients that does not appear to affect efficacy.[54-57] Most treatment cessations are associated with local or regional symptoms of irritation. We have used a modified regimen of administration at 3, 6, 12, 18, 24, 36, and 60 months. Anecdotally, this regimen has been better tolerated. Although low-grade fever is common and increases in incidence with successive maintenance doses, this complication has not been found to be related to cessation of therapy.[56]

Purified Protein Derivative Conversion

A positive purified protein derivative (PPD) skin test result occurs in approximately 34% of patients treated with intravesical BCG and should not be considered a complication of BCG therapy.[58] Although favorable responses to treatment have been shown to occur more frequently in patients with PPD conversion, this factor has not been shown to be a reliable indicator or either prognosis or tolerance of therapy.[29,30,59]

Contraindications

Classic contraindications to BCG therapy include human immunodeficiency virus infection, leukemia, lymphoma, transplantation, pregnancy, breast-feeding, active tuberculosis, and intractable UTIs.[60] Yossepowitch and Dalbagni and their colleagues[61] evaluated the use of BCG induction therapy in 24 "immunocompromised patients" with lymphoma, chronic obstructive pulmonary disease, or steroid therapy and found a response rate of 58% overall; only a single patient experienced a self-limited febrile illness (≤39.3°C for 48 hours after his third BCG cycle). BCG therapy also has been safely given in patients with renal transplant.[62] These results occurred in small case series of highly selective patients, however, and severely immunocompromised patients should not undergo BCG therapy.

Another area of debate is transmission of BCG by sexual intercourse. Even though no cases of sexual transmission have been reported, use of a condom is generally advised during sexual intercourse for 1 week after BCG therapy.

BCG may be given to patients with vesicoureteral reflux without significant risk of complication.[63] Some investigators have advocated resection of the ureteral orifices to induce reflux before BCG therapy to increase the proportion of urothelium in contact with the BCG. Only one case of necrotic pyelonephritis has been reported. When patients do develop severe febrile reactions to BCG, consideration should be given to BCG pyelonephritis or renal abscess.

No contraindication exists to giving BCG therapy to patients with valvular heart disease. However, antibiotic prophylaxis for bacterial endocarditis should be administered before urethral instrumentation is undertaken.[30]

Interferons

IFNs are proteins with antiviral, antiproliferative, and immunomodulatory properties. Three classes of IFNs are recognized.[64] IFN-α, IFN-β, and IFN-γ derive from leukocytes, fibroblasts, and lymphocytes, respectively. IFNs stimulates macrophages for antigen presentation, promote cytokine release, enhance natural killer cell activity, and indirectly activate T and B lymphocytes.[65]

The best studied IFN is IFN-α. When it is used alone, this agent is well tolerated, with minimal local inflammatory effects or low-grade fever.[66] Efficacy depends on dose (range, 10 million to 100 million U). IFN-α is less effective and more expensive than BCG, and therefore its primary use is in salvage intravesical therapy for BCG-refractory tumors.[67-69] In patients with CIS and BCG treatment failure, the complete response to IFN-α is 15% to 20% at 1 year, with a durable response rate of 12% by 2 to 3 years.[23] The combination of 50 million U IFN-α and low-dose BCG had a higher success rate than did BCG alone in single institution study at 1 to 2 year follow-up.[18]

Complications

Most side effects of IFN are the result of the systemic inflammatory response generated by lymphokine release. Acute IFN toxicity consists of flulike symptoms, which occur in 0% to 27% of patients and include chills, fever, headache, malaise, and myalgia.[66,70] Chronic toxicities include fatigue, weight loss, and anemia. Some patients develop local cystitis and hematuria (0%-10%).[71] Most adverse events resolve with expectant management within 24 to 48 hours of onset or on discontinuation of therapy. Acetaminophen can be used as a supportive agent to reduce fever and myalgia. Although treatment is generally symptomatic, dose reduction can aid in the completion of therapy.

O'Donnell and colleagues conducted a phase II randomized trial comparing IFN alfa-2b with BCG and found systemic side effects in 5.3% of patients.[19] The use of lower-dose BCG showed a trend toward decreased severe inflammatory and infectious events.

Although most toxicities associated with intravesical IFN are mild, transient, and completely reversed on discontinuation of therapy, on occasion these symptoms can interfere with patient compliance and completion of therapy. Dose reduction (25 or 10 million U, if necessary) offers a potential means of continuing therapy.

Intravesical Chemotherapy

Intravesical chemotherapy is an important class of therapeutics for treatment of Ta and T1 bladder carcinoma. The most commonly used drugs are mitomycin C

TABLE 8-2	Toxicity of Intravesically Administered Mitomycin C							
Study (year)	No. Patients	Induction Dose	Dose Frequency	Chemical Cystitis	Bladder Capacity Reduction	Contact Dermatitis	Leucopenia	Thrombocytopenia
Nissenkorn et al[77] (1981)	29	8 × 40 mg/mL	Weekly induction; every	3 (10%)	None	3 (10%)	None	None
Prout et al[72] (1982)	28	8 × 40 mg/mL	Weekly induction	9 (32%)	None	None	None	None
Issel et al (1984)	60	8 × 40 mg/mL	Weekly induction	33%	None	7 (12%)	3 (5%)	1 (2%)
Huland et al[75] (1990)	209	20 mg/20 mL, every 2 wk × 1 yr	Every 4 wk × 1 yr; every 3 mo × 1 yr	25%	None	None	None	None
	96	20 mg/20 mL, every wk × 8 wk	Every mo × 3 yr	12%	None	None	None	None
	75	20 mg/20 mL weekly × 20 wk		18%	None	None	None	None
Eijsten et al[76] (1990)	75	2 × 20 or 30 2 doses in first wk	Every 2 wk × 6 mo; every mo × 6 mo; every 2 mo × 1 yr	None	17 (23%)	None	None	None
Rintala et al[59] (1996)	93	5 × 20-40 mg	Weekly induction; every mo × 1 yr; every 3 mo × 1 yr	3 (3%)*	None	3 (3%)	None	None
Bohle et al[57] (2003)	776			39.2%				

(MMC), epirubicin, doxorubicin, and valrubicin. Given the high molecular weight of chemotherapeutic drugs, the risk of absorption is low; consequently, systemic toxicity is less than with BCG. Furthermore, the use of intravesical chemotherapy eliminates the risk of sepsis and death associated with BCG therapy.

Mitomycin C

MMC is an antibiotic chemotherapeutic alkylating agent that acts by inhibiting DNA synthesis.[72-74] Because of its high molecular weight, MMC is not easily absorbed and has a lower incidence of systemic reactions. This agent has been used in 20- to 60-mg doses for 8 weeks, although the usual dose is 40 mg in 40 mL of saline or water intravesically for 8 weeks followed by monthly maintenance therapy for 1 year in most studies. Table 8-2 summarizes the different schedules of intravesical MMC therapy and their associated side effects.

Chemical cystitis, the most common side effect of MMC therapy, has an incidence of 3% to 33%.[75,76]

Symptoms generally respond to phenazopyridine and anticholinergics, but ≤3% of patients may require discontinuation of therapy because of severe cystitis.[59] Common symptoms include dysuria, suprapubic discomfort, and urinary frequency or urgency. UTI should be ruled out before palliative therapy is instituted; before discontinuation of therapy, consideration should be given to reducing the dose. Toxicity partly depends on the dose administered, but cystitis can occur even at low doses.

Eczema-like desquamation of the skin of the palms, soles of the feet, perineum, chest, and face is another side effect of MMC. Other investigators have reported a generalized rash.[59,77] The incidence of dermatologic toxicity ranges from 4% to 12% in most series. Two causes are contact dermatitis resulting from a delayed hypersensitivity reaction and direct contact of the drug with the skin.[78] Delayed hypersensitivity was postulated as a cause after deGroote and colleagues[78] reported on six patients, all of whom developed rash after their second instillation, a finding suggesting that MMC sensitization was required for the dermatitis to occur.

Dermatologic toxicity may be prevented by careful cleansing of the hands and genitals after voiding. Topical steroids can sometimes suppress the reaction enough to continue therapy.[78] When rash does arise, MMC therapy is generally discontinued. In most cases, repeat treatment results in recurrence of the dermatitis. Some investigators have suggested skin testing patients with a 0.1% MMC petroleum patch to see whether a systemic response occurs, but this approach has not gained favor.[79]

Myelosuppression after intravesical MMC therapy is rare. Multiple investigators have reported rare accounts of myelosuppression following intravesical MMC therapy.[80] In general, patients appear to have coexisting risk factors for leukopenia, thus making it difficult to assess the causative factor. Myelosuppression is rare enough that routine monitoring is not necessary.

A relatively infrequent complication of MMC instillation is bladder contracture.[76] Although a reduction in bladder capacity has been reported by numerous investigators, interpretation of the finding is difficult because in most cases, pretreatment bladder capacity is not measured. In patients with a severe reduction in bladder capacity, it appears that MMC administration at the time of resection is the major risk factor, and the most likely contributor is extravasation. Selecting patients carefully based on the extent and depth of resection, and particularly avoiding administration in the setting of perforation, may decrease the risk.

MMC may cause peritonitis, pelvic pain, fibrosis, and necrosis if bladder perforation and extravasation occur.[81-83] Urologists must constantly be aware of the depth of transurethral resection, and if perforation is suspected, MMC should be withheld until a cystogram is done to confirm bladder integrity. In rare instances, extravasation may be a direct effect of MMC-induced transmural muscle necrosis.[82]

Thiotepa

Thiotepa was used in the past for high-risk superficial bladder tumor recurrence resulting from multifocality, frequent recurrence, or high-grade disease associated with urothelial atypical cancer or CIS. The drug was appealing because of its low cost, but it lost appeal because of the availability of anthracycline compounds and because of the relatively increased risk of systemic absorption and myelosuppression. Unlike MMC, thiotepa has a low molecular weight, which allows as much as one third of the drug to be absorbed through the urothelium when it is retained in the bladder for 3 hours.[74] Because of the low molecular weight, the high rate of absorption, and the potential for bone marrow suppression associated with thiotepa, the treating physician should be extremely cautious when administering this agent (Table 8-3).

Doxorubicin and Epirubicin

Doxorubicin, epirubicin, and valrubicin are anthracycline antibiotics. Doxorubicin is used primarily in treatment of pTa and pT1 tumors for treatment and prophylaxis. BCG is better for treating CIS, but doxorubicin may be used in patients who cannot tolerate BCG. Because of its large molecular weight, doxorubicin is minimally absorbed and has few systemic complications. Local toxicity, however, is far more common (Table 8-4).

Chemical cystitis manifesting as dysuria, frequency, urgency, and suprapubic pain is seen in 13% to 56% of patients.[74] Management is symptomatic, and urine cultures should be obtained to rule out bacterial infection.

TABLE 8-3	Toxicity of Intravesically Administered Thiotepa						
Study (year)	No. Patients	Induction Dose	Dose Frequency	Leucopenia	Thrombocytopenia	Deaths	Irritative Voiding Symptoms
Abbassian and Wallace (1996)	13	4 × 90 mg/50 mL	Every 4 days	7 (54%)	None	2	9 (69%)
Gavrell et al (1978)	22	6 × 30 mg/60 mL, or 30 mg/60 mL	2/day every mo × 1 yr	2 (9%)	None	None	3 (14%)
Hollister and Coleman (1980)	29	60 mg/30 mL	Weekly, biweekly, or monthly × 1 yr	5 (17%)	9 (31%)	2	
Heney et al[63] (1988)	73	8 × 30 mg/30 mL	Every wk	15 (21%)		None	22 (30%)
Martinez-Pineiro et al (1990)	56	4 × 50 mg/mL	Every mo × 11 mo	None	None	None	8 (14%)
Bouffioux et al (1992)	103	4 × 50 mg/mL	Every week; every mo × 1 yr	None	1 (1%)	None	2 (2%)

TABLE 8-4	Toxicity of Intravesically Administered Doxorubicin				
Study (year)	No. Patients	Dose Induction	Dose Frequency	Chemical Cystitis	Systemic
Schulman et al (1984)	110	6 × 50 mg/50 mL	2 × 1st wk; every mo × 1 yr; every 3 mo × 1 yr	29 (26%)	None
Garnick et al (1984)	27	8 × 60-90 mg/ 40-50 mL	Every 3 wk; every 6 wk × 2; every 12 wk × 2	15 (56%)	None
Huland et al[75] (1990)	39	None; 50 mg/ mL?	Every 2 wk × 1 yr; every mo × 1 yr; every 3 mo × 1 yr	48%	Unknown
Martinez-Pineiro et al (1990)	53	50 mg/50 mL weekly × 4 wk	Every mo × 1 yr	13%	None
Ali-el-Dein et al[85] (1997)	60	50 mg/mL weekly × 8 wk	Every mo × 1 yr	22 (37%)	3 (5%)

Local treatment with phenazopyridine and anticholinergics provides relief of mild symptoms. Systemic side effects are uncommon and occur in <5% of patients in most series. Rare systemic side effects include gastrointestinal upset, fever, and rare hypersensitivity reactions. In very rare reported instances, hypersensitivity reactions manifested with tachypnea and bronchospasm and were treated with diphenhydramine; in one case, subcutaneous epinephrine was required.[84,85]

Epirubicin is similar to doxorubicin but has become more popular, especially in Europe, because of comparable or improved efficacy when compared with doxorubicin and decreased toxicity. Numerous investigators have verified the efficacy of epirubicin in the treatment of superficial bladder cancer.[86-91] Theo and colleagues[86] randomized 168 patients to either 50 mg epirubicin or 81 mg BCG for CIS. The clinical response rate was not statistically significant for the two agents; however, time to tumor recurrence after initial clinical response was longer in patients treated with BCG than in those treated with epirubicin (5.1 versus 1.4 years). More CIS recurrences were noted with epirubicin than with BCG therapy (45% versus 16%).[86] Side effects were more common in the BCG-treated group. Because of side effects, 26 patients stopped treatment in the BCG group, as opposed to only 8 patients in the epirubicin group.

Valrubicin is a semisynthetic analogue of doxorubicin. It has demonstrated antitumor activity in the treatment of superficial bladder cancer and was shown to have superior efficacy and less contact and cardiac toxicity than doxorubicin in animal models.[92] Valrubicin has claimed an important role in BCG-refractory CIS in patients who are not candidates for cystectomy. Local bladder symptoms may occur in ≥90% of patients during at least a portion of the treatment. Urinary frequency, urgency, and dysuria occurred in approximately 60% of patients in the largest study. Overall symptoms are mild to moderate in severity and do not typically cause cessation of therapy. Other less common side effects include UTI, asthenia, urinary retention, and foul-smelling urine with or without passing of tissue.

CONCLUSION

The management of superficial bladder cancer is greatly aided by the use of intravesically administered adjuvant therapies. The use of these therapies is generally safe, and through the use of careful techniques of administration, patient selection, and patient observation, long-term sequelae should be minimal. Thorough knowledge of the individual toxicity profile of each agent is essential for the practicing urologist. Similarly, although various agents carry different risks of toxicity, adherence to the standard treatment principles of intravesical therapy, outlined in this chapter, will minimize the likelihood of complications.

KEY POINTS

1. The local and systemic inflammatory toxicities of BCG are usually short-lived and can be managed symptomatically.
2. Prevention of systemic absorption and infectious toxicity of BCG relies on healing of the bladder wall and avoidance of trauma at the time of instillation.
3. Prompt recognition and treatment of BCG sepsis is essential, given its potential for mortality.
4. MMC is the least likely absorbed intravesical chemotherapeutic agent, given its molecular weight.
5. Toxicity of MMC is usually related to irritation of the bladder and resolves with time. Nonetheless, instillation should be avoided in the setting of bladder perforation, large resection defects, or ureteral orifice resection.
6. Although MMC is frequently given perioperatively, BCG should not be given until bladder wall healing is achieved following transurethral resection.

REFERENCES

Please see www.expertconsult.com

Chapter 9

COMPLICATIONS OF HORMONAL TREATMENT FOR PROSTATE CANCER

Mischel G. Neill BHB, MBChB, FRACS
Consultant Urologist, North Shore Hospital, Auckland, New Zealand

Neil E. Fleshner FRCSC, MD, MPH
Chief of Urology, Princess Margaret Hospital, University Health Network; Associate Professor, University of Toronto, Toronto, Ontario, Canada

Surgical castration as a treatment for enlargement of the prostate first appeared in the medical literature in 1896.[1] However, the modern era of manipulation of the hormonal axis of the prostate to modify prostate cancer behavior began in 1941 with the landmark observation that men with metastatic prostate cancer had symptomatic improvement following orchiectomy.[2] Since that time, hormonal therapy has provided the mainstay of treatment for this group of patients.

In the 1960s and 1970s, studies performed by the Veterans Administration Co-operative Urological Research Group identified the significant cardiovascular mortality associated with medical castration using estrogens.[3,4] As understanding of the hormonal cascade influencing prostate cancer has been refined, medical alternatives to surgical castration or estrogens have increasingly appeared. With each modality comes morbidity, which may be viewed as a composite of side effects of changes in the hormonal milieu and side effects of the drugs themselves.

Because of the trend toward earlier treatment, the cumulative morbidity over time has become greater. Further evaluation of the effects of these therapeutic approaches on adverse treatment-related events and overall survival are ongoing. This chapter aims to review the more commonly experienced side effects of hormonal treatment for prostate cancer and management options to alleviate these effects.

OPTIONS FOR AND ADVERSE EFFECTS OF HORMONAL TREATMENT

Figure 9-1 is a simplified representation of the hormonal pathways of primary importance to benign and malignant prostatic epithelial cell growth. Interruption of these pathways is associated with degeneration of prostatic capillaries, alterations in gene expression, and cellular apoptosis.[5] Reductions in prostate gland size of between 30% and 60% may result.[6,7] Subtle differences

in effect and side effect may result, depending on the point at which the hormonal pathway is interrupted. These differences, in turn, may be used to tailor treatment to patients in whom a preponderance of one type of symptom is observed.

MEDICAL CASTRATION

Medical castration may be achieved by estrogens, luteinizing hormone–releasing hormone (LHRH) agonists, or LHRH antagonists. Because testosterone levels are reduced dramatically, these treatments also induce the androgen withdrawal syndrome. However, each treatment method has its own additional adverse effects. Symptoms associated with androgen deprivation are shown in Table 9-1.

Estrogens

Although the androgen withdrawal syndrome is associated with estrogen use, these agents cause markedly fewer vasomotor-related hot flashes and may induce less of the osteoporotic and cognitive changes seen with other forms of androgen deprivation therapy (ADT).[8-10] The two significant problems that have relegated estrogen use largely to historic interest are cardiovascular toxicity and, to a lesser extent, gynecomastia. Veterans Administration studies from the 1960s demonstrated similar overall survival outcomes for those men with metastatic prostate cancer who were taking 5 mg/day of diethylstilbestrol (DES) compared with those men undergoing orchiectomy with placebo as treatment.[3] However, this hormonal treatment was associated with a 36% increase in deaths from causes other than prostate cancer. These events were largely cardiovascular, specifically sudden cardiac death, cerebrovascular accident, and pulmonary embolus. Dose reduction to 1 mg DES decreased but did not eliminate this observation, as did concurrent administration of warfarin or aspirin.[11-13]

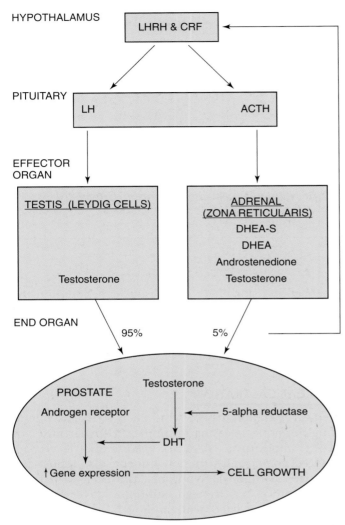

HYPOTHALAMUS

PITUITARY

EFFECTOR ORGAN

END ORGAN

95%   5%

PROSTATE
Androgen receptor
Testosterone
5-alpha reductase
DHT
↑Gene expression ⟶ CELL GROWTH

Figure 9-1 A simplified schematic representation of the hormonal axis influencing prostatic epithelial cell growth. ACTH, adrenocorticotropic hormone; CRF, corticotropin-releasing factor; DHEA, dehydroepiandrosterone; DHEA-S, dehydroepiandrosterone sulfate; DHT, dihydrotestosterone; LH, luteinizing hormone; LHRH, luteinizing hormone–releasing hormone.

TABLE 9-1	Symptoms Associated With the Androgen Deprivation Syndrome
Aspect	**Specific Changes**
Sexual function	Loss of libido, erectile dysfunction, reduced penile length and volume
Osteoporosis	Bone mineral density reduction and fracture risk
Hot flushes/flashes	Vasomotor instability causing sensation of heat, flushing, sweats, and nausea
Gynecomastia	Breast growth with or without pain (mastodynia)
Anemia	1-3 g/dL reduction in hemoglobin levels
Weight gain	Fat body mass gain ≤10% at 1 year of combined androgen blockade
Muscular strength loss	Lean body mass reduction ≤3% at 1 year of combined androgen blockade
Cognitive/mood	Attention and memory impairment, depression
Cardiovascular effects	Increased risk of cardiac events and mortality resulting from hypertension, lipid changes, insulin resistance, and electrocardiographic abnormalities
Health-related quality of life	Functional decline in multiple domains
Fatigue	Severe fatigue in 14% at 3 months that is multifactorial
Metabolic syndrome	Adverse changes in lipid profile and insulin resistance

Gynecomastia, the abnormal enlargement of male breast tissue, occurs in approximately 40% of men treated with DES.[14] It is thought to result from an excess of estrogens relative to androgens and is seen regardless of the route of estrogen delivery.[15] Gynecomastia causes mild to moderate distress in ≤80% of affected men.[16] Although a prominent feature of estrogen treatment, gynecomastia is seen with other forms of ADT and management is therefore discussed later in the chapter.

Luteinizing Hormone–releasing Hormone Agonists

As would be expected from the mechanism of action of these drugs, initial hyperstimulation of the LHRH receptors in the pituitary induces a surge of LH and therefore of testosterone. This surge translates in turn into a *tumor flare* phenomenon whereby tumor growth is acutely accelerated until the testosterone peak subsides. It is usually noted by 48 hours and peaks at 7 to 10 days. Far from being a theoretical risk in the patient with widespread metastatic disease, tumor flare frequently results in exacerbation of cancer-related bone pain and can cause paraplegia resulting from spinal cord compression. It can induce ureteric obstruction or urinary retention and was the precipitating factor leading to death in 2% of patients in a review of the phenomenon.[17] Complication prevention in this setting is eminently preferable to management, and patients with known metastatic disease are prescribed antiandrogen treatment 1 to 2 weeks before they begin taking LHRH agonists. This regimen is continued for a further 2 to 4 weeks, thereby blocking the effects of higher circulating testosterone levels.[18,19] In patients with biochemical disease progression only, however, the relevance of tumor flare is questionable, and most clinicians routinely omit prophylactic antiandrogen regimens when these patients start taking LHRH agonists.[20]

Should metastatic progression occur during the flare period, management of the specific complication may be undertaken simultaneously with instigation of antiandrogen blockade or surgical castration. Exacerbations of bone pain are relieved with combinations of nonsteroidal anti-inflammatory drugs, steroids, neuromodulators such as gabapentin, regional anesthesia, and opiates. Site-directed external beam radiation therapy may also be useful. The diagnosis of spinal cord compression should be considered in any patient with an acute exacerbation of back pain, changes in bowel and bladder function, or new-onset neurologic changes in the lower limbs or perineum. High-dose intravenous (IV) dexamethasone is administered while an emergency confirmatory magnetic resonance imaging scan of the spinal cord is obtained. Surgical decompression may be necessary for demonstrated spinal cord compression, although external beam radiation therapy may suffice for incipient cases. Urinary retention may be managed with temporary indwelling catheterization or intermittent self-catheterization. α-Blockade may be useful if it is not contraindicated.

Luteinizing Hormone–releasing Hormone Antagonists

To avoid the tumor flare response, LHRH antagonists were developed. These agents work by directly inhibiting LHRH from binding to its pituitary receptor. This therapy appears to achieve testosterone and prostate-specific antigen (PSA) responses equivalent to those observed with LHRH agonists, at least in the short term, but is limited by a 3.6% anaphylactic response rate.[21,22] Currently, because of the availability of other means of ADT, indications for the use of LHRH antagonists are few.

ANTIANDROGENS

The effects of antiandrogenic agents result from blockade of the action of testosterone on the cells of end organs, including prostate cancer cells. The group may further be subdivided into steroidal and nonsteroidal forms, a difference important in that it distinguishes the effect and side effect profile. Broadly speaking, nonsteroidal forms work purely by competitive inhibition of the androgen receptor. As a result they induce positive feedback to the hypothalamic-pituitary axis that increases circulating testosterone. Steroidal antiandrogens, by contrast, competitively inhibit the androgen receptor but also provide negative feedback to the hypothalamic-pituitary axis, with resulting reductions of circulating testosterone.

Nonsteroidal Antiandrogens

Although the "pure" antiandrogens share a similar mode of action, side effects vary among individual drugs, and this variability has important therapeutic consequences. If one agent must be discontinued for reasons of toxicity, this does not necessarily preclude others as alternatives. The agents have different half-lives, ranging from 6 hours (flutamide) to 1 week (bicalutamide), with correspondingly different dosing intervals. Less frequent dosing intervals may favor compliance with treatment. Of the three agents in this group, nilutamide is not recommended by its manufacturer for use as single-agent treatment and is less extensively evaluated in clinical trials.

One of the leading reasons for interest in antiandrogens is the potential to preserve sexual function. Nonsteroidal agents have a theoretical advantage over steroidal forms in that circulating testosterone levels are generally preserved. Sexual function is more complex than just hormonal levels, and one of the interesting findings from Scandinavian bicalutamide studies was the decline in sexual function in the placebo arm of the trials that was commensurate with the diagnosis of prostate cancer.[23] In this study, at almost 1 year after randomization, 63% of men receiving 150 mg of bicalutamide had remained sexually active, as opposed to 78% in the placebo arm of the study.

Multiple small trials have evaluated the effect of flutamide on sexual function; however, results vary widely. Perhaps the best designed of these studies compared flutamide with the steroidal antiandrogen cyproterone acetate (CPA) and showed a surprisingly high (78%) loss of sexual activity.[24] Studies of flutamide in men with benign prostatic hypertrophy estimated a less than 10% loss of sexual function.[25] In a small, methodologically suspect trial, 58% of men receiving nilutamide retained their potency.[25] Overall, although no direct assessment has been undertaken and the trials in general are limited, preservation of sexual function would seem to be best achieved by bicalutamide in this group.

Hot flashes are thought to relate to the vasomotor instability that results from changes in circulating hormone levels, although the exact mechanisms have not been fully elucidated.[26] They can induce significant morbidity to the point of interfering with daily function and causing sleep disturbance.[27] The progestational effects of CPA mean that this agent is frequently used as a treatment for hot flashes following castration. However, these effects are not shared by nonsteroidal antiandrogens. Generally, the incidence of hot flashes with this group is not nearly as marked as that seen with castration, as a result of the preservation of circulating testosterone. A pooled analysis of two trials comparing bicalutamide with castration by orchiectomy or goserelin showed the incidence of hot flashes to be 13% and

50%, respectively.[28] Flutamide had similarly low hot flash rates of 7% as opposed to 26% in comparison with orchiectomy.[29] Once again, direct comparisons among agents with a standardized instrument for assessment have not been made, but as a class, nonsteroidal antiandrogens do not appear to differ widely in the rate at which they induce hot flashes.

During treatment with nonsteroidal antiandrogens, circulating estrogen levels rise because of aromatization of testosterone in peripheral tissues, and this is thought to be the underlying mechanism for the development of gynecomastia.[30] Why this complication should affect some men and not others and should be associated with pain in some men but not in others is not fully understood. Higher rates of gynecomastia are seen with DES therapy and combined androgen blockade (CAB) (40%-50%) than with LHRH agonists alone (25%), orchiectomy (10%), or CPA (<10%).[31-33] Gynecomastia is one of the most frequent and troubling side effects seen during treatment with nonsteroidal antiandrogens. The incidence appears comparable with each of the agents; it ranges widely but averages approximately 50%.[34]

Changes in bone mineral density (BMD) are commonly seen with ADT at rates ≤5% per year on CAB, as opposed to 1% in men not receiving ADT.[35] Bicalutamide monotherapy is thought to maintain BMD over a 2-year period and shows a reduction in biochemical markers of bone turnover compared with medical castration.[36,37] Similar evidence for other antiandrogens is lacking at this time.

All antiandrogens have been associated with hepatotoxicity to some degree and induce the cytochrome P-450 system. This feature may lead to multiple drug interactions such as with warfarin.[38] Liver function tests (LFTs) and PSA monitoring are recommended after treatment with these agents is initiated. Generally, although not without exception, hepatotoxicity is mild to moderate, and abnormalities of blood values are reversible on discontinuation of the drug. Flutamide may induce liver enzyme abnormalities in ≤25% of patients and has an estimated incidence of significant and potentially fatal hepatotoxicity of 3 in 100,000.[38,39] The incidence of LFT elevations with bicalutamide in the Early Prostate Cancer Program was 3.1%.[40]

Agent-specific side effects in the nonsteroidal antiandrogen group are not insignificant. These side effects are important to recognize as drug related in the management of patients with prostate cancer, to optimize care and to avoid overinvestigation. Flutamide has bothersome gastrointestinal side effects, particularly diarrhea, in more than one third of users. Nilutamide use is associated with visual impairments of dark adaptation in 30%, alcohol intolerance in 19%, and interstitial pneumonitis in 1% of patients.[38,41] Bicalutamide has perhaps the most favorable side effect profile and has the added advantage of once-daily dosing, although painful gynecomastia is significantly limiting for many men receiving this treatment. Whether this complication is a greater problem for men receiving bicalutamide than for men taking the other nonsteroidal antiandrogens has not been formally assessed in a randomized controlled trial (RCT).

Steroidal Antiandrogens

CPA, the main agent in this group, is not available in the United States but is widely used elsewhere; megestrol acetate has similar attributes. The synthetic derivative of hydroxyprogesterone, CPA has progestational effects that reduce serum testosterone levels to approximately 25% of normal, and this action has numerous subsequent effects in terms of symptoms.[21] In a small RCT, CPA was shown to reduce the number of hot flashes following orchiectomy.[42] Gynecomastia is relatively infrequent, and although CPA was used previously for "sexual delinquency," libido and sexual function are ablated less than with LHRH agonists or surgical castration.[22] Although improvements in bone preservation relative to castration may theoretically be predicted, this possibility has been inadequately evaluated in the medical literature to date such that firm conclusions may not be drawn.

Hepatotoxicity is seen rarely and is generally mild to moderate. This effect is usually reversible on discontinuing the drug. Monitoring of serum LFTs and of PSA response is recommended for patients receiving CPA. Case reports exist of fatalities from fulminant hepatic failure and of new-onset hepatocellular carcinomas.[34]

Dyspnea is not infrequently seen with cyproterone (as with nonsteroidal antiandrogen) use. In the case of CPA, dyspnea is thought to represent stimulation of the respiratory center by progestational effect and is seen particularly in patients with preexisting respiratory dysfunction.[43]

The European Organisation for Research and Treatment of Cancer protocol 30892 compared monotherapy with flutamide with monotherapy with cyproterone as first-line agents for metastatic prostate cancer.[24] The trial was underpowered to show any difference in survival between the two arms and did not, although significant differences in side effects between the drugs were demonstrated. CPA had significantly reduced rates of painful gynecomastia and gastrointestinal adverse events and resulted in approximately 2.5 times fewer treatment cessations. Conversely, sexual activity was preserved in 11.8% of men taking CPA and in 21.9% taking flutamide, with median time to loss being 8.9 and 12.9 months, respectively.[44] These results were not significantly different, and potency at the start of the trial was on the order of only 25% for each group. With increasingly early detection, primary treatment, and biochemical failure, a growing subgroup of relatively young men having greater initial potency will be considering the use of hormonal ablation. This group represents men for whom the absolute percentages seen in this study are unlikely to apply.

INHIBITORS OF STEROID SYNTHESIS

Historically, surgical hypophysectomy and adrenalectomy were used to ablate the roughly 10% of androgen production contributed by the adrenal glands. Subsequently, these very morbid interventions were replaced by drugs that either suppressed adrenocorticotropic hormone release from the hypophysis, such as corticosteroids, or interfered with the metabolic function of the adrenal cortex, such as ketoconazole, aminoglutethimide, and spironolactone. These drugs are no longer used routinely as front-line agents in management of metastatic prostate cancer, but they do have some demonstrated efficacy. Contemporary management of hormone-refractory prostate cancer has moved toward clinical trials of chemotherapeutic agents such as taxanes either because of limited response rates and duration or because of significant toxicity or both. In select circumstances, such as the inability to access relevant trials and patient motivation to persist with further treatment, these agents remain a valid therapeutic option.

Ketoconazole

Ketoconazole is an imidazole antifungal that interferes with the cytochrome P-450–mediated hydroxylation reactions of the adrenal cortex (and testis) and ablates adrenal androgen production in this manner. For absorption to occur, gastric acidity is required; therefore, supplemental vitamin C, cola, or orange juice at the time of administration may be useful, especially if the patient is taking histamine (H_2) antagonists or proton pump inhibitors. If it is uncertain that the drug is being absorbed, blood levels may be monitored (usually taken 4 hours after the morning dose). Dosage must be adjusted for patients with significant hepatic dysfunction. Castrate level serum testosterone values are reached within 48 hours of initiating ketoconazole.[45] When urgent androgen ablation is required and surgical orchiectomy is contraindicated or unavailable, ketoconazole represents a viable therapeutic option.

The action of ketoconazole is not specific to the adrenal, and toxicity from the drug is significant. Even in the setting of well-motivated patients with good medical support in an RCT, the discontinuation rate resulting from toxicity approaches 20%.[46] In addition to adrenal suppression, ketoconazole may induce wide-ranging gastrointestinal upset, particularly diarrhea, nausea, and vomiting, as well as dyspepsia, abdominal pain, and gastrointestinal hemorrhage. It rarely induces serious hepatic dysfunction; however, mild LFT derangement is seen more commonly and should be tested for

specifically while patients undergo treatment. A disulfiram-like response to alcohol is commonly seen, with vomiting, headache, and flushing the predominant features. Skin reactions such as dermatitis and alopecia may be seen, as may all the features of androgen deprivation. Among the most common and debilitating side effects of ketoconazole are profound fatigue, subjective weakness, and objective loss of strength; some investigators stress the importance of muscle-building exercise programs.[47] Small studies using lower doses of ketoconazole (200 or 300 mg three times daily) have shown comparable biochemical responses. However, toxicity is still seen in more than one third of patients, and 15% of patients in one study withdrew from the trial as a direct result.[47,48]

Complications of the use of ketoconazole are prevented to some degree by the prophylactic use of steroid replacement (20 mg hydrocortisone twice daily or 7.5 mg prednisone once daily with 0.3 mg fludrocortisone once daily). Addisonian crisis results from adrenal insufficiency and often manifests following a physical stressor (e.g., infection) with agitated confusion, abdominal pain, fever, and orthostatic hypotension that progresses to refractory circulatory collapse. Patients have associated hyponatremia, hyperkalemia, and hypoglycemia. This condition is treated with aggressive fluid management with normal saline and correction of biochemical abnormalities. IV hydrocortisone (200 mg) is given as soon as venous access is established, and then a regimen of 100 mg every 8 hours is commenced. This approach represents a "stress dose" that is gradually tapered down to the physiologic dose described earlier. Hydrocortisone can be used as a single agent because it has both glucocorticoid and mineralocorticoid properties, but if prednisone is to be used, this should be supplemented with fludrocortisone to avoid the biochemical changes that will otherwise eventuate.[48]

Less profound side effects of ketoconazole may be managed prospectively with simple analgesics, antiemetics, and antidiarrheals. Avoidance of alcohol and the use of regular muscle mass–preserving exercise programs may be beneficial. Patients should undergo regular liver enzyme assessment in addition to PSA monitoring. Ultimately, ketoconazole is usually discontinued for toxicity or failure of treatment benefit.

MANAGEMENT OF HORMONAL THERAPY–RELATED TOXICITY

Three approaches may be taken to the management of hormone therapy related toxicity:

1. Therapeutic maneuvers can be undertaken preemptively to prevent or at least lessen the expected impact of the therapy
2. Further treatment can be commenced in response to specific side effects as they arise

3. Therapy can be avoided, or, more specifically, the timing of therapy can be manipulated to reduce patient exposure to it and therefore the degree of symptoms. This option underlies the debates on early versus delayed intervention and the concept of intermittent androgen deprivation (IAD).

Management of Specific Toxicities

Interest is growing in the prevention and management of many of the consequences of ADT that have a direct impact on health and quality of life. Chief issues among these currently are sexual function, bone health, and the cardiovascular sequelae of metabolic changes.

Sexual Function

Definitive treatments of prostate cancer have well-documented negative impacts on sexual function; however, men who then undergo ADT fare even more poorly in this regard.[49] Testosterone is an important component of the incompletely understood complex that is male sexual function. Although testosterone has a profound impact on libido, it has several peripheral effects that contribute to sexual function as well. Testosterone has been shown to have a direct effect on cavernosal nerve size and function.[50] Investigators have observed that penile length and volume are reduced during ADT, possibly from reductions in penile tissue oxygenation and fibrosis.[51] Additionally, when considering the impact of hormonal treatment, the seemingly self-evident statement that not all men start with good sexual function must be borne in mind. Factors such as age, preexisting low testosterone levels, psychogenic causes, and medications and the comorbidities for which they are taken may all contribute to impaired sexual function.

The Prostate Cancer Outcomes Study addressed the impact of 1 year of ADT alone on sexual function in men with prostate cancer.[52] No sexual interest was reported by 63.6% of men who underwent orchiectomy and by 58% of men undergoing LHRH agonist treatment, up from 27.6% and 31.7%, respectively, at the start of the study. No spontaneous erections were reported by 78.6% of patients who had undergone orchiectomy and by 73.3% of patients who had received LHRH agonists. Men who underwent orchiectomy reported rates of sexual activity at 1 year that were similar to rates in men receiving LHRH agonist treatments, 17.2% versus 19.8% (down from 52.1% and 55% at entry into the study). Despite the much discussed impact of orchiectomy on cosmesis and self-image, no significant differences in sexual activity were reported between the groups at 1 year. Also of interest is the point that libido and sexual function are not simply direct correlates of testosterone level.

In the approximately 40% of men who preserve their libido despite ADT, standard options for the management of erectile dysfunction may be pursued. Having determined that help is being sought for erectile dysfunction rather than for an absence of libido, a full initial history and examination are followed by stepwise progression through treatment options. Further questioning should focus on sexual understanding and expectations, additional problems such as pain or curvature with erections suggestive of Peyronie disease, and medications the patient is taking and the comorbidities for which they are taken. This assessment offers the opportunity to assess blood parameters such as PSA, testosterone levels, and LFTs (if indicated, depending on the type of ADT). Increasingly realized as directly relevant to urologic treatment and general well-being, lipid profile and blood glucose control (glycosylated hemoglobin [HbA$_{1c}$]) should be incorporated into the laboratory screening at this time as well.

Oral phosphodiesterase inhibitors have become the accepted front-line option, and most urologists suggest trials of different agents within the same drug class if this approach is initially unsuccessful. Other options for oral medications include apomorphine hydrochloride and various agents in complementary and alternative medicine (CAM). Failure of oral agents is then followed by local nonsurgical treatments such as intraurethral alprostadil or intracavernosal injections, most commonly using a combination of papaverine, alprostadil, and phentolamine. Mechanical vacuum constriction devices that use a vacuum pump and ring deployed at the base of the penis are simple and effective, and they achieve good patient satisfaction levels. If each of these options fails or is contraindicated and the patient is suitably motivated, surgical implantation of a penile prosthesis remains. Contemporary management usually involves the insertion of a three-piece inflatable prosthesis; however, many variations exist. Patient satisfaction with this device is generally high, although many patients require surgical revision with time.[53]

When patients have no sexual interest, attempts to treat them with increasingly invasive therapeutic options for erectile dysfunction have little benefit. As mentioned previously, the male libido is a composite of more elements than just the serum testosterone level. Psychogenic factors related to cancer diagnosis and treatment combine with partner opinion and are overlaid on the physiologic environment. Sexual counseling may be of value in this regard. Otherwise, preservation of libido focuses mainly on manipulating the form and timing of ADT. Delaying the commencement of ADT is an option that should be discussed with the patient. Although immediate ADT has clear benefits over delaying treatment until disease progression, choice of a point of intervention between the two extremes based on an arbitrary PSA value has not been adequately addressed to allow a clear recommendation. Alternatively, the stratagem of IAD offers promise and allows the return of potency for many men during the drug holiday interval.

Hot Flashes

Hot flashes, a term interchangeable with *hot flushes*, occur suddenly but may last anywhere from a few seconds to an hour and may occur every day or only once a week. Patients note a sensation of heat that affects the face, neck, upper chest, and back and may be associated with facial flushing, profuse sweating, and nausea. Hot flashes vary in intensity from mild (well tolerated) to severe (interfering with everyday activity and sleep). They may decline in frequency and severity with time but equally may persist unchanged. Episodes can be provoked by consumption of hot liquids, changes in body position, stress, or heat, or they may occur spontaneously.[54] Investigators have theorized that the pathologic mechanism for hot flashes results from decreased testosterone (or estrogen in women) feedback at the hypothalamus. The subsequent reduction of endogenous peptide production, in turn, promotes local catecholamine generation. This process intermittently stimulates the nearby thermoregulatory center, induces instability, and results in symptoms.[54,55]

The incidence of hot flashes varies with the type of ADT. Up to 66% of men taking LHRH agonists are affected to some degree with hot flashes, and up to one fourth of patients find them very distressing.[56,57] A pooled analysis of two trials comparing bicalutamide with castration by orchiectomy or goserelin showed the incidence of hot flashes to be 13% and 50%, respectively.[28] Flutamide had a similarly low hot flash rate of 7% as opposed to a 26% rate associated with orchiectomy.[29] Unlike other forms of ADT, estrogens are used in the treatment of hot flashes, as are steroidal antiandrogens because of their stabilizing progestational effects (Table 9-2).

DES, one of the oldest forms of hormonal manipulation in prostate cancer management, has the additional advantage of treating hot flushes when they are induced by other forms of ADT.[58] As mentioned previously, because of the significant cardiovascular toxicity and, to a lesser extent, the high gynecomastia rates seen with this medication, it is no longer being used frequently, and in some countries it is not even available. Rates of approximately 70% (complete) and 20% (partial) response may be seen with even low doses of DES.[59] Parenteral estrogens avoid cardiovascular side effects and prevent hot flushes at the expense of significant gynecomastia.[60] Transdermal estrogens represent a more promising delivery mode, with 83% of patients reporting some improvement in their symptoms; the higher dose (0.1 mg twice a week) is approximately three times more effective than is the low dose (0.05 mg twice a week) but is associated with significantly more gynecomastia.[61]

Megestrol acetate is a progestin that was shown to decrease hot flashes by ≤85% in a placebo-controlled crossover trial using 20 mg twice daily.[62] Its side effect profile includes chills in 54%, weight gain in 12%, and

TABLE 9-2	Treatment Options and Dosing Schedule for Troublesome Hot Flashes
Agent	**Dosing Schedule**
Megestrol acetate	20 mg PO daily or bid
Medroxyprogesterone acetate	400 mg IM monthly
Cyproterone acetate	50 mg PO daily
Venlafaxine hydrochloride	37.5 mg PO daily initially increased to 75 mg PO daily PRN
Estrogen	Transdermal patch 0.1 mg applied twice weekly
	Oral DES 1 mg PO daily
Gabapentin	300 mg PO daily (titrate upward base on pain control)
Soy	75 mg PO daily (or general increase in dietary consumption)
Vitamin E	150 IU PO daily (not >400 IU/day)
Black cohosh	160 mg PO daily
Acupuncture	Weekly PRN

bid, twice daily; DES, diethylstilbestrol; IM, intramuscularly; PO, orally; PRN, as needed.

exacerbation of carpal tunnel–related symptoms in 4%. Megestrol is thought to be of no benefit in the prevention of osteoporosis. Perhaps most concerning, however, was a widely cited case report of biochemical disease progression that then reversed on discontinuation of the drug.[34] If megestrol acetate is prescribed for hot flushes, PSA monitoring should be frequent, and discontinuation of the drug with assessment of PSA response should be undertaken before further alterations are made in the ADT regimen if PSA progression occurs.

Medroxyprogesterone acetate (MPA) also known as Depo-Provera, is given intramuscularly, once a month at a 400-mg dose. Timing of the injections may be titrated out further than monthly, depending on the response. Response rates were high in a small retrospective study; 90% of patients had some response, approximately half completely responded, and some responses persisted after the medication was stopped.[63] Further evaluation of efficacy is required with a prospective RCT. The side effect profile appeared minimal, although it was not particularly well assessed in the study quoted. Certain potential problems with this agent in female patients have been identified in the literature. Salt and fluid retention may exacerbate congestive heart failure; as with megestrol, increased appetite and weight gain are often seen, and concern exists about the loss of BMD in women using this drug for contraception. As the authors of the foregoing study suggest, until further information is available in the context of ADT and prostate cancer, "it would be prudent to follow their bone mineral density closely during the first few years of MPA treatment."

The steroidal antiandrogen CPA, although not available in the United States, is widely used elsewhere in the hormonal manipulation of prostate cancer. One of its favorable attributes is its significant impact on hot flash occurrence. When CPA is given in doses of 50 mg daily, hot flashes may be reduced by ≤80%, in line with the other progestational agents reviewed earlier.[64] The side effect profile is discussed earlier in this chapter.

For the patient troubled by hot flashes concurrent with depressive symptoms, selective serotonin reuptake inhibitors may represent a good treatment option. Venlafaxine hydrochloride is the best evaluated of these drugs, although paroxetine has been studied as well. Venlafaxine is started at 37.5 mg daily and is increased to 75 mg daily if needed and well tolerated. The side effect profile is usually minimal, although dry mouth, tremor, drowsiness, constipation, and sexual dysfunction may be bothersome. As with most antidepressants, mood changes do not tend to occur before 2 weeks of use. Small trials with placebo controls demonstrated efficacy exceeding 50% for hot flashes.[65,66]

In a meta-analysis of two well-designed RCTs, the anticonvulsant gabapentin showed a 20% to 30% improvement in menopausally related hot flushes in women; however, experience with this drug in men receiving ADT is limited to case reports.[67] Given that this medication is used frequently in chronic pain management, it represents an option worth considering in the patient with metastatic prostate cancer in whom pain is an issue and hot flash control has been suboptimal. Although clonidine showed a 13% to 26% improvement in hot flashes in four out of seven RCTs in women with a benefit indicated at meta-analysis, a well-designed RCT for men after orchiectomy failed to show any benefit.[67,68]

CAM use is popular and increasing rapidly.[69] Many CAM therapies have been suggested for the treatment of hot flushes, and because they are perceived as "natural," they are often of greater appeal to patients. As with CAM in other fields of medicine, rigorous scientific evaluation is generally lacking. It is difficult to know how to advise men with a strong preference for CAM with regard to treating hot flushes. Currently, no high-level evidence supports the use of these agents, and any effects on symptoms are likely to be largely if not entirely those that would be seen with placebo. Conversely, many men experiment with CAM regardless, and with the burgeoning interest in soy and vitamin E in prostate cancer chemoprevention as well as the serum lipid level–altering properties of soy products, perhaps these may be acceptable first-line CAM suggestions.[70,72]

Gynecomastia and Mastodynia

Traditionally, *gynecomastia* (abnormal enlargement of male breast tissue) and *mastodynia* (breast tenderness or pain) have been well-recognized complications of ADT; however, the incidence has proved more difficult to determine. Hypogonadism predisposes patients to gynecomastia, and as such the incidence of this condition is increased in elderly men not receiving ADT as compared with younger men.[16] Moreover, information collected in ADT trials on adverse events is often incomplete or fails to use a standardized instrument to quantify symptoms in a way that allows comparison among studies. Most authors either use the Marshall-Tanner puberty staging system or simply measure the amount of palpable breast tissue.[73] Gynecomastia is thought to result from an excess of estrogens relative to androgens and causes mild to moderate distress in ≤80% of affected men.[16,73] The incidence associated with DES has been reported at 40%, although recorded rates in more recent studies of parenteral estrogens were in the order of 70%.[13,31] Rates of gynecomastia following orchiectomy and with CPA have consistently been ≤10%.[42,43,74] Although gynecomastia is associated with LHRH agonists in approximately 25% of patients, the development of nonsteroidal antiandrogen monotherapy, especially with high-dose bicalutamide, has rekindled interest in this subject because gynecomastia occurs in approximately 50% of patients.[28,42]

Gynecomastia most frequently manifests as bilateral change, and any unilateral swelling, particularly if hard, warrants further evaluation for malignancy with mammography and biopsy. Gynecomastia appears to have a time-dependent aspect of reversibility. Patients whose bicalutamide therapy was stopped within 6 months had resolution of their symptoms 64% of the time as opposed to 29% if the treatment had been ongoing for 18 months.[75] This effect is hypothesized to reflect chronic tissue changes such as fibrosis and hyalinization.[76] Treatment of gynecomastia should therefore be initiated early. Treatment options range from prophylactic breast irradiation through medical therapies to surgical excision with subareolar mastectomy or liposuction (Table 9-3).

TABLE 9-3	Treatment Options for Gynecomastia and Mastodynia
Option	**Treatment Details**
Prophylactic radiation	10-15 Gy as a single fraction
Tamoxifen	20 mg PO daily
Anastrazole	1 mg PO daily
Liposuction	Outpatient based (under local anesthetic)
Subareolar mastectomy	Outpatient based (under local anesthetic)

PO, orally.

Prophylactic irradiation of breast tissue reduces the incidence of gynecomastia when radiation is delivered before ADT with flutamide, bicalutamide, and estrogen.[76-79] The dose that has been given in RCTs of radiation therapy ranges between 10 and 15 Gy, usually given as a single fraction. In the flutamide study of 253 men at 1 year of follow-up, rates of gynecomastia (28% versus 71%) and mastodynia (43% versus 75%) were both significantly better when breast tissue was irradiated before patients started ADT.[80] Overall improvements are seen in 30% to 40% of men. Therapeutic radiation is effective for some men in relieving mastodynia (more so than gynecomastia), a finding reflecting chronic breast tissue changes that occur with time.[76] Adverse effects are reported as minimal.[76]

Pharmacologic attempts at preventing glandular proliferation have been focused on competing with estrogenic stimulation at the receptor level. An RCT based on bicalutamide therapy compared placebo with tamoxifen (20 mg orally once daily) or anastrozole (1 mg orally once daily) over a 48-week period.[81] Gynecomastia was seen least in the tamoxifen group (10%) and most in the placebo group (73%), with the anastrozole group intermediate (51%). Mastodynia rates followed similar trends (6%, 39%, and 27%, respectively), and both results were statistically significant. An RCT of 102 patients receiving 150 mg bicalutamide as adjuvant treatment following radical prostatectomy compared a control group (no intervention) with a tamoxifen group (10 mg once daily) with a prophylactic radiation group (12 Gy). With a minimum follow-up of 1 year, both gynecomastia and mastodynia rates favored the tamoxifen group (8% and 7%) over the radiation group (34% and 30%) over the control group (67% and 58%). No statistically significant differences were noted in quality of life between the radiation and tamoxifen groups.[82] Therefore, of the nonsurgical options for treatment of gynecomastia, tamoxifen appears the most promising, with the one caveat of uncertainty about whether it influences overall survival rates.

Surgical techniques for the relief of established gynecomastia are numerous.[83] These form the main therapeutic option for established gynecomastia, particularly if it is of long standing (>18 months) or extensive (Marshall-Tanner grade ≥3). Current practice involves either subareolar mastectomy or liposuction.[84] These techniques may be performed on an outpatient basis, often with the use of a local anesthetic. Complications most commonly seen include hematoma or seroma formation, which may require prolonged drainage, and infection, which usually responds to antibiotics and drainage. Cosmetic difficulties with skin reduction and residual glandular tissue may be problematic.

Osteoporosis

The loss of BMD is a significant problem with some forms of ADT, and the long-term consequences have come under increasing scrutiny. Investigators have estimated from longitudinal and cross-sectional studies that BMD loss occurs at approximately 4% per annum.[85] This finding compares with approximately 1% per annum for men in a similar age group without ADT.[86] A study based on Surveillance, Epidemiology and End Results (SEER) and Medicare databases in the United States looked at the risk of fracture for >50,000 men with prostate cancer as a function of whether they received ADT.[87] The risk of fracture for men who received ADT was 19.4% as opposed to 12.6% for men who did not. The risk increased in direct proportion to the number of doses of LHRH agonist administered. The number needed to harm (i.e., to cause a fracture) over a 1- to 5-year period was 28 for men receiving LHRH agonists and 16 for men who underwent orchiectomy. Men in their first year of ADT were 1.5 times as likely to sustain a fracture and 1.7 times as likely to require hospitalization as a result. Most fractures occur predominantly at femoral neck, vertebral, and distal forearm sites.[86] The effects on BMD are detectable within 9 months of starting LHRH agonists and 6 months of orchiectomy.[88] Most bone loss appears to occur in the first year but continues beyond that at a slower rate. Osteoporosis is thought to be less of an issue with estrogen or antiandrogen monotherapy, although studies are few.[13,35,73,89]

Osteoporosis is defined as 2.5 or more standard deviations below normal levels for young adults. *Osteopenia* is 1 to 2.5 standard deviations below normal. For women, each standard deviation below normal corresponds to a twofold increase in fracture risk.[90] A retrospective study of 181 men with prostate cancer who were receiving ADT and a median of 47 months of follow-up reported a risk of osteoporotic fracture five times higher than in age-matched healthy controls, with a 20% incidence by 10 years.[86] The retrospective nature of the study made it difficult to assess the relative contribution of ADT to these skeletal events, however. More interestingly, the following risk factors were identified from this study: the duration of ADT, race (European at higher risk than African American), and body mass index <25 kg/m².

Diagnosis of osteoporosis is based on screening with radiologic testing of sites such as the hip, lumbar spine, and forearm. Of the two most commonly used radiologic techniques for evaluating BMD, dual-energy x-ray absorptiometry (DXA) is generally preferred to quantitative computed tomography (QCT) for reasons of cost, accessibility, and reduced radiation exposure. Spondyloarthropathy, facet joint disease, and aortic calcification may all artificially elevate spinal BMD and therefore for practical purposes femoral neck DXA is used routinely for diagnosis, whereas spinal and total hip BMDs are used for monitoring BMD over time.[85,91] Ideally, all men commencing ADT should undergo bone densitometry studies, but especially men with any of the identified risk factors. This testing should be repeated at regular intervals throughout treatment. Although optimal timing for this testing has not been established, the initial follow-up imaging should probably be within the first 1 to 2 years, when the rate of BMD loss is greatest.

All men with a diagnosis of incurable prostate cancer should be encouraged to undertake lifestyle changes to improve their bone health because even men not receiving ADT are at increased risk of osteoporosis. These general measures include smoking cessation, moderation of alcohol consumption, and regular weight-bearing exercise. Dietary supplements of 400 to 800 IU/day vitamin D (to keep serum 25 hydroxyvitamin D level >15 ng/mL or > 50 nmol/L) and calcium to maintain a daily intake of 1200 mg/day are suggested.[90-92]

Much interest has been displayed in the bisphosphonate drug class for maintenance of BMD. These drugs work by binding to the bone mineral surfaces in areas of high bone turnover, are then ingested by and inhibit the activity of osteoclasts, and subsequently achieve reduced osteolysis and bone resorption (Table 9-4).[93] Several studies showed alendronate to preserve BMD and reduce fracture rates in men with osteoporosis.[94,95] A retrospective cohort study suggested BMD gains from alendronate in men with prostate cancer.[96] Alendronate is associated with erosive esophagitis, and absorption is reduced if the drug is taken with food and other medica-

tions. Therefore, the manufacturers recommend that alendronate be taken in the morning with water on an otherwise empty stomach with the patient in the upright position for at least 30 minutes. This drug is the subject of ongoing trials in the context of ADT.

Etidronate was previously shown to prevent BMD loss in ADT in a small, open-label study, although the other two IV agents have been the more intensively studied.[85] Pamidronate, 60 mg given every 12 weeks, prevents bone loss in men receiving ADT for prostate cancer; however, bone turnover marker fluctuations suggested that this dosing regimen may have been suboptimal.[97,98] These studies did not address whether treatment had an effect on the incidence of skeletal-related events.

Zoledronic acid, a third-generation bisphosphonate with greatly increased in vitro potency, has been evaluated in RCTs for the prevention of both BMD loss and of skeletal-related events resulting from metastatic prostate cancer. Specifically, the drug was evaluated in the prevention of BMD loss in men with prostate cancer who were starting ADT in a multicenter randomized study of 106 patients who received the 4-mg dose every 3 months for 1 year.[99] BMD at the lumbar spine increased by 5.6% (and to a lesser extent in the femoral neck and total hip assessments) compared with a 2.2% decrease on placebo, and this finding was statistically significant ($P < .001$).

Bisphosphonates must be taken with vitamin D and calcium supplements to be effective, these drugs and have certain side effects that deserve mention.[100-102] Bisphosphonates are often associated with flulike symptoms and gastrointestinal side effects such as esophagitis, ulceration, epigastric pain, nausea, and constipation. Anemia and hypophosphatemia should be tested for, as should renal function, which is particularly affected by zoledronic acid at higher doses (8 mg) in more concentrated infusions.

Injection site reactions and osteonecrosis of the jaw have been observed. Several hundred case reports of osteonecrosis of the jaw have been published, and the osteonecrosis is thought to represent an avascular phenomenon related to antiangiogenic properties of the drug class.[103] This complication manifests as ulceration with the exposure of underlying visibly necrotic bone that may or may not be painful and occurs usually 1 to 3 years after the institution of treatment.[103] The risk has been estimated at 1% to 10% with long-term bisphosphonate use.[104] Prevention is important because, once established, this problem is difficult to eliminate. Before starting bisphosphonates, the patient should be screened for dental problems by a dentist, and any necessary work should be performed. Education on the importance of dental hygiene should be undertaken as well. Once the disorder is established, treatment of osteonecrosis of the jaw includes discontinuation of bisphosphonate therapy, long-term antibiosis, and surgical

TABLE 9-4	Summary Table for the Recommended Doses of Agents Useful in the Prevention of Osteoporosis for Men on Hormonal Treatment of Prostate Cancer
Agent	**Recommended Dosing**
Calcium supplements	To maintain daily dietary intake of 1200 mg/day
Vitamin D	400-800 IU/day
Exercise	Weight bearing 3 times/wk
Deferred treatment	
Intermittent androgen deprivation	
Bicalutamide	150 mg daily as monotherapy
Transdermal estradiol	6 × 0.1 mg patches replaced every 7 days
Alendronate	70 mg PO q1wk (taken upright with water; vitamin D and calcium supplements required as well) or 10 mg OD
Pamidronate	60 mg q12wk slow IV infusion (vitamin D and calcium supplements required as well)
Zoledronate	4-8 mg q12wk slow IV infusion (vitamin D and calcium supplements required as well)

IV, intravenous; OD, once daily; PO, orally.

débridement, although this therapy is regarded as palliation rather than cure of the problem.[104]

Body Composition and Metabolic Changes

Serum testosterone has a direct bearing on fat and muscle mass, and replacing testosterone deficiency increases lean body mass, protein synthesis, and muscle strength.[105-108] These effects may be mediated at least in part by insulin-like growth factor I and growth hormone.[109] Men receiving ADT gain weight, with an increase in the percentage of body fat and a decrease in the percentage of body muscle. Prospective (although uncontrolled) studies comparing body composition before and 6 to 12 months after the initiation of ADT showed increases in body mass index between 1.6% and 2.4%.[105,110,111] In addition, fat body mass increases of 9.4% and lean body mass decreases of 2.7% after 1 year of CAB have been demonstrated.[112] Further studies using CAB have shown median weight gain of 6 kg and loss of muscle strength with long-term use.[112,113] Fat deposition is both subcutaneous and visceral and results in abdominal obesity.[112]

As would be expected with these changes in body composition, certain serum lipid changes develop. In one of the previously mentioned studies, increases in total cholesterol by 9% and triglycerides by 26.5% were accompanied by increases in high-density and low-density lipoproteins (11.3% and 7.3%, respectively).[114] A cross-sectional study comparing men with prostate cancer who were receiving ADT with men with prostate cancer who were not receiving ADT and with age-matched controls without prostate cancer identified a significant negative correlation between testosterone levels and markers of the metabolic syndrome, including fasting glucose levels, insulin levels, leptins, and an index for insulin resistance.[113] A further study from the same researchers identified a >50% incidence of metabolic syndrome in men receiving long-term ADT.[114] Both LHRH agonists and orchiectomy increase the likelihood of a diabetes mellitus diagnosis.[115] Insulin resistance is thought to result from increases in adipokines that have, in turn, increased because of visceral fat accumulation.[116] Insulin resistance and the metabolic syndrome are independent predictors of cardiovascular mortality.[117-119]

The loss of muscle mass and the issue of patient-identified weakness are common problems with potential for improvement. Exercise in the form of strength training with either an isometric or an isokinetic focus leads to improvements in both type 1 slow-twitch (oxidative) and type 2 fast-twitch (glycolytic) muscle fiber populations.[120] Many studies have demonstrated the benefits of strength training for elderly persons.[121-124] The benefits in muscle strength combined with weight and glycemic control, as well as preservation of cardiovascular and bone health, make this a logical intervention.[123,124]

The growing evidence of adverse metabolic changes on ADT that predispose patients to cardiovascular complications emphasizes the importance of screening and prevention that have until recently remained unaddressed. Monitoring of serum lipid profiles, glycemic control (e.g., fasting glucose and HbA_{1c} levels), blood pressure, waist circumference, and weight are simple office-based assessments that would enable early recognition and effective management of metabolic complications. Advice on exercise, cessation of smoking, and dietary modification should be offered and combined with early referral to a cardiologist for antihypertensive and statin-based treatment or an endocrinologist for diabetes control.

In addition to fat and muscle mass changes that occur with ADT, many men notice changes in the nature, growth rate, and distribution of their hair.[125] Some patients have an increase in their scalp hair but a dramatic loss of body hair. Beards may grow less rapidly and become less coarse, so men may need to shave less frequently.

Anemia and Fatigue

Anemia in men receiving ADT is generally normocytic and normochromic. It is thought to result from decreased testosterone and dihydrotestosterone (DHT) stimulation of renal erythropoietin production and of bone marrow erythroid precursors.[126] Hemoglobin may start to decline measurably within 1 month of ADT commencement but usually takes 6 months to reach a stable low level. Patients often experience hemoglobin declines of 1 to 3 g/dL; almost everybody has a reduction of 10%, and an eighth of patients have a reduction of 25% or more.[126] Patients receiving nonsteroidal antiandrogen monotherapy appear to experience anemia as well but to a lesser extent.[27] Patients in whom ADT is discontinued usually recover pretreatment hemoglobin levels within 6 months, but levels may take >1 year to normalize.[111,126] Several options exist for the management of symptomatic anemia, which occurs in approximately 13% of patients.[126] These options include the following:

1. Administration of exogenous steroids, which stimulate increased production of erythroid precursors and lengthen erythrocyte survival
2. Administration of recombinant erythropoietin, which is effective but expensive
3. Blood transfusion, with the risk of accompanying adverse reactions and infectious phenomena (Table 9-5)

Fatigue is a common complaint of men receiving ADT but also of men with advanced cancer. *Cancer fatigue* is defined as the unusual, persistent, subjective sense of tiredness that is related to cancer or cancer treatment and interferes with usual functioning.[127]

TABLE 9-5	Treatment Options for Anemia and Fatigue
Option	**Treatment Details**
Exercise	3 times/wk
Psychotherapy and support groups	
Deferred treatment	
Intermittent androgen deprivation	
Bicalutamide	150 mg PO every day as monotherapy
Prednisone	40 mg PO every day
Dexamethasone	8 mg/day × 2 wk
Methylphenidate	5-10 mg PO bid morning and lunchtime
Modafinil	100 mg PO daily increased to 200 mg daily
Megestrol acetate	80 mg PO qid
Fluoxetine (or similar SSRI)	20 mg PO daily
Ferrous gluconate	300 mg PO once to three times a day
Recombinant erythropoietin	100 µg/kg/wk SC
Blood transfusion	Number of units titrated to hemoglobin

bid, twice daily; PO, orally; qid, four times daily; SC, subcutaneously; SSRI, selective serotonin reuptake inhibitor.

Health-related quality of life studies have identified fatigue as one component contributing to reduced quality of life in men receiving ADT as opposed to those deferring treatment.[128] Some 14% of patients receiving ADT develop severe fatigue within 3 months of starting treatment, and this is not the result of psychological distress alone.[129]

Depression, social isolation, and other psychological factors including treatment for an incurable disease with increasing PSA values may combine with physical factors such as cancer pathophysiology, sleep deprivation, medication side effects and interactions, muscle mass and strength loss, pathologic fractures, anemia, and insulin resistance to contribute to fatigue. Given the multifactorial origin of ADT-related fatigue, multiple therapies may be required, and this complication may prove difficult to treat. Resistance training exercise was shown to reduce the extent to which self-reported fatigue interferes with activities of daily living.[122] It was also associated with statistically significant improvements in health-related quality of life. Given the many areas of health that may benefit from regular exercise, this should form a central role in patient care. Cognitive interventions from counseling, support groups, and education through to medication for depressive disor-

ders should also be offered. Strategies for replacement of falling hemoglobin levels as discussed previously may be used if anemia is thought to be a contributing factor. Adequate diabetes and pain control with simultaneous medication rationalization to avoid unwanted interactions may all be helpful.

Finally, some evidence indicates that medications may be of use in the treatment of cancer fatigue. The psychostimulant methylphenidate (Ritalin), used for the treatment of attention-deficit/hyperactivity disorder (ADHD) in the young, opiate-related drowsiness in palliative care, and depression in elderly patients, may be beneficial in treating fatigue in patients with cancer.[130-133] So far, no studies have been published in men with advanced prostate cancer who are receiving ADT, but studies are currently under way, and the role in advanced cancer in general is evolving.[134] In patients with cancer, RCTs have been performed or are being performed to study corticosteroids, megestrol acetate, L-carnitine, modafinil (a psychostimulant), and donepezil (a cholinesterase inhibitor used in Alzheimer disease), but results will require further refinement with respect to dosing and indications.[135-137]

Cardiovascular Complications

Cardiovascular disease is the second leading cause of death in men with prostate cancer and the leading cause of non–cancer-related death.[138,139] Rates of non–cancer-related death in men with a diagnosis of prostate cancer are higher than are those in men without prostate cancer.[140,141] Rapidly accumulating evidence suggests that hormonal manipulation may contribute to cardiovascular disease in that it promotes atherogenesis and in some cases hypercoagulability.[138] In addition, low testosterone is thought to result in reduced systemic arterial compliance, with consequent hypertension.[142]

Testosterone deficiency may prolong the QT interval of the electrical cardiac cycle, which may, in turn, predispose men to arrhythmia and sudden cardiac death. This effect appears to be independent of drug type because abarelix, bicalutamide, and leuprolide have all been associated with QT prolongation. It is recommended that men with baseline QT >450 msec or men who are taking class 1a or 3 antiarrhythmics avoid these modes of ADT if possible.[138,144]

A large population-based observational study of Medicare patients in the United States looked at the incidence of diabetes, coronary heart disease, myocardial infarction, and sudden cardiac death in patients receiving either LHRH agonists or orchiectomy for the treatment of prostate cancer.[117] Those treated with orchiectomy (only 6.9% of the population) had an increased risk of developing diabetes (hazard ratio, 1.34) but not of the other three outcomes assessed. Those treated with LHRH agonists had a statistically significant increased risk of all four outcomes, with hazard ratios ranging between 1.11 and 1.44. LHRH agonists are expensive relative to such other treatments as orchiectomy and estrogens (oral, IV, or transdermal), and they now account for one third of all expenditure from the Medicare prostate cancer budget.[139]

Screening for risk factors and prevention of disease are more likely to be beneficial than trying to close the cardiovascular gate after the horse has bolted. Monitoring of serum lipid profiles and determinations of glycemic control (e.g., fasting glucose or HbA_{1c} levels), blood pressure, weight, and girth are important screening tools. Advice with referral to specific programs for exercise, cessation of smoking, and dietary modification should be offered. These measures should be combined with early referral to a cardiologist for antihypertensive and statin-based treatment or an endocrinologist for diabetes control when indicated. Despite the common sense extrapolation of these measures from general medical practice, long-term studies of the cost effectiveness of such interventions on the outcome of patients with prostate cancer who are taking ADT are entirely lacking and require further investigation.

Gastrointestinal Complications

Gastrointestinal side effects are generally minor considerations with most forms of treatment but may be particular features of flutamide and ketoconazole use. Diarrhea has been recorded at a rate of 17% in men taking the flutamide, and more than one third have either diarrhea or significant nausea.[24] Generally, diarrhea may best be managed by discontinuation of the agent and by trials of alternative hormonal therapies; however, anticholinergic medications such as hyoscine may be useful alternatives, as may codeine, if pain control is also an issue.

Hepatotoxicity and LFT derangements are particularly common with antiandrogens because of induction of the cytochrome P-450 enzyme system. Again, flutamide is the principal offender; LFT abnormalities are noted in one fourth of patients, and potentially fatal hepatotoxicity occurs in 3 in 100,000 patients.[29,30] Generally with other antiandrogens, hepatotoxicity is seen at a rate of ≤5%.[27,43] Fulminant hepatic failure and new-onset hepatocellular carcinoma have been described in case reports of people receiving CPA.[125] Appropriate management of hepatic enzyme induction abnormalities involves regular monitoring of LFTs (e.g., concurrent with PSA) to allow timely detection and discontinuance of the agent if identified. More significant abnormalities or those that fail to resolve require referral for specialist gastroenterologic evaluation.

Cognitive and Emotional Changes

The effect of hormonal manipulation for prostate cancer on cognition has long been neglected, although some studies have begun to address this issue. The effect of LHRH agonists particularly on memory was identified at least a decade earlier in women and was found to be reversible to some degree with estrogen supplementation.[145,146] Hypogonadal men with "andropause" show improvements in spatial ability, verbal memory, and fluency with testosterone supplementation.[147] A randomized study of 82 men to ADT with LHRH agonists or CPA versus no ADT demonstrated a decline in performance of attention and memory based tests in half of the men receiving ADT but no corresponding decline in any men deferring treatment.[148] A smaller English study corroborated this finding and noted that spatial memory and ability were particularly affected.[149] Another study attempted to relate a decline in the cognitive powers of men starting ADT to the sudden fall in sex hormone levels.[150] These investigators found that declines in estradiol were associated with selective cognitive impairments in the domains of visual fluency, visual recognition, and visual memory. Some evidence of recovery was present at 1 year despite persistent estradiol reduction, and the investigators did not extrapolate their findings to the point of recommending estradiol supplementation, as others have.[151] Long-term evaluation of cognitive decline during ADT has not been published to date.

Although the beginnings of cognition deficit quantification in ADT are under way, a dearth of investigation exists with regard to prevention and management in this area. A small study found no curative effects from the administration of supplemental transdermal estradiol.[152] The role of pre-ADT transdermal estrogen as well as IAD, antiandrogen monotherapy, cognitive exercises, socialization, and depression management awaits further definition. Currently, it seems reasonable to warn patients that cognitive decline is possible during hormonal manipulation therapies and to present the strategies of deferred treatment, IAD, and antiandrogen monotherapy as potential although not proven options that may have less impact in this regard. Patients should be encouraged to participate in prostate cancer support groups and other social interactions to avoid isolation as well as the pursuit of activities with a cerebral focus.

The Advanced Cognitive Training for Independent and Vital Elderly (ACTIVE) study showed that cognitive training results in less functional decline for elderly persons, and this effect was sustained out to 5 years.[153] Although formalized cognitive training programs are not yet widely used, their combined use with prophylactic neuropharmaceuticals offers promise for the future.[154] There seems little detriment to recommending mental as well as physical exercise to the patient starting ADT. This may take the form of crossword puzzles, Sudoku, or educational courses that require focused learning of material.

Emotional lability often accompanies ADT. Patients may experience moodiness and may become prone to feeling upset or anxious, and depressive symptoms are prominent.[155] Symptoms may be worsened by, but also contribute to, social isolation, as is often reported by spouses.[156] Although men diagnosed with prostate cancer may have up to eight times the frequency of depression by comparison with the general public, this finding seems to be independent of ADT.[22] After correcting for age and comorbidity, a study based on SEER data found little difference in rates of depression between men with prostate cancer treated with or without ADT.[157] Recognition of and early intervention for depression may have significant benefits in terms of a patient's quality of life. Therapy may have further benefits beyond those expected in general health, sleep, fatigue, diet, and treatment compliance.[158] Education and social enrichment with prostate cancer group interaction may be invaluable in helping to prevent and identify these symptoms. Depressive symptoms should be inquired about at clinic follow-up. Unfortunately, many of the physical expressions of depression are seen as side effects of ADT, and thus the diagnosis may be difficult to make.

ACKNOWLEDGMENT

We wish to thank Assistant Professor Linda Lee, Department of Dentistry, Princess Margaret Hospital, Toronto for her contribution to this chapter.

KEY POINTS

1. The androgen deprivation syndrome is a composite of multiple organ system dysfunctions resulting from inhibition of the growth and regulatory effects of sex hormones on a range of tissues.

2. Different forms of ADT have different side effect profiles that result from predictable hormonally related changes and agent-specific characteristics.

3. Bilateral orchiectomy is a simple, inexpensive, and effective form of treatment. Adverse effects are limited not only to those of surgery and hormone deprivation but also to those of altered body self-image.

4. Oral estrogens are associated with hypercoagulability and an increased risk of non–prostate cancer–related death because of the hepatic first-pass effect with induction of liver enzymes following intestinal absorption. This effect may be bypassed by using different methods of administration, but the efficacy of these approaches requires further evaluation.

5. Tumor flare is associated with the commencement of LHRH agonists and results from a transient increase in circulating testosterone. This condition can induce symptomatic disease progression if androgen receptor blockade is not administered concurrently.

6. Significant changes in lipid profile, coagulation, and insulin resistance may occur with forms of ADT that predispose patients to increased cardiovascular morbidity. Screening of weight, blood pressure, and blood values (lipid profile, glucose tolerance) is important to detect and allow intervention for these changes, to minimize the risk of a premature cardiovascular event.

7. Bone health declines in association with some forms of ADT, which lead to osteoporosis and pathologic fractures. All men should be screened for osteoporosis risk factors, started on supplemental vitamin D and calcium, and advised about the benefits of regular exercise in preventing loss of BMD. The role of bone densitometry has yet to be defined, but this technique should be considered for high-risk individuals before bisphosphonate treatment is begun.

8. Sexual functioning is significantly affected by most forms of ADT and should be enquired about specifically. Monotherapy with nonsteroidal antiandrogens may represent a treatment alternative that minimizes this effect.

9. Hot flashes result from vasomotor instability following testosterone withdrawal. They may be severe, interfering with everyday activities. Although treatment options exist, they mostly reduce rather than eliminate symptoms.

10. Gynecomastia and mastodynia are thought to result from increases in the estrogen-to-androgen ratio with ADT. These disorders are particularly prominent in treatments based on estrogen and nonsteroidal antiandrogen. Prophylaxis is preferable to surgical cure, and in this regard tamoxifen shows early promise.

11. Cognitive changes, fatigue, and depression are probably underappreciated in ADT for men with prostate cancer but may have profound impacts on health-related quality of life.

12. Variations in the timing of ADT such as deferred or intermittent treatment may allow minimization of the side effects of therapy.

REFERENCES

Please see www.expertconsult.com

Chapter 10

TOXICITIES OF CHEMOTHERAPY FOR GENITOURINARY MALIGNANCIES

Bruce Montgomery MD
Associate Professor, Department of Medicine, University of Washington/Seattle Cancer Care Alliance; Attending Physician, Veterans Administration Puget Sound Health Care System, Seattle, Washington

Daniel W. Lin MD
Associate Professor and Director of Urologic Oncology, Department of Urology, University of Washington/ Seattle Cancer Care Alliance; Attending Physician, Veterans Administration Puget Sound Health Care System, Seattle, Washington

The use of systemic chemotherapy carries important benefits in the treatment of genitourinary cancers. For patients presenting with clinically localized disease, systemic therapy can reduce disease burden when this treatment is given before definitive local therapy, thus optimizing local disease control. Neoadjuvant and adjuvant therapy in localized disease may also eliminate micrometastatic disease that may otherwise lead to relapse despite effective local therapies. For patients with metastatic genitourinary cancer, systemic chemotherapy can effect a cure in a majority of patients with testis cancer and in a small proportion of patients with other histologic tumor types. More commonly, the focus of therapy is to provide palliative benefits for patients with clinically apparent metastatic disease by enhancing duration and quality of survival. For the majority of genitourinary cancers, chemotherapy involves combinations of drugs that optimize tumor response by targeting the many tumor-associated mechanisms that generate drug resistance and block cell death.

These potential benefits of chemotherapy come at a cost to the patient in the form of toxicity, both acute and delayed, which can have a substantial impact on quality of life. In addition to the critical aim of improving duration of survival and cure, preventing and effectively treating the toxicities of therapy will optimize outcomes for patients. In the remainder of the discussion, the term *chemotherapy* is used to refer to both cytotoxic agents and a newer class of drugs, the multikinase inhibitors, which are now being widely used in the treatment of renal cell carcinoma. Considerable progress has been made in the use of agents that prevent some of the most feared complications, and the rapidly developing field of targeted therapeutics holds promise for more effective and less toxic treatment in the future. This chapter reviews the mechanisms of action of these agents, the regimens in which they are most commonly used in the treatment of genitourinary cancer, and the most frequent toxicities that are considerations in the multidisciplinary management of these patients.

SYNDROMES OF TOXICITY

The universal language of toxicity is the National Cancer Institute's Common Toxicity Criteria for Adverse Events (CTCAE). Adverse events or effects are graded on a scale of 0 to 5, with 0 indicating no toxicity, grade 1 being mild, grade 2 moderate, grade 3 severe, grade 4 life-threatening, and grade 5 fatal. The current version is CTCAE v3.0 and is available on the Cancer Therapy Evaluation Program Web site (www.ctep.cancer.gov/ protocolDevelopment/electronic_applications/ctcaev3. pdf). The use of this grading system allows standardization of reporting and modification of therapy across multiple studies and cooperative groups. Despite these well-defined criteria, distinctions among adverse effects of chemotherapy, complications of malignant disease, and toxicities of other supportive drugs are often not clearly defined, and other causes of complications must always be considered.

Nausea and Vomiting

Although many toxicities of therapy may last longer and constitute a greater threat to life, few are as feared by patients as nausea and vomiting. Control of nausea and emesis is critical to completion of treatment, and prophylactic agents should be tailored to the expected potential for chemotherapy-associated nausea. Patterns of nausea and emesis may vary. Anticipatory nausea and emesis may manifest before chemotherapy as a form of conditioned response in patients who have experienced nausea with previous cycles of chemotherapy. Acute nausea usually occurs within several hours after chemotherapy administration, and delayed nausea, particularly associated with medications such as cisplatin, may occur 24 to 120 hours after drug administration.

Chemotherapy-induced nausea has been proposed to be controlled by several sites, including the lateral reticular formation of the medulla in the brainstem, the area postrema in the floor of the fourth ventricle (the chemoreceptor trigger zone), and the nucleus tractus solitarius. The process begins when chemotherapy directly stimulates the chemoreceptor trigger zone and thus promotes release of serotonin from cells lining the gastrointestinal tract. Serotonin then may bind receptors within the chemoreceptor trigger zone and other sites within the central nervous system (CNS). These centers then feed impulses to the nucleus tractus solitarius and the reticular formation within the CNS and stimulate emesis. Dramatic advances in the prevention and control of nausea have been made with the recognition of the central role of 5-hydroxytryptamine (5-HT$_3$) and neurokinin-1 receptors within the chemoreceptor trigger zone, and antagonists have been developed to each of these receptors. The relative risk of emesis in the absence of prophylaxis for select agents is given in Table 10-1.

The use of selective antagonists of 5-HT$_3$ receptors, including ondansetron, granisetron, and palonosetron, has allowed administration of numerous cisplatin-containing regimens in an outpatient setting. The neu-rokinin-1 antagonist aprepitant has also shown significant activity when it is combined with 5-HT$_3$ antagonists in patients with highly emetogenic regimens.[1] Corticosteroids are an important component of regimens for patients receiving therapy at a high risk of inducing emesis because corticosteroids consistently add significant efficacy to both 5-HT$_3$ and neurokinin antagonists.[2] These agents have changed the face of chemotherapy-associated nausea and vomiting and have made outpatient administration a viable strategy in the treatment of advanced cancers.

Myelosuppression

For the majority of cytotoxic agents, myelosuppression is the most common toxicity, and it results from the rapid proliferation of bone marrow and consequent sensitivity to drugs that inhibit or kill rapidly proliferating cells. Both cytotoxic agents and tyrosine kinase inhibitors may suppress bone marrow function, with resulting leukopenia, anemia, or thrombocytopenia. The circulating half-life of the relevant cell determines the expected duration of these toxicities. Neutrophils, with a half-life of <10 hours, are often the most severely suppressed cells, and for most agents, the nadir count occurs 7 to 14 days after a single administration of chemotherapy, with recovery by 28 days. The incidence of the most significant complication, febrile neutropenia, varies dramatically from agent to agent, ranging from 3% for docetaxel to >75% for testicular salvage regimens (Table 10-2).

The complications of myelosuppression include infections and bleeding and account for the majority of hospital admissions in patients with cancer who are receiving systemic chemotherapy. Hematopoietic

TABLE 10-1	Relative Risk of Emesis for Commonly Administered Agents in Genitourinary Malignancies	
Risk Level	**Frequency of Emesis (%)**	**Agents**
High	>90	Cisplatin >50 mg/m^2
Moderate	30-90	Carboplatin Cisplatin <50 mg/m^2 Doxorubicin Ifosfamide
Low	10-30	Docetaxel Etoposide Gemcitabine Mitoxantrone Methotrexate Paclitaxel Sorafenib Sunitinib
Very low	<10	Bleomycin Vinblastine Vincristine Vinorelbine

Adapted from Kris MG, Hesketh PJ, Somerfield MR, et al. American Society of Clinical Oncology guideline for antiemetics in oncology: update 2006. *J Clin Oncol.* 2006;24:2932.

TABLE 10-2	Risk of Neutropenia for Commonly Administered Agents in Genitourinary Malignancies	
Risk Level	**Frequency of Febrile Neutropenia (%)**	**Agents/Regimens**
High	>20	TIP (paclitaxel, ifosfamide, cisplatin) VIP (vinblastine, ifosfamide, cisplatin)
Moderate	10-20	MVAC (methotrexate, vinblastine, doxorubicin, cisplatin) BEP/EP (etoposide, cisplatin, bleomycin)
Low	<10	Docetaxel, prednisone Gemcitabine, cisplatin Mitoxantrone, prednisone Sunitinib Sorafenib

growth factors, such as granulocyte colony-stimulating factor (G-CSF), erythropoietin, and darbepoetin, are used extensively to prevent complications and relieve fatigue in patients treated with chemotherapy. Guidelines from the American Society of Clinical Oncology and the National Comprehensive Cancer Network for the use of myeloid growth factors suggest that primary prophylaxis is indicated if the risk of febrile neutropenia is >20%, prophylaxis may be considered if the risk is 10% to 20%, and it is not indicated if the risk is <10%.

Secondary prophylaxis may be considered in the setting of febrile neutropenia or a dose-limiting neutropenic event, which is generally considered to be neutropenia lasting >7 days or infection (www.nccn.org).[3] The use of erythroid growth factors is generally considered to preclude the need for transfusion and it usually targets hemoglobin to levels between 10 and 12, to avoid the documented cardiovascular toxicities when the hemoglobin is targeted to levels >12.[4,5] In addition, prior chemotherapy, prior pelvic or spinal radiation, age, and other factors must be considered when determining risk for febrile neutropenia.

Pulmonary Toxicity

Multiple drugs can induce pulmonary complications, particularly when they are combined with other agents or radiation therapy. Methotrexate, doxorubicin, gemcitabine, and docetaxel have all been reported to cause acute and chronic interstitial pneumonitis.[6-8] However, bleomycin pneumonitis and fibrosis are the best described and most closely monitored pulmonary complications of chemotherapy. Bleomycin toxicity can be acute, manifesting as acute chest pain during infusion, probably as a result of hypersensitivity, or more commonly it occurs weeks to months after initiation of therapy with cough, dyspnea, or chest pain. The incidence of bleomycin-related pneumonitis is most clearly associated with the total dose, although age, renal function, and radiation have been identified as additional risk factors.[9,10] The specificity of bleomycin for the lung is related to very low tissue levels of hydrolase activity, which inactivates the drug. When the total dose reaches >450 to 500 U, the incidence of pulmonary toxicity may reach 17%.[10] The reported fatal pulmonary toxicity after three cycles of BEP (bleomycin, etoposide, cisplatin) is <1%, and after four cycles it is 1% to 2%.[11,12] Idiosyncratic pulmonary toxicity may occur at much lower doses, although this complication is rare.

To prevent the development of fatal complications, multiple different approaches have been considered, although few have been tested in a prospective manner and practices vary substantially. These approaches range from discontinuation of bleomycin if the diffusing capacity of the lung for carbon monoxide measured at the beginning of each cycle declines to <60% of pretreatment baseline to limiting the administration to 10 weeks of therapy. At other institutions, pretreatment evaluation is used to determine whether bleomycin is appropriate, but no additional function testing is performed in the absence of clinical signs or symptoms.[13]

Early investigators documented that some patients who were previously treated with bleomycin developed fatal acute respiratory distress when they were exposed to high oxygen tension intraoperatively.[14] Other studies disputed this finding and suggested that judicious fluid management is the most critical aspect of care.[15] Current practice takes both mechanisms into consideration, and patients with previous bleomycin exposure receive oxygen tension adequate to prevent hypoxia while their fluid needs are closely monitored. Corticosteroids remain the foundation of treatment in patients with established pneumonitis.

Cardiovascular and Thrombotic Complications

The acute and chronic vascular complications of genitourinary chemotherapy have been best described in patients with curatively treated testicular cancer. In one single-institution series, venous thromboembolism and arterial thrombosis occurred in 8% of patients. The presence of hepatic metastases, the use of high-dose corticosteroids, and a high body mass index were associated with a greater risk of thrombotic events.[16,17] The complication of vascular hypersensitivity or Raynaud phenomenon may also occur during or for several years after conclusion of chemotherapy for testicular cancer. Retrospective analyses have suggested that each of the agents used—cisplatin, bleomycin, and vinblastine—plays a role in development of the syndrome. The mechanisms by which the drugs may mediate this effect remain unclear, but >30% of patients in some series developed symptoms within 3 years of therapy.[18] Supportive measures and the use of calcium channel blockers have shown some efficacy in reducing the frequency of these episodes,[19] and early studies with phosphodiesterase inhibitors appear promising.[20]

The use of chemotherapy is also associated with a greater than twofold increase in the incidence of cardiovascular disease (angina, myocardial infarction, or sudden death) in long-term cancer survivors after chemotherapy,[21] radiation therapy, or both. The mechanisms by which chemotherapy may cause cardiovascular morbidity include vasospasm (similar to Raynaud phenomenon), increases in body mass index and the metabolic syndrome, and changes in electrolyte levels. At present, no data are available regarding the efficacy of aggressive management of blood pressure and dyslipidemia, but regular screening and intervention when appropriate are strongly recommended.[22]

Secondary Malignant Diseases

The increased use of alkylating agents and adjuvant therapy has revealed that certain agents commonly place otherwise curatively treated patients at risk for a second malignant disease. The best defined of these is the development of leukemia after exposure to etoposide, which induces gene rearrangement at the MLL locus, particularly after prolonged exposures in children and young men.[23] For men treated with standard doses of EP (etoposide and cisplatin) or BEP, and <2000 mg/m^2 of etoposide, the incidence of secondary leukemia is less than 0.5%.[24] Mitoxantrone provides palliation in men with prostate cancer, and in adjuvant studies of patients with breast and prostate cancer, the risk of secondary leukemia after the use of this drug was 0.6% to 2.2% for myelodysplasia and acute leukemia.[25]

Fertility

Chemotherapy targets rapidly dividing cells, and disrupted spermatogenesis is a common side effect of systemic chemotherapy. Alkylating agents, such as cisplatin and carboplatin, effect spermatogenesis in a dose-dependent manner.[26] The effects of chemotherapy on spermatogenesis have been studied most extensively in testicular cancer. Patients with testis cancer in these studies have had profoundly abnormal semen parameters at baseline, with 60% azoospermia or oligospermia.[27-29] Although systemic chemotherapy has well-documented adverse effects on semen quality and gonadal function, these abnormalities are not always permanent, and normalization of gonadal (both endocrine and spermatogenic) function can be expected in the majority of cases.[30,31]

One large single-institution review found improved semen parameters in ≤80% of patients 5 years after chemotherapy; 58% of these patients achieved normal sperm counts.[32] Higher pretreatment sperm counts, use of carboplatin versus cisplatin, and normal follicle-stimulating hormone levels have been correlated to recovery of normal semen parameters.[26,33] Despite encouraging recovery of spermatogenesis, we advocate a detailed discussion of sperm cryopreservation and assisted reproductive technologies before initiation of chemotherapy.[34]

SPECIFIC AGENTS

Table 10-3 is an overview of specific chemotherapy regimens by disease subtype.

Bleomycin

Bleomycin, a water-soluble antibiotic, induces cytotoxicity by induction of single-strand breaks in DNA through formation of a bleomycin-DNA complex. This complex chelates ferrous iron and allows reduction of oxygen to reactive species, which induce strand breaks.

Cytotoxicity appears to be specific to the G$_2$ phase of the cell cycle. Renal metabolism accounts for the major-

TABLE 10-3	Chemotherapy Regimen by Disease Subtype	
Regimen	**Agent**	**Dosing**
Testis Carcinoma		
BEP	Bleomycin	30 U days 1, 8, 15
	Etoposide	100 mg/m^2 days 1-5
	Cisplatin	20 mg/m^2 days 1-5
		Duration: 3-4 cycles every 21 days
EP	Etoposide	100 mg/m^2 days 1-5
	Cisplatin	20 mg/m^2 days 1-5
		Duration: 4 cycles every 21 days
VIP	Vinblastine	0.11 mg/kg days 1, 2
	Ifosfamide	1.2 g/m^2 days 1-5
	Mesna	1.2 g/m^2 days 1-5
	Cisplatin	20 mg/m^2 days 1-5
TIP	Paclitaxel	250 mg/m^2 continuously day 1
	Ifosfamide	1.5 g/m^2 days 2-5
	Cisplatin	25 mg/m^2 days 2-5
Bladder Carcinoma		
	Gemcitabine	1000 mg/m^2 day 1, 8, 15
	Cisplatin	70 mg/m^2 day 2
		Every 28 days
GC	OR	
	Gemcitabine	1250 mg/m^2 day 1, 8
	Cisplatin	70 mg/m^2 day 2
		Every 21 days
MVAC	Methotrexate	30 mg/m^2 day 1, 15, 22
	Vinblastine	3 mg/m^2 day 2, 15, 22
	Doxorubicin	30 mg/m^2 day 2
	Cisplatin	70 mg/m^2 day 2
		Every 28 days
HD-MVAC	Methotrexate	30 mg/m^2 day 1
	Vinblastine	3 mg/m^2 day 2
	Doxorubicin	30 mg/m^2 day 2
	Cisplatin	70 mg/m^2 day 2
		Every 14 days
Prostate Carcinoma		
DP	Docetaxel	75 mg/m^2 day 1
	Prednisone	5 mg bid continuously
		Every 21 days
MP	Mitoxantrone	12-14 mg/m^2 day 1
	Prednisone	5 mg bid continuously
		Every 21 days
Renal Carcinoma		
	Sunitinib	50 mg/day days 1-28, every 42 days
	Sorafenib	400 mg bid continuously

bid, twice daily.

ity of drug elimination, and significant renal insufficiency prolongs the drug's half-life, thereby requiring dose adjustments for patients with a glomerular filtration rate <50 mL/minute. The total dose is usually kept to <400 U to attempt to offset the risk of pulmonary toxicity (see "Pulmonary Toxicity," earlier). The drug is inactivated by a tissue hydrolase that is sparse in lung tissue and skin, and the result is the relatively organ-specific toxicity seen in patients who receive bleomycin regimens.

In addition to interstitial pneumonitis, bleomycin may cause an acute hypersensitivity reaction characterized by fever and chills, and premedication with hydrocortisone is often considered. Rarely, an acute anaphylactoid reaction occurs, with hypotension, wheezing, and angioedema.

Dermatologic complications occur in 50% of patients. Erythema, hyperpigmentation, edema, and hyperkeratosis and nail changes are the most common findings. Palms and soles are preferentially affected. Bleomycin is used as a critical component of regimens for patients with testicular cancer in combination with cisplatin and etoposide.

Carboplatin

Carboplatin is a cisplatin analogue that also induces DNA adduct formation and interstrand cross-linking. Despite a similar mechanism of action to cisplatin, the toxicity profile is significantly different, with myelosuppression being the dose-limiting toxicity. Thrombocytopenia may be more prominent that neutropenia, although all lineages may be suppressed in combination therapy. Emesis and chemical hepatitis may occur in greater than 25% of patients, and renal insufficiency and neuropathy in less than 10%. Carboplatin is dosed in most cases according to glomerular function, targeting a specific area under the curve.

Acute hypersensitivity reactions occur in <5% of patients but can be dramatic, including flushing, rashes, itchy palms, nausea, dyspnea back pain, hypotension, and tachycardia. For patients with severe reactions, and those with recurrent milder reactions, desensitization protocols which incorporate prolonged infusions over approximately 6 hours have allowed patients in whom carboplatin is required to receive drug without further complication.[35] Carboplatin is used in the adjuvant treatment of seminoma and as a component of high dose regimens for patients with high risk or relapsed testicular cancer.

Cisplatin

Although the toxicity of cisplatin (*cis*-diamminedichloroplatinum, CDDP) is daunting, it is among the most effective chemotherapeutics used in oncology. Cisplatin covalently binds to DNA, inducing adduct formation and interstrand cross-linking that result in DNA damage and cell killing. The extensive use of cisplatin has defined a wide range of toxicities that can result in reversible and irreversible organ damage. The incidence of nausea and emesis decreased substantially with the development of $5\text{-}HT_3$ and neurokinin antagonists, but emesis still occurs in 20% to 40% of patients[36] receiving cisplatin regimens.

Renal insufficiency and magnesium and potassium wasting necessitate the use of intravenous hydration with electrolytes before and after therapy. Measured glomerular filtration rates <60 mL/minute are considered relative contraindications to the use of cisplatin.

Peripheral neuropathy is dose and duration dependent, and high-frequency hearing loss occurs in ≤25% of patients. Both these neurotoxicities are only partially reversible and may be dose limiting. Myelosuppression also occurs commonly, although the need for prophylactic myeloid growth factors depends on the dose and regimen. Cisplatin is the most effective agent in combination regimens used for patients with bladder cancer (gemcitabine, cisplatin, MVAC [methotrexate, vinblastine, doxorubicin, cisplatin]) testicular cancer (EP and BEP), and less common histologic types such as urethral, penile, and scrotal cancers.

Docetaxel

Docetaxel is a semisynthetic taxane that binds to the β-tubulin component of cellular microtubules and thus induces cytotoxic and apoptotic cell death at the G_2-M phase of the cell cycle. The principal toxicities are edema, neuropathy, diarrhea, emesis, chemical hepatitis, weakness, myalgia, interstitial pneumonitis, and acute hypersensitivity, the last of which requires corticosteroid premedication. Grade 3 or 4 neutropenia occurs in approximately 30% of patients, although febrile neutropenia occurs in <5%.[37] Less frequently, patients may suffer hyperlacrimation, particularly when docetaxel is administered weekly.

When docetaxel is given every 3 weeks, premedication with dexamethasone 12 hours, 3 hours, and 1 hour before docetaxel administration has been effective at minimizing hypersensitivity and peripheral edema. The principal indication is for patients with castration-resistant metastatic prostate cancer in conjunction with daily prednisone, and docetaxel is being more widely used as an alternative to cisplatin-containing regimens for advanced bladder cancer.[37,38]

Doxorubicin

Doxorubicin is the most widely used anthracycline antibiotic. Its mechanism of action appears to be intercalation into DNA and inhibition of topoisomerase II activity, thus blocking DNA synthesis and causing both cytotoxic and apoptotic cell death. The dose-dependent development of cardiomyopathy in patients receiving >450 mg/m^2 necessitates pretreatment evaluation of myocardial ejection fraction in the majority of patients. If the left ventricular ejection fraction is ≤40%, doxorubicin is often withheld. Inflammation of the gastrointestinal tract is common and manifests as mucositis, emesis, diarrhea, and esophagitis. Neutropenia is dose limiting, and both anemia and thrombocytopenia may also occur.

The other remarkable toxicity common to all anthracyclines is the induction of acute myeloid leukemia in curatively treated adult and pediatric patients; the risk of this complication is 1% to 3%.[25] Dose adjustments are required for patients with significant hepatic dysfunction as manifested by elevated total bilirubin or transaminases. Doxorubicin is most commonly used in neoadjuvant, adjuvant, and palliative regimens for bladder cancer (MVAC and HD-MVAC).[39,40]

Etoposide

Etoposide is a podophyllotoxin derivative that inhibits DNA topoisomerase II, with resultant DNA strand breaks and induction of cytotoxic and apoptotic cell death. Etoposide is relatively cell cycle specific, and it affects cells in the S and G$_2$ phases of cell division. The dose-limiting toxicity is myelosuppression, with neutropenia the principal form of hematologic toxicity. Mild thrombocytopenia, mucositis, nausea, alopecia, and emesis are common. Rarely, anaphylactoid reactions may occur. Hypotension occurs with high doses during rapid infusion, but this effect is uncommon in the doses used for the treatment of testicular cancer.

Secondary myelodysplastic syndrome and acute leukemia are associated with the characteristic 11q23 mutation related to etoposide use.[23] With the cumulative doses of ≤2000 mg/m^2 administered with BEP and EP, the risk of leukemia appears to be <0.5%.[24] Etoposide is used in combination with bleomycin and cisplatin or with cisplatin alone in the treatment of testicular carcinoma.

Gemcitabine

Gemcitabine is a pyrimidine antimetabolite that is phosphorylated to monophosphates, diphosphates, and triphosphates that are incorporated into DNA and block DNA polymerase and ribonucleotide reductase. Most studies have used weekly dosing and have reported dose-limiting toxicities of thrombocytopenia and neutropenia. Chemical hepatitis has also been dose limiting in some studies, whereas renal insufficiency, emesis, and peripheral edema occur less frequently. Noninfectious fever has been reported intermittently and must be considered in the differential diagnosis in febrile patients.

GC (gemcitabine and cisplatin) is currently the most widely used regimen for patients with metastatic bladder cancer and is equal in efficacy to standard MVAC.[41]

Ifosfamide

Ifosfamide is an alkylating agent that, when metabolized to 4-hydroxyifosfamide and to the ultimate alkylating agent ifosforamide mustard, causes DNA cross-linking that inhibits DNA and protein synthesis. Myelosuppression is the dose-limiting toxicity. Additional risks are emesis, and neurotoxicity characterized by altered mental status, seizures, cerebellar dysfunction, and aphasia. The high incidence of hemorrhagic cystitis resulted in the routine use of mesna and hydration. Significant renal and hepatic dysfunction is generally considered an indication for dose adjustment or consideration of other agents. Ifosfamide is used primarily in patients with relapsed testis cancer after initial etoposide-based regimens.[42]

Mitoxantrone

Mitoxantrone is an anthracenedione, or anthracycline analogue, and has similar anthracycline mechanisms of action, with intercalation into DNA and inhibition of topoisomerase II activity Myelosuppression is the most commonly observed toxicity, although the incidence of febrile neutropenia is <5%. Alopecia, mild hepatic dysfunction, and cardiomyopathy are significantly less frequent than similar complications associated with the other anthracyclines. The incidence of acute myeloid leukemia in curatively treated adult and pediatric patients ranges from 0.5% to 2.2%.[25]

Dose adjustments are required for patients with significant hepatic dysfunction as manifested by elevated total bilirubin or transaminases. Although mitoxantrone has been approved for the use in palliation of metastatic prostate cancer,[43] this drug has been largely supplanted by docetaxel in the treatment of men with castration-resistant metastatic prostate cancer.

Sorafenib

Sorafenib is an oral kinase inhibitor that was designed to inhibit the Raf kinase family oncogenes. This drug was found to inhibit multiple kinases in addition to Raf, including platelet-derived growth factor receptor (PDGFR), vascular endothelial growth factor receptor (VEGFR), and c-kit. The inactivation of Von Hippel–Lindau gene function in a significant proportion of renal cell carcinomas, with subsequent upregulation of hypoxia inducible factor (HIF) and HIF induction of angiogenesis-related proteins such as PDGF and VEGF, provided a rationale for the activity seen in early-phase studies in patients with renal cell carcinoma.[44,45]

A phase III study of sorafenib for clear cell carcinoma with good to intermediate prognosis in patients whose disease had progressed despite one prior systemic therapy regimen demonstrated improved progression-free survival and a borderline improvement in overall survival.[46] The recommended dose is 400 mg twice daily, with potential dose reduction to daily or every other day in the event of significant toxicity.

The most common grade 3 or 4 toxicity is hand-foot cutaneous eruptions, followed by hypertension, fatigue, diarrhea, and dyspnea. At present, sorafenib is indicated as a sole agent in the treatment of advanced renal cell carcinoma, although multiple comparisons of combinations of targeted agents are awaiting completion and analysis.

Sunitinib

Sunitinib (SU011248) is another oral tyrosine kinase inhibitor that also exhibits potent antiangiogenic activity and potency against the receptor tyrosine kinases VEGFR, PDGFR, and c-kit. A phase III study of sunitinib for patients with untreated clear cell carcinoma with good to intermediate prognosis demonstrated improved progression-free survival, and preliminary analysis of overall survival appears statistically significant.[47] The recommended dose is 50 mg daily, 4 weeks on, 2 weeks off.

The most common toxicity is fatigue, followed by diarrhea, emesis, hypertension, and the hand-foot syndrome. Skin discoloration occurs in >20% of all patients treated with sunitinib and is reversible in all patients. Other rare but significant complications include decreases in ejection fraction in 10% and hypothyroidism in up to one third of patients. At present, sunitinib is indicated as a sole agent in the treatment of advanced renal cell carcinoma, although combined therapy with other targeted agents is being tested in randomized studies.

Temsirolimus

Temsirolimus (CCI-779) inhibits the mammalian target of rapamycin (mTOR) kinase through binding to FKBP-12 and complexing with mTOR. Signaling through mTOR induces HIF, angiogenesis, and cell cycle progression and provides multiple antineoplastic effects for mTOR inhibitors. The toxicities associated with temsirolimus are similar to those of other targeted agents for renal cell carcinoma. Anemia is the most common grade 3 or 4 toxicity, followed by fatigue, hyperglycemia, and infection, all of which have occurred in ≥5% of patients.[48] Some level of grade 3 or 4 toxicity has occurred in 67% of patients treated with temsirolimus. Temsirolimus is now indicated as first-line therapy of patients with poor risk metastatic renal cell carcinoma.[48]

Vinblastine

The vinca alkaloids achieve cytotoxic effects by binding to β-tubulin at a site distinct from that of the taxanes. The effect of vinca alkaloids is mediated by inhibition of microtubule assembly and by tubulin self-association, leading to cell death. All the vinca alkaloids have similar effects on microtubules; these drugs suppress both microtubule growth and shortening by binding at high-affinity sites on the ends of microtubules, with resulting inhibition of microtubule assembly and cell death. The dose-limiting toxicity of vinblastine is myelosuppression, most commonly neutropenia. Although paralytic ileus occurs most commonly with vincristine, this difficult clinical situation can occur in 2% to 4% of patients receiving vinblastine.[41]

All the vinca alkaloids can cause hyponatremia resulting from the syndrome of inappropriate antidiuretic hormone, and all are vesicants that require care in administration. Dose adjustments are necessary in the presence of hepatic dysfunction related to impaired excretion. Vinblastine is used primarily in the treatment of locally advanced and metastatic bladder cancer and relapsed testicular cancer.[40,42]

CONCLUSION

Advances in the treatment of genitourinary cancer have dramatically changed the field and have resulted in lower relapse rates and better palliation for patients with locally and systemically advanced disease. Minimizing the acute and chronic toxicity of currently used chemotherapeutic agents while maintaining their clinical efficacy remains a critical focus of research, even in the age of targeted therapy. More effective management of chemotherapy-induced toxicities will, we hope, lead to fewer hospitalizations and better use of health resources for patients dealing with genitourinary cancers.

KEY POINTS

1. New drugs and combinations of existing drugs have resulted in better survival and less toxicity for most patients with genitourinary malignancy.
2. Duration of therapy should be informed by potential acute and chronic toxicities of therapy.
3. Patients who have been exposed to agents in the adjuvant setting or as treatment for testicular cancer are at the greatest risk of developing leukemia and pulmonary and cardiac complications in the long term.

REFERENCES

Please see www.expertconsult.com

Chapter 11

COMPLICATIONS OF RADIATION THERAPY FOR UROLOGIC CANCER

David A. Berger MD
Fellow in Urologic Oncology, Division of Urologic Surgery, Washington University School of Medicine, St. Louis, Missouri

Steven B. Brandes MD
Professor of Urologic Surgery, Division of Urologic Surgery, Washington University School of Medicine, St. Louis, Missouri

Jeff M. Michalski MD
Professor of Radiation Oncology, Division of Radiation Oncology, Washington University School of Medicine, Alvin J. Siteman Cancer Center, St. Louis, Missouri

Adam S. Kibel MD
Professor of Urologic Surgery, Division of Urologic Surgery, Washington University School of Medicine, Alvin J. Siteman Cancer Center, St. Louis, Missouri

The treatment of urologic malignant diseases often requires the integration of multiple modalities including radiation therapy (RT). Patients with testicular, bladder, and prostate cancers are frequently treated with RT. As such, the practicing urologist is often asked about the potential complications of treatment. In addition, other common malignant diseases, such as cervical and rectal carcinoma, often require RT, and the urologist is often called on to manage complications ranging from hematuria to secondary malignancies. It is therefore critically important for the practicing urologist to be familiar with the cause and management of RT-induced complications.

RT is not uniform. The dose and field used vary substantially by indication. Not surprisingly, the complications of treatment are influenced by these variables. Organs within a field are at risk, and higher doses increase risk. The use of conformal beam RT (CRT) and intensity-modulated RT (IMRT) have sculpted RT to minimize exposure to surrounding organs; however, not all medical centers have these technologies, patients may have received treatment years or decades before they present with complications, and fields often need to be expanded to treat more aggressive malignant diseases.

In this chapter, we outline the cause and treatment of RT-induced complications. The focus is on cancers treated by the urologist. However, given that urologic complications can result from the treatment of other diseases, these complications are addressed as well.

RADIOBIOLOGY

Radiation causes cell death in multiple ways, and active investigation is still under way to understand this process fully. Radiation damage can act directly by ionization or indirectly by free radical formation when radiation interacts with intracellular water. The ultimate effect is damage to DNA that impairs replication and protein synthesis. The effect of ionizing radiation on normal tissues depends on total dose, dose fraction size, total volume treated, and time over which therapy is delivered.

Radiation causes both acute and chronic effects on tissue. Acute effects usually occur within 2 to 3 weeks of therapy, whereas chronic effects can manifest months and, indeed, years later. Tissues with rapid cell turnover such as skin and mucous membranes are most susceptible to the acute effects of radiation. Chronic tissue damage is characterized by cell ischemia and fibrosis. Multiple theories have been postulated to explain chronic effects, which include microvascular damage and stem cell injury. The result is vascular damage characterized by endothelial proliferation and obliterative endarteritis leading to ischemia and fibrosis of the affected and surrounding tissue.

The onset of subacute and chronic complications typically occurs 6 to 24 months after RT. However, some chronic complications, such as bleeding, fibrosis, and scarring can occur even decades later. In general, some of the comorbid conditions that predispose patients to

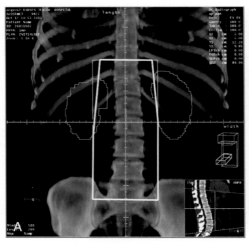
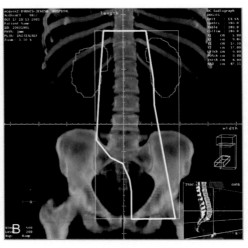

Stage 1, Paraaortic field

Stage 1 or 2, "Dog-leg" field

Figure 11-1 **A** and **B**, Radiation fields for seminoma.

RT complications and vascular damage are diabetes mellitus, hypertension, cardiovascular disease, prior surgical procedures, and concomitant radiation-sensitizing chemotherapy.

Tremendous advances in tumor localization with RT have been made since the late 1980s. Originally, radiation oncologists used skeletal anatomy to guide the radiation beams. Prostate cancer was treated by aiming the beams at the area between the pubic symphysis and the femoral heads. Computed tomography (CT) scanning, more widely used in the 1990s, allowed three-dimensional visualization of the target organ. This led to a more advanced technique, *CRT,* which employs sophisticated software to allow the radiation to conform to the shape of the target organ. The end result of these advances is to maximize cancer control while greatly limiting the amount of radiation delivered to surrounding organs.

Prostate brachytherapy (BT) achieves a high radiation dose to the prostate with a rapid dose decline in the juxtaposed and interposed adjacent normal tissue. Seeds are typically placed in a distribution to spare the prostatic urethra. The number and percentage of men treated with BT have increased dramatically since the 1990s. Complications of BT are detailed in Chapter 15. IMRT, the most current and advanced form of CRT, uses a combination of CT scanning and computer software to deliver an unprecedented level of radiation to the target tissue while minimizing exposure to surrounding organs.

RETROPERITONEAL RADIATION THERAPY

Retroperitoneal RT is used to treat a variety of malignant diseases including testicular, endometrial, and ovarian carcinomas and soft tissue sarcomas.[1,2] In advising patients about treatment options, the most common tumor encountered by the practicing urologist is testicular seminoma.

At present, most patients with stage I and low-volume stage II seminomas receive approximately 25 Gy of external beam RT (**Fig. 11-1**). Reports suggest that adjuvant RT to the para-aortic and pelvic fields results in 10- and 20-year relapse-free survival rates of 91% and 95%, respectively.[3,4]

Acute Toxicity

Acute morbidity after abdominal RT is primarily gastrointestinal (GI) and hematologic. Acute toxicity can include nausea, vomiting, and increased bowel frequency as well as neutropenia and thrombocytopenia.[5,6] The acute complications tend to be self-limited, and although patients sometimes require antiemetics and antidiarrheal agents, they usually require little supportive care. This does not mean that these side effects are not bothersome to the patient, and efforts to control symptoms have focused on limiting radiation exposure.

Gastrointestinal Toxicity

GI symptoms are common during retroperitoneal RT. Yeoh and colleagues[7] evaluated early GI toxicity and found that 90.9% of the patients experienced at least one GI side effect. Malas and associates[8] found a 66% incidence of nausea or vomiting and a 59% increase in bowel frequency in patients undergoing RT for seminoma. Although bowel frequency was directly related to dose, nausea and vomiting were independent of both the dose and volume of RT received.[8] Fernandez-Banares and colleagues[9] examined patients with a variety of malignant tumors who were receiving abdominopelvic RT and reported that 92% of patients exhibited symptoms consistent with acute RT enteropathy, primarily diarrhea. Other groups have reported substantial lower rates of GI toxicity for retroperitoneal RT ranging from 7.6% to 54.7%.[5,10]

Radiation enteritis is believed to be secondary to RT damage to the gut mucosa. This results in malabsorption and decreased transit time. Fernandez-Barnares and colleagues found that lactose malabsorption following RT results in accelerated orocecal transit, which likely contributes to the severity of the diarrhea.[9] Yeoh and coworkers compared a cohort of seminoma patients treated with RT to healthy volunteers and demonstrated that gastric emptying was more rapid in patients receiving RT. None of the other objective parameters were statistically different between the cases and controls.[11] In addition, RT-induced nausea and vomiting is believed to be related to the release of serotonin from enterochromaffin cells in the gut.[12]

Management of acute GI toxicity primarily requires the use of 5-hydroxytryptamine (5-HT$_3$) antagonist antiemetics. Many investigators showed that use of these agents reduced nausea by up to twofold in randomized studies.[13-15] The National Cancer Institute of Canada showed that dexamethasone was effective at reducing RT-induced nausea and vomiting in another randomized clinical trial.[16]

Limiting the radiation fields is another way to decrease the risk of GI complications substantially. Fossa and associates[17] evaluated the difference between GI complications and RT field. Para-aortic radiation was associated with a statistically significant improvement in nausea or vomiting and diarrhea as compared with the para-aortic plus ipsilateral pelvic nodes (dog leg). Additional GI acute symptoms such as dyspepsia and colic were also improved.[17] A second similar study showed the same results.[18]

Hematologic Toxicity

Acute hematologic toxicity is rarely dose limiting in patients treated for seminoma. Although the bone marrow responsible for hematologic function is in the radiation fields, at the relatively low volumes employed in this young population, the toxicity is rarely significant, and limiting the field and dose is the primary method of prevention. Fossa and colleagues[17] evaluated the rates of acute hematologic toxicity in the cohorts of patients treated with traditional fields (n = 242) or para-aortic fields only (n = 236). Overall, the incidence of adverse hematologic consequences was reduced in patients receiving para-aortic RT only (P < .0001). The incidence of grade 1 leukopenia (leukocyte count, 1.5-1.9) in the para-aortic and traditional fields was 14% and 29%, respectively, whereas the incidence of grade 2 leukopenia (leukocyte count, 1.0-1.4) was 5% and 12%, respectively. Grade 3 leukopenia (leukocyte count, 0.5-0.9) did not occur in the patients receiving para-aortic RT only, but it did occur in 1% of the patients receiving RT with traditional fields.[17] However, in general, no supportive measures to maintain leukocyte counts are necessary. No risk of infection or bleeding was associated with these radiation volumes.

Delayed Toxicity

Gastrointestinal Toxicity

Delayed GI complications are a significant burden in patients receiving infradiaphragmatic RT, particularly patients with preexisting GI disease. The primary late GI complications include peptic ulceration, chronic diarrhea, hemorrhage, and intestinal obstruction.

Coia and colleagues[19] examined the complications of 1026 patients treated with infradiaphragmatic RT for a wide variety of malignant diseases, including 386 patients with seminoma. These investigators found a clear correlation between chronic GI complication rates and the total RT dose. Although many of the major complications (60%, 21 of 35) were of GI origin, the absolute incidence of GI complication was relatively low. Limiting the dose of RT may decrease side effects; 3% of patients had chronic GI toxicity at doses >35 Gy compared with 1% at doses <35 Gy (P = .03).[19] Glanzmann and colleagues[20] examined 289 patients who received 30 to 35 Gy and found no relationship between RT and incidence of GI morbidity, such as peptic ulcer disease.

The true impact of GI complications may be higher than reported in the literature. Often, toxicity is reported based on physician assessments using the Radiation Therapy Oncology Group (RTOG) or National Cancer Institute Common Toxicity Criteria for Adverse Events scales. When patient-reported outcomes are measured, the rates of side effects are commonly greater. This is true for both surgical treatment and RT. Fossa and colleagues[21] examined physician-reported and patient-reported delayed GI complications. Although only 4% of the physicians' charts documented GI complications, 41% of patients reported GI morbidity.[21]

Cardiac Toxicity

Cardiac toxicity following RT for seminoma was particularly a problem when supradiaphragmatic RT was routinely used, and as a result this technique has been largely abandoned. However, patients who were irradiated in the 1960s and 1970s are now approaching an age at which cardiovascular events are frequent, and therefore the practicing urologist should be aware of this potential complication.

Van den Belt-Dusebout and colleagues[22] studied 2512 patients with testicular cancer including both seminomas and nonseminomatous germ cell tumors. This report found that mediastinal RT was associated with an elevated myocardial infarction risk (relative risk [RR], 3.7), whereas infradiaphragmatic RT was not. Chemotherapy, notably the BEP (bleomycin, etoposide, cisplatin) and PVB (cisplatin, vinblastine, and bleomycin) regimens, was also associated with an increased RR of 1.5 and 1.9, respectively.[22] Other investigators have reported that cardiac risk after mediastinal RT is associated with smoking habits, age, and depth of RT penetration on multivariate analysis ($P = .047$).[23] A review of 477 men treated at MD Anderson Cancer Center in Houston over a 48-year period revealed that adjuvant RT predisposes patients to a higher likelihood of cardiac-related death.[24]

Although cardiovascular disease is clearly related to mediastinal radiation, infradiaphragmatic RT still carries a substantial risk. One study examined 992 patients who received either surgical treatment alone, chemotherapy alone, RT alone, or combined chemotherapy and RT. At a median of 10.2 years, the RR of cardiovascular complications in patients receiving any RT, including the majority (only infradiaphragmatic RT) and the minority (additional mediastinal), was 2.61 (95% confidence interval [CI], 1.23-5.56; $P = .013$). When the 30 patients receiving supradiaphragmatic RT were excluded, the increased risk remained statistically significant ($P = .012$).[25]

As a result of this heightened risk in the setting of RT and certain chemotherapy regimens, management should be focused on decreasing risks for developing cardiovascular disease. These risk modifiers, including cessation of smoking and heart-healthy lifestyle choices, are recommended. Additional changes that could affect cardiotoxicity include a low-fat, low-cholesterol diet and regular exercise.

Secondary Cancers

The risk of a secondary malignant disease following RT is elevated. RT functions as a DNA-damaging agent and as such injures normal as well as malignant tissue. Normal tissues in the RT field may therefore be affected; however, most of the DNA damage does not result in tumor formation. Secondary tumors associated with RT and with at least twice the standard risk in the general population include lesions from a variety of sites and are presented in Table 11-1.[26] Although the literature has many studies that demonstrated no association between RT and secondary malignant diseases, follow-up in these studies with negative results was short. With extended follow-up, the risk clearly increases.

Chao and colleagues[27] from Washington University in St. Louis described 128 patients who underwent orchiectomy and adjuvant RT for low-stage seminoma and analyzed the RR of developing a secondary tumor. Nine patients within the cohort developed a secondary lesion after a median follow-up of 11.7 years. When the cohort was examined in its entirety, the increased risk compared with an untreated control population was not statistically significant (RR, 2.09; 95% CI, 0.39-3.35). However, analysis of the subgroups with longer follow-up, 11 to 15 years after RT, demonstrated an elevated risk that was statistically significant (RR, 4.45; 95% CI, 1.22 to 11.63). In a similar study, the cumulative incidence of second extratesticular malignant disease was 0.4% at 4 years, 1.3% at 9 years, 4.5% at 14

TABLE 11-1	Standard Incidence Ratios for Secondary Lesions After Seminoma	
Secondary Neoplasm	**SIR (%)**	**95% CI**
Bladder	2.27	1.91-2.68
Gallbladder/bile duct	2.17	1.12-3.79
Kidney	2.02	1.53-2.60
Myeloid leukemia	2.39	1.41-3.77
Nonmyeloid, nonlymphoid leukemias	3.48	2.03-5.57
Pancreas	2.45	1.87-3.15
Small intestine	2.52	1.01-5.19
Soft tissue sarcoma	2.01	0.96-3.70
Stomach	2.25	1.82-2.75
Thyroid	3.06	1.63-5.23

CI, confidence interval; SIR, standard incidence ratio.
From Richiardi L, Scelo G, Boffetta P, et al. Second malignancies among survivors of germ-cell testicular cancer: a pooled analysis between 13 cancer registries. *Int J Cancer.* 2007;120:623.

years, 6.3% at 19 years, 7.5% at 24 years, 15.6% at 29 years, and 23.6% at 35 years.[20] Multiple large retrospective studies have reinforced this relationship with an increased risk of cancer with longer follow-up.[26-28]

Among 22,424 patients with seminoma with a cumulative 36% rate of malignant disease at 40 years of follow-up, the RR of secondary neoplasm formation according to treatment received was greater among patients who received chemotherapy in addition to RT than among those received either modality alone.[29] This study demonstrated an association between younger age at the time of diagnosis and increased risk of secondary malignant diseases.[29] Because younger age at onset is often a sign of a hereditary predisposition, one possible explanation for this finding is that younger patients are predisposed to secondary malignant diseases.

Although the overall risk of secondary malignant disease does increase with time, specific cancers become clinically evident at different time intervals of follow-up. For example, the peak occurrence of lymphoma and leukemia is within 4 years, and GI cancer and bladder cancer develop after 10 years.[30-32]

One proposed method to decrease secondary malignancies is to limit the radiation field or dose. However, it is unclear if this has an impact. However, it is unclear if this has an impact. Hanks and colleagues[33] reported that the size of the irradiated field did not impact the rate of second cancer formation. Fatigante and associates[34] evaluated stage I-II seminoma over 30 years and actually found an increased risk (RR, 2.8; $P = .015$) of secondary malignancies with lower doses (<4000 cGy) of RT.

Clearly, patients receiving RT are at increased risk for malignancy. Clinicians need to minimize exposure by limiting radiation fields and doses. In addition, clinicians need to warn patients about the risk of secondary malignancies occurring years after the initial diagnosis.

Infertility

Infertility is a significant problem in patients with testicular cancer that is related to both treatment and the underlying disease itself. This population of men often has not had children, and patients in the younger age groups may lack the emotional maturity to realize the implications of lost reproductive capacity.

It is well known and described that RT has effects on the testis itself, which has the capacity to disrupt functions. Spermatogonia are some of the most radiation-sensitive cells in humans. Radiation doses as low as 50 cGy may cause temporary oligospermia. In 1974, Rowley and colleagues[35] used human subjects to determine the intra-RT and post-RT absorption of radiation, as well to monitor sperm parameters such as motility, morphology, volume, and concentration. These findings were later corroborated by a second study that reported a 30% decrease in fertility in a combined cohort of 451 patients with testicular cancer who received RT alone or chemotherapy alone.[36] Huyghe and colleagues[36] found that the effect of RT was considered much more deleterious than chemotherapy on fertility rates after treatment for seminoma ($P < .01$). The pre-RT conception rate among men who were trying to conceive was 91.2%; post-treatment rates decreased to 67.1%.

In the majority of patients, semen parameters return to normal after treatment. Nalesnik and colleagues[37] surveyed 73 patients with stage I or IIa seminoma treated with RT. These investigators found that 11 of 73 patients had tried to conceive and 7 of the 11 were successful, with a mean time to pregnancy of 3.5 years after treatment. Infertility in the 4 remaining patients was the result of female infertility, erectile dysfunction, history of vasectomy, and unknown factors.

Limiting dose is probably the best method to maintain fertility. The first study describing the use of a testicular shield was written in the late 1950s, and this approach was described later by others.[38,39] An original study performed in 1982 that evaluated the RT scatter affecting the contralateral healthy testicle showed that 1.6% of the prescribed dose reached the contralateral testis.[40] This percentage was reduced to 0.1% if one used a 10-cm thick lead scrotal block just superior to the scrotum. Eliminating the pelvic component of prophylactic RT further reduces the amount of internal radiation scattered to the testicle, and more recent data have suggested that eliminating the pelvic portion of the radiation field for stage 1 seminoma does not decrease disease-free or overall survival.[17,41]

Given the risk of decreased fertility following treatment of testicular tumors in general and specifically with RT, it is prudent to advise patients to undergo sperm banking. Unfortunately, this option is not offered or used frequently. Nalesnik and colleagues[37] found that this option was offered only to16 of 73 (22%) of respondents to the questionnaire within their cohort. Although 50% of the patients did regain normal semen parameters in this study, clearly many of the remaining patients could have benefited from sperm banking.

Limiting Radiation Therapy

Although an individual recommendation to address each specific complication is possible, the best way to limit toxicity in general is to reduce fields or to decrease exposure. For this reason, significant interest has been expressed in limiting or eliminating RT for the treatment of low-risk disease. A key aspect of this approach is maintaining the high cure rates of standard treatment.

The first step in this direction was elimination of iliac nodal and supradiaphragmatic irradiation. The traditional field irradiates both the para-aortic nodes and the iliac nodes.[17] In an effort to limit toxicity while maintaining cure, it has become standard practice to irradiate only the para-aortic nodes. Santoni and colleagues[10] evaluated the overall survival of patients receiving RT limited to the para-aortic nodes or a more traditional approach irradiating the iliac nodes as well and found similar survival rates (98% and 96%, respectively) at 10 years. As outlined previously, this approach has been found to decrease morbidity for several parameters, particularly GI. In addition to dropping the iliac nodal RT, supradiaphragmatic RT for seminoma has been abandoned because of long-term cardiac toxicity.[24]

The practice of decreasing the radiation field, taken to its logical extreme, involves eliminating radiation treatment entirely and using surveillance or chemotherapy for low-risk disease.[42-44] Tyldesley and associates[45] studied patients with stage 1 seminoma and found the 5-year actuarial relapse-free survival rate was 78%. The vast majority of failures were salvaged with RT or chemotherapy, resulting in a 5-year disease-specific survival for the entire cohort of 96%. Observation protocols have not been as popular in North America as in Europe, primarily due to difficulty monitoring the patient given the lack of serum markers with seminoma and the relatively low toxicity of RT. Furthermore, inconsistent insurance portability poses problems for patients who are managed with active surveillance.

Other groups have turned to low-dose chemotherapy as an alternative for RT. Although the short-term side effects of low-dose chemotherapy appear to be less severe than in RT, the long-term complications and usefulness as cancer control remain to be determined. Oliver and colleagues[43] found that the relapse-free sur-

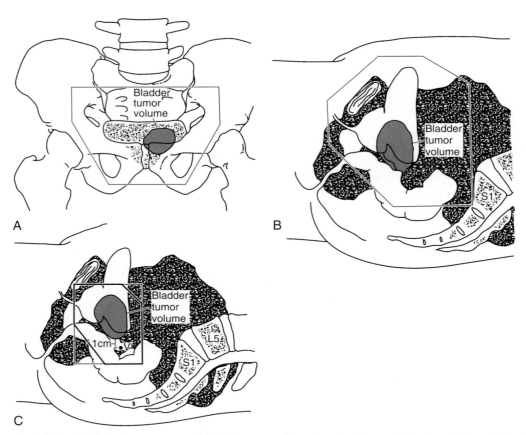

Figure 11-2   A to **C,** Radiation fields for the treatment of bladder cancer. *(From Coen JJ, Zietman AL, Kaufman DS, et al. Benchmarks achieved in the delivery of radiation therapy for muscle-invasive bladder cancer.* Urol Oncol. *2007;25:76.)*

vival rates for RT and for carboplatin were similar (95.9% and 94.8% at 3 years, respectively), but they reported that patients in the chemotherapy arm were less likely to be lethargic and more apt to return to work faster than patients in the RT arm.

Not all studies support an improved toxicity profile with alternatives to RT. Miyake and associates[46] evaluated a cohort of 130 patients that consisted of surveillance (*n* = 40), cisplatin-based chemotherapy (*n* = 64), and infradiaphragmatic RT (*n* = 26) to find out if there was a difference in health-related quality of life. The authors reported that there was no discernible difference in quality of life among the three subsets; however, patients receiving high-dose chemotherapy were noted to have worsened mental health in comparison with the other groups.

PELVIC RADIATION THERAPY

Pelvic RT is used for a variety of malignant diseases, the most common of which are bladder, prostate, cervical, and rectal carcinomas. Because of the doses and the fields used, the complications are similar but not identical. Once again, because urologists manage bladder cancer and prostate cancer much more frequently, an understanding of the complications associated with

treatment is critical. However, because urologists are commonly asked to manage RT-induced complications of other diseases, an understanding of the complications of pelvic RT in general is important.

Although pelvic RT has similar acute complications, because of the delivery of radiation to surrounding normal structures, the dose, the fields, and the use of concurrent chemotherapy drugs differ significantly. These differences can result in complication rates that vary slightly in incidence. In addition, the evolution of RT to more accurate fields using three-dimensional CRT, IMRT, proton beam RT (PBRT), and improved daily target localization has made many of the side effects, particularly chronic side effects, much less frequent.

Whereas the treatment of bladder cancer in the United States focuses on intravesical agents for superficial disease and radical cystectomy for locally invasive disease, RT does play a prominent role in the management of this disease (**Fig. 11-2**). Patients unfit for radical cystectomy, patients desiring bladder preservation, and patients with local disease recurrence often receive RT as part of their treatment.[47,48] As such, urologists must be aware of the acute complications associated with the treatment of this disease.

RT for bladder cancer is usually accompanied by radiation-sensitizing chemotherapy, which increases

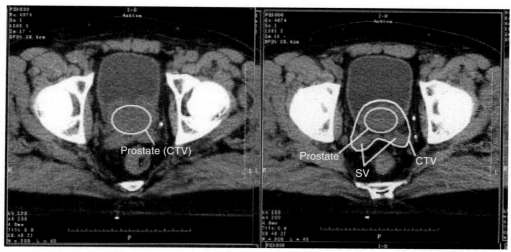

Figure 11-3 Radiation fields to the prostatic bed vary by stage. Patients with low-risk disease have more limited fields and therefore lower dose to surrounding organs. In comparison, the fields of higher-risk patients include seminal vesicles and periprostatic regions and therefore higher dose to surrounding tissues. CTV, clinical target volume; SV, seminal vesicle. *(From Boehmer D, Maingon P, Poortmans P, et al. Guidelines for primary radiotherapy of patients with prostate cancer. Radiother Oncol. 2006;79:259.)*

the risk of side effects and complications. Colquhoun and associates[49] reviewed the literature on radiosensitizing agents in bladder cancer. These investigators concluded that efforts to improve efficacy of radiation-sensitizing agents would allow safer and more efficacious RT for treating bladder cancer. Although standard therapy currently consists of cisplatin, some investigators have proposed that alternatives such as paclitaxel, which has both chemotherapeutic and radiosensitizing properties, may be more efficacious and better tolerated.[50] The side effects of the radiosensitizer must also be considered when treatment is planned.

The most common malignant disease that urologists manage during RT is prostate cancer. RT is commonly used as primary treatment, as adjuvant RT for adverse pathology at the time of surgery, or for salvage after prostate-specific antigen failure. The dose and fields vary significantly by stage and indication. Patients with high-risk disease often receive treatment to the seminal vesicles or whole pelvic radiation, whereas patients with low-risk disease have a treatment field that is much more closely tailored to the prostate (**Fig. 11-3**).[51] In addition, total dose varies significantly by indication and stage of disease, with adjuvant RT ranging from 60 to 70 Gy compared with primary therapy being between 70 and 80 Gy. Not surprisingly, complication risks are affected by these parameters.

Complications of pelvic RT for are primarily related to the genitourinary (GU) and GI tracts as a result of exposure of the bladder, urethra, small bowel, and rectum to radiation fields. Not surprisingly, bladder complications are slightly higher in bladder cancer RT because the organ is deliberately included in the radiation field. Technologic advances hopefully will have an impact on complication rates.

In a randomized clinical trial of two-dimensional versus three-dimensional CRT techniques, Tait and colleagues[52] showed a significant reduction in the incidence of acute toxicity with three-dimensional CRT. Using standard prostate RT, the RTOG documented that ≥34% of patients had acute toxicity, primarily limited to grade 1 and 2, and toxicity resolved spontaneously in 80% of the patients.[53] More recent studies examining three-dimensional CRT demonstrated very similar acute side effects. Chou and colleagues,[54] examining 198 patients with localized prostate cancer, demonstrated grade 1 and 2 toxicity in 40% and 33% of men, respectively. Chronic complications of RT remain a significant problem for patients. These complications include erectile dysfunction, hematuria, chronic irritative voiding complaints, rectal urgency, and rarely ulceration or fistula formation.

Acute Toxicity

The primary acute toxicity of pelvic irradiation is radiation cystitis or urethritis. Mild toxicity is generally limited to irritative bladder. Moderate toxicities typically consist of marked bladder irritation and hematuria, whereas severe complications include severe bladder irritation, painful hematuria, stranguria, and dysuria. Rectal complications are usually limited to diarrhea; however, rectal urgency and bleeding can become a problem.

Using a validated questionnaire, Talcott and colleagues[55] examined 182 patients for changes in bladder, bowel, and sexual function at baseline and at 3, 12, and 24 months following RT by (**Fig. 11-4**). Incontinence was not increased with RT. At 3 months, however, shortly after completion of RT, urinary obstruction or irritation was increased. Although reported bowel dysfunction was minimal before treatment, by 3 months, bowel problem scores had risen significantly. In particular, the proportion of men reporting at least occasional diarrhea had risen from 17% at baseline to 43%, and 13% of patients reported diarrhea at least several times a week.[55] With further follow-up, these acute side effects diminish in severity and frequency (Table 11-2).

Three-dimensional CRT and IMRT are reported to decrease acute complication rates, but these rates remain

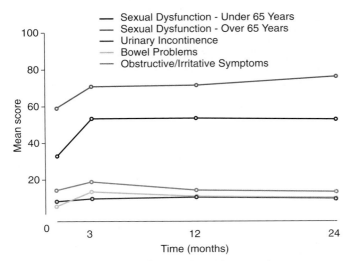

Figure 11-4 Time course of urinary incontinence, urinary obstruction or irritation, bowel problems, and sexual dysfunction for patients who underwent external beam radiation therapy. *(From Talcott JA, Manola J, Clark JA, et al. Time course and predictors of symptoms after primary prostate cancer therapy. J Clin Oncol. 2003;21:3979.)*

substantial. Rates of moderate or severe acute toxicity accompanying dose escalation were low in the RTOG dose escalation trial for early-stage prostate cancer.[56-58] Michalski and colleagues[56] reported that 53% to 60% of men had either no or only grade 1 acute GI or GU toxicity. Another 36% to 45% of patients experienced grade 2 toxicity, which is managed by short-term medical intervention. Only 2% to 4% of patients experienced any grade 3 toxicity, and no patients experienced toxicity worse than grade 3.[56] Dearnaley and colleagues[59] reported slightly higher acute bladder and bowel toxicity. Rates of grade 1 or 2 bladder and bowel toxicity were 75% and 79%, respectively. Grade 3 toxicity occurred in 1% and 2%, respectively, and no patients had grade 4 toxicity.[59]

Similar problems have been encountered with RT to the bladder. Zietman and colleagues[60] examined the records of 49 patients who participated in a bladder preservation protocol and identified bladder outlet obstruction in one third of men and involuntary detrusor contractions in 30% of women following treatment. Furthermore, these investigators reported urinary incontinence (19%) and bowel urgency (14%) and suggested that the incidence of these acute adverse effects should improve with more modern treatment techniques.[60]

Hyperfractionated RT may allow dose intensification by delivering multiple smaller fractions of radiation. *Hyperfractionation* allows the delivery of higher radiation doses without an increase in late effects. Another fractionation schema, *accelerated fractionation (AF)*, compresses the overall treatment time while maintaining a similar total dose prescription. Both hyperfractionation and AF involve multiple treatments per day. Although

TABLE 11-2	Radiation Therapy Oncology Group Toxicity Definitions				
Toxicity	**Grade 0**	**Grade 1**	**Grade 2**	**Grade 3**	**Grade 4**
Genitourinary	No change	Frequency of urination or nocturia twice pretreatment habit; dysuria, urgency not requiring medication	Frequency of urination or nocturia that is less frequent than every hour; dysuria, urgency, bladder spasm requiring local anesthetic	Frequency with urgency and nocturia hourly or more frequently; dysuria, pelvic pain, or bladder spasm requiring regular, frequent narcotics; gross hematuria with or without clot passage	Hematuria requiring transfusion; acute bladder obstruction not secondary to clot passage, ulceration, or necrosis
Lower gastrointestinal tract including pelvis	No change	Increased frequency or change in quality of bowel habits not requiring medication; rectal discomfort not requiring analgesics	Diarrhea requiring parasympatholytic drugs (e.g., Lomotil [atropine and diphenoxylate]); mucous discharge not necessitating sanitary pads; rectal or abdominal pain requiring analgesics	Diarrhea requiring parenteral support; severe mucous or blood discharge necessitating sanitary pads, abdominal distention (flat plate radiograph demonstrating distended bowel loops)	Acute or subacute obstruction, fistula or perforation; gastrointestinal bleeding requiring transfusion; abdominal pain or tenesmus requiring tube decompression or bowel diversion

the acute side effects may be worse, the late side effects should be lessened with this approach. Horwich and associates[61] studied 229 patients with cT2-T3 bladder cancer; in this prospective randomized trial, 129 patients received AF and 100 received conventional RT. The investigators concluded that AF did not improve the efficacy of treatment but did incur additional acute toxicity risk beyond conventional RT. Evaluation of specific toxicity end points demonstrated that bowel toxicity was increased in the patients receiving hyperfractionated RT (44%) compared with those receiving standard RT (26%; $P = .0001$).[61]

RT for rectal cancer is predominantly given as a short course before surgical treatment. As such, whereas the perioperative complication rate is slightly increased, the acute and chronic complications seem to be limited and well tolerated.[62] Korkolis and colleagues[63] found that significant perioperative complications, such as hemorrhage, pelvic or abdominal wound infections, ileus, urinary tract infection, and anastomotic leak, were similar in patients who did or did not receive preoperative RT. The incidence of long-term complications may be slightly increased. Pollack and colleagues[64] studied 252 patients randomized to preoperative RT versus no RT and evaluated the incidence of long-term complications. These investigators found an increased rate of overall complications ($P = .002$) and specific increases in cardiovascular disease, fecal incontinence, and urinary incontinence ($P = .032$, 0.013, and 0.023, respectively).[64]

Acute GI and bowel toxicity may limit treatment. If not severe, acute irritative bladder and bowel complications can be managed pharmacologically. Bowel hypermotility generally resolves spontaneously but can be managed with standard combinations of antidiarrheal and anticholinergic medications such as diphenoxylate and atropine. Bladder urgency can also be managed with bladder-specific anticholinergics such as tolterodine or oxybutynin.[55]

Delayed Toxicity

Chronic toxicity following pelvic radiation is a significantly greater problem because it may be irreversible. Common complications include urinary urgency, lower GI complaints, erectile dysfunction, fistula formation, increased risk of second malignant disease, and hematuria. Of particular concern to the urologist is the patient who requires subsequent pelvic surgical intervention.

Urinary Toxicity

The risk of acute and chronic toxicity is not insignificant but is manageable following RT for prostate carcinoma. Peeters and colleagues[65] reported 40% grade 1 or 2 and 12% grade 3 late toxicity rates. High-dose RT (78 Gy) did not seem increase the risk of grade 1 or 2

or grade 3 toxicity to significantly compared with low-dose RT (68 Gy).[65] Similar late GU toxicity was reported by Michalski and colleagues,[56] with 39% of patients reporting grade 1 or 2 toxicity. Grade 3 toxicity was limited to hematuria in 3% of patients.[56] Patient-reported studies have given a similar picture. Questionnaires were mailed out to 200 patients 24 to 56 months after RT for prostate carcinoma and to 200 age-matched controls to determine the incidence of urinary complications. The RT group experienced increased leakage (22% versus 33%), urgency (19% versus 42%), and difficulty initiating a urine stream (11% versus 32%) compared with the control population.[66]

The study by Talcott and colleagues[55] demonstrated that urinary symptoms returned to baseline after 3 months. The difference in studies may reflect that fact that Peeters and Michalski and their colleagues were examining multiple toxicity parameters, whereas Talcott and associates were focused on obstructive and irritative symptoms. Widmark and associates[66] identified patients after treatment, whereas Talcott and associates performed the study prospectively. Possibly this approach biased the results. In addition, Talcott and colleagues were examining patient bother. Patients with grade 1 or 2 symptoms may be satisfied, given that they would trade a small amount of urinary toxicity for cancer cure.

Expertise in the management of urinary toxicity is important for the practicing urologist. Most long-term urinary complications seem to be well tolerated. Treatment should be focused on controlling symptoms that are bothersome to the patient. Anticholinergics can be particularly useful in controlling irritative symptoms; however, because many patients also have obstructive symptoms, it is important to use the medications judiciously to avoid urinary retention.

Ureteral Obstruction

Although ureteral obstruction can occur following all forms of pelvic RT, the association with cervical carcinoma seems to be particularly strong. The reasons are the relatively high doses (≥ 80 Gy) and the close proximity of the cervix to the ureters. McIntyre and associates[67] studied 1784 patients over a 3-decade period and found that 29 of 1784 developed an RT-induced ureteral stricture with an incidence of 1.0%, 1.2%, 2.2%, and 2.5% at 5, 10, 15, and 20 years of follow-up, respectively. The actuarial risk rises each year by 0.15%. The investigators further stated that in the first 5 years after RT, the most common cause of ureteral stricture is recurrent disease, although future onset of stricture may be related to initial latent radiation injury.[67,68]

Radiation Cystitis

Cystitis induced by pelvic RT may be seen after treatment for prostate cancer (3%-5%) and cervical cancer (3%-6.5%).[69,70] Given that the bladder is deliberately included in the RT field for bladder cancer, the risk appears to be higher in this patient population. Tonoli and colleagues[71] found the 5-year actuarial incidence of bladder toxicity to be 52%, with rates of grades 1, 2, 3, and 4 toxicity of 30%, 18%, 8%, and 2%, respectively. The timing of RT cystitis varies and can occur from 6 months up to 10 years after pelvic irradiation.[72]

Hematuria can be acute or chronic and is often associated with other cystitis symptoms including urinary frequency, urgency, and dysuria. If possible, discontinuation of anticoagulants such as aspirin may resolve the problem. When bleeding from the bladder is diffuse, as is typical for radiation cystitis, intravesical therapy is often required. In the acute setting, complete evacuation of clots is essential. Once the bladder has been cleared, continuous bladder irrigation and correction of all medical bleeding or coagulopathy (i.e., stop nonsteroidal anti-inflammatory drugs, warfarin [Coumadin], heparin, aspirin) may resolve the problem.

In many cases, instillation of agents into the bladder is required to control refractory bleeding. The typical first-line agent is alum (aluminum sulfate and either ammonium or potassium). Alum is an astringent that causes protein precipitation and induces clot formation over the belling epithelium. Although this agent is useful in controlling moderate bleeding, the precipitate often clogs the catheters with a thick, adherent paste. One percent alum is infused as a continuous bladder irrigation through a three-way Foley catheter. Alum can be absorbed systemically; therefore, in patients with renal insufficiency, the potential exists for aluminum, potassium, or ammonia toxicity, depending on the solution used. Because encephalopathy and acidosis have been reported, aluminum levels need to be monitored in patients with mental status changes.[73]

Another common bladder instillation agent is 0.5% to 1.0% silver nitrate. Silver nitrate needs to be mixed in water and causes protein precipitation in the bladder, which induces clotting. Silver nitrate causes only minor discomfort and can be instilled at the bedside, typically for periods of 10 to 20 minutes. Multiple instillations may be necessary, and the effects are often short-lived.[74,75]

Formalin instillation works by hydrolyzing proteins and coagulating bleeding from the mucosa and submucosa. Formalin is essentially a 37% solution of formaldehyde (i.e., 10% formalin = 3.7% formaldehyde), so it is important to clarify the nomenclature with the pharmacist. Formalin instillation is particularly painful and thus needs to be performed using spinal or general anesthesia. Because reflux of formalin into the ureters can result in papillary necrosis, ureteral stricture, and hydronephrosis, a cystogram needs to be performed in *all* patients *before* formalin instillation. When reflux is evident on the cystogram, occlusive Fogarty or ureteropelvic junction balloon catheters need to be placed.[76,77]

Formalin is typically instilled under gravity, and the Foley catheter is clamped for 10 minutes. A 1% to 4%

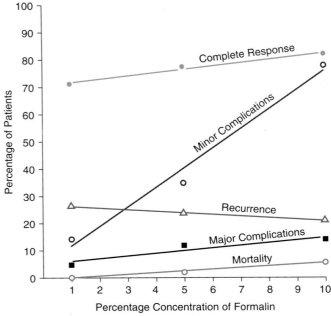

Figure 11-5 Response rates and complications are affected by concentration of formalin. *(From Donahue LA, Frank IN. Intravesical formalin for hemorrhagic cystitis: analysis of therapy. J Urol. 1989;141:809.)*

solution is typically used, and after drainage, the bladder is irrigated with normal saline. In a meta-analysis by Donahue and Frank[78] of 235 cases in 32 reports, the response rates were dependent on solution concentration; 10% formalin effected a cure in 83% of patients, 5% effected a cure in 78%, and 1% effected a cure in 71%. Furthermore, complications were also directly proportional to the concentration of the solution instilled (**Fig. 11-5**).[78] For 5% and 1% formalin, rates of major complications are 7% and 5%, respectively, whereas rates of minor complications are 40% and 12%, respectively.

Other techniques that have been reported over the years but are less commonly used and have had variable results are intravesical hydrostatic pressure techniques, oral or intravenous conjugated estrogens, oral pentosan polysulfate sodium (Elmiron), intravesical prostaglandins, phenol (carbonic acid) argon beam coagulator,[79] and intravesical ice water irrigations.[80]

In the very rare instance in which all the foregoing methods fail, options include selective embolization of the hypogastric arteries. As long as embolization is distal to the superior gluteals, the risk of buttock claudication is remote. Bladder necrosis after embolization is possible, yet it is extremely rare. The last heroic options are salvage cystectomy and open packing of the bladder.

Urethral Stricture and Bladder Neck Contracture

The overall incidence of bulbomembranous urethral stricture or bladder neck contracture following RT is approximately 3% to 16%.[81] Time to presentation is typically 12 to 36 months (mean, ≈24 months), and the typical presentation occurs with obstructive and irritative voiding symptoms. However, at longer follow-up and the inclusion of significantly greater numbers of patients, stricture disease has been documented ≤6 years after BT. Elliot and colleagues,[81] in their analysis of the CaPSURE database (mostly community practices), noted that the post-RT stricture incidence was initially very low, but over time increased at a steady rate from an initial almost 0% to 5% rate to 16% by 4 years, depending on the subpopulation examined. This finding suggests that the effects of RT on the urethra and bladder neck are typically delayed.

Bladder neck contracture can occur with RT alone; however, it primarily occurs with RT after radical prostatectomy. Thompson and colleagues[82] found that adjuvant RT in high-risk patients increased the risk of urethral strictures (17.8% versus 9.5%) and of total urinary incontinence (6.5% versus 2.8%) compared with controls. Multiple risk factors for the development of strictures have been examined. A history of transurethral resection of the prostate (TURP) before RT has been implicated as a cause of stricture and bladder neck contracture.[83]

Overall, the bladder neck contracture rate with RT alone is 3.7%, whereas the rate in patients with prior TURP increases significantly to 5.8%.[81,83] Seymore and colleagues[84] noted that 72% of the patients who developed bladder neck contractures after RT to 68 Gy had a prior TURP. The risk appeared to be highest when RT was delivered immediately following TURP. The likely mechanisms of stricture formation are ischemia and microfibrosis following cautery use (especially at the bladder neck), resulting in a relative inability of the area to repair endothelial damage caused by radiation. To reduce the risk of such strictures, these investigators recommended an interval between TURP and prostate RT of ≥6 weeks. Numerous other studies that also noted that prior TURP increased the incidence of RT-induced strictures.

Management of Urethral Strictures In general, radiation impairs the healing potential of tissues, particularly as a result of end arteritis hypovascularity, decreased intrinsic cellular vitality, and interstitial fibrosis. RT-induced urethral strictures typically have an unhealthy or "washed leather" appearance on cystoscopy and have varying degrees of local tissue induration or dense fibrotic scarring.

In general, urethral strictures after external beam RT are typically minor and can be managed by endoscopic dilation or incision. More complex stricture disease can be more of a management dilemma. The devastating complications of rectourethral fistula (RUF), vesicorectal fistula, and obliterative strictures of the prostatic or membranous urethra occur after BT. Merrick and colleagues[85] noted that 29 of 1186 patients developed a membranous or proximal bulbar urethral stricture after prostate BT. All 29 strictures were initially managed by dilation or urethrotomy. Approximately one third (9 of 29) of these patients had recurrent strictures requiring repeat urethrotomy and intermittent self-catheterization to prevent restenosis. Of these 9 patients, 3 developed obliterative and refractory strictures and thus were eventually managed with suprapubic urinary diversion. Thus, approximately one third of BT-related urethral strictures are recurrent, and of these, one third of them are devastating, requiring a urinary diversion. Of all the BT-treated patients, the need for supravesical diversion translates to a 0.25% incidence.

Ragde and colleagues[86] noted a 12% rate of bulbomembranous strictures at median follow-up of 69 months. Most of the urethral strictures were short and were managed by urethral dilation with and without self-catheterization.

Devastating obliterative strictures are recurrent and refractory to endoscopic means. Typically, such strictures require open reconstruction and supravesical urinary diversions, whether by suprapubic tube, by urinary conduit or enterocystoplasty and continent catheterizable stomas, or by salvage cystoprostatectomy and urinary diversion.[87]

Flexibility in treating complex urethral strictures is critical. Refractory RT-induced strictures may need to be treated with urethrotomy and intermittent self-catheterization, off-label use of the UroLume endourethral prosthesis (American Medical Systems, Minnetonka, Minnesota), anastomotic urethroplasty, salvage prostatectomy with anastomotic urethrovesical urethroplasty, combined abdominal-perineal urethroplasty, onlay flap urethroplasty, or supravesical urinary diversion surgery.

If urethroplasty is employed for RT-induced strictures, excision and primary anastomosis (for short bulbar strictures) or an onlay flap should be the primary mode of repair. Grafts should be avoided in the radiated field because grafts rely on the host bed for vascularity (imbibition and inosculation), and this bed is typically compromised in the patient who has undergone pelvic RT. Instead, a pedicle island skin flap is a good method for reconstructing the radiated stricture because it has its own blood supply and can be sewn into place as a readily available onlay flap. Another option for urethral reconstruction is the use of extragenital skin that has been grafted onto a gracilis muscle flap and then used as an onlay flap.

Hyperbaric oxygen (HBO) therapy has been shown to help stimulate angiogenesis, which can help to repair the baseline obliterative endarteritis–induced ischemia physiologically. Treatment typically requires breathing 100% oxygen at two atmospheres of pressure for 2 to 3 hours per day for a total of 40 to 60 sessions. HBO has been used with varying results with bladder complications and with fair results in patients with grade 2 and 3 rectal complications. Theoretically, HBO could be used as an adjunctive method to promote angiogenesis of the urethra and thus could improve the success of a subsequent urethroplasty or a staged reconstruction. However, Theodorescu and associates[88] reported on the uniform failure of HBO for grade 4 RTOG urinary complications. The practical value of HBO for urethral stricture surgery thus appears to be minimal.

Urinary Fistulas

Urinary fistulas are uncommon in association with external RT alone. These fistulas tend to occur in the setting of a procedural intervention following RT. The practicing urologist needs to be cognizant of this potential complication before treating a patient who has undergone pelvic RT.

By definition, a *fistula* is an extra-anatomic, epithelialized channel between two hollow organs or between a hollow organ and the body surface. Acquired RUFs are uncommonly associated with pelvic RT and are typically associated with iatrogenic injury during pelvic surgical procedures (e.g., laparoscopic and open radical prostatectomy or abdominal perineal resection), transrectal biopsy of a rectal ulcer, or overly aggressive transurethral resection of bladder neck contracture after prostatectomy.

With the increased use of brachytherapy (BT) and its combination with external beam RT boost, particularly devastating fistulas can occur. RUFs after BT are reported in ≤0.4% to 0.8% of cases, and for BT plus EBRT, in ≤2.9%.[89,90] Such RT-induced fistulas are more common when RT is used as salvage therapy or when the anterior rectal wall has been sampled for biopsy after RT. Transanal rectal wall or rectal ulcer biopsies (through a sigmoidoscope) in the patient who has undergone pelvic RT are unwise and have a high chance of eliciting an RUF. The reported average time from last RT session to RUF diagnosis is approximately 2 years. The mean time from a rectal procedure to the diagnosis of RUF is 4 months.[89,91]

To decide on the proper management of bladder or urethral urinary fistula, the clinician must know or determine the cause of the fistula, the integrity of the anal and external urethral sphincters, the functional status of the bladder, the extent of rectal radiation damage, the size and location of the urinary fistula, and the overall performance and nutritional status of the patient. Small, nonradiated fistulas are often successfully managed by the transanal or York-Mason approach. Complex fistulas that are large or are caused by RT are best managed by primary repair, buttressed with a gracilis interposition flap, or by proctectomy and coloanal pull-through. Few surgeons have had extensive experience with RUF, and thus no clear standard surgical repair approach is recommended.

Because radiated fistulas have a poor blood supply and tissue planes are distorted, interposition of well-vascularized, nonradiated tissue is essential. In general, a redundant surgical approach is wise. In other words, the success of fistula repair can be maximized by fecal

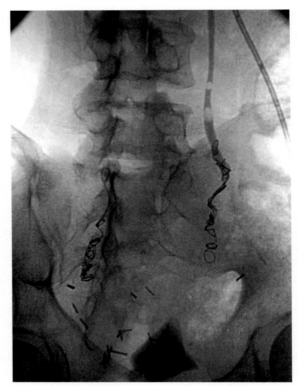

Figure 11-6 Ureteral embolization for a radiation-induced urethrorectal fistula and urinary incontinence in a patient with poor performance status. Note the deployed Gianturco coils in the distal ureters.

and urinary diversion, tension-free and watertight closure of the fistula, multiple layers of nonoverlapping suture lines, and interposition of vascularized tissue flaps.

When considering surgical repair of RT-associated urinary fistulas or incontinence, patients should have good performance status, to tolerate the necessary major surgical reconstruction. Patients with multiple comorbidities and who are thus poor surgical candidates with limited life expectancy have few options for managing their urinary fistulas. Typically, a suprapubic tube is initially placed to divert the urine away from the urethral-rectal or urethral-perineal fistula, as long as the internal urinary sphincter is intact. However, if the bladder neck is open or the urinary fistula is in the bladder, then the only noninvasive method that will successfully divert the urine is often bilateral percutaneous nephrostomy tube placement. Although in most cases nephrostomies can divert the urine, in some instances the majority of the urine still travels down the ureters. Bilateral transureteric embolization of the distal ureters with a combination of Gianturco coils (steel coils) and Gelfoam (gelatin sponge) can often resolve this problem (**Fig. 11-6**). However, this approach should be used as definitive management only in patients with a limited life expectancy (<1 year) because it is irreversible.[92]

Vesicovaginal Fistulas

Most RT-induced vesicovaginal fistulas, when low lying and not associated with the ureter or bowel, can be repaired transvaginally with the interposition of a Martius flap or gracilis muscle flap. When the surgeon anticipates that vaginal mucosa will be inadequate to close the Martius flap, an island of skin can be raised with it. Occasionally, bilateral Martius flaps need to be raised for adequate coverage of the fistula. If the patient has an associated ureteral or bowel RT injury or if the fistula is very cephalad or particularly close to the ureteral orifices, then omentum or a combination of gastric and omental segments can be raised based on the left gastroepiploic arteries. Patients with a frozen pelvis who are not judged suitable for primary repair should be managed with supravesical diversion.[93]

Gastrointestinal Toxicity

RT-related GI toxicity appears to affect long-term quality of life more often than does urinary toxicity. Several reports have noted RT toxicity resulting from three-dimensional CRT techniques in prospective clinical trials. Peeters and colleagues[65] reported a 29% rate of grade 1 or 2 late toxicity and a 5% rate of grade 3 toxicity. No significant difference was reported between high-dose (78 Gy) and low-dose (68 Gy) arms of this trial.[65] In another publication from the same trial, Michalski and colleagues reported that the incidence of grade 1 or 2 bowel toxicity was 38% to 40% with a dose of 78 Gy in 39 fractions. The incidence of grade 3 complications was 2.3% when the high dose was delivered with 1.8 Gy/day and 5.9% when it was delivered with 2.0 Gy/day. The rates of grade 4 toxicity were <2% and consisted of severe proctitis and an RUF fistula requiring surgical intervention.[56,58]

Increasing the volume treated does raise the rate of GI complications, presumably by increasing the dose to the rectum and other bowel structures. In a prospective clinical trial examining a total dose of 79.2 Gy, Ryu and colleagues[58] found GI toxicity in 21% of patients receiving a smaller treatment volume compared with 38% in patients receiving a larger treatment volume.

Using a patient reported outcome questionnaire, Widmark and associates[66] conducted a comparison of healthy, nonirradiated controls and a group of patients with prostate cancer who were receiving pelvic RT. Not surprisingly, the patients with prostate cancer were at increased risk of general GI symptoms (14% and 59%), specifically increased mucus production (4% versus 38%), cramps (5% versus 14%), stool leakage (2% versus 27%), and bloody stools (2% and 36%) compared with the control population.[66] Using a validated quality of life questionnaire, Talcott and colleagues[55] found that bowel complaints in general retuned to baseline by 24 months, even though individual symptoms continued to be a problem. Although diarrhea returned to baseline, tenesmus and bowel urgency continued to be prob-lematic. The rate of rectal bleeding increased significantly from 5% before treatment to 25% at 2 years.[55]

Delayed GI complaints are very common following pelvic RT for bladder carcinoma. GI symptoms can be quite disruptive to post-RT recovery. A retrospective analysis of >400 patients with T1-T4, N0-X, M0 disease sought to determine any late effects of RT only for managing bladder cancer.[71] The 5-year cumulative risk of bladder toxicity was 14%. Grade 1, 2, 3, and 4 toxicity was 11%, 2%, 1%, and 2%, respectively. GI morbidity is one of the primary complaints of patients. Although dose reduction is an attractive possible remedy, randomized trials have not demonstrated an improvement in outcome, and concern about loss of efficacy clearly exists. Quilty and colleagues,[94] randomizing patients to high-dose and low-dose RT, found no improvement in GI symptoms.

Minor GI complications such as diarrhea can be managed conservatively with anticholinergic medications and stool bulking agents such as psyllium (Metamucil). A cohort of patients who had undergone pelvic RT were randomized to receive or not receive an antidiarrheal, and prophylactic use of this medication was found to be associated with statistically significant decreased incidence and severity of RT-induced diarrhea.[95] More significant problems such as stool incontinence and persistent bleeding require referral to a gastroenterologist. As with hematuria, one should not assume that abnormalities are only the result of RT. Patients may require colonoscopy to exclude other causes of lower GI bleeding, including malignant disease. Rarely patients may require bowel diversion secondary to GI toxicity.

Erectile Dysfunction

Pelvic RT in general is associated with decreased sexual function as a result of the radiation injury to the neurovascular bundles. Pelvic RT is usually associated with decreased sexual function. The incidence of erectile dysfunction ranges from 23% to 56% at 2 years following RT.[96,97] Fransson and Widmark[97] used a sexual function questionnaire to evaluate 199 patients who were treated with RT for prostate carcinoma. At 48 months of average follow-up (range, 24-56 months), 56% of the patients who had received RT alone and 87% of patients who had received RT with androgen deprivation complained of impotence.[97] A study by Fowler and colleagues,[96] examining 691 patients enrolled in the Surveillance, Epidemiology, and End Results (SEER) registry, found that 23% of patients developed erectile dysfunction following RT at 3 years.

Comparisons with surgical treatment are often performed. In a study by Talcott and colleagues,[55] after 2 years the erectile dysfunction in men undergoing RT and radical prostatectomy is similar. However, patients undergoing RT generally have worse performance before treatment.[55]

Erectile dysfunction is not an immediate problem during treatment but develops gradually afterward. Mantz and colleagues[98] studied 287 men who underwent three-dimensional CRT for localized prostate cancer. Potency decreased from 96% at 1 month to 75% at 20 months, to 59% at 40 months, and to 53% at 60 months after therapy.[98] Partial loss of function can also occur and decrease quality of life. Helgason and colleagues[99] found that 77% of patients had decreased sexual desire, 34% had erections insufficient for intercourse, and 77% reported decreased tumescence. Overall, half of the men reported that their quality of life had decreased as a direct result of their erectile dysfunction.[99]

Data on erectile function are most frequently studied in prostate carcinoma, but this complication remains an issue for patients with other diseases treated with RT. Patients with bladder cancer are older and frequently have significant smoking histories that add to their difficulties with sexual function following RT. Lynch and colleagues[100] reported the sexual intercourse rate after RT to be 41%. A more recent report by Zietman and colleagues[60] examined men who had undergone bladder preservation using RT and chemotherapy; 36% of these patients reported full erections, and 54% had erections sufficient for vaginal penetration.

The management of erectile dysfunction is identical to standard management. A history and physical examination should be performed to ensure that the patient does not have a more serious cause of impotence. Initial treatment uses phosphodiesterases, but prostaglandin E_1 or even a penile prosthesis may be necessary in some cases.

Cancer Risk

As outlined in the earlier section on retroperitoneal RT, a long-term complication of RT is increased risk of secondary malignant disease in the radiation fields. The primary organ at risk in the pelvis is the bladder. A review of the literature found no evidence of an increased risk of prostate, testis, or cervical carcinoma related to radiation exposure. Rectal and uterine carcinomas are inconsistently linked to exposure; some studies report positive results and others negative. Bladder cancer is the one pelvic malignant disease that seems to be associated with both low-dose and high-dose RT.[101]

Brenner and colleagues[102] examined 51,584 men in the SEER data registry who were treated with RT. These investigators found that 3549 developed a second malignant disease. The comparison group was 70,539 patients with prostate cancer who were treated surgically, of whom 5055 developed a second malignant disease. The increased risk with RT was 6%, but at 5 years it had reached a more substantial 15%, and it was 34% at 10 years. Carcinomas of the bladder, rectum,

and lung as well as in-field sarcomas contributed most to the increased risk.[102]

A similar study was performed by Moon and colleagues,[103] who examined SEER data records comparing men who received RT with men who did not. Using multivariant logistic regression analysis, these investigators found an increased risk of secondary cancers at sites within the RT field such as the bladder (odds ratio [OR], 1.63; 95% CI, 1.44-1.84) and rectum (OR, 1.60; 95% CI, 1.29-1.99). In contrast to the previous study, Moon and colleagues also found an increase in secondary malignant diseases outside the RT field such as cecum (OR, 1.63; 95% CI, 1.10-1.70), transverse colon (OR, 1.85; 95% CI, 1.30-2.63), brain (OR, 1.83; 95% CI, 1.22-2.75), stomach (OR, 1.38; 95% CI, 1.09-1.75), melanoma (OR, 1.29; 95% CI, 1.09-1.53), and lung and bronchus (OR, 1.25; 95% CI, 1.13-1.37) (**Fig. 11-7**).[103]

The first time the SEER data were analyzed to answer this question, only an increased risk of bladder cancer was identified.[104] Only with longer follow-up was the true risk determined. In addition, single-institution studies frequently fail to find an association.[105] This reason may be the smaller sample size, which is insufficiently powered to find the association. Alternatively, the larger studied identify an association with limited clinical impact. Brenner and colleagues[102] found fairly high increases in risk, although the RR of secondary cancers was still relatively low. It increased from 1 in

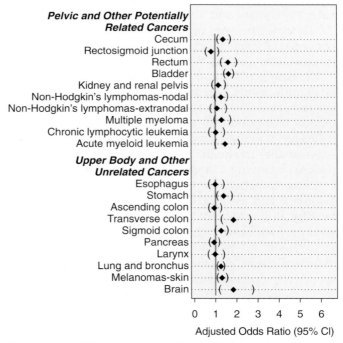

Beam Radiation Versus No Radiation

Pelvic and Other Potentially Related Cancers
- Cecum
- Rectosigmoid junction
- Rectum
- Bladder
- Kidney and renal pelvis
- Non-Hodgkin's lymphomas-nodal
- Non-Hodgkin's lymphomas-extranodal
- Multiple myeloma
- Chronic lymphocytic leukemia
- Acute myeloid leukemia

Upper Body and Other Unrelated Cancers
- Esophagus
- Stomach
- Ascending colon
- Transverse colon
- Sigmoid colon
- Pancreas
- Larynx
- Lung and bronchus
- Melanomas-skin
- Brain

Adjusted Odds Ratio (95% CI)

Figure 11-7 Risk of secondary malignant diseases in men who underwent external beam radiation therapy. *(From Moon K, Stukenborg GJ, Keim J, et al. Cancer incidence after localized therapy for prostate cancer. Cancer. 2006;107:991.)*

TABLE 11-3	5-Year Cumulative Risk of Fracture: Patients After Radiation Therapy Versus Patients With No Radiation Therapy				
Cancer Type	**No. Patients (Cases; Controls)**	**5-Yr Fracture Rate After RT (Cases)**	**5-Yr Fracture Rate After No RT (Controls)**	**Hazard Ratio From Receiving Pelvic RT**	**95% CI**
Anal	399; 157	14.0%	7.5%	3.16	1.48-6.73
Cervical	1139; 466	8.2%	5.9%	1.66	1.06-2.59
Rectal	1317; 2116	11.2%	8.7%	1.65	1.33-2.05

CI, confidence interval; RT, radiation therapy.
Data from Baxter NN, Habermann EB, Tepper JE, et al. Risk of pelvic fractures in older women following pelvic irradiation. *JAMA*. 2005;294:2587.

290 patients for all survivors to 1 in 70 for those who received RT at 10 years.[102]

Patients who receive RT should be made aware of the late risk of cancer induction and should be encouraged to follow healthy lifestyles and avoid activities that further increase their risk such as tobacco abuse. They should also practice vigilant cancer screening for common malignant diseases of the lung, breast, and GI tract.

Fracture Risk

RT can adversely affect bone structure in the radiation fields and is associated with an increased risk of fracture. Although this risk has not been documented with GU malignancies, urologists should be aware of this problem. Bone mineral loss and in increase in adverse skeletal events are particularly important in light of the association between hormone therapy and bone loss. Baxter and colleagues[106] evaluated the association between RT and fracture in the SEER database with 2855 RT cases and 3573 controls. Patients with anal, cervical, and rectal cancer were included (Table 11-3). Overall, an increase in fracture rate was reported and was limited to bone structures within the radiation field.[106]

A similar study examining gynecologic malignant disease found an 11% risk of pelvic fracture over an 11-year span. The peak of incidence occurred in women within the first year of menopause, a finding emphasizing the interactions among disease, RT, and the hormonal axis.[107] For this reason, an emphasis on bone health should be a priority in men undergoing hormone ablation who have been treated with RT. This includes vitamin D and calcium supplementation. Bisphosphonates should be used if patients demonstrate bone loss on imaging.

CONCLUSION

RT is an important component of the treatment options for a variety of malignant diseases including testis, prostate, bladder, cervical, and rectal carcinoma. Unfortunately, side effects and complications exist. The urologist often advises the patient about the efficacy and side effects of RT and is also asked to manage many of the complications of this treatment. As such, the practicing urologist needs to be familiar with the risks and treatment considerations of RT.

KEY POINTS

1. Limiting dose, duration, and fields of RT is the best way to decrease complications.
2. Acute toxicity is usually self-limiting and can be managed pharmacologically.
3. Secondary malignancies occur following RT; therefore, patients need regular cancer screening after RT.
4. Some forms of RT have increased levels of cardiac toxicity; therefore, a heart healthy lifestyle should be encouraged.
5. Hemorrhagic cystitis and stricture disease can result from pelvic radiation.
6. Fistulas need to be managed with flap reconstruction because radiated fields have poor vasculature.

REFERENCES

Please see www.expertconsult.com

COMPLICATIONS OF MINIMALLY INVASIVE UROLOGIC PROCEDURES

Chapter 12

COMPLICATIONS OF THERAPEUTIC RADIOLOGIC PROCEDURES

Steven S. Raman MD

Associate Professor of Radiology, Division of Abdominal Imaging and Cross Sectional Interventional Radiology, David Geffen School of Medicine, University of California–Los Angeles; Director, Abdominal Imaging Fellowship, Radiological Sciences, University of California–Los Angeles, Los Angeles, California

Sachiko T. Cochran MD

Professor Emeritus, Division of Abdominal Imaging and Cross Sectional Interventional Radiology, David Geffen School of Medicine, University of California–Los Angeles, Los Angeles, California

Advances in imaging and interventional techniques have transformed the diagnosis and management of a variety of common urologic disorders. Since the mid-1990s, the intravenous urogram has essentially been replaced by the computed tomography (CT) scan or magnetic resonance urogram. Similarly, percutaneous treatment of renal stones is now routinely performed by precise placement of a 20- to 30-Fr sheath into the renal calyx to enable laser or sonographic disruption of a renal stone with evacuation. Since the last edition of this textbook, percutaneous radiofrequency ablation or cryoablation of small renal cell carcinomas has become well established. This chapter discusses the complications of percutaneous and vascular therapeutic procedures performed by radiologists.

PERCUTANEOUS NONVASCULAR PROCEDURES

General Considerations

Before performing any percutaneous procedures, we ask that patients refrain from taking antiplatelet agents such as aspirin, ibuprofen for 5 to 7 days, or anticoagulants such as clopidogrel (Plavix) for 3 days. We also obtain a serum hemoglobin determination, hematocrit, and platelet count and a basic assessment of the patient's coagulation including the prothrombin time and partial thromboplastin time. When elevated, the prothrombin time is corrected to <1.5 times normal, and the platelet count is augmented to at least 50,000 to minimize bleeding complications. Hypertension is also controlled. Informed consent is obtained for the procedure, and a bleeding history is obtained. Intravenous antibiotics tailored for expected flora are prophylactically given during placement of percutaneous nephrostomies or stents and during percutaneous ablation procedures. If the procedure is performed on an outpatient basis, the patient is admitted to an observation unit for 2 to 3

hours after the procedure and is discharged with specific written instructions regarding the procedure, the symptoms and signs that may indicate that a complication has occurred, and the necessary steps to take should any of the described symptoms appear.

Percutaneous Nephrostomy for Obstruction

Percutaneous nephrostomy tube placement is the most common therapeutic radiologic procedure in urology. Azotemia resulting from bilateral obstruction and obstruction of a solitary functioning kidney are the most common indications. In some cases, percutaneous nephrostomy tube placement is a temporizing measure until sepsis, electrolyte imbalance, or renal failure is corrected before definitive surgery, to decrease the risk of operative morbidity and mortality. In patients with cancer, this procedure may temporize while waiting for hormonal therapy, chemotherapy, or radiotherapy (RT) to take effect. In many malignant obstructions of one or both ureters, as can occur with cervical cancer, percutaneous nephrostomy allows the kidneys to function normally and permits continuing treatment with chemotherapy. It may also allow time for the resolution of postoperative edema at the ureteral anastomosis or for the passage of a ureteral calculus. Percutaneous nephrostomy is also used to divert the urine stream temporarily when the patient has an anastomotic urine leak distally or in the presence of hemorrhagic cystitis.

The success rate for percutaneous nephrostomy varies from 83% to 100%, depending on the skills of the operator.[1] Major complications are reported to occur in 5% to 7% of percutaneous nephrostomy procedures and minor complications occur in 15% to 28%.[2-4] Complications include infection, colon perforation, hemorrhage, and urinoma. Complications related to the catheter include dislodgment and obstruction. For experienced radiologists who use cross-sectional image guidance such as CT or ultrasonography (US) in the creation of the tract and fluoroscopy to place the tube, virtually no major complications have been reported, and minor complications have been reported to occur in 2% of patients, with catheter dislodgment in 1%.[5] In a review of >1200 nephrostomy tube placements, Stables and colleagues[2] reported 2 deaths (0.2%). Four deaths have been reported in the literature from hemorrhage. This finding is in contradistinction to the mortality rate from surgical nephrostomy, which ranges from 6% to 8% and which in septic patients may reach 12%.

Infection

Sepsis has been reported to occur in 1.5% to 21% of patients. Patients undergoing percutaneous nephrostomy for pyonephrosis and patients with infected renal calculi are particularly prone to septicemia. Transient bacteremia during percutaneous nephrostomy for infected obstruction is unavoidable because the passage of needles, dilators, and catheters through the infected parenchyma and collecting system inoculates bacteria into the bloodstream. Shaking, chills, or hypotension may develop, and the patient may be mistakenly diagnosed as experiencing postprocedural hemorrhage. Appropriate intravenous antibiotic treatment before the procedure is essential in a known infected system. Prophylactic intravenous antibiotics are advisable for all percutaneous nephrostomy procedures because patients may develop signs of sepsis even when they are at low risk.[6]

Elevation of intrarenal pressure during percutaneous nephrostomy tube placement heightens the risk of sepsis. Therefore, antegrade pyeloureterography should be postponed until the urine is clear. If the organism is unknown, a useful regimen is ampicillin, 1 g administered intravenously, to cover *Enterococcus* and *Proteus,* given in combination with an aminoglycoside, such as gentamicin, 80 mg intravenously, to cover all gram-negative organisms except *Enterococcus*. A single dose given 1 hour before the procedure is sufficient for prophylaxis. Alternatively, a first-generation cephalosporin, such as cefazolin, can be used relatively inexpensively. In cases of allergy to penicillin, vancomycin and ciprofloxacin can be used. Perinephric abscess is a rare complication of percutaneous nephrostomy in patients with infected urine or in patients with small infected stone fragments that may be extruded into the perinephric space (**Fig. 12-1**).

Hemorrhage

Major hemorrhage that requires specific treatment or prolongs hospitalization occurs in 4% to 5% of percutaneous nephrostomy procedures; this finding is in comparison to 25% of surgical nephrostomies. Major hemorrhage is more likely to occur in patients with coagulopathies. Transient hematuria clearing in 24 hours occurs in almost all patients after percutaneous

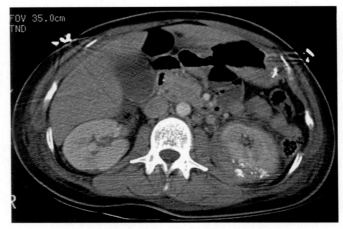

Figure 12-1 Extruded stone fragments in the left posterior perinephric space after percutaneous nephrostomy tube removal that caused a perinephric abscess.

nephrostomy tube placement and is not regarded as a complication.

CT scan demonstrates hematoma in 13% of tube placements. To minimize the risk of hemorrhage, understanding the renal vascular anatomy and its relation to the collecting system is important. Obstruction from the blood clot can occur (**Fig. 12-2**). Intermittent flushing with 5 to 10 mL of sterile normal saline maintains patency of the catheter until the bleeding abates and the urokinase in the urine begins to lyse the clot. Persistent hematuria requiring transfusions or pulsatile bleeding during the procedure should raise the possibility of an arterial fistula, in which case embolization may be necessary. Massive hemorrhage from major injury to the renal vein has been reported to be treated by inflation of a Councill-tip balloon catheter.[7]

Colon Perforation

Because the normal relationship of the kidneys to adjacent visceral organs varies, occasional puncture of these organs during percutaneous nephrostomy is possible. Reports of iatrogenic colon perforation are rare (<1%). The colon can lie in the path of a percutaneous nephrostomy tract that originates near the posterior axillary line. This far posterolateral position of the colon appears more commonly in patients with little retroperitoneal fat (e.g., women). Occasionally, the colon can even lie in a retrorenal position. Perforation of the colon is virtually eliminated when the procedure is performed using modern US or spiral CT guidance for access needle placement.

When the complication does occur, a nephrostomy tube is usually discovered to be going through the colon at the time of a nephrostogram (**Fig. 12-3**). Presenting symptoms include fever, fecaluria, abdominal pain, and leukocytosis.[8] Appropriate parenteral antibiotic coverage should be started and the tube should be removed. To prevent a fistula from occurring, a double-J stent

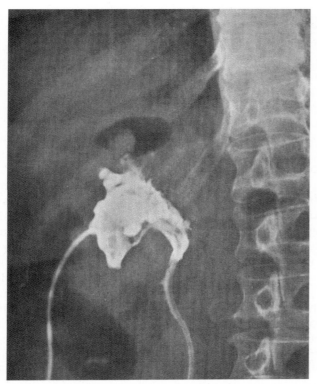

Figure 12-2 Blood clot. Antegrade pyelouretrography through a nephrostomy tube. The entire lumen of the right renal pelvis is filled with a blood clot. The irregular appearance of the contrast along the medial aspect of renal pelvis suggests that some contrast is outside the renal pelvis and perforation may be present. The ureteral stent is in place, apparently filled with clot and nonfunctional. Within 24 hours, most blood clots lyse and disappear.

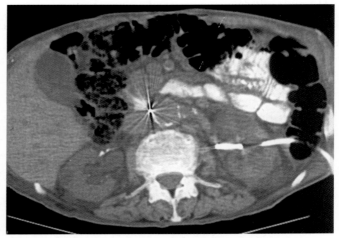

Figure 12-3 Colon perforation. The nephrostomy tube was discovered going through the colon at the time of a CT scan.

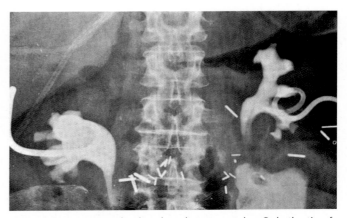

Figure 12-4 Improperly placed nephrostomy tube. Only the tip of the left nephrostomy tube is in the renal pelvis. The remainder is probably coiled in the perinephric space.

should be placed to ensure that no urinary obstruction is present, and the misplaced nephrostomy tube should be pulled back in stages: first into the perinephric space, then a day later into the colon, then a day later pericolonically, and then the last day removed. The tract usually seals without sequelae.

Urinoma

Persistent urine leak from the collecting system has been reported in 0.6% to 2% of percutaneous nephrostomy procedures. Small leaks are usually of no consequence. Massive leaks may lead to peripelvic fibrosis. Extravasation of infected urine may produce an abscess. Urinoma can occur when the catheter is placed through the collecting system and is inadvertently looped in the renal sinus or perinephric space (**Fig. 12-4**). Such misplacement may not be immediately recognized because the system will continue to drain if any of the side holes of the catheter remain in the collecting system.

Dislodged Catheter

The complication of catheter dislodgment is much less common when self-retaining catheters are used. The Cope loop catheter has a self-retaining loop that is

formed within the renal pelvis by pulling on an anchoring suture at the distal end of the catheter that is connected to the proximal tip of the catheter. The 10- and 12-Fr catheters are the most useful if the catheter is to remain for any length of time. Because these catheters are self-retaining, anchoring the catheter to the skin should not be necessary except in the most uncooperative patient. In the setting of critical drainage for infection or long-term drainage, skin sutures may be useful until the nephrostomy tract matures.

When the catheter becomes dislodged, the ease of reinsertion of a new catheter depends on the maturity of the tract, the size of the catheter, and the time elapsed since dislodgment. When attempting reinsertion, the collecting system should be opacified, and a 5-Fr catheter used in conjunction with a floppy guidewire may facilitate reentry into the system. On rare occasions, a catheter may break at the entry point to the skin and migrate. Biplane fluoroscopy may be needed to localize the catheter and to retrieve it with forceps.

Obstructed Catheter

The catheter usually clears with vigorous irrigation. This procedure should be performed with caution so as not to cause excessive pressure in the collecting system that could lead to forniceal rupture and sepsis. If this fails, inserting the stiff end of a guidewire into the catheter, under fluoroscopic control, often clears the tube of debris. If the obstruction is not relieved, a mature tract usually allows a guidewire to be passed into the collecting system alongside the obstructed catheter. If this fails, the catheter can still be replaced without repuncturing by using the sheath-over-catheter method, in which a Teflon sheath is advanced over the obstructed nephrostomy catheter into the collecting system. The nonfunctioning tube is then removed through the sheath, contrast material is injected to check sheath position, and a new catheter is inserted through the sheath.

As prophylaxis for tube obstruction, nephrostomy tubes should be changed every 2 to 3 months. Routine daily flushing of the catheter may need to be taught to patients whose urine easily encrusts the catheter.

Other Catheter Problems

Occasionally, removal of a self-retaining catheter is attempted by someone unfamiliar with its mechanics. The catheter may be removed with the loop in locked position, and pain and hemorrhage may result. The incomplete removal of the anchoring suture of a Cope nephrostomy tube may result in calcification of the foreign body.[9]

Nephrostomy tract tumor seeding after nephrostomy in the presence of transitional cell carcinoma has been described.[10] Scarring of the renal parenchyma and traumatic cysts also occur in the area of nephrostomy placement (**Fig. 12-5**).

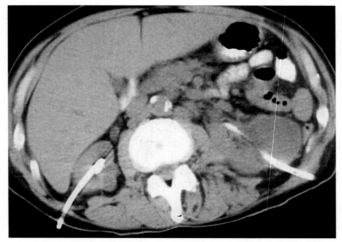

Figure 12-5 Traumatic cyst developed in the left kidney secondary to nephrostomy tube placement.

Antegrade Ureteral Stent Placement

When long-term urinary diversion is needed, an internalized ureteral stent is preferable to a nephrostomy tube and drainage bag. Retrograde insertion of an internal stent is generally attempted first but may be unsuccessful when the ureter is severely stenosed, is markedly tortuous, or has been anastomosed to bowel. With the advances made in flexible ureteroscopy, failure of retrograde stenting is unusual. Consequently, antegrade stenting is now a less common procedure.

Antegrade ureteral stent placement is usually performed in patients who have an existing nephrostomy tube and in whom conversion to internal urinary drainage is desirable.[11-13] The success of stent placement depends on properly chosen access. Percutaneous entry into the midcalyceal group allows for better torque control of the catheter than that into the lower pole calyx. If difficulty is encountered in advancing a stent through a region of stenosis by way of an existing nephrostomy tube tract because of buckling in the renal pelvis, it may be necessary to establish a new tract that offers better leverage. A stiff wire may have to be used with force to traverse a tight obstruction, which may result in ureteral or renal pelvis perforation. Continued nephrostomy tube diversion of urine allows the perforation to heal.

If passing a stent through the region of stenosis is difficult, balloon dilation of the stricture may be necessary (**Fig. 12-6**). Occasionally, both antegrade and retrograde attempts at stent placement are unsuccessful, and only the guidewire traverses the stenosis. In these instances, we have had success using a combined approach with the urologist in which a long, 240-cm guidewire is passed into the bladder from the antegrade direction and a ureteral stent is advanced from the retrograde direction over the guidewire. With both ends of the guidewire available, maximal leverage is possible for placement of a stent from below (**Fig. 12-7**).[14]

Irritative bladder symptoms may occur if the ureteral stent is too long. If the chosen stent is too short, the distal or proximal end may not drain properly into the bladder or may become lost in the tract before proper seating. The proper length of the stent is determined at the time of internalization by using the guidewire as a measuring stick. The tip of the guidewire is placed at the ureterovesical junction, and the guidewire is crimped where it exits the catheter. The guidewire is then withdrawn until the tip reaches the renal pelvis, and a second crimp is made. The distance between the two kinks is the ureter length. If the stent is not changed at regular intervals, it may become occluded or calcified (**Fig. 12-8**). The stent may become brittle and fracture. Lost or broken stents and catheter fragments may be retrieved percutaneously after tract dilation and sheath placement to accommodate an endoscope and grasping forceps (**Fig. 12-9**).[15,16]

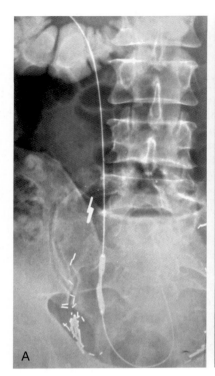
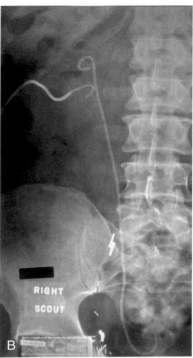

Figure 12-6 Balloon dilation of stricture. A tight stricture at the distal ureter makes antegrade stent placement difficult. **A,** The area of narrowing is balloon dilated before passing the stent in antegrade fashion. **B,** Both the stent and nephrostomy tube are left in place until proper function of the stent has been established.

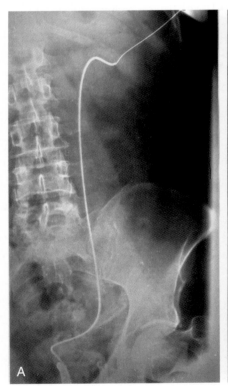
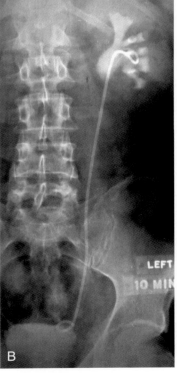

Figure 12-7 Combined antegrade and retrograde approach to stent placement. After failed retrograde and antegrade ureteral stent placement for a midureter leak secondary to ureterolithotomy, a combined approach was used. **A,** Long, 240-cm guidewire is passed from the nephrostomy tube tract and is brought out of the bladder. The double-J stent is then passed over the guidewire from below. **B,** Intravenous pyelogram several days later demonstrating good positioning of double-J stent and good function of the kidney.

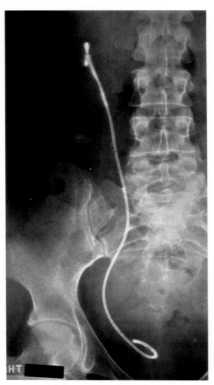

Figure 12-8 Calcified stent.

Another complication of antegrade ureteral stent internalization is obstruction of the stent either by blood clots or because of the tight fit of the stent through the area of ureteral stenosis. To minimize the risk of obstruction by blood clots, ureteral stents are not usually placed at the time of percutaneous access into the collecting system. Instead, if internalization of a stent is the final goal, a percutaneous nephrostomy tube is placed by a route that maximizes ureteral access. After the tract has matured a few days, antegrade ureteral stent internalization is performed. A nephrostomy tube is also left in the renal pelvis, which is clamped but can be opened for drainage should the ureteral stent fail to provide proper drainage. In a couple of days, when good drainage through the stent has been established, the nephrostomy tube can be safely removed.

If an internalized stent occludes, the percutaneous access will no longer exist, and the urologist can attempt catheter exchange from the retrograde direction. This exchange is generally successful as long as access to the upper tract is maintained with a guidewire.

It is possible to place or exchange a ureteral stent from the retrograde direction without cystoscopic assistance.[17,18] In women with a short urethra, the radiologist can use an Amplatz snare to pull the distal end of the stent out of the bladder by using fluoroscopic control, so that a guidewire can be threaded through the stent and exchanged.[19] The average fluoroscopy time is 3 minutes, and the procedure can be performed with the patient under intravenous sedation. This technique is not successful when the trigone is distorted.

Fluid and Abscess Drainage

Percutaneous drainage of fluid collections can usually be safely achieved using US or CT for guidance (**Fig. 12-10**).[20-22] Drainage procedures are performed either for definitive treatment or as a temporizing procedure until surgery can be safely performed. Bleeding diathesis is a relative contraindication, and abnormal bleeding parameters should be corrected before the procedure. Lack of a safe route for puncture precludes drainage. In the abdominal cavity, it is important to find an access route into the fluid collection that avoids puncturing the surrounding bowel. When a fluid collection is loculated, multiple drainage catheters may have to be placed. In the pelvis, a variety of approaches including US-guided intracavitary approaches (transrectal or transvaginal) may be used. In all cases, one must avoid the bowel, bladder, and seminal vesicles in men and the uterus and ovaries in women. If using a transgluteal approach, the sciatic nerve, sacral plexus, and gluteal vessels must be avoided.[23]

In the urinary tract, the most common complications of percutaneous drainage of renal and perinephric abscess are bacteremia and subsequent sepsis resulting from manipulation of an infected fluid collection.[24,25] These complications may be minimized by avoiding unnecessary manipulation and using appropriate prophylactic antibiotic coverage. An investigation for an underlying treatable cause of an abscess should be undertaken several days after the abscess pocket has had a chance to drain. Sinograms and fistulograms of the abscess cavity should not be performed on the day of drainage. Another complication of abscess drainage is spread of infection to a previously sterile contiguous compartment, such as the pleural space. Pain can be a problem, particularly when the entry point for tubes into or around the kidney is between ribs. Other complications include injury or fistula to adjacent organs.[26]

Lymphoceles may develop after lymph node dissection or renal transplantation. Most lymphoceles resolve spontaneously, but when they cause symptoms or present a dilemma in diagnosis, aspiration, drainage, or sclerosis may be entertained. More than 50% of lymphoceles do not recur after a single percutaneous image-guided aspiration or catheter drainage. Repeated aspirations because of recurrence and indwelling catheter drainage increase the possibility that the lymphocele will become infected. Lymphoceles have been successfully sclerosed with povidone-iodine, tetracycline, and ethanol.[27] Complications are rare. Infection of a lymphocele after initiation of sclerotherapy can be treated with antibiotics; if unresponsive, surgical drainage and marsupialization may be necessary. Catheter dislodgment can also occur during the treatment period.

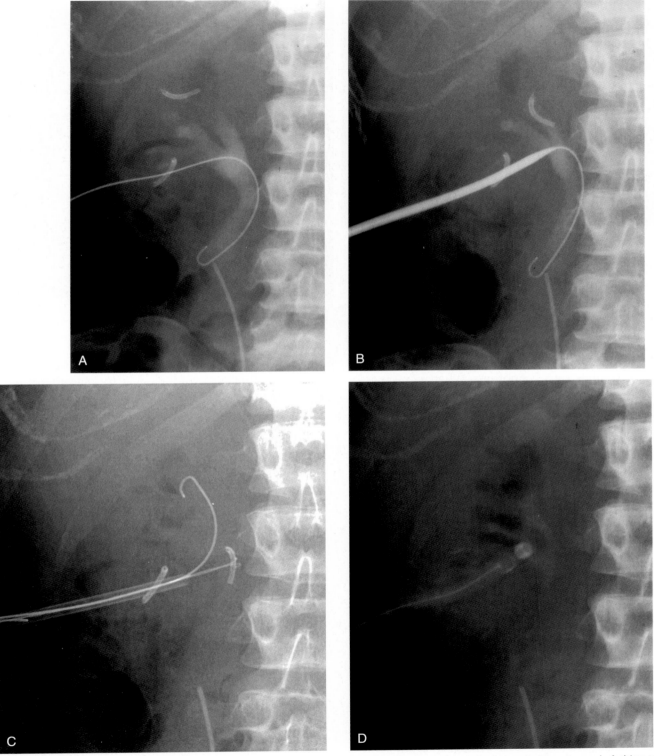

Figure 12-9 Percutaneous removal of fractured double-J stent fragments. **A,** Straight ureteral catheter is inserted in retrograde fashion to opacify the system. A guidewire is inserted into the collecting system after percutaneous access. **B,** Dilation of the nephrostomy tube tract. **C,** Grasping forceps are used through a sheath to remove catheter fragments. **D,** A catheter is left in place after removal of fractured stent fragments.

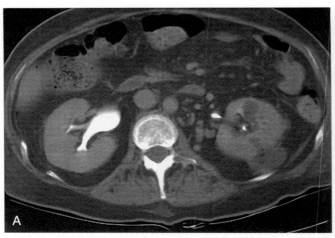
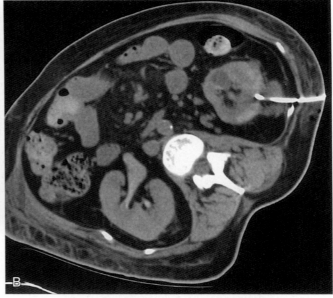

Figure 12-10 CT-guided perinephric abscess drainage. **A,** Perinephric abscess in posterior aspect of left kidney. **B,** The patient is placed in the supine oblique position to access the abscess under CT guidance, and a small drainage tube is left in place.

Cyst Ablation

Renal cysts rarely cause symptoms. When a cyst is associated with flank pain, hypertension, proteinuria, calyceal obstruction, or erythrocytosis, therapeutic cyst puncture and ablation may be necessary. Because the potential complication of ablation includes extravasation of the sclerosing agent into the perinephric or periureteral tissue, therapeutic cyst puncture is usually performed first to determine whether the particular symptom is relieved by decompression. If the cyst recurs, as it does in 40% of cases, permanent treatment is attempted by instilling a sclerosing agent, such as 95% ethanol, into the cyst.[28]

Complications of cyst puncture and cyst ablation are rare. Major complications occur in 1.4% and minor complications occur in 6.5% of cases.[29,30] Transient hematuria and flank pain are the most common complaints. Severe flank pain may indicate retroperitoneal bleeding, which can be confirmed by CT scan and serial hematocrit determinations. Severe or prolonged hematuria may indicate an arteriovenous fistula, which may require selective renal angiography and transcatheter embolization to remedy. If the cyst is located in the upper pole of the kidney, pneumothorax is a potential complication that may require a chest tube for treatment. Laceration of adjacent organs, such as the spleen, liver, or bowel, is a potential complication that is virtually eliminated by using a spiral CT scanner to guide cyst puncture.

Percutaneous Renal Biopsies

Thin-walled needle aspirations and core biopsies are frequently performed under fluoroscopic, US, or CT scan guidance. Imaging guidance allows for accurate tissue sampling and avoids damage to adjacent organs.[31] Percutaneous biopsies are widely and safely performed for two major types of indications: renal tumors and renal parenchyma. Biopsy of renal tumors is performed to establish a diagnosis of the subtype of renal cell carcinoma before tumor ablation or to establish an alternative diagnosis such as lymphoma, metastasis, or transitional cell carcinoma. Biopsy of renal parenchyma is performed to establish a diagnosis of diffuse renal diseases such as membranous glomerulonephropathy.

Complications are reportedly rare and include hemorrhage, infection, pneumothorax, and tumor seeding along the needle tract. Overall, significant complications such as hemorrhage following image-guided percutaneous biopsies are rare (<1%).

Percutaneous Image-Guided Tumor Ablation of Renal Cell Carcinoma

Since the late 1990s, image-guided renal tumor ablation has become an established alternative to open or laparoscopic simple or partial nephrectomy for treatment of small renal cell carcinomas (<3 cm) in patients unable or unwilling to undergo more established procedures. Various thermal technologies have been developed and applied including cryoablation, radiofrequency ablation, and microwave ablation. Other techniques include laser ablation and irreversible electroporation, which is currently under development. All these techniques may be performed by open, laparoscopic, or percutaneous approaches.

Of all these techniques, cryoablation and radiofrequency ablation have been the most widely used for the treatment of small renal cell carcinomas. Although no multicenter randomized trials have been conducted to compare the two methods, in experienced hands both techniques appear to treat small lesions with high efficacy and low rates of complications.[32,33] Individual lesions best treated with these procedures include small, exophytic renal cancers away from the renal hilum or collecting system. Lesions near the renal hilum tend to be more resistant to either heat-based or cold-based therapy because of the presence of a strong heat sink effect in which large surrounding hilar renal arteries and veins draw away thermal energy and preclude complete ablation.

VASCULAR PROCEDURES

Vascular Embolization

Renal Artery

Transcatheter embolization of the renal artery is performed for renal carcinoma to reduce tumor vascularity preoperatively. It is used palliatively for inoperable renal carcinoma when the patient is having extreme pain, hematuria, or hypercalcemia. Subselective intrarenal embolization is also used to occlude arteriovenous malformations and fistulas, to treat renal vascular hypertension, and to occlude aneurysms or bleeding vessels, such as those found in angiomyolipomas. Percutaneous renal ablation is occasionally performed for end-stage renal disease when the patients have intractable hypertension or significant proteinuria.

An expected consequence of embolization is *post-infarction syndrome,* which includes fever, flank pain, leukocytosis, hematuria, transient hypertension, and occasionally nausea and ileus. The severity and duration depend on the amount of tissue that is infarcted, and the syndrome usually lasts 3 to 5 days. Symptoms are treated with narcotics and sedation.[34] Symptoms of prolonged fever and flank pain raise the possibility of complicating abscess formation within the infarcted tissue. An infectious complication is more likely if the kidney has an underlying infection; in these cases, embolization should not be attempted.[35] Bubbly gas shadows within the kidney confirm this complication; however, gas can been seen in the parenchyma 4 to 8 days after embolization in patients who have neither symptoms nor infection.[36]

Complications of embolization include reflux of embolic material into the aorta, possibly resulting in distal embolization (e.g., spinal cord, bowel, testicles, skin) and its complications, and contralateral renal artery embolization.[37-43] These complications can be avoided by careful placement of the catheter tip deep into the renal artery or use of an occlusive balloon to prevent reflux.[43]

Hypogastric artery embolization is performed for severe bleeding from trauma in patients with pelvic fractures or bleeding from an infiltrating pelvic tumor. Skin necrosis over the buttocks has been described as a complication.

Varicocele Embolization

Symptomatic varicoceles occur in 4% to 15% of the male population. Indications for treatment include pain and infertility. Varicoceles can be treated on an outpatient basis by sclerotherapy or embolization.[44-47] Local thrombophlebitis of the testicular vein has been seen in 2% of patients after sclerotherapy. This is usually the result of the sclerosing agent's reaching the pampiniform plexus.

The recurrence rate of varicocele after embolization is 4% to 11%.[48] The lower recurrence rate is seen when the level of occlusion is in the inguinal region and all collateral veins are occluded.[49] Recurrences after surgical ligation are successfully treated by embolization. Perforation of the spermatic vein can cause retroperitoneal hematoma. Inadvertent migration of embolization material into the pulmonary artery is a rare complication but is without permanent sequelae. Overall, spermatic vein embolization is a procedure with few complications, and sclerotherapy and embolotherapy appear to be equally safe.

Renal Artery Angioplasty

Percutaneous transluminal angioplasty is used in renal artery stenosis when >50% of the arterial lumen is stenosed and when a systolic pressure gradient of >15% is present. This procedure can preserve renal function and can improve renal function in some patients with azotemia. Both fibromuscular and atherosclerotic stenotic lesions have been dilated by percutaneous transluminal angioplasty. Transplanted kidneys are also amenable to this procedure.

Complications of renal artery angioplasty are few and easy to manage.[47] They are estimated to occur in 5% to 10% of cases. Peripheral embolization by cholesterol debris, plaque fragments, or thrombus has not proved to be important. Although it occurs frequently, peripheral embolization is usually clinically symptomatic in only 1% of cases.

Irregularity of the intima at the angioplasty site immediately after balloon dilation is an expected result. Remodeling takes place, and the intima appears smooth on the follow-up arteriogram performed weeks or months later. Intimal dissection at the site of angioplasty may frustrate the procedure. If the true lumen can be reentered, repeat balloon dilation is performed to push the lifted intima back against the media. Dissection leading to thrombosis precludes further attempts at dilation (**Fig. 12-11**). Local thrombolytic therapy should be considered, particularly when vascular surgical reconstruction is not feasible.

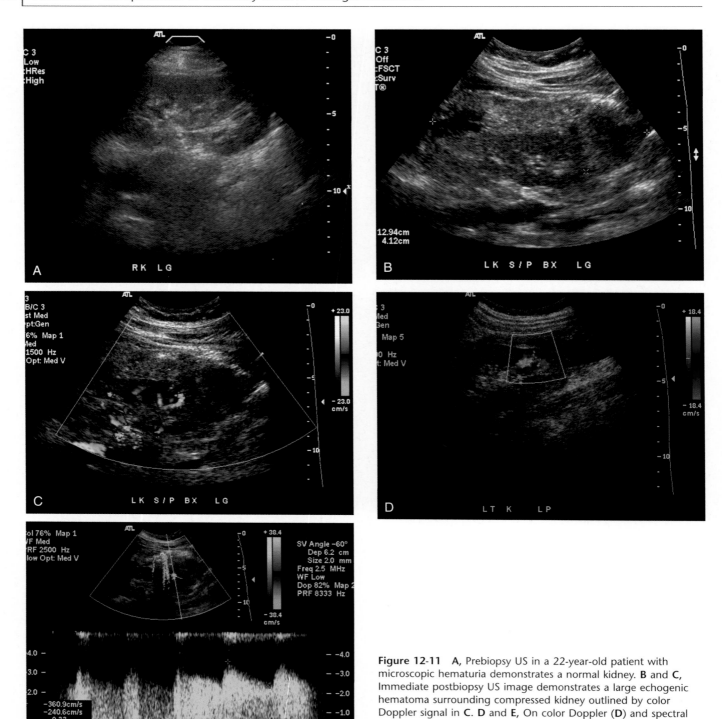

Figure 12-11 **A,** Prebiopsy US in a 22-year-old patient with microscopic hematuria demonstrates a normal kidney. **B** and **C,** Immediate postbiopsy US image demonstrates a large echogenic hematoma surrounding compressed kidney outlined by color Doppler signal in **C**. **D** and **E,** On color Doppler (**D**) and spectral Doppler (**E**), a biopsy-related arteriovenous fistula was demonstrated.

Vessel spasm from guidewire and catheter manipulation is not uncommon (**Fig. 12-12**). Calcium channel blockers, such as verapamil or nifedipine, can be administered just before angioplasty to decrease susceptibility to spasm. Vessel perforation may also occur when the guidewire crosses a region of stenosis and is usually of no consequence. Renal artery rupture is a rare complica-tion, occurring in <1% of cases. The patient usually has severe and persistent back pain. This complication is more likely to occur in patients receiving steroid medi-cation and in the presence of fibromuscular disease. Once the complication is identified, the balloon cath-eter should be inflated across the rupture site. Immedi-ate open surgical correction is necessary.[50]

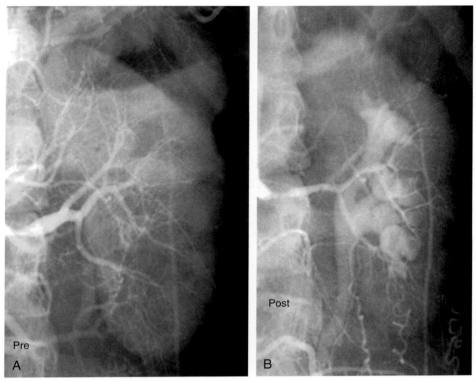

Figure 12-12 Vessel spasm after PTA. **A,** Before PTA, the patient had stenosis of the left renal artery. **B,** After balloon dilation, spasm of the renal artery has occurred. Note how all the branches are smaller compared with the predilation angiogram.

At the puncture site, hematoma occurs in 2% to 4% of cases. Hypertension, obesity, size of the catheter, and anticoagulation contribute to increased risk. False aneurysm is rare and is more likely to occur at the site of a large hematoma. Doppler US is used to detect its presence and to occlude it. Arteriovenous fistula is also rare and occurs in conjunction with through-and-through femoral artery and vein puncture. It, too, is diagnosed by Doppler US. Balloon burst resulting from faulty manufacturing or inadvertent overinflation may occur. If segments of the balloon detach, they can be retrieved angiographically or by open surgical methods. A burst balloon may be difficult to remove from the vessel at the site of entry, and surgical cutdown may become necessary.

KEY POINTS

1. Thermoablative technologies were introduced to minimize the morbidity of partial nephrectomy particularly in infirm, elderly patients with multiple comorbidities.
2. Inadvertent ablation with either modality in proximity of the ureteropelvic junction may result in urinary extravasation and stricture formation even in the absence of direct piercing of the ureteropelvic junction.
3. Injection of a gelatin sponge or other hemostatic agents into the probe tract following percutaneous renal cryoablation may reduce the incidence of postoperative bleeding.
4. Bleeding after LCA is frequently the result of premature needle extraction and renal parenchymal fractures, which can be prevented by ensuring that cryoneedles enter the tumor at a right angle.
5. Significant bleeding causing hemodynamic instability can be treated by selective embolization of the bleeding vessel, whereas patients with stable vital signs can be treated conservatively with strict bed rest and frequently repeated blood counts.
6. Treatment of urine leak consists of draining the collecting system percutaneously or with a ureteral stent for 4 to 6 weeks because most leaks will seal by that time.

REFERENCES

Please see www.expertconsult.com

Chapter 13

COMPLICATIONS OF EXTRACORPOREAL SHOCK WAVE LITHOTRIPSY

Rahul A. Desai MD
Surgeon, Urology, The Polyclinic, Seattle, Washington

Dean G. Assimos MD
Professor of Surgical Sciences, Department of Urology, Wake Forest University School of Medicine, Winston-Salem, North Carolina

Extracorporeal shock wave lithotripsy (SWL) revolutionized treatment for patients afflicted with nephrolithiasis. Many patients have benefited from this technology, but the energy that causes stone fragmentation may result in trauma to the targeted tissue and surrounding structures. This trauma usually has limited clinical impact, but there is potential for serious acute and chronic complications. In addition, other untoward events may occur, such as peritreatment infections and renal obstructive complications, which may lead to adverse sequelae. These complications and prevention methods are reviewed in this chapter.

HEMATOMA

The delivery of shock wave energy to the kidney results in some degree of acute renal injury, including interstitial bleeding and disruption of small to medium renal arteries and veins.[1,2] This may result in intrarenal bleeding (hematoma), which may extend into the perinephric tissue. Some degree of such bleeding may be commonly detected on posttreatment imaging, but it is rarely clinically significant.[3-6] **Figure 13-1** shows a computed tomography (CT) image of a left perirenal hematoma that developed after SWL.

The reported incidence of renal hematoma varies between 0.28% and 4.1% in large series.[3-6] The risk factor most commonly associated with the development of hematoma is hypertension, especially when it is poorly controlled. Other risk factors include older age, obesity, diabetes mellitus, and vascular disease.[7,8] Knapp and associates reported a 0.66% overall incidence of hematoma after SWL: a 2.5% incidence for patients with well-controlled hypertension and a 3.8% for patients with poorly regulated hypertension.[9]

Clinical signs of hematoma include intense flank or abdominal pain, tachycardia, hypotension, and anemia. Hematoma generally is self-limited, and patients respond to supportive measures such as hydration, analgesics, and transfusion. Intervention is rarely necessary

and renal loss is exceedingly rare.[3-6] If one suspects that hematoma has developed, upper tract imaging (CT, magnetic resonance imaging [MRI], or ultrasonography) should be performed to establish the diagnosis.

Most hematomas resolve spontaneously over time. Krishnamurthi and Streem followed 19 patients with 21 post-SWL hematomas for up to 5 years, with a mean follow-up of 19.6 months. During the follow-up, 85.7% of the hematomas completely resolved, 9.5% became smaller, and 4.8% did not change size. No patient without pre-existing hypertension became hypertensive.[10] Collado Serra and colleagues, however, found that 36% of post-SWL hematomas remained at 18 months after SWL.[3]

Hematomas can be prevented by using shock wave energy judiciously and ensuring that patients have well-controlled blood pressure and are free of any coagulation or platelet functional disturbances. Administering a small number of lower energy shock waves to the ipsilateral or contralateral renal unit before delivering therapeutic energy doses has been shown to dramatically attenuate hemorrhagic injury in an animal model.[11] It is hypothesized that the lower energy shock waves induce reduced renal blood flow in both kidneys and thus limit injury. This response is thought to be modulated by renal nerves.[12]

STEINSTRASSE

Steinstrasse, the accumulation of stone fragments in the ureter, after SWL usually occurs in patients with larger stones, typically >2 cm, and the reported incidence varies between 2% and 10%.[13-15] A CT image of steinstrasse is seen in **Figure 13-2**.[16] Patients may have symptoms such as flank or abdominal pain, nausea, and emesis. However, a significant number may be asymptomatic. Weinerth and associates reported that 5 of 19 patients with *large steinstrasse* (defined as stone fragments occupying greater than one third of total ureteral length) were asymptomatic.[17] Almost three quarters of

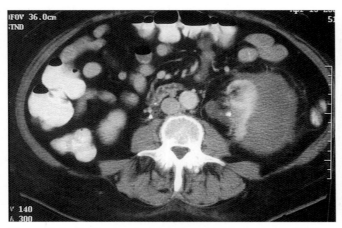

Figure 13-1 A CT scan of a left perirenal hematoma after SWL.

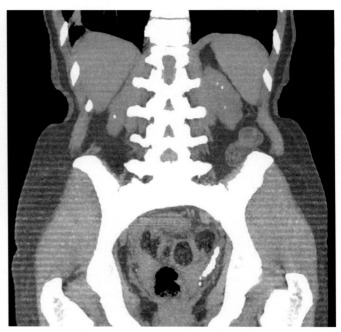

Figure 13-2 A coronal CT scan of steinstrasse of the left distal ureter after SWL.

large steinstrasse occur in the distal portion of the ureter.[16] **Figure 13-2** shows a coronal CT image of steinstrasse of the left distal ureter.

If the patient has no or minimal symptoms, is without signs of sepsis, has adequate renal function, and is not at risk for permanent renal damage, close observation is recommended because 48% to 63% of steinstrasse resolve spontaneously.[18,19]

Percutaneous nephrostomy is a viable treatment option for those who have persistent steinstrasse or refractory symptoms; 75% of steinstrasse passed in one series, solely with percutaneous nephrostomy.[20] Percutaneous nephrostomy is recommended if the patient has signs of sepsis or renal functional deterioration.

Repeat SWL is another approach and has been reported to be 80% to 90% successful.

Ureteroscopic management of patients with steinstrasse after SWL is the most definitive treatment, and success rates approach 100%, although it is not often required.[18,19]

The administration of α_1-blockers has not been demonstrated to eradicate steinstrasse. However, patients receiving such agents may have better pain control.[21]

The occurrence of steinstrasse can be limited by carefully selecting patients and choosing alternative treatments for patients with stones >2 cm. Ureteral stent placement may limit the risk of steinstrasse in patients with stones <3 cm but is ineffective for those with larger stones and is not associated with higher stone-free rates.[13,15] In addition, stented patients generally have significant bothersome symptoms.[22] Stent placement must be considered strongly in those patients with anatomically or functionally solitary kidneys.

SEPSIS

The risk of sepsis after SWL is higher in patients who have had previously treated or untreated urinary tract infections (UTIs) and especially those with infection stones. Li and colleagues found that the risk of sepsis was higher in those with larger stones, especially staghorn calculi. Sepsis risk is expected in the staghorn cohort in which the majority of patients have struvite or carbonate apatite stones. Li and colleagues reported that the urine in patients with larger stones more frequently contained endotoxin, which was associated with a higher risk of sepsis.[23] Similar findings were noted by Orenstein and coworkers.[24] A study by Yilmaz and associates compared bacteremia risks of 75 patients with either calcium or infection stones; all of these patients had sterile urine cultures before SWL. Bacteremia developed in 2.6% of those with struvite stones after SWL as compared with 1.3% of those with calcium stones after SWL. An elevation of the inflammatory mediatory, C-reactive protein (CRP), also has been identified as a predictor of bacteremia.[25,26]

Controversy exists regarding whether or not to administer prophylactic antibiotics at the time of SWL to patients who had sterile pre-treatment urine. A meta-analytic study by Pearle and Roehrborn demonstrated that there was a significant decrease in the development of post-SWL UTI in patients who received prophylactic antibiotics.[27]

Patients with UTI should receive appropriate antibiotic therapy before SWL. Those suspected of harboring infection stones should receive broad spectrum antibiotic therapy because there may be discordance between stone and urine cultures.[28] These prophylactic measures lessen the risk of sepsis.

CARDIAC ARRYHTHMIAS

Cardiac arrhythmias have been reported with both gated and ungated SWL, being more prevalent with the latter. Zanetti and colleagues reported that the incidence of cardiac arrhythmia was 8.8% among 269 consecutive patients without a history of cardiac arrhythmia who underwent ungated SWL. Although 59% who developed arrhythmia converted back to normal sinus rhythm with temporary halting of shocks and remained so after resumption of ungated SWL, 36% required gating to prevent arrhythmia recurrence and <1% (1 patient) required atropine to manage persistent bradycardia. There was no correlation found with the side of treatment with SWL, the number or strength of shocks, or the anesthetic agents delivered.[29]

Greenstein and associates reported asymptomatic premature ventricular contractions in 18.4% of 125 ungated SWL procedures. No correlations were found with age or gender of patient, presence of heart disease, size or location of stone, presence of ureteral catheter or nephrostomy, mode of anesthesia, and number of shocks delivered. Interestingly, arrhythmia was seen more often during right-sided procedures.

The immediate postprocedure course of patients undergoing ungated SWL was studied by Winters and colleagues. Of 82 patients, 21% developed arrhythmias. All but 2 arrhythmias were benign and all reversed with subsequent gating. No arrhythmias occurred with shock energies lower than 20 kV. No electrocardiogram changes were seen up to 1 hour after the procedures were completed.[30]

Gating and ungating during the same procedure were compared by Ounnoughene and colleagues. Twenty-five patients with no cardiac history underwent SWL and Ounnoughene and coworkers delivered shocks gated and ungated. During the gated phase, no arrhythmias developed. During the ungated phase, 7 of the 25 patients developed arrhythmias, but all were asymptomatic and the arrhythmias regressed spontaneously after the procedure was completed.[31]

A comparison of 3288 patients with and without a history of arrhythmia was performed by Cass. In this unique study, ungating was used in patients with known arrhythmias and gating was used in patients without known arrhythmias. In the group with no known pre-existing arrhythmias, 1 patient developed a malignant arrhythmia during the ungated procedure.[32]

Rhee and colleagues, in a study of children, showed no development of arrhythmia during ungated SWL in eight children.[33]

These findings indicate that the development of cardiac arrhythmia is mainly associated with ungated SWL. The consequences of cardiac arrhythmia appear minimal, however, because most arrhythmias are benign and resolve with gating; therefore, gating is advocated in the presence of arrhythmia.

VASCULAR INJURY

Rupture of abdominal aortic aneurysms (AAAs) has been reported after SWL.[34,35] It is not clear whether the shock wave energy promoted rupture or was unrelated.

The impact of shock wave energy on atherosclerotic vessels has been assessed in an in vitro study. Vasavada and associates found minimal histologic changes in aortic aneurysmal tissue subjected to shock wave energy.[36] There have been reports of patients with AAAs undergoing uneventful SWL; however, the aneurysm size was modest in these series, all <5.5 cm.[37] Patients with calcified renal artery aneurysms and vascular grafts also have undergone successful SWL.[38,39] Despite reported successes with the use of SWL in patients with AAAs, the clinical safety has not yet been established.

There also have been reports of patients developing venous thrombosis after SWL, affecting the portal vein and iliac vein. Exact cause of the venous thrombosis could not be determined in these cases, however.[40,41]

PULMONARY INJURY

Shock waves may traverse the lungs during SWL and inflict damage. This has been demonstrated to produce blast injury in rat and rabbit models.[42,43] Children appear most susceptible to this type of injury, but it also may occur in adults.[44] There have been reports of pulmonary contusion with SWL,[45] which typically manifests with hemoptysis or hypoxemia. Styrofoam has been applied to the chest area of children, and air vests have been worn by children to prevent such occurrences.

MUSCLE DAMAGE

Skeletal muscle can be traversed with shock waves during SWL. Although studies have demonstrated increases in muscle-derived enzymes in the serum and urine of patients subjected to SWL, we are unaware of any reports of clinically significant muscle damage or rhabdomyolysis after treatment.[46,47] In fact, shock wave energy may have beneficial therapeutic effects in patients suffering from certain musculoskeletal disorders such as plantar fasciitis and calcific tendonitis.[48,49]

INJURIES OF THE LIVER, SPLEEN, AND PANCREAS

A mild degree of hepatic injury is not uncommon after SWL of renal and proximal ureteral stones. Apostolov and colleagues reported that an increase in serum glutamate dehydrogenase, a marker for hepatocellular injury, is common after SWL[50]; however, significant injuries are extremely rare and include subcapsular hematoma and hepatic fracture.[51-53] The symptoms and signs of subcapsular hematoma and hepatic fracture include hypotension, tachycardia, anemia, abdominal pain, and ileus. Imaging studies (ultrasonography, CT, MRI) should be obtained if hepatic injury is suspected. Patients with subcapsular hematoma are observed closely, whereas an active intervention may be required if hepatic fracture has occurred.

A few cases of injuries to the spleen and pancreas have been reported in patients who received SWL to

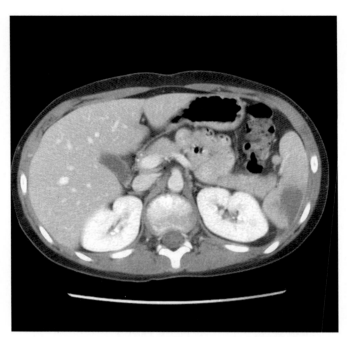

Figure 13-3   A CT scan of a splenic injury after left-sided renal SWL.

treat renal stones, although these complications are rare and manifestations vary. In one case report, a man developed shock after SWL of an 18-mm left upper pole stone. CT demonstrated splenic rupture and the patient underwent splenectomy.[54] A similar event occurred in a woman who received SWL for a 2-cm stone in the left renal pelvis. The initial clinical diagnosis was renal hematoma, but CT demonstrated splenic rupture requiring splenectomy.[55] Infectious sequelae can arise with such injuries. A man underwent SWL of a left lower pole renal stone and subsequently developed anemia, leukocytosis, and fever. He was found to have a perisplenic hematoma and abscess, requiring splenectomy and abscess drainage.[56] Although a select group of patients with spleen and pancreas injuries from SWL can be managed with observation, a death from anemia and sepsis with this wait and see approach has been reported.[57] **Figure 13-3** shows a CT scan of a splenic injury that occurred after left-sided SWL.

The pancreas also can be injured when SWL is used to treat upper urinary tract stones. Pancreatitis has been reported after SWL of renal calculi.[58] The occurrence of pancreatitis is higher with SWL of pancreatic duct stones, as anticipated.[59] In addition, more severe pancreatic injuries can occur. A man with a right renal pelvic stone treated with SWL developed peritonitis and elevated serum pancreatic enzymes shortly after treatment. Imaging demonstrated areas of necrosis in the body and tail of the pancreas and a peripancreatic fluid collection. The patient was treated successfully with percutaneous drainage of the fluid collection.[60] The signs of injuries also may manifest later. A man devel-

oped persistent abdominal pain 1 year after SWL of right renal pelvic stones. He was found to have a large pseudocyst of the head of the pancreas, which required open surgical correction. The occurrence of the pseudocyst was attributed to his SWL procedure because he had none of the usual risk factors for pancreatic disease.[61]

Both splenic and pancreatic injuries resulting from SWL are extremely rare. Patients with both splenic and pancreatic injuries may have varying signs and symptoms including abdominal pain, peritonitis, sepsis, and shock. The diagnosis is best established with CT or MRI. Splenic injury is more common with treatment of the left renal unit, whereas pancreatic injury typically occurs after right-sided procedures. Although some patients can be managed with observation, others may require an open surgical intervention.

GASTROINTESTINAL INJURIES

The stomach, duodenum, small and large bowel may be injured during SWL. In a literature review, Maker and Layke found 10 reported bowel perforations in 3423 patients (0.34%) who underwent SWL. There were 6 small bowel perforations, 3 colonic perforations, and 1 dehiscence of a gastrojejunal anastomosis. All 10 patients required open surgical correction.[62]

A left ureterocolic fistula in a patient with an impacted stone was also noted in this review; the patient was treated with nephroureterectomy. An additional 12 patients had evidence of less severe injury not requiring surgery including ulcerations of the cecum, colonic hematoma, and hematochezia.[62] The potential for upper gastrointestinal injury with SWL was assessed by Al Karawi and colleagues who performed esophagogastroduodenoscopy in 40 patients before and after SWL. New gastric or duodenal erosions were identified in 32 (80%) after SWL.[63]

Patients who undergo SWL may sustain significant bowel injury including perforation. Those who are treated in the prone position may be at higher risk for this occurrence. Although this complication is extremely rare, one needs to suspect this complication in any patient who develops peritonitis after SWL. Prompt evaluation and treatment are mandatory.

URINARY FISTULAS

There have been scattered reports of patients developing fistulas after SWL including pyelocutaneous, pyeloduodenal, ureterocolic, and ureterovaginal. The majority of these fistulas occurred in patients with staghorn stones or undiagnosed xanthogranulomatous pyelonephritis. Nephrectomy was undertaken in most of these cases. The primary renal problem was the most likely inciting factor in these cases.[64-69]

HYPERTENSION

There is ongoing debate as to whether or not SWL causes hypertension. This association was first reported in the late 1980s, and numerous conflicting studies have been published in subsequent years. The respective studies that address this matter are profiled in Table 13-1.[70-80]

Certain patient factors and treatment approaches have been demonstrated to be associated with the development of hypertension. Janetschek and colleagues reported that older age was a risk factor for the development of new onset hypertension. They reported that patients older than 60 years were at higher risk. They also found that older age correlated with an increase in the renal resistive index measured with Doppler ultrasonography.[76]

In the study with the longest follow-up (19 years), Krambeck and associates reported that hypertension developed more commonly in SWL-treated patients than in a case-controlled group of patients who had had stones but had not received to SWL. They found that those subjected to bilateral SWL were at higher risk for

developing hypertension but that this hypertension was not related to the number of shocks delivered or shock wave intensity.[80] Others have not found this association, however. Krambeck and associates also reported that that those who received SWL were more prone to developing diabetes mellitus and that there was a positive correlation to the numbers of shocks delivered and shock wave intensity, whereas the side of the involved renal unit had no influence.[80]

The literature review indicates that the association between SWL as a risk factor for developing hypertension is not uniformly confirmatory. This, most likely, is due to several factors such as study design and inadequate controls. In addition, hypertension is a multifactorial disease, and association does not always equate with causation. Furthermore, patients who formerly had stones, as a group, have been demonstrated to be more at risk for developing hypertension.[81-85]

RENAL INSUFFICIENCY

The kidney sustains some degree of acute injury after it has received shock wave energy. The reduction in renal blood flow that occurs with delivery of shock wave energy to the kidney may produce renal ischemia, which could lead to renal injury.[86] Animal models have demonstrated that this results in the generation of oxygen free radicals, which may further promote injury.[86] Direct shock wave trauma also plays a role in acute renal dysfunction. Koga and colleagues examined canine kidneys after repeated SWL treatments and positively correlated degree of tissue hypoxia and rupture of interstitial capillaries with number of shocks delivered.[87]

While stone formers are at risk of developing renal insufficiency (RI), there is no current evidence to suggest that SWL promotes it. Krambeck and associates did not find increased rates of RI after long-term follow-up in patients treated with SWL.[80] The majority of the patients in the aforementioned study received one or two SWL treatments. The impact of repetitive SWL on renal function has not been adequately addressed at this time.

Although animal models have demonstrated that the smaller or undeveloped kidney appears to be more susceptible to shock wave injury, a number of longitudinal studies performed on children who received SWL demonstrated no reduction in renal function or growth over time.[88] However, Lifshitz and associates reported that children subjected to SWL had attenuated renal growth.[89]

There have been a few reports of patients developing renal failure after SWL, and renal biopsies demonstrated the presence of complement fixation and anti-glomerular basement membrane antibodies.[90,91] Westman and colleagues questioned whether SWL played a role in the development of renal failure because they did not find an increased number of autoantibod-

TABLE 13-1	Reports of Hypertension and Extracorporeal Shock Wave Lithotripsy		
Study (year)	Length of Study (mo)	Incidence of HTN	Diastolic BP
Liedl et al[70] (1989)	40	No change	Not recorded
Williams et al[71] (1988)	21	Increased	Increased
Puppo et al[72] (1990)	12	No change	No change
Montgomery et al[73] (1989)	29	Increased	No change
Lingeman et al[74] (1990)	—	No change	Increased
Yokoyama et al[75] (1992)	19	NR	Increased
Janetschek et al[76] (1997)	26	Increased (60-80 years of age)	Increased
Jewett et al[77] (1998)	24	No change	No change
Strohmaier et al[78] (2000)	24	Increased	Increased
Elves et al[79] (2000)	26	No change	No change
Krambeck et al[80] (2006)	228	Increased	NR

BP, blood pressure; HTN, hypertension; NR, no record.
Data based on Wein AJ, Kavossi LR, Peters CA, et al. *Campbell-Walsh Urology*, 9th ed. Philadelphia: WB Saunders; 2007.

ies associated with glomerulonephritis in 59 consecutive patients who underwent SWL.[92]

Shock wave lithotripsy in patients with pre-existing renal insufficiency or a solitary kidney has also been studied. Chandhoke and colleagues found stable renal function after SWL in patients with solitary kidneys or serum creatinine levels <3 mg/dL. Only patients with serum creatinine levels >4 mg/dL continued to have worsening renal function after SWL, suggesting continued insult from the primary renal disease.[93]

There is no question that shock wave energy induces renal trauma, yet it appears that, in the majority of patients, this renal trauma has no significant impact on renal function. Better designed longitudinal studies are needed to assess the impact of repetitive SWL, especially in patients more susceptible to renal injury. The judicious use of SWL should help limit any reduction in renal function. This includes close monitoring for obstructive complications. Other approaches may be taken to limit renal damage and the risk for RI with SWL. Some have advocated the administration of free radical scavengers such as allopurinol, nifedipine, verapamil, and mannitol to limit acute renal injury.[94-97] The experience with pharmacologic protection is too limited to advocate its use at this time. Others have shown in animal studies that pretreatment with lower energy shock waves may reduce renal injury through vasoconstriction, but no human studies have yet been published.[98]

FERTILITY EFFECTS

Shock wave energy delivered to distal ureteral stones can theoretically injure gonadal tissue. Animal models have been used to determine the acute effects of delivering shock wave energy to the ovary. Recker and colleagues demonstrated minimal subcapsular bleeding, desquamation of superficial cells, and loss of microvilli immediately after shock wave energy was delivered to the rat ovary. However, these were not persistent changes and had resolved by 35 days.[99] McCullough and associates demonstrated normal reproductive ability in rats that had shock wave energy delivered to the ovaries. In addition, there were no teratogenic effects noted in the progeny.[100]

Studies of female patients have focused on the subjects' ability to reproduce after SWL. Erturk and colleagues evaluated women who underwent SWL for distal ureteral stones and noted no fertility problems or genetic abnormalities in their children.[101] In another study, Vieweg and associates found similar results.[102]

Male gonadal function also has been assessed in patients subjected to SWL. Perisinakis and coworkers compared the radiation dose to gonadal tissue between SWL of proximal and distal stones and found four times

higher radiation exposure to the testes during SWL for distal stones. They postulated that this would result in a four times higher genetic defect risk in the children of patients, although the overall risk still is thought to be exceedingly rare.[103] Martinez and colleagues found a worsening in semen parameters in men who underwent SWL for distal ureteral stones. However, the effects were self-limited and parameters returned to baseline within 3 months.[104] Reports of transient hematospermia in men who have been subjected to SWL for distal ureteral stones are reflective of the potential temporary perturbation of the male reproductive tract.[105]

There is ongoing controversy regarding the use of SWL to treat girls or women of reproductive age harboring distal ureteral stones. This issue remains controversial due to the current medicolegal environment in the United States.

CONCLUSION

SWL is generally a safe and effective treatment for patients with nephrolithiasis. However, complications may result. Their occurrence can be limited with proper patient selection, good preparation, and correct technique.

KEY POINTS

1. Hypertension, especially poorly controlled, is a risk factor in post-SWL hematoma.
2. Steinstrasse often resolves with observation, but management depends on the patient's clinical status and the presence of sepsis or renal deterioration.
3. Sepsis is more common after SWL of infection stones, but preprocedure antibiotic choice should be broad spectrum because stone and urine cultures are often discordant.
4. Cardiac arrhythmias are associated with ungating, and they usually spontaneously revert with gating.
5. Pulmonary injuries are seen mostly in children and can be prevented by prophylactic padding of the torso.
6. Splenic injuries may require splenectomy.
7. Although gastric and duodenal erosions are common, those gastrointestinal injuries requiring intervention are extremely rare.
8. Hypertension caused by SWL is a controversial topic and may be seen more in older patients and those who have undergone bilateral procedures.

REFERENCES

Please see www.expertconsult.com

Chapter 14

COMPLICATIONS OF RENAL TISSUE ABLATION

Ilia S. Zeltser MD
Instructor, Department of Urology, University of Texas Southwestern Medical Center at Dallas, Dallas, Texas

Jeffrey A. Cadeddu MD
Ralph C. Smith, MD, Distinguished Chair in Minimally Invasive Urologic Surgery; Professor, Department of Urology, University of Texas Southwestern Medical Center at Dallas, Dallas, Texas

Between 1995 and 2005, the diagnosis rate of renal cell carcinoma (RCC) increased significantly due to widespread use of cross-sectional imaging techniques. Most incidentally discovered renal tumors are small, locally confined, and represent a low-stage RCC (T1a).[1] Long-term oncologic outcomes of open partial nephrectomy have demonstrated that these small tumors (<4 cm) can be successfully treated with nephron-sparing surgery (NSS) techniques while providing cancer cure that is equivalent to that of radical nephrectomy.[2] Since development of laparoscopic partial nephrectomy (LPN) in 1993, several centers of excellence have successfully used this technique to treat small renal masses. In fact, recent data of the 5-year outcomes of LPN revealed disease-free survival rates of >90% with minimal compromise of renal function.[3]

Yet despite the excellent outcomes of NSS, the widespread adoption of this technique by the urologic community outside of the centers of excellence has been slow. A recent survey of the Surveillance, Epidemiology, and End Results (SEER) cancer registries showed a significant underuse of NSS in the treatment of small renal masses.[4] Only 42% of the tumors <2 cm were treated with NSS from 2000 to 2001, and a mere 20% of tumors 2 to 4 cm were treated with NSS. One potential reason for this trend is the technical complexity of NSS. LPN is especially challenging because it requires surgeons to be adept at laparoscopic suturing, which is often complicated by the time constraints of warm renal ischemia. Compared with open partial nephrectomy, LPN is associated with a longer renal ischemia time and higher urologic complication rate, even in the most experienced hands.[5]

Thermoablative technologies were introduced to minimize the morbidity of partial nephrectomy, particularly in infirm, elderly patients with multiple comorbidities.

Cryoablation (CA) and radiofrequency ablation (RFA) are the two most commonly used energy sources, and both can be applied percutaneously or laparoscopically.[5] The main limitation of in situ ablation is that the tumor is not excised; therefore, there is no pathologic confirmation of complete tumor removal. Instead, the adequacy of ablation is confirmed by the absence of tumor on follow-up imaging. Despite this limitation, excellent midrange oncologic efficacy of both CA and RFA has been demonstrated. Gill and colleagues showed a 98% cancer-specific survival in 51 patients undergoing laparoscopic CA (LCA) for a unilateral sporadic renal tumor. In a subset of patients with a median follow-up of 6 years, they demonstrated a 5-year overall survival of 80%.[6] With a mean follow-up of 25 months, Park and associates demonstrated a 98.5% cancer-specific survival and a 92.3% overall survival in 78 patients (94 renal masses) treated with percutaneous radiofrequency ablation (PRFA) and laparoscopic radiofrequency ablation (LRFA).[7]

Other ablative modalities currently available include high-intensity focused ultrasound, laser thermal ablation, chemoablation, microwave thermotherapy, and gamma knife radiosurgery. Clinical experience with these modalities is in its infancy; further studies are needed to define the role of these modalities in the minimally invasive treatment of renal tumors and to evaluate their potential morbidities.

Presently, the morbidity of RFA and CA compares favorably with that of LPN. If the long-term cancer control of CA and RFA remain excellent and as the population ages, these modalities may supplant LPN as the procedures of choice for the treatment of small renal masses. However, thorough knowledge of potential complications and proper technique are critical to achieving excellent oncologic efficacy while minimizing morbidity. This chapter reviews the mechanism of action of CA and RFA, outlines the technical nuances of their clinical applications, and discusses potential complications of ablation observed both in experimental models and clinical practice.

MECHANISM OF ACTION

Radiofrequency Ablation

RFA uses a monopolar alternating electrical current using the frequency within the radio segment of the electromagnetic spectrum. The current flows between the grounding pad and the RFA probe. Heat is generated as a result of ionic agitation of the tissue around the probe, and cell death is achieved when the temperature within a tumor and a small rim of the surrounding tissue rises to >60°C. High temperatures produce occlusion of the microvasculature and destruction of the cellular cytoskeleton, causing tissue ischemia, impaired DNA replication, and ultimately resulting in a predictable zone of coagulation necrosis around the radio frequency electrode.[8]

Based on the type of the feedback loop modulating energy delivery to the probe, there are two types of radiofrequency generators: impedance-based (Valleylab, Boulder, Colorado; Boston Scientific, Natick, Massachusetts) and temperature-based (RITA Medical Systems, Mountain View, California). The feedback loops are designed to prevent an overly rapid tissue heating which would produce charring and increase tissue resistance, thus decreasing the ablation zone.

To minimize tissue charring, multiple probe designs have been developed. There are single- and multiple-tined electrodes, which are subdivided further into wet, dry, or cooled tip probes. Multiple tines distribute the electrical current over a larger surface area than do single tines, allowing more energy to be delivered to the tissue before charring occurs. Wet probes (StarBurst XLi-Enhanced and StarBurst Talon, AngioDynamics, Queensbury, New York) infuse conductive fluid into the treated tissue, thus decreasing resistance and permitting deeper penetration of the current, which enables ablation of a larger lesion. The cooled tip probe (Cool-tip, ValleyLab) is a single-tine electrode, which minimizes tissue charring by circulating cooling liquid within the probe to decrease its surface temperature and allow more energy to be delivered into the tissue.

Cryotherapy

Cell death secondary to rapid severe freezing occurs by several mechanisms. Extracellular ice formation results in movement of water out of the cell and leads to changes in intracellular pH, protein denaturation, and mechanical disruption of the plasma membrane followed by intracellular ice formation.[9] Delayed tissue effects are caused by injury to the microvasculature

resulting in tissue hypoxia, endothelial cell damage, edema, platelet aggregation, and thrombosis, and these delayed tissue effects culminate in coagulative necrosis.[10] Recently, apoptosis and gene-regulated cell death were identified as other mechanisms of tissue disruption following freezing.[11]

It is generally accepted that a temperature of −40°C must be achieved to ensure cytotoxic effects of CA. Animal studies have shown that a double freeze cycle creates a larger cryolesion as compared to a single freeze.[12] It is not clear whether passive thawing between freezing cycles has greater tissue effects than active rapid thawing; however, it is generally accepted that a double freeze-thaw cycle with ice ball extension beyond the tumor margin should be used in clinical practice.

Since the 1960s, CA probes have evolved from large 5-mm to 3.4-mm probes to the currently available 1.47-mm (17 g) IceRod needles (Galil Medical, Yokneam, Israel). Smaller probes were designed to allow nontraumatic placement through the body wall and the renal capsule, more precise tumor targeting, and minimal bleeding following cryoprobe removal. The third generation machines use argon for freezing and helium for active thawing.

PATIENT SELECTION

Irreversible coagulopathy is an absolute contraindication to RFA and CA. Large tumors, cystic tumors, and tumors located in the hilum or adjacent to the uretero-pelvic junction (UPJ) are relative contraindications. Generally, thermoablation is indicated for contrast enhancing (>10-12 Hounsfield units) small renal masses (<4 cm). Additional indications include tumors in a solitary kidney and bilateral tumors in a patient with renal insufficiency. Both RFA and CA can be used to treat exophytic as well as completely endophytic renal masses, and a percutaneous approach can be used in an outpatient setting. Selection of the approach (laparoscopic versus percutaneous) depends on tumor location, patient's health status, and the surgeon's expertise. A percutaneous technique is suitable for patients with posterior or laterally located renal masses and those who cannot tolerate abdominal insufflation because of cardiac or pulmonary disease. Laparoscopic ablation is generally performed under general anesthesia; however, percutaneous ablation can be performed under either general anesthesia or intravenous (IV) sedation.[13] We prefer general anesthesia for the percutaneous approach because it prevents patient movement and allows for a controlled respiratory expansion, thus stabilizing kidney location. We believe that these advantages provide for more precise and expedited tumor targeting.

In addition to intolerance of abdominal insufflation, contraindications to a laparoscopic approach include multiple adhesions secondary to previous abdominal surgery and history of peritonitis. The percutaneous approach is contraindicated in patients with anteriorly located tumors and those unable to lie prone. Relative contraindications include morbid obesity precluding computed tomography (CT) or magnetic resonance imaging (MRI), large spleen or liver interfering with probe positioning, tumor location immediately adjacent to the renal pelvis or ureter, and presence of bowel within 1 cm of the tumor.

TECHNIQUE

Laparoscopic Radiofrequency Ablation

Following abdominal insufflation, laparoscopic renal ultrasound is used to define tumor margins. Ultrasound is imperative in helping to identify and define the margins of partially or completely endophytic renal tumors. Perinephric fat is dissected off to expose the tumor. The location on the abdominal wall that allows the most perpendicular path of the probe to the tumor is identified. The probe is inserted through the abdominal wall, and the kidney is then manipulated so that the probe enters the lesion at a right angle to the most exophytic point of the tumor. The probe is inserted into the tumor and the tines are deployed to encompass a diameter extending 5 to 10 mm beyond the measured margin of the tumor. Tine placement is confirmed with laparoscopic ultrasound. The generator is then activated and the target temperature is maintained, depending on the size of the tumor and manufacturer's recommendations. Once ablation is completed the probe is removed and biopsies of the tumor are performed. The biopsy site on the surface of the kidney is examined, and usually no or minimal bleeding results. If bleeding is encountered, it can be controlled by application of TISEEL and Floseal (Westlake Village, California), hemostatic sealants, or argon beam coagulation.

Percutaneous Radiofrequency Ablation

PRFA can be performed under CT, MRI, or ultrasound guidance. It is important to emphasize that expansion of the ablation zone cannot be imaged in real time, and the margins of ablation are defined by the position of the tines. CT is our modality of choice for PRFA, and the Starburst XL RFA probe and RITA 1500X Generator are our preferred tools. We favor general anesthesia.

Following induction of general anesthesia or IV sedation, the patient is secured in a prone or flank position on the CT table and all the pressure points are carefully padded. Two radiofrequency grounding pads are placed per manufacturer recommendation. A CT of the abdomen is performed with a one half normal contrast dose to accurately identify the lesion.

Following the initial scan, the best percutaneous route to the tumor is planned to ensure that the probe will avoid the surrounding structures such as liver, spleen, colon, and pleura. The RFA probe is inserted

---

BOX 14-1 Potential Complications of Renal Tumor Ablation

Minor
Elevated serum creatinine
Hematuria
Minor hemorrhage (small perinephric hematoma)
Minor urinary extravasation
Pain or paresthesia at the probe site
Urinary tract infection
Wound infection
Liver burn/freeze

Major
Bowel injury
Ileus
Open conversion
Pancreatic injury
Renal failure
Significant hemorrhage (large or expanding hematoma)
Significant urinary extravasation (large urinoma)
Ureteropelvic junction obstruction

---

percutaneously and directed toward the lesion. Correct placement is confirmed with repeated CT imaging, and adjustments are made to ensure that the deployed tines fully encompass the tumor and that the ablation zone will extend at least 5 mm beyond the tumor margin. Successful deployment must be confirmed on CT before ablation. Core needle biopsies of the tumor can be performed once the correct probe position is verified. It is important to position the probe before placing the biopsy needle because bleeding from the biopsy may change the contour of the lesion and obscure its margins. Ablation protocol is the same as for LRFA. See potential complications in Box 14-1. Following tumor ablation, track ablation is performed as the tines are withdrawn and the probe is simultaneously pulled back 5 to 10 mm. Postablation CT with one half dose of IV contrast is obtained to confirm successful tumor ablation.

Percutaneous Cryoablation

Percutaneous CA (PCA) can be performed with CT, MRI, or ultrasound guidance.[6,14,15] Unlike RFA, expansion of the ice ball can be monitored with imaging in real time. The growing ice ball appears as an enlarging hyperechogenic curvilinear surface with posterior acoustic shadowing on ultrasonography, as a signal void on T1-weighted MRIs, and as a markedly hypoattenuated area with smooth sharp borders on CT. The temperature at the leading margin of the ice ball is about 0°C; therefore, to achieve complete ablation, it is critical to ensure that the ice ball extends 1 cm beyond the tumor margin.

Following induction of general anesthesia or IV sedation and placement of a Foley catheter, a patient is placed prone and the tumor is localized with imaging. Three of four cryoablation probes are placed at the periphery of the tumor and their position is verified with imaging. Biopsies of the tumor can be performed before or after cryoprobe placement. The cryosystem is activated and a 1-minute freeze is initiated while the growth of the ice ball is monitored in real time to ensure that the collecting system is not involved. Two freeze-thaw cycles are performed while imaging to ensure that the ice ball engulfs the tumor with a 5-mm to 1-cm margin of normal parenchyma. The cryoprobes are removed following the second thaw cycle.

Laparoscopic Cryoablation

Depending on the tumor location, prior abdominal surgery, and patient habitus, either retroperitoneal or transperitoneal laparoscopic access can be established. The kidney is mobilized within Gerota's fascia, and the perirenal fat surrounding the tumor is submitted for histologic examination. The kidney is imaged with a laparoscopic ultrasound probe to define the margins of the tumors and the location of the collecting system. Biopsies of the tumor are performed, and three or four cryoprobes are inserted under sonographic guidance. Two freeze-thaw cycles are performed, and freezing is continued until the ice ball extends about 1 cm beyond the tumor margin. After the second thaw cycle, the cryoprobes are removed and FloSeal (gelatin-thrombin matrix) may be applied into the puncture sites to help with hemostasis.

Follow-up

The Working Group on Image Guided Tumor Ablation, after reviewing patterns of tumor persistence or recurrence in 616 patients treated with RFA or CA, recommended a minimum of three to four imaging studies in the first year after ablative therapy.[16] Our protocol following RFA consists of follow-up imaging with MRI or CT with IV contrast at 6 weeks, 6 months, 12 months, and every 12 months thereafter for 5 years. For biopsy-proven benign lesions, the imaging is done at 6 weeks and then yearly thereafter. Imaging at 6 weeks after RFA is critical to confirm success of RFA (**Fig. 14-1**).

Following LCA, Gill and colleagues described serial MRI with or without gadolinium enhancement on day 1 postablation; at 1, 3, 6, 12, 18, and 24 months; and annually thereafter for 5 years.[17] Additionally, at 6 months a CT-guided core needle biopsy of the cryoablated lesion was performed. Shingleton followed his patients after PCA with a contrast-enhanced CT or MRI at 1 month and 3 months and then every 6 months for 5 years.[18,19]

Lack of contrast enhancement within the tumor and a margin of normal parenchyma is the hallmark of successful ablation. MRI appearance of successful cryoablation shows lack of gadolinium enhancement within the cryolesion; however, a small rim of enhancement may be seen on early scans. This rim gradually disappears and is thought to represent reactive changes in the area

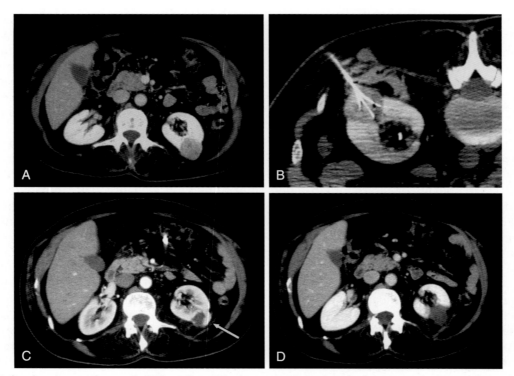

Figure 14-1 **A,** Left enhancing renal mass. **B,** PRFA probe within the tumor. **C,** Persistent enhancement in the periphery of the tumor at 6 weeks, indicating incomplete ablation. **D,** CT at 6 months following re-treatment.

of sublethal injury and interstitial hemorrhage along the periphery of the cryolesion.[20]

Following cryoablation, some cryolesions demonstrate gradual reduction in size with a mean decrease in diameter of 75% at 3 years. In contrast, RFA lesions persist on follow-up scans, although they may contract slightly. Endophytic lesions may retract from the renal parenchyma, with a narrow rim of fat infiltrating the margin. Lesions treated with PRFA may exhibit a peri-tumor halo in the perinephric fat surrounding the tumor probably caused by fibrosis at the margin of ablation zone.[21] Characteristic MRI appearance of successful RFA consists of high signal intensity on T1-weighted images, low signal intensity on T2-weighted images, and an absence of gadolinium enhancement. The peri-tumor halo after PRFA is seen as a rim of low signal intensity on T1- and T2-weighted images.[22]

Tumor recurrence following percutaneous ablation usually can be successfully reablated using the percutaneous approach and the same tumor targeting and ablation techniques. Recurrence in anterior lesions following laparoscopic ablation is difficult to re-treat, however. Most of these tumors require a formal excision with a partial or radical nephrectomy, and a partial nephrectomy in this setting is usually very difficult secondary to severe fibrosis and scarring around the ablated tumor.

COMPLICATIONS OF ABLATION

Experimental Experience

Multiple animal studies have been conducted to evaluate potential complications of CA and RFA injury to vital renal structures.[10,23-29] These experiments consisted of deliberate targeting and ablation of the renal collecting system, UPJ, and renal vasculature. Because of inconsistencies in study design and inherent limitations of animal models, it is difficult to endorse clinical recommendations from the results of these studies. General guidelines can be inferred, however.

First, RFA and CA of renal tissue adjacent to the intraparenchymal collecting system appear to be equally safe and will not result in fistula formation and urinary extravasation; however, direct puncture of the collecting system must be avoided. Second, inadvertent ablation with either modality in proximity of the UPJ may result in urinary extravasation and stricture formation even in the absence of direct piercing of the UPJ. Third, retrograde renal cooling may protect the collecting system from RFA injury and reduce potential complications. Although retrograde cooling without hilar occlusion does not affect medullary and cortical temperatures, theoretical concerns for creation of a heat sink, which could reduce the RF lesion size and compromise oncologic treatment efficacy, are not resolved. Conversely, retrograde renal warming has not been shown to provide any cryoprotective advantage to the calyx at risk. Finally,

injection of a gelatin sponge or other hemostatic agents into the probe tract following percutaneous renal cryoablation may reduce the incidence of postoperative bleeding.

Clinical Complications

Current evidence indicates that both renal RFA and CA have low morbidity and are associated with few complications, most of which are minor. In a multi-institutional study, Johnson and associates found a complication rate of 11.1% in 271 patients undergoing renal RFA and CA.[30] Complications occurred after 14.4% of CA cases and 7.6% of RFA cases, with the most common complication being paresthesia or pain at the percutaneous probe insertion site for both modalities. Major complications in the RFA group included ileus, UPJ obstruction requiring a delayed nephrectomy, and a urinary system leak. Significant hemorrhage necessitating a transfusion and an open conversion were the major complications of CA. One patient with poor overall health, obstructive pulmonary disease, congestive heart failure, and pulmonary histoplasmosis died following RFA secondary to aspiration pneumonia. The death was not attributed to the ablation technique but rather to the patient's overall poor health. In the subgroup of 90 laparoscopic procedures, complications attributable to the laparoscopic technique occurred in 3.3%, the ablation procedure in 4.4%, and 1.1% were iatrogenic.

In a series of PRFA of 100 renal tumors, Gervais and associates found that hemorrhage (5 patients) was the most common complication.[31,32] Two of the 5 patients experienced major hemorrhage requiring, in 1 patient, red blood cell transfusion and stent placement for ureteral obstruction and, in the other patient, red blood cell transfusion for a subcapsular hematoma. In all 5 patients, hemorrhage was diagnosed at the end of ablation and no delayed bleeding was observed; 3 of these 5 patients had central tumors.

Other major complications included a ureteral stricture treated with stenting and ureteral injury with urinoma formation managed with percutaneous drainage. Minor complications consisted of first- and second-degree burns at the grounding pad site and transient neuropathic pain along the distribution of the lumbar plexus. One patient developed an asymptomatic inflammatory mass in the posterior abdominal wall. Interestingly, all complications were detected at the time of ablation or within 24 hours of ablation. There were no cases of bowel injury or tumor seeding.

Clinical experience with CA has also shown low complication rates and minimal morbidity. In 56 patients undergoing LCA, Gill and coworkers reported two major and two minor complications.[33] The major complications included a splenic hematoma managed conservatively in one patient and heart failure in another. The minor complications included a pleural effusion and herpetic esophagitis. CA had a minimal impact on renal function. The preoperative and postoperative creatinines were comparable in both the entire study group and the subset of patients with a solitary kidney. Even in 13 patients with a preexisting renal insufficiency no significant change in renal function occurred following CA.

In a series of 37 patients undergoing LCA, 3 patients were found to have bleeding complications secondary to renal fracture.[34] Perinephric hematomas were seen in 2 patients and gross hematuria developed in 1. All 3 patients were managed conservatively. Interestingly, this was the first series to show delayed UPJ obstruction resulting from CA. This patient was treated successfully with a pyeloplasty at 8 months after CA.

Cryoinjury to the pancreas has been reported in a single patient undergoing retroperitoneal LCA.[35] The injury was not apparent intraoperatively, and the patient had a delayed presentation with abdominal pain and guarding. CT revealed cryoinjury to the pancreas. Abdominal exploration showed no bowel injury, and drains were placed around the pancreas. The patient recovered without further morbidity and was discharged on the postoperative day 9.

The impact of renal ablation on renal function and blood pressure (BP) has been evaluated clinically for both RFA and CA. Carvalhal and associates followed 22 patients for at least 6 months following LCA. No differences were found between the preoperative and the postoperative serum creatinine, between the systolic and diastolic BP values, or in the estimated creatinine clearance.[36] The dose of antihypertensive medication did not change for any patient. The BP and serum creatinine values also did not change in the 3 patients with a solitary kidney after a minimum follow-up of 6 months. Similarly, Johnson and colleagues found that no patient experienced new onset of hypertension or worsening of existing hypertension following PRFA or LRFA after a minimum follow-up of 6 months.[37] No changes in mean serum creatinine or estimated creatinine clearance were observed. The one patient with a solitary kidney demonstrated stable renal function after undergoing RFA. From these two studies it appears that both RFA and CA preserve renal function and do not affect the BP at least in the short term but this issue should be revisited once the long-term data become available.

MANAGING COMPLICATIONS OF ABLATION

Hemorrhage

Most perinephric hematomas following PRFA and PCA are diagnosed using the immediate postablation imaging done to document the adequacy of ablation. These are usually small and often are not clinically relevant. However, severe hemorrhage can occur. Significant bleeding causing hemodynamic instability can be treated by selective embolization of the bleeding vessel. Patients with large hematomas but stable vital signs can be treated conservatively with strict bed rest and frequently repeated blood counts. Prevention of bleeding complications following PCA consists of avoiding large vessels and possibly injecting a hemostatic agent into the cryoprobe tract following ablation.

Bleeding after LCA is frequently due to premature needle extraction and renal parenchymal fractures, which can be prevented by ensuring that cryoneedles enter the tumor at a right angle. It is important to wait until the thawing is complete before attempting to remove the cryoneedle to avoid large cracks in the tumor or renal parenchyma. If bleeding occurs, FloSeal can be placed into the defect and is often sufficient to achieve hemostasis. Hemorrhage following LRFA is uncommon because RFA effectively coagulates the vessels within the tumor and a rim of normal parenchyma. In fact, biopsies and even excision of the entire tumor following LRFA can be done without much bleeding.[38]

Injury to the Collecting System/Urine Leak

Urine leaks following ablation result from either direct caliceal puncture or unintended extension of the ablation zone into the collecting system. There is, however, clinical evidence suggesting that it may be safe to involve the intrarenal collecting system within the ice ball, as long as this extension does not exceed 3 mm.[39] Nevertheless, until the long-term data is available, we recommend careful avoidance of the collecting system with either modality. Both RFA and CA have been shown to cause UPJ obstruction; therefore, tumors within 1 cm of the UPJ should not undergo ablation unless, during LRFA or LCA, the UPJ can be safely manipulated away from the ablation zone.

If urine leak is suspected, CT of the abdomen with IV contrast is usually diagnostic and will show contrast extravasation into a perinephric urinoma. In patients with renal insufficiency or contrast allergy antegrade or retrograde pyelography can help establish the diagnosis. Treatment consists of draining the collecting system percutaneously or with a ureteral stent for 4 to 6 weeks as most leaks will seal by that time.

Pain or Paraesthesia at the Probe Insertion Site

With CA, pain or paraesthesia occurs secondary to cryoinjury to the sensory nerves at the body surface. The entire cryoneedle is cooled during CA; therefore, take care to avoid freezing the skin at the insertion site. Place a warm, saline-soaked gauze around the cryoneedle; this is usually sufficient to prevent freezing of the skin. With RFA, the active portion of the probe is positioned within the kidney, but the injury to the sensory nerves in the skin may occur if the probe absorbs and conducts the heat to surrounding tissues. Track ablation is usually the final step of PFRA. It is used to decrease bleeding and prevent tumor seeding. The generator is activated as the probe is slowly withdrawn through the renal parenchyma and the perinephric fat. It is important to deactivate the generator before withdrawing the probe beyond Gerota's fascia because thermal injuries to psoas muscle can result in pain and paraesthesias. Most of these are self-limited and will resolve after a few days; however, significant sensory or motor deficits may require a neurologic consultation.

Injuries to Adjacent Organs

Injuries to the bowel and other adjacent organs are the most serious complications of renal ablation. Fortunately, these complications are rare, and currently there are only two reports of colonic injury following PRFA.[40] During laparoscopic RFA and CA, colon is usually reflected off the kidney before ablation. If the probe is positioned correctly and is monitored carefully during ablation to ensure that the bowel never comes in contact with it, colonic injury should never complicate laparoscopic RFA or CA.

Significant changes in bowel proximity to the tumor can occur between the diagnostic CT examination and the localizing CT at the time of ablation; therefore, careful preoperative planning and appropriate patient selection are critical to prevent bowel injuries and pleural transgression during percutaneous renal ablations. When planning a percutaneous approach, a CT or MRI in a prone or flank position is very helpful in defining the caudal extent of the pleural cavity and proximity of the bowel to the needle path and the tumor. As a general rule, presence of bowel within 1 cm of the ablation zone that cannot be manipulated with changes in patient position should preclude percutaneous ablation. However, various techniques of bowel displacement during PRFA have been described.[31,32,41] Hydrodissection involves instilling 50 to 200 mL of sterile water to displace the colon, and repeated instillations may be necessary during ablation because the water diffuses into the tissues. Using this technique, Gervais and colleagues[31,32] reported no bowel complications following CT and ultrasound-guided PRFA ablation of 100 renal masses under IV sedation, despite the fact that 27 tumors were within 1 cm of bowel. Recently, a technique of unilateral ventilation to prevent traversing the pleura during PCA has been described.[42]

CT of the abdomen and pelvis with oral contrast has very high sensitivity for diagnosis of a bowel injury and should be obtained immediately if bowel injury is suspected. If CT is indicative of a bowel perforation, an immediate exploration with bowel repair and/or resection is often necessary.

Pneumothorax can result from inadvertent lung injury during percutaneous insertion of an ablation probe. The diagnosis is made with a chest radiograph. Small pneumothoraces can be followed with repeated chest radiographs, and treatment with oxygen is frequently sufficient. However, large, expanding pneumothoraces or those causing respiratory compromise will require a chest drain for resolution.

CONCLUSION

RFA and CA are promising technologies and can be used effectively to treat small renal masses. They can be used percutaneously and laparoscopically and provide a viable treatment option for patients who are poor candidates for surgical extirpation. Careful preoperative planning, proper patient selection, and meticulous technique will ensure excellent cancer control with minimal morbidity.

KEY POINTS

1. Large tumors, cystic tumors, and tumors located near the hilum or adjacent to the UPJ are relative contraindications to CA and RFA.
2. Percutaneous approach to ablation is suitable for posteriorly or laterally located renal masses and for those patients who cannot tolerate laparoscopy. The percutaneous approach is contraindicated for anterior tumors.
3. Lack of contrast enhancement within the tumor and a margin of normal parenchyma is the hallmark of successful ablation.
4. The most common complication of tumor ablation is paresthesia or pain at the percutaneous probe insertion site.
5. Hemorrhage from the tumor or probe path is an uncommon complication, although it is more common in cryoablation. In laparoscopic cryoablation, a topical hemostatic agent can be placed in the probe tract to minimize this risk. If bleeding occurs after percutaneous ablation, selective embolization may be required.
6. Although rare, urine leaks after tumor ablation are generally associated with collecting system puncture by the ablation probe.

REFERENCES

Please see www.expertconsult.com

Chapter 15

COMPLICATIONS OF INTERSTITIAL SEED IMPLANTATION

Gregory R. Hanson MD
Surgeon, Metro Urology, Maple Grove, Minnesota

R. Alex Hsi MD
Section Head, Radiation Oncology, Virginia Mason Medical Center, Seattle, Washington; Adjunct Assistant Professor, University of Pennsylvania School of Medicine, Philadelphia, Pennsylvania

John M. Corman MD
Medical Director, Virginia Mason Cancer Institute, Virginia Mason Medical Center; Associate Clinical Professor of Urology, University of Washington School of Medicine, Seattle, Washington

Since the late 1950s, interstitial brachytherapy for prostate cancer has developed from an inexact retropubic placement of radioactive sources to a precise, percutaneous, guided outpatient procedure. As technique has evolved, brachytherapy for prostate cancer has emerged as an effective, well-tolerated treatment for clinically localized prostate cancer (**Figs. 15-1 and 15-2**). For such localized disease, in many urologic practices, brachytherapy is the treatment of choice in >50% of patients. The primary rationale for a patient's selection of this technique is the perception that this treatment has a lower impact on quality of life issues, particularly voiding function, sexual function, and fecal bother, when compared with radical prostatectomy or external beam radiation. In fact, morbidity associated with brachytherapy is frequent. Although grade 1 toxicities typically resolve with time, more profound complications are not uncommon. Management of such issues is the emphasis of this chapter.

For the purpose of the ensuing discussion, gastrointestinal and urologic complications common to brachytherapy are categorized according to the Radiation Therapy Oncology Group (RTOG) Acute and Late Radiation Morbidity Scoring Criteria morbidity grading system (Table 15-1). Side effects relevant to erectile function, ejaculatory function, and seed migration are discussed separately.

URINARY MORBIDITY

Obstructive Voiding Symptoms

Acute urinary retention (AUR) that requires catheterization during the first postoperative year has been reported in 2% to 32% of patients undergoing brachytherapy, with a median of 55 days required for drainage.[1] The pathophysiology of AUR is multifactorial but is thought likely to be secondary to prostatic edema, bladder neck irritation, and detrusor hyporeflexia resulting from overdistention during surgery. Chronic urinary retention (CUR) is far less common after brachytherapy and is more likely associated with urethral stricture disease and underlying voiding dysfunction. Table 15-2 is an overview of reports of AUR following brachytherapy.

As prophylaxis against AUR, most centers treat patients who undergo brachytherapy with α-blockade in the immediate perioperative period. In our practice, a urethral catheter is left in place for 24 hours postoperatively as prophylaxis against AUR, particularly in those patients receiving regional anesthesia. Patients are asked to remove their catheter on postoperative day 1 and to continue taking a selective α-blocker for 3 months postoperatively. Patients with persistent urinary retention despite medical intervention are prescribed intermittent self-catheterization. After 6 months of urinary retention, urodynamic studies are obtained to elucidate the cause of the retention. Transurethral resection of the prostate (TURP) is entertained only after 12 months have passed.

The following predictive factors are widely regarded to increase the risk of AUR after brachytherapy: elevated preoperative International Prostate Symptom Score (IPSS) score, preoperative urinary retention, and enlarged prostate volume.[2,3] Specifically, patients with a gland volume of >35 cm^3 have been shown to have a higher rate of obstructive voiding complaints and retention.[4] Such patients are typically managed with early, preoperative medical therapy (α-blockade or combined block-

TABLE 15-1	**Radiation Therapy Oncology Group Morbidity Grading System**				
	Acute and Late Radiation Morbidity Scoring Criteria				
	0	**1**	**2**	**3**	**4**
Acute GU	No change	Frequency of urination or nocturia twice pretreatment habit; dysuria, urgency not requiring medication	Frequency of urination or nocturia that is less frequent than every hour; dysuria, urgency, bladder spasm requiring local anesthetic (e.g., phenazopyridine [Pyridium])	Frequency with urgency and nocturia hourly or more frequently; dysuria, pelvis pain, or bladder spasm requiring regular, frequent narcotic; gross hematuria with or without clot passage	Hematuria requiring transfusion; acute bladder obstruction not secondary to clot passage
Acute GI	No change	Increased frequency or change in quality of bowel habits not requiring medication; rectal discomfort not requiring analgesics	Diarrhea requiring parasympatholytic drugs (e.g., diphenoxylate and atropine [Lomotil]); mucus discharge not necessitating sanitary pads; rectal or abdominal pain requiring analgesics	Diarrhea requiring parenteral support; severe mucus or blood discharge necessitating sanitary bags; abdominal distention (flat plate radiograph demonstrates distended bowel loops)	Acute or subacute obstruction, fistula or perforation; GI bleeding requiring transfusion; abdominal pain or tenesmus requiring tube decompression or bowel diversion
Late GU	None	Slight epithelial atrophy; minor telangiectasia (microscopic hematuria)	Moderate frequency; generalized telangiectasia; intermittent macroscopic hematuria	Severe frequency and dysuria; severe generalized telangiectasia (often with petechiae); frequent hematuria; reduction in bladder capacity (<150 mL)	Necrosis; contracted bladder (capacity <100 mL) Severe hemorrhagic cystitis
Late GI	None	Mild diarrhea; mild cramping; bowel movement 5 times daily; slight rectal discharge or bleeding	Moderate diarrhea and colic; bowel movement >5 times daily; excessive rectal mucus or intermittent bleeding	Obstruction or bleeding requiring surgery	Necrosis; perforation; fistula

GI, gastrointestinal; GU, genitourinary.
Data from Radiation Therapy Oncology Group, http://www.rtog.org/members/toxicity/late.html.

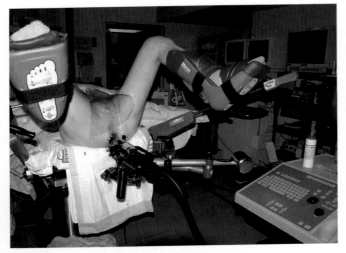

Figure 15-1 Position for seed implantation.

ade with 5-α-reductase inhibitor). The use of certain radioactive sources (e.g., palladium-103 [^{103}Pd]), in multivariate analysis, has been shown to be predictive of AUR. Such agents are therefore routinely avoided in patients believed to be at increased preoperative risk. Additionally, the number of needles used to place seeds as well as the use of neoadjuvant hormonal therapy may be correlated with an increased need for catheterization after implantation.[5] Although luteinizing hormone–releasing hormone agonist therapy is useful in downsizing the prostate before brachytherapy, in our experience it has not been useful in treating urinary retention after brachytherapy.

As an alternative to preoperative pharmacologic intervention, patients with severe preoperative outflow obstructive symptoms may elect to proceed with TURP before brachytherapy. Such patients must wait at least 4 months following TURP before proceeding with

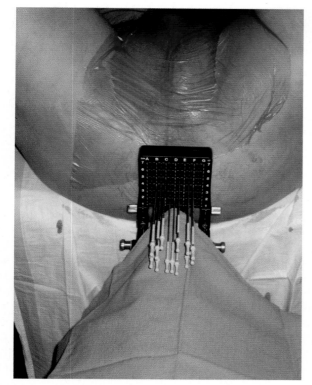

Figure 15-2 Needle insertion.

TABLE 15-3	Rates of Transurethral Resection of the Prostate for Urinary Retention After Implantation		
Reference	Technique	Agent	Patients (%)
Tsui et al[13] (2005)	Seattle	[125]I	1
Merrick et al[14] (2000)	Seattle	[125]I and [103]Pd	1.2
Gelblum et al[4] (1999)	Seattle	[125]I and [103]Pd	4.7
Wallner et al[46] (1996)	CT based	[125]I	8

CT, computed tomography.

TABLE 15-4	Comparison of Isotopes Used in Brachytherapy	
	Half-life (days)	Energy (kev)
Iodine-125	60	28
Palladium-103	17	22
Cesium-131	9.7	29

TABLE 15-2	Comparison of Rates of Urinary Retention		
Reference	Technique	Agent	Acute Urinary Retention (%)
Tsui et al[13] (2005)	Seattle	[125]I	5.8
Sarosdy[1] (2004)	Peripheral isodose plan	[125]I and [103]Pd	24
Zelefsky et al[26] (1999)	CT planning		3
Blasko et al[20] (1991)		[125]I	7
Wallner et al[46] (1996)	CT planning	[125]I	14

CT, computed tomography.

brachytherapy and must be counseled regarding an increase likelihood of urinary incontinence following their treatments. Stone and associates[6] found no increase in morbidity in patients who had undergone previous TURP and in whom a real-time peripheral loading brachytherapy technique was used. However, the preponderance of data infers that patients who have had previous TURP are at significantly higher risk of long-term incontinence.[7,8] In our practice, patients with severe outflow obstructive symptoms typically undergo radical prostatectomy or external beam radiation treatments rather than seed implantation.

Postimplant Transurethral Resection of the Prostate

The rate of urinary retention necessitating TURP is typically reported to be <10% at a median of 12 months after implantation (Table 15-3).[1,9] Postimplantation TURP should be delayed at least until the seeds have given off the majority of their radiation dose, a period that varies from 2 months for [103]Pd seeds to 6 months for iodine-125 (^{125}I) (Table 15-4). General considerations for performing this operation include minimizing the volume of tissue resected, preserving apical tissue, and limiting the use of cautery. Invariably, some of the inferior seeds will be resected, and these should be disposed of properly by a radiation safety officer.

All patients should be counseled regarding the risk of urinary incontinence following postimplantation TURP, a risk that can approach 20%.[4] The cause of urinary incontinence following post-brachytherapy TURP is likely related to urethral ischemic changes secondary to the effects of both radiation and electrocautery. Patients should be counseled about the possibility of requiring a second TURP procedure for post-brachytherapy AUR. Staging such therapy, in our clinical experience, can reduce the ultimate risk of incontinence.

Irritative Voiding Symptoms

Lower urinary tract irritative symptoms including dysuria, frequency, urgency, and nocturia are all common following brachytherapy for prostate cancer. Most patients experience grade 1 (37%) or grade 2 (37%)

toxicities, although 21% present with no urinary complaints.[10]

Henderson and colleagues[11] and Kleinberg and associates[12] reported irritative urinary symptoms in 80% of men who received transperineal brachytherapy; these symptoms typically peaked at 6 weeks after implantation. Forty-five percent of patients experienced such symptoms up to 1 year after treatment.[12] Overwhelmingly, most symptoms improve over the first year, but some patients report symptoms that do not return to baseline at >3 years after implantation.[4,13,14]

Merrick and colleagues[14,15] suggested that prophylactic use of selective α-blockers can reduce irritative symptoms in the postoperative period and can permit a return to baseline symptoms at a median of 6 weeks. In comparison, patients who do not receive α-blockers after implantation have delayed resolution of their symptoms for ≤2 years after implantation.[16] Up to one third of these patients will continue to use α-blockade for ≤3 years after implantation.[13] The prophylactic use of α-blockers before implantation has shown efficacy in reducing the time to return to baseline IPSS scores.[17] Patients with mild (RTOG grades 1 and 2) symptoms are typically managed with local anesthetic agents, hydration, and anticholinergic therapy. Patients with grade 3 symptoms are often treated with narcotic analgesics and belladonna alkaloid suppositories.

Cystitis and hemorrhagic cystitis (HC) are common early morbidities associated with brachytherapy. HC can, however, occur 6 months to 10 years following exposure to radiation. In patients with grade 1 or grade 2 HC, the primary treatment modality is observation or bladder irrigation after cystoscopy and upper urinary tract studies rule out other causes of bleeding. Oral and intravenous agents such as aminocaproic acid, estrogens, and pentosan polysulfate sodium (Elmiron) have been tried with limited success. Intravesical treatments with alum silver nitrate, prostaglandins, or formalin are sometimes employed if bleeding persists. Finally, selective embolization of the hypogastric arteries, urinary diversion, and cystectomy may be used as necessary in the most severe cases.

Hyperbaric oxygen (HBO_2) has emerged as a primary option in the management of grades 3 and 4 HC. In our experience HBO_2 results in improvement or resolution of symptoms in 80% to 86% of patients.[18,19] The treatment course is rigorous, with the protocol calling for an initial course of 40 treatments over 20 to 40 days. HBO_2 appears to be an efficacious and economical approach to the treatment of radiation-induced HC. It is the only therapy that has been demonstrated to promote healing in this condition.

Urinary Incontinence

Urinary incontinence following brachytherapy has a reported incidence of 0% to 85%.[20,21] Talcott and col-

TABLE 15-5	Rates of Urinary Incontinence After Brachytherapy	
Reference	**Incontinence (%)**
Clark et al[59] (1999)	15
Blasko et al[20] (1991)	0
Stone and Stock[60] (2007)	1.2
Benoit et al[24] (2000)	6.6

leagues[21] reported that approximately 13% of patients treated with brachytherapy had worn a pad for urinary leakage in the preceding week. Wei and associates[22] noted that 52% of men within the 1-year follow-up after implantation reported occasional urinary dribbling with a 3% total incontinence rate (Table 15-5). These series noted an increased rate of incontinence in patients who had undergone previous TURP. Early series reported a 17% to 50%[20] risk of urinary incontinence following brachytherapy in patients who had received previous TURP. This risk appears highest in patients who had a uniform loading pattern of seeds, although peripherally loaded implants have not definitely demonstrated an improved rate of continence in patients after TURP.[6,23]

All patients who have complaints of persistent urinary incontinence after implantation are evaluated with a thorough voiding history as well as a postvoid residual evaluation to rule out overflow incontinence. Initially, most patients are given a trial of oral anticholinergic therapy, and urodynamic evaluation is considered for those patients who fail to show improvement. Only rarely in our practice have our patients required placement of an artificial sphincter for control of incontinence. This finding is consistent with nationally reported figures.[24]

Urethral Stricture

The incidence of urethral stricture following brachytherapy ranges from 0% to 12% and represents a later cause of urinary obstruction.[25-27] In a large series, Merrick and colleagues[28] found a stricture rate of 3.6% with a mean presentation at 2.6 years after implantation (Table 15-6). Post-brachytherapy strictures invariably are found at the bulbomembranous urethra. In the series reported by Merrick and associates,[29] a statistically greater urethral radiation dose was associated with stricture development.

Similarly, patients who have undergone previous TURP are at higher risk for stricture development. In this circumstance, the mechanism of injury is likely vascular compromise of the underlying tissue. The risk of recurrent stricture has been shown to approach almost 30%, and many of these strictures have refrac-

TABLE 15-6	Rates of Urethral Stricture Following Monotherapy Seed Implantation	
Reference	Agent	Patients (%)
Allen et al[61] (2005)	[125]I and [103]Pd	0
Merrick et al[28] (2006)	[125]I and [103]Pd	3.6
Albert et al[27] (2003)	[125]I	0
Zelefsky et al[62] (2000)	[125]I	10
Ragde et al[7] (1997)	[125]I	12

tory to conservative measures. Ragde and associates[7] found that 2.5% of these patients ultimately necessitated urinary diversion secondary to dense stricture disease.

In our practice, all patients who are seen for postoperative evaluation after implantation are queried regarding their urinary symptoms. Patients who have complaints of a decreased urinary stream are evaluated for possible urinary stricture by flexible cystoscopy followed by a retrograde urethrogram if indicated.

Initial treatment depends on the length and density of the stricture, but it usually entails dilation or internal urethrotomy using direct visualization with the patient under anesthesia. Most patients perform temporary intermittent catheterization to reduce the rate of restenosis. More invasive therapy including urethroplasty or formal urinary diversion may be required in selected cases. Patients who develop strictures after multimodality therapy often have disease that is refractory to minimally invasive management.

SEXUAL DYSFUNCTION

Erectile Dysfunction

Classically, interstitial brachytherapy was thought to have fewer effects on erectile function compared with either external beam radiation therapy or radical prostatectomy. More recent studies, however, indicated that post-brachytherapy erectile dysfunction is seen in ≤90% of patients.[30] Most early studies were complicated by the lack of validated quality of life instruments, hence the large variation in reported rates of impotence. Merrick and colleagues[31] evaluated post-brachytherapy erectile dysfunction by use of patient-administered International Index of Erectile Function (IIEF) questionnaires. The reported rate of erectile preservation in these patients was 39% at 6 years, a rate that improved to 92% with the use of oral phosphodiesterase inhibitors. Other investigators have corroborated these findings and have shown that many brachytherapy recipients respond favorably to oral phosphodiesterase therapy.[32] Most studies have shown a median time to the onset of erec-

tile dysfunction after brachytherapy of approximately 6 months.[31]

The origin of erectile dysfunction after brachytherapy is thought to be multifactorial but likely incorporates arteriogenic and vascular compromise, psychogenic concerns, and postimplantation swelling and trauma to the neurovascular bundles.[33] Radiation dosage to the neurovascular tissue itself has not been shown to compromise erectile function,[34,35] but the dosage delivered to the bulb of the penis has been shown to increase the risk of impotence.[36] To minimize this impact, several investigators have recommended limiting the half-maximal inhibitory dose (D_{50}) of the bulb to ≤50 Gy.[37]

The strongest predictor of post-brachytherapy erectile dysfunction is preimplantation impotence.[31,38] In addition, patients who receive adjuvant radiation therapy during the course of brachytherapy have impaired sexual function outcomes. Diabetes has also been shown to be a significant predictor of erectile dysfunction following implantation.[31] Similarly, age-related changes in erectile function must be considered.[20]

In our series, after brachytherapy, patients are evaluated with an IIEF questionnaire during their course of treatment. We do not typically obtain penile flow or other tumescence studies in patients with postimplantation erectile dysfunction. Patients with new-onset sexual dysfunction are initially treated with oral phosphodiesterase therapy. Those who do not respond are typically offered a vacuum erection device or intracavernosal penile injection therapy. Motivated patients in whom these therapies fail are offered a penile prosthesis.

BOWEL COMPLICATIONS

Rectal Complications

Rectal complications after brachytherapy can be a significant cause of morbidity in the postoperative period. The more common complications include rectal bleeding, tenesmus, proctitis, and decreased bowel function scores. The majority of these complications are low grade (1 and 2). More than 70% of these complications manifest between the first and second year after implantation.[39]

Radiation proctitis, a common complication of brachytherapy, has been shown to correlate with the radiation dose to the anterior rectal wall. Proctitis typically manifests with rectal pain, urgency, diarrhea, frequency, or bleeding and is reported in ≤10% of brachytherapy recipients.[40] Ninety-five percent of radiation-induced proctitis is RTOG grade 1 or 2, temporary, and self-limiting; most symptoms peak at 8 months. Rectal bleeding has been seen in approximately 20% to 26% of patients assayed by patient-administered questionnaires; the peak of this complication occurs within 36 months.[13] In patients with low-grade complaints, early treatment consisting of corticosteroid enemas, dietary modification, and anti-inflammatory agents may alleviate these symptoms.

In contrast to well-documented outcomes with urinary symptoms, fecal-related symptoms after brachytherapy have not been as thoroughly delineated. Merrick and associates[41] detailed bowel function of a large series of patients after implantation and found no significant long-term changes in bowel function. Although overall objective bowel function scores were worse after brachytherapy, almost 20% of patients felt that their bowel function was subjectively worse.

Up to 5% of patients will experience grade 3 to 5 toxicities refractory to conservative management and will require more aggressive therapy.[42] These complications are more commonly seen in patients who have undergone combined therapy and consist of severe bleeding, ulceration, or fistula formation. These patients often have had an antecedent evaluation for lower-grade toxicities and have undergone biopsy or fulguration of the rectal wall. Such biopsies should be discouraged after brachytherapy. Grade 3 to 5 radiation-induced proctitis represents a particular therapeutic challenge because it greatly affects the patient's quality of life and causes considerable life-threatening morbidity.

Traditional treatment options described for radiation-induced proctitis consist of a variety of oral medications and rectal suppositories including steroids, sulfasalazine, aspirin products, sucralfate (oral and rectal), and formalin.[43] HBO_2 therapy has a well-defined role in treating chronic wounds, osteomyelitis, HC, and necrotizing fasciitis and has emerged as a treatment option for radiation-induced proctitis refractory to other attempts at management.[44] By increasing the partial pressure of oxygen in the affected tissues, HBO_2 delivery promotes angiogenesis and thus nutrient influx and ultimately repair of damaged, poorly vascularized tissue.[45]

Twenty-seven patients with radiation-induced proctitis were treated with HBO_2 therapy at Virginia Mason Medical Center in Seattle, Washington (**Fig. 15-3**). All patients had RTOG acute grade 3 or 4 or chronic grade 2 to 4 toxicities and all had undergone unsuccessful primary medical or endoscopic management. All patients had endoscopically confirmed injuries to their rectum. Patients received 100% oxygen in a multiplace hyperbaric chamber at a pressure of 2.4 atmospheres absolute for 90 minutes 5 to 7 days per week for an average of 36 sessions (range, 29-60). Responses to therapy were graded as good, partial, or failure based on change in symptoms, amount of rectal bleeding, need for further management, and post-HBO_2 endoscopic evaluation of treatment response.

In this study, 48% of patients with bleeding showed complete resolution after therapy, whereas 28% reported

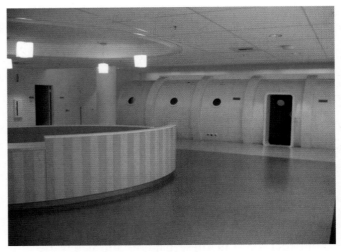

Figure 15-3 Hyperbaric oxygen chamber.

significantly fewer bleeding episodes. Of 4 patients with fecal urgency, 2 noted complete resolution, whereas 1 patient described some improvement. Of the 8 patients with pain, 6 noted some improvement after therapy; however, no patients reported complete resolution of rectal pain. Only 2 of 14 patients with rectal ulceration showed complete resolution of the ulcer on post-treatment endoscopy, whereas 5 showed evidence of improvement; 6 of the patients had no change or worsening of their rectal ulcers. Sixty-seven percent of patients had a partial to good response overall, although 33% showed either no response or progression of their condition. Of the 9 patients in whom HBO_2 therapy failed, 6 had worsening of their preexisting ulcers and 1 developed severe ulceration during therapy. There were 2 patients who had failed treatment with worsening symptoms or persistent rectal bleeding. Of the 9 patients showing no response to therapy, 7 ultimately required diverting colostomy for management of their symptoms.

Urinary Fistula

Perhaps the most serious complication of brachytherapy is the formation of a fistula. Although the incidence ranges from 0.3% to 3%,[8,46] this complication is one of the most feared morbidities encountered with brachytherapy. The most commonly encountered fistula is from the rectum to the urethra, but rectovesical or vesicocutaneous fistulas have been reported (**Fig. 15-4**).[47] Most patients present with urine in their stool, fecaluria, or recurrent urinary infection. In addition, pain appears to be a major complaint in men who present with this complication.

Predisposing factors for the development of a rectourethral fistula include a combination of seed implant and external beam radiation therapy radiation, as well

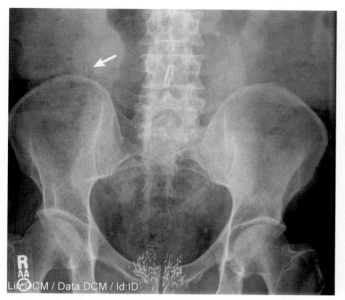

Figure 15-4 Rectourethral fistula following brachytherapy.

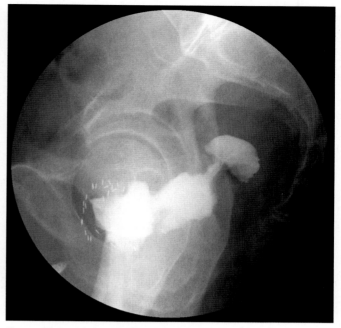

Figure 15-5 Seed migration to right kidney.

as rectal biopsy and electrocautery for rectal bleeding.[48]

Although most authorities recommend a trial of conservative therapy if a fistula is asymptomatic, most fistulas ultimately require intervention. Typically, definitive repair with primary anastomosis in the presence of a radiated field fails. Most patients need either fecal diversion or urinary diversion for alleviation of their symptoms.[49]

HEALTH-RELATED QUALITY OF LIFE

As brachytherapy techniques have evolved and long-term oncologic outcomes have improved, contemporary research has focused on patient-reported health-related quality of life (HRQoL) outcomes. Although much of the reported morbidity consists of physician-reported rates, some efforts have focused on patient-reported outcomes and validated questionnaires.

Miller and colleagues[50] evaluated >700 men treated for prostate cancer with a median follow-up of >6 years. Whereas brachytherapy recipients described early irritative voiding symptoms, this complication appeared to improve over time, consistent with physician-reported data. Surprisingly, incontinence complaints appeared to worsen over time, in contrast to previous physician-reported data on quality of life symptoms.[51] The clinical relevance of these data is unclear because these HRQoL questions may reflect patients who had urinary dribbling or poor stream and not stress or urge incontinence. As validated quality of life questionnaires are used in larger patient groups with long-term outcomes, this approach will evolve as the standard means of assessing patient outcomes following brachytherapy.

SEED MIGRATION AND OTHER COMPLICATIONS

In patients who have undergone brachytherapy implantation, several minor complications have been described including infection and migration of implanted seeds. The overall risk of perioperative infection with brachytherapy varies between 1% and 2%.[52] Some evidence suggests that postimplantation antibiotic prophylaxis may not be necessary.[53] Symptomatic urinary tract infections have been reported in approximately 1% of patients. Epididymitis is an uncommon entity following brachytherapy that occurs in approximately 1% of patients and appears unrelated to the use of prophylactic or perioperative antibiotics.[54] Most patients respond to conservative therapy including antibiotics and anti-inflammatory agents.

Systemic migration of the seeds during brachytherapy can be a common event, but the clinical significance is unknown. Systemic migration is most often seen in the lungs or kidneys (**Fig. 15-5**). The reported rate of pulmonary migration varies from 5.9% to 72.5%,[55,56] although contemporary experience suggests a significantly lower rate. One such study assessed the use of polyglactin 910 (Vicryl)–linked seeds in their peripheral placement technique that reduced the rate of pulmonary seed embolization to the lungs to 0.7%.[57] The true incidence of migration likely is higher than reported because not all patients undergo routine imaging after implantation.

No data suggest that recovery of migrated seeds is warranted.[58] The dose of a single migrated source to the lungs or other organs results in no functional impairment.

CONCLUSION

Brachytherapy is a common treatment for clinically localized prostate cancer that appears to offer adequate long-term oncologic control for ≤10 years in appropriately chosen patients. Complications of brachytherapy can affect urinary, sexual, and bowel function and are often most pronounced in the first several years after implantation. Although implanting techniques have been modified to reduce radiation dosage to adjacent structures, the side effects can still have a significant effect on a patient's quality of life. Therefore, close attention must be paid to the placement of seeds regardless of technique used. Postoperative assessment of seed placement provides appropriate feedback to the implanter and helps guide technique modifications to minimize toxicity. It is imperative that both the urologist and the radiation oncologist examine the results of their work to provide the best possible outcomes for their patients. Further long-term follow-up studies using validated quality of life instruments should lead to more accurate assessment of the morbidity associated with these procedures.

KEY POINTS

1. The use of α-blockers in the perioperative period may reduce the risk of AUR and irritative voiding symptoms.
2. HBO₂ therapy has been shown to be efficacious for patients suffering from HC and proctitis.
3. The majority of rectal morbidity is low grade and often responds to conservative management.
4. Erectile dysfunction following brachytherapy is a common complaint during longer follow-up.
5. Diabetic patients, men who are >70 years old, and those with preoperative erectile dysfunction are more likely to have postsurgical erectile impairment.
6. Rectal fistulas, although rare, often necessitate fecal and urinary diversion for definitive treatment.
7. Seed migration appears to be a common event following brachytherapy, with apparently minor clinical implications.
8. Infection is a relatively uncommon complication of brachytherapy.

REFERENCES

Please see www.expertconsult.com

Chapter 16

COMPLICATIONS OF CRYOSURGICAL ABLATION OF PROSTATE

Katsuto Shinohara MD

Professor, Department of Urology, University of California–San Francisco, San Francisco, California

In the United States, the incidence of prostate cancer more than doubled between the late 1990s to 2008, and 218,890 new cases were expected to be detected in 2007.[1] The treatment of prostate cancer, however, remains controversial, and no consensus has been established regarding appropriate treatment for any stage of disease, especially for localized cancers. Radical prostatectomy, radiation therapy, and watchful waiting all have their advocates, and the risks and benefits of these approaches are frequently discussed.

Cryosurgery as a treatment for localized prostate cancer has seen renewed interest because of promising reports citing low morbidity, minimal blood loss, and short hospital stay as a result of technologic advances. Cryotherapy has its earliest antecedent in 19th century London, where Arnott applied ice-salt mixtures to breast and cervical cancers.[2] Modern cryotherapy began in 1966 with the advent of probes cooled by liquid nitrogen in closed circulation.[3] One of the first applications of this technology was the transurethral cryoablation of benign prostatic hyperplasia,[4] followed shortly by the use of cryoablation to treat prostate cancer through an open perineal approach.[5] The transperineal approach was introduced in 1974, initially using a single cryoprobe that was guided digitally and repositioned as needed during the procedure.[6] In 1984, Onik and colleagues[7] demonstrated that the frozen area could be seen ultrasonographically as a well-marginated hyperechoic rim with acoustic shadowing.

Transrectal ultrasound (TRUS) technology was in widespread use in the 1990s for the early detection of prostate cancer, and a transperineal, percutaneously introduced, multiple cryoprobe system for prostate cancer treatment was developed.[8] In addition, a urethral warmer using a continuous irrigation system was developed for protection of the urethra, to minimize the risk of urethral tissue sloughing and stricture formation. The first clinical application of such a system was reported in 1993.[9] Major advances in the use of cryotherapy for prostate cancer at that time included the following:

1. Real-time TRUS monitoring of probe placement and freezing[10]
2. Simultaneous use of multiple cryoprobes
3. Use of urethral warming catheters[9]

A significant, more recent development was the introduction of a second-generation cryotherapy system based on argon gas rather than on liquid nitrogen. By the Joule-Thompson principle, rapidly expanding argon gas cools the probe tip to −150°C and can be quickly exchanged for helium to induce an active thawing phase, thus significantly speeding two-cycle treatment.[11] The much smaller diameter of the more recently developed third-generation gas-based cryotherapy system permits direct percutaneous transperineal insertion, avoids the need for tract dilation, and facilitates conformal cryosurgery by allowing more probes to be placed (Table 16-1).[12]

MECHANISM OF TISSUE ABLATION BY CRYOTHERAPY

Cellular damage during freezing is the product of many mechanisms. After reaching a tissue temperature of <0°C, the extracellular fluid begins to crystallize. This process increases the osmotic pressure of the unfrozen portion of fluid in the extracellular compartment and causes water to shift from the intracellular space to the extracellular space. As a result, cells become dehydrated. Cellular pH also changes, leading to the denaturing of cellular proteins.[13] With further temperature drops, water in the intracellular space crystallizes and mechanically breaks down the cellular membrane. On thawing, extracellular fluid shifts back into the intracellular space and causes cells to burst. The blood vessels around the targeted tissue initially dilate after thawing, and hyperpermeability of the vessel wall occurs. After a few hours of this hyperemic state, microthrombi form on the damaged vessel wall and lead to ischemia of the tissue.

	Manufacturer							
TABLE 16-1		**Cryotherapy Technologic Improvement**						
Generation	(System Name)	Cryogen	No. Probes	Probe Diameter	Probe Placement	Temperature Monitor	Active Thawing	Other Characteristics
1st	Cryomedical Services (AccuProbe)	Liquid nitrogen	5	3 mm	Tract dilation required	No	No	1. TRUS guided and monitored 2. Urethral warming device
2nd	Endocare (Cryocare)	Argon gas	8	3 mm/2.4 mm	Direct puncture with 2.4-mm probe	Yes	Yes	1. Template guidance 2. Computerized planning system 3. Autofreeze control 4. Variable freezing length probe
3rd	Galil Medical (SeedNet)	Argon gas	30	17 gauge	Direct puncture	Yes	Yes	1. Template guided 2. Variable freezing length probe

TRUS, transrectal ultrasound.

Factors Affecting Tissue Ablation

Two parameters correlate with the degree of cell destruction achieved during cryotherapy: (1) the cooling rate during the freezing process and (2) the lowest temperature achieved. A faster freezing rate and slower thawing rate also result in more cellular destruction.[13] The duration of freezing is also an important factor in tissue destruction. More cellular destruction is achieved by prolonged freezing at a low temperature. In a clinical setting, however, the number of freezing cycles, the lowest temperature achieved, and the existence of heat sinks caused by large blood vessels may be more important factors in cancer cell destruction.

Investigators have long known that repeated freeze-thaw cycles create more extensive tissue damage than does a single cycle.[14] Tatsutani and colleagues[15] described that cells not completely destroyed by initial freezing to −20°C were completely destroyed with a second freezing cycle. Larson and associates[16] reported that cryoablation results in two tissue zones, a central zone of complete cellular necrosis surrounded by a peripheral zone of less extensive cell damage. These investigators reported that the central zone of complete cellular necrosis could be significantly enlarged by a second freezing cycle.[16] This finding has important clinical implications for the urologist performing cryosurgery. After starting circulation of cryogen through the probe, a sphere of frozen tissue, called an *ice ball,* begins to form at the tip of the probe. The hyperechoic edge of the ice ball visualized during procedures has a temperature of 0°C to −2°C, and temperatures as low as −20°C to −40°C exist inside this edge. Therefore, one has to extend the ice ball well beyond the edge of the prostate to ensure adequate tissue abla-

tion. The urologist must also be aware that large blood vessels may act as heat sinks. Such areas may not achieve target temperatures even though they are completely enclosed in the treatment area.

PATIENT SELECTION

Primary Therapy

As with any other treatment for prostate cancer, appropriate patient selection is critical to the success of cryotherapy. Patients with low-risk tumor features (i.e., serum prostate-specific antigen [PSA] ≤10 ng/mL, diagnostic biopsy Gleason score ≤6, and clinical stage T1c or T2a) have the best cryotherapy outcomes. Patients with higher-grade tumors or higher PSA levels are at increased risk for localized extension of disease or metastatic spread. In most clinical series, cryotherapy is associated with higher rates of impotence than are other localized treatment alternatives. Consequently, patients for whom preservation of erectile function is a high priority are less appropriate candidates for cryosurgery. Cryoablation has also been used for local disease control in patients with known metastatic disease who are receiving systemic therapy but require palliative maneuvers for local symptoms.[17]

Salvage Treatment

Few localized treatment alternatives exist for patients who experience a rising PSA level after radiation therapy and who are found to have biopsy-confirmed residual disease. Additional radiation therapy in the form of brachytherapy[18,19] or radical prostatectomy[20,21] is an option. Most patients in this position, however, receive systemic androgen deprivation therapy. This approach may control the cancer for up to several years but does not offer the possibility of definitive cure.

Cryotherapy has been established as a viable treatment alternative for patients after failure of radiation treatment. Tumor cells that are resistant to radiation therapy, androgen deprivation, and chemotherapy may remain vulnerable to the physical trauma of freezing and thawing.

Patients who may be candidates for salvage treatment with cryotherapy should be carefully selected. If the goal is cure of disease, the treating physician must be reasonably confident that the PSA elevation is attributable to persistent or recurrent local disease and not to occult metastatic disease.

Most reported series of patients who undergo salvage cryotherapy have included imaging tests—nuclear scintigraphy and pelvic cross-sectional imaging (computed tomography [CT] or magnetic resonance imaging [MRI])—to rule out metastases to the bones and pelvic lymph nodes, respectively. The sensitivity of these tests, however, particularly for lymph node involvement, is <50%,[22] and a positive test result in the presence of a low PSA reading is unlikely.[23] Some investigators have confirmed the presence of viable, treatable, localized disease by prostate biopsy.[24] In patients with high-risk features such as a preradiation PSA >20 ng/mL, Gleason score 8 to 10, or a rapidly rising PSA level after radiation therapy, pelvic lymphadenectomy may be considered to rule out metastatic disease.

The patient should have a life expectancy independent of prostate cancer of ≥10 years and should understand the increased risk of adverse side effects associated with salvage therapy. Most reported cases have been performed in patients in whom external beam radiation therapy has failed, but success has also been reported in patients who have failed to respond to brachytherapy.[24]

Anatomic Considerations

Even with a multiprobe cryotherapy device, a large prostate gland may be difficult to treat because of prolonged freezing time. A gland >50 cc may be best treated with neoadjuvant hormone therapy to reduce the target volume before the procedure. Other relative contraindications include the following:

1. Prior transurethral resection of the prostate
2. Large tissue defects in the prostate that are likely to lead to tissue sloughing of the urethra despite the use of a urethral warming catheter
3. Active inflammatory disease of the rectum
4. Severe anal stricture
5. Prior abdominoperineal resection of the rectum

PREOPERATIVE CONSIDERATIONS

Neoadjuvant Hormone Therapy

A large prostate volume (>50 cc) can limit the technical feasibility of complete cryoablation. Neoadjuvant androgen ablation using a 3-month depot injection of a luteinizing hormone–releasing hormone agonist usually reduces the prostate to 60% to 70% of its original size.[25] Androgen ablation may also reduce the tumor burden in patients with stage T3 disease (gross extracapsular extension or seminal vesicle involvement). The use of neoadjuvant androgen ablation has not been prospectively evaluated in the context of cryotherapy. In subset analysis of a retrospective series of patients, however, this strategy was not shown to improve outcomes.[26] Indeed, in one large analysis, patients receiving neoadjuvant therapy had poorer biochemical outcomes that did those receiving cryotherapy alone, although the patients in the neoadjuvant therapy group also tended to have more aggressive tumor characteristics.[27]

Lymph Node Dissection

Patients contemplating cryosurgery who are at high risk for lymph node metastasis but who have had negative results of cross-sectional imaging studies may undergo regional lymphadenectomy to identify lymph node metastases that would relatively contraindicate aggressive localized therapy for prostate cancer. Lymphadenectomy may be performed laparoscopically or by mini-laparotomy, with low morbidity.[28] Patients with significant risk factors for lymph node metastases, such as a PSA >20 ng/mL or a Gleason score of 8 to 10, are associated with localized treatment failure, even if removed lymph nodes prove to be free of disease.

PROCEDURE

Preoperative Preparations

Patients should discontinue anticoagulant or antiplatelet medications before cryotherapy. Light bowel preparation is recommended before the procedure and consists of administration of oral magnesium citrate the day before treatment and an enema the morning of treatment.

Cryotherapy Procedure

Cryosurgery may be performed using general or regional anesthesia. After anesthesia is induced, the patient is placed in the lithotomy position. A Councill-tip catheter is placed in the urethra, and the bladder is distended with saline solution to displace the peritoneal contents away from the treatment area. A TRUS probe is inserted into the rectum, and the anatomic configuration of the prostate and tumor, if ultrasonically identifiable, are confirmed.

Current cryotherapy uses small-gauge, needle-shaped probes that can be placed directly into the prostate gland through the perineum. Probe placement is carried out under TRUS guidance and can be performed with a freehand technique or with a perineal template. The Cryocare system usually requires six probes, two placed anteriorly and four posteriorly. The SeedNet system uses 17-gauge, needle-shaped probes, more than six of which may be placed to achieve a more conformal freezing pattern by means of a perineal template.[12] After cryoprobe placement, thermosensors are placed to monitor temperature at the gland apex and the external sphincter, along Denonvilliers' fascia, at the neurovascular bundles, and at the edge of the tumor. After completing these punctures, the Councill-tip urethral catheter is exchanged over a guidewire for a urethral warmer, and warm saline irrigation is started through the warming catheter.

Once freezing is initiated, ice within the prostate casts a dense acoustic shadow that obscures all anatomic detail anterior to the ice. For this reason, the anterior probes must be activated first. The anterior ice balls are extended posteriorly and laterally, including a 2- to 4-mm margin into the lateral periprostatic tissues and beyond the gland apex. If tumor extracapsular extension is suspected, the ice is propagated further laterally on the involved side. The anterior probes are then allowed to thaw, and the posterior probes are activated. The posterior ice balls are extended into, but not beyond, the rectal muscularis propria (**Fig. 16-1**). If the apex is inadequately frozen, the probes may be withdrawn toward the apex and reactivated. If seminal vesicle involvement is suspected, probes may be placed deeper into that organ.

Once freezing is completed, the ice is allowed to thaw actively by circulating helium instead of argon gas through the probe. Two freeze-thaw cycles are generally carried out, as stated earlier, after which the cryoprobes and cannulas are removed. The urethral warmer remains in place until all thawing is completed; it is then exchanged for a Foley catheter or is removed with suprapubic catheter placement.

Postoperative Care

Cryotherapy is usually performed as an outpatient procedure. A urethral or suprapubic catheter should be left in place for 1 to 3 weeks following treatment until urinary retention resolves. Some investigators have reported leaving the urethral warming catheter in place for several hours after the procedure in an attempt to minimize injury to the urethra,[11] but the efficacy of this maneuver has not been well studied.

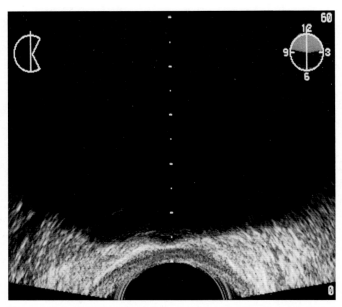

Figure 16-1 TRUS image of the prostate during freezing. The ice ball is seen as an area with acoustic shadow completely encroaching the gland. The leading edge of the ice ball touches the rectal wall muscle.

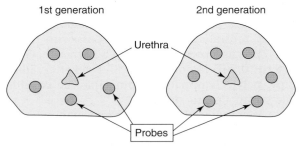

Figure 16-2 The first-generation cryosurgery machine had only five probes simultaneously operable. The probe in the midline just posterior to the urethra is always close to the urethra, thus leading to urethral damage. The second-generation machine can operate more than five probes simultaneously, and posterior medial probes can be placed away from the urethra. This improvement has resulted in safer procedure.

COMPLICATIONS

Complications associated with cryotherapy are listed in Tables 16-2 and 16-3. Improved understanding of the risks of overfreezing, the importance of urethral protection, and technologic advances have reduced complications associated with cryoablation significantly. In particular, the introduction of built-in thermosensors and the development of second- and third-generation machines with more than five probes have allowed us to perform cryoablation more safely (**Fig. 16-2**).

Complications of cryosurgery are generally observed at least a few weeks after the procedure when patients start to void spontaneously. Overfreezing and incomplete protection of surrounding tissue are the main

TABLE 16-2	Complications Associated With Primary Cryotherapy in Selected Publications						
Reference	No. Patients	Generation of Cryosystem	Impotence (%)	Incontinence (%)	Fistula (%)	Urinary Obstruction (%)	Rectal Pain (%)
Bahn et al[48] (1995)	210	1st	41	9	2.4	3	NA
Shinohara et al[45] (1996)	102	1st	86	15	1	23	3
Cohen et al[29] (1996)	239	1st	4	0.4	2.2	3	0.4
Wake et al[52] (1996)	100	1st and 2nd	NA	NA	0	22	NA
Long et al[35] (1998)	145	1st and 2nd	88	88	1.3	17	2.3
Badalament et al[53] (1999)	290	2nd	85	85	0.4	NA	12
Long et al[27] (2001)	975	1st and 2nd	NA	NA	0.5	13	NA
Cohen[40] (2004)	865	1st	NA	8.6	2	NA	NA
	98	2nd		3.2	0	NA	
		3rd		0	0	NA	
Prepelica et al[54] (2005)	65	2nd	NA	3.1	0	1.5	NA
Ellis et al[39] (2007)	416	2nd	60.9	4	0	NA	0

NA, not available.

TABLE 16-3	Complications Associated With Salvage Cryotherapy in Selected Publications						
Reference	No. Patients	Generation of Cryosystem	Impotence (%)	Incontinence (%)	Fistula (%)	Urinary Obstruction (%)	Rectal Pain (%)
Pisters et al[17] (1997)	150	1st	72	73	1	67	NA
Chin et al[24] (2001)	118	2nd	NA	6.7	3.3	8.5	NA
Ghafar et al[41] (2001)	38	3rd	NA	7.9	0	4	NA
de la Taille et al[11] (2000)	43	2nd	NA	9	0	5	26
Han et al[38] (2004)	29	3rd	NA	9	0	3	NA

NA, not available.

causes of various complications associated with this procedure.

The management of patients who have local disease recurrence following radiation is associated with an increased risk of complications following cryosurgery.[29-31] Irradiated tissues surrounding the prostate are already damaged and are slow to repair when additional injury occurs. Alternately, radiation therapy appears to be given safely for local recurrence after cryosurgery.

Impotence

Impotence after cryotherapy is common. Cryotherapy impairs the penile arterial blood supply[32] and damages the cavernosal nerves responsible for erectile function.[33] This combined neurovascular insult results in impotence in 41%[34] to 88%[35] of treated patients. Rates depend on such factors as the use of multiple freeze-thaw cycles, the size of the ice ball generated, preoperative potency, instruments used to assess potency, and time elapsed since treatment.

Because nerve and vascular regeneration is possible after surgery or radiation therapy, some patients have reportedly recovered erectile function as long as 2 years after treatment. Bahn and colleagues[34] reported that 95% of the patients who were potent before cryotherapy became impotent, and 5% regained their potency at a mean of 16 months after treatment. Donnelly and associates[36] reported that 47% of their patients had return of erectile function at 3 years. These investigators hypothesized that cryotherapy does not sever nerves and maintains a potential recovery route.

Long and colleagues[27] conducted a pooled analysis of 975 patients treated at 5 institutions between 1993 and 1998 and reported an impotence rate of 93%. However, Robinson and associates[37] found that 3 years after cryoablation, 13% of 38 patients had regained potency, and an additional 34% of patients were potent with the help of erectile aids.

Advanced cryotherapy equipment has significantly reduced other complications, but the impotence rate appears to remain high even with second- or third-generation equipment. Han and colleagues[38] reported an 84% rate of impotence among their patients when a third-generation device was used. These investigators stated that to eradicate the tissue completely at the edge of the gland, ablation of neurovascular bundle was necessary.[38]

Postprocedural potency is an important quality of life issue, and cryotherapy remains clearly inferior by this measure compared with other localized treatment modalities for prostate cancer. Until outcomes in this area improve, high post-treatment impotence rates will continue to constitute an impediment to wider use of this treatment approach among patients for whom erectile function is important.

Ellis and colleagues[39] reported a penile rehabilitation program with regular use of a vacuum erectile device after cryotherapy. These results showed potency rates of 41.4% and 51.3% at 1 and 4 years, respectively, after treatment and suggest a substantial increase in potency by the use of rehabilitation.[39]

Incontinence

Reported rates of incontinence depend greatly on the definitions of continence and the methods of assessment. Another factor is the number of patients treated without a urethral warming device. Rates vary from 0%[29] to 27%[30] for patients who received cryotherapy as primary treatment. In one of the largest single series of patients who underwent primary cryotherapy, Bahn and associates[34] reported that 4.3% of patients required at least one urinary pad per day, and 11.6% had lesser degrees of incontinence. The analysis by Long and colleagues[27] reported a 7.5% incontinence rate.[27] Cohen and associates[40] reported an incontinence rate of 3.2% among patients treated using first- and second-generation devices, but the rate fell to 0% when the third-generation machine was introduced.[40]

Among patients undergoing cryotherapy for salvage treatment after failure of radiation therapy, the prevalence of incontinence is higher, ranging from 6.7%[24] to 73%[17] in the largest series. Approximately one third of the patients reporting incontinence had nearly total or total incontinence.[24] The large salvage cryotherapy series by Pisters and colleagues[17] reported an incontinence rate of 73%, but this series contains large numbers of patients who were treated before the urethral warming catheter became available. Using modern equipment and a urethral warming device, incontinence rates for salvage cryotherapy are between 6.7% and 9%.[24,38,41]

Tissue Sloughing

Cryosurgery induces necrosis in the treated prostate tissue (**Fig. 16-3**). If the urethra freezes during treatment, its mucosal barrier will fail, thus exposing the necrotic prostate tissue to the urinary tract and to a risk of infec-

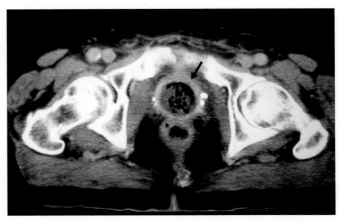

Figure 16-3 CT scan of the prostate area after cryosurgery. The prostate gland is necrotic and is surrounded by a thick, fibrous tissue (*arrow*).

tion. This tissue may then slough into the urethra, typically 3 to 8 weeks after treatment, and may produce irritating and obstructive voiding symptoms, pyuria, and occasionally urinary retention. The use of urethral warming devices significantly reduces the risk of this complication.[42,43] However, a urethral warming device protects the urethra only where it is in direct contact.

The catheter is relatively stiff, and the floor in the middle of the prostatic urethra may not be protected (**Fig. 16-4**). This situation results in partial necrosis of the urethra. In their pooled analysis, Long and colleagues[27] similarly reported obstruction requiring transurethral resection of the prostate in 10% of patients who had received urethral warming through an approved catheter, compared with 44% in patients who did not undergo urethral warming. In one clinical series, the overall rate of sloughing ranged from 3.8%[31] to 23%[44] for patients receiving primary cryotherapy and from 5%[11] to 44%[17] for those undergoing salvage treatment. Cohen and colleagues[40] reported tissue sloughing in 14% of patients treated by first- and second-generation machines, yet only 2% patients treated with the third-generation machine had tissue sloughing.

Conservative treatment of sloughing-related complications includes antibiotics and urinary drainage. Continuous intermittent self-catheterization may help dislodge obstructing tissue. In some cases, however, transurethral removal or resection of necrotic tissue may be required. Because nearly 50% of patients requiring transurethral resection after cryotherapy develop incontinence,[45] use of this approach should be as limited as possible.

Pelvic and Rectal Pain

Pelvic or rectal pain is occasionally encountered after cryotherapy. One percent[46] to 11%[30] of patients receiv-

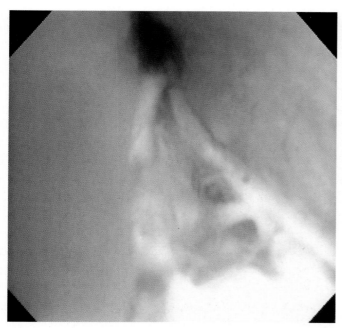

Figure 16-4 Cystoscopic finding of a patient complaint of urethral pain 4 weeks after salvage cryoablation. White necrotic tissue is seen over the floor of the prostatic urethra.

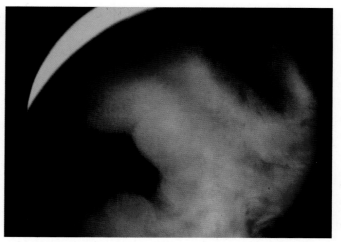

Figure 16-5 Cystoscopic finding of the prostatic urethra. Matured rectourethral fistulas with complete epithelial coverage are seen.

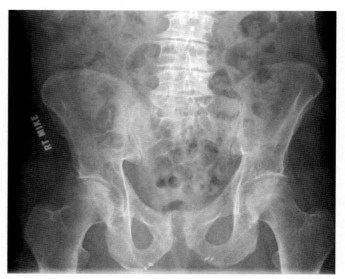

Figure 16-6 Pelvic radiograph of a patient with severe pelvic pain after cryosurgery. Note the pubic bone destruction over the midline. Freezing too anteriorly resulted in freezing of the pubic bone.

ing primary cryotherapy and 26%[11] to 77%[47] of those receiving salvage therapy for radiation therapy failure report pelvic or rectal pain. The origin of this pain is unclear but may include rectal wall ischemia, freezing of the pelvic floor musculature or pubic bone, and extravasation of urine into the periprostatic tissues. Urinoma or abscess must be ruled out in these patients. The pain is best managed with anti-inflammatory medications.

Penile Numbness

Some patients treated with cryotherapy develop penile numbness attributable to injury to the dorsal nerve of the penis in the pelvis by probe insertion. This numbness usually resolves spontaneously.[46]

Fistula

Complete freezing of tissues posterior to the prostate including rectal wall, with urinary extravasation and possible subsequent infection, can lead to rectourethral fistula formation, which is reported in 0%[31,35] to 2.4%[48] of patients undergoing cryotherapy as their primary treatment. In their series of 590 patients, Bahn and associates[34] reported only 2 cases of fistula. Similarly, Long and colleagues[27] reported a 0.5% rate of fistula among 975 patients. Rates may be higher among patients receiving salvage therapy (≤11% in one report).[35] In a large series of patients receiving salvage therapy, however, only 4 cases of fistula were reported among 118 patients.[24] This complication may occur as long as several months after treatment and typically manifests with watery diarrhea or pneumaturia. Diagnosis is confirmed with a voiding cystourethrogram (**Fig. 16-5**) or CT scan. Conservative treatment consists of Foley catheter drainage, which may be facilitated by fistula tract fulguration when the tract is mature (**Fig. 16-6**). Any formal fistula repair should be delayed 4 to 6 months to allow the inflammatory process to subside. A transperineal approach[49] and a posterior approach[50] to close have been described.

Although it is rare, urethrocutaneous fistula has been reported in the literature.[51] Cryoprobes are insulated with the vacuum chamber at the main shaft. If the probe is defective and the vacuum insulation is not perfect, freezing of the entire shaft can occur. This situation creates perineal tissue necrosis and possible fistula formation. Observation of the ice pattern on probes at test freezing initially and of perineal skin condition during the procedure will alert the clinician to the presence of a defective probe.

Urethral Stricture

Urethral stricture results from extensive tissue sloughing, usually at the bladder neck or even in the middle of the prostatic urethra. In their multiple-institute pool study, Long and colleagues[27] reported stricture in 3.4% of their patients. This is a rare complication when urethral warming is employed; it usually can be managed successfully with transurethral incision or balloon dilation.

Small Bowel Obstruction

Small bowel obstruction after cryotherapy is rare. This complication probably occurs when the ice ball extends to the cul de sac of the peritoneal cavity. Careful TRUS examination can show the level of the cul de sac behind the bladder. Distention of the bladder cavity with normal saline solution during the procedure generally prevents this complication.

Hydronephrosis

Hydronephrosis is not a common complication associated with cryosurgery. However, overfreezing of the bladder neck area or placement of the probe deep into the seminal vesicle may result in freezing of the ureteral orifices or ureters. Bales and associates[47] reported hydronephrosis in 36.4% of patients treated with cryosurgery for recurrent prostate cancer after radiation therapy. However, Pisters and associates[17] did not report this complication. Careful observation of the trigone area by TRUS generally shows the location of the ureteral orifices. If the seminal vesicles or bladder neck need to be treated, localization of the ureteral orifices before the freezing is important.

Osteitis Pubis

Excessive anterior freezing at the apex may cause osteitis pubis. A CT scan and bone scan may show bone

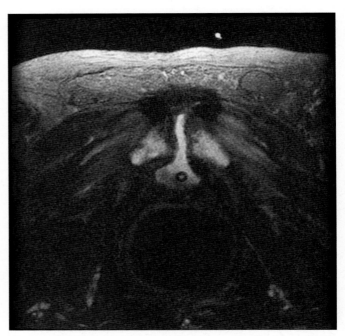

Figure 16-7 This patient underwent salvage cryoablation for local disease recurrence after radiation therapy. The patient complained of urinary incontinence, pelvic pain, and gait disturbance. MRI shows pubic bone destruction with extravasations of urine at the anterior part of the membranous urethra.

destruction in the area of the pubis (**Fig. 16-7**). Tenderness over the pubic bone and pain at the base of the penis are common. Again, conservative treatment with nonsteroidal anti-inflammatory medication and rest is recommended. If pain persists despite conservative therapy, osteomyelitis or extravasation of urine resulting in secondary infection must be excluded.

CONCLUSION

Advances in technology and clinical algorithms may be expected to improve cryotherapy outcomes. Varying the intensity and extent of cryoablation should allow patients and physicians to contemplate tradeoffs between quality of life and the certainty of cancer control. Finally, expertise in ultrasound imaging, careful control of the freezing zone, and protection of the urethra are the keys for prevention of common complications after cryosurgical ablation of the prostate. Experience of the surgeon who performs the procedure likely contributes greatly to the success of the cryosurgical ablation.

KEY POINTS

1. Cryosurgery as a treatment for localized prostate cancer has seen renewed interest because of promising reports citing low morbidity, minimal blood loss, and short hospital stay with advances in technologies.

2. A urethral warmer using a continuous irrigation system was developed for protection of the urethra to minimize the risk of urethral tissue sloughing and stricture formation.

3. A large prostate gland may be difficult to treat because of prolonged freezing time. A >50-cc gland may be best treated with neoadjuvant hormone therapy to reduce the target volume before the procedure.

4. The posterior ice balls should be extended into, but not beyond, the rectal muscularis propria.

5. Overfreezing and incomplete protection of surrounding tissue are the main causes of various complications associated with cryosurgery.

6. Cryotherapy impairs the penile arterial blood supply and damages the cavernosal nerves responsible for erectile function.

7. Among patients undergoing cryotherapy for salvage treatment after failure of radiation therapy, the prevalence of incontinence is higher, ranging from 6.7% to 73% in the largest series.

8. Nearly 50% of patients requiring transurethral resection after cryotherapy develop incontinence, so its use should be as limited as possible.

REFERENCES

Please see www.expertconsult.com

Chapter 17

COMPLICATIONS OF MINIMALLY INVASIVE PROCEDURES FOR BENIGN PROSTATIC HYPERPLASIA

Rajiv Saini MD
Clinical Assistant Professor of Urology, Weill Medical College of Cornell University, New York; Attending Urologist, Voiding Dysfunction, Brookdale University Hospital and Medical Center, Brooklyn, New York

Richard Lee MD
Urology Resident, Weill Medical College of Cornell University, New York, New York

Alexis E. Te MD
Associate Professor of Urology and Director, Brady Prostate Center, Weill Medical College of Cornell University, New York, New York

The management of benign prostatic hyperplasia (BPH) has undergone substantial change in recent years. The objectives of treatment, however, have remained constant: to decrease bladder outlet obstruction by either medical management or physical removal of obstructing prostatic tissue.[1,2] This treatment entails creating an open channel for voiding and thereby relieving symptoms attributed to the obstruction. Methods of relieving outlet obstruction from BPH have evolved from more invasive (open prostatectomy) to less invasive. Transurethral resection of the prostate (TURP) is considered a second-generation treatment after open surgery. It was considered the first available minimally invasive alternative to open surgery.

Both open prostatectomy and TURP are considered the gold standards for treatment. Open prostatectomy and TURP have proven to be both efficacious and durable. Long-term data have shown improvements in American Urological Association Symptom Index (AUASI), peak flow rate (Qmax), and quality of life (QoL) score. Although it is effective, TURP is associated with substantial potential morbidity, as well as the need for anesthesia and possible hospitalization.[3] These factors have provided the impetus for the development of new, minimally invasive therapies, such as transurethral microwave thermotherapy (TUMT) and transurethral needle ablation of the prostate (TUNA). These minimally invasive therapies seek to offer a cost-effective alternative to TURP while achieving substantial improvement in QoL with a lower risk of complications.

Complications of TURP include hemorrhage (6%), blood transfusion (8%), cardiovascular events (5%), urinary retention (5%), urinary tract infection (UTI) (6%), retrograde ejaculation (65%), erectile dysfunction (10%), urinary incontinence (3%), bladder neck contracture or urethral stricture (7%), and transurethral resection (TUR) syndrome (2%).[4] The risk of transfusion-requiring hemorrhage events is approximately 4% to 8%.[3,5,6] Although death is also a possibility, the overall mortality rate remains low, approximately 0.4% to 2.5%, depending on age.[7]

Intraoperative and perioperative complications (3% overall) of TURP include irrigant absorption and bladder perforation. TUR syndrome, caused by absorption of irrigating solution and leading to dilutional hyponatremia, mental confusion, visual disturbances, nausea, vomiting, bradycardia, and hypertension, can occur in 2% of patients.

Postoperative complications of TURP include failure to void after catheter removal, clot retention, infection including UTI, and irritative symptoms (15%). Late complications include bladder neck contracture or urethral stricture, urinary incontinence, ejaculatory dysfunction, and erectile dysfunction, as well as a 5% retreatment rate.

THERAPEUTIC MODALITIES AND THERMAL EFFECTS ON THE PROSTATE

The success of each modality depends on its clinical efficacy and safety profile compared with TURP. The focus of this chapter is to compare the complications and potential advantages of each technique for treatment of BPH. Although many technologies are available, this chapter discusses those more easily available in the clinical practice of today's urologists. In addition, the complications are discussed based on the difference in equipment and technology for each alternative. Specifically, this chapter focuses on TUMT, TUNA, interstitial laser coagulation (ILC), and laser procedures including photoselective vaporization of the prostate (PVP).

The successful management of BPH with minimally invasive thermal therapies depends on the temperature-time relationship for tissue destruction. Combinations of duration and temperature applied to prostate tissue have been studied to determine the effect on tissues. The threshold for causing heat necrosis in the prostate is 60 minutes at 45°C, 30 minutes at 50°C, 5 minutes at 55°C, 2 minutes at 60°C, and 1 minute at 70°C. Therefore, higher temperatures can cause equivalent destruction despite shorter time intervals when compared with lower temperatures and longer time intervals.[8]

Many modalities use the tissue ablative effect of heat on prostate tissue to obtain a TURP-like clinical effect while decreasing operative and postoperative morbidity. In general, these therapeutic heat effects can be divided into three general categories:

1. Therapeutic temperatures <45°C do not induce irreversible tissue destruction, and these "hyperthermia" procedures have become obsolete.
2. Temperatures in the range of 47°C to 100°C lead to tissue destruction through gradually irreversible coagulation necrosis. The temperature range of 47°C to 60°C produces gradual tissue atrophy, whereas that between 60°C and 100°C produces immediate larger cystic cavities comparable to post-TURP defects.[9] Procedures with this range of temperatures are called *thermotherapy* or *thermoablation*.
3. Temperatures >100°C lead to tissue vaporization and therefore immediate removal of tissue.

Given the foregoing temperature subdivisions, technologies can be categorized into coagulators or vaporizers. Standard TURP loop resection, laser vaporization (e.g., PVP), and electrovaporization of the prostate employ vaporization heat to achieve the desired clinical effect, whereas TUMT, TUNA, high-intensity focused ultrasound (HIFU), ILC, and visual laser ablation of the prostate (VLAP) employ coagulative temperatures to gain their desired effects. Each technique possesses specific risks, morbidities, and clinical advantages.

In the evaluation of all BPH therapies, two major tenets are important to consider in the development of a successful treatment modality. The first is to decrease subjective symptoms of BPH. The second is to relieve obstruction by anatomically widening the channel through the prostatic urethra. Although many studies have failed establish a causal relationship between the two, it is often accepted that relieving obstruction will improve symptoms. However, considerable variability is noted with regard to symptoms, and a significant placebo effect exists. At present, invasive surgical therapies such as open prostatectomy and TURP do not always improve symptoms despite improvement in outlet obstruction. This factor is especially significant in a symptom-driven disease process such as BPH.

TRANSURETHRAL MICROWAVE THERMOTHERAPY

TUMT represents an effort to treat BPH in minimally invasive fashion by delivering microwave energy to heat and thereby destroy prostatic tissue. Transurethral catheters use oscillating magnetic and electrical fields to radiate electromagnetic energy, with frequencies ranging from 300 to 1300 MHz. As microwaves propagate through tissue, the resulting heat destroys surrounding tissue by inducing coagulation necrosis.[10-14] Thermal injury is related in a linear fashion to time but exponentially to temperature, a feature implying that small increases in temperature may lead to large increases in heat-induced cell necrosis.

TUMT has undergone an evolution from a low-energy modality causing minimal damage, referred to as *microwave hyperthermia,* to a high-energy (HE-TUMT) modality causing significant coagulative necrosis, often referred to as *microwave thermotherapy.* Lower frequencies were initially used, resulting in lower peak temperatures but greater penetration of energy; later, frequencies were increased, resulting in higher peak temperatures but diminished energy penetration. For example, microwave hyperthermia typically generates heat <45°C, insufficient for tissue destruction. Thermotherapy, in contrast, uses high microwave frequencies generating heat >50°C. The rate-limiting factor in frequency (i.e., energy) selection is the maintenance of safe temperatures at the outer zone of treatment. With current modalities, temperatures can reach 60°C in the prostatic stroma while remaining <45°C in the urethra and rectum.[13,15,16] The actual overall temperature profile, however, is influenced by several factors in TUMT device design.[17,18]

Several factors govern the effectiveness of microwave heating in the tissue. First, tissue with low water content such as fat does not absorb microwave energy as well as does tissue with high water content. Second, microwave penetration is inversely related to the frequency of the energy. Third, microwaves can be refracted, reflected, and dispersed, thus causing effectiveness to vary secondary to tissue heterogeneity. Finally, tissue perfusion factors may affect the heat conduction and convection characteristics in the prostate and therefore the overall temperature able to be generated by microwave energy.

Current microwave thermotherapy produces an optimal concentric heating distribution limited to the borders of the prostate and concentrated in the transition zone areas of the prostate without affecting more distal structures such as the rectal wall. Temperature and time are varied in combinations higher than the minimal thresholds of 45°C and 30 minutes for cytotoxic destruction of prostate tissue.[19]

All current TUMT devices use a catheter-based system containing a microwave antenna for energy delivery. The catheter contains a balloon that is inflated in the bladder to secure proper positioning during therapy. Additionally, many devices employ a catheter with a water channel for cooling during therapy to protect the urethra. The use of a cooling system, in addition to antenna and catheter design, level of frequency or energy, and overall duration of energy application, allows one to generate specific intraprostatic temperatures with specific heating geometries.

TUMT devices are also equipped with temperature probes to monitor areas such as the rectum, penis, and urethra. These devices act in concert with built-in safety mechanisms to shut down microwave radiation should temperature limits be exceeded in adjacent areas. Damage to the urinary sphincters, for instance, can lead to urinary incontinence, whereas damage to the penis can lead to erectile dysfunction. Damage to the rectum, specifically the anal sphincter, can lead to fecal incontinence.

Most procedures are performed on an outpatient basis and require only local anesthesia or local prostatic block. Current contraindications to TUMT include the following:

- Cardiac pacemakers or defibrillators
- Genitourinary implants
- Metallic implants in the pelvis or hip
- Urethral stricture
- Peripheral arterial disease with intermittent claudication or Leriche's syndrome
- Large, protruding intravesical median lobes
- Prostate cancer or bladder cancer

Optimal prostate size should be between 30 and 100 g, although patients with smaller prostates have occasionally been treated.

Clinical Experience

Several TUMT devices are approved by the U.S. Food and Drug Administration (FDA). These include TMx-2000 (TherMatrx, American Medical Systems), Prostatron (Urologix, Inc., Minneapolis), Targis (Urologix, Inc.), Cooled ThermoCath (CTC, Urologix, Inc.), CoreTherm (Prostalund, Inc.), and Prolieve (Boston Scientific Corp.). No studies have examined FDA-approved TUMT devices in a prospective, comparative fashion.

Initial data regarding the efficacy of TUMT used low-energy protocols, mostly with the Prostatron device using Prostasoft 2.0 software (Urologix, Inc.).[20-22] As efficacy data matured, HE-TUMT was developed to increase tissue destruction and theoretically to yield greater improvements in voiding ability.[22] Initially, these newer devices included Prostatron 2.5 and Targis (Urologix, Inc.) and the Urowave (Dornier Medical Systems, Inc., Wessling, Germany). Data from one manufacturer's device cannot be applied to other manufacturers' devices, however, because each device has unique power delivery characteristics that result in differing levels of tissue destruction. In fact, total power delivery from one technology to another can vary vastly and therefore can produce very different amounts of coagulation necrosis. Only certain microwave technologies with higher-power delivery have demonstrated efficacy with patients in urinary retention, and efficacy in patients with urinary retention at lower microwave powers has not been well demonstrated.

TMx-2000

The TMx-2000 system represents a low-power (23-W) TUMT device operating at 915 MHz that uniquely lacks a cooling mechanism. It is designed to attack the adjacent urethral wall and nearby prostatic tissue.[23] The catheter offers variable radiating helical coil lengths to match the length of the prostatic urethra. Currently, it is contraindicated in patients who have received pelvic radiation.

The TMx-2000 system was studied in a controlled trial of 200 patients.[24] Statistically significant declines in AUASI were seen from 22.4 to 11.9 at 12 months, although recatheterization was required in 16.8% of patients. No major adverse events were noted. This device is currently FDA approved for symptomatic improvement only. Efficacy in patients with urinary retention has not been demonstrated.

Prostatron

The updated version of the Prostatron antenna employs an active urethral cooling system. It operates at a frequency of 1296 MHz and is capable of generating powers of up to 80 W. Several studies have demonstrated variable efficacy of this device.

Francisca and associates[25] randomized 147 patients to treatment with Prostatron 2.5 TUMT or TURP. Whereas TURP demonstrated greater efficacy in improving Qmax, postvoid residual (PVR), International Prostate Symptom Score (IPSS), and prostate volume, TUMT demonstrated a statistically significant lower rate of sexual side effects, such as retrograde ejaculation (63% in TURP arm versus 33% in TUMT arm) at 1 year. Laguna and colleagues[26] studied 388 patients treated with Prostatron 2.5 or 3.5. An improvement of ≥50% was observed in IPSS, QoL, and Qmax in 57%, 62%, and 44% of patients, respectively.

The broadest Prostatron experience was that of Vesely and associates,[27] who reported an 11-year follow-up of 841 patients treated with Prostasoft 2.0 or 3.5. With version 2.0, 67% of patients were satisfied with the results of treatment; 18% of patients experienced complications, 25% had transient UTIs, and 16% had urinary retention. Secondary treatment was needed in 32% of patients. IPSS and QoL decreased from 15.9 and 2.9 to 12.0 and 2.1, respectively. With Prostasoft 3.5, 82% of patients were satisfied over 11 years. A total of 17% of patients experienced complications, 25% had UTIs, and 26% had urinary retention. Only 7% required additional treatment. IPSS and QoL decreased from 19.8 and 3.8 to 11.2 and 1.5, respectively.

Targis

A second-generation microwave device, the Targis system uses a dipole antenna capable of impedance matching by tuning the operating frequency in the range of 902 to 928 MHz.[19] As a result, backheating effects are minimal. The catheter balloon in the Targis system is inflated with static water and is positioned 0.4 cm away from the end of the antenna. Targis is unique in that it uses cooling water at 8°C during therapy to protect the urethra and bladder neck. Contraindications to Targis include a prostate urethral length of <3 cm and middle lobe enlargement.[28]

Djavan and associates[29] studied the effects of 51 patients treated with Targis TUMT and 52 treated with α-blockers. Whereas mean IPSS, Qmax, and QoL improved in statistically significant fashion for both groups, the TUMT-treated group demonstrated greater magnitude of improvement. Between-group differences were 35%, 22%, and 43% superior, respectively, in the TUMT group, whereas the actuarial treatment failure rate in the medical management group was sevenfold greater. These effects were maintained for ≥18 months.

In a prospective trial in which 200 patients were treated with Targis TUMT, Thalmann and colleagues[30] demonstrated that the median Qmax increased from 6 mL/second at baseline to 13, 12, and 13 mL/second at 6, 12, and 24 months, respectively.[3] In addition, median PVR decreased from 170 mL before treatment to 17, 20, and 27 mL after similar time periods. IPSS decreased from 23 to 3, also over similar time periods. Two years after treatment, 59 of the original 200 patients agreed to undergo repeat urodynamic evaluation: pressure flow studies revealed a persistently decreased median minimal urethral opening pressure from 70 to 38 cm H_2O at 24 months. Similarly, median detrusor pressure at Qmax decreased from 86 to 58 cm H_2O at 2 years.

Miller and associates[31] studied the durability of Targis TUMT over 3 centers in 150 patients for 5 years. AUASI improved 11.5 (53%) and 10.6 (47%) points at 1 and 5 years. Qmax improved by 3.4 (48%) and 2.4 (37%) over similar time periods. However, 4 patients required repeat TUMT, whereas 27 required subsequent invasive treatments. Additionally, 5-year follow-up existed for only 59 of the original 150 patients.

Berger and colleagues[32] studied Targis TUMT in a high-risk population with acute urinary retention with a mean follow-up of 34 months. Sixty-eight (87.1%) of

these patients were able to void subsequent to therapy, although 5 (7.3%) of these patients experienced repeat urinary retention within 2 years. Mean Qmax improved to 11.1 mL/second, whereas mean PVR decreased to 46 mL.

Kellner and associates[33] studied 39 patients with BPH with chronic urinary retention. After treatment with TUMT, 32 (82%) patients were able to void after a mean of 4.1 weeks of postprocedure catheterization. At 18 months, statistically significant improvements in IPSS (27.5-13.7), PVR (720-58 mL), and Qmax (0-7.3 mL/second) were seen.

The largest prospective Targis trial involved 345 patients treated over 9 institutions.[34] In this study, Kaplan and colleagues[34] demonstrated that 65% of patients showed a ≥50% reduction in symptom scores the first year, with a mean IPSS improvement of 11.1 points. In the 85 patients available for follow-up at 5 years, absolute IPSS improvement was maintained at 8.4 points. Flow rates improved from 7.5 to 10.5 mL/second at 3 years.

Cooled ThermoCath

This third-generation update to the Targis design employs an expandable urethral balloon in addition to changes in the device catheter to cool the urethral surface more effectively during treatment, thus allowing greater energy delivery to the prostate while protecting adjacent tissues. Treatment time has therefore been decreased from 60 to 28.5 minutes with Cooled ThermoCath.

Huidobro and associates[35] conducted the first multicenter trial with the Cooled ThermoCath. Forty patients were followed for 12 months after treatment; 36 patients demonstrated a decreased prostate volume (8%) versus Targis (21%), QoL (44% versus 58%), AUASI (41% versus 60%), and increased Qmax (28% versus 55%).

CoreTherm

CoreTherm represents the only TUMT device to use an interstitial probe with three sensors to monitor the intraprostatic temperature and thereby provide a mechanism by which a clinician can control and adjust the volume of tissue ablation.[36] This technique is known as the ProstaLund Feedback Treatment (PLFT).[37] With PLFT, treatment is usually stopped when approximately 55°C has been measured in any part of the treatment zone. PLFT is thought to compensate for the interindividual and intraindividual differences in prostatic blood flow; this feature is in contrast to standard TUMT devices, which do not take into account the cooling influence of prostatic blood flow, thus possibly leading to theoretical overtreatment and undertreatment in different areas of the prostate. CoreTherm uses 915-MHz microwaves with three different length catheters and is capable of delivering up to 100 W of power. The heat distribution of the system reflects the backheating component of the system, in which an exposed inner conductor is positioned at the tip of a coaxial cable.

Many clinical studies have been performed with a significant number of patients. de la Rosette and associates[38] studied 180 patients pooled from 3 prospective clinical trials who were followed for 12 months. Statistically significant improvements in prostate volume reduction (52 to 34 mL), Qmax (7.7 to 16.1 mL/second), and IPSS (20.9 to 6.4) were seen. Prostate volume reduction correlated with changes in Qmax and voiding pressure.

Wagrell and associates[39] summarized the 3-year experience of PLFT versus TURP in 146 patients treated in a prospective trial. No statistically significant differences were found in Qmax or QoL between the study groups, although IPSS was different at 36 months (8.2 for TUMT group versus 5.0 for TURP). The most frequent side effects of TUMT were impotence (8%), prostate-specific antigen increase (5%), and hematuria (4%).

Schelin and colleagues[40] studied the efficacy of PLFT in 54 patients with chronic urinary retention versus 52 treated with TURP in a prospective trial. Both groups were catheter free at 3- and 6-month follow-up. Mean catheterization time was 34 days in the TUMT-treated group versus 5 days in the TURP-treated group. IPSS at 6 months was significantly less in the TURP group (4.4) than in the TUMT group (7.3). Qmax at 6 months was 18.0 mL/second in the TURP group versus 13.4 mL/second in the TUMT group.

Mattiasson and associates[41] described the 5-year experience with TUMT (103 patients) versus TURP (51 patients). Ninety-six (62 TUMT, 34 TURP) patients were available for follow-up at 60 months. Ten percent of TUMT-treated patients required additional BPH treatment, whereas 4.3% of the TURP-treated patients required retreatment. IPSS decreased from 21.0 to 7.4 for TUMT and from 20.5 to 6.0 for TURP; QoL decreased from 4.3 to 1.1 and from 4.2 to 1.1 in the same groups. Qmax increased from 6.7 to 11.4 mL/second for TUMT and from 7.9 to 13.3 mL/second for TURP. PVR decreased from 106 to 70 mL for TUMT and from 94 to 51 mL for TURP. No statistically significant differences were found between the two groups, although 80 complications were seen in the TUMT group, whereas 39 were seen in the TURP group.

Prolieve

The Prolieve system uses a frequency of 915 MHz with a monopolar antenna. It contains an expandable urethral balloon that inflates with circulated water maintained at 34°C ± 0.5°C. Despite the expected loss of energy that would be anticipated from heat dissipation by this large volume of cooling water, the system is capable of running at a moderate power of 50 W for a treatment period of 45 minutes to achieve interstitial temperatures of 41°C to 46°C.

Larson and associates[42] reviewed the temperature mapping experience with the Prolieve system in 10 patients undergoing TUMT. Interstitial temperature reached an average peak of 51.8°C an average of 7 mm away from the urethra. As expected, subtherapeutic temperatures were seen adjacent to the urethra.

Bock and colleagues[43] reviewed the 1-year clinical experience with the Prolieve system in a multicenter, randomized trial. Treatment with Prolieve TUMT in 94 patients was compared with therapy with finasteride alone in 31 patients. Fewer than 20% of patients required catheterization after TUMT. AUASI improved significantly more in the TUMT-treated group than in the finasteride-treated group at 6 months. The magnitude of improvement was similar among patients with prostates ≤50 g versus >50 g. Efficacy with patients in urinary retention has not been demonstrated.

Morbidities

Safety represents the most common reason that minimally invasive treatments such as TUMT are assuming a larger role in treating BPH. As mentioned previously, the gold standard, TURP, possesses several well-known and established risks, including hemorrhage requiring blood transfusion, TUR syndrome, and death. In contrast, no reports of hemorrhage, TUR syndrome, or death have ever been reported after TUMT.

TUMT, however, does destroy prostatic tissue by coagulative necrosis, thus causing mainly irritative symptoms and acute urinary retention in the immediate post-procedure period, albeit less frequently than in TURP. The most common side effects are urinary retention leading to prolonged postoperative catheterization, UTI, and post-treatment dysuria. The highest rates of retention have occurred in studies in which transurethral catheters or suprapubic tubes were not placed after the procedure.

In a report of 5-year data from a prospective randomized multicenter trial comparing TUMT with CoreTherm versus TURP, Mattiasson and associates[41] reviewed their short- and long-term complications with TUMT. These included impotence (7.5%), hematuria (6.3%), bladder stones (2.5%), urinary retention (2.5%), urinary urgency (2.5%), and urinary frequency, incontinence, and epididymitis at 1.3% each. Table 17-1 reviews complications associated with TUMT from several studies.[6,25,26,33,38,42,44-54]

Although more serious adverse events have not been encountered with TUMT in major multicenter trials, the FDA[55] did issue a public health notification entitled "Serious Injuries from Microwave Thermotherapy for Benign Prostatic Hyperplasia" in October of 2000. The FDA reported a total of 16 unexpected TUMT procedure-related thermal injuries since marketing of these devices began in 1996. Of these injuries, 10 resulted in fistula formation, whereas 6 resulted in clinically significant

TABLE 17-1	Selected Adverse Events of Transurethral Microwave Thermotherapy	
	TUMT	TURP
Acute urinary retention	2%-40%	6.5%-13%
Hematuria	0-24%	100%
Urinary tract infection	0-45%	2%-10%
Erectile dysfunction	0-5%	11%
Ejaculatory dysfunction	0-17%	20%-98%
Stricture	0	0-12%
Incontinence	0-6%	13%
Transfusion	0	4%
Postoperative catheter time	0-6 wk	3 days-2 wk
Invasive re-treatment	≤66% at 5 yr	5% at 5 yr

TUMT, transurethral microwave thermotherapy, TURP, transurethral resection of the prostate.

tissue damage to the penis or urethra. Although these injuries were not apparent at the time of treatment and sometimes took days to develop, many patients required colostomies, partial amputation of the penis, or other invasive treatments. Likely risk factors included incorrect catheter placement, catheter migration, failure of physician supervision during treatment, failure to stop treatment when pain was experienced, oversedation of the patient that inhibited the ability to express pain, and history of prior pelvic radiation. The FDA also issued a list of recommendations that are now available on the website (http://www.fda.gov/cdrh/safety/bph.html).

TRANSURETHRAL NEEDLE ABLATION OF THE PROSTATE

The TUNA procedure represents a heat-induced coagulative necrosis procedure similar to TUMT. It was initially designed to be performed in an outpatient setting and to use minimal anesthesia. It was therefore deemed ideal for men in poor health or those with multiple comorbidities. In addition, TUNA has been shown to reduce voiding symptoms, subjectively and objectively, in men with BPH.[56,57]

TUNA uses high-energy thermotherapy. A visually inserted transurethral pair of needles delivers monopolar radiofrequency current to heat and destroy targeted prostate tissue. The device consists of a special 22-Fr transurethral delivery system attached to a radiofrequency generator. It differs from TUMT in that it is a site-specific modality that allows the surgeon to select where treatment will be delivered. Under direct vision with a 0-degree lens, two needles are placed through the urothelium into selected areas of prostatic tissue. The exact position of the needle tip can be visualized by transrectal ultrasound (TRUS). Several areas are treated in one session from approximately 1 cm distal to the bladder neck to 1 cm proximal to the verumontanum. Low-level, 490-kHz monopolar radiofrequency energy is delivered by the needles to heat tissues to ≤110°C, thus creating necrotic lesions approximately 1 cm in size. Each treatment cycle takes approximately 3 to 5 minutes. Because the needles are in protective sheaths, the temperature in the prostatic urethra is maintained at <46°C, to minimize urethral damage and patient discomfort. The numbers of lesions and treatment cycles depend on the size of the prostate.[58,59]

After the procedure, many urologists leave a urethral catheter in overnight, although others have advocated longer catheterization of ≤7 days. TUNA requires local anesthesia ranging from intraurethral or intravesical lidocaine to locally injected prostate blocks. Currently, two patient groups are ideal candidates for TUNA: (1) patients with predominant irritative voiding symptoms and a moderate obstruction and (2) high-risk patients who can be treated only with local anesthesia.[60]

Medtronic, Inc. (Minneapolis) is the only manufacturer producing an FDA-approved TUNA device. The following review of TUNA is based on this device.

Clinical Experience

Several prospective clinical trials have compared TUNA with the gold standard TURP. However, the studies are limited by several factors, including the small number of patients enrolled and the relatively high attrition rate of patients at follow-up (e.g., ≤60%).

Cimentepe and associates[61] demonstrated favorable results for TUNA when compared with TURP. Eighteen months after the treatment, no statistically significant differences were found between the IPSS and QoL values of the TUNA and TURP groups, whereas the improvement in Qmax achieved with TURP was significantly greater than that seen with needle ablation (17.7 versus 23.3 mL/second).[61]

With 5-year follow up, Hill and colleagues[56] demonstrated significant improvements in IPSS, QoL, and PVR from baseline at the end of every year with TUNA. The data demonstrated that TURP was superior to TUNA for all parameters, especially Qmax. However, given the decreased morbidity with TUNA, these investigators concluded that TUNA represented an effective option for men with bothersome voiding symptoms.

Morbidities

Most studies of TUNA show the procedure to be well tolerated. TUNA can protect the prostatic urothelium, thereby preventing injury to this pain sensitive area and also limiting the need for spinal or general anesthesia.[62] However, reports have noted both minor and major adverse events.

TABLE 17-2	Selected Adverse Events of Transurethral Needle Ablation of the Prostate	
Adverse Event	**No. Events**	**Total Patients (%)**
Hematuria	463	Mild, 28; severe, 1
Transient urinary retention	279	23
Dysuria	167	14
Irritative symptoms	117	10
Urinary tract infection	43	4
Pain during procedure	15	Moderate, 0.9; severe, 0.3
Postoperative perineal pain	13	1
Epididymo-orchitis	11	0.9
Urethral stricture	4	0.3
Erectile dysfunction	4	0.3
Retrograde ejaculation	4	0.3

In a meta-analysis of 35 studies, Bouza and associates[63] reviewed the efficacy and complications of TUNA in >1200 patients. In noncomparative studies, the most common complication seen with TUNA was hematuria, ranging from mild (28%) to severe (1%). A complete list of these complications appears in Table 17-2.[63] Postprocedure myocardial infarction and cerebrovascular events have also been reported; however, these events occurred 6 weeks and 8 months after TUNA, respectively.[64] In the same meta-analysis, Bouza and associates[63] showed that TUNA has a lower overall side effect profile than does TURP, with the exceptions of longer duration of dysuria and a higher rate of post-therapy urinary retention.

Despite initially favorable results, the retreatment rate with TUNA is significant. A meta-analysis of 26 noncomparative studies indicated an overall risk of retreatment of 19%, with a wide range among various studies. Most of these patients underwent subsequent TURP, and very few had repeat TUNA. Contributing factors include patient selection, prostate volume, poor improvement of symptom scores, inadequate procedure (i.e., not enough lesions created in prostate), and inadequate temperature attained during treatment.[64]

In summary, TUNA is a minimally invasive procedure that provides adequate short-term improvements in both symptoms and urinary flow rates with minimal morbidity; long-term effectiveness is mixed, however. TUNA can be performed as an outpatient, office-based procedure, a feature that makes it an appealing option to patients and physicians.

INTERSTITIAL LASER COAGULATION

ILC of the prostate is a minimally invasive coagulative technique using an 830-nm diode laser system. Commercial systems, such as the Indigo LaserOptic (Johnson & Johnson, Cincinnati) and Fiber Tome (Dornier, Munich), are compact, readily transportable, and low power, with diode laser devices using a 15- to 20-W variable power source.

ILC is performed as an office-based technique using local anesthesia. The laser fiber is introduced by a transurethral approach directly into the prostate. In the current Indigo system, the laser transmits through the fiber to a 2-cm long, light-diffusing tip for 90 seconds. The principle of ILC is to shrink the prostate by generating intraprostatic necrosis without damaging the urethra. An ellipsoid lesion of tissue coagulates around the axis of the fiber. The affected area has a diameter of 1.5 to 2 cm and a length of 2 cm corresponding to the length of the energy-diffusing fiber tip.

Clinical Experience

Limited randomized controlled trials are available. However, several published series suggest moderate improvements in BPH parameters, with the most improvement seen with longer follow-up.[65]

In a 60-month follow-up of patients who had undergone ILC, Terada and associates[66] demonstrated improvements in mean IPSS from 19.7 at baseline to 7.9 at 3 months and 13.3 at ≥60 months (32% reduction). QoL improved from 4.5 to 1.8 at 3 months and 2.7 at ≥60 months (40% reduction). Qmax increased from 6.9 mL/second at baseline to 11.3 mL/second at 3 months and 8.5 at ≥60 months (23% improvement), as did mean PVR, from 108.0 mL at baseline to 37.6 at 3 months and 56.0 at ≥60 months (48% reduction). Postoperative catheter time was 2 to 3 days, and retreatment rate was 35%, with the majority of such patients undergoing TURP.[66]

In a comparative study with 2-year follow-up, Kursh and associates[67] compared ILC with TURP. These investigators showed that the ILC group had improvements in Qmax (9.2 mL/second to 13.9), PVR (81 mL to 57.7), AUASI (24 to 9), and QoL (11 to 3).[67] Postoperative catheter time was 1 week, and retreatment rate was 16%.

Morbidities

Studies show that ILC induces no clinically important changes in hematologic, blood chemistry, or urinalysis variables at any follow-up period. The major complication in most studies is UTI, ≤65% reported in one study.[68]

Overall, the advantages of ILC lie in its minimally invasive nature coupled with its minimal anesthesia requirements. Short-term clinical outcomes are moderate, although only limited trial data are available. Disadvantages include long catheterization times, lack of immediate symptomatic relief, high incidence of UTI, and an unsatisfactory retreatment rate.

LASER PROSTATECTOMY

In the surgical treatment of symptomatic BPH, lasers have slowly evolved from theory to practical application over the last few decades. Advances in laser technology and growing clinical experience have refined the use of lasers in the treatment of outlet obstruction.[69]

Laser therapy promised several advantages over standard TURP, including technical simplicity and the absence or minimization of complications such as intraoperative fluid absorption, bleeding, retrograde ejaculation, impotence, and incontinence. Laser therapy also promised a potentially shorter hospital stay and quicker recovery. Hemostasis and limiting of irrigant absorption, especially hypotonic, hyponatremic solutions, have allowed clinicians to use laser prostatectomy to treat larger prostates and patients at high surgical risk with less physiologic stress and fewer adverse events.[70,71] Not surprisingly, estimates indicate that increasing numbers of practicing urologists are in fact already performing laser prostatectomies on patients with symptomatic BPH, and this number is rising.

The predominant effect of laser energy on tissue is the conversion of laser energy to heat in a process known as *photothermolysis*, which results in the elevation of target tissue temperature. Laser tissue effects may be subsequently categorized as either coagulation, or *photopyrolysis*, followed by delayed tissue sloughing or vaporization *(photovaporolysis)*, with resulting immediate tissue ablation.

Coagulation represents the process of raising the temperatures of organic compounds to the point of molecular breakdown, usually >50°C. Once tissue has been coagulated and further laser energy is applied, absorption does not appear to be affected, but scattering may be doubled. The backscatter and reflection cause greater diversion of energy and therefore a wider and longer zone of coagulation. This feature may be useful if a limited depth of penetration with a wider field of laser effect is desired. For BPH tissue ablation, however, the use of coagulation alone makes tissue removal imprecise and can be especially hazardous when one is working close to the external urethral sphincter.

Vaporization refers to the change from solid to gaseous state of a given material. Human tissue requires approximately 2500 joules/g to change its temperature from 37°C to 100°C. With laser prostatectomy, gaseous vapors and tissue proteins are converted to smoke, which is then washed away with irrigation. The kinetic energy of escaping vapor also causes miniexplosions within tissue and further adds to mechanical rupture of membranes.

The overall rate of tissue ablation is determined by the rate of laser energy deposition into tissue, a rate that, in turn, is thought to be driven by the laser light wavelength. In laser prostatectomy, one attempts to deliver a sufficient amount of energy per unit volume of tissue quickly to bring cells to vaporization temperature. If the cells are brought only to coagulation temperature, they then become half as penetrable to laser energy, thus increasing backscatter and surrounding coagulation and thereby halting the forward progress of ablation. This finding directly implies that applying laser light energy at lower-power densities for increasing periods of time will result only in a greater depth of coagulation and possible periprostatic injury rather than in creation of a channel defect.[72]

The penetration depth of laser energy depends on its wavelength as well as the absorption coefficient and composition of the receiving tissue. Penetration is often described by *extinction length*, the depth of penetration of an incident beam beyond which only 10% of the initial beam energy is left (i.e., 90% absorption). With its longer extinction length, the 1064-nm neodymium-doped:yttrium-aluminum-garnet (Nd:YAG) laser has energy that penetrates tissue 10 times more deeply than does the 532-nm potassium-titanyl-phosphate (KTP) laser. The greater degree of penetration leads to more coagulative necrosis and less vaporization of tissue.

A standard Nd:YAG, holmium:yttrium-aluminum-garnet (Ho:YAG) laser or KTP laser source is used to provide energy for laser prostatectomy. This laser should be capable of at least 40 W of power output and continuous laser emission without interruption. Some older machines may also require an external water source attachment for cooling; newer machines with internal cooling mechanisms, which do not require an external water source attachment, are generally much more convenient and versatile. Generally, standard 21- to 22-Fr rigid cystoscopes have been used to perform laser prostatectomy. Continuous flow cystoscopes with a beaked-tip can aid in holding the opposite prostate lobe away from the site of lasing. The KTP laser beam is fully transmitted through the aqueous irrigant but highly absorbed by oxyhemoglobin in the tissue, allowing selective tissue absorption by organs such as the prostate. The end result is a laser that is targeted and more efficient for prostatic tissue vaporization, leading to the term *photoselective vaporization of the prostate.*

The KTP laser has gained widespread utilization. It is commercially marketed as the GreenLight Laser (American Medical Systems, Inc., Minnetonka, Minnesota), with subsequent evolution to an advanced 120-W system, dubbed GreenLight High-Power System (HPS).[70]

Other modalities for laser prostatectomy include VLAP, holmium laser ablation of the prostate (HoLAP) and holmium laser enucleation of the prostate (HoLEP).

VLAP, using Nd:YAG energy and HoLAP, using Ho:YAG energy, involve direct laser application to tissue to cause ablation. HoLAP works in a near-contact mode to create a channel within the prostatic fossa to relieve the patient of BPH symptoms. This technique requires longer operative time patients in larger prostates. The HoLEP technique was subsequently developed to decrease operative time with larger prostates. HoLEP differs in that it is used to vaporize as well as enucleate adenomatous prostate tissue. Enucleated tissue is then pushed into the bladder for subsequent removal by morcellation.

A high-frequency modulation of laser light generates a continuous stream of short micropulses with a duration of 4.5 msec and a peak power of 280 W (i.e., 3.5 times the average laser power of a regular 80-W laser). The short duration of the micropulses does not allow time for heat to diffuse from the superficial layer, thus confining energy to a small volume of tissue, in a situation referred to as *thermal confinement*. As each micropulse generates a very fast temperature increase inside tissue, the tissue water is not only rapidly vaporized but also the surrounding tissue matrix is torn apart, thus allowing for efficient removal of prostatic tissue. Continuous bladder irrigation is required to cool the tissue as well as to provide a clear aqueous medium for laser light to transmit to target tissue without loss of energy.

The current technique of PVP as described by Malek and associates[73] employs a side-to-side sweeping technique with the side fire laser moving from the area of the bladder neck to approximately the level of the verumontanum in a clockwise-counterclockwise fashion to create an open TUR-like channel. An important sign of vaporization efficiency is observation of bubble formation, which signifies vaporization of tissue. Without bubbles, the predominant effect is coagulation necrosis. To maintain maximum delivery of light energy to target tissue, a distance of ≤ 0.5 mm (near contact) is recommended to maximize efficiency of vaporization.

At the conclusion of laser prostatectomy, a urinary catheter is left in place to provide drainage. A suprapubic catheter may be left in place to facilitate early or repeated voiding trials if desired. Catheter drainage is required for most patients treated with the Nd:YAG laser because its effects essentially represent a burn injury to the prostatic parenchyma and are therefore associated with an acute phase of tissue edema that tends to cause urinary retention.

Many patients who undergo laser prostatectomy are discharged following complete recovery from anesthesia, thus making it an outpatient procedure. Catheter drainage to a urinary leg bag if necessary can be maintained and easily mastered by most patients. Patients with a history of preoperative urinary retention or detrusor hypocontractility with a large preoperative residual urine volume may require longer catheterization times. Postoperative management with suprapubic catheter drainage in these individuals may be ideal to allow easy or repeated voiding trials if needed.

When the urinary catheter is removed, patients should receive a 5- to 7-day course of a broad-spectrum oral antibiotic to clear the urine of any bacterial colonization that may have occurred during catheterization. Following catheter removal, immediate improvement in voiding may not occur, especially with the VLAP or HoLAP techniques. Patients may experience little or no change in voiding during the first 1 to 2 weeks postoperatively; they may in fact experience slightly worse symptoms while the treated prostatic transition zone sloughs. During this time, patients may notice that their urine looks cloudy or white as a result of proteinaceous material from the dissolving prostate; others may note the passage of minute particulate matter. This phase of active tissue dissolution can be associated with symptoms of mild dysuria, which are usually relieved by nonsteroidal anti-inflammatory drugs as needed. Phenazopyridine, a urinary tract analgesic, may also be used as needed.

Patients with intractable dysuria usually have pyuria requiring appropriate antibiotic therapy. By 4 to 6 weeks, most patients begin to notice a significant improvement in their voiding pattern. Improvement continues in most men for an additional 6 to 12 weeks, when maximum voiding outcome is usually achieved. By 3 months, voiding outcomes are similar to those expected after electrocautery TURP.

Because of the superior surgical hemostasis associated with laser prostatectomy, no restrictions on physical activity are needed, even in the immediate postoperative period. After catheter removal, sexual intercourse is also allowed immediately if desired. Patients should be warned of the possibility that the ejaculate may be temporarily dark or bloody.

Clinical Experience

This section briefly reviews the experience with KTP laser prostatectomy. The first experiments with the 80-W KTP laser began with ex vivo animal models.[74] KTP laser resection was compared with high-frequency current (i.e., TURP-like resection). The 80-W KTP laser technique showed a statistically significant decrease in hemorrhage ($P < .0001$) compared with traditional TURP-like resection, a finding demonstrating that essentially bloodless ablation of tissue could occur. The slower ablation performance of the KTP laser compared with electrocautery (100 versus 20 seconds/16 cm^3) seen in the series could be attributed to the particular drag speeds, sweeping modes, and repetition of applications chosen for the KTP laser in the experiment.

Hai and Malek[75] presented the first human experience with 80-W KTP laser prostatectomy. Ten patients were followed for 1 year after their prostatectomy in a pilot study. Patients experienced statistically significant improvements in AUASI (23.2 to 2.6), QoL (4.3 to 0.5), Qmax (10.3 to 30.7 mL/second), and PVR (137.6 to 3 mL). No patient experienced postoperative urinary retention, infection, incontinence, or erectile dysfunction; none subsequently developed bladder neck contractures or urethral stricture. Two patients in fact did not require postoperative catheterization at all. One patient, who was receiving active anticoagulation, experienced mild transient postoperative hematuria requiring recatheterization for 24 hours.

Te and associates[76] presented the largest and more recent series on the use of 80-W KTP in laser prostatectomy for 45 patients. Significant and durable improvements in AUASI, QoL, Qmax, and PVR were demonstrated ≤12 months postoperatively. Mean AUASI declined from 24 to 1.8 at 12 months; mean QoL improved from 4.3 to 0.4, Qmax from 7.7 to 22.8 mL/second, and PVR volume from 114.2 to 7.2 mL. Mean prostate volume, as determined by ultrasound, decreased from 54.6 to 34.4 mL. Mean operative time was 36 minutes, and no patient required a blood transfusion. More than 30% of patients were sent home without a catheter; those with postoperative catheters had them removed in a mean of 14 hours. Reported morbidities were generally minor: 8% experienced mild to moderate dysuria lasting >10 days, 8% had transient hematuria, and 3% had postoperative urinary retention. Among the 56 men who were potent before the procedure, 27% experienced retrograde ejaculation, but none experienced impotence.

One of the advantages with the 80-W KTP laser lies in the ability to perform laser prostatectomy on larger glands with decreased bleeding and irrigant absorption. Sandhu and associates[77] detailed large prostate volume resection with the 80-W KTP laser. Sixty-four men with BPH whose prostates had volumes of ≥60 mL and in whom medical therapy had failed underwent prostatic resection with the 80-W KTP laser. The mean preoperative prostate volume was 101 mL, with a mean operative time of 123 minutes. IPSS decreased from 18.4 to 6.7 at 12 months; Qmax increased from 7.9 to 18.9 mL/second, whereas PVR decreased from 189 to 109 mL. No transfusions were required, nor evidence of postoperative hyponatremia noted. All 64 patients were discharged within 23 hours. This was the first evidence that the 80-W KTP laser could be used as a safe and effective means for prostatic resection with durable results for large-volume prostatectomy.

The final safety aspect of the 80-W KTP laser to be studied in detail was its use in anticoagulated patients at high risk for clinically significant bleeding. A series of 24 anticoagulated patients with BPH who were treated with laser prostatectomy using the 80-W KTP laser was studied.[78] Of these patients, 8 were receiving warfarin, 2 were receiving clopidogrel, and 14 were taking aspirin. Eight (33%) of these patients had a previous myocardial infarction, 7 (29%) had cerebrovascular disease, and 7 (29%) had peripheral vascular disease. No patients

developed clinically significant hematuria postoperatively, and none developed clot retention. No transfusions were required, and no thromboembolic events were reported. One patient had transient postoperative urinary retention requiring discharge with a catheter, 2 patients developed retrograde ejaculation, and 2 patients experienced postoperative UTIs. Mean operative time was 101 minutes. Follow-up revealed a decrease in IPSS from 18.7 to 9.5 as well as an increase in Qmax from 9.0 to 20.1 mL/second at 12 months. PVR decreased from 134 to 69 mL at 1 month but was not statistically significant beyond that time point. In this study, all patients underwent PVP safely without any adverse thromboembolic or bleeding events. Significantly, more energy and time were used for lasing per gland size in these patients. Additionally, the major difference between anticoagulated patients and those not receiving anticoagulation lay in the safe and effective use of the perineal prostate block instead of regional anesthesia, which was contraindicated by anticoagulation status.

Clinically, PVP KTP laser prostatectomy appears to possess many advantages. Its efficacy appears to be equivalent or nearly equivalent to that of standard TURP because an instant tissue defect can be created with excellent hemostasis, without absorption of hypotonic fluid. The use of normal saline irrigation also removes the risk of dilutional hyponatremia. The procedure can be performed with a range of anesthesia from a prostate block with intravenous sedation to regional anesthesia to general anesthesia. It can be used in high-risk patients such as those anticoagulated with heparin, warfarin, nonsteroidal anti-inflammatory drugs, and aspirin. Often, no postoperative irrigation is required, and catheter time is relatively short. Many patients do not even require postoperative catheters.

Morbidities

All reported studies have noted markedly less morbidity associated with laser prostatectomy compared with traditional surgical approaches. Bleeding is the main complication of traditional electrocautery TURP, often necessitating transfusion and causing associated problems such as clot retention, premature termination of the procedure, and inadequate relief of obstruction.[6] Bleeding can also result in the need for continuous catheter irrigation and complications such as stricture secondary to traction on the Foley catheter. Rarely, uncontrolled bleeding can even require open packing of the prostatic fossa. Poor visibility because of bleeding is also thought to be a cause of sphincteric damage and incontinence resulting from TURP. The incidence of hemorrhage requiring blood transfusion is 3.9% and increases twofold when the amount of resected tissue is >45 mL or the resection time is >90 minutes. In contrast to TURP, which cuts across the prostatic parenchyma and opens prostatic venous sinuses, laser prostatectomy seals blood vessels as it coagulates the transition zone, thereby preventing both absorption of irrigating fluid and hemorrhage.[79,80]

Irrigant fluid absorption during electrocautery TURP results in a 2% incidence of TUR syndrome because of dilutional hyponatremia, glycine-induced ammonia intoxication, or the direct toxic effect of glycine.[6] As with bleeding, fluid absorption increases in patients with larger glands and longer resection times. Laser prostatectomy minimizes this complication through its sealing zone effect on tissue, which prevents fluid absorption.

The incidence of urethral stricture after electrocautery TURP is 3.1%; if bladder neck contractures are included, this figure approaches 5%.[6] Stricture formation is thought to be secondary to trauma induced by the large size of the resectoscope as well as the use of low-intensity, coagulating current, which penetrates deeper into tissue than cutting currents. Because laser procedures do not use electrical current, the cystoscopes are smaller, and the overall operative time is usually shorter, the incidence of stricture is lower following laser procedures.[81,82] The incidence of reoperation for residual obstructive tissue is difficult to determine because most published series of laser prostatectomy have documented initial, short-term experiences with this technology, which involves not only a learning curve factor but also a relatively short postoperative follow-up (i.e., generally ≤1 year).

Postoperative infections may also occur after TURP. The incidence of UTI following TURP is 15.5% (median), whereas epididymitis occurs in 1.2%.[6] UTIs have been reported in 1% to 20% and epididymitis in 5% to 7% of patients following laser prostatectomy.[83-85] Treatment of such infections may be more problematic in VLAP-type prostatectomies secondary to the residual necrotic prostate tissue that remains in situ for several weeks after laser coagulation. Although postoperative UTI may occur as uncomplicated cystitis, the coagulated and necrotic prostate may also become infected. When this occurs, the most common manifestation is subacute prostatitis, characterized by significant and persistent irritative voiding symptoms, with mild prostatic or epididymal tenderness on examination, persistent pyuria, and positive urine cultures. Two cases of frank urosepsis have in fact been reported following laser prostatectomy; both patients required TURP to remove infected necrotic prostate tissue.[86] Aggressive antibiotic therapy is therefore warranted in these patients.

Historically, residual necrotic prostate tissue was a problem related to laser procedures with the Nd:YAG wavelength procedures and was responsible for the 20% to 32% incidence of postoperative urinary retention, which may last from for a few days to several weeks after VLAP treatment. This incidence far exceeds that of the 6.5% incidence of urinary retention following electro-

cautery TURP.[6] To overcome this problem, some investigators have resorted to higher power or the use of absorbable urethral stents in the postoperative phase following VLAP.[87] However, infection and prolonged chronic dysuria continued to make the procedure unpopular. In comparison with current, more contemporary technology, postoperative urinary retention is not an issue with the high-power 532-nm wavelength-driven PVP, with which the incidence was noted to be as low as 3%.[77]

Another complication unique to VLAP is the high incidence of irritative voiding symptoms during the initial few weeks following surgery, again the result of both coagulated necrotic tissue that has not yet sloughed and raw and unepithelialized mucosa.

HoLEP has been associated with prostatic capsule perforations secondary to the use of the transurethral tissue morcellators that cut and aspirate pieces of prostate tissue as well as from the cutting laser technique.[88] In addition, this technique uniquely predisposes patients to bladder mucosal injury and bladder perforation because of direct injury from the morcellators. This situation was seen in >6% of patients in one study.[89] Perforation often requires an open cystotomy closure, which frequently involves moving the patient from a cystoscopy suite to an operating room.

The newer GreenLight HPS has an improved laser beam quality resulting in a tighter and more confined beam profile over a greater distance. This feature allows the surgeon to lase at a greater distance without a loss of vaporization efficiency. Unlike the standard PVP, in which laser application at a distance of 1 to 3 mm may result in increase coagulation necrosis, vaporization efficiency is maintained with the HPS. Consequently, the potential exists to lase deeply into the bladder wall inadvertently when the fiber is pushed into passed bladder neck; this situation may result in potential bladder perforation or injury to ureteral orifices. Additionally, stationary laser application at high powers should be avoided because of the potential to create deep unwanted defects quickly in the treated area. Deep penetration of the prostatic tissue may lead to bleeding, which can be troublesome. An offsetting feature of the HPS therefore lies in the dual-mode power pedal that allows instant selection of a lower power setting for coagulation without vaporization. This feature allows the surgeon to address bleeding areas quickly with low-power application to attain hemostasis.[70] The application of the coagulation setting should be the main modality to control bleeding; this clearly differs from the standard PVP technique with the GreenLight HPS laser.

Finally, retrograde ejaculation, another potential side effect of electrocautery TURP, occurs in ≤90% of patients. The most recent 80-W KTP laser data show that retrograde ejaculation also represents a potential problem in laser prostatectomy (i.e., 27% incidence).[77] Similarly, the incidence of impotence following electrocautery TURP ranges from 4% to 13%.[6] Such impotence is thought to result from either (1) the diffusion of electrical current into the cavernosal nerves, which travel close to the prostatic apex, or (2) interference with penile arterial flow, which occasionally depends in part on prostatic vascularity. The overall incidence of impotence following all forms of laser prostatectomy is rare. Norris and associates[90] reported that of 108 patients who underwent VLAP, 56 were sexually active before the procedure (intercourse more than once a month) and 37 patients were sexually active at 3 to 6 months afterward. The outcome in the remaining 19 patients was not specified. Other VLAP studies cited a 4.3% to 9.5% rate of impotence.[91-94] In contrast, KTP data show no loss of potency in patients.[77]

CONCLUSION

Current minimally invasive procedures for BPH have attempted to replicate the clinical and objective results of traditional more invasive procedures, such as TURP and open prostatectomy. Although most of these minimally invasive procedures cannot completely duplicate the extent of adenomatous tissue removal from the prostate, they do offer at least reasonable short-term therapeutic effects to justify their continued use. This is especially true when the lower rates of adverse effects and complications associated with these procedures are considered. By far, these minimally invasive options offer a safer and easier, if less effective, way to improve the symptoms of obstruction seen in men with BPH. As technology improves and these procedures become even less invasive, the choice of these alternatives by both patient and physicians will increase despite the lack of TURP-like efficacy. This situation was noted in a survey in which urologists who were closer to the completion of residency were more likely to offer a minimally invasive treatment option to a patient for symptomatic BPH.[95]

In addition, it may be more prudent to subject patients to a procedure associated with less morbidity to obtain a satisfactory, yet less clinically effective, result. In fact, by having a less invasive procedure associated with less morbidity, many patients who would otherwise be treated by medical therapy may choose these alternatives instead. In selecting the optimal therapy to treat BPH, consideration of the many risks and benefits must be weighed by both the patient and the surgeon.

KEY POINTS

1. The most common side effects of TUMT include urinary retention leading to prolonged postoperative catheterization, UTI, and post-treatment dysuria.
2. The highest rates of retention following TUMT occur when transurethral catheters or suprapubic tubes are not placed after the procedure.
3. The most likely risk factors for severe adverse events with TUMT include incorrect catheter placement, catheter migration, failure of physician supervision during treatment, failure to stop treatment when pain was experienced, oversedation of the patient that inhibits the ability to express pain, and history of prior pelvic radiation.
4. Most studies of TUNA show it to be well tolerated.
5. Studies show that ILC induces no clinically important changes in hematologic, blood chemistry, or urinalysis variables at any follow-up period. The major complication in most studies is UTI, ≤65% reported in one study.
6. All reported studies have noted markedly less morbidity associated with laser prostatectomy compared with traditional surgical approaches.
7. The PVP KTP laser prostatectomy can be safely used in high-risk patients such as those anticoagulated with heparin, warfarin, nonsteroidal anti-inflammatory drugs, and aspirin.

REFERENCES

Please see www.expertconsult.com

Chapter 18

COMPLICATIONS OF LASERS IN UROLOGIC SURGERY

Gaurav Bandi MD

Assistant Professor, Department of Urology, Jefferson Medical College, Thomas Jefferson University, Philadelphia, Pennsylvania

Stephen Y. Nakada MD

Professor and Chairman, Division of Urology, Department of Surgery, University of Wisconsin School of Medicine and Public Health, Madison, Wisconsin

Since theorized by Einstein in 1917 and brought to fruition by Maiman in 1960,[1] lasers have become an important and prevalent technology in medicine. In 1968, Mulvaney and Beck[2] first described the urologic application of a laser when they used the ruby laser in attempting to fragment urinary calculi. Significant improvements made since 1990 in endoscopic technology and laser delivery systems have enabled the urologic surgeon to perform various procedures using the unique characteristics and intense energy of different lasers. Since their first description, applications of lasers in urology have expanded to include intracorporeal lithotripsy and treatment of benign prostatic hypertrophy (BPH), transitional cell carcinoma (TCC), urethral stricture, and other urologic conditions. However, the same unique properties of lasers may also be a source of significant hazard in the operating room. Understanding the physical characteristics of the laser, laser-tissue interactions, and the complications associated with the use of laser can enable the urologist to minimize these complications.

LASER PHYSICS

What Is a Laser?

The word *laser* was initially coined as an acronym for *light amplification by stimulated emission of radiation*. Not found ordinarily in nature, a laser is an intense beam of light generated under very specific conditions. Light is considered part of the electromagnetic spectrum found in the universe. This spectrum includes wavelengths of energy that vary considerably in wavelength from the very short waves in the ultraviolet end of the spectrum (γ rays and x-rays) to the very long waves in the infrared extreme of the spectrum (television waves,

radio waves, and microwaves). In between are the intermediate wavelengths of the visible spectrum (400-700 nm).

Light consists of individual energy packets known as *photons*. These photons have specific wavelengths and have wavelike properties with peaks and troughs. These waves can be *in phase*, in which peaks and troughs of adjacent waves are synchronized, or *out of phase*, with the peak of one and the trough of an adjacent wave canceling out each other. Laser light has three unique properties (**Fig. 18-1**). Unlike ordinary light, which scatters quickly, laser light is *collimated*, meaning the beam travels in a single direction without divergence over a long distance. Collimated light can produce the most intense light ever created, and this property imbues lasers with their potential power. Unlike ordinary light, which is composed of many different wavelengths, laser light is *monochromatic*, with all waves having the same wavelength. This characteristic allows lasers to be more specific in their application because their effect on tissue depends on the targeted tissue's inherent sensitivity to particular wavelengths. Finally, light is *coherent*, with all waves in phase. These three unique physical properties create an intense, focused, precise, and directional energy beam with a predictable and reproducible effect on target tissue.

The process of photon energy release from excited atoms is called *spontaneous emission of radiation*. Spontaneous emission of radiation is uncoordinated, and therefore photons released are out of phase of each other. In 1917, Einstein postulated the phenomena of *stimulated emission*. By stimulating an atom with photons of a specific wavelength, he deduced that the photons generated would be identical to those used to stimulate them and would travel in the same direction (**Fig. 18-2**).

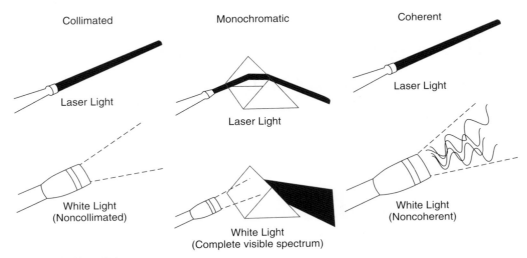

Figure 18-1 Characteristics of laser light.

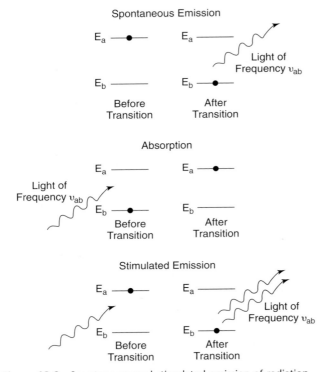

Figure 18-2 Spontaneous and stimulated emission of radiation. Light emission and absorption by atoms. The *black dots* represent the atoms in different energy levels (E_a and E_b). The *wavy lines* represent electromagnetic radiation.

A laser system consists of three main parts:

1. The medium that is stimulated and produces the photons
2. The excitation source that provides the energy for stimulation
3. A resonator system that produces the collimated beam of light

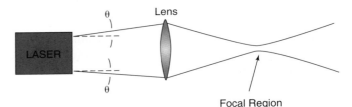

Figure 18-3 Focusing of laser using an optical lens.

The medium determines the wavelength of the laser light and can be solid, liquid, or gas.

Laser Beam Characteristics

At the point of exit from the resonator, a laser beam is large and somewhat diffuse and must be concentrated through a focusing lens. At its focal length, the beam diameter is at its smallest. Beyond this it diverges and increases in diameter (**Fig. 18-3**). *Power density*, a term that reflects the amount of energy delivered to the tissue at the beam-target interface, is determined by dividing the energy setting of the laser (in joules) by the square of the spot diameter (in centimeters). Maximum power density is achieved when the probe-to-target distance is identical to the laser's focal length. This measurement is important because each laser has a critical power density at which optimal tissue ablation and minimal thermal damage occur. Lasers of the same type can have different properties. *Power intensity* of a laser depends on the size of the laser medium (e.g., 20 and 100 W holmium:yttrium-aluminum-garnet [Ho:YAG] laser). Intensity distribution within the laser beam is measured by *spot size*, which is defined as the radius of the aperture that transmits 86% of the beam intensity. The same laser can also be delivered in either a *continuous* or a *pulsed* form. The application of pulsed energy results in

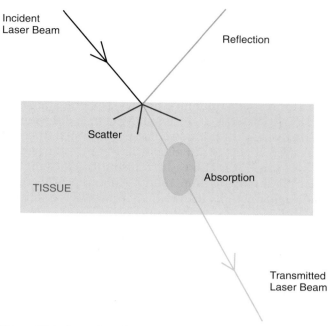

Figure 18-4 Laser-tissue interactions.

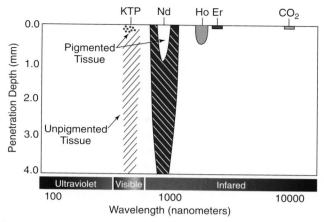

Figure 18-5 Depth of penetration of various lasers in pigmented and unpigmented tissues.

high power density at the target tissue but little heat dissipation.

Delivery of the laser beam can be accomplished using a series of mirrors, flexible fibers (usually made of quartz or glass), a contained tube, or a slit lamp. The fibers delivering the laser can deliver the energy in either an *end-firing* or a *side-firing* mechanism. Side-firing fibers use a reflective system (e.g., gold-plated mirror, solid gold tip) or a refractive system (e.g., glass prisms) to deflect the beam. The angle of reflection varies from 45 to 105 degrees, with 90 degrees the most common. This angle is important because it determines the power density by establishing the size of the laser spot on the target tissue. In the development of medical lasers, the manufacturers' ability to deliver the generated laser energy in a reliable, safe, and effective manner has been more technically challenging than has generation of the laser itself. Because many laser wavelengths are not in the visible spectrum, such lasers are commonly coupled with a parallel helium:neon (He:Ne) laser that emits red light to facilitate tissue targeting.

Laser-tissue Interaction

When laser energy strikes a tissue surface, four possible primary interactions can occur: *reflection, scatter, absorption,* or *transmission* (**Fig. 18-4**). The predominant interaction of lasers is absorption, which causes tissue heating and is the mechanism by which lasers generally exert their clinical effect. Although some reflection and scattering of light at the tissue surface as well as some transmission may take place, these are generally insignificant and little heating of surrounding tissues occurs.

The differences of clinical effects among lasers are largely attributable to the degree to which the individual laser's wavelength is absorbed by the target tissue. When less energy is absorbed by the target tissue, more laser energy is transmitted beyond the target. This situation can lead to inadvertent heating of deeper tissues and clinically significant thermal damage. Each tissue has its own specific optical properties (absorbs light of specific wavelengths), which depend on the components (water, pigments, protein) of the individual tissue.

Because most human tissues are predominantly made of water, the depth of penetration of various laser wavelengths is a direct consequence of the absorption coefficient in water (**Fig. 18-5**). Lasers that are highly absorbed by water (carbon dioxide [CO_2] and Ho:YAG) primarily produce surface effects like cutting and vaporization, whereas those minimally absorbed by water (neodymium:YAG [Nd:YAG] and potassium-titanyl-phosphate [KTP]) produce deep tissue effect of thermal coagulation. Because most endourologic procedures are performed in a water-based medium, the absorption of a specific wavelength by water also affects the safety profile of the laser. Both Nd:YAG and KTP lasers are transmitted through irrigation fluid without much loss of energy until they strike soft tissue, which may lead to unintended tissue injury.

The different tissue effects produced by a laser also depend on the duration of contact of laser energy with tissues (interaction time) and the power density of the laser at the point of contact. With decreasing interaction time and high power density, absorption of the laser energy by the tissues leads to *photothermal effect,* wherein the laser energy is transformed into heat. Depending on the tissue temperature attained, various biologic effects can be seen (Table 18-1). This effect is used for tissue ablation, incision, coagulation, and welding. With extremely long interaction times and low power density, a *photochemical effect* is seen with absorption of light and no heating of tissues. The best example is photosensitized oxidation, in which selective photo-activation of a specific drug (photosensitizer) leads to its transformation into a toxic compound. *Photomechanical* and *photoionizing effects* are seen with lasers with short interaction time and very high power densities, wherein the strong laser light is converted to kinetic energy.

Tissue effects also depend on the energy density at the target tissue. By moving the laser fiber closer (focusing) or farther away (defocusing) from the target tissue, the power density can be varied. For example, tissue vaporizing can be achieved with high power density in close proximity to the tissue, whereas coagulation may be achieved by moving the delivery fiber away from the target.

LASERS COMMONLY USED IN UROLOGY

Table 18-2 is an overview of lasers commonly used in urologic surgery.

Holmium:yttrium-aluminum-garnet Laser

The Ho:YAG laser is the most commonly used laser in urologic surgery. It is available in low-power (20 W) and high-power (60-100 W) versions for use in laser lithotripsy and treatment of BPH, respectively. The Ho:YAG laser has a wavelength of 2120 nm with a pulse duration of 250 to 350 μsec. The optical absorption coefficient for water at this wavelength is approximately 40 cm^{-1},

so it is strongly absorbed by water in the superficial tissue. This property allows the laser to perform superficial cutting. Dissipating heat with a high-power laser can cause tissue vaporization. The zone of thermal injury associated with laser ablation ranges from 0.5 to 1 mm and ensures adequate hemostasis during ablation even for vessels >1 mm in diameter. The pulse duration of Ho:YAG laser is short enough so that diffusion of thermal energy of low-power lasers is minimal (thermal relaxation time for soft tissues has been estimated to be 310 msec). It is also easily transmitted efficiently by silica fibers ranging from 150 to 940 μm in diameter, a feature that permits its use in endoscopic procedures.

Neodymium:yttrium-aluminium-garnet Laser

The Nd:YAG laser is an invisible solid-state laser with a wavelength of 1020 nm. The optical absorption coefficient for water at this wavelength is between 2 and 10 cm^{-1}, a level that is weakly absorbed and easily scattered by the tissue, with consequent tissue heating and a wide zone of thermal injury or coagulative necrosis of 4 to 6 mm. Because the energy density in tissue is low, the heating of tissue remains lower than the boiling point, and coagulative necrosis results. This laser is excellent for coagulating tissue and for hemostasis, but it has no cutting properties. The coagulated tissue turns white and subsequently sloughs over a period of 4 to 8 weeks. Vaporization can be performed if power density is increased; however, heat is generated continuously, and this feature makes it difficult to control and predict the depth of thermal necrosis.

Potassium-titanyl-phosphate Laser

The KTP laser is generated by passing a rapidly pulsed Nd:YAG beam through a KTP crystal, which halves the wavelength to 532 nm. This laser provides an intermediate level of coagulation and vaporization. Compared with the Nd:YAG laser, only half the depth of tissue penetration is reached. Because the laser is also effi-

TABLE 18-1	Tissue Effects of Photothermal Ablation at Various Temperatures	
Temperature	**Physical Effect**	**Optical Effect**
40°C-50°C	Protein denaturation	None
60°C-140°C	Protein coagulation	Blanching
100°C-300°C	Water vaporization	"Popcorn" effect
300°C-1000°C	Carbonization, tissue vaporization	Charring, smoke, ablation

TABLE 18-2	Lasers Commonly Used in Urologic Surgery					
Laser Properties	**Ho:YAG**	**Nd:YAG**	**KTP**	**FREDDY**	**Indigo**	**CO₂**
Wavelength (nm)	2120	1020	532	532/1064	800-850	10,600
Power (W)	20-100	5-100	80-120	3.2	2-20	0.3 to 1.5 μsec
Operation mode	Long pulse	CW	CW	Short pulse	CW	CW
Pulse length (μsec)	250-350	NA	NA	0.3-1.5	NA	NA
Applications	Lithotripsy Stricture BPH	BPH TCC	BPH	Lithotripsy	BPH	Condyloma

BPH, benign prostatic hypertrophy; CO₂, carbon dioxide; CW, continuous wave; FREDDY, frequency-doubled double-pause neodymium:yttrium-aluminium-garnet; Ho:YAG, holmium:yttrium-aluminum-garnet; KTP, potassium-titanyl-phosphate; NA, not applicable; Nd:YAG, neodymium:yttrium-aluminum-garnet; TCC, transitional cell carcinoma.

ciently absorbed by hemoglobin, hemostasis is excellent and the depth of penetration (0.3-1mm) is shallow, with a coagulation zone of approximately 2 mm. High-powered (80 and 120 W) rapid-pulse versions of the KTP laser have been popularized for laser treatment of BPH.

Frequency-Doubled Double-Pause Neodymium:yttrium-aluminium-garnet Laser

By incorporating a KTP crystal into the resonator of an Nd:YAG laser, the frequency-doubled double-pause Nd:YAG (FREDDY) laser produces two pulses, one at 532 nm and another at 1064 nm simultaneously using pulse durations of 0.3 to 1.5 μsec. FREDDY laser fragments stone by a photoacoustic mechanism. Laser light at 532nm initiates plasma formation at the stone surface, whereas light at 1064 nm heats the preformed plasma and causes expansion and contraction. A few studies have shown that FREDDY laser is capable of lithotripsy without any significant effects on normal tissues; however, treatment of hard urinary calculi can be difficult.

Diode Laser (Indigo Laser)

The Indigo laser is a diode laser with a wavelength of 800 to 850 nm and a radially diffusing optical fiber for interstitial laser coagulation of the prostate in BPH. The laser provides 2 to 3 mm of optical penetration in the tissue and produces coagulative necrosis through thermal diffusion of the absorbed laser radiation.

Carbon Dioxide Laser

The CO_2 laser is an invisible laser with an infrared wavelength of 10,600 nm. The optical absorption coefficient for water at this wavelength is approximately 800 cm^{-1}, which is significantly greater than that of Ho:YAG laser. This feature results in very superficial tissue penetration of approximately 0.05 mm with a thermal coagulation zone of approximately 0.5 mm. This laser can ablate or make precise incisions by vaporizing tissues with high water density. Although this level of penetration produces a very precise cut with an extremely narrow zone of thermal damage, the residual thermal energy is not enough to provide hemostasis in vascularized tissues. The CO_2 laser is frequently used for the treatment of superficial genital warts.

COMPLICATIONS RELATED TO UROLOGIC APPLICATIONS OF LASERS

Laser Lithotripsy

The surgical management of nephrolithiasis has undergone dramatic changes since the mid-1980s. Developments in radiographic equipment, endourologic devices, and intracorporeal lithotrites have resulted in more effective stone comminution, more efficient stone removal, and increased stone-free rates, combined with a significant reduction in operative morbidity compared with the open surgical alternatives.

The initial laser lithotrites (pulsed dye, Q-switched YAG, and alexandrite) fragmented stones through generation of a shock wave. The pulsed-dye laser was first used for the fragmentation of ureteral calculi in 1986.[3] This laser delivers short, 1-μsec pulsations at 5 to 10 Hz that are produced from a coumarin green dye. The 504-nm wavelength laser is selectively absorbed by the stone (except cystine) and not by the surrounding ureteral wall.[4] Because the energy is delivered in short pulses, minimal heat is generated, thus protecting the ureteral mucosa. Initial experience yielded stone fragmentation rates of 64% to 95%. Failures have been related to equipment malfunction (4%-19%) or more often to stone compositions that are resistant to lithotripsy (cystine, calcium oxalate monohydrate). In addition, the coumarin laser requires approximately 20 minutes before it is ready to function, and the required eye protection (amber glass) makes visualization of the stone and laser fiber difficult. Along with the foregoing limitations, its large size, high initial cost, and high maintenance cost of toxic disposables resulted in its decreasing use.

The Ho:YAG laser was first introduced for lithotripsy in 1995.[5,6] The holmium laser works by a dual mechanism: photoacoustic effect and photochemical effect. Like the previous lasers, the short-pulsed laser induces rapid formation of a spherical plasma cavitation bubble that expands symmetrically to a maximum size and then collapses violently. Bubble collapse leads to the generation of a shock wave that, on impingement on the targeted stone, comprises the primary mechanism of fragmentation referred to as a *photoacoustic effect* or *photomechanical effect.*[4] The long pulse duration of the Ho:YAG laser produces an elongated cavitation bubble that generates only a weak shock wave. In addition, the cavitation bubble generated is asymmetrical. As a result, different portions of the bubble collapse at slightly different times, thus giving the effect of multiple shock waves generated from a single bubble. The shock waves generated by the Ho:YAG laser are much weaker than are those generated by short-pulsed lasers and electro-hydraulic lithotripsy (EHL) probes,[7-9] a finding suggesting additional mechanisms of stone formation. This theory is further supported by evidence that Ho:YAG laser stone fragmentation starts before the collapse of the vapor bubble.[8]

The Ho:YAG laser also works by a *photothermal mechanism* that involves the direct absorption of the laser energy by the stone. In other words, the stone is literally melted.[8,10] Support for this theory arises from the findings that Ho:YAG laser stone fragmentation increases with increased stone temperature and that thermal byproducts for all stone compositions tested are found on the surfaces of the craters and in the irrigation solution during Ho:YAG laser lithotripsy. The photothermal mechanism of action of the Ho:YAG laser has several clinical implications, most of which favor the Ho:YAG laser over other intracorporeal lithotrites. The absence of a very strong shock wave minimizes stone retropulsion,[11] which is thought to be directly proportional to laser fiber diameter, pulse width, and total pulse energy output.[12-14] It also minimizes the risk of scatter damage to adjacent tissues (e.g., ureteral wall) and endoscopic equipment, encountered more commonly with EHL energy.[11,15-18]

Because the Ho:YAG laser energy is absorbed by all stone compositions, this laser can be used to fragment all stone types, including the harder cystine and calcium oxalate monohydrate stones.[19,20] Another advantage of Ho:YAG laser lithotripsy over other lithotrites is production of significantly smaller fragments, which can be easily irrigated, thus reducing the need for extraction of the fragments with basket or grasping devices.[15]

The biggest advantage of the Ho:YAG laser is that laser energy can be delivered to the target using silica fibers ranging from 150 to 940 μm in diameter. This characteristic allows its use in endoscopic procedures. However, even though the 200-μm fiber is quite flexible, one can still lose anywhere from 10 to 45 degrees of tip deflection of a 7.5-Fr flexible ureteroscope when it is placed through the working channel.[21,22] This feature may limit access to lower pole of the kidney, especially in the presence of hydronephrosis or when the ureteral-infundibular angle is >170 degrees. Transposition of the stone to an upper pole calyx using a stone basket may be required in this situation.

Lithotripsy efficiency correlates with energy density and depends on the pulse energy output and the diameter of the optical delivery fiber.[23] Although energy density increases with decreasing fiber diameter, in vitro studies demonstrated that peak lithotripsy occurred with 365- and 550-μm fibers, whereas the 200-μm fiber can act as a fine drill, which is less effective.[24] To maximize lithotripsy efficiency, the treating physician should move the laser fiber over the stone surface in a "painting" fashion, thus vaporizing the stone rather than fragmenting it; the physician should avoid drilling into the stone, thus fracturing the fiber tip, or drilling past the stone, thereby damaging the urothelium.[25] Compared with some of the soft tissue applications of the Ho:YAG laser, the power used for stone fragmentation is considerably lower. In general, pulse energies of 0.6 to 1.2 J and pulse rates of 5 to 15 Hz are used. Because high pulse energy narrows the safety margin and may increase stone retropulsion as well as fiber damage, it is recommended that treatment be commenced with low pulse energy (e.g., 0.6 J) with a pulse rate of 6 Hz and that pulse frequency be increased (in preference to increasing pulse energy) as needed to speed fragmentation.[25]

Other advantages of the Ho:YAG laser include a compact machine that requires minimal maintenance and is ready for use 1 minute after it is turned on. The required eye protection for the Ho:YAG laser does not compromise the endoscopic view of the surgeon, and energy levels used for stone disease (i.e., <15 W) would be harmful to the operator's cornea only if the eye were positioned at a distance of ≤10 cm from the fiber.[26]

As long as the Ho:YAG laser is fired away from the urothelial mucosa, soft tissue damage is not observed because much of the laser energy is absorbed by the medium (usually water) between the laser fiber and the mucosa. Urothelial injury is highly unlikely if the distance between the fiber and the urothelium is >0.5 mm.

Complications are few and most often result from anesthesia, limitations in endoscopic technology, and the clinical situation, not the laser. Because the Ho:YAG laser can cut and coagulate tissue, it is very important that the entire procedure be done under direct vision. If the stone dust begins to obstruct the operator's vision, lithotripsy should be halted until the irrigation has an opportunity to clear the operating field.[26] If the laser comes in contact with the urothelial mucosa, the depth of thermal injury is 0.5 mm.[27-29] The typical injury is a small mucosal defect or a small perforation the size of the laser fiber.

Clinical studies have shown low perforation and strictures rates with the use of the Ho:YAG laser for lithotripsy.[30] Most perforations are minor, can be managed by ureteral stenting, and do not require open conversion. One must also be cautious about drilling through the stone to the backside where tissue damage can occur blindly. Finally, because the laser is capable of cutting through metal, it is important not to direct the laser energy directly at wires or baskets. Moreover, the laser fiber should always be extended at least 2 mm beyond the tip of the endoscope to avoid damage to the lens.

Studies have found that the photothermal breakdown of uric acid stones produces cyanide in linear proportion to the total holmium energy employed.[31,32] Cyanide is highly soluble in water and is readily absorbed from intact or injured urothelium.[32] Until this toxicity profile is better defined, the Ho:YAG laser should be used cautiously for the treatment of large uric acid stones, especially in the presence of soft tissue trauma (e.g., percutaneous lithotripsy, traumatic ureteroscopy), which can enhance the systemic absorption of cyanide.

Laser Treatment of Transitional Cell Carcinoma

The ablative and hemostatic properties of the lasers have also been employed for the treatment of TCC within the urinary tract.[33,34] Laser ablation of bladder tumors is best reserved for small papillary tumors in patients with a history of recurrent superficial, low-grade cancer. Treatment of invasive bladder tumors is associated with higher recurrence rates and should be reserved for patients too ill to undergo radical cystectomy.

Either a coagulating or a cutting technique can be employed. To coagulate, the fiber is placed within 1 to 2 mm of the tumor and is then activated. This technique is useful for treating tumors with no defined stalk. Cutting is performed by placing the fiber in contact with the tissue during activation and can be used for tumors on a stalk. Both Nd:YAG[35,36] and Ho:YAG[37,38] lasers have been used for laser ablation of bladder tumors.

In a randomized study, Nd:YAG laser–treated stage T1 and T2 tumors had a lower recurrence rate compared with tumors treated with standard electrocautery (5% versus 32%).[39] Similar recurrence rates were seen in another study.[40] However, the Nd:YAG laser is rarely used now because of its unpredictable depth of penetration. Perforation of urinary tract and adjacent structures beyond the tumor (e.g., intestine) has been reported.[41,42] Bowel injury can occur in the absence of gross bladder perforation as a result of the penetration of laser energy. The Ho:YAG laser has a higher safety margin; however, ablation of larger tumors can be quite slow and tedious. Although more tissue can be ablated with larger-diameter fibers and higher energy settings, the greater movement of the tissue may make the ablation more difficult.[43]

A study comparing Ho:YAG laser and transurethral resection of superficial bladder cancer in high-risk patients showed shorter catheterization time and hospital stay with the Ho:YAG laser.[44] Most procedures can be performed with a flexible endoscope on an outpatient basis without the need for postoperative catheterization.[45,46] Because of the superficial depth of invasion of the Ho:YAG laser, complications such as perforation and obturator reflex are rare. The disadvantages of laser ablation include an absence of material for histologic examination and the inability to determine the precise depth of tissue destruction.

Endourologic treatment of upper tract TCC is a reasonable alternative to nephroureterectomy in highly selected patients (low-stage and low-grade tumors, solitary kidney, renal insufficiency, poor surgical candidates). Both Nd:YAG and Ho:YAG lasers have been used ureteroscopically and percutaneously to fulgurate and ablate tumors in the ureter and renal pelvis.[34] The superficial depth of invasion of Ho:YAG laser is especially advantageous for treatment of ureteral tumors because it allows precise ablation with low risk of injury to neighboring structures. Keeley and associates[47] recommended use of Nd:YAG laser to coagulate the tumor before ablation with the Ho:YAG laser.

Several reports have confirmed successful treatment results and the absence of complications with the proper use of endoscopic therapy with electrocautery and laser for the conservative management of superficial TCC.[34]

Ureteroscopy has been used successfully, with recurrence rates ranging from 31% to 65% and disease-free rates of 35% to 86%. Disease progression and metastatic disease are rare in appropriately selected patients and correlate with tumor grade. Similarly, percutaneous approaches have been shown to have good results in patients with low-grade tumors; recurrence rates and disease-specific survival rates are 26% to 28% and 96% to 100%, respectively.[34] Percutaneous treatment is generally favored for larger tumors located proximally in the renal pelvis or proximal ureter. Because of high recurrence rates, it is imperative that all patients treated with endoscopic therapy undergo strict surveillance. The surveillance protocol may be very labor and resource intensive and requires a motivated patient for optimal outcome.

Complication rates are low in most ureteroscopic series. Because of the limited degree of holmium energy tissue absorption, the risk of perforation is greatly reduced. The rate of ureteral perforation from technical errors with endoscopes, guidewires, baskets, or lasers is 1% to 4%.[34] The stricture rates approach 9%, and this complication is becoming less common.[34] Some investigators have suggested that rates of scarring and stricture formation are lower after the use of lasers versus electrofulguration for the treatment of upper urinary tract disease.[48,49] Ureteral stricture is not always caused by technical factors and may represent disease recurrence in ≤40% patients.[50] Ureteroscopic treatment has also been shown not to increase the risk of progression or spread of disease to other urothelial surfaces or metastatic sites.[51,52]

Percutaneous resection is associated with higher complication rates than is the retrograde approach. Transfusion rates were 20% to 50% in several series.[34] Less common complications include ureteropelvic junction (UPJ) stricture, pleural effusions and tract seeding. Complications tend to be related to the location of the access and the extent of resection performed. Although multiple cases of nephrostomy tract infiltration in patients with high-grade tumors have been reported, percutaneous tract seeding is rare in patients with low-grade disease. Using a human kidney model, Low[53] showed that placing the sheath in the collecting system as opposed to the parenchyma during resection reduced intrapelvic pressures by half. Additionally, using a sheath of ≥30 Fr limits pyelolymphatic backflow. These techniques may reduce the potential risk of tumor seeding.

Photodynamic therapy (PDT) was introduced for treatment of bladder cancer in mid-1990s. After intravenous administration of a photosensitizer, the bladder is subject to laser light, which leads to destruction of malignant cells that retain the photosensitizer. Although some promising results were seen in patients with superficial bladder carcinoma refractory to standard therapy, the high incidence of complications resulted in loss of interest in the procedure. Complications included severe and prolonged irritative urinary symptoms, associated with detrusor injury and fibrosis, as well as transient leg edema from toxicity in the pelvic lymphatic system. Cutaneous photosensitization can lead to skin damage if patients are exposed to sunlight within 4 to 6 weeks after PDT. However, novel second- and third-generation photosensitizers with improved tissue selectivity and target cell destruction capabilities have had successful outcomes with lower morbidity, thus renewing interest in PDT as an alternative, minimally invasive approach for management of TCC.[54-57]

Management of bladder hemangioma seems to be the only absolute indication for laser therapy in urology because endoscopic resection of these lesions has been associated with uncontrollable bleeding. Successful treatment of this condition has been achieved with the use of the Nd:YAG laser.[58,59]

Laser Incision of Urethral and Ureteral Strictures

Lasers can be used to make precise endoscopic incisions of strictures in the urethra and the ureter. Although surgical reconstruction of the urethra remains the gold standard, various lasers have been used as minimally invasive alternatives to cold knife incision and balloon dilation. More recent studies have used the Nd:YAG[60,61] and Ho:YAG lasers[62-65] for urethral incision or core-through urethrotomy. The Ho:YAG laser has also been used for the treatment of post–radical prostatectomy anastomotic strictures[63,66] and pediatric urethral atresia.[67] Overall, outcomes of laser therapy have been suboptimal because of stricture recurrence, presumably caused by thermal damage to adjacent tissue and subsequent scar formation. Experimental studies using the erbium:YAG (Er:YAG) suggested that this laser is capable of performing precise incision of urethral tissues with minimal peripheral thermal damage.[68-70]

Open pyeloplasty has been considered the gold standard treatment of UPJ obstruction, with success rates of >90%.[71] Modern endoscopic instrumentation and techniques have directed the treatment of UPJ obstruction toward minimally invasive procedures such as endopyelotomy and laparoscopic pyeloplasty. These techniques share the advantages of short operative time, minimal morbidity, decreased postoperative pain, shorter hospitalization, and early recovery. The basic principle of endopyelotomy is a full-thickness incision of the narrow segment followed by stenting. The incision could be carried through antegrade or retrograde routes.[72,73]

Laser energy has been used as an alternative to electrocautery to incise the UPJ. The high energy produced by laser leads to tissue vaporization and results in a precise incision. In contrast, low energy produced by electrocautery leads to tissue coagulation at the periphery and results in a compromised blood supply. The second advantage of laser is the small diameter and flexibility of laser fibers that enable its passage through small-diameter ureteroscopes[74,75] permit treatment of UPJ obstruction in a retrograde fashion.

Two laser energy sources have been used: Nd:YAG and Ho:YAG. Although a success rate of 85% using the Nd:YAG laser was observed by Renner and colleagues,[76] a high recurrence rate of 45% was reported by Gallucci and associates.[77] Coagulating laser wavelengths (e.g., Nd:YAG and KTP) when used at higher settings to make incisions tend to produce extensive thermal energy to surrounding tissues and may actually promote recurrence. Therefore, the Nd:YAG laser was considered not ideal for endoscopic incision.[78] With the Ho:YAG laser, a precise incision can be performed with minimal bleeding because of its ablative and hemostatic properties. Controlled endoscopic incision can be performed in a "what you see is what you get" fashion because the depth and direction of the cut can easily be controlled.[78] A laser energy setting of 1 to 2.5 J at a rate of 10 to 20 Hz is used and a full-thickness lateral or posterolateral incision is made. Success rates have ranged from 73% to 85%.[79] Hospital stays of <24 hours have been reported. Early treatment failures are usually detected within 1 year; however, long-term follow-up is recommended to detect late failures.[78] In addition, failed endopyelotomy did not jeopardize the success of subsequent open pyeloplasty.[80]

The complications of ureteroscopic endopyelotomy have decreased dramatically and are usually minor in comparison with earlier series.[74,79,81] Reasons include improvements in ureteroscopic instruments, use of laser energy, increasing experience, and exclusion of patients with crossing vessels.[82] Reported rates of complications of laser endopyelotomy range between 8.5% and 12.5%.[79]

Possible iatrogenic complications of ureteroscopy include ureteral perforation, stricture, false passage, ureteral avulsion, bleeding from the ureteral mucosa or adjacent structures, infection, and sepsis. Several studies reported an overall complication rate associated with ureteroscopy of between 1% and 15%.[83] Complications associated with incision of the UPJ include bleeding from adjacent aberrant vessels, fracture of the guidewire, stent migration through the UPJ incision, and recurrent UPJ obstruction.

Massive bleeding requiring nephrectomy is no longer reported because of the routine use of preoperative radiographic studies to identify aberrant vessels and the use of a complete lateral incision at the UPJ to avoid injuries to those vessels. Bleeding requiring blood transfusion was reported in <2% patients, and the need for embolization to control severe bleeding is extremely rare in contemporary series.[79]

Other minor complications include proximal stent migration, stent intolerance, bleeding, perirenal urinoma or hematoma, pyelonephritis, and urinary tract infection. Most of these complications can be managed conservatively.[78,82,84,85] Some surgeons recommend using a ureteral stent one size longer than anticipated to prevent downward migration of the renal coil into the incised UPJ.[82] Stent-related symptoms are usually alleviated after removal of the indwelling stent. The use of antispasmodic and anesthetic drugs must be considered while the stent is in place. In a prospective randomized comparison of retrograde laser and Acucise endopyelotomy (Applied Medical Resources Corp., Rancho Santa Margarita, California), the incidence of complications was higher with the Acucise technique (10% versus 25%).[84] Significant postoperative hematuria resulting in prolonged hospital stay and hemoglobin decrease developed only in the Acucise-treated group. In addition, subjective and objective success was better in the laser endopyelotomy group (85% versus 65%).

The Ho:YAG laser has also been used for the treatment of ureteral and ureterointensinal strictures, with reasonable success rates.[86-90] For the endoureterotomy to be successful, a clean cut must be made from 1 cm above to 1 cm below the stricture, down to the retroperitoneal fat.

Laser Ablation of External Genitalia Lesions

Condylomas refractory to medical therapy require surgical intervention. For multifocal small lesions, the CO_2 laser gives excellent cosmetic results because of its superficial vaporizing properties.[91,92] The Ho:YAG laser can also be used, but it produces more splatter of body fluids and thus raises concerns about transmission of infectious agents. Large lesions are treated by fulguration or local excision. The Nd:YAG laser can be used to coagulate these lesions, which subsequently slough over several days. Because depth of penetration is difficult to judge, destruction of normal tissue can occur, leading to ulcers and urethral injuries. These ulcers are slow to heal, can become infected, and should be treated as full-thickness burns. Skin grafting may occasionally be required for very large ulcers. The surgeon should err on the side of undertreatment to avoid these complications. Laser treatment can also be used for treatment of recurrent urethral condylomas,[93,94] with a low stricture rate.

Laser treatment can be used in patients with Tis and small T1 squamous cell carcinoma of the penis and in patients with manageable T2 tumors who refuse more aggressive surgical treatment. Laser therapy has the potential advantage of eliminating the primary tumor with preservation of surrounding tissues and penile function. However, because a histologic specimen is lacking, accurate diagnosis and staging may be problematic.

The CO_2 laser is has been most often used as monotherapy for ablation of dysplastic lesions and squamous cell carcinoma in situ.[95,96] However, a local recurrence rate of ≤33% has been reported.[96] This laser can also be used to excise small superficial lesions of the penis.[97] In this study, surgical specimens were adequate for pathologic examination in 87% of cases. Healing time varied from 5 to 8 weeks, and one patient had significant arterial hemorrhage controlled by cautery. Cosmetic appearance was good in all cases, and no meatal stenosis was noted.

The Nd:YAG laser is the most commonly used laser to coagulate squamous cell carcinoma; local recurrence rates are approximately 20% when this laser is used for carcinoma in situ and T1 lesions.[98-103] The Nd:YAG laser can also be used after surgical resection to coagulate the base and margins of the defect.[98,100,102] Attempts to decrease the recurrence rate have been made by preparation of the genital skin with 5% acetic acid and by photodynamic diagnosis with 5-aminolevulinic acid autofluorescence.[95,99] Postoperative healing requires 8 to 12 weeks for Nd:YAG laser and can be potentially difficult in patients who are obese, immunocompromised, or receiving anticoagulation therapy.[95,99] Overall cosmetic results are good; in one study, 7% of patients had minor postoperative bleeding, and erectile function was unaltered in 72% of patients.[104] Because data on long-term follow-up, recurrence, and survival are scant, close follow-up is mandatory.

LASER SAFETY

Safety considerations in the medical applications of lasers are of prime importance to physicians, patients, and support personnel in the operating room. Because most laser wavelengths are readily transmitted through the air, laser safety precautions must extend beyond the operative field to the entire operating room. Disruption of the laser fiber with stray laser light emission outside the operative field (from any point between the laser source and the operating end of the delivery fiber used) is the most commonly occurring accidental event.

The main considerations are ocular, cutaneous, and electrical. Because of the directional and coherent nature of laser beams, lasers can produce significant and permanent ocular damage if they come in contact with the eye. Depending on the wavelength of the laser, it can be absorbed by the cornea or the lens or focused on the retina and can lead to significant injury. Current laser safety standards follow the practice of categorizing all laser products in several hazard classes, and control measures are specified for each class depending on the specific hazard posed by the laser beam. Based on their safety profile, lasers are grouped into four hazard classes.

Class 1 laser products are considered eye-safe and do not emit potentially hazardous laser radiation to pose any health hazard. Most lasers that are totally enclosed (e.g., laser compact disk recorders) are class 1. No safety measures are required for class 1 lasers.

Classes 2 through 4 pose an increasing hazard to the eye and skin. Class 2 (e.g., laser pointers) refers to visible lasers that emit with a very low power (<1 mW) that would not be hazardous even if the entire beam power entered the human eye and was focused on the retina. The eye's natural aversion response (blink reflex, eye rotation, and head movement) to viewing bright light protects the eye against retinal injury in such cases.

In the last few years, two new classes, class 1M and 2M, were introduced. These laser are effectively eye-safe unless the beam is directly viewed with magnifying optical instruments.

Class 3 lasers pose a hazard to the eye because the aversion response is not fast enough to limit retinal exposure to a momentarily safe level or because damage to other structures of the eye (e.g., corneal and lens) could take place. Skin hazards normally do not exist for incidental exposures. Examples of class 3 lasers are many research lasers and military laser rangefinders.

Class 4 lasers may pose a potential fire hazard, a significant skin hazard, or a diffuse-reflection hazard. Virtually all surgical lasers and material processing lasers used for welding and cutting are class 4 if they are not enclosed. All lasers with an average power output exceeding 0.5 W are class 4. If a higher-power class 3 or 4 laser is totally enclosed so that hazardous radiant energy is not accessible, the total laser system could be class 1.

General Laser Safety Principles

All operating room windows should be covered with opaque material to prevent stray emission of laser light. All portals of entry to the operating room should be appropriately marked with signs that include the type of laser and its safety class, wavelength, and energy. Access in and out of the operating room should be limited during laser usage. The configuration of the operating room must be optimized for laser surgery to ensure that the laser is close to the operative field.

Operative Field

The operative field should be prepared with noninflammable preparation solutions. Flammable paper drapes should be avoided as well. During open surgery, all exposed surfaces that are not to be treated should be protected by wet surgical drapes. A basin of water can be kept on an instrument table as a final line of defense to douse a laser-induced fire. Reflective steel instruments should be avoided because they may reflect the laser beam in unpredictable directions. For laser ablation of virally induced external genitalia lesions, additional protection of the surgeon and operating room personnel is necessary to prevent viral transmission. A high-volume suction device to evacuate all smoke and virus-filtering face masks should be used in such cases.

While using the laser endoscopically, metallic guidewires and baskets should be avoided or covered or replaced with plastic ureteral catheters when possible because the laser is capable of disrupting them or reflecting off them. Special care should also be taken while using flexible endoscopes to ensure that no significant laser energy is being absorbed into the distal tip of the scope. Such absorption can lead not only to photoacoustic scope damage, but also to ignition and potential flash fires. The tip of the laser fiber should always be under direct vision beyond the tip of the scope to prevent these complications.

Laser Source Handling

A commonly overlooked consideration of lasers is their electrical safety. Laser power supplies produce lethal voltages and currents, and only trained service personnel should be allowed to service or work inside a laser system. Routine maintenance and repair of the laser source along with calibration on a regular basis are also key to ongoing safe operation. The total laser energy use during an operation should be monitored and recorded as well.

Laser Fiber Handling

Lasers equipped with fiberoptic delivery systems should be handled with extreme care. The laser source should be placed as close as possible to the operating field to minimize accidental disruption of the laser fiber by operating room personnel. Even though the light emitting from the fiber is in a divergent geometry, its intensity can be significant enough to cause ocular and other tissue damage The fiber should always be elevated off the floor and should not cross obvious footpaths or interfere with access to other equipment. The foot pedal should be close to the laser surgeon in the operative field and away from other foot traffic to avoid inadvertent depression. Whenever the laser is not in active use, the safety shutter should be in the closed position.

Eye Protection

Laser eye protection becomes of great importance when engineering controls fail or accidental firing occurs, to ensure that potential optical exposure will not exceed the maximum permissible levels. For these reasons, it is required that *all persons* in the room in which the laser is operating wear protective eyeglasses or goggles. The goggles required depend on the type of laser in use and should be explicitly marked with regard to the specific wavelengths to which they provide a barrier. Modern laser safety goggles are lightweight, provide protection against various wavelengths, and produce little or no distortion of the surgeon's vision.

Skin Protection

Although laser-induced eye injuries can produce permanent disability, accidental cutaneous laser burns occur much more commonly. Other than general laser safety principles, careful attention to location and aiming of the laser delivery device along with care in preventing breakage of the laser fiber from undue mechanical trauma or overflexing should be ensured. A laser-induced cutaneous injury should be treated like a burn injury. Although most cutaneous injuries are limited to a superficial burn in a single spot, deeper injuries may happen at higher power settings.

CONCLUSION

Lasers are intense beams of energy generated through the stimulation of radiation. Clinical effects occur through tissue heating by absorption of laser energy. The clinical appeal of lasers in urologic applications is based on preferential absorption by water-containing tissues and easy delivery through endoscopes. Lasers represent an attractive alternative to many invasive and minimally invasive techniques; however, laser surgery is a constantly evolving discipline and requires appropriate understanding of basic principles to ensure the best outcomes. The knowledge and skill of the operating surgeon are the most important factors in preventing complications during the use of lasers. With proper employment and appropriate precautions, lasers can be the safest and most versatile energy sources for surgical use.

KEY POINTS

1. Lasers are intense beams of monochromatic, coherent, and collimated light.
2. Laser-tissue interaction varies depending on the energy density and wavelength of the laser and on the composition of the tissue in contact.
3. The Nd:YAG and KTP lasers have deeper penetration than do the Ho:YAG and CO_2 lasers.
4. The Ho:YAG laser is the most versatile laser and can be used for multiple urologic indications including treatment of BPH, intracorporeal lithotripsy, incision of ureteral or urethral strictures, and ablation of urothelial cancers.
5. The Ho:YAG laser can be used for precise tissue cutting (e.g., endoureterotomy, endopyelotomy, enucleation of the prostate).
6. The Ho:YAG laser can break all types of stones and has a high safety margin and a low incidence of stone retropulsion.
7. Laser treatment of penile and urothelial cancer should be reserved for compliant patients with small-volume, low-stage, and low-grade cancers.
8. Lasers carry a significant amount of energy can cause serious damage to eye and skin. Appropriate laser safety precautions should always be followed.

REFERENCES

Please see www.expertconsult.com

COMMON SURGICAL CONSIDERATIONS

Chapter 19

ASSESSING QUALITY OF CARE IN UROLOGIC SURGERY

Elizabeth A. Soll PhD
Research Associate, Division of Urologic Health Services Research, Department of Urology, University of Michigan Medical Center, Ann Arbor, Michigan

Simon P. Kim MD, MPH
Resident, Division of Urologic Health Services Research, Department of Urology, University of Michigan Medical Center, Ann Arbor, Michigan

John T. Wei MD, MS
Associate Professor, Division of Urologic Health Services Research, Department of Urology, University of Michigan Medical Center, Ann Arbor, Michigan

Whether we are aware of it or not, every evaluative act depends on antecedent criteria, implicit or explicit or both.
—Donabedian, 1986

In the United States, health care costs in 2005 exceeded $2.0 trillion, an estimated 16.0% of the annual gross domestic product, with approximately $10,000 spent per citizen.[1] Despite outspending all other industrialized countries, markers of health such as newborn mortality rate have ranked poorly against our peer industrialized nations. Disparities in patient outcomes, prevalence of medical errors, and variation in practice patterns have brought attention to the need to examine more closely the quality of care (QOC) in the United States. QOC initiatives initially focused on poor outcomes and higher complications associated with differences in health care structure, such as hospital, provider, and patient characteristics. An Institute of Medicine (IOM) report brought attention to the pervasiveness of medical errors and complications.[2] Medical errors have been associated with medical injury during hospitalization, longer length of stays, and significant health care costs.[3] Higher mortality rates, attributed to limited access to specialists and technology, have been reported for many common conditions.[4]

QOC research has also been useful in the evaluation of surgical outcomes based on hospital and surgeon characteristics. Decreased mortality rates and fewer complications have been well documented in hospitals with high surgical volume, a finding that supports the concept of centers for excellence.[5-10] Although surgical subspecialties have remained largely insulated from quality improvement efforts, reports have noted a similar pattern of improved outcome with high surgical volume. Medical centers with low volumes of radical prostatectomies (RPs) have reported higher morbidity rates relative to hospitals performing high rates of such surgical procedures.[11] Similar outcomes, including shorter length of stay and lower mortality rates, have been demonstrated by hospitals and surgeons performing high volumes of radical cystectomies.[12]

Observing that a salient gap between ideal and actual medical care existed, the IOM released a report addressing the need to close the "quality chasm."[13] The IOM recognized the need for national leadership in spearheading QOC initiatives by standardizing performance measures, ensuring data collection, evaluating the impact of pay for performance, and reporting methods.[14] Indeed, the increasing importance of the IOM policy was illustrated by the Centers for Medicare and Medicaid Services plan to incorporate financial incentives for demonstrating QOC, the Physician Quality Reporting Initiative (PQRI).[15,16] Thus, it behooves urologists to recognize the growing influence and importance of improving patient outcomes and help lead QOC initiatives in urology. This chapter reviews the conceptual framework and background of QOC, methodology for measuring QOC, and QOC assessment in surgery. QOC methodology is applied to prostate cancer and benign prostatic hyperplasia (BPH) because some progress has already

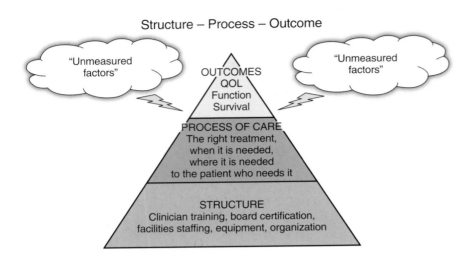

Structure – Process – Outcome

"Unmeasured factors"

"Unmeasured factors"

OUTCOMES
QOL
Function
Survival

PROCESS OF CARE
The right treatment,
when it is needed,
where it is needed
to the patient who needs it

STRUCTURE
Clinician training, board certification,
facilities staffing, equipment, organization

Figure 19-1   Donabedian's structure-process-outcome model. QOL, quality of life.

been made toward QOC initiatives for these common urologic conditions.

BACKGROUND FOR QUALITY OF CARE

The advancement of QOC assessment in medicine is often attributed to the life's work of Avedis Donabedian. In his landmark 1966 article, Donabedian defined quality in medical care as a judgment made relative to the goals and values of practitioners and society.[17] He later specified that this definition of quality depends on who and what are to be assessed. Health care may be evaluated at the system, practitioner, or patient level, each of which has a certain degree of associated responsibility.[18] Other investigators defined QOC in a rather subjective manner, as meeting "acceptable" standards.[19] The IOM defined QOC as "... the degree to which health services for individuals and populations increase the likelihood of desired health outcomes and are consistent with current professional knowledge."[20] The IOM noted the importance of considering patient preferences and the application of the most recent empirical evidence. More recently, Campbell and associates[21] stressed the need to include treatment accessibility and effectiveness in the definition of QOC. Indeed, effectiveness is clearly the dominant component throughout the QOC literature.[21-24]

Relevance, equity, acceptability, accessibility, economy, continuity, comprehensiveness, patient-centered focus, and efficiency were all suggested to be important components of QOC models.[23-25] All these paradigms were based on Donabedian's structure-process-outcome model, a then novel approach of delineating quality indicators, or criteria, and their interrelationships.[17,18,25-27] *Structure* refers to physical and organizational components, including medical staff expertise. *Process* is the application of medical care based on current knowledge and care standards[26] and may be viewed as consisting of interpersonal and technologic components.[21] Campbell and associates[21] defined

outcome as a tangible result of interactions among health care providers, patients, and the health care system. Structure, process, and outcome are causally related, and the strength of these relationships determines the validity and usefulness of the quality indicator selected.[25] This relationship was described as progressively reliant, outcome dependent on process, which is contingent on structure.[27] Thus in ideal world, quality care assessments would involve measuring elements of structure, process, and outcome (**Fig. 19-1**).

Structural Component of Quality Defined

Structural quality measures are those that measure the physical, environmental, organizational, and staffing components of an institution.[26] Such indicators represent health system or institutional resource use required for the process of care. Mainz[28] described the application of structural indicators as a "judgment" of how well the institutional conditions uphold standards. Although structural measures were the basis for quality ratings used in accreditation,[29] such indicators have been largely ignored in favor of process and outcome indicators. However, investigators have increasingly recognized the important role that structure plays in QOC assessment.[30] In fact, in the late 1990s the Performance Measurement Coordinating Council (PMCC) designed specific criteria for structural QOC indicators.[31] Meyer and Massagli[30] addressed relatively unexplored knowledge areas of structure quality criteria partially based on the PMCC report. The need for consideration of the aesthetic environment was echoed by Fowler and colleagues,[32] who conducted focus groups to determine what was most important to patients from different types of health care settings. This patient-focused priority was further supported by the creation of the Leapfrog Initiative, a group of large businesses directed toward using structural criteria to inform health care consumers better and ultimately to improve health care quality.[33] As new structure criteria are beginning to be developed, priorities need to be set and relevance, validity, and feasibility must be considered for each measure. In addition, the association with process and outcome must not be neglected when structural quality indicators are developed.[30]

Process Component of Quality Defined

Process measures assess patient care, what was actually planned or performed.[28] Such indicators measure components of or the entire treatment course and involve the application of appropriate technical and interpersonal skills.[18,34] Brook and associates[35] considered process measures to be the most difficult and the most appropriate quality assessments to conduct for the majority of medical settings. Process measures have been regarded as simple to comprehend and direct measures of care quality.[36] According to Rubin and colleagues,[37] the development and implementation of process criteria require a team effort in defining purpose, selecting the appropriate specific clinical event to assess, evaluating the indicator psychometrically to establish feasibility, and formalizing rating and analytic requirements. Treurniet[38] and associates also proposed important requirements for the proper application of health care process indicators, including the establishment of a validated relationship between process and outcome and the use of established clinical databases as well as prospective data collection to understand case mix.

Depending on the medical condition and treatment, processes of care may be simple or complex, involving one or many health care providers. Processes may be evaluated by review of treatment documentation in medical records or administrative data. Thus, data collection relies on the completeness and comprehensiveness of chart notes or billing data. Some variables are documented routinely, whereas others are difficult to find, must be retrieved from multiple data sources, or are not recorded at all. This may not be an issue if a quality assurance plan is in place that requires providers to document specific process components for future evaluation.

Outcome Component of Quality Defined

Outcome is the presumed result of core processes and is often considered the quality indicator of most value to the patient.[29] Mainz[28] suggested that an optimal outcome indicator measures the effect of the care process on patient health and well-being. He described "the five Ds" often used to represent health care outcome as discomfort, dissatisfaction, disability, disease, and death. Mainz also defined intermediate outcome criteria as evidence-based physiologic variables that change with time depending on disease process. In addition, he provided examples of end result outcomes in addition to morbidity and mortality: functional and work status, quality of life, satisfaction, and health status. Variables

purported as important for determining outcome, aside from structural and process measures, included the following: patient demographics, lifestyle, and compliance; illness severity and comorbidities; treatment competence, evidence-based application, equipment, accuracy, and efficacy; and organizational cooperation, application of clinical standards of care, and efficiency.[28]

The outcomes management movement optimized patient care quality through assessment of outcome. al-Assaf[29] described the outcome management procedure as collecting and analyzing data, evaluating results, developing practice guidelines, informing practitioners, and improving outcomes. He saw this as a progressive, continuous circle of steps.[29] Indeed, with the ultimate goal of quality improvement, outcome measures relate to QOC by providing information to guide structural and process changes.[39]

Quality assessments need to be based on the actual care provided regardless of the ultimate outcome.[18] Therefore, measuring outcome without evaluating process bypasses this important level. Donabedian[25] examined the complexities of assessing medical care quality by measuring outcome as the sole criteria. He noted that that this approach requires a large sample because of the reliance on inferences. In addition, outcome encompasses provider, patient, and other less closely related variables. Factors not directly related to health care play roles in treatment outcome and these variables must be controlled for (i.e., case mix).[35] In addition, appropriate time frame selection is critical when measuring outcome.[25] A shorter time window may be effective if the potential exists for outcome modification. A more extended time frame may limit the amount and usefulness of the data collected but may capture outcomes that occur in a delayed fashion.[35] Use of a long time window makes it difficult to identify specific errors that influenced a poor outcome. Thus, when outcome is used alone to measure care quality, the potential for misinterpretation of assessment results is great.

Taken together, the structure, process, and outcome components of quality are each necessary to the provision of optimal care. The *quality pyramid* is built on a foundation of structural elements that permits some, if not all, aspects of process to take place. The outcome component is the result of processes of care that, in and of themselves, may be subject to many unidentified and therefore unmeasured factors (see Fig. 19-1).[27] Thus, health care quality and assessment are complex, multifaceted, and not fully operationalized phenomena.

MEASURING QUALITY OF CARE

Appropriate QOC assessment requires selection of criteria, norms, and standards.[26] According to Donabedian,[27] selection and application of criteria to QOC assessment require consideration of approach, source, referents, specification, format, and evaluation. *Approach* refers to the selected criteria, structure, process, outcome, or any combination thereof. If results are the criteria of interest, the selected outcome must be relevant to the intervention to allow for meaningful comparison.[25] Independent of the selected criteria, the degree of causality among structure, process, and outcome must be established before assessment. In addition, referents or medical conditions and situations must be congruent with the selected criteria. Criteria may be implicit or explicit and may be weighted based on relative importance for quality assessment. *Implicit criteria* depend on the reliability of expert opinion and the judgment associated with such a process. The reasoning behind the judgment may or may not be conveyed by those conducting the QOC assessment. *Explicit criteria* are based on empirical data and are, theoretically, concrete, consistent, and independent of individual judgment. Ironically, subjectivity may prevent development of completely explicit criteria because scientific creativity is the basis for empirical knowledge.[40]

Another important decision in selection of criteria is *format* (**Fig. 19-2**). The *linear format* is typically applied to diagnostic criteria. The *partially branched format* divides criteria into that which must be applied to all cases and that which should never appear in any case. The *fully branched* or *criteria maps* categorize cases into increasingly homogeneous groups using decision trees and a series of steps to apply more specific criteria. Evaluation of criteria and the QOC assessment plan involve determining validity, relevance, importance, case adaptability, stability, and screening efficiency.[27]

According to Mainz,[28] because QOC is a multidimensional concept, quality measures by themselves only indirectly assess quality. He specified criteria for the optimal indicator as follows:

1. Clearly operationalized by consensus
2. Applicable for comparisons
3. Highly specific and sensitive
4. Reliable and valid
5. Discriminative
6. Representative of the defined clinical procedure
7. Based on empirical evidence[28]

Indeed, other experts in the field suggested that criteria development relies on scientific evidence and consensus of expertise ideas.[22,28,41] Selection of referents, standards, specifications, norms, and pilot testing follows quality indicator definition.[27,28] The criteria must be quantifiable, and a level must exist at which the standard is considered good.[26] McGlynn[41] described the lack of standardization as one of the major impediments to implementation of health care quality assessment. Other challenges include creating an accountability framework, establishing consensus of care quality within a health care system, selecting and implementing a set of empirically based and relevant quality indicators, designing a quality monitoring information system, and minimizing conflict between incentives and quality care objectives.[41]

Donabedian[18] suggested additional considerations for the assessment of care quality that included cost, measurement methods and sample selection, relevance of measures to care objectives, accuracy, completeness and

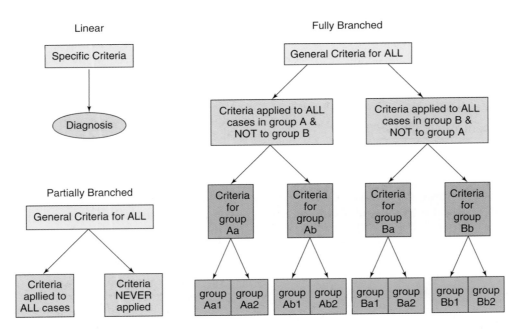

Figure 19-2 Examples of quality of care assessment formats.

reliability of data collected or extrapolated, and expected outcome. He stipulated that when evaluating treatment cost, cost and care are confounded, and he suggested two methods of dealing with this issue: (1) the *maximalist approach*, providing the maximum amount of care possible independent of cost; and (2) the *optimalist approach*, providing care until the point at which it is no longer cost effective.[18] Selection of appropriate quality indicators and assessment tools depends on clearly operationalized questions.[41] Similarly, sampling and data collection methods rely on the particular quality indicators selected. Sampling techniques include stratification, the *tracer method*, and adverse outcome case selection. Stratification requires use of the most appropriate variable. The tracer method selects cases that represent a specified classification.[18] Thus, developing a QOC assessment initiative requires careful planning and meticulous attention to detail and steps.

As conceived by Donabedian,[18] within the provision of health care are three levels of quality assessment: technical, interpersonal, and aesthetic. *Technical quality* is based on use of empirical evidence to apply the appropriate treatment in a skillful manner. *Aesthetics* and amenities are institutional attributes. *Interpersonal quality* refers to the rapport between practitioner and patient. This level of quality assessment is based on human factors, intuition, preferences, and social standards and is therefore more difficult to measure compared with technical and institutional aspects of care. Donabedian[18] suggested other important factors to assess including access to care, quality of provider-patient interface, and patient and family contribution. Take BPH medical management, for example. A health care provider may be very skilled at applying the proper care and communicating treatment options to the patient. However, if the patient fails to follow through on behavior modifications and medical therapy, then he will not have good long-term outcome. Thus, QOC measurement would be incomplete if provider skills and facility amenities were evaluated without considering patient contributions.

In addition to QOC assessment indicators, clinicians have practice guidelines and consensus statements to aid in achieving superior care quality. Both resources are usually generated by professional societies or governmental agencies and serve to consolidate medical information rather than to measure QOC.[42] Clinical practice guidelines (CPGs) are evidence-based practice recommendations that may be used by health care providers in creating or gauging individual treatment plans. These guidelines are geared toward quality improvement and minimization of treatment variation. Users may interject clinical judgment and seek to improve on the knowledge contained in such guidelines. Thus, CPGs are an internal mechanism used to strive for optimal care. Conversely, QOC measures are sets of carefully selected and specific indicators designed to evaluate particular care components of interest. QOC indicators are generally used externally, either outside of a department or an institution, to make performance ratings and to compare such ratings with other departments or institutions.[43] Standardization is critical for quality assurance comparison purposes. The goal of QOC assessment is to improve any structure, process, or outcome criteria deemed less than adequate. Thus, if CPGs are being used routinely, QOC assessment may measure some CPG components.

Arguably one of the earliest and best-known QOC initiatives, the Health Plan Employer Data and Information Set (HEDIS), was established in 1989 by a coalition of private health care providers and large companies.[31,44,45] As the first of its kind, HEDIS uses measures from the National Committee of Quality Assurance (NCQA) to prepare quality report cards on chronic medical conditions for privately insured patients.[46] The attributes measured in HEDIS include health care access, effectiveness, patient satisfaction with experience of care, health care plan stability, use of service, and care cost. Examples of the effectiveness of care evaluated include the following: adulthood and childhood immunization rates; screening for colorectal, cervical, and breast cancers; control of high blood pressure and β-blocker treatment after an acute myocardial infarction; and comprehensive diabetes care. Service use measures include well-child visits, chemical dependency and mental health care use, frequency of selected procedures, and rate of hospitalization. Although HEDIS measurements focus on common chronic medical conditions, BPH and other urologic conditions have not been included.

QUALITY OF CARE ASSESSMENT IN SURGERY

Results on the effects of surgeon and hospital volume have been equivocal and appear to depend on data sources. Studies using administrative databases have generally found relationships between hospital or surgeon volume and outcome. Birkmeyer and colleagues[8] studied the relationship between mortality rates and surgeon as well as hospital volumes for cardiac and cancer surgical procedures reported in Medicare databases. Mortality was inversely related to hospital volume for all 14 surgical procedures studied. However, even when comparing very low-volume to very high-volume hospitals, the strength of that relationship varied immensely among surgical procedures.[8]

With further study, Birkmeyer and associates[7] found that it was actually surgeon volume that was responsible for hospital volume effects. Surgeon volume was significantly related to mortality rates for all eight surgical procedures studied ($P = .003$ for lung resection and $P < .001$ for all other procedures).[7] Furthermore, high surgeon volume related to positive outcomes for coronary artery bypass graft (CABG) surgery,[47,48] whereas high hospital volume related to decreased mortality for CABG[49] and cancer[50] operations as well as for RP.[51] Significant effects of both high surgeon and hospital volumes on decreased mortality were detected in the need for CABG with percutaneous coronary interventions (PCIs),[52] CABG,[53,54] and cancer operations.[55-57] Although CABG mortality rates decreased with increased hospital volume, Peterson and colleagues[49] emphasized that the large variability among similar-volume hospitals in risk-adjusted mortality may have limited the strength of the volume-outcome relationship.

Although the strength of the volume-outcome argument continues to be debated, Joudi and Konety[58] concluded that support continues to grow for the theory that better outcomes occur at high-volume versus low-volume hospitals. However, the results of the majority of the studies evaluated were based on administrative databases. Thus, the weight of these studies in the volume debate may be limited.

An example of a surgical QOC assessment program is the National Surgical Quality Improvement Program (NSQIP) of the U.S. Department of Veterans Affairs Health Administration, which was implemented in 1995.[59] The goal of this program is facility-wide QOC improvement.[60] Evidence-based, reliable, and valid quality indicators are applied to the measurement of care quality. The NSQIP uses presurgical risk factors, prospective surgical care processes, and risk-adjusted outcomes for 30-day morbidity and mortality as QOC indicators.[59] This program also provides self-assessment tools, structured site visits, performance assessment, outcome based, site-specific and comparative reports, and provision of best practice information.[61] Applicability to nonfederal hospitals was demonstrated.[62,63] As the lead investigators from the NSQIP, Khuri and Henderson[64] pointed out the inherent problems in using administrative databases to evaluate outcome, including limited case-mix information, missing or incomplete data including that on comorbidities, lack of follow-up and functional status information, and lack of surgical risk data (i.e., cancer grade and stage, albumin level, and hypotension).[53,65] Scott and colleagues[66] stressed the importance of risk adjustment and demonstrating validity of indicators based on administrative data. These investigators stated that any diagnostic indicator of systematic variation must not be attributed to factors other than case-mix and random error. Such indicators need to be validated with risk adjustment before they are applied to the determination of hospital care quality.

Structural indicators, other than surgeon and hospital volume, and relation to outcome have been explored as surgical quality indicators. Researchers investigated the effects on outcome of hospital credentialing, hospital type, and presence of specialty clinics and services as well as surgeon age, degree of specialization, Board certification, and experience. Again, most of the studies used administrative databases and thus the results should be validated with prospective study before specific conclusions are reached. Although Simunovic and colleagues[50] found no difference in cancer surgical outcomes between teaching hospitals and nonteaching hospitals, Yuan and associates[67] demonstrated a mortality hierarchy (osteopathic → teaching public → public [nonteaching] → for-profit → not–for-profit [nonteaching]) when hospitals were grouped based on both type and financial status. For 10 common surgical procedures, 30-day and 6-month mortality rates were superior in teaching not–for-profit hospitals when compared with all other hospital types.

Hospital credentialing did not affect morbidity or mortality of surgical outcomes.[68] Surgical mortality rates were higher for older surgeons, who generally perform fewer CABG surgical procedures when compared with their younger counterparts.[69] Specialized surgeons treating ovarian cancer had better outcomes than did general surgeons performing the same operations.[70] Prospective studies indicated that full-time trauma surgeons had better surgical outcomes for head injury than did surgeons serving part time on a trauma service[71] and that the percentage of Board-certified surgeons was inversely related to mortality rates for transurethral resection of the prostate (TURP).[72] Wennberg and colleagues[4] found that patients in a nonemergency situation who received PCIs at hospitals without an onsite CABG surgery unit were more likely to die than were patients at a hospital with such a unit ($P < .001$). The majority of deaths occurred at hospitals where physicians performed <50 Medicare PCIs annually. Silber and associates[73] ranked hospitals based on predetermined characteristics thought to influence care quality. Complication and mortality rates were only weakly associated with hospital quality. Daley and colleagues[74] found that, based on site visits, hospitals with less than expected morbidity and mortality rates had significantly more and technologically better equipment and superior QOC when compared with hospitals with greater than expected poor outcomes.

Research has been relatively limited on the use of process indicators for the evaluation of surgical care quality. Stevenson and colleagues[75] conducted a prospective study of admissions to an acute surgical service. These investigators focused on process indicators, including documentation, general management, and processes specific for admission diagnosis, during the initial 24 hours following admission. Quality of a sample of specific processes was also measured. A baseline composite process score was calculated without staff knowledge. Then, following a brief period of observation, three interventions were conducted: active observation (staff members were informed that they were being observed), increasing awareness (through questionnaire), and provision of job descriptions. Results demonstrated overall process quality improvement when compared with baseline ($P < .001$). Only the second and third interventions affected process quality ($P < .001$ for all three major processes). The investigators concluded that processes involved in acute surgical care are measurable quality indicators.[75]

In 1997, Ashton and associates[19] conducted a meta-analysis of studies on process indicators and patient-specific readmissions. Less than acceptable standards were associated with a 55% increased risk of readmission when compared with normal or acceptable processes. QOC was associated with readmission when the process of care was actually studied.

QUALITY OF CARE ASSESSMENT IN UROLOGY

Prostate Cancer

Prostate cancer remains the most commonly diagnosed noncutaneous malignant disease and leads to as many male cancer-related deaths as does colon cancer.[76] Since the late 1980s, therapies for localized prostate cancer have proliferated, but RP and radiation therapies remain the mainstays. Although randomized clinical trials examining the efficacy of such therapies have been limited,[77] the general paucity of level I clinical evidence for various definitive therapies has resulted in significant variations in the utilization of RP, a situation that raises important questions regarding quality discrepancies.[78-81]

To date, several studies of Medicare data have attempted to measure RP quality.[82] Using data from the first half of the 1990s, Yao and coworkers[83] reported serious complications, defined by author consensus, in 26% to 31% of cases despite an overall mortality rate of <1%. Although definitions vary, other investigators have reported complications following prostatectomy to be in the same range.[84]

In 2002, Begg and colleagues[85] presented a highly publicized study in which Surveillance, Epidemiology and End Results (SEER) Medicare-linked data were used to evaluate postprostatectomy urinary strictures and incontinence. Based on the records of >11,000 cases between 1992 and 1996, the researchers empirically demonstrated that higher hospital and surgeon volumes were associated with fewer postoperative urinary complications.[85] Recognizing that such variation may be explained, at least partially, by confounding patient and disease characteristics, the investigators specifically included case-mix adjustment. The findings suggested that the disparate outcomes may have reflected differences in QOC. This study was a wake-up call for urologists who had largely been complacent when it came to QOC self-assessment. Given the large number of patients who select active treatment, the need for formal evaluation of QOC for localized prostate cancer is particularly relevant.

Initial efforts at QOC assessments for localized prostate cancer were led by Mark Litwin and colleagues at the University of California–Los Angeles (UCLA) and the RAND Corporation,[86] who used established methodology to develop a comprehensive set of quality indicators. The RAND indicators were designed to assess the spectrum of early-stage prostate cancer care, to evaluate multiple practitioners accountable for patient care, and to allow for aggregation of the quality measures at the systems level. Using methodology and infrastructure previously developed at RAND and based on the Donabedian paradigm, the investigators employed literature review, patient focus groups, expert interviews, and a RAND consensus panel to establish a measurement framework with a group of indicators proposed for use in quality assessment.[87] Table 19-1 summarizes the RAND quality indicators for prostate cancer. Candidate quality indicators included measures of structure (e.g., hospital volume and Board certification of providers), process (e.g., pretreatment referrals and preoperative testing), and outcome (e.g., multiple survival end points, as well as patient assessment of post-therapy urinary, bowel, and sexual function using validated instruments).

Once developed, it was imperative that this set of indicators be field tested before wider dissemination. Feasibility and sensitivity of this set of proposed quality indicators were empirically examined in different clinical settings across several institutions.[88] Miller and colleagues[88] found that compliance measurement was generally feasible for 19 of the 22 (86%) quality indicators assessed. Measurement of compliance was possible for several of the structural indicators (e.g., number of patients treated, availability of conformal radiation therapy) because such indicators simply reflect available institutional resources and services. For most of the remaining structure, process, and outcome measures, assessment of compliance was feasible using a combination of thorough explicit official medical record or institutional electronic database review. Significant differences in compliance were detected for five indicators between the 1995 and 2000. In sum, this study established that measurement of a subset of the RAND quality indicators for localized prostate cancer is realistic in a clinical hospital setting. Furthermore, the demonstration of variation in compliance with several indicators between 1995 and 2000 exemplifies the presumed ability of such indicators to detect QOC changes over time.[88]

In a separate setting, Krupski and colleagues[89] examined the feasibility of measuring RAND indicators in a convenience sample of men with prostate cancer drawn from IMPACT (IMProving Access, Counseling, and Treatment for Californians with prostate cancer), a program funded by the California Department of Public Health. Using a combination of chart review, administrative documents, and patient questionnaires, the researchers concluded that measurement was feasible for most of the RAND indicators.

TABLE 19-1 RAND Prostate Cancer Quality of Care Indicators

Indicator Class	Indicators	Definition of Indicator Compliance or Outcome
Structural Resources	≥1 Board-certified urologist	Hospitals with ≥1 Board-certified urologist
	≥1 Board-certified radiation oncologist	Hospitals with ≥1 Board-certified radiation oncologist
	Conformal radiation therapy available	Hospitals with 3-dimensional conformal radiation facilities
	Psychological counseling available	Hospitals with psychological counseling services available on site
	Treatment at a center with high prostate cancer case volume (top quartile)	Hospitals in the top quartile of total prostate cancer case volume
Processes of Care	DRE	Documentation of DRE by treating physician within 6 mo before treatment date
	PSA blood test	Documentation of pretreatment PSA test result by treating physician within 6 mo before treatment date
	Pathologic grading with Gleason sum	Documentation of biopsy Gleason grade/sum by treating physician within 6 mo before treatment date
	Clinical stage	Documentation of clinical stage by treating physician within 6 mo before treatment date
	Family history of prostate cancer	Documentation of family history of prostate cancer (positive or negative) by treating physician within 6 mo before or 3 mo following the treatment date
	Comorbidity	Documentation of comorbid diseases by treating physician within 6 mo before treatment date
	Urinary function	Documentation of pretreatment urinary function by treating physician within 6 mo before treatment date
	Sexual function	Documentation of pretreatment sexual function by treating physician within 6 mo before treatment date
	Bowel function	Documentation of pretreatment bowel function by treating physician within 6 mo before treatment date
	Communication with PCP	Documentation by treating physician or PCP of communication between them 6 mo before or 6 mo following treatment date
	Discussion of treatment options	Documentation of discussion of treatment options between patient and treating physician within 6 mo before treatment date
	Discussion of risks of treatment	Documentation of discussion of risks of planned treatment between patient and treating physician within 6 mo before treatment date
	2+ follow-up office visits	Documentation of at least 2 follow-up office visits to treating physician within 6 mo following completion of treatment
	Tumor size	Documentation of primary tumor size by pathologist in surgical pathology report
	Tumor location	Documentation of primary tumor location by pathologist in surgical pathology report
	Pathologic stage	Documentation of pathologic stage by pathologist in surgical pathology report
	Pathologic Gleason sum	Documentation of pathologic Gleason sum by pathologist in surgical pathology report
	Surgical margins	Documentation of surgical margin status by pathologist in surgical pathology report
	Seminal vesicle involvement	Documentation of presence or absence of seminal vesicle invasion by pathologist in surgical pathology report
	Capsular penetration	Documentation of presence or absence of capsular penetration by pathologist in surgical pathology report
	Total radiation dose ≥70 Gy (conformal)	Documentation of total radiation dose administered >70 Gy for conformal external beam radiation
	CT planning	Documentation of results of a CT scan of the pelvis performed specifically for the purpose of radiation treatment planning
	Patient immobilization	Documentation that patient was immobilized during administration of external beam radiation
	Rectal protection (conformal)	Documentation that shaping of the radiation beam for conformal radiation therapy selectively spared the rectum
	High-energy accelerator	Documentation that the linear accelerator used for radiation therapy exceeded 10 MV
Outcomes	High estimated blood loss	
	Prolonged length of stay	
	Any surgery complication	
	Surgery treatment failure	
	Any radiation complication	
	Radiation treatment failure	

CT, computed tomography; DRE, digital rectal examination; PCP, primary care physician; PSA, prostate-specific antigen.

Adapted from Litwin M, Steinberg M, Malin J, et al. *Prostate Cancer Patient Outcomes and Choice of Providers: Development of an Infrastructure for Quality Assessment.* Monograph MR1227. Santa Monica, CA: RAND Corporation; 2005.

Taking an important step toward the objective of validating a measurable set of quality indicators for prostate cancer treatment, the American College of Surgeons (ACOS), in collaboration with investigators from University of Michigan and UCLA, approved a special study, the first of its kind, designed to assess quality, as measured by a subset of the RAND indicators, on a national level. This ongoing investigation is supported both financially and administratively by the Commission on Cancer of the ACOS. The purpose of this study is to measure QOC for localized prostate cancer across a national sample of ACOS-accredited cancer programs using a subset of the RAND candidate quality indicators.

More recently, the American Urological Association (AUA) served as lead organization for the development of prostate cancer measures through the Physician Consortium for Performance Improvement (PCPI) of the American Medical Association (AMA). This effort was informed by prior work summarized earlier and by the AUA's *Guideline for the Management of Clinically Localized Prostate Cancer: 2007 Update*.[90] These prostate cancer indicators, now approved by the AUA Board and the Ambulatory Quality Alliance (AQA), are available at http://www.prostateline.com/treatment-guidelines/18265?itemId-2617494&nav-yes. This physician performance measurement set consists of five accountability measures for evaluation, diagnosis, and specific treatments of prostate cancer and one quality improvement measure. Calculations for individual performances are described for each measure and may be applied to individual physicians, practices, and institutions.

Benign Prostatic Hyperplasia

The prevalence of BPH and its significant economic costs to the U.S. health care system have led to increasing scrutiny in QOC and patient outcomes for this condition. Much literature has been devoted to the description of practice pattern variation and associated suboptimal outcomes.

The Veterans Affairs NSQIP, a prospective assessment of noncardiac surgical procedures, allowed for risk-adjusted morbidity and mortality by patient presurgical risk factors and process of care during surgery to enhance surgical quality.[59] In this study, TURP was the most common operation performed. Similarly, another NSQIP study demonstrated prolonged length of stay for TURP that was related to identified preoperative risk factors such as nonwhite race, poor functional status, prostate-specific antigen levels of 3 or 4, older age, and prolonged operative duration.[91]

Such variations in practice patterns and complication rates have led to research and assessment of candidate quality indicators and outcome measures for BPH. Some investigators have also proposed risk-adjusted outcomes suited for assessing surgical quality.[92] Operative mortality is a readily available and validated risk factor that has been used to measure quality. However, risk-adjusted surgical mortality may have limited application to BPH treated with TURP, given the low BPH-associated mortality rate. Moreover, the natural progression of BPH rarely affects overall survival rate. Therefore, BPH treatment decisions are typically driven by quality of life considerations.

In surgical procedures with low operative mortality, such as TURP, risk-adjusted functional outcome assessment is arguably a more appropriate method for assessing surgical quality compared with operative mortality. Functional outcome assessments focus on patient satisfaction and cost effectiveness of surgical care as quality measures. Such assessment is also generalizable to BPH treatments with differing costs, disease progression, and quality of life.[93] Moreover, if poor surgical quality results in increased mortality, the ever rising cost of health care will be viewed as a critical component of quality.

The Assessing the Care of Vulnerable Elders (ACOVE) project, a collaboration between RAND Health and Pfizer, is a one of a kind initiative with a goal to develop quality assessment tools for elderly patient care.[94] Specifically, the ACOVE project was formulated with the following objectives: to improve care for *vulnerable elders*, defined as community-living individuals >65 years of age; to identify important and common medical conditions, including BPH, with effective available prevention and management options; to develop evidence-based QOC; and to design validated methods for implementing and measuring the quality indicators. In the ACOVE study, clinical guidelines and care indicators were designed for each of 22 conditions. Initially, experts on each condition provided content feedback as well as suggestions for QOC criteria. Validation was conducted with extensive review of relevant literature.

Other resources used in the creation of clinical guidelines included the Computerized Needs-Oriented Quality Improvement (CONQUEST),[95] DEMPAQ: A Project to Develop and Evaluate Methods to Promote Ambulatory Care Quality,[96] the AMA Directory of Clinical Practice Guidelines,[97] HEDIS,[98] the National Guideline Clearinghouse, the National Library of Healthcare Indicators of the Joint Commission,[99] the Administration on Aging, the Agency for Healthcare Policy and Research, the Centers for Disease Control and Prevention, the Health Care Financing Administration, and the National Committee for Quality Assurance. Potential quality measures were framed as *if-then-because* models. The *if* specified condition-specific clinical characteristics, the *then* referred to the process of obtaining the quality indicator, and the *because* reflected the outcome of the quality indicator. An example of the structure of this fully branched criteria format is displayed in **Figure 19-2.** Thus, the ACOVE methodology employed the Donabedian model of QOC with an emphasis on the process and outcome criteria.

Once potential quality indicators were fitted into the if-then-because format, a literature review was completed to support the link between the quality indicator and outcome. Emphasis to support the relationship between process and outcome criteria was based on randomized controlled trials and prospective studies. Using the modified RAND/UCLA Appropriateness Method,[100,101] the potential quality indicators were rated for scientific validity. The final set of quality indicators was then based on expert panel consensus.

Three phases of ACOVE have been completed to date. Urinary incontinence was one of the 22 conditions covered in ACOVE-1. Process criteria domains included screening, prevention, diagnosis, treatment, follow-up, and continuity.[102] The ACOVE-2 study focused on the development of tests and interventions to aid physicians in adhering to specific quality indictors, including that for urinary incontinence.[103] With ACOVE-3,[104] the number of conditions was expanded to 26, including BPH. Quality indicators were proposed for diagnosis and treatment of BPH in individuals ≥65 years old at risk of functional decline and death. Candidate indicator development for BPH was based on review of clinical guidelines and expert opinion. Criteria were exclusively process measures that, by prespecification, demonstrated significant impacts on patient outcome. A process similar to that used in creation of the original 22 quality indicators was applied toward the development of BPH criteria. Tables 19-2 and 19-3 summarize the final set of quality indicators for BPH evaluation and treatment, respectively, constructed in ACOVE-3.[104]

CONCLUSION

Surgeons have been reporting complications since morbidity and mortality conferences were first introduced. However, complications as an outcome, although undeniably important, represent just one component of quality assessment. It is possible to provide good-quality care and still have complications. Historically, surgeons reported risk-adjusted[105] outcomes as the sole QOC element. This was largely because outcomes are easy to measure and data may typically be obtained from hospital databases. Although problematic for most procedures because of low prevalences, morbidity and mortality are the most frequently used surgical outcome indicators.[106] However, other outcome indicators may be more applicable for the majority of urologic and other surgical procedures.

Access to care, quality of life and functional status,[41] patient satisfaction,[41,107] cost effectiveness, and resource use have been mentioned as more expansive outcome measures that could be applied to surgery.[108] Treurniet and associates addressed the use of health-related quality of life indicators to measure outcome.[109] These investi-

TABLE 19-2	Assessing the Care of Vulnerable Elders: Three Quality of Care Indicators for Benign Prostatic Hypertrophy Evaluation

Initial LUTS Evaluation
Complete medical history, including:
   Dietary history
   Neurologic disease evaluation
   Surgical history (urologic, neurologic, orthopedic, and general)
Medication list
UA
AUASI score

Additional Testing by History
LUTS and complex medical history
   PVR >300 mL: refer for urodynamic testing and cystoscopy
LUTS and history of lower urinary tract surgery
   Refer to urologist
LUTS and microscopic hematuria
   Repeat UA in 1 mo
   Positive 2 of 3 UA: refer to urologist
   Serum creatinine
   Upper urinary tract imaging
   Urine cytology

AUASI, American Urological Association Symptom Index; LUTS, lower urinary tract symptoms; PVR, postvoiding residual; UA, urinalysis.
Adapted from Shekelle PG, MacLean CH, Morton SC, et al. Assessing care of vulnerable elders: methods for developing quality indicators. *Ann Intern Med.* 2001;185(8 Pt 2):647-652.

TABLE 19-3	Assessing the Care of Vulnerable Elders: Three Quality Indicators for Benign Prostatic Hypertrophy Treatment

AUASI Score	Treatment
≤7	Watchful waiting
>7 (no bother)	Watchful waiting
>7 + bother	Medical therapy (α-blockers, 5α-reductase inhibitors) Surgical treatment (radical prostatectomy, transurethral prostatic resection)

AUASI, American Urological Association Symptom Index.
Adapted from Shekelle PG, MacLean CH, Morton SC, et al. Assessing care of vulnerable elders: methods for developing quality indicators. *Ann Intern Med.* 2001;185(8 Pt 2):647-652.

gators stressed the importance of establishing a validated relationship between process and outcome as well as the use of prospectively collected data to augment that of clinical databases.

According to Peskin,[109] QOC assessment has been particularly difficult for surgeons. The importance of understanding relationships among structure, process, and outcome to creating a valid quality indicator is well understood. However, most researchers have not yet established the strength of such associations when measuring surgical care quality. Structure and process indicators have been largely ignored, whereas outcomes based on morbidity and mortality have been the primary QOC measures for surgical procedures.[109] Hammermeister and associates[110] noted the inadequacies of relying solely on outcome-based quality indicators, mortality in particular, in assessing quality of surgical care, including the small number of deaths providing limited power for statistical analyses, the difficulty in measuring nonfatal outcomes, and the chance of failing to capture long-term outcomes. Nevertheless, most QOC research to date in urology has focused only on hospital and surgeon volume indicators.

With the current exponential growth of health care costs, we should anticipate that interest in health services delivery, as a major cost center, will only increase. By participating in larger efforts such as PCPI and PQRI, urologists will have greater input on national policies related to health care delivery. Failure by urologists to participate in the development and implementation of QOC programs could result in significant financial penalties to individual physicians and institutions. More importantly, if urology as a specialty ignores the impending QOC trends and national efforts, it is likely that other nonurologic specialty interests will prevail and will increasingly dictate urologic care.

KEY POINTS

1. Decreased mortality rates and fewer complications have been well documented in hospitals with high surgical volume, a finding that supports the concept of centers for excellence.
2. Outcome is the presumed result of core processes and is often considered the quality indicator of most value to the patient.
3. Studies using administrative databases have generally found relationships between hospital or surgeon volume and outcome.
4. The general paucity of level I clinical evidence for various definitive therapies has resulted in significant variations in the utilization of RP, a finding that raises important questions regarding quality discrepancies.
5. BPH treatment decisions are typically driven by quality of life considerations.

REFERENCES

Please see www.expertconsult.com

Chapter 20

COMPLICATIONS OF THE INCISION AND PATIENT POSITIONING

Matthew K. Tollefson MD
Fellow in Urologic Oncology, Department of Urology, Mayo Clinic, Rochester, Minnesota

Stephen A. Boorjian MD
Fellow in Urologic Oncology, Department of Urology, Mayo Clinic, Rochester, Minnesota

Bradley C. Leibovich MD
Associate Professor, Department of Urology, Mayo Clinic, Rochester, Minnesota

Successful surgical therapy depends on proper healing of the surgical wound. Problems with wound healing can lead to seromas, hematomas, surgical site infections (SSIs), dehiscence, and incisional hernias. In addition, nerve injuries related to patient positioning or retractor placement may affect postoperative mobility. All these complications increase morbidity and can contribute to mortality in surgical patients.

Complications related to the incision are important for all surgeons to be aware of because they are among the most common complications following operative procedures. Often, these complications are relatively minor and may resolve with conservative management (e.g., simple wound seromas or hematomas). However, at times they may be expensive and time-consuming (e.g., complicated wound infection), may require additional surgical procedures (e.g., incisional hernia), or may cause permanent disability (e.g., postoperative neurapraxia). Therefore, management of these complications is focused on prevention, as well as prompt recognition and appropriate treatment. The objective of this chapter is to review common complications of the incision with respect to their pathogenesis, clinical features, prevention, and management.

SEROMA

Pathogenesis and Clinical Features

One of the most common and likely underreported complications following operative procedures is the development of a wound seroma. Although typically a benign finding, when not treated, seromas may lead to more serious wound infections, wound breakdown, or potentially skin necrosis. A *seroma* is a collection of sterile, clear, ultrafiltrated serum, lymphatic fluid, or liquified fat.[1] The fluid is usually clear, amber, and slightly viscous. Seromas are located under the incision, above the fascial layer, and directly beneath the dermis of the skin. They are more likely to occur when large tissue flaps are mobilized or when extensive lymphadenectomy is performed, such as during axillary[2] or inguinal lymph node dissection.[3] Thus, efforts to limit the extent of dissection where feasible without compromising cancer control such as sentinal lymph node procedures[4] or preservation of the saphenous vein during inguinal lymphadenectomy[5,6] may reduce the risk of seroma formation.

Prevention and Management

Most postoperative seromas are discovered incidentally and require no active intervention. However, when large or symptomatic, seromas can be evacuated by opening the overlying skin edges, packing the wound with sterile saline-soaked gauze, and allowing the wound to heal by second intention. Seromas that develop under flaps (i.e., after inguinal lymph node dissection), however, may be more difficult to manage because these have the potential to damage the delicate vascular supply to the flap. Therefore, in incisions that involve extensive skin flaps, placement of closed-suction drains is typically performed and recommended. These drains are left in place until their output decreases to a minimal amount (typically <30 mL in a 24-hour period). Pressure dressings may be useful postoperatively when seroma formation is of concern. Occasionally, premature removal of the drains may allow a seroma to develop, and percutaneous aspiration or drain placement may be required.

HEMATOMOA

Pathogenesis and Clinical Features

A *hematoma* is a collection of blood in or near a recent surgical incision. Hematomas typically occur in the subcutaneous space, but they may also occur deeper in the incision, such as in the rectus sheath. Wound hematomas are most often caused by inadequate hemostasis after the skin has been closed. Many factors contribute to the formation of hematomas. First, hemostasis at the time of wound closure may be inadequate. Extra care should be taken in patients who are hypotensive or in shock at the time of wound closure. Additionally, the use of epinephrine may mask small bleeding vessels during closure. Postoperatively, anticoagulants such as aspirin, nonsteroidal anti-inflammatory drugs, heparin, and warfarin also increase the likelihood of postoperative bleeding and therefore should be used with care in the perioperative period. Finally, a host of disease processes may be present that may predispose patients to the development of hematomas, including myeloproliferative disorders, renal or hepatic insufficiency, deficiency of clotting factors, and platelet dysfunction.

Hematomas usually manifest by ecchymosis of the overlying skin, localized wound swelling, pain or pressure, and drainage of blood from the surgical site. These hematomas can often track significant distances from the surgical site. The diagnosis can be confirmed by inspection, palpation, and gentle probing of the wound. If these measures prove insufficient, ultrasound evaluation can be useful to delineate the hematoma.[7] In addition, large rectus sheath hematomas may manifest with signs of significant hemorrhage, including hemodynamic shock. Often these hematomas result in large ecchymoses that track subcutaneously a long distance from the patient's surgical site. Large hematomas that collect in the retroperitoneum or rectus sheath may cause paralytic ileus, anemia, and ongoing bleeding resulting from the consumption of coagulation factors. One of the most common problems associated with the development of a surgical hematoma is the risk of secondary infection. Blood is a good medium for growth of bacteria that may infiltrate the hematoma and result in a substantial SSI.

Prevention and Management

The most important factor in the prevention of wound hematoma is meticulous hemostasis at the time of closure of the subcutaneous tissue. Prevention is also facilitated by correction of all clotting abnormalities preoperatively and by discontinuing all medications that can prolong the bleeding time. In addition, wounds that involve large skin flaps or those with large potential spaces in which blood could collect should be drained with a closed-suction surgical drain until the output of these drains decreases. Management of wound hematomas is similar to management of wound seromas, discussed earlier.

SURGICAL SITE INFECTION

Since the development of modern surgical technique and the innovations of Joseph Lister, surgeons have battled microbial infection. However, despite advances in antimicrobial therapy, aseptic technique, and perioperative patient management, SSIs continue to be the most common infectious complications suffered by surgical patients. Monitoring for these complications is even more complex because shorter hospital stays, outpatient surgery, and the mobility of patients who often see several physicians during the recovery period may affect the rates of complication reporting.[8] In healthy, nonobese patients, the overall SSI rate is estimated at 2.5% of all open surgical procedures, whereas this rate can be many-fold higher in patients with additional risk factors.

The impact of these infections is not insignificant. From an economic standpoint, patients with SSI often require extended hospital stays, additional nursing care, wound supplies, and possibly additional surgical procedures.[9] The estimated cost of this additional care can exceed $30,000 in patients with complicated infections.[10] Moreover, SSIs have significant quality of life implications for patients who may require weeks to months of additional treatment following a surgical procedure. Finally, some series have linked SSIs to an overall increase in postoperative mortality.[11,12]

Definition

The term *surgical site infection* distinguishes a postoperative infection from a traumatic wound infection. The Centers for Disease Control and Prevention (CDC) developed a universal nomenclature for SSIs that involves categorization according to the depth of infection (**Fig. 20-1**).[13] Infections that are confined to the skin and subcutaneous tissue (above the fascia) are considered *superficial incisional SSIs*. These infections account for the majority of all SSIs. Infections that involve the deep soft tissue (below the fascia) are termed *deep incisional SSIs*. Deep incisional SSIs include postoperative necrotizing fasciitis and osteomyelitis. Finally, an infection that involves an organ space that was manipulated during a procedure is termed an *organ space SSI*. Organ space SSIs may include peritonitis or other infections that involve the cavitary space entered during the procedure. By definition, these infections are diagnosed within 30 days of the procedure. An exception to this rule is the case of implanted material, when SSIs are recorded up to 1 year from the surgical procedure and appear to be related to the operation.[13]

Risk Stratification

The development of an SSI depends on complex interactions between the pathogenic organism and the host's local and systemic defense mechanisms. Factors influencing the pathogenic organism include the virulence of the contaminating organism itself and the number of organisms inoculated into the wound. In 1964, the National Research Council (NRC) of the National Academy of Sciences reported on a study designed to evaluate the effect of ultraviolet irradiation on postoperative infections.[14] Although this study did not reach its desired end point, it was the first effort to categorize incisions based on the estimated degree of bacterial contamination. The four categories of incision described by the NRC (Table 20-1) remain the most widely accepted classification of surgical wounds to date, and the system remains useful to estimate the risk of SSI, predict pathogens, and determine the need for antimicrobial prophylaxis. This effort represented the first connection between the contaminating flora at various surgical sites and the subsequent infecting pathogens.

Class I, or clean, wounds: Those wounds in which only skin flora are likely to contaminate the operative field because no hollow viscus has been entered. The risk of infection in these cases is low (0.5%-2%). A subset of class I wounds, class I_D, consists of wounds in which prosthetic material is implanted. These wounds are classified differently because although the incidence of infection is also low, the consequences of the infection can be dire and may obviate the entire purpose of the procedure.

Class II, or clean-contaminated, wounds: Those wounds in which a hollow viscus likely to harbor bacteria is entered under controlled circumstances. In these cases, both skin flora and microbes within the viscus may contribute to the SSI and thus the incidence of infection is higher (2%-5%).

Class III, or contaminated, wounds: Those wounds in which substantial microbial contamination exists and the risk of infection is even greater (5%-15%), particularly if the skin is closed.

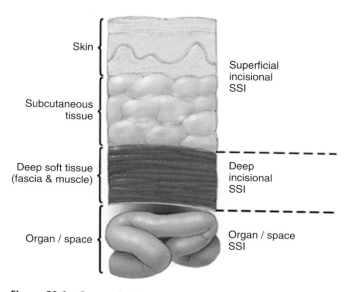

Figure 20-1 Centers for Disease Control and Prevention classification of SSI. Superficial incisional SSIs are limited to skin and subcutaneous tissues and deep incisional SSIs involve muscle and fascia, whereas organ space SSIs include infections within the cavitary space of the procedure. (Copyright © 2007, Mayo.)

TABLE 20-1	Surgical Wound Classification		
Classification	**Wound Description**	**Example**	**Definition**
Class I	Clean	Varicocele ligation; herniorrhaphy	An uninfected operative wound in which no inflammation is encountered and the respiratory, alimentary, or uninfected genitourinary tract is not entered; in addition, clean wounds are primarily closed and, if necessary, drained with closed drainage
Class I_D	Clean; prosthetic material implanted	Penile prosthesis implantation	Same as class I (clean), with the exception of placement of prosthetic material
Class II	Clean-contaminated	Radical prostatectomy	Operative wounds in which the respiratory, alimentary, or genitourinary tract is entered under controlled circumstances and with minimal contamination
Class III	Contaminated	Radical cystectomy with stool spillage	Open, fresh, accidental wounds; in addition, wounds with a major break in sterile technique or gross spillage from the gastrointestinal tract and incisions in which acute nonpurulent inflammation is encountered
Class IV	Dirty/infected	Perineal débridement for Fournier's gangrene	Old, traumatic wounds with devitalized tissue and those in which purulent infection is encountered

Class IV, or dirty/infected, wounds: Those wounds in which the wound is infected preoperatively and the organisms causing the postoperative infection are presumed to be present before the surgical procedure.

In an effort to improve this risk stratification for SSIs, the CDC introduced the National Nosocomial Infection Surveillance (NNIS) risk index.[15] The NNIS risk index incorporates additional patient- and procedure-related factors into the previously described wound classification. It is operation specific and assigns points based on patient-related risk factors (as defined by the American Society of Anesthesiologists preoperative assessment score), the duration of the operation, and the degree of microbial contamination of the incision. The duration of the operation is important because lengthy procedures may result in increased exposure to microbial contamination as well as compromised local defenses resulting from dessication, hypothermia, and lower concentrations of prophylactic antibiotics.

Since the NNIS risk index was produced, additional risk factors for SSIs have been identified. For example, hypothermia has been identified as an independent risk factor for infection, and therefore maintenance of normothermia is an important aspect of intraoperative and postoperative care.[16] Strict glucose control has been independently associated with decreased wound infection rates as well as with decreased mortality in an intensive care setting.[17] Serum albumin level has long been identified as an important risk factor because it reflects a wide range of comorbid conditions that contribute to wound healing.[18] Other important risk factors are age, vascular insufficiency, diabetes, radiation, preoperative smoking, and obesity.

Microbiology

Endogenous pathogenic organisms implicated in SSI most commonly come from the patient's skin, alimentary tract, or genitourinary tract. The patient's microflora may be altered by preoperative admission to the hospital. In fact, a demonstrable shift in the microbial environment toward more resistant bacterial species occurs within 48 to 72 hours of hospital admission.[9,19] Exogenous contamination can be minimized by strictly following aseptic technique and maintaining a sterile operating room environment.

The most common organisms isolated from surgical sites remain gram-positive cocci, specifically *Staphylococcus aureus* (Table 20-2). However, gram-negative infections are common in class II wounds. It is important to recognize the type of infection associated with various operative sites to select appropriate antimicrobial prophylaxis.

TABLE 20-2	Prevalence of Organisms Isolated From Surgical Sites	
Organism	**Percentage (%)**
Staphylococcus aureus	26.9
Escherichia coli	18.8
Streptococcus epidermidis	10.1
Pseudomonas aeruginosa	9.6
Enterococcus faecalis	3.8
Enterococcus faecium	3.8
Proteus mirabilis	3.4
Candida albicans	3.0
Klebsiella pneumoniae	1.5

Prevention

Preoperative and Intraoperative Techniques

Prevention of infection in the surgical wound begins by reducing the potential number of microbial contaminants that have access to the wound. Therefore, whenever possible, one should identify and treat all infections before surgical intervention. As discussed earlier, lengthy preoperative hospitalizations can increase bacterial antimicrobial resistance and can make any future SSIs more difficult to manage.[19] Patients should be encouraged to stop use of tobacco products for ≥30 days before the operation.[20]

The value of preoperative bowel preparation for reducing SSIs has been debated because several randomized trials[21-24] and meta-analyses[25] demonstrated an increased rate of anastomotic leakage and wound complications when mechanical bowel preparations were used. Indeed, evidence indicates that preoperative bowel preparation is associated with increased stool spillage intraoperatively.[26] Adequate bowel preparation, however, decreases operative time by improving bowel handling during construction of the anastomosis and reducing the need for intraoperative bowel cleaning. Additionally, it may be helpful in patients who require abdominal exploration for identification of metastatic sites of malignant disease. Therefore, we continue to employ mechanical bowel preparation for all intra-abdominal procedures and may use an antibiotic preparation as well when an intestinal surgical procedure is planned (i.e., urinary diversion).

When the patient reaches the operating room, surgical preparation should consist of an appropriate antiseptic agent for skin preparation. Removal of hair at the surgical site can create nicks and cuts in the skin that may become colonized and increase postoperative infection rates.[27] The CDC recommends that hair not be removed unless excess hair at the operative site would interfere with the operation.[13] When necessary, hair removal should be performed with clippers, rather than razors, because razors are associated with more frequent epithelial damage. Some evidence indicates that the hair should be removed as close to the surgical time as possible.

Intraoperative strategies to prevent wound infection include aseptic technique to reduce the microbial inoculum as well as good surgical practice to minimize dead space and devitalized tissue. An adequate preoperative surgical scrub of at least 2 to 5 minutes should be performed for surgical procedures. Instruments should be adequately sterilized, and efforts should be made to avoid breaks in aseptic technique. During the procedure, gentle handling of the tissue minimizes desiccation and necrosis that may serve as a nidus of infection. Electrocautery was thought to increase the incidence of wound complications because of devitalized tissue. However, more recent studies[28,29] did not show a relationship, and electrocautery may be used according to the surgeon's preference. Foreign bodies such as staples and sutures may provide a nidus of infection, and their use must be weighed against the risks of poor hemostasis and hematoma formation.

Antimicrobial Prophylaxis

The purpose of antimicrobial prophylaxis is to reduce microbial contamination of the incision and to decrease the incidence of SSI. Surgeons have recognized the importance of antimicrobial prophylaxis in the prevention of SSI for many years.[30-32] For optimal prophylaxis, an antibiotic with a targeted spectrum should be administered at sufficiently high concentrations in serum, tissue, and the surgical wound during the entire time that the incision is open and at risk for bacterial contamination.[33]

To optimize the effectiveness of antibiotic prophylaxis, the antibiotic should be given approximately 60 minutes before surgical incision. This antibiotic should be administered in appropriate doses because patients who are severely obese or have a high volume of distribution may require increased doses. Similarly, small patients or pediatric patients may require dose reductions. In lengthy cases, the antibiotic will need to be readministered approximately every two half-lives of the drug, at which point only 25% of the drug remains in active circulation. In cases with excessive blood loss, an additional dose should be given for every 4 U of estimated blood loss.

Antibiotics, when given in a prophylactic setting, should be discontinued within 24 hours of the procedure.[34] Antibiotics given too late (<30 minutes before surgical incision) do not reach effective tissue concentrations and are less effective in the prevention of SSI,[35] whereas antibiotics given too long afterward (>24 hours after the procedure) increase the incidence of bacterial

resistance[36] and raise the economic cost of therapy[37] without decreasing the rate of SSI.

Prophylaxis is recommended for all class II (clean-contaminated) wounds and for class I$_D$ (clean) wounds in which prosthetic material or a vascular graft is implanted because the consequences of infection are serious in these instances. The routine use of prophylactic antibiotics is less clear in elective class I cases with no prosthetic material. In addition, patients with class III or IV wounds are considered to have an infected wound, and most of these patients are treated with antibiotics empirically.

Diagnosis and Management

Most SSIs manifest within 4 to 8 days of the surgical procedure. However, they may manifest within 30 days of the operation or up to 1 year in cases with implanted prosthetic material. This finding implies that, in the current medical environment of outpatient surgery or early discharge, most of these infections occur in the outpatient setting.[8] This implication emphasizes the importance of patient education in the postoperative period. Patients should be aware of the signs and symptoms of SSI and should know when to seek additional care.

The diagnosis of SSI is clinical and has been described for as long as surgical procedures have been performed. Classically, the most common symptoms have been described (in Latin) as *rubor* ("erythema"), *dolor* ("pain"), *tumor* ("induration"), and *calor* ("warmth"). Some patients may also note drainage from the wound or separation of the skin closure. If the SSI is not treated, systemic symptoms may develop, including fever (38°C-39°C), fatigue, leukocytosis, and increased heart rate.

The management of SSI depends on the extent and type of infection. Drainage and débridement have been and remain the cornerstones of management. Superficial SSIs are treated by opening the incision to provide adequate drainage. A small piece of saline-soaked gauze may be placed in the wound to serve as a wick and to prevent closure of the skin while allowing deeper aspects of the wound heal by second intention. Wet-to-dry dressing changes have been a staple of wound care after SSI, although it may take several weeks to months for the wound to heal by second intention. A culture and Gram stain may identify the offending organism, although these methods are not always necessary. In the setting of superficial SSI, antibiotics need be given only when patients are at risk for systemic dissemination of the infection. Severe infections, such as necrotizing fasciitis, represent surgical emergencies and patients should be taken immediately back to the operating room for wide débridement. The identification of only "dishwater" pus, subcutaneous crepitus, or sepsis should alert the clinician to the possibility of necrotizing fasciitis.

These infections progress rapidly and are caused by either *Clostridium perfringens* or group A β-hemolytic streptococci.

The development of vacuum-assisted closure has eased the process of multiple daily dressing changes. Vacuum-assisted closure was designed to promote healing of large wounds by constant or oscillating application of negative pressure. This negative pressure promises to increase local blood flow, control exudates, and reduce edema of the surrounding tissue.[38-40] In our experience, these negative pressure techniques have proved useful in treating large, chronic wounds. However, their use should be limited when wounds are near conduits, anastomoses, and neobladders because in our experience, they may be associated with an increased rate of cutaneous fistula formation.

WOUND DEHISCENCE

Pathogenesis and Clinical Features

Surgical wound dehiscence is one of the most alarming complications faced by abdominal surgeons. Put simply, a *dehiscence* represents the mechanical failure of wound healing and is defined as a separation of the facial layers early in the postoperative period. *Evisceration*, in turn, is a related term referring to the extrusion of peritoneal contents through the dehisced wound. Dehiscence is of great concern because it may rapidly lead to evisceration. Abdominal dehiscence with evisceration has been associated with a mortality rate nearing 50%.[41] When diagnosed early in the postoperative period, complete wound dehiscence almost always requires a return to the operating room for fascial closure or repair. However, small partial wound dehiscences that are diagnosed >2 weeks postoperatively may often be watched with delayed repair of the resultant incisional hernia, because the risk of evisceration is very low in such patients.

Unfortunately, wound dehiscence frequently occurs without warning. Up to 80% of the time, it manifests as sudden, dramatic drainage of a large volume of clear, serous fluid from the incision. Patients may also note a pulling or ripping sensation. This often occurs when the patient is standing or changing positions, because the pressure on the incision is greatest at these times. The diagnosis is then confirmed by gently probing the incision with a sterile, cotton-tipped applicator to determine the integrity of the fascia. If clinical suspicion remains despite equivocal physical examination findings, imaging studies such as ultrasound or computed tomography can be used. When a large segment of the incision is open, immediate plans for closure in the operating room should be made. In the event of evisceration, the eviscerated intraperitoneal contents should be covered with a sterile saline moistened towel until an emergency operation can be performed.

TABLE 20-3	**Risk Factors Associated With Wound Dehiscence**
Preoperative Risk Factors	**Intraoperative and Postoperative Risk Factors**
Malnutrition	Technical error with fascial closure
Anemia	Emergency procedures
Hypoproteinemia	Wound complications (infection, seroma, hematoma)
Obesity	
Comorbid disease (e.g., diabetes, renal failure, chemotherapy, irradiation)	
Increased intra-abdominal pressure (e.g., coughing, straining, ascites)	
Advanced age	
Long-term corticosteroid use	

Numerous factors can contribute to wound dehiscence (Table 20-3). However, despite advances in suture material and perioperative care, the incidence of abdominal fascial dehiscence has remained steady at nearly 1% of abdominal wounds.[42,43] Other factors that contribute to wound dehiscence remain. Obesity, for example, is associated with increased difficulty in identifying the fascia and in closing the incision. Corticosteroids, over long periods, can decrease the tensile strength of healing wounds.[44] Patients with cancer are more likely to have problems with wound healing, because these patients are more likely to have a contaminated wound and have undergone previous irradiation or chemotherapy.[45] Radiation causes obliterative sclerosing endarteritis that can decrease the microvascular arterial supply to the wound.[46] Malnourished patients nearly uniformly have decreased protein synthesis and turnover, which lead to poorer fascial integrity. Finally, diabetic patients encounter more healing problems than do patients without diabetes and have a greater risk of wound dehiscence.[41] The likely reason is that diabetic patients have less collagen synthesis and deposition, decreased wound breaking strength, and impaired leukocyte function.

Suture Selection and Technique

Wounds have <5% of normal tissue strength during the first postoperative week and may not ever develop normal tensile strength. In fact, studies have demonstrated that abdominal fascia regains 50% to 59% of this original tensile strength at 7 weeks and 70% to 90% at 20 weeks but may never exceed 93% of uninterrupted fascia.[47,48] Therefore, initial postoperative wound security depends solely on suture strength and technique of closure.[49] As such, the choice of suture material is of critical importance in closing abdominal surgical wounds. The suture material should be strong enough to reapproximate the tissue and keep the wound intact during normal postoperative activity.

Numerous suture materials are available for wound closure. These sutures can be classified as natural or synthetic as well as rapidly absorbable, slowly absorbable, and nonabsorbable. Synthetic material has the advantages of being more uniform, inducing less tissue reaction, having greater tensile strength for a given diameter, and eliminating the risk of disease transmission. In 2001, the United Kingdom eliminated the use of catgut suture because of the risk of transmission of bovine spongiform encephalopathy (BSE, or mad cow disease).

Nonabsorbable sutures have been widely used to close abdominal incisions for many years. However, stainless steel wire and braided silk, once commonplace, have been replaced by more modern suture materials. Nonabsorbable monofilament sutures are associated with less tissue reaction[50] and more resistance to infection[51] than are absorbable sutures. However, they are associated with a higher incidence of sinus formation and long-term wound pain.[52-55] The primary benefit of nonabsorbable suture is that it maintains tensile strength throughout the process of wound healing.

Absorbable suture is designed to reapproximate the fascia through the initial phases of wound healing until the fascia itself has regained enough tensile strength. Rapidly absorbable suture is not recommended for closure of abdominal incisions because this suture type has been demonstrated to have a higher incidence of wound dehiscence[56] and postoperative hernia formation[55,57] when compared with nonabsorbable suture. However, slowly absorbable sutures, such as polydioxanone (PDS) and polyglyconate (Maxon) have been shown to cause less incisional pain and suture sinuses, with no effect on the long-term hernia rate. Additionally, these newer-generation monofilament sutures are more resistant to infection than are multifilament sutures.[58,59] They are degraded by hydrolysis and are not as subject to enhanced absorption resulting from bacterial enzymatic activity.[60]

When a suture is placed through the fascia in the operating room, wound dehiscence has three potential causes:

1. The suture may break.
2. The knot may slip.
3. The suture may cut through the tissue.

Several studies have demonstrated that suture breakage and knot failure are rarely the source of wound dehiscences, and in ≤95% of wounds that have dehisced, the suture and knots are intact but the suture has torn through the fascia.[49,61] This finding brings to light the importance of suture diameter because smaller-diameter sutures are associated with a greater likelihood of tearing through tissue.[43,62,63] Therefore, most sutures used for abdominal wound closure are number 0 or larger. Additionally, continuous running looped suture has gained popularity as a method to increase the speed and tensile strength of wound closure. A double-looped closure has been demonstrated to be the strongest method of wound closure, but it has been associated with increased pulmonary complications, potentially because of decreased abdominal compliance.[43]

Surgical dictum states that sutures should be placed ≥1 cm from the fascial edge while advancing ≤1 cm with each throw. This recommendation results from concern for thermal injury related to the use of electrocautery on the fascial edge. Jenkins[64] demonstrated that the length of a midline laparotomy can increase ≤30% in the postoperative period as a result of elasticity and increased intra-abdominal pressure. Therefore, it is important when closing using a running suture that the suture is of adequate length. Investigators have demonstrated that wounds that have been closed with a suture length that is twice as long as the wound have a higher rate of wound dehiscence[64] than do wounds closed with suture that is four times the length of the wound. This concept is referred to as the *suture-to-wound length ratio*, and a ratio of at least 4:1 provides good wound security.[65-68] Theoretically, this approach affords adequate approximation of the fascial tissues while minimizing the ischemic effects of increased tension along the suture line.

Layered Versus Mass Closure

Layered closure of the abdominal wound involves separate closure of each of the distinct fascial layers with or without closure of the peritoneum. *Mass closure*, or Smead-Jones closure, is the closure of all layers of the abdominal wall, except the skin, as a single structure. Classically, this approach involved interrupted sutures. However, no benefit has been demonstrated over a continuous suture technique. Layered closure was believed to decrease intraperitoneal adhesions, increase wound strength, and promote hemostasis. These effects were especially noted with paramedian incisions,[69-71] which currently are used less frequently than are muscle-splitting midline incisions. However, several prospective, randomized studies[54,72] and large meta-analyses[57,73,74] demonstrated that layered closure is associated with higher rates of dehiscence and prolonged operative times as compared with mass closure. Separate peritoneal closure, in particular, has been associated with more intraperitoneal adhesions, increased operative times, and obscured fascial closure.[75-77] Furthermore, evidence indicates that the peritoneum re-epithelializes within 48 to 72 hours without closure,[78] and separate closure of this layer is unnecessary.

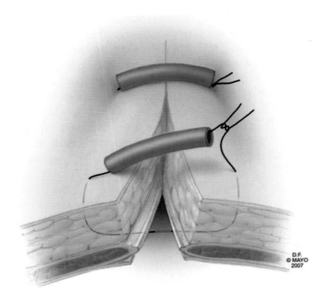

Figure 20-2 Retention sutures are placed through all layers of the abdominal wall and are secured around rubber tubing. (Copyright © 2007, Mayo.)

Retention sutures are sutures that are placed through all layers of the abdomen, including skin. They are often secured around a piece of rubber tubing and tied down (**Fig. 20-2**). Although historically they were used to decrease the incidence of abdominal dehiscence in patients at high risk, more recent studies did not demonstrate a beneficial effect on the rate of dehiscence. These sutures have also been associated with increased pain and inconvenience.[79]

NERVE/PLEXUS INJURIES

Nerve injury during urologic surgery may be caused by direct surgical trauma (i.e., nerve transection) or by stretch and compression of nerves from improper patient positioning or retractor placement. With regard to injuries caused by surgical trauma, all surgical incisions risk division of cutaneous sensory nerves and thereby may result in abdominal wall neuralgias or sensory deficits.[80] These complications are likely underreported by physicians, and therefore the incidence of such events is difficult to quantitate. The following discussion is a review of nerve injuries resulting from stretch and compression.

Improper patient positioning or retractor placement may cause stretch and compression of nerves that manifests as a deficit in postoperative neurologic function. In addition, ischemic injury compromising the blood supply of a nerve (i.e., ischemia of the intraneural vasa nervorum) may result in nerve injury as well.[81] Anesthetized patients have reduced muscle tone and are unable to report the discomfort of improper positioning, factors that place these patients at particular risk of injury. Although such nerve injuries are usually temporary, they significantly affect patients' quality of life and may

result in permanently debilitating complications. For example, nerve injuries may limit postoperative ambulation and thereby increase the risk for thromboembolic events. Therefore, a thorough understanding of the risk factors, presentation, and management of nerve injuries associated with common urologic procedures is essential for the urologic surgeon.

Although nerve injuries may occur during any of a variety of urologic procedures, the most common circumstances in which we have encountered these events involve brachial plexus injuries after surgery in the flank position, femoral nerve injuries from radical pelvic surgery, and lower extremity nerve injury from procedures in the lithotomy position. Therefore, these injuries are the focus of this section.

Upper Extremity Nerve Injuries

Upper extremity nerve injuries during urologic surgery most often are the result of injuries to the brachial plexus, which contains the C5-T1 nerve roots and runs between the prevertebral fascia and the axillary fascia of the arm. This plexus supplies multiple nerve branches including the musculocutaneous, axillary, radial, median, and ulnar nerves. The brachial plexus is particularly vulnerable to injury because of its lack of mobility, being fixed to the vertebrae, prevertebral fascia, and axillary fascia, as well as its proximity to bony structures, including the first rib, clavicle, coracoid process, and the head of the humerus.[82] Injuries to the brachial plexus may be the result of direct trauma, excessive stretching, external pressure, or a combination of these factors. In our experience, although brachial plexus injuries have been reported to result from excessive extension and external rotation during surgical procedures in the supine position, including radical prostatectomy,[83] most brachial plexus injuries occur during procedures in the flank position, which is commonly used for procedures involving the kidney and retroperitoneum.

Given that the flank position is one of the most common positions for urologic surgery, we describe here our technique of flank positioning, which aims to achieve optimum operative exposure while avoiding neurologic injury. After general anesthesia is established, patients should be placed in the lateral decubitus position with the nonoperative side against the operating table. The lower leg is then flexed at the knee and hip, the upper leg is kept straight, and pillows are placed between the knees to prevent contact of potential pressure points. Heels and knees are padded, and the patient is secured to the operating table using either cloth tape or Velcro straps. The head is padded as well to prevent angulation of the neck. Indeed, excessive dorsal extension or lateral flexion of the neck risks stretching of the brachial plexus to the opposite side of the patient between the fixed points at the transverse processes of the cervical vertebrae and the axillary fascia of the upper arm.[81]

The downside arm is then placed at an approximately 90-degree angle to the table and is secured to the armboard. Suspension of the upside arm (i.e., from an anesthesia screen, from a bar anchored to the operating table, or on blankets placed over the downside arm) must be done with care because excessive tension or abduction may stretch the brachial plexus around the clavicle and compress the nerves against the tendon of the pectoralis minor muscle.[81] A somewhat misnamed "axillary roll," which should more correctly be considered a chest roll, is then placed just beneath the true axilla. In fact, placement of this roll (we use a blanket) within the true axilla may result in compressive injury to the brachial plexus or vascular obstruction of the upper extremity.

After securing the patient to the bed, we then flex the operating table and raise the kidney rest, which should lie just above the iliac crest, until the muscles of the flank become tight.[81] This maneuver maximizes separation of the costal margin and iliac crest for surgery while minimizing the risk of vena caval compression.

Despite vigilant attention to patient positioning, injuries to the brachial plexus may occur during procedures in the flank position. Injuries to the brachial plexus of the downside arm during flank positioning, for example, are most often compressive, although stretch injuries may occur if the dependent arm shifts position during the surgical procedure.[81] Brachial plexus injuries of the upside arm in the flank position, meanwhile, are most often the result of abduction, extension, and external rotation of the humerus that stretch the plexus around the clavicle, the tendon of the pectoralis minor, and the head of the humerus.[84]

The presentation of brachial plexus injuries varies somewhat with the level of injury but most often involves some degree of weakness of the affected upper extremity, including the deltoid, supraspinatus, biceps, brachioradialis, and triceps muscles, as well as the wrist and finger flexors and extensors.[82] Patients may also report decreased pinprick sensation along a dermatomal (i.e., C7-T1) distribution. Deep tendon reflexes of the biceps and brachioradialis muscles are characteristically absent on physical examination. Peripheral branches of the brachial plexus may be injured after their exit from the axilla, and these injuries may manifest as isolated nerve deficits; for example, the median and ulnar nerves can be damaged if the arm is allowed to hang unsupported over edge of the operating table, whereas the radial nerve of the downside arm may be injured if the arm is pushed cephalad against the vertical bar of the anesthesia screen, thus compressing the nerve between the humerus and the bar.[81] The role of electromyography in the evaluation of patients with a suspected nerve injury is discussed further later in the section on femoral nerve injuries.

Management of a suspected brachial plexus injury includes careful neurologic examination, protection of potentially hypesthetic skin from injury, and physical therapy consultation to prevent muscle wasting.[82] Other treatments including intermittent galvanic stimulation to the affected muscle and surgical repair have been described.[82,85] We have seen considerable variability in the course of recovery of function after brachial plexus injury, from hours to months. Nevertheless, we, as others,[82,86] have noted that sensation consistently returns before motor function, and that the lower nerve roots recover function before the upper nerve roots.

Lower Extremity Nerve Injuries

Various injuries to the nerves that innervate the lower extremities have been described during urologic procedures. These injuries include direct trauma to the nerves, such as intraoperative transection, injuries that relate to patient positioning, and injuries that result from retractor compression. Here, we separate the discussion into injuries of the femoral nerve, which may occur by any of these mechanisms but are most commonly the result of compression from retractor placement, and nerve injuries related to the lithotomy position that may involve the femoral nerve but often affect other nerves of the lower extremity.

Injuries to the Femoral Nerve

The femoral nerve, which arises from the second through the fourth lumbar nerve roots, represents the largest branch of the lumbar nerve plexus. The femoral nerve is formed within the body of the psoas major muscle and then passes inferolaterally within the psoas before emerging just superior to the inguinal ligament, in a groove between the psoas and iliacus muscles.[87] The blood supply to the extrapelvic portion of the femoral nerve is the lateral femoral circumflex artery, whereas the intrapelvic component of the femoral nerve is supplied by the iliolumbar and deep circumflex iliac arteries.[88] A more extensive collateral blood supply to the right femoral nerve has been demonstrated,[89] a finding suggesting that the left femoral nerve may be more susceptible to ischemic injury than the right.[88]

The femoral nerve contains both sensory and motor components, including the sensory branches of the anterior and medial femoral cutaneous nerve, as well as the long saphenous nerve. Motor innervation from the femoral nerve is provided to the psoas, iliacus, quadriceps femoris, pectineus, and sartorius muscles. Therefore, injury to the femoral nerve may result in weakness of hip flexion, knee extension, adduction, and external rotation.[88,90,91] Clinically, femoral nerve injuries usually manifest as difficulty with ambulation in the early postoperative period. Patients whose injuries are not recognized before discharge commonly report difficulty in climbing stairs at home.[91] In addition, patients may report numbness and paresthesias of the anteromedial thigh.[92] On physical examination, weakness of the quadriceps muscles and diminished or absent deep tendon reflexes at the knee (patellar reflex) are consistent findings.

Femoral nerve injuries may result from patient positioning, retractor-related compression, or direct operative trauma. Direct injury is usually suspected intraoperatively, and careful inspection along the course of the nerve is recommended in such cases. Positioning-related femoral nerve injuries in urology have most consistently been reported from procedures in the lithotomy position,[93,94] and they are discussed in the next section.

The most common mechanism for femoral nerve injury during urologic procedures, however, is compression of the nerve by self-retaining retractors. This situation typically occurs during prolonged abdominal cases such as radical cystectomy, although injuries have been reported after radical prostatectomy and even perineal prostatectomy.[95] Retractor injuries occur when the blades of the retractor are placed directly on the psoas muscle, where they may compress the nerve directly or indirectly by trapping the nerve against the lateral pelvic wall (**Fig. 20-3**).[88] In addition, retractor blades may compromise the blood supply to the femoral nerve by compressing the iliolumbar artery.[92] Thin patients, in whom the retractor blades are more likely to compress the psoas muscle, are at particular risk for femoral nerve injury from retractor compression.[96] Moreover, the length of time of retraction has been correlated with the severity of nerve injury.[97] Therefore, care should be taken to ensure that retractor blades retract only the rectus muscle and do not sit directly on the psoas

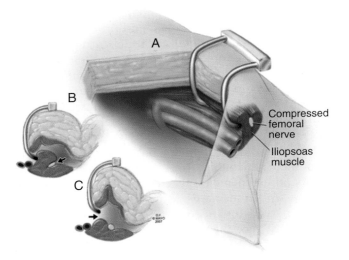

Figure 20-3 Common mechanism of femoral nerve injury by retractor placement. **A** and **B**, Compression of the femoral nerve by placement of the retractor along the iliopsoas muscle. **C**, Correct position of the retractor to retract the rectus muscle only. (Copyright © 2007, Mayo.)

muscle. Periodic inspection of retractor placement during the surgical procedure by placing the surgeon's fingers beneath the blades to ensure clearance off the psoas muscle is mandatory to avoid inadvertent compression injury.

The initial evaluation of a suspected femoral nerve injury includes careful documentation of the neurologic findings, along with physical therapy consultation. Immediate physical therapy helps to prevent muscle atrophy and may decrease the risk of thromboembolic complications associated with prolonged bed rest.[96] Ambulation may be facilitated in the case of femoral nerve injury by locking the ipsilateral knee to compensate for the associated thigh muscle weakness.[88] Although most femoral nerve injuries in our experience are caused by retractor-related compression, nerve compression from pelvic or retroperitoneal hematomas have been described.[88,98] Therefore, if one clinically suspects bleeding, three-dimensional imaging should be obtained as well.

In the setting of a persistent postoperative nerve deficit clinically consistent with a femoral nerve injury, neurologic consultation and an electromyogram to evaluate for anatomic denervation are warranted. Electromyography should be performed ≥3 weeks from the time of injury to maximize its prognostic value.[99] Although the recovery process may be prolonged, compression-related nerve injuries usually resolve over time, and patients regain nerve function. Early return of function has been thought to correlate with full recovery,[91] and sensory lesions are more frequently transient than are motor lesions.

Prevention of femoral nerve injury is paramount because the consequences may significantly affect patients' quality of life. Vigilant attention to patient positioning, limiting surgical time, and periodically inspecting retractor placement are key to avoiding these injuries.

Injuries Resulting From Lithotomy Position

Standard lithotomy position requires the patients' legs to be separated from the midline into 30 to 45 degrees of abduction, with the hips flexed until the thighs are angled between 80 and 100 degrees. The patient's legs are placed into stirrups, with the knees bent such that the lower legs are parallel to the plane of the torso.[100] The lithotomy position is used for a variety of open and endoscopic urologic procedures. Therefore, an understanding of potential postoperative complications related to this position is essential to the care of these patients. In addition to neurologic complications, which are discussed here, other complications that have been reported after procedures in the lithotomy position include lower extremity compartment syndrome, venous thrombosis, and rhabdomyolysis.[101,102] The frequency of perioperative complications may increase with an exaggerated or "high" lithotomy position because the angle of the hips and lower extremities in this position is even more pronounced.[103]

Neurologic injuries related to the lithotomy position may affect the femoral, sciatic, and common peroneal nerves. One series found that the most common lower extremity neuropathies associated with procedures in the lithotomy position were common peroneal (81%), sciatic (15%), and femoral (4%).[104] Other, less commonly injured nerves include the obturator and femoral cutaneous nerves. A study of 1170 patients operated on in the lithotomy position found postoperative neurapraxic complications in 1% of patients.[103] Age >70 years, operative time >180 minutes, and improper positioning were cited as risk factors for neurologic injury.[103] These findings were supported by a separate investigation, which noted lower extremity neuropathies in 1.5% of 991 patients undergoing procedures in the lithotomy position and found that prolonged (>2 hours) positioning in the lithotomy position was a risk factor for injury.[105] A previous study reported postoperative neurapraxia in 21% of patients undergoing perineal prostatectomy using the exaggerated lithotomy position.[106]

Positioning-related nerve injuries in the lithotomy position have been attributed to overflexion of the hips and knees, which causes stretching and compression of the nerves. For example, hyperabduction of the thighs with external rotation of the hips may lead to injury of the femoral nerve secondary to ischemia from compression of the nerve beneath the inguinal ligament. Presentation, management, and prevention of femoral nerve injuries have been discussed. The sciatic nerve, meanwhile, is the largest nerve in the body and arises from the fourth lumbar through the third sacral nerve roots of the lumbosacral plexus.

The sciatic nerve then exits the pelvis through the sciatic foramen and travels through the thigh before dividing in the popliteal fossa into the common peroneal and tibial nerves. The sciatic nerve functions to provide cutaneous innervation to the foot and leg, as well as motor innervation of the biceps femoris (hamstring muscle), leg, and foot.[107]

Excessive stretching of the sciatic nerve by overflexion of the hip and extension of the knee during establishment of the lithotomy position or by shifting of the patient during the procedure may result in injury. In particular, investigators have suggested that excessive hip flexion in the lithotomy position may compress the nerve as it passes through the sciatic notch, thus potentially resulting in ischemic neuropathy.[108,109] The potential sequelae of sciatic depend on the location of the insult along the course of the nerve. Injury to the thigh portion of the sciatic nerve, for example, results in difficulties with flexion of the leg, whereas disruption of the tibial nerve abolishes the ankle jerk reflex.

The common peroneal nerve, meanwhile, arises from the sciatic nerve behind the knee and then wraps around the head of the fibula before separating into the superficial peroneal, which provides sensory innervation to the lateral leg, and the deep peroneal, which provides motor innervation to the tibialis anterior that allows dorsiflexion of the foot. Because this nerve is very superficial when it crosses the head of the fibula, it may easily be compressed and injured at this point (i.e., by direct contact of the leg against an immobile, hard support). Therefore, padding the lateral leg supports during positioning for lithotomy procedures is recommended. Injury to the peroneal nerve most commonly manifests as foot drop, resulting from an inability to dorsiflex the foot. In addition, patients may experience numbness of the lateral aspect of the lower leg and dorsum of the foot.[109]

Overall, nerve injuries during procedures in the lithotomy position may be minimized by careful attention to proper patient positioning, including padding of exposed peripheral nerves, avoiding unnecessary tension on the hips and knees by checking to see that the muscles of the lower extremity are not taut after the lithotomy position is established, and minimizing operative times. Modifications in stirrup design have also been proposed to help minimize the complications of lithotomy positioning.[110]

KEY POINTS

1. Large hematomas that collect in the retroperitoneum or rectus sheath may cause paralytic ileus, anemia, and ongoing bleeding resulting from the consumption of coagulation factors.
2. Wounds that involve large skin flaps or those with large potential spaces in which blood could collect should be drained with a closed-suction surgical drain until the output of these drains decreases.
3. Intraoperative strategies to prevent wound infection include aseptic technique to reduce the microbial inoculum as well as good surgical practice to minimize dead space and devitalized tissue.
4. Antibiotic prophylaxis is recommended for all class II (clean-contaminated) wounds and for class I_D (clean) wounds in which prosthetic material or a vascular graft is implanted because the consequences of infection are serious in these instances.
5. Severe infections, such as necrotizing fasciitis, represent surgical emergencies and patients should be taken immediately back to the operating room for wide débridement.
6. The use of vacuum-assisted closure should be limited when wounds are near conduits, anastomoses, and neobladders because this technique may be associated with an increased rate of cutaneous fistula formation.

7. If clinical suspicion of dehiscence remains despite equivocal physical examination findings, imaging studies such as ultrasound or computed tomography can be used.
8. Investigators have demonstrated that wounds that have been closed with a suture length that is twice as long as the wound have a higher rate of wound dehiscence than do wounds closed with suture that is four times the length of the wound.
9. Although brachial plexus injuries have been reported to result from excessive extension and external rotation during surgical procedures in the supine position, including radical prostatectomy, most brachial plexus injuries occur during procedures in the flank position, which is commonly used for procedures involving the kidney and retroperitoneum.
10. Retractor injuries to the femoral nerve occur when the blades of the retractor are placed directly on the psoas muscle, where they may compress the nerve directly or indirectly by trapping the nerve against the lateral pelvic wall.

REFERENCES

Please see www.expertconsult.com

Chapter 21

MANAGEMENT OF VASCULAR COMPLICATIONS

Venkatesh Krishnamurthi MD
Director, Kidney/Pancreas Transplant Program, Glickman Urological Institute, Cleveland Clinic, Cleveland, Ohio

Rodrigo Frota MD
Fellow, Glickman Urological Institute, Cleveland Clinic, Cleveland, Ohio

Burak Turna MD
Fellow, Glickman Urological Institute, Cleveland Clinic, Cleveland, Ohio

Knowledge of the management of vascular problems is a fundamental requirement for all surgeons. Although most urologic operations are not performed to correct vascular conditions, familiarity with the specific vascular complications that can arise during abdominal and pelvic surgery is essential.

The best approach to managing vascular complications is to prevent them. This principle is best accomplished by thorough knowledge of the operation, relevant anatomy, and application of precise surgical technique. Occasionally, unexpected vascular complications arise and require intraoperative attention and correction. The objective of this chapter is to review the common vascular complications that occur during abdominal and pelvic urologic procedures and their respective management. The techniques described herein are not the only available methods but are chosen based on our (Krishnamurthi's) personal observations and experiences in practice in urologic and transplantation surgery.

VASCULAR INSTRUMENTATION

Proper instruments and fine suture needles are paramount to the performance of successful vascular reconstruction. Although the specific instrument is a matter of individual preference, instrumentation for vascular surgical procedures should include the following:

1. Noncrushing vascular clamps designed for blood vessel occlusion
2. Forceps with fine tips designed to atraumatically grasp vessel walls as well as suture needles
3. Needle holders with fine tips to grasp small needles, yet, prevent unwanted needle movement

4. An assortment of Silastic vessel loops and umbilical tapes for atraumatic vessel manipulation

Vascular clamps are designed to occlude blood vessels in a noncrushing, atraumatic fashion. They are manufactured in a variety of shapes and sizes, and their selection depends on the size of the vessel to be occluded and the desired direction of vessel wall occlusion (longitudinal, transverse, or oblique). The jaws of vascular clamps should have rows of interdigitating teeth that allow vessel wall apposition without endothelial damage. Vascular clamps should be applied by compressing the jaws only to the point necessary for blood flow cessation. Overaggressive application can result in endothelial damage and subsequent dissection.

For small, delicate vessels or relatively inaccessible areas, spring-loaded (Bulldog) clamps are useful devices. These also come in a variety of sizes, strengths, and shapes. Additionally, plastic varieties with soft padded jaws may be useful for extremely delicate vessels.

Vascular forceps must have tines that are in direct apposition, and the tips should be fine enough to grasp the vascular adventitia as well as a suture needle. Forceps with rows of interdigitating teeth serve to accomplish both of these purposes. In contrast, forceps designed for stable needle grasp such as diamond jaw forceps do not allow for reliable manipulation of tissue.

Vascular needle holders should have fine tips to grasp fine suture needles. The two common choices in vascular needle holders are a ring-handled type (Scanlan or Ryder) needle holder and the spring-loaded type (Castroviejo or Jacobson needle holder) (**Fig. 21-1**). Needle holder selection, again, is a matter of individual preference; however, spring-loaded needle holders generally allow for precise needle placement without large degrees

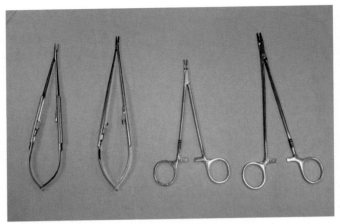

Figure 21-1 Needle holders commonly used for vascular repairs.

of wrist rotation. Ring-handled needle holders enable a more stable needle grasp and facilitate accurate placement in deep structures or through densely calcified vessels.

To some degree, the selection of vascular suture is also matter of individual preference. The caliber of the suture should be as fine as possible, without risking suture line disruption, to minimize bleeding through suture holes. In most cases, suture sizes ranging between 2-0 and 7-0 are applicable for vascular procedures in the abdomen and pelvis. At the level of the aorta, 2-0 or 3-0 suture should suffice, and 4-0 is almost always suitable for the inferior vena cava (IVC). As one progresses to smaller vessels, including the common and external iliac arteries and veins, 5-0 and 6-0 suture is most often satisfactory. Repair of small vessels, such as segmental renal arteries, may require 7-0 suture.

Nonabsorbable sutures are most often selected for vascular procedures. Although silk suture has favorable handling and tying characteristics, its popularity waned with the development of synthetic, nonabsorbable sutures such as polypropylene. In comparison with silk, synthetic monofilament sutures are relatively inert in tissue, have a low coefficient of friction thereby resulting in less tissue drag, and tend to retain a greater amount of tensile strength over time. Vascular sutures are swaged onto fine, one-half–circle or three-eighths–circle needles. The vascular needle should be large enough to penetrate tissue yet small enough not to cause hemorrhage from the needle holes. A common practice in vascular repair is to use a continuous suture with needles swaged onto both ends. This construction allows for greater flexibility in accomplishing the repair (e.g., closure from both directions). In select instances, specifically in pediatric vascular surgery, absorbable monofilament suture with a long half-life (e.g., polydioxanone suture) can be used to allow anastomotic growth.

BASIC VASCULAR TECHNIQUES

General Principles of Vascular Dissection

In planned vascular operations, exposure and control of blood vessels are typically the first orders of business. Both electrocautery and sharp dissection can successfully be used to expose blood vessels. Knowledge of the vascular anatomy and of the characteristic appearance of the correct dissection plane greatly facilitates proper vascular exposure. Blood vessels are enwrapped in a loose periadventitial sheath. Separation of this sheath from the vessel wall, which is identified by the characteristic vasa vasorum on the arterial wall, allows for circumferential dissection of the artery. In general, arteries should be exposed along the anterior surface because major branches are unlikely to arise from this direction. The artery can then be circumferentially exposed, and encirclement with a vessel loop will permit atraumatic mobilization of the vessel for division of its posterior attachments. While handling arteries, it is advisable to grasp only the adventitial tissues with forceps rather than compressing the part or all of the lumen. Traumatic application of forceps to the arterial lumen may result in intimal disruption with dissection or distal embolization of loose atheromatous plaques.

Major veins often run adjacent to arteries and can be dissected in similar fashion. Grasping part (or all) of the vein wall is, in general, a safe maneuver and can greatly facilitate dissection of the vein from the surrounding tissues.

Control of Hemorrhage

Unlike planned vascular operations, urologic procedures during which vascular complications occur require exposure of blood vessels in unplanned situations. Perhaps the most important principle in managing unexpected bleeding is that properly applied digital pressure can control virtually all abdominal and pelvic bleeding. Multiple attempts to use instruments, such as vascular clamps and hemostats, in a poorly exposed operative field carry significant risks of causing additional vascular injury and worsening the ongoing hemorrhage. Digital pressure should be applied by the first assistant while the primary surgeon and others obtain improved exposure by suctioning the field, focusing the lights, extending the incision, and repositioning the retractor. Once exposure has been improved, attention should be directed toward obtaining proximal and distal vascular control. After inflow and outflow vessels are identified and are suitably exposed, vascular clamps should be placed, and digital pressure on the area of hemorrhage should be slowly released such that the site of vessel wall injury can be inspected.

If hemostasis has not been satisfactorily achieved to allow for suitable inspection, these steps should be repeated until the site of injury can be fully examined. Attempts to place suture through poorly exposed tissues pose the risk of inadvertent injury to adjacent structures.

If hemostasis is satisfactory and the site of vessel wall injury can be directly examined, irregular tissue should be excised and the type of vascular repair required should be determined. Two principles should be considered when conducting vascular repairs: (1) hemostasis and (2) preservation of the normal luminal caliber to maintain flow.

Before conducting the vascular repair, the surgeon should determine the need for systemic anticoagulation and proximal and distal embolectomy. Following prolonged occlusion (>30 minutes), thrombi may form along the occluded end of major vessels. Therefore, the surgeon should anticipate the length of time between vessel occlusion and restoration of flow and accordingly administer systemic anticoagulation and/or perform proximal and distal thromboembolectomy. These issues are not a consideration when the vessel is simply ligated and distal flow is terminated.

Systemic anticoagulation is achieved with the administration of intravenous heparin. The anticoagulant effect of heparin generally occurs within 5 minutes and reaches peak activity at approximately 90 minutes following administration. Restoration of a normal coagulation profile can be accomplished by administering protamine sulfate at a milligram for milligram equivalent dose, thus allowing for the temporal decay of heparin that was given earlier. Caution must be exercised with the administration of protamine because it (1) may cause hypotension if it is injected too rapidly and (2) may result in hypocoagulability if it is administered in excessively high doses. In general, because most repairs of vascular complications can be accomplished fairly quickly, a safer practice is to administer smaller doses of heparin (60-70 U/kg) and to allow enough time for the effects simply to dissipate.

It is essential to remove intravascular thrombus before restoring the flow. Failure to do so may result in distal embolization and distal ischemia, with potentially catastrophic consequences. Thrombi within the arterial system can be removed with an Edwards Fogarty arterial embolectomy catheter (Edwards Life Sciences, Irvine, California). These catheters range in length from 40 to 100 cm. The diameter of the inflated balloon should approximate that of the vessel in which the catheter is inserted. Inflated balloon diameters range from 4 mm (2-Fr catheter) to 14 mm (7-Fr catheter). After selecting the smallest balloon that will accomplish the task required, the catheter should be advanced with the balloon deflated. Should resistance be met, further advancement should not be attempted. The balloon should then be inflated using "only" the volume of liquid required to inflate the balloon and the catheter should be withdrawn.

During catheter withdrawal, if the surgeon meets resistance, the balloon should be allowed to deflate slightly before another attempt is made to withdraw again. Should clot be removed, additional passes should be accomplished until no further clot remains. It is essential to consider embolectomy in both the proximal and distal circulations. Additionally, overinflation of the balloon and forcible withdrawal of the catheter may result in intimal damage and extraction of intima that will leave a segment of vessel with a denuded endothelium.

Attempts to remove thrombi in the venous system can also be made using a Fogarty venous thrombectomy catheter. These 80-cm catheters have balloons ranging in inflated diameters of 12 to 19 mm (6-Fr to 8-Fr catheter). From the standpoint of urologic procedures, venous thrombectomy is relevant in the setting of thrombus formation in the infrarenal IVC or common and external iliac veins. Simple ligation of these vessels may be a satisfactory consideration, rather than potentially incomplete thrombectomy.

As mentioned previously, vascular repairs may involve simple ligation or vessel wall closure with maintenance of luminal patency. When restoration of flow is not required, as in the pelvis, which has a rich collateral circulation, vessels can be ligated with ties or clips. For larger vessels (>4 mm), a transfixion technique such as suture ligature or oversewing of the vessel walls effects a more reliable closure than does simple ligature. When restoration of flow is intended, the vessel should be repaired such that the ≥50% of the original luminal diameter is maintained. Greater reductions are likely to result in flow disturbances with hemodynamically significant consequences.

Short lacerations (≤4 mm) in the vessel wall can be repaired by direct closure with continuous or interrupted suture. In general, transverse closure (perpendicular to the direction of blood flow) preserves the luminal diameter better than does longitudinal closure. For arterial lacerations >4 mm, luminal diameter can be maintained by closing the defect with an elliptical autogenous (usually venous) or synthetic vascular patch. The patch is trimmed to match the size of the defect. One apex of the patch is then anchored, and the sides of the patch are approximated to the arterial wall. The opposite end of the patch can be trimmed or the arteriotomy can be extended to complete the patch closure.

In the setting of vascular disruption or significant luminal compromise by a ligature or a clamp, excision and reanastomosis of the vessel may be required. As with other anastomoses, the fundamental principle of constructing a relaxed, tension-free anastomosis should be followed. When the ends of the vessel can be reapproximated in this manner, a simple end-to-end anastomosis can be constructed using either interrupted or continuous suture.

Our preference has been to perform this procedure with a double-armed suture placed along the posterior aspect of the anastomosis. We then use each needle to sew along both sides of the vessel walls. Concerns that this technique will result in purse-string–type narrowing of the anastomosis can be minimized by purposefully tying a small air knot. An alternative is to complete the anastomosis and just before tying the suture, gently open the clamps (distal followed by proximal) to allow for expansion of the anastomosis. The clamps can then be reapplied and the suture can be tied. Placement of interrupted sutures has a theoretical advantage of avoiding a purse-string type constriction; however, this is generally not a clinically relevant problem for larger abdominal and pelvic vessels.

When the two vessel ends cannot be reapproximated in a tension-free manner, an interposition graft must be used. The selection of autogenous versus synthetic conduits is discussed later in this chapter. In general, when using a synthetic conduit, synthetic monofilament nonabsorbable suture (polypropylene) should be used for the anastomosis.

When constructing an end-to-end anastomosis between small vessels (<4 mm), the ends of the vessels should be spatulated to prevent anastomotic narrowing. The vessels should be spatulated 180 degrees opposite each other, and the heel and toe of the anastomoses should be matched to the corresponding points. A similar concept can be applied to the construction of an end-to-side anastomosis. The end of the vessel (synthetic or autogenous conduit) is spatulated, and the anastomosis is begun at the heel (most inaccessible point) and is continued around to the toe.

Finally, several points regarding vascular suture technique should be followed when conducting vascular repairs. It is imperative that the suture passes through all the layers of the vessel wall, a goal accomplished by placing the needle perpendicular to the vessel wall. Incorporation of all the layers results in optimal coaptation and minimizes the risk of pseudoaneurysm formation. For normal vessels, sutures placed at approximately a 1-mm distance and with 1-mm bites should provide satisfactory hemostasis. When one is sewing arteries with significant calcific disease or loose, flaky intima, larger bites are often necessary. Additionally, placement of the needle in an inside-out direction (inside the lumen to outside the lumen) should be considered to avoid lifting an intimal flap and causing intimal dissection.

VASCULAR SUBSTITUTES

Vascular substitutes, composed of grafts (conduits) and patches, have extended the scope of the therapy for vascular injuries. Any segmental loss of vessel >2 cm is generally an indication for vascular interposition. In cases of partial loss of a vessel wall, an appropriately sized and shaped patch preserves luminal patency over primary closure.

Vascular substitutes may be derived from synthetic materials or from autogenous tissues. Expanded polytetrafluoroethylene (ePTFE) is the primary component of vascular substitutes used for arteriovenous access. ePTFE offers the advantages of strength, resistance to significant dilatation, ability to be implanted without preclotting, and theoretical advantage of being less thrombogenic.[1] ePTFE grafts may also be more resistant to infection than textile grafts because of their smoother surface, which makes bacterial adherence difficult.[2]

Dacron grafts are textile grafts composed of yarn, which is either woven or knitted to form the fabric. Woven grafts, tighter and less porous than knitted grafts, are recommended for situations in which hemostasis, without time consuming preclotting, is required. Knitted grafts require preclotting and are believed to promote faster and more complete healing and incorporation. Dacron grafts have very high patency rates for large vessel reconstruction.

The selection of a suitable vascular substitute depends largely on the clinical situation. Substitution of arterial defects with native arteries is preferential. For large arteries, such as the aorta and the common iliac and external iliac arteries, autogenous vessels are generally not readily available, and therefore Dacron and ePTFE are most often employed. For smaller arteries, such as the main or segmental renal artery, a suitable arterial conduit is the hypogastric artery. This vessel can be harvested, with its terminal branches, as a free graft and can be fashioned as an interposition graft or patch. For small segmental renal arteries, the inferior epigastric artery may be similarly used.

In patients with advanced atherosclerosis that precludes the use of an autogenous arterial substitute, autogenous veins can serve as acceptable conduits. When a vein is used as an arterial conduit, it is imperative to check for venous valves and accordingly reverse the direction of the vein. The saphenous vein is readily available in most patients and has been used extensively as a bypass conduit for patients with renal artery disease.[3] Although the gonadal vein is similar in diameter to the renal artery, the thin wall of the gonadal vein predisposes it to aneurysmal degeneration when it is used as a bypass graft. Substitution of larger-caliber arteries, such as the aorta and iliac vessels, can be accomplished by using the superficial femoral vein.[4] Nearly any vein that can serve as an arterial conduit can function well as a patch.[5]

The presence of collateral venous drainage greatly minimizes the need for venous substitutes. When substitutes are required, however, autogenous veins are preferred but are hampered by mismatches in size. Common clinical situations that may require preservation of venous drainage involve the renal vein (particularly the right renal vein), the IVC, and the iliac veins. The saphenous vein can be fashioned as a spiral graft and matched to the main renal vein.[6] For patients with IVC tumor thrombi that extend to the right atrium, autogenous pericardium is an excellent caval substitute.[7]

If use of an autogenous vein for venous replacement is not feasible, externally supported (ring-reinforced) ePTFE grafts may function acceptably. These grafts are preferred over Dacron secondary to their ability to resist respiratory compression and thus avoid graft collapse. The graft should have a diameter slightly smaller than that of the native vessel so the blood flow velocity is increased, thereby potentially decreasing the risk of thrombosis. Eight- to 12-mm grafts are suitable for ilio-femoral replacement, and 16- to 20-mm grafts serve well as IVC grafts. A PTFE patch can function well for partial replacement of the IVC (**Fig. 21-2**). The need for long-term anticoagulation with synthetic venous grafts and patches remains unclear.

When neither autogenous vessels nor synthetic materials are suitable as vascular replacements, cadaveric vessels have been routinely used in organ transplantation. An assortment of arterial and venous conduits should always be procured with liver and pancreas grafts. If not used at the time of transplant, these grafts can be kept in cold storage in preservation solution (4°C) for ≤1 week and used in the intended recipient if necessary. As a final effort, third-party vascular grafts have been used to salvage kidneys for transplantation.[8] Extension of this practice beyond the transplant recipient is inadvisable because of the need for immunosuppression and the risk of viral transmission. Additionally, blood group compatibility and viral serologic status must be verified before implantation of cadaveric vessels.

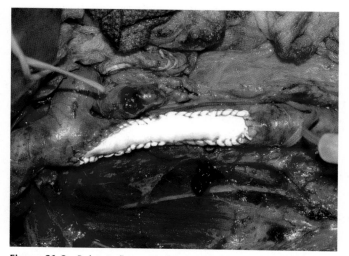

Figure 21-2 Polytetrafluoroethylene patch replacement of the infrarenal inferior vena cava.

MANAGEMENT OF SPECIFIC VASCULAR COMPLICATIONS

This section is devoted to the management of complications that occur along anatomically distinct vascular structures. Although specific urologic procedures may be associated with injuries to specific vessels, this relationship is not absolute because numerous operations can have the same vascular complication.

Arterial System

Aortic Injury

Injuries to the aorta can occur during operations for large retroperitoneal masses. Most cases of aortic injury involve left-sided procedures (retroperitoneal lymphadenectomy, left nephrectomy, or left adrenalectomy) and are undoubtedly the result of proximity of the operative disease to the aorta.

Almost all cases of aortic injury occur during excision of a mass that is closely adherent to the aortic adventitia. With current computed tomography imaging, the relationship between the mass and the aortic wall should be appreciated by careful review of preoperative computed tomography scans. If aortic involvement or adherence is suspected on preoperative imaging, consideration should be given to concomitant aortic replacement during mass excision. Intraoperative determination for the potential of aortic injury should occur when the "normal" aortic wall is not apparent. As mentioned previously, the surgeon should appreciate the vasa vasorum that identify the correct periadventitial layer. As is commonly noted in postchemotherapy retroperitoneal lymphadenectomy, a subadventitial plane can be easily developed; this plane results in a weakened aortic wall with the potential for catastrophic hemorrhage. Another situation in which aortic injury can occur is during left nephrectomy, particularly if the renal artery is ligated and divided in an extreme proximal location. The mistake in this situation is to maintain the dissection too close to the aorta, and the result is too little proximal renal artery after ligation and division.

When significant hemorrhage from the juxtarenal aorta is encountered, initial treatment attempts should not include clamping the aorta. The suprarenal aorta is covered by a thick network of neural and lymphatic tissue and the overlying diaphragmatic crural fibers. Attempts to divide this tissue to identify the aorta just above the renal artery are fraught with difficulty and risk the potential of additional injury. The first attempt to control aortic hemorrhage along this location should be directed toward compressing the aorta at the level of the esophageal (diaphragmatic) hiatus. At this location the distal thoracic aorta can be accessed by retracting the stomach caudally and the left lateral segment of the liver toward the patient's right; then, by opening

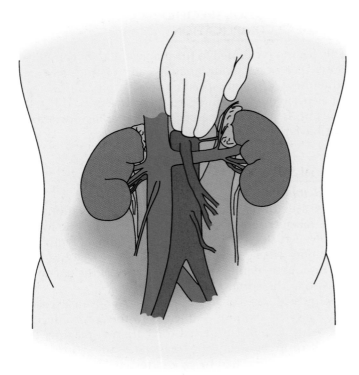

Figure 21-3 Schematic depicting compression of the distal thoracic/supraceliac aorta.

the lesser omentum, the aorta can be compressed in this location (**Fig. 21-3**). Once the aorta is compressed and the site of hemorrhage is identified, the previously described methods can be employed to control bleeding.

Visceral Artery Injury

Superior mesenteric artery (SMA) and celiac artery injuries likely occur more often than the few reported cases in the literature. The highest reported incidence was that seen by Ritchey and colleagues,[9] in which approximately 2% of children undergoing nephrectomy for Wilms' tumor with venous involvement had SMA injury. Other sporadic cases of SMA injury have been reported, but these undoubtedly are an extremely small proportion of all (unreported) SMA injuries.[5,10]

Nearly all cases of inadvertent SMA ligation or division involve the resection of large left-sided tumors. These neoplasms may displace structures from their expected position and distort the normal anatomic relationships. The close proximity of the SMA and left renal vein is well known and clearly plays a role in the mistaking of the SMA for the renal artery. In the majority of reported cases of SMA injury, the injury was recognized intraoperatively either after direct visualization of the transected SMA or by recognition of ischemic-appearing small intestine. Once the injury is recognized, immediate attempts to revascularize the SMA should be undertaken, through direct reanastomosis, placement

of an interposition graft, reimplantation into the aorta, bypass with the splenic artery, or construction of patch angioplasty following thromboembolectomy.[5,9,10]

Several points deserve mention to avoid inadvertent SMA injury. First, the surgeon should be certain to stay on the (left) lateral aspect of the aorta. This relationship can become distorted, particularly when the patient is placed in a left thoracoabdominal or left flank position. However, reassessment and recognition of the lateral aspect of the aorta are imperative to avoid visceral artery injury. Second, nearly all major arteries to the left kidney lie posterior to the left renal vein (with the exception of a retroaortic left renal vein). Before ligating any large (>2 mm) artery during excision of a left-sided mass, the relationship of this artery and the left renal vein should be verified, and the previously mentioned relationship should be noted. Inadvertent ligation of a large vessel anterior to the renal vein carries the risk of visceral artery ligation. Third, and particularly when the two prior principles are not apparent, the renal artery can be approached from a posterior direction. The entire kidney can be mobilized and rotated medially (toward the patient's right), and the major renal vessels can be palpated from the posterior location. Following identification and verification that these vessels are posterior to the main renal vein, these arteries can be ligated. In cases of anomalous venous drainage, such as a circumaortic or retroaortic vein, the major renal artery may in fact be anterior to the renal vein. This relationship should be noted from careful review of the preoperative imaging, and the principle of staying on the left lateral aspect of the aorta should be followed.

Injuries to the celiac axis are also rare; only one has been reported in the literature.[10] The celiac axis arises only a few millimeters proximal to the SMA, and injuries to this vessel occur in a manner identical to SMA injuries. Inadvertent ligation of both the SMA and celiac axis is extremely poorly tolerated because it likely results in loss of collateral vessels to the distal SMA through the splenic artery and intrapancreatic collateral vessels. The presence of thick fibrous tissue (neural and lymphatic tissue) surrounding a major artery should suggest inadvertent dissection of the SMA or celiac axis. These vessels are surrounded by thick neural and lymphatic tissue much more so than the renal artery, and recognition of this anatomic relationship should aid in avoiding inadvertent ligation.

Lumbar Artery

Hemorrhage from lumbar arteries can occur during resection of lymphatic tissue posterior to the aorta. The important principle when dissecting lumbar arteries is to avoid keeping the dissection too close to the aorta. In this case, inadvertent bleeding from the lumbar artery can be controlled by simply grasping each end and applying an effective hemostatic maneuver. When bleeding occurs from the origin of the lumbar artery, one often has insufficient vessel to grasp, and hemostasis involves directly suturing the aorta. The important principle in this situation is to mobilize the posterior surface of the aorta adequately so that the sutures can be placed with good visualization.

External Iliac Artery

Injuries to the external iliac artery can occur during pelvic lymphadenectomy procedures or organ transplantation procedures. Because the external iliac artery is an end artery, the surgeon should always attempt to maintain prograde blood flow when repairing this vessel. If this is not feasible, vascular surgical consultation for construction of an extra-anatomic bypass (femoral-femoral or axillofemoral bypass) should be pursued as soon as possible. Techniques to control hemorrhage from the external iliac artery are identical to those previously mentioned in this chapter.

Two special considerations deserve mention. If the displacement between the two ends of the external iliac artery necessitates placement of an interposition graft, a native hypogastric artery may be a suitable and readily available conduit. This vessel can be procured and fashioned as a free interposition graft or patch, or conversely, prograde blood flow can be restored by ligation of the distal hypogastric artery and anastomosis of the proximal hypogastric artery to the distal external iliac artery.[11] In most cases, the hypogastric artery provides only a short interposition graft and generally does not meet the caliber of the external iliac artery. For long disruptions of the external iliac artery, a synthetic interposition graft may be used. One other option is use of the patient's external iliac vein, which can be procured and then placed in a reversed configuration as a vascular conduit.

Venous System

Significant hemorrhage during urologic procedures is much more likely to occur from venous structures.

Malignant renal diseases induce the formation of new blood vessels, and most urologists have encountered large renal tumors with a parasitizing network of veins. Additionally, many of these veins are extremely thin walled and fragile. Tumor extension into the major renal veins from adrenal veins and the IVC is seen with malignant tumors of the kidney and adrenal gland, and knowledge of the management of tumors involving the venous system is essential during procedures on the kidney.

Renal Vein/Interior Vena Cava Thrombus Extraction

Malignant renal diseases involve the renal vein and IVC in approximately 5% to 10% of cases. These tumors can extend within the lumen of the venous system up to the level of the right atrium. Although locally advanced, renal cell cancers with venous involvement are considered localized disease, and surgical resection of these cancers is intended to be curative.

The surgical technique for management of cancers involving the renal veins or IVC directly depends on the level of extension. The techniques presented in this chapter are based on the classification scheme proposed by Neves and Zincke (**Fig. 21-4**).[12]

Tumor thrombi involving the renal vein and those protruding just into the IVC through the renal vein orifice can be managed without complete IVC occlusion. Our approach is to mobilize the entire kidney after early arterial ligation. Following this maneuver, the renal vein is circumferentially dissected. As a result of renal vein obstruction from the tumor thrombus, the development of thin-walled venous collateral vessels may pose challenges to obtaining circumferential control.

Once the renal vein has been isolated, the surgeon should carefully palpate the tumor thrombus within the vein and determine whether it can be safely retracted back toward the kidney. With the thrombus retracted toward the kidney, a tangentially occluding clamp, such

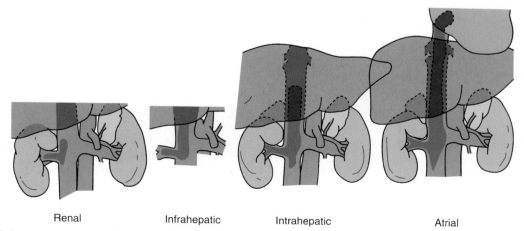

| Renal | Infrahepatic | Intrahepatic | Atrial |

Figure 21-4 Inferior vena cava tumor thrombus classification scheme. *(Adapted from Neves RJ, Zincke H. Surgical treatment of renal cancer with vena cava extension. Br J Urol. 1987;59:390-395.)*

as a Cooley clamp or a Satinsky clamp, can be placed partially across the IVC. It is important to mobilize the posterior aspect of the IVC before placing the clamp so that the walls of the IVC can be reapproximated without undue tension. Once the clamp has been placed, a small cuff of the IVC can be resected with the renal vein. The surgeon can inspect the portion of the IVC within the clamp to ensure adequate tumor resection. If tumor resection is incomplete, the clamp should be left in place and the kidney should be removed. Circumferential control of the IVC and left renal vein, which are reviewed subsequently, is then required for further tumor extraction.

During removal of a renal cell carcinoma with level I thrombus, we tend to leave the division of the vein as the final step. In this setting, the entire kidney has been mobilized, thus allowing for maximum retraction of the kidney and unobstructed placement of the partially occluding clamp. Another caveat is that by leaving the venous dissection for the last step, one ensures that all sources of inflow have been ligated and divided. In the event that arterial inflow to the kidney remains, placement of the clamp will potentially result in outflow obstruction, venous hypertension, and new areas of venous bleeding. Closure of the vena cava can be performed with 4-0 or 5-0 polypropylene suture. In most instances, the IVC walls are fairly thick and are satisfactorily apposed with 4-0 suture. Our preference is to begin a suture at each apex of the vena cavotomy and run these continuously to the midpoint where the sutures are secured. We have not found that an over-and-back technique is necessary for low-pressure venous systems.

Management of level II and level III tumor thrombi requires control of the infrarenal and suprarenal IVC as well as all tributaries, such as the contralateral renal vein, lumbar veins, and adrenal veins. Our approach is to encircle the contralateral renal vein and infrarenal vena cava and then address the suprarenal vena cava.

From an operative perspective, the principal distinction between a level II and a level III thrombus is the need to mobilize the liver so that the IVC can be encircled above (cephalad to) the level of the thrombus. For level II thrombi, the liver does not need to be mobilized and the caudate lobe can be retracted cephalad, thereby exposing a greater length of the suprarenal IVC. Occasionally, small venous branches that drain the caudate lobe directly into the IVC need to be divided. These veins tend to be short, wide, and occasionally fragile. Our approach is to ligate both sides of these small veins before division; however, occasionally, the very short nature of the vein does not permit double ligation, and small clips can be placed on the hepatic side of these veins before division. If one encounters hemorrhage from the hepatic side, a suture ligature (polypropylene or silk) can often control the hemorrhage. These small veins tend to retract into the liver parenchyma and thus

hemostasis is best accomplished by incorporating some of the surrounding hepatic parenchyma. Once the IVC cephalad to the thrombus is exposed, it can be encircled with a vessel loop or umbilical tape. Our preference is to use umbilical tapes because their relative inelasticity allows for better upward retraction of the IVC.

For level II thrombi, once all segments of the IVC have been encircled, the kidney can be addressed with the standard approach to a radical nephrectomy. We typically attempt to gain early arterial control and then completely mobilize the entire kidney in a perifascial manner. All attachments except for the tumor-filled renal vein should be divided. At this point, control of the IVC is obtained by first occluding the contralateral renal vein, then the infrarenal IVC followed by the suprarenal (cephalad to the thrombus) IVC. The IVC is carefully palpated, and if the occluded segment becomes distended, the surgeon needs to consider the possibility of uncontrolled venous tributaries. The clamps should be released and additional dissection of the IVC should be conducted. In most instances, the uncontrolled tributaries are posteriorly inserting lumbar veins.

In our experience, we have not encountered lumbar veins along the suprarenal IVC. The only significant posterior branch above the level of the renal vein is the right adrenal vein. Once the caval segment is satisfactorily occluded, a vena cavotomy is made along the renal vein ostium. We generally prefer to make the vena cavotomy along the anterolateral aspect of the IVC and extend this to a degree that allows complete visualization of the caval lumen at the level of the tumor thrombus. Most often, the vena cavotomy should be made only large enough to allow extraction of the thrombus.

Once the thrombus has been extracted, the lumen of the IVC can be inspected and the vena cavotomy can be enlarged accordingly. At this point, the entire lumen of the cava should be both visually and digitally inspected. Any adherent areas of tumor should be managed with resection of the IVC wall. The remaining IVC can be reapproximated with 4-0 polypropylene suture. As stated previously, we prefer to place one suture at each apex and run this continuously until the midpoint is reached.

Controversy exists regarding the need to vent the IVC. We do attempt to avoid entrapping a large amount of air in the IVC before unclamping. Any entrapped air can be expelled by releasing the clamps before tying the suture. The clamps are released in the following sequence: suprarenal IVC, contralateral renal vein. The retrograde flow of blood within the IVC generally expels any entrapped air and the suture can be tied. At this point, the clamp on the infrarenal IVC can be released, thereby restoring prograde blood flow.

With level III thrombi, more extensive liver mobilization is necessary for suprarenal caval control. For thrombi near the level of the hepatic veins or just above the hepatic veins, we completely mobilize the liver. Following standard exposure of the retroperitoneum, we divide the falciform ligament and left triangular ligament to expose the suprahepatic IVC. We then mobilize the right lobe of the liver. Initially, several small venous branches that drain the caudate lobe can be divided in the manner described previously. The posterior aspect of the right hepatic lobe should then be carefully freed from the kidney. In many instances, right-sided tumors can result in dense adherence to the posterior aspect of the right hepatic lobe, and the correct plane of separation is identified by gently retracting on the liver and kidney. Vigorous retraction on the liver can result in a laceration to the liver that will be accompanied by troublesome bleeding.

Once the attachments between the liver and kidney are completely divided, the right triangular ligament can be addressed. In our experience, the best approach to releasing the right hepatic lobe is to have the surgeon stand on the left side of the patient and gently retract the right lobe of the liver toward the patient's left. The assistant can then free the attachments between the right lobe and the diaphragm (right triangular ligament), which can be divided with the electrocautery. Anterior and posterior leaflets to the right triangular ligament are present, and each needs to be divided to release the liver from the diaphragm. Division of the triangular ligament should generally proceed in a lateral to medial direction.

Once the right hepatic lobe is completely mobilized off the diaphragm, the right hepatic vein and right aspect of the suprahepatic vena cava become visible. With progressive release of the right hepatic lobe, retraction on the right lobe displays additional veins draining directly into the IVC. As one proceeds up the IVC

toward the major hepatic veins, the tributaries draining the caudate and right lobe tend to become wider and more difficult to control with simple ties.

For veins >5 mm in width, we prefer to divide these vessels after placing small vascular clamps such as a spoon clamp or angled or straight DeBakey clamp on each side of the vein. After placing these clamps, the vein is divided, and the venous stump can be oversewn with a polypropylene suture. We leave more vein on the IVC side so that a suitable portion of the vein wall remains to reapproximate. For the hepatic end of the vein, a figure-of-eight–type stitch that incorporates some hepatic parenchyma can be placed around the clamp and secured just after releasing the clamp.

Full mobilization of the liver enables reliable control of the suprahepatic IVC. We make every attempt to mobilize the liver off the IVC all the way to the level of the hepatic veins. The IVC just below the hepatic veins is palpated, and if this segment appears free of thrombus, we encircle the IVC in this location. In many instances, the cephalad extent of the thrombus can be retracted below the portion of the IVC to be clamped (**Fig. 21-5**). The advantage of clamping below the hepatic veins is that hepatic outflow is not obstructed, thus making control of the hepatic inflow unnecessary.

In the setting of thrombi above the level of the hepatic veins but still below the diaphragm, the IVC must be occluded along its suprahepatic segment. The inflow to the liver must also be occluded by clamping the porta hepatis (portal vein and hepatic artery) with an atraumatic vascular clamp (Pringle's maneuver). Level III thrombi are addressed identically to level II in that the relevant segment of the IVC and all significant tributaries are isolated and controlled. The kidney is then mobilized by dividing all attachments except for

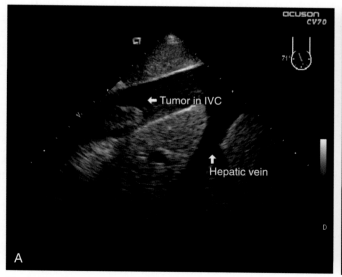 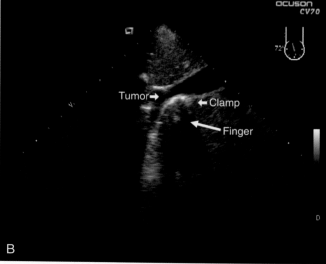

Figure 21-5 **A,** Echocardiographic images of the inferior vena cava with level III tumor thrombus. **B,** The tumor thrombus is being retracted by the surgeon's fingers just before application of the clamp.

the thrombus-filled renal vein. The IVC is then controlled and opened, the tumor is extracted, the IVC is closed, and flow is reestablished as described previously.

Two points deserve special mention. In our experience, left-sided tumors require a slightly different approach. For left-sided tumors with vena caval thrombi (levels II-IV), we complete the left nephrectomy before addressing the IVC. The renal vein is divided and we close the renal vein stump, which is filled with tumor thrombus, with a running polypropylene suture. Occasionally, the renal vein stump is expanded with tumor and is difficult to close. In this situation, we sew a small section of a surgical sponge over the vein end. Because this vein will subsequently be resected, the closure needs only to be hemostatic to prevent overt tumor spillage.

We then expose the IVC by turning our attention to the right side of the retroperitoneum. The duodenum is mobilized through a standard Kocher maneuver. The left renal vein stump is then dissected and is brought over toward the patient's right. The usual landmark of the aorta posterior to the left renal vein serves as a consistent reminder that no significant posterior branches to the left renal vein are present at this level. Once the renal vein stump has been brought over to the patient's right side, additional mobilization can be gained on the left lateral and left posterior aspect of the IVC, and the caval portion of the operation can proceed in the previously described manner.

Another important distinction between right-sided and left-sided tumors is the need for arterial inflow control to the contralateral kidney. For right-sided tumors, occlusion of the left renal vein at its entry into the IVC generally does not result in venous hypertension because the left renal vein has collateral drainage through adrenal, gonadal, and lumbar branches.

For left-sided tumors, occlusion of the right renal vein may result in venous hypertension, acute tubular necrosis, and renal insufficiency. Occlusion of the right renal vein without inflow control can be tolerated if the caval portion of the operation is fairly short. However, if the thrombus is adherent to the IVC wall and removal of the tumor from within the IVC is protracted, it is helpful to occlude the right renal artery as well. In the majority of the cases, the right renal artery rises from the aorta just posterior to the left renal vein. As the left renal vein stump is mobilized toward the patient's right, the lymphatic tissue posterior to renal vein is carefully divided, thus enabling identification of the proximal aspect of the right renal artery. The artery is encircled with a vessel loop and isolated for later occlusion. It is imperative to dissect the right renal artery very gently because, in most cases, it supplies the only functioning kidney.

One final point in the management of IVC tumor thrombi relates to the placement of the suprarenal IVC

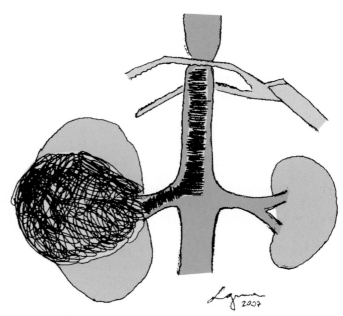

Figure 21-6 Schematic depicting the direction of clamp application along the suprarenal IVC. The thrombus can be retracted inferiorly and the clamp is applied so that the anterior wall of the IVC is compressed against the posterior wall.

clamp. We prefer to occlude the suprarenal IVC with a clamp that is placed in an anterior to posterior direction. The anterior aspect of the IVC is compressed against the posterior aspect of the IVC (**Fig. 21-6**). The clamp is best applied by the surgeon, standing on the right side of the table, and is done by retracting the thrombus with the left hand and then applying the clamp with the right hand. The importance of placing the clamp in this direction relates to the possibility of needing to place a vascular graft should IVC resection become necessary.

If the IVC is resected, the suprarenal portion can be transected by leaving a suitable cuff of tissue within the clamp. The anterior and posterior walls are more easily identified and approximated to a tube graft than are the lateral walls, as would be seen with a clamp placed in a straight up-and-down manner. Because the thrombus generally does not involve the infrarenal IVC, the clamp along this portion of the IVC can be placed further from the cut edge, thereby making an anastomosis more straightforward.

Level IV (supradiaphragmatic or atrial) thrombi are approached in conjunction with a cardiothoracic surgical team. Because the tumor is controlled from within the chest, extensive mobilization of the liver is not necessary. The caudate lobe of the liver should be mobilized off the IVC enough to allow for a vena cavotomy of adequate length. Similar to the situation described previously, we complete the nephrectomy and mobilize the IVC and control all tributaries before the institution of cardiopulmonary bypass (CPB). Because the patient will be maximally anticoagulated while undergoing

CPB, it is imperative to have meticulous hemostasis following the nephrectomy. Once the patient has been placed on CPB, the cardiothoracic and urologic surgeons can work simultaneously to open the IVC and atrium and extract the tumor thrombus from both directions.

We previously preferred to use deep hypothermic circulatory arrest (DHCA) to aid in resection of level IV thrombi.[13] However, this technique can be associated with significant perioperative complications. More recently, we prefer to extract atrial thrombi with a cardiopulmonary bypass type approach. Venous blood from the infrarenal IVC and superior vena cava is directed toward the CPB circuit, which is then returned through an aortic cannula. When the IVC is opened and the tumor thrombus is extracted, the surgeon encounters significant bleeding from the hepatic venous return, but this bleeding can be controlled and returned to the bypass circuit with vacuum-assisted venous drainage. The suction rate can be set to match the rate of bleeding from the liver, to enable the surgeon to inspect the IVC lumen adequately. The advantage of cardiopulmonary bypass (over DHCA) lies in the ability to resect intracaval tumors adequately under normothermic CPB and without needing to arrest the heart. DHCA may still be required for massive tumors within the atrium.

Inferior Vena Cava Hemorrhage

As many urologists may have encountered, hemorrhage from the IVC can be associated with massive blood loss. In our experience, the best way to prevent significant IVC hemorrhage is first to obtain control of the IVC and significant tributaries, as described previously. Once control has been obtained, bleeding from the IVC can easily be terminated by occluding the isolated segment. For small lacerations in the IVC, we prefer to obtain immediate control simply with digital pressure. After the adjacent cava has been adequately mobilized, a small clamp (e.g., a spoon-type clamp) can be placed such that the IVC is atraumatically apposed in this location. Lacerations can be closed in the previously described manners. Other surgeons have had success with Allis clamps in these situations, and we think this technique is acceptable for surgeons experienced with placing these clamps. Occasionally the IVC or renal vein can become very thin, and attempts at placing Allis clamps can result in tearing and more vigorous bleeding.

Whenever possible, we prefer to decrease the pressure within the IVC by controlling inflow and outflow before we attempt to close a laceration. It is difficult to control flow at the IVC bifurcation, and injuries to this extremely thin-walled location can result in catastrophic hemorrhage. Dissection in this area must be undertaken with extreme care and is ill-advised without obtaining control of the iliac veins as well as the IVC. Despite control of the external iliac veins and infrarenal IVC, several large posterior branches along the common iliac segment can cause significant bleeding. If significant bleeding from posteriorly located branches persists during attempts to close an injury to the caval bifurcation, closure of the injury can be attempted; however, this may be fraught with additional tearing. In this situation, it is best to close the laceration with the aid of pledget.

Lacerations to the IVC bifurcation that extend under the common iliac arteries can be very difficult to visualize because of the overlying arteries. These vessels can be mobilized and retracted; however, these maneuvers may still limit visualization of the full extent of the laceration. Occasionally, intentional division and subsequent reanastomosis of the artery are necessary to fully appreciate hemorrhage from the IVC bifurcation.

Lumbar Vein Hemorrhage

Lumbar vein hemorrhage can also occur during operations on the IVC. In our experience, the best method for controlled division of lumbar veins involves first obtaining control of the IVC. We prefer to encircle the IVC with umbilical tape, and with upward traction, the posteriorly draining lumbar veins can be identified. These veins can then be dissected and doubly ligated before dividing. Occasionally, the veins are too short to place two ties and therefore the distal aspect of the vein can be controlled with clips. We prefer to place a tie on the IVC side and leave a reasonable cuff on this side. If hemorrhage occurs from the IVC side, the previously obtained control of the IVC can aid to decrease bleeding.

Hemorrhage from the distal side (lumbar side) can be troublesome because the vein tends to retract into the posterior body wall musculature. The bleeding from this location can be controlled with a fingertip, and then a long, slender instrument, such as a tonsil clamp, can be used to grasp the vein edges after the digital pressure has been slowly released. Once the edges are grasped, the vein can be occluded by twisting the clamp. If the vein cannot be grasped, a figure-of-8 stitch (2-0 or 3-0 polypropylene on a large half-circle needle) incorporating some of the posterior body wall musculature can also be successful in controlling the bleeding.

Hypogastric (Internal Iliac) Venous Hemorrhage

Hemorrhage from the hypogastric or internal iliac veins can be encountered during renal transplantation or pelvic lymphadenectomy procedures. Injuries to these large veins can result in substantial hemorrhage. Often, three hypogastric veins insert posteriorly into the external iliac vein. At least one of these veins is fairly wide, a feature that can make dissection and subsequent ligature placement fairly difficult. In comparison with lumbar vein hemorrhage, bleeding from the hypogastric veins tends to be more severe and more difficult to control. Accordingly, dissection of these veins should be approached in a very meticulous manner.

Our approach to exposing and dividing the hypogastric veins starts with mobilizing the common, external, and (proximal) internal iliac arteries and retracting these vessels medially. The external iliac vein is then circumferentially mobilized all the way to the insertion of the first hypogastric branch. We then circumferentially dissect the common iliac vein and encircle this with an umbilical tape or vessel loop. Again, if substantial bleeding from the hypogastric veins occurs, the inflow and outflow of the iliac veins can be controlled. We now dissect the hypogastric veins after retracting up on the vascular loops on the common and external iliac veins. Additionally, the hypogastric veins can most often be exposed from a lateral direction. With the artery mobilized medially, the vein can be further mobilized to a medial direction that allows a somewhat unobstructed access to the hypogastric veins. The psoas muscle can be retracted laterally with a handheld-type retractor to provide improved exposure. Each hypogastric vein is circumferentially dissected, doubly ligated, and divided. Similar to lumbar veins, these veins can be very short, and placement of two separate ligatures can be difficult. In these situations, we have found that clips placed on the distal aspect (segment of vein away from the iliac vein) can accomplish satisfactory hemostasis. After each internal iliac vein is divided, the iliac vein is now completely mobilized and can be placed lateral to the iliac artery.

Occasionally, the ligature on the iliac vein side cannot be placed. In these cases, we control the distal vein and then gain control of the iliac vein by occluding proximally and distally. The hypogastric veins can then be divided, leaving the portion of the vein entering the external iliac vein uncontrolled. If the external iliac vein has been fully mobilized, this vein can be readily flipped over and the uncontrolled branches on the posterior aspect can be sutured. Given that the external iliac and common iliac veins have been previously controlled, no bleeding should occur during this maneuver.

Hemorrhage from the hypogastric or internal iliac vein can be considerable, and bleeding from the distal end is particularly is very difficult to control. The approach to controlling the distal end is similar to that described for control of lumbar vein hemorrhage. Immediate control is gained with digital pressure, and a long, slender instrument or suture ligature that incorporates adjacent tissue can establish more definitive control.

External Iliac Vein Hemorrhage
In relative terms, hemorrhage from the external iliac vein is more readily controlled than is hemorrhage from the vena cava or internal iliac vein. The reason is the lack of branches and relative ease in which to encircle the external iliac vein. Occasionally, an obturator branch can insert along the posterior aspect and can result in troublesome bleeding. The external iliac vein can be grasped with forceps and flipped over, and the branch point of a tributary can be suture ligated.

Renal Vein Hemorrhage
Hemorrhage from the renal veins can be associated with large quantities of blood loss. The right renal vein, in particular, can be extremely thin walled. Occasionally, while encircling this vein, a posteriorly inserting branch (infrequent) or the posterior wall can be injured. Bleeding from the renal vein can be immediately controlled with digital pressure. Once this is applied, the next steps relate to the intended operation. If the injury occurs during nephrectomy, pressure can be maintained on the vein until the renal artery is ligated, after which the vein can be ligated and divided. If the artery cannot be readily controlled, attempts to fix the laceration in the renal vein while the kidney is perfused are extremely difficult and will undoubtedly result in large volumes of blood loss. An alternative approach is to place a large clamp across the renal pedicle and remove the kidney. The transected edges of the renal artery and vein are then identified and suture ligated with fine polypropylene suture (4-0 or 5-0). Placement of a pedicle-type clamp on the right side must be done with the appreciation of the short right renal vein. The hilum must be transected in a manner that maintains tissue within the clamp. If this is not considered, the tissue within the jaws of the clamp may retract, thereby resulting in ongoing bleeding.

KEY POINTS

1. In general, arteries should be exposed along the anterior surface because major branches are unlikely to arise from this direction.

2. Perhaps the most important principle in managing unexpected bleeding is that properly applied digital pressure can control virtually all abdominal and pelvic bleeding.

3. Two principles should be considered when conducting vascular repairs: hemostasis and preservation of the normal luminal caliber to maintain flow.

4. Before conducting vascular repair, the surgeon should determine the need for systemic anticoagulation and proximal and distal embolectomy.

5. The close proximity of the SMA and left renal vein is well known and clearly plays a role in mistaking the SMA for the renal artery.

6. Nearly all major arteries to the left kidney lie posterior to the left renal vein (with the exception of a retroaortic left renal vein).

7. Occlusion of the left renal vein at its entry into the IVC generally does not result in venous hypertension because the left renal vein has collateral drainage through adrenal, gonadal, and lumbar branches.

8. Occlusion of the right renal vein may result in venous hypertension, acute tubular necrosis, and renal insufficiency. If ligation or resection of the suprarenal vena cava is required, reconstruction of the right renal vein is required.

9. The best way to prevent significant vena caval hemorrhage is to first obtain control of the IVC and significant tributaries.

REFERENCES

Please see www.expertconsult.com

Chapter 22

MANAGEMENT OF BOWEL COMPLICATIONS

Phuong M. Pham MD

*Surgical Resident, Department of Surgery, David Geffen School of Medicine, University of California–
Los Angeles, Los Angeles, California*

Oscar Joe Hines MD

*Professor of Surgery, Department of Surgery, David Geffen School of Medicine, University of California–
Los Angeles, Los Angeles, California*

Urologists are often faced with clinical and operative decisions that involve the bowel. The bowel can be invaded by urologic tumors, may be used as a urinary conduit, and simply may be in the way of complex urologic procedures. The approach to some common problems associated with operating in the abdominal cavity and the management of potential complications associated with the gastrointestinal (GI) tract are outlined in this chapter.

ILEUS

Ileus, or intestinal paralysis, is experienced by most patients following an intraperitoneal procedure and can also be exhibited following an extraperitoneal procedure. This condition is a normal physiologic response of diminished bowel motility and function following an operation and is characterized by abdominal distention, lack of bowel sounds, delayed passage of flatus and defecation, and accumulation of gas and fluids in the bowel that may result in nausea and vomiting. However, prolonged ileus lengthens the patient's discomfort, increases the need for parenteral nutritional support, and constitutes the most common reason for delayed discharge after abdominal surgery. The economic impact of ileus is estimated to be $750 million to $1 billion in the United States annually.[1]

The pathophysiologic mechanism of ileus is incompletely understood but appears multifactorial involving neurogenic, inflammatory, and pharmacologic mechanisms. Increased sympathetic outflow inhibits bowel motility by preventing the release of acetylcholine from excitatory fibers located in the myenteric plexus. In addition, catecholamines released during an operation are associated with inhibited motility,[2] and β-adrenergic blockade improves motility in animals.[3] Intestinal manipulation elicits a local inflammatory response with the release of nitric oxide, prostaglandins, and interleukins by macrophages.[4] It appears that these inflammatory mediators interact with numerous neurotransmitters and hormones such as vasoactive intestinal polypeptide, calcitonin gene–related peptide, substance P, and corticotropin-releasing factor to result in ileus.[5] Pharmacologically, opioids used postoperatively contribute to ileus by their depressant effects on GI transit.[4]

Following abdominal surgical procedures, each section of the GI tract recovers at a different rate. The small intestine first regains function within 24 hours, the stomach in 24 to 48 hours, and the colon in 3 to 5 days. Therefore, once the patient has experienced flatus following an operation, the physician can assume that the colon and the remaining GI tract have recovered. During this period, it is unlikely the patient will want to take anything by mouth, and in fact this may prolong the ileus. The bowel should be given a period of rest before starting oral intake.

The mainstay of treatment for postoperative ileus has been nasogastric decompression. However, the use of this technique during this period has become somewhat controversial. In fact, a meta-analysis of 26 studies concluded that routine nasogastric decompression after elective laparotomy results in significantly increased rates of pulmonary complications such as fever, atelectasis, and pneumonia.[6] The same study also found that selective decompression resulted in fewer wound complications and shorter hospital stay. Thus, nasogastric decompression may benefit the patient in selected cases. If bowel anastomosis was performed, it probably shows good judgment to use a nasogastric tube. However, many colorectal surgeons have successfully stopped using a nasogastric tube for left colonic anastomoses. If no bowel anastomosis is performed, one can reliably not use a nasogastric tube. If the patient does become distended, experience nausea or vomiting, or complains of heartburn (a sign of poor gastric function, reflux, and a prodrome of vomiting in the postoperative patient), a nasogastric tube should be placed.

Several abnormalities can initiate and propagate ileus. Simple electrolyte abnormalities including hyponatremia, hypokalemia, and hypo-osmolarity can usually be corrected and may aid in correction of this motility problem. Excessive use of narcotic analgesia prolongs ileus, and a non-narcotic approach to pain relief should be considered. Ileus, however, can be a sign of more severe conditions including sepsis and acute blood loss. If postoperative bowel function is not progressing as one would expect, the clinician should look for sources of infection including intra-abdominal abscess, bowel leak, urinary tract infection, or pulmonary infection. Finally, the acute withdrawal or accelerated taper of steroids in the postoperative period is known to prolong or even precipitate ileus and is corrected with bolus steroid administration.[7] After these problems have been corrected, the ileus should resolve without much delay.

In some patients, ileus may last significantly longer than normal. In such a case, the use of a nasogastric tube is advised. Parenteral nutrition should be started if it is anticipated that prolonged ileus will continue (>7-10 days). Once bowel obstruction has been ruled out and the correctable abnormalities listed earlier have been addressed, a trial of prokinetic agents may be started. Several agents are available including cisapride, metoclopramide, bethanechol, and erythromycin.

Some investigators have attempted to improve problems of ileus by the use of prokinetic agents in the immediate postoperative period. Unfortunately, the use of metoclopramide or cisapride in a prospective manner does not appear to shorten the length of ileus or discharge to home.[8,9] Erythromycin is a motilin receptor agonist in human GI smooth muscle and induces migrating motor complexes,[10] but studies have shown mixed results with regard to its effects on ileus. One study showed that erythromycin shortened the time to oral intake and hospital stay following pancreaticoduodenectomy,[11] whereas another study showed that the drug did not alter clinically important outcomes related to postoperative ileus in patients undergoing resection for colorectal cancer.[12]

The most appropriate treatment for ileus maybe a multimodal approach because of the multifactorial origin of this condition. The use of nonsteroidal anti-inflammatory drugs may help improve ileus by reducing the amount of opioid given postoperatively. Thoracic epidural blocks with bupivacaine hydrochloride have been shown to reduce ileus significantly as opposed to systemic opioid therapy in patients undergoing abdominal surgical procedures.[13] Early postoperative ambulation has not been shown to expedite GI tract function recovery, but it is encouraged for its benefits in reducing thromboembolism and pulmonary complications. Laparoscopic procedures have been shown to decrease the duration of ileus because of reduced tissue trauma, which results in the release of lower levels of inflammatory cytokines.

Finally, the most important factor determining correction of ileus may be the power of suggestion and the doctor-patient relationship. Autonomic activity, the major mediator of ileus, is subject to control by suggestion. One study examined the effect of preoperative instructions for the early return of GI motility and compared this group of patients with a group who received an equal-length of interview offering reassurance and nonspecific instructions. The group receiving the specific preoperative instruction returned to normal intestinal motility in 2.6 versus 4.1 days and had a 1.5-day shorter hospital stay and a $1,200.00 cost savings.[14] This simple 5-minute intervention may significantly affect your practice.

BOWEL OBSTRUCTION

Intra-abdominal adhesions are the most common cause of bowel obstruction in the United States. Other potential causes include both internal and external herniation, carcinomatosis, and radiation. The incidence of postoperative obstruction varies with the approach and procedure performed. The percentage of obstruction ranges from 0.7% to 14.9%[15,16] for ureteroileal conduit diversion and 5%[17] for retroperitoneal lymph node dissection. In general, bowel obstruction rates are higher for pelvic procedures. Trocar site intestinal herniation must also be considered for patients who have undergone a laparoscopic procedure.

Intestinal obstruction in the early postoperative period must be distinguished from ileus. Ileus is associated with many intra-abdominal and extra-abdominal processes that interfere with normal bowel motility, and it resolves spontaneously once the provoking source has been abolished.

Most patients with bowel obstruction exhibit abdominal pain, nausea, vomiting, obstipation, and abdominal distention. Alternatively, if bowel function never returns postoperatively, the patient may also have a bowel obstruction. Pain is usually intermittent and may become constant if the bowel becomes compromised. However, pain severity may decrease over time as a result of bowel fatigue and atony. The periodicity of pain can be a clue to the level of obstruction: pain from proximal intestinal obstruction has short periodicity (3-4 minutes), and distal small bowel or colonic pain has longer intervals (15-20 minutes) between episodes of nausea, cramping, and vomiting. When pain and tenderness begin to localize in a more somatic pattern, one should be concerned with bowel ischemia and peritonitis with attendant parietal peritoneal irritation. Vomiting is earlier and more bilious if the obstruction is high, and later and more feculent if the obstruction is low. Abdominal distention may be prominent if the

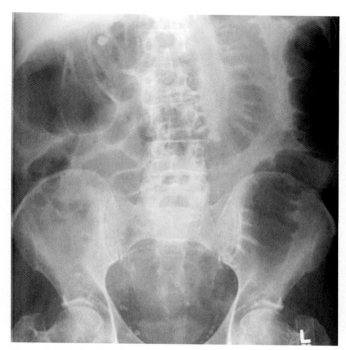

Figure 22-1   Supine plain film of the abdomen demonstrating dilated loops of small and large intestine and a large bowel obstruction.

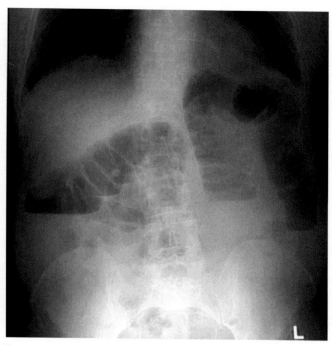

Figure 22-2   Upright plain film of the abdomen demonstrating air-fluid levels of the large intestine and a large bowel obstruction.

obstruction is low and minimal if the obstruction is high.

Patients usually become profoundly intravascularly depleted manifested by orthostatic hypotension, tachycardia, and low urinary output. In addition, laboratory findings may include an elevated hematocrit and blood urea nitrogen. Eventually, patients manifest hypokalemic, hypochloremic metabolic alkalosis secondary to gastric loss of hydrogen and chloride and the renal compensation of potassium wasting.

The essential test in diagnosing bowel obstruction is supine and upright radiographic views of the abdomen. A chest radiograph should also be obtained to exclude a pneumonic process and to look for subdiaphragmatic air. Supine views demonstrate distended loops of bowel (**Fig. 22-1**). Upright views characteristically show multiple air-fluid levels (**Fig. 22-2**). In contradistinction to ileus, which may also produce air-fluid levels, gas is not seen through the entire GI tract, especially distal to the point of obstruction. In early or partial bowel obstruction, gas can be seen distal to the point of obstruction. In addition, if the patient has had a rectal examination, gas may be identified in the rectal vault.

The use of contrast studies to diagnose or confirm bowel obstruction is sometimes useful. If the bowel is massively distended with air and it appears that large bowel obstruction is present, a barium enema is indicated. It is rare, however, for a patient with an obstruction in the immediate postoperative period to harbor a large bowel obstruction.

In patients with suspected bowel obstruction and equivocal abdominal films, other radiologic modalities are indicated. Multiple studies have demonstrated computed tomography (CT) scanning to have sensitivity and specificity of >90% for small bowel obstruction[18]. In addition, CT scanning is capable of detecting the cause as well as the presence of closed-loop obstruction and strangulation and therefore usually the first radiologic examination performed. The use of upper GI contrast studies to establish the diagnosis of small bowel obstruction is more controversial. Many published series in the radiologic literature have documented the accuracy of this approach. Again, barium should be used because Gastrografin dilutes as it travels through the GI tract and makes this medium less reliable. However, some physicians believe that an upper GI series can lead to overdiagnosis or underdiagnosis of obstruction and does not predict which patients will ultimately need reoperation. An upper GI series is indicated, however, if the diagnosis of bowel obstruction is unclear.

The most important initial step in treating a patient with bowel obstruction is to replace intravascular volume. Balanced salt solutions of normal saline or lactated Ringer's may be used. The patient may require several liters of fluid before rehydration is complete. Rehydration should be monitored with a Foley catheter and, if indicated, measurement of central venous pressure or Swan-Ganz perimeters. In addition, serum electrolytes should be monitored and adjusted as indicated.

Antibiotics should not be used unless the patient is to go to the operating room or ischemic bowel is contemplated. Finally, a nasogastric tube should be placed to decompress the stomach and prevent aspiration.

Differentiating partial from complete bowel obstruction is important. *Complete bowel obstruction* is defined by the complete lack of passage of stool or flatus and the absence of evidence of gas distal to the site of obstruction on plain abdominal films. Some patients with early complete bowel obstruction are still passing some gas but soon this ceases. Many cases of partial obstruction resolve with conservative management; however, most cases of complete obstruction will not. Nearly 80% of patients with complete obstruction will require an operation. Therefore, surgical intervention should occur earlier in patients with complete bowel obstruction. Similarly, in approximately 80% of patients, partial bowel obstruction resolves on its own.[19]

Some physicians have used a long intestinal tube or Levin tube to decompress to bowel. This approach is believed to be more effective than that using an ordinary nasogastric tube because it decompresses the bowel directly at the site of the obstruction, improves circulation, and leads to faster resolution. Unfortunately, the studies examining the utility of this approach have found that patients treated with a Levin tube have a longer period of preoperative treatment, a higher incidence of ischemic bowel, and a longer period of postoperative care.[20-22] Therefore, the routine use of Levin tubes cannot be advocated, and in most cases, decompression with a standard nasogastric tube is sufficient.

Strangulation of the bowel is a potential complication of obstruction and must be quickly corrected to avoid a poor outcome because it carries a much higher mortality rate than does simple obstruction. The diagnosis of bowel strangulation is made by a combination of signs and laboratory findings. The patient may have a fever, unexplained tachycardia, nausea, and vomiting. Physical examination reveals localized tenderness. Laboratory findings corroborating strangulation include a rising white blood cell count and elevated serum lactic acid or amylase levels.

Some clinicians have attempted to correlate specific findings with the diagnosis of strangulated bowel, without much success.[23] Even the use of formulas to predict the presence of compromised bowel based on preoperative data has failed to reach sufficient predictive ability.[24] If fever, tachycardia, localized pain, and leukocytosis are all absent, the likelihood that the patient is harboring ischemic bowel is near zero.[25] When strangulated bowel is suspected, an expedited trip to the operating room is mandatory following adequate resuscitation.

Bowel obstruction in the immediate postoperative period almost always resolves with conservative treatment. The initially aggressive nature of adhesions usually improves and leads to resolution of symptoms.

In nearly 90% of these patients, the condition resolves with nasogastric decompression. Two thirds of these bowel obstructions resolve within 7 days and the remainder resolve within 14 days.[26] During this period, parenteral nutrition should be considered. If the condition has not resolved after 2 weeks of conservative measures, reoperation is likely indicated.

Reoperation

Once a determination has been made that reoperation is necessary to relieve obstruction, the patient should be prepared with perioperative antibiotics and careful induction of general anesthesia to avoid aspiration. The incision is best made away from any previous incision because adhesions are likely present in the undersurface of the previous incision. A midline incision is preferable for adequate exposure. Special care should be taken while entering the abdomen to avoid injury to the intestine.

On entering the abdomen, the surgeon should note the character of the peritoneal fluid. Turbid or dark fluid is an indication of ischemic bowel. The entire intestine should be freed of adhesions using sharp dissection from the ligament of Treitz to the sigmoid colon. Blunt dissection tends to remove serosa from the bowel. The bowel should be repaired if the mucosa is visible. A point of transition between proximal dilated and distal decompressed bowel should be identified and the inciting cause corrected. If one determines that completely dissecting the bowel free of adhesions is dangerous, a bypass of the segment should be considered.

Determining the viability of the intestine can be difficult. The intestine should be examined for coloration, presence of motility, and arterial pulsations. In addition, Doppler examination can be used to identify arterial flow. If the viability is still in question, one ampule of intravenous fluorescein can be administered. Viable bowel will glow with the use of Wood's lamp. If dead bowel is identified, a segmental resection should be performed as well as primary anastomosis. Alternatively, the bowel maybe left in place if the suspected bowel segment is long and there is concern of short gut syndrome after resection. However, these patients should undergo repeat exploration within 24 hours and any nonviable bowel should be removed.

Milking the bowel to remove the intraoperative contents should be avoided. Sometimes it is necessary to perform this maneuver to close the abdomen. If the bowel is milked, the surgeon can be assured that this will cause transient bacteremia and the potential complications of infection.

The abdomen should be closed in a standard fashion. The skin may be closed in most circumstances unless significant contamination is present. Occasionally, the abdomen cannot be closed because of edema. In this circumstance, a piece of prosthetic material (Gore-

Tex) should be placed. The patient can undergo reoperation for primary fascial closure once the edema has resolved.

Laparoscopy offers the potential for minimally invasive approach for diagnostic as well as therapeutic intervention. Several clinical studies have demonstrated that patients with bowel obstruction who underwent laparoscopic management of bowel obstruction had fewer postoperative complications, quicker recovery of bowel movements, and a shorter hospital stay than those who underwent conventional laparotomy.[27-29] However, complications such as perforations were more common overall in the laparoscopic group, and patients with two or more previous laparotomies had higher rates of these complications.[29] Thus, when perform by a skilled surgeon on selected patients, laparoscopic management is both feasible and safe.

Prevention

Unfortunately, current surgical practices are not very effective in preventing adhesions. Careful surgical technique, avoidance of tissue ischemia, minimization of the use of foreign material, and minimal manipulation of the bowel are recommended.

Many substances have been investigated in an attempt to prevent adhesions. Heparin, kinases, fibrinolysin, steroids, nonsteroidal prostaglandin antagonists, and dextran have all been used in animal models and in some patients. In addition, the use of prokinetics, especially cisapride, has been tried.[30] None of these agents seem to prevent adhesion formation reliably.

Newer products have been developed that show some value and are now commercially available. Seprafilm (Genzyme, Cambridge, Massachusetts) and INTERCEED (Ethicon, Cincinnati, Ohio) are two absorbable physical barriers that are approved by the U.S. Food and Drug Administration for the prevention of adhesions. Seprafilm is a membrane made of hyaluronate and carboxymethylcellulose and is applied intraoperatively. The application of Seprafilm was demonstrated by several randomized trials to reduce the incidence and severity of adhesions after surgery.[31-33] INTERCEED, a membrane composed of oxidized regenerated cellulose, has also been shown to reduce the incidence, extent, and severity of postoperative adhesions significantly.[34-35] However, its effectiveness is reduced in the presence of blood.[36] Whether the application of these absorbable barriers will translate into a lower rate of bowel obstructions has yet to be determined, but the initial results are promising.

ENTEROCUTANEOUS FISTULA

An *enterocutaneous fistula* is defined as an abnormal communication between the bowel and skin. This is a serious condition with a mortality rate still ≤15%. The approach to a patient who develops an enterocutaneous fistula requires stringent attention to detail and patience.

Enterocutaneous fistulas can generally be classified as spontaneous or postoperative. Most enterocutaneous fistulas (75%-85%) result from operative intervention, whereas spontaneous enterocutaneous fistulas account for the remainder and are associated with inflammatory bowel disease.[37] The most common operations leading to enterocutaneous fistulas include procedures performed for malignant disease, inflammatory bowel disease, or adhesiolysis. The major risk factor appears to be poor nutritional status of the patient. Patients who have lost 10% to 15% of body weight over a short period of time, have a serum albumin level of <3.0 g/dL and a transferrin level <220 mg/dL, have anergy to injected recall antigens, or are unable to perform normal daily tasks because of weakness are at highest risk. Poor nutritional status leads to a greater possibility of anastomotic leak, poor wound healing, and inadequate response to infection. Finally, a history of radiation therapy and of an emergency appears to increase the risk for enterocutaneous fistula.

The three most important actions that can be taken to prevent the complication of fistula are as follows:

1. Improve the nutrition of malnourished patients.
2. Use mechanical and antibiotic bowel preparation.
3. Perform careful surgical technique.[38]

In addition to the factors already mentioned, patients who are generally septic, have renal failure or diabetes, or who are taking immunosuppressive medications such as steroids or chemotherapy agents are at increased risk for fistula formation. A multivariate analysis of factors that lead to anastomotic leaks also found that chronic obstructive pulmonary disease and the use of >2 U of red blood cells in the perioperative period increased the risk.[39]

When an enterocutaneous fistula develops postoperatively, the usual clinical situation is a temperature spike at about day 4 to day 7 accompanied by elevated white blood cell count and a wound infection. The wound appears cellulitic and requires opening for treatment. On opening the wound, the clinician may find pus and obvious enteric contents in the wound. Alternatively, the appearance of enteric contents on the dressing may not be noted for 12 to 24 hours. The initial treatment of a new enterocutaneous fistula does not include reoperation. If this approach is used, the best case situation is that the patient will continue to have a fistula and the worst is that a poor outcome will result.

The initial problems a new fistula presents are sepsis, electrolyte imbalance, and malnutrition. Each of these must be effectively addressed to ensure a good result. Local and systemic sepsis should be treated within the first 24 to 48 hours after a fistula is diagnosed. The patient may need replacement of intravascular volume

TABLE 22-1	Electrolyte Composition of Gastrointestinal Tract Effluent			
	Electrolyte (mEq/dL)			
Bowel Segment	**Na^+**	**K^+**	**Cl^-**	**HCO_3^-**
Stomach	60	10	100	—
Duodenum	140	5	80	50
Ileum	130	10	110	30
Colon	60	30	40	20

Cl^-, chloride; HCO_3^-, bicarbonate; K^+, potassium; Na^+, sodium.

TABLE 22-2	Categorization of Enterocutaneous Fistula
Type	**Volume**
Low-output fistulas	<200 mL/24 hr
Moderate-output fistulas	200-500 mL/hr
High-output fistulas	>500 mL/24 hr

TABLE 22-3	Predicting the Likelihood of Spontaneous Enterocutaneous Fistula Closure	
Favorable	**Unfavorable**
Gastrointestinal continuity maintained	Complete disruption
End fistula	Lateral fistula
No abscess	Abscess
Healthy adjacent bowel	Diseased adjacent bowel
Jejunal	Ileal, gastric
Fistula tract >2 cm	Fistula tract <2 cm
Bowel defect <1 cm	Bowel defect >1 cm
Well-nourished patient	Malnourished patient

with crystalloid and blood as appropriate. Broad-spectrum antibiotics covering normal enteric flora should be instituted. Antibiotics should be used only when a specific indication exists, however. Patients with fistulas are routinely overtreated with antibiotics, and superinfections or resistant organisms develop. The presence of an intra-abdominal abscess should be identified with the use of an abdominal CT scan. An abscess, if present, can be treated with percutaneous drainage and the content can be sent for microbiologic culture.

Local sepsis and skin care need to be addressed early. This care involves controlling the fistula and protecting the skin. The use of a nasogastric tube does not seem to affect the long-term outcome for patients with a fistula and is not part of routine practice. The fistula should be locally controlled with the use of a sump tube or Robinson catheter. The surrounding skin should be treated like an ostomy; thus, an enterostomal nurse should be asked to evaluate the patient. Karaya gum powder, cement, and resin are useful. DuoDERM (ConvaTec, Skillman, New Jersey) application may be very helpful and can be cut the fit the defect.

The most common electrolyte disturbances, depending on the normal output of the segment of bowel affected (Table 22-1), involve potassium and sodium. In addition, patients may have problems with acid-base status and magnesium or phosphorous. These conditions should be monitored closely because patients may require surprisingly large amounts of replacement.

Patients with enterocutaneous fistulas are often malnourished because of the lack of food intake, the hypercatabolism of sepsis, and the loss of protein-rich enteral contents. In general, the patient with an enterocutaneous fistula should not be allowed any oral intake, Therefore, nutrition is delivered parenterally. Full support is achieved with central total parenteral nutrition. This approach diminishes bowel output and helps to control the fistula. Patients with fistulas have increased calorie and protein requirements. In general, the patient should be feed at 1.3 to 1.5 the basal calorie requirements. The goal of nutritional therapy is to restore nitrogen balance and protein synthesis to aid in healing.

If it is possible, the GI tract is preferable for nutritional support. Enteral feedings, even small amounts, may help preserve the integrity of the mucosal barrier and the immunologic and hormonal functions of the gut and to improve hepatic protein synthesis. Sometimes a feeding tube may be introduced per os or radiologically so the bowel can be used. Finally, for some patients, feeding by mouth does not significantly affect the volume output from the fistula or the electrolyte disturbances, and this route can be used.

Once sepsis, metabolic derangements, and nutrition are addressed, measures to diminish fistula output should begin. Fistulas are often categorized by output volume, and this approach helps to predict outcome and treatment (Table 22-2). Although decreasing fistula output does not seem to increase the chances of spontaneous closure, for those fistulas that are going to close, decreasing output shortens the time to closure (Table 22-3).

The patient should receive a histamine receptor (H_2) antagonist or proton pump inhibitor, which will not only reduce the chance of peptic ulceration in these very ill patients but also decrease gastric secretion and therefore pancreaticobiliary and small intestinal secretion.[40] The use of somatostatin analogues to diminish output and hasten closure is somewhat controversial. Somatostatin is a peptide that slows intestinal transit and decreases pancreatic and intestinal secretion. The initial enthusiasm for this treatment waned through the years. If somatostatin is used, it can be expected that output will fall by half within the first 24 hours. The use of somatostatin does not increase the number of fistulas that will close spontaneously, but it significantly cuts the number of days until closure (10 days versus 50 days).[41] Negative pressure vacuum-assisted closure systems have been used by physicians for many years to promote wound healing. Several case reports[42-44] have documented the successful use of vacuum-assisted closure systems in the management enterocutaneous fistulas. The patients in these case reports had either spontaneous closure of the fistula or significantly decreased output.[45]

After 7 to 10 days of care and stabilization, the patient should undergo fluoroscopic fistulography with the use of water-soluble contrast (**Fig. 22-3**). The fistula is intubated with a small-caliber tube, and the site of entry into the bowel, the nature of the adjacent bowel, and the presence of intestinal continuity are assessed. The passage of dye distally should be seen because a fistula will not close in the presence of distal obstruction.

The goals of treatment for these patients are restoration of intestinal continuity and resumption of oral intake. In 60% to 80% of patients, they occur spontaneously with the measures outlined earlier. For the remaining 20% to 40%, timing of operation remains questionable. If a fistula has not closed within 6 weeks with adequate nutrition and no infection, the fistula is unlikely to close. If the patient does not improve with conservative management and sepsis continues, operation may be mandatory and should address sites of intra-abdominal infection. Repair of the fistula is not usually undertaken early, and diversion should be considered.

Definitive operation should occur no earlier than 6 weeks from the initial diagnosis, preferably postponed as long as tolerable. Fistula-related infection leads to significant adhesions. Therefore, waiting before surgical repair ensures a safer and technically easier procedure. When the operation is performed, segmental resection and hand-sewn anastomosis lead to the lowest rates of recurrence and the lowest incidence of complications.

Postoperatively, the patient should be maintained on nutritional support until he or she is able to take the caloric requirements by mouth. This phase may take some time if the patient as been on "nothing by mouth" orders for a while. Finally, encouragement and emotional support from the medical team are very important.

INTRA-ABDOMINAL ABSCESS

An *intra-abdominal abscess* represents a walled-off infection and collection of bacteria, pus, blood, and possibly foreign material. Most intra-abdominal abscesses develop in the postoperative period. The diagnosis should be suspected in a patient who is not progressing adequately following an operation. Ileus, abdominal distention, and anorexia are common symptoms. Spiking fevers are common but may be masked in immunosuppressed patients, in elderly patients, and in patients receiving antibiotics. This abscess is accompanied by leukocytosis with a shift to the left.

Diagnosis is made by ultrasound or CT scan (**Fig. 22-4**).[46] Both methods are effective in identifying an intra-abdominal abscess and may be used therapeutically. Once an abscess has been identified, antibiotic treatment is not adequate; the abscess must be drained. For most intra-abdominal abscesses, a percutaneous approach should be attempted before operative intervention.[47,48] On occasion, the location of the abscess is such that it cannot be drained by that approach. The advantages of percutaneous drainage include a lack of contamination of the remainder of the peritoneal cavity, avoidance of general anesthetic, and a lower incidence of inadequate drainage. Periprocedural antibiotics should be administered. The success rate of this approach ranges from 80% to 90%. In general, a pigtail catheter should be left in to the assess cavity and removed when drainage has subsided. Some physicians choose to irrigate the catheter with saline solution daily to keep it open.

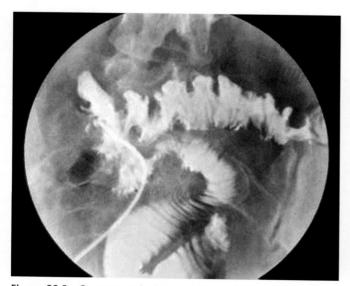

Figure 22-3 Contrast study demonstrating an enterocutaneous fistula (fistulogram).

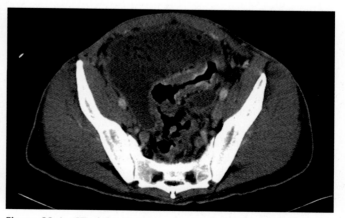

Figure 22-4 CT of the abdomen demonstrating a well-organized intra-abdominal abscess.

The indications for open surgical drainage include failure of percutaneous drainage, inability to drain percutaneously, and the presence of interloop abscesses. Closed-suction drains can be placed and left until output diminishes. Some physicians assess the abscess cavity with a contrast study through the drain before pulling the tube to be assured that the cavity has collapsed.

Antibiotic use should be directed by culture information until signs of infection have resolved. It is not necessary to continue antibiotics for long periods because the treatment is drainage. If the patient does not improve within 24 to 48 hours, one can assume that the abscess was not adequately drained and the patient should undergo reimaging. Reasons for failure include thick material in the cavity, a multiloculated cavity, or multiple abscesses.

Patients can present with an abscess in a variety of intra-abdominal locations. Patients with a subphrenic abscess may also complain of shoulder and back pain. In addition, diaphragmatic irritation may lead to intractable hiccups. Multiple interloop abscesses require exploration for treatment but rarely require drainage catheters to be placed. Abscesses located in the pelvis can often be drained through the vagina, rectum, or ureteral stump after cystectomy.

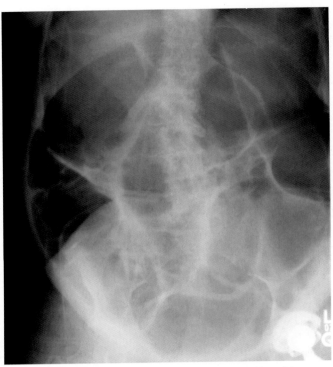

Figure 22-5   Plain film of the abdomen revealing a sigmoid volvulus.

VOLVULUS

Volvulus occurs when a segment of the bowel twists along its longitudinal axis and contorts the mesentery in the process. Although volvulus of all individual segments of the colon has been reported, sigmoid volvulus is by far the most common, followed by cecal volvulus. Volvulus leads to acute bowel obstruction and can progress to strangulation, necrosis, and perforation.

Volvulus is the third most common cause of large bowel obstruction in the United States. Gangrene results in 10% of patients with sigmoid volvulus and in 33% of patients with cecal volvulus.[49]

Sigmoid volvulus most often occurs in elderly, nursing home patients, patients with Parkinson's disease, and those receiving phenothiazine tranquilizers. Patients complain of sudden onset of abdominal pain and obstructive symptoms including massive distention, nausea, and vomiting. A plain film of the abdomen classically reveals an "inner tube" sign or an "upside-down U" sign (**Fig. 22-5**). If the diagnosis is unclear and no chance of necrosis is present, a contrast enema may be obtained that will show a "bird's beak" sign.

The initial approach to the patient with sigmoid volvulus consists of intravenous hydration and rigid sigmoidoscopy. Sigmoidoscopy is not only diagnostic but often also therapeutic. One can correct the twist of the bowel with the use of the scope, and the segment will decompress, often with an impressive result. At that time, a rectal tube can be placed to assist with decompression and to stent the colon so that torsion does not recur.

If the patient has signs of peritonitis, emergency laparotomy should be performed. The bowel is untwisted and viability is assessed. Nonviable bowel or perforation requires resection. If the bowel is viable, the sigmoid colon can be fixed in placed or resected. Patients with sigmoid volvulus have a 90% recurrence rate. Elective sigmoid colectomy should be performed to prevent recurrence. This can usually be performed during the same hospital admission following colonoscopic decompression and bowel preparation.

Cecal volvulus is much more uncommon than sigmoid volvulus and rarely can be addressed colonoscopically.[50] The symptoms of cecal volvulus are similar to those of small bowel obstruction. Plain films reveal a distended kidney bean–shaped loop of bowel in the left upper quadrant. Laparotomy and detorsion constitute the initial approach to cecal volvulus. Resection and primary anastomosis can be safely performed, even in the presence of unprepared bowel, and ensure permanent treatment. Some surgeons employ additional procedures such as cecopexy and cecostomy to prevent recurrence. *Cecopexy* involves anchoring the right side of the colon to the parietal peritoneum to reduce hypermobility and cecostomy involves placement of a cecostomy tube through a cecal wall incision and bringing the tube to the skin. Some researchers advocated cecopexy, claiming a lower mortality and recurrence rate of 13%.[50]

OGILVIE'S SYNDROME

Ogilvie's syndrome, or colonic pseudo-obstruction, was first described by Sir William Ogilvie in the *British Medical Journal* in 1948. This condition manifests by colonic distention that appears mechanical but is actually functional. It is thought that this condition results from an autonomic imbalance leading to increased sympathetic tone or excessive parasympathetic suppression. The precise physiologic mechanism, however, is still poorly understood.

Ogilvie's syndrome rarely occurs in patients who have undergone an intra-abdominal procedure. It is much more common in patients who are long-term residents of a nursing home or psychiatric ward. Conditions associated with this disease include stroke, dementia, orthopedic procedures, sepsis, neuroleptic use, narcotic use, electrolyte abnormalities, gynecologic surgery, prostate and bladder procedures, and renal failure.

Most patients present with massive abdominal distention and few other complaints. Patients rarely complain of much pain, and when they do, the clinician should suspect another diagnosis or pending perforation of the colon. Physical examination reveals a distended and tympanic abdomen with diminished bowel sounds. Fever and leukocytosis are rare. The presence of marked abdominal pain, fever, and leukocytosis should alert the physician to ischemia or perforation. When ischemia or perforation is present, the mortality rate is ≤40% compared with 15% in patients with viable bowel.[51]

The diagnostic process begins with flat and upright abdominal radiographs, which demonstrate a massively dilated colon beginning in the cecum and extending no farther than the splenic flexure. One must be sure that volvulus or bowel obstruction is not the cause of the colonic distention. A gentle enema contrast study can be ordered to rule out these causes and confirm the diagnosis. Ischemic bowel can also have a similar appearance on plain films, but these patients have significant abdominal complaints and are usually much sicker.

For most patients, treatment is conservative. Electrolyte abnormalities should be corrected and the medication list reviewed. Patients with a cecum measuring <12 cm should receive nothing by mouth, and a nasogastric tube should be placed. These patients should be monitored with serial examinations and abdominal films.

Patients who do not show improvement with conservative management may respond to neostigmine, a reversible acetylcholinesterase inhibitor. Neostigmine, administered intravenously, results in stimulation of muscarinic parasympathetic receptors and contraction of the affected colon. A randomized, double-blind, placebo-controlled trial found that 10 of 11 patients who received neostigmine had colonic decompression but none in the placebo group did.[52] Because neostigmine can cause bradycardia, bronchoconstriction, and tremors, close monitoring of cardiorespiratory status is required, and any toxicity should be treated with atropine.

When conservative and pharmacologic management fails, colonic diameter measures >12 cm, colon size is increasing rapidly, or the duration is >3 days, the colon should be decompressed colonoscopically with placement of a long rectal compression tube.[53] Surgical management is indicated in patients with ischemia or perforation or when pharmacologic methods and decompression have failed. Cecal perforation is reported in approximately 10%. The mortality rate is approximately 50%. According to Laplace's law, the most tension in a hollow viscus occurs in the portion of the colon with the greatest diameter: the cecum. Tension on the bowel wall diminishes blood flow and leads to necrosis and perforation. In the case of perforation, the entire segment of diseased colon is resected. Alternatively, tube cecostomy can be performed in patients without ischemia or perforation. This procedure can be performed using local anesthesia with high success and relatively low morbidity.

STAPLING COMPLICATIONS

Hungarian surgeon Hültl first conceived of the concept of stapling as an alternative to suturing tissues in 1908. These devices were not generally accepted until the 1950s, when surgeons in the Soviet Union began using them more frequently for all types of procedures. Today, stapling devices are widely used in the United States, especially for GI tract surgery and creation of urinary conduits and for reconstitution of GI continuity if resection is required for en bloc excision of tumors.

Numerous staplers exist and, when used properly, provide an anastomosis as reliable as that of hand-sewn reconstruction. The most commonly used staplers are the GI anastomosis stapler and the thoracoabdominal stapler. In addition, the end-to-end anastomosis stapler has been used for construction of the intestinal conduit stoma.[54] This type fires two circular rings of staples creating an anastomosis between two lumina. All these staplers fire a thin wire through two intestinal walls and are compressed to form a B shape. The shank length of the staple determines the thickness of the tissue after application of the instrument. Thus, a longer staple shank should be chosen for thicker tissue. Small vessels may course through the eye of the B, thereby allowing excellent vascular supply but sometimes poor hemostasis.

When the same principles of hand-sewn anastomosis, including adequate blood supply, lack of tension, and well prepared intestine, are applied, a stapled anastomosis appears as safe as that of a sewn one[55,56]

TABLE 22-4	Sewn Versus Stapled Anastomosis			
	Complications		Mortality	
Reference	Sewn (%)	Stapled (%)	Sewn (%)	Stapled (%)
Hedberg and Helmy[55] (1984)	15	4	2	0
Reiling et al[56] (1980)	16	18	0	5

TABLE 22-5	Sewn Versus Stapled Anastomosis			
	Operating Room Time (min)		Anastomotic Time (min)	
Reference	Sewn	Stapled	Sewn	Stapled
Didolkar et al[57] (1986)	154	170	19	9
Cajozzo et al[59] (1990)	—	—	14	14.3
Seufert et al[60] (1990)	194	180	—	—

(Table 22-4). This is true despite carcinomatosis, adhesions, prior chemotherapy and radiation therapy, bowel obstruction, anemia, and low leukocyte count or albumin value.[57] Some surgeons avoid a stapled anastomosis in the patient who has edematous, thickened, or attenuated bowel or who is taking steroids.

Most clinicians would agree that at the time of the anastomosis, an attempt at inspection for hemostasis along the staple line should be performed both inside and outside the bowel. This is especially true because a well-placed staple line on the intestine should not be completely hemostatic. Unrecognized massive bleeding has been reported and may require repeat exploration.[58] The surgeon should be sure to inspect the inside of a side-to-side anastomosis performed with an anastomosis stapler before it is closed.

Many surgeons have claimed that the use of stapling devices save time. Nonetheless, studies that specifically addressed this issue found the operative times to be quite similar (Table 22-5).[58-60] Certainly, the cost associated with the use of disposable devices is higher.

Allergic reactions to skin staples have been reported, including dermatitis from nickel allergies or chronic urticaria from tantalum staples, but allergies do not appear to be a issue for anastomotic staple application. A unique potential complication in urology appears to be the formation of calculi around a staple nidus.[61,62] Brenner and Johnson[62] noted a 4.2% incidence in patients who had ileal conduit diversions. The management of such stones is discussed in detail in a separate chapter. These few incidents of calculi formation appear to occur early after surgery and require no intervention.

VESICOENTERIC FISTULA

Vesicoenteric fistula, or the abnormal communication between bladder and bowel, is rare. Most of these fistulas are a consequence of inflammatory and neoplastic processes of the bowel. Diverticulitis alone accounts for ≤50% of these fistulas, whereas colonic malignant disease, granulomatous bowel disease, and radiation therapy make up the majority of the remainder.[63]

Patients with vesicoenteric fistulas primarily present with urologic symptoms rather than with symptoms related to the bowel. The presence of pneumaturia (passage of gas) and fecaluria (passage of feces) per urethra is pathognomonic and occurs in ≤83% of cases.[63] Patients may also exhibit bladder irritation, frequency, urgency, dysuria, and hematuria. Abdominal symptoms such as abdominal pain, diarrhea, constipation, intestinal obstruction, and acute abdomen also occur, but to a much lesser extent. Because of higher colonic pressure, passage of urine per rectum is not seen unless the patient has severe bladder obstruction or a diverting colostomy.

The diagnosis of vesicoenteric fistula is sometimes difficult to make on clinical grounds alone, and confirmatory studies are necessary. The most sensitive diagnostic modality is cystoscopy, which may show mucosal abnormalities, feces, and particulate matters. In a series[64] of 76 patients diagnosed and treated for vesicoenteric fistulas, investigators found that cystoscopy was sensitive in 60% of the cases. Alternatively, one can perform cystography to document the presence of contrast material in the bowel. CT scan, magnetic resonance imaging, and barium enema are not sensitive when used alone and are commonly used in combination with cystoscopy and cystography. CT scan before bladder instrumentation can provide evidence of air in the bladder, thereby confirming the presence of an enteric fistula, although it may not define the location in the absence of associated phlegmon. In this regard CT scan is the most sensitive modality for confirmation of a fistula, and cystoscopy may allow localization.

Once the diagnosis of vesicoenteric fistula is made, surgical therapy is the management of choice in most cases. Whether the approach is a one-stage or two-stage procedure is controversial, and the surgeon must make that decision based on the individual patient. In general, a one-stage repair is indicated in patients with the following factors: younger age, good general condition, small fistula, no involvement of a third organ, and absence of pericolonic or peri-intestinal abscess. In contrast, patients who have larger fistulas with possible involvement of a third organ and who may not tolerate the long surgical procedure well should undergo a two-stage repair.

In a one-stage repair, the surgeon resects the diseased bowel and portion of the involved bladder then primary bowel anastomosis is achieved and the bladder closed.

During the procedure, urinary diversion can be attained by a urethral catheter or a suprapubic catheter. A two-stage repair involves creating a diverting colostomy to control the inflammatory process and avoid infection and sepsis. A second operation is then performed weeks later in which the diseased bowel and involved bladder are resected follow by bowel anastomosis, bladder closure, and closure of the colostomy. To promote healing, it is advisable to fill the potential dead space between the bladder and bowel with vascularized tissue. This can be accomplished with an omental flap by fixing it between the bladder and bowel or creating a pedicle flap.

INTERNAL HERNIAS

Internal hernias are protrusions of a viscus through a normal or abnormal peritoneal or mesenteric aperture within the confines of the peritoneal cavity. Their overall incidence is <1%, but these hernias are responsible for up to 5.8% of all small bowel obstructions.[65] Many different types have been described, and paraduodenal hernias account for 53% of all internal hernias. Pericecal, foramen of Winslow, transmesenteric and transmesocolic, intersigmoid, and retroanastomotic hernias make up the remainder. When a patient presents with a bowel obstruction and a history of prior operation, an internal hernia should be considered and almost always requires operative intervention to reduce and prevent recurrence.

The surgeon can help to decrease the chance of internal herniation if care is taken to close mesenteric defects created by bowel resections. This can be accomplished by reapproximating the mesentery with interrupted silk suture. Defects located behind the descending colon generally do not need to be addressed.

BOWEL INJURY

If you operate in the abdomen, it is inevitable that at some point you will cause an inadvertent bowel injury. This can be avoided by careful technique, but one is faced with how to handle this in the moment. If your patient has had bowel preparation, then it is less likely that a complication of infection will occur. A simple serosal injury should be oversewn with Lembert-type suture, usually 3-0 silk. If the bowel is perforated, the approach varies depending on the size of the injury. When a majority of the circumference of the bowel is violated or the segment does not appear viable, segmental resection should be performed. The small bowel can safely be reconnected. The large bowel can probably be reconnected as long as fecal impaction or spillage is minimal.

One may consider diverting a colonic resection if the patient is immunocompromised or the surgeon has another reason to suspect that the anastomosis will not heal. If the bowel is perforated but the perforation does not appear to involve a large segment or circumference, primary repair in two layers with an inner layer of 3-0 polydioxanone (PDS) and an outer layer of interrupted 3-0 silk suture can be used. Closing the injury transverse to the longitudinal access of the bowel should be considered so that the luminal diameter is not compromised.

KEY POINTS

1. Prolonged ileus lengthens the patient's discomfort, increases the need for parenteral nutritional support, and constitutes the most common reason for delayed discharge after abdominal surgery.
2. Following surgical procedures, the small intestine first regains function within 24 hours, the stomach in 24 to 48 hours, and the colon in 3 to 5 days.
3. The most important initial step in treating a patient with bowel obstruction is to replace intravascular volume.
4. Nearly 80% of patients with complete obstruction will require an operation. Therefore, surgical intervention should occur earlier in patients with complete bowel obstruction. Similarly, in approximately 80% of patients, a partial bowel obstruction will resolve on its own.
5. The three most important actions that can be taken to prevent the complication of fistula are (1) improve the nutrition of malnourished patients, (2) use mechanical and antibiotic bowel preparation, and (3) perform careful surgical technique.
6. Once an intra-abdominal abscess has been identified, antibiotic treatment is not adequate; the abscess must be drained.
7. When conservative and pharmacologic management of Ogilvie's syndrome has failed, colonic diameter measures >12 cm, colon size is increasing rapidly, or the duration is >3 days, the colon should be decompressed colonoscopically with placement of a long rectal compression tube.
8. Patients with vesicoenteric fistulas primarily present with urologic symptoms rather than with symptoms related to the bowel.

REFERENCES

Please see www.expertconsult.com

Chapter 23

MANAGEMENT OF URINARY FISTULAS

Priya Padmanabhan MD, MPH
Instructor, Department of Urologic Surgery, Vanderbilt University School of Medicine, Nashville, Tennessee

William Lea MD
Resident, Department of Surgery, Indiana University School of Medicine, Indianapolis, Indiana

Harriette Scarpero MD
Associate Professor, Department of Urologic Surgery, Vanderbilt University School of Medicine, Nashville, Tennessee

Descriptions of urinary fistulas exist in the ancient writings of Hippocrates and Rufus. Today, surgeons in the Western world encounter fistulas as a result of surgery or radiation for other medical conditions. Repair can be challenging but success is common. The World Health Organization estimates that in developing regions such as West Africa, approximately 2 million women suffer from obstetric fistula, and 50,000 to 100,000 new cases occur annually around the world. The prevention and correction of obstetric fistula are therefore humanitarian issues of significant proportion. Despite differences in origin and patient demographics, optimal fistula repair adheres to several basic surgical tenets (Box 23-1).

URETHROVAGINAL FISTULA

Etiology

Urethrovaginal fistula is an uncommon disorder that may be the consequence of various pathologic situations. Historically, dystocia was one of the chief contributory factors. Cephalopelvic disproportion can cause ischemic necrosis of the bladder and urethra from prolonged intense pressure of the fetus or forceps pressure on the symphysis pubis. With the avoidance of traumatic vaginal deliveries and prolonged labor in the developed world, obstetric trauma is now a much less common cause of urethrovaginal fistulas.

Young women in the developing world, particularly in Africa, are still at high risk of developing urethrovaginal fistula because of inadequate obstetric care.[1] In Nigeria, 350 of every 100,000 deliveries are complicated by fistula formation. These patients suffer from the *obstructive labor delivery complex,* including complex urethrovesical fistulas, rectal injuries (17%), foot drop (20%), and amenorrhea with infertility (63%).[2] Today, the most common cause of urethrovaginal fistulas is iatrogenic, from a surgical procedure in the area of the urethra, such as urethral diverticulectomy or anterior colporrhaphy. These two procedures contribute 15% to 45% of reported urethrovaginal fistulas.[3-7] Other surgical procedures that confer risk for urethrovaginal fistula include bladder neck suspension, Kelly plication, vulvectomy, and anti-incontinence surgery (periurethral injection, pubovaginal sling). Significant nonsurgical risk factors are radiation therapy, trauma, genital tumors, and congenital conditions.[1,8]

Presentation

Urethrovaginal fistulas can manifest with vaginal voiding from a pinpoint lesion or total incontinence from complete loss of the urethra (**Fig. 23-1**). The clinical presentation depends on the location and size of the fistula and the competency of the bladder neck. Distal fistulas are usually asymptomatic but can create a spraying or split urine stream, recurrent urinary infections, or vaginal voiding. Midurethral and proximal fistulas usually manifest with abnormal urine stream, vaginal pooling of urine, perineal skin irritation, vaginal fungal infections, intermittent positional wetness, and possible stress urinary incontinence (SUI). Forty-nine percent of continent menopausal women have an incompetent bladder neck mechanism and therefore rely on an intact proximal urethral mechanism and external sphincter to maintain continence. When the bladder neck mechanism is competent in a patient with a proximal urethral fistula, incontinence may not occur.[8,9]

The onset of symptoms relates to the mechanism of the fistula formation. Anterior vaginal wall laceration from trauma or obstetrics usually manifests ≤24 hours or immediately after Foley catheter removal. Ninety percent of fistulas associated with pelvic surgery are symptomatic within 7 to 30 days postoperatively (after catheter removal). Radiation-induced urethrovaginal fistulas are associated with slower progressive devascu-

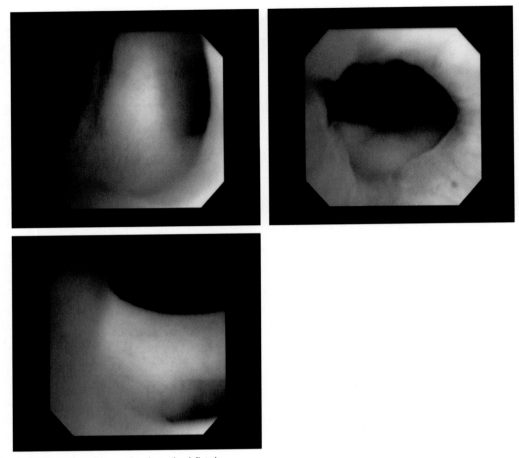

Figure 23-1 Three photographs of a proximal urethral fistula.

BOX 23-1 **Principles of Fistula Repair Technique**

Optimal exposure of the fistula
Wide mobilization of tissues
Tension-free approximation of the tissues
Watertight closure
Multilayer repair with no overlapping suture lines
Use of vascularized interposition grafts

---

larization necrosis and may manifest 30 days to many years later.[9,10]

Diagnosis

The differential diagnosis of urethrovaginal fistula includes vesicovaginal fistulas (VVFs) and ureterovaginal fistulas, severe SUI, and occasionally simple vaginal discharge.[11] Evaluation must begin with a comprehensive history and physical examination, including information of previous surgery, trauma, or radiation. Diagnosis is usually not difficult, and identification by a vaginal speculum examination and cystourethroscopy is often sufficient. Cystoscopy helps identify the size and location of the fistula tract and enables the urolo-

gist to evaluate the bladder for evidence of bladder neck or trigone involvement. Voiding cystourethrogram (VCUG) and intravenous pyelogram (IVP) are not required to make the diagnosis of a urethrovaginal fistula, but these studies are of paramount importance in excluding VVF and ureterovaginal fistula, respectively. The urologist must have a high index of suspicion for associated injuries. Older series reported a 19% incidence of concomitant VVFs.[3] In patients with concurrent SUI, videourodynamic study (VUDS) is helpful in identifying patients who may benefit from an incontinence procedure at the time of the fistula repair.[9,10] Urodynamic studies have detected a higher incidence of SUI and detrusor instability with fistulas involving the urethra or bladder neck than with fistulas solely into the vaginal vault.[12]

Prevention

Surgical technique during transvaginal procedures is crucial in preventing the formation of a urethrovaginal fistula. Surgical dissection should be performed carefully to preserve the periurethral fascia and to avoid the risk of injuring the urethral spongiosum, which is highly vascular and associated with fibrosis when injured. In urethral dissection, Bovie cautery should be avoided and bipolar cautery should be used preferentially because of the risk of penetrating, full-thickness injury. Before closure of urethral and anterior vaginal repairs, a small-diameter Foley catheter (14 or 16 Fr) should be placed to prevent local ischemic damage and pressure.

Management

Repairing urethrovaginal fistulas requires careful assessment of the health and integrity of the tissues surrounding the fistula. Often, urethrovaginal fistulas are associated with significant scarring and insufficient surrounding tissues to achieve a tension-free multiple-layer closure. Therefore, the interposition of well-vascularized tissue is often required to ensure adequate healing. In the absence of tissue for interposition, some series report a 100% failure rate.[7,9] Additionally, it is important to determine whether patients have concurrent SUI, which can be treated simultaneously with an autologous fascial sling. The fascial sling has the added benefit of providing an extra layer of tissue between the urethral repair and vaginal closure. Synthetic slings are contraindicated at the time of urethrovaginal fistula repair secondary to the risk of erosion.

The optimum timing of surgical correction remains a point of discussion. Repair is usually delayed for >2 months after the initial injury to allow the inflammation to resolve. When the fistula is a result of radiation therapy, repair is usually delayed for ≥1 year until the fistula tract has time to mature and the ischemic injury has stabilized.[9,7,13] Radiation-related fistulas should undergo biopsy before repair to rule out local tumor recurrence. During this period before repair, postmenopausal atrophic tissue should be treated with estrogen cream to improve the quality of the tissue and to maximize the potential for a successful repair.[11]

The complexity and choice of repair depend on the location of the fistula: small, medial to distal fistulas versus large, proximal urethral fistulas with bladder neck or trigone involvement. A common approach for fixing smaller, distal fistulas has been described.[8] An inverted-U–shaped incision is made proximal to the urethrovaginal fistula to circumscribe but not excise the fistula. Anterior and posterior vaginal wall flaps are mobilized and the fistula is closed in a two-layer, watertight closure with 3-0 absorbable suture material. When concern exists regarding integrity of tissue near the fistula (e.g., radiation, previous repair), a Martius labial fat pad flap is an important adjunctive procedure. The Martius flap is secured over the fistula repair. An important surgical tip is to avoid making the fat pad too thick because it becomes difficult to close the vaginal incision if the fat pad is bulky.

When the gold standard, the Martius labial fat pad, fails or when a large proximal fistula involves the bladder neck or trigone, the method of repair is more complicated. Additional tissue flaps have been described to achieve proper repair: gracilis flap, peritoneal flaps, gluteal skin flaps, omental flaps, and lyophilized dura mater patches.[14] The disadvantages of the other flaps are that they frequently require extra operations and they may be deforming. The pedunculated rectus flap has been described as useful in treating both the fistula and the SUI related to intrinsic sphincter deficiency.[15] This flap operation requires a combined vaginal and retropubic approach. Although it is helpful to know of alternative methods to provide healthy tissue interposition, we find that most cases of iatrogenic urethrovaginal fistulas are amenable to correction with primary closure, Martius labial fat interposition, and an autologous pubovaginal sling in select cases. Another important caveat is that any foreign body material such as mesh must be completely removed before closure.

In some cases, such as in patients with significant loss of urethral tissue necessitating urethral reconstruction or a neourethra fistula involving the bladder neck or trigone, described techniques fall into the following three categories:

1. Anterior bladder flaps[16]
2. Posterior bladder flaps[17,18]
3. Vaginal flaps

Blaivas and Heritz[19,20] simplified a vaginal approach enabling both fistula repair and a concomitant incontinence procedure. An inverted-U–shaped incision is made in the anterior vaginal wall, through the fistula site, thus circumscribing the fistula and closing the site with absorbable suture. The neourethra is created by making two parallel incisions in the anterior vaginal wall on both sides of the Foley catheter; this maneuver creates flaps that are then tubularized around the catheter. In a patient who has undergone radiation, the use of rectus or gracilis flap is advisable. These well-vascularized grafts provide a new blood supply to the neourethra and allow the defect to be closed in a tension-free manner. Sexual function may be preserved because vaginal stenosis is unlikely to occur.[21]

Following repair of urethrovaginal fistulas, urinary drainage is usually maintained for 1 to 3 weeks, depending on the location and complexity of the repair. Both suprapubic and urethral catheters (8 or 10 Fr) are often inserted. Because the suprapubic tube is placed under the direct vision of the cystoscope, this tube is generally placed at the start of the procedure. If the surgeon has already decided to use an autologous pubovaginal sling, it will be harvested and the sutures passed before fistula closure. The rationale for completing these tasks before urethrovaginal fistula closure is that doing so reduces the need to pass a scope over the delicate urethral repair. Occasionally, a urethral catheter is avoided to prevent ischemia or pressure to the repair, especially in the case of middle or distal urethrovaginal fistulas. Oral anticholinergics are always given and may be discontinued 24 hours before a postoperative VCUG is obtained. The VCUG is performed by filling through the suprapubic tube and removing the urethral catheter. When extravasation is present, the suprapubic tube is returned to drainage, and VCUG is repeated in 1 week. The urethral catheter is usually not replaced because of the risk of disturbing the delicate suture lines.[8]

Sequelae

Multiple autologous, other biologic, and synthetic options for sling material have been described for treating SUI. Most proximal fistulas involve the intrinsic continence mechanism, and therefore these patients benefit from concomitant sling surgery at the time of fistula repair if SUI is demonstrated on the preoperative VUDS evaluation. The incidence of incontinence following all urethrovaginal fistula repairs is 20% to 70%.[4,22,23] In one study, Pushkar and colleagues[9] reported that 37 of 71 (52%) patients developed SUI following urethrovaginal fistula repair. These patients were treated with a combination of fascial slings, other autologous tissue slings, or tension-free vaginal tapes (retropubic or obturator). Only 8% remained incontinent or were dissatisfied with the results. Blaivas and Heritz[20] found three cases of refractory SUI following fistula repair and bladder neck suspension that were cured with pubovaginal slings. A synthetic sling should never be used in an incontinence procedure at the time of a urethrovaginal repair. Periurethral tissue is fragile and a fibrotic reaction is associated with initial injury and repair. Therefore, we prefer to use autologous rectus fascia for all slings in urethrovaginal fistula repair. The role of bulking agents is unclear.[24]

VESICOVAGINAL FISTULA

Etiology

The underlying cause of VVF formation is tissue ischemia from pelvic floor injury. VVF can be a result of obstetric trauma, surgery (hysterectomy, anti-incontinence procedures), congenital anomalies, or malignant disease or its treatment (radiation). With advances in obstetric care, most VVFs in developed countries (90%) occur after surgical procedures for "benign disease," and total abdominal hysterectomy accounts for 70% of these fistulas.[3] VVF in developing countries remains associated with prolonged labor and traumatic delivery. Current estimates are that 1 in 3 of every 1000 deliveries in West Africa will result in a VVF (**Fig. 23-2**).[25]

Even though numerous predisposing factors have been identified in the development of postoperative fistulas (infection, ischemia, arteriosclerosis, pelvic inflammatory disease, previous uterine surgery, uterine leiomyomas, radiation, diabetes), most fistulas occur following normal operative circumstances.[26] In cases associated with malignant disease (cervical, uterine, ovarian, rectal), the VVF could be a result of a surgical complication, radiation treatment, or the presence of cancer. Surgical procedures performed for cancer are usually more radical and thus are more likely to cause tissue hypovascularization, which predisposes to the formation of a fistula.[27] Radiation causes chronic vascular changes with a field effect leading to a loss of microcirculation, mucosal atrophy, ulceration, and fistula formation. The incidence of fistula formation induced by radiation is 1% to 5%.[28,29] VVF may also be caused by direct invasion of the tumor through the vagina or bladder.

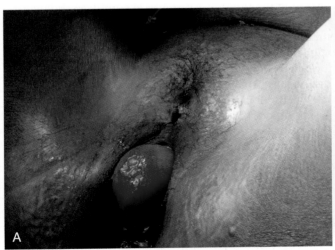
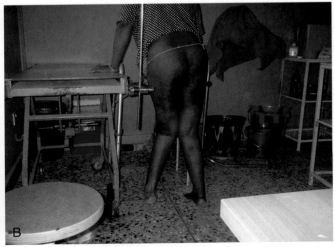

Figure 23-2   A, Complete prolapse of bladder mucosa through a large vesicovaginal fistula secondary to obstructed labor. **B,** Demonstration of the foot drop that accompanies these obstetric fistulas in 20% of cases. *(Courtesy of Dr. Alyona Lewis and the West Africa Fistula Foundation.)*

Presentation

The clinical presentation and onset of VVF vary depending on the cause. VVFs that form after pelvic surgery rarely manifest with immediate fever, ileus, abdominal discomfort, hematuria, or bladder irritability, because of urine leakage into the peritoneum. Most patients present with the complaint of vaginal leakage of urine 3 to 7 days after Foley catheter removal; 10% to 15% of these patients present later, 10 to 30 days after the procedure. Patients with a small fistula or a fistula located high in the vaginal vault may void normally. They may note being dry at night while supine and voiding large volumes in the day despite frequent leakage. With larger fistulas, the bladder does not store any appreciable urine, and patients complain of minimal voids with large, continuous leakage. The differential diagnosis includes urethrovaginal fistula, ureterovaginal fistula, and vaginal discharge.[21,11] When radiation is the cause of the VVF, presentation may be delayed from 5 months up to 30 years after treatment, and 25% of these patients may be asymptomatic for >5 years. Irritative lower urinary tract symptoms have been reported to be relieved by the sudden appearance of the VVF. Occasionally patients present with vaginal flatulence or feces, and these patients should be evaluated for concomitant rectovaginal fistula.[30,31]

Diagnosis

A complete history and physical examination, including a thorough pelvic examination, are necessary in evaluating for a VVF. In acute fistulas, the mucosa around the VVF tract can be inflamed and erythematous, thus concealing the opening. In mature fistulous tracts, a small opening may be visualized in the vaginal wall. If one is in doubt, fluid collecting at the vaginal apex can be sent for urea and creatinine concentrations to confirm the presence of urine but this is usually not necessary. A simultaneous rectal examination in cases of posterior vaginal distortion by inflammation and edema should be performed to rule out rectal involvement.[21] If examination results are highly suggestive of rectal involvement, proctoscopy should be performed.

A *tampon test* using a combination of phenazopyridine (Pyridium) and diluted methylene blue provides preliminary evidence of a VVF or a ureterovaginal fistula. Patients are given phenazopyridine, which colors the urine orange. A tampon is inserted into the vagina before the phenazopyridine is administered. The bladder is also distended with diluted methylene blue before placement of the tampon. The patient then ambulates for 15 to 30 minutes. If the tampon is orange, a ureterovaginal fistula and a VVF are likely. If the tampon turns blue, this finding supports a VVF. Although a classic and frequently described test, it is imperfect. A ureterovaginal fistula cannot be confirmed without imaging. In our

experience, proper cystoscopic and radiologic staging is prerequisite for diagnosis.

Radiologic examination should include an IVP or retrograde pyelography, to rule out ureterovaginal fistula, which is present 10% of the time in patients with VVF. With an IVP, ureteral involvement often appears as extravasation or hydronephrosis. A persistent column of contrast material in the ureter may be the only sign of ureteral involvement. Bilateral retrograde pyelography is the most accurate method for determining concomitant ureteral involvement and also for localizing it.[21] Cystoscopy with vaginal manipulation is essential in elucidating the size, number, and location of fistulas in relation to the ureteral orifices, vaginal cuff, and trigone (**Fig. 23-3**). Passage of a 0.35-mm sensor wire through the fistula helps in identification when one of the openings is unidentifiable. VVFs that occur after hysterectomy usually are located along the anterior vaginal vault and the interureteric ridge.

Fistulas that occur after radiation are often located in the caudal position of the trigone, distal to the interureteric ridge.[32] VUDS is a useful adjunct in evaluating these patients preoperatively. VUDS helps identify patients with SUI who would benefit from a concomitant anti-incontinence procedure at time of VVF repair. Moreover, patients who have received radiation should be evaluated for their bladder capacity and compliance to consider augmentation cystoplasty during fistula repair. VVF in patients with a history of gynecologic malignant disease should always be examined by biopsy preoperatively, to rule out recurrence of malignancy.

Prevention

A VVF generally results from simultaneous injury to the bladder and vagina, most commonly occurring during abdominal hysterectomy. Bladder injury usually occurs during sharp and blunt dissection of the cervix from the bladder, especially when the procedure is complicated by prior radiation therapy, obesity, or prior surgery. Injuries take a few forms: direct laceration of the bladder during dissection, excessive cautery producing full-thickness necrosis, and placement of sutures at the vaginal cuff that accidentally incorporate the bladder. Prevention of VVF formation depends on surgical technique and postoperative urinary drainage. The surgeon must maintain a high index of suspicion following dissection, and in cases of suspected bladder or ureteral injury the urologist should be consulted intraoperatively. If the surgeon is a urologist, filling of the bladder with dilute methylene blue can reveal a bladder injury, whereas the intravenous injection of indigo carmine can assist in the diagnosis of a ureteral injury.

Technical points in closing a bladder injury include watertight bladder anastomosis, tension-free repair, and interposition of healthy tissue (between bladder repair and vaginal cuff closure). Postoperatively, adequate

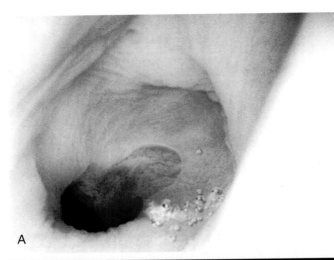

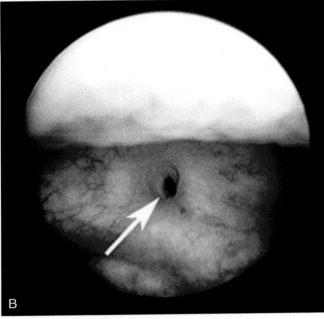

Figure 23-3 **A** and **B,** Two cystoscopic photographs of vesicovaginal fistula from within the bladder.

Timing of repair
Choosing an approach (vaginal versus abdominal)
Ruling out associated injuries (ureteral involvement)
Assessing the health of tissues (infection, estrogenization, recurrent cancer, extent of radiation change)
Planning concomitant procedures (ureteral surgery, stress incontinence surgery, or augmentation cystoplasty)

urinary drainage should be accompanied by maximal detrusor relaxation induced by anticholinergic medication, and a confirmatory cystogram should be performed before the urethral catheter is removed.[11] The repair and management of ureteral injuries are discussed in the later section on ureteral fistulas.

Management

VVFs are classified according to their size and origin. Simple fistulas are small (<0.5 cm), single, and not irradiated. Complex fistulas include previously failed fistula repairs or large fistulas (>2.5 cm), often the result of chronic disease or radiation. Intermediate-size fistulas (0.5 to 2.5 cm) are often categorized as complex fistulas.[27] Treatment options are based on the origin and

complexity of the VVF and on the timing of repair. Options range from conservative management (bladder drainage, fulguration) to surgical therapy (transvaginal versus transabdominal repair). Conservative treatment has been attempted in simple fistulas 2 weeks to 2 months after injury, with success rates ranging from 0% to 100%.[33] No prospective study has correlated the duration of drainage with the chance for spontaneous healing, and often this is based on personal experience. At most, one third of small fistulas will close with catheter drainage.[11] Another conservative option for closure of VVF is electrofulguration with or without injection of bovine collagen and fibrin glue. The bladder is subsequently drained for ≤4 weeks.[34,35] We find that this approach has very limited utility and rarely use it.

Most conservative methods are ineffective; therefore, surgery remains the primary method for repair. Surgical planning includes decisions on timing, approach, the need for fistula tract excision, and the use of interpositional flaps (Box 23-2). Surgical repair is best performed when the edema and inflammation have subsided and no infection is present. Traditionally, a 3- to 6-month waiting period has been recommended to allow the fistula tract to mature. Some studies showed that fistulas may be closed within weeks of diagnosis.[36,37] Zimmern and associates[38] observed that surgical repair performed 2 to 3 weeks after injury had no associated increased morbidity or failure results. Contraindications to early closure include multiple unsuccessful closures, associated enteric fistula with pelvic phlegmon, and previous radiation. These types of fistulas are usually repaired after a 4- to 8-month waiting period.[29] Ultimately, the timing of surgery should be based on the preference of the surgeon and the patient.

Traditionally, an abdominal approach was used for supratrigonal fistulas, whereas a vaginal approach was used for infratrigonal, bladder neck, and proximal urethral fistulas. Current practice among experienced transvaginal surgeons is a vaginal approach in cases of VVF with a few exceptions. The advantages of a vaginal approach include patient comfort and recovery time.[21] Contraindications to a vaginal approach include severely indurated vaginal epithelium around the fistula, small capacity or poorly compliant bladder requiring augmentation, repair requiring ureteral reimplantation, involvement of other pelvic structures, vaginal stenosis, or the inability to obtain proper exposure.[36]

The classic transvaginal repair for uncomplicated small fistulas was perfected by Raz.[38,39] An inverted-J– or U–shaped incision is made circumferentially around the fistula and flaps are dissected, thus mobilizing the vaginal epithelium away from the fistula. The margins of the fistula are trimmed and closed using absorbable suture. It is up to the surgeon to decide whether to excise the fistula. The advantage of excision is achieving a mucosa-to-mucosa closure of healthy tissue. The disadvantage is that the fistula size increases, the hyperemic surrounding tissue bleeds, and that the friable bladder may not hold the stitches. Because the fistula tract also provides extra strength to the closure, most surgeons do not excise simple fistula tracts.[11] The perivesical fascia is then closed with absorbable sutures in a perpendicular fashion (over the fistula tract), with the edges inverted. The bladder is filled with diluted methylene blue at this point to check for a watertight closure. Finally, the vaginal wall is closed in a third layer, in a nonoverlapping absorbable suture line. Usually, a suprapubic tube and a Foley catheter are left for straight drainage, and anticholinergics are given liberally. We often remove the urethral catheter before hospital discharge on the first postoperative day. A cystogram is performed 2 to 3 weeks postoperatively and if no extravasation is seen, the suprapubic tube is removed.

Complex fistulas including those associated with eroded mesh or radiation require the use of tissue interposition between vesical and vaginal suture lines (**Fig. 23-4**). Generally, a Martius flap is used for distal fistulas and a peritoneal flap is used for proximal fistulas (high in the vaginal vault). The selection of autologous tissue depends on the size of the fistula, its location, the quality of patient tissues, and the surgeon's preference. The Martius flap is reliable, but it requires a separate incision and may not reach fistulas high in the vaginal vault. The vagina may be shortened during attempts to extend the flap from the labia to the vagina.

Peritoneum is a suitable alternative in these high fistulas. The peritoneal flap is well vascularized and readily available, and it can be harvested with only one incision.[37] Raz and colleagues[37,40] reported success rates with a peritoneal flap of 91% and, more recently, 96%. To prepare a peritoneal flap, the peritoneum is mobilized in the cul de sac sharply and is advanced over the repair, between the second and third layers of the basic repair.[37,40] Another option is a deepithelialized vaginal wall flap.

The abdominal approach may be extraperitoneal or transperitoneal, with or without opening the bladder. An abdominal approach is easily reproducible and successful, yet it has the associated risks, complications, and longer convalescence associated with laparotomy. An abdominal approach is required when vaginal exposure is difficult, when concomitant bladder augmentation or

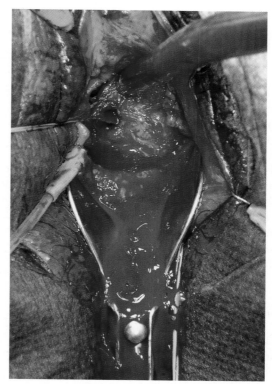

Figure 23-4 A rare form of vesicovaginal fistula created by incorrect placement of a polypropylene sling through the detrusor. Note the sling material being excised from the fistula tract.

ureteral reimplantation is necessary, or when it is the surgeon's preference. The bladder and vagina are sharply dissected apart, and each opening is closed in single layers. A flap of peritoneum or omentum is placed in between to prevent recurrence or creation of a fistula.[11] The traditional abdominal approach, the *O'Conor technique,*[41] is a transperitoneal, transvesical operation in which the bladder is bivalved down to the fistula. The fistulous tract is excised and the bladder is mobilized off the vagina. The vaginal and vesical walls are repaired separately, and omentum or peritoneum is interposed between the two. The incidence of bladder spasms is usually more pronounced followed abdominal repairs and the standard use of a suprapubic tube. Urethral catheters and anticholinergics are maintained until a cystogram is performed 3 weeks postoperatively.

The success rates in the literature for repair of VVF, independent of the access route and tissue conditions, approach 90%. In addition to showing no appreciable improvement in success rates with delaying surgical repair, Blaivas and colleagues[36] found that, in expert hands, VVF repairs were equivalent whether they used an abdominal or a vaginal approach. The most difficult fistulas to repair are those caused by radiation and therefore the success rates for these repairs should not be compared with rates for nonradiated fistulas. The success rate of nonradiated VVF repair varies from 70% to 100%, with a mean success rate of 92%.[23,42-45] Most of these operations were performed using a transvaginal approach. Conversely, the success rate of radiation-induced VVF repairs is between 40% and 100%.

Some surgeons advocate urinary diversion instead of repair of a radiated fistula. The highest success rates have been noted with procedures performed using an abdominal approach or a combined approach with rectus or omental and gastric flaps based on the right gastroepiploic artery.[28,44,46-50] At our institution, a tertiary referral center for many complex, recurrent VVFs, we find that use of only one approach is not practical. The surgical approach is based on the surgeon's appraisal of each individual case: the location and size of the fistula, the quality of the surrounding tissue, the number of prior repairs, the mobility of the vaginal tissues, the necessary concomitant procedures, and the patient's comorbidities.

Sequelae

Even in cases of successful fistula repair, voiding dysfunction with de novo frequency, urgency, and incontinence may result and may be a considerable burden to the patient. The rates of long-term voiding dysfunction after fistula repair are not commonly reported and very few series address them specifically, nor does a clear consensus exist on what causes postoperative irritative symptoms. The fistula itself and not the repair may be responsible.[51,52] Another theory is that bladder capacity may be compromised if repair is delayed, thus resulting in voiding dysfunction. We believe that postoperative voiding dysfunction is multifactorial and is related to the inciting operation, surgical complexity, timing of repair, number of repairs, and adjunctive procedures. In our own series of 48 fistula repair patients from April of 1998 through July of 2006, de novo urgency and frequency were seen postoperatively in 21 (48%). Symptoms may be controlled with anticholinergics or sacral neuromodulation in refractory cases.

URETERAL FISTULAS

Ureteral fistulas are rare, but the diagnosis has become more common with the development of advanced and extensive options for pelvic and abdominal disease, endourologic procedures, and vascular reconstruction. Ureteral fistulas are associated with high morbidity. In certain ureteral fistulas, misdiagnosis leads to a 100% mortality rate. This section reviews the etiology, presentation, diagnosis, prevention, management, and sequelae of ureterovaginal, ureteroenteric, and ureteroarterial fistulas.

Etiology

The formation of ureteral fistulas depends on injury to the ureter that can expose the ureteral lumen or result

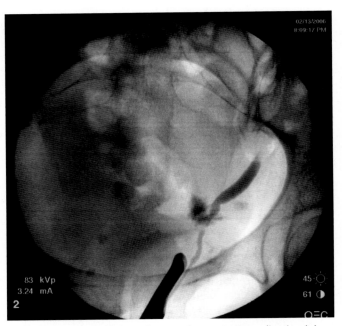

Figure 23-5 Retrograde pyelogram demonstrating a ligation injury and obstruction of the ureter at the time of hysterectomy. This type of injury may lead to ureteral ischemia and potentially a ureteral fistula or stricture.

in delayed necrosis of a portion of the ureter, thus leading to subsequent urine extravasation.[53] This injury may be acute or insidious in onset. Acute ureteral injury, as in the case of iatrogenic injuries (suture ligation, incision or transection, avulsion, or crushing) or trauma is immediately apparent. A delayed change in ureteral patency is seen in iatrogenic devascularization, heat therapy or cryoablative therapy, radiation, or vascular grafting.[54]

The course and blood supply of the ureter are fundamental to an understanding of common sites of ureteral injury (**Fig. 23-5**). The ureter travels caudally through the retroperitoneum, along the anterior psoas muscle, posterior to the colonic mesentery, and lateral to the gonadal vein. The complex blood supply to the ureter arises from the renal artery, gonadal artery, lumbar arteries, and aorta proximally and from the internal iliac artery and branches distally. The small arteries, intimate with the peritoneum, approach the ureter medially in the abdomen and laterally in the pelvis,[54,55] and they direct the surgical approach of the ureter.

Ureteral fistulas may occur as complications of colorectal surgery, vascular surgery, other urologic procedures, obstetric care, or penetrating trauma, but most arise following gynecologic surgery. The incidence of iatrogenic ureteral injuries during gynecologic surgery is 0.4% to 2.5%, and these numbers probably underestimate the true incidence.[56,57] Many injuries are missed at time of operation until they become symptomatic.[58] The ureterovaginal fistula is the most common ureteral fistula. Most ureterovaginal fistulas are caused by one procedure—

hysterectomy. The risk of ureteral injury is greatest during laparoscopic hysterectomy, followed by abdominal hysterectomy and finally by vaginal hysterectomy. With the introduction of laparoscopy and minimally invasive techniques, the incidence of iatrogenic gynecologic ureteral injuries is increasing.[59,60] Risk factors for the development of ureterovaginal fistulas include endometriosis, obesity, pelvic inflammatory disease, radiation therapy, and pelvic malignant disease.[58] Most ureterovaginal fistulas occur during procedures for benign indications,[61] usually hysterectomy, but also cesarean section, pelvic organ prolapse repair, and other pelvic operations during which surgical injury of the distal third or pelvic portion of the ureter occurs (**Fig. 23-6**).

Ureteroenteric fistulas are extremely rare, with fewer than 15 cases reported in the literature since 1918.[62] Most cases reported are ureteroduodenal fistulas secondary to chronic renal infection, ureteral calculi, duodenal ulcer disease, roundworm infection of the urinary tract, iatrogenic injury, trauma, or ingestion of foreign body.[63-65] As in most fistulous formation, the presence of ureteroenteric fistulas is often associated with radiation or ureteral ischemia.

Ureteroaortic fistulas are also uncommon. Approximately 90 cases have been reported in the English-language literature, mostly since 2000.[66] The increased incidence is related to the greater numbers of vascular reconstructions, treatments of pelvic malignant disease, and long-term use of ureteral stents. This is the only type of ureteral fistula that has a 100% mortality rate if it is left undiagnosed and untreated. Ureteroaortic fistulas most commonly involve the middle to distal ureter where the ureters cross the pelvic brim, most commonly involving the common iliac artery,[67] but they may also involve the external iliac artery, internal iliac artery, and aorta.[68,69] Ureteroaortic fistulas are classified into three categories according to causes: primary, secondary (iatrogenic), and pregnancy related.[66] Primary fistulas represent <15% of ureteroaortic fistulas and are usually found in association with aortoiliac aneurysmal disease.[70,71] Secondary fistulas account for 85% of ureteroaortic fistulas and usually manifest after pelvic surgery for malignant disease, often in association with radiation, retroperitoneal fibrosis, and ureteral stenting, or after vascular surgery with synthetic grafting.[56,72,73]

Three cases[74-76] of ureteroaortic fistula were reported during pregnancy in the late 1930s; all three patients had urinary tract infections with sepsis and hematuria. All three patients eventually died, and the diagnosis was made post mortem. Two of the patients required ureteral stent placement during pregnancy for hydronephrosis. Pregnancy-related ureteroaortic fistulas have not been reported since that time with the advent of soft, flexible ureteral stents and more effective antibiotic therapy.[73] The pathophysiology of ureteroaortic fistula formation is still uncertain. It is believed that these fistulas are related to inflammation or ischemic injury

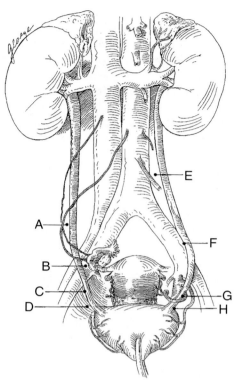

Figure 23-6 Common sites of ureteral injury. *A,* Division of the gonadal vessels and infundibulopelvic ligament. *B,* Resection of adnexal masses adherent to the ureter within the broad ligament. *C,* The apex of the obturator fossa in pelvic lymphadenectomy. *D,* Division of the lateral ligaments of the rectum in abdominoperineal resection. *E,* Division of the inferior mesenteric vessels in sigmoid resection. *F,* The pelvic brim during vascular bypass procedures. *G,* Division of the uterine artery during hysterectomy. *H,* The lateral vaginal fornix, entry into the trigone of the bladder during hysterectomy and vaginal procedures. *(From Payne CK, Raz S. Ureterovaginal and related fistulas. In: McAninch JW, ed. Traumatic and Reconstructive Urology. Philadelphia: WB Saunders; 1996:213.)*

to the ureters, iliac vessels, or both. Surgery, radiation, and urine leakage can disrupt the vasa vasorum. This disruption leads to changes in the media and adventitia of the large arteries and makes them more susceptible to rupture and necrosis. Inflammation and fibrosis then fix the ureter to the artery or vascular graft. A ureteral catheter acts as a counter brace that facilitates transmission of arterial pulsations into the ureteral wall.[73,77-79]

Presentation

Ureterovaginal fistulas most commonly manifest with a sudden onset of persistent urinary incontinence 1 to 4 weeks after surgery.[61] This complication may be associated with or preceded by flank pain, nausea, prolonged ileus, or fever, related to a urinoma or renal obstruction.[80] Flank pain is often limited by postoperative analgesics. Unlike patients with large VVFs, these patients maintain normal voiding patterns as the bladder continues to be filled by the contralateral collecting system.

The type of ureteral injury does often determine the timing of presentation. Lacerations and partial excisions of the ureter usually lead to urinary extravasation and related symptoms ≤48 hours postoperatively. Ischemic injuries (ligation, clamping, partial ligation, or stripping of periureteral blood supply) may initially be associated with obstruction, followed by stricture formation, necrosis, and fistula formation. Therefore, presentation may not occur for 1 to 3 weeks. In radiated patients and in the setting of chronic ischemia, ureterovaginal fistulas appear late, approximately 5 weeks postoperatively.[55]

Ureteroenteral fistulas are usually associated with chronic or recurrent urinary tract infections. Patients commonly present with fever, flank pain, and pneumaturia. The most common initial clinical findings are pyuria and hematuria.[64]

In ureteroaortic fistula, the most common symptom is gross hematuria, usually intermittent. This feature usually relates to the degeneration of clot by proteolytic enzymes interchanging with formation of clot. Initially, patients present with bleeding ranging from microscopic hematuria to life-threatening hemorrhage with associated hypotension and shock. Bleeding is usually provoked or worsened by provocative maneuvers (stent exchange).[66,72,78,81] Occasionally, patients may complain of flank pain, related to the formation and passage of clots in the renal pelvis and ureter. A few patients have experienced symptoms of urinary tract infection or pyelonephritis.[73]

Diagnosis

The diagnostic workup of a patient who presents with persistent incontinence is summarized at length in the earlier discussion of VVF. Ureterovaginal fistulas are unique in their association with urinoma or ureteral obstruction, and therefore upper tract imaging with computed tomography (CT) is valuable in patients who present with flank pain, fever, nausea, or prolonged ileus. These patients may need percutaneous drainage of a urinoma or abscess. Most of these patients should undergo an intravenous urogram, retrograde pyelogram, and cystoscopy.

On initial evaluation of a patient with an unknown ureteroenteral fistula, ultrasound and CT imaging are usually the first modalities pursued, in light of the flank pain and hematuria. Hydroureteronephrosis is frequently present, a finding that encourages further radiography for clarification. Antegrade or retrograde pyeloureterography often demonstrates contrast material outlining a segment of the involved bowel or a clear connection between the ureter and bowel, hydronephrosis, and a delayed nephrogram on the involved side.[64,65]

Demonstrating a ureteroaortic fistula is challenging and requires a high degree of suspicion to treat expediently. In earlier studies, retrograde pyelography and cystoscopy were thought to have the greatest sensitivity of diagnosis, between 45% and 60%.[72,81] Cystoscopy is extremely useful and sensitive in localizing hematuria to one ureteral orifice, yet it is not specific for ureteroaortic fistula. Retrograde pyelography is useful in demonstrating extravasation when only a pressure gradient from the ureter to the artery exists, a finding that is unlikely during episodes of pronounced bleeding. Urography and ureterography usually show only nonspecific findings of intraluminal blood clot and irregularity of the middle to distal ureter.[73] Ureteroscopy is not recommended because the fistula may tear or a tamponading clot may be dislodged, leading to massive hemorrhage.[77] When severe pulsatile bleeding from the ureteral orifice is encountered during cystoscopy or ureteroscopy, a balloon catheter may be used temporarily to block the hemorrhage.[82,83]

Selective iliac arteriography has been considered the most sensitive technique of diagnosis, with rates <50%. However, false-negative results usually occur when the ureteroaortic fistula is quiescent. When selective iliac arteriography is performed, it is essential that multiple oblique images be taken to identify small pseudoaneurysms that may otherwise be overlooked.[84] Provocative measures such as high-pressure balloon occlusion pyeloureterography, arteriography during ureteral stent removal, or production of friction with ureteral stent or ureteroscopy to dislodge occluding thrombus do increase the sensitivity of finding a ureteroaortic fistula. Provocative angiography increased the sensitivity to 100% in one series.[85] However, this technique must be approached with caution and with the ability to tamponade bleeding quickly by reinflating an occlusion balloon or replacing a stent. An operative team must be available to operate, in case these temporizing measures are unsuccessful and the patient becomes unstable.[81] Negative results of a provocative angiogram do not exclude the diagnosis of a ureteroarterial fistula.[77]

Prevention

Many ureteral iatrogenic injuries occur during blind cauterization or clipping to gain hemostasis or dissection without respect for location and direction of the ureteral blood supply. Essential to limiting formation of ureterovaginal fistulas and ureteroenteric fistulas is a sound understanding of the ureteral blood supply and anatomy and careful dissection without blind attempts at control during times of significant bleeding. The use of intraoperative stents to delineate the course of the ureter for dissecting large tumors has been controversial over the years. Stenting can add time, morbidity, and cost to the procedure. No objective evidence indicates that ureteral stenting decreases ureteral complication rates.[55]

Ureteroaortic fistulas are more common in situations of prolonged use of ureteral stents, in patients receiving radiation therapy after pelvic surgery, in urinary extravasation following ureterolithotomy, in patients surgically managed for pelvic malignant diseases, and in patients undergoing vascular reconstruction. To avoid this morbid and potentially fatal complication, long-term treatment with rigid ureteral stents should be avoided, especially in a previously irradiated patient. Surgical principles may be altered, such as placement of the ureter in front of the graft during aortofemoral reconstruction with synthetic graft, to prevent the ureter from being crushed between the graft and the involved artery.[66]

Management

Management of a ureterovaginal fistula depends on time of diagnosis, location, nature, and extent of injury. Intraoperative detection and repair are ideal, with excellent results and fewer complications. At that time, the tissues are typically in their best condition. In general, minimally invasive techniques for repair are favored over open repair except in cases of extensive ureteric damage, complete transection, or significant delay in recognition of injury. Ligation of the ureter is usually managed with immediate intraoperative removal of the ligature or surgical clip and observation because damage is usually minimal as a result of the inclusion of other tissue. If the surgeon is in doubt about ureteral integrity, a stent should be placed. If recognition of the condition is delayed, retrograde pyelogram and attempt at stent should be performed. A successfully placed stent is maintained for 4 to 6 weeks.[86,87]

When retrograde stenting fails, antegrade stenting through a percutaneous nephrostomy tract is often successful. We routinely clear patients for both procedures and consult our interventional radiology colleagues preemptively in difficult cases. Patients who present with sepsis are better managed with nephrostomy tube placement and simultaneous drainage of a present urinoma.[55] Most ureteric injuries during vaginal surgery are ligation injuries that result from attempts to achieve hemostasis and are detected after the operation. In all these cases, ureteric patency should be assessed with intravenous indigo carmine before completion of the procedure. If efflux of indigo carmine is not noted, the ureter may be kinked or ligated.[88,89] Complete ureteric obstruction during cystocele, enterocele, or bladder neck suspension surgery is managed with removal of offending sutures and confirmation of efflux. If any doubt exists about the integrity of the ureter, a retrograde pyelogram may be done and a stent placed. Following vaginal hysterectomy or vaginal vault reconstruction, obstructing ureteral sutures are typically not removed and the ureter is reimplanted.[86]

Ureteral crush injuries (by a clamp) usually take several days for the ischemic injury to manifest. The severity of injury depends on the size of the clamp, the length of time it was applied, and the amount of tissue actually crushed. Stenting the involved portion is a minimal requirement, but if ureteric viability is in question, the involved ureter should be resected, débrided, and reanastomosed over a double-J stent. Devascularization injuries (i.e., thermal injury, skeletonization, gunshot wounds) similarly should be excised to the level of healthy tissue and reapproximated over a double-J stent. Partial transection (iatrogenic or penetrating trauma) usually can be managed with primary sutured closure of spatulated ureteral ends after intraoperative passage of retrograde flexible guidewire followed by double-J stent. If more than half the ureteral diameter is lacerated, ureteric division followed by a ureteroureterostomy or reimplantation is required over a double-J stent.

General principles of ureteric reconstruction include ureteral mobilization preserving adventitia, débridement of devitalized tissue (to bleeding edge), mucosa-to-mucosa spatulation (tension free, watertight), ureteric drainage, and isolation of anastomosis from associated injuries (omental or peritoneal coverage).[86,90,91] Management of ureteric injuries during vascular graft surgery has been controversial since the late 1980s. Historically, nephrectomy was the treatment of choice during ureteral injury (with normal contralateral kidney) sustained at the time of concomitant vascular graft surgery. In a series of eight patients with sterile urine, ureteric repair at time of vascular grafting (with omental wrap and ureteral drainage) did not increase vascular graft infection or failure rates.[86,92,93]

Traditional recommendation was that repair of fistulas with delayed presentation should not be attempted for 3 to 6 months. However, fistulas diagnosed ≤2 weeks postoperatively can be immediately repaired because inflammation is minimal. In the range of 2 to 6 weeks, some controversy exists, but most surgeons proceed with operative repair at 6 weeks. Delayed repair continues to be followed when fistulas are associated with radiation or pregnancy, as a result of concerns over delayed ischemic necrosis. Repair in patients presenting with sepsis or abscess formation are also delayed until drainage and complete abscess treatment are achieved.[55] More recent studies have found similar outcomes for immediate and delayed repairs. Gilberti and associates[56] reported an 88% cure rate for patients managed endoscopically with similar operative rates for delayed and immediate repair of 90% and 87%, respectively.

The location of injury and fistula usually dictates the choice of open repair. Most fistulas that occur within the middle or upper ureter and abdominal ureter (above the iliac artery bifurcation) are managed with a ureteroureterostomy.[86,94,95] Injuries to the distal third of the ureter or within the intramural tunnel are usually repaired with reimplantation by a refluxing anastomosis or a tunneled, nonrefluxing technique. When the involved segment is long (>2 cm), a psoas hitch or Boari flap may be required. The psoas hitch is preferred in conjunction with reimplantation when the distal third of the ureter (caudal to the iliac vessels) is involved.[86,96-101] When additional length is required (lower two thirds of ureter is involved), a Boari flap and psoas hitch may be used. Boari flaps are avoided in patients who received prior pelvic radiation or who have neurogenic bladder dysfunction.[60,86,99,102] More complicated open repairs, such as transureteroureterostomy, ureterocalicostomy, ileal transposition, or renal autotransplantation, are very rare and are used only in selected circumstances.[86]

Management of ureteroenteral and ureteroaortic fistula requires treatment of the enteral or vascular and urologic disorders associated with the fistula. In the case of a ureteroenteral fistula, management of the ureteral portion depends on the patient's renal function. With normal renal function, ureteroureterostomy, excision of fistulous tract, and repair or excision of bowel is performed. If ipsilateral kidney function is poor, nephrectomy may be required.[63-65]

Until the 1990s, open surgery and radiographic embolization were the only options for treatment of the arterial component in a ureteroaortic fistula. Since then, the use of endovascular procedures, aside from embolization (balloon occlusion or endovascular stent grafts), has increased.[66,103] The choice of arterial repair is affected by associated local infections, the presence of aneurysmal or occlusive disease, collateral circulation to the ipsilateral leg, and the presence of an arterial graft. Options for vascular repair include local reconstruction (arteriorrhaphy, patch closure, interposition graft, bypass), ligation with or without extra-anatomic bypass, and ligation of the internal iliac artery.[66]

The addition of endovascular stent grafts is promising because these devices permit complete closure of the fistula and maintenance of antegrade blood flow through the iliac artery without direct arterial or ureteral surgery and they avoid subsequent revascularization of the lower extremities.[73,104] The potential exists for stent graft occlusion or infection, a complication that can lead to persistent hemorrhage, occlusion, or recurrent fistulization. In such cases, extra-anatomic vascular reconstruction may be required.[105] The ureteral defect can be managed with ureteral stenting, nephrectomy with ureteral ligation or nephroureterectomy, nephrostomy tube placement, ureteral resection, and primary anastomosis or creation of an ileal ureter. Ureteral repair without arterial repair often leads to increased morbidity and mortality rates without substantial effects on control of hematuria.[72,81,82,106] In the largest single-institution series of ureteroaortic fistula, Krambeck and colleagues[77] proposed a systematic treatment strategy based on a patient's renal function and suitability for surgery (**Fig. 23-7**).

RECTOURETHRAL FISTULAS

Etiology

Rectourethral fistula (RUF) may be congenital, associated with imperforate anus, or acquired. The causes of acquired RUF include iatrogenic rectal injury during pelvic surgery, anterior rectal wall biopsy, inflammatory or infectious conditions, trauma, and brachytherapy or external beam radiation therapy. RUF is a condition encountered in men almost exclusively because in female patients, the vagina sits between the urethra and the rectum and thus protects against RUF. The most common causes of RUF are prostatectomy by any surgical approach (suprapubic, transurethral, and radical retropubic) and radiation therapy for prostate cancer.[107-113] The incidence of rectal injury at the time of radical prostatectomy is between 0.5% and 9%.[114-116] The incidence when using laparoscopic or robotic access is 1% to 2.7%.[117-121] Although RUF is a rare complication of radiation therapy for prostate cancer, as rates of brachytherapy and external beam radiation treatment for prostate cancer have increased, so has the prevalence of radiation-associated RUF. Success of RUF repair in cases of radiation injury and Crohn's disease tends to be lower than in patients with other causes of RUF.

Management of Intraoperative Rectal Injury

The prevention of a serious complication of rectal injury rests with the surgeon's attention to preoperative preparation of the patient and to surgical technique. All patients should receive a bowel preparation before radical prostatectomy. The extent of this bowel preparation regimen may vary according to the surgeon's preference from a clear liquid diet with magnesium citrate the day before the operation to clear liquids with a full gallon of polyethylene glycol or more until all effluent is clear. Our preference is for the latter, particularly in irradiated patients or in patients who have had many prior abdominal surgical procedures. Oral antibiotics are generally given as well.

The mechanism and management of rectal injury are discussed in detail elsewhere in the text. When a rectal injury occurs, the options for treatment include primary repair if the operative field is clean or diverting colostomy if the field is contaminated. Rectal injury from thermal energy is rarely recognized intraoperatively and usually manifests a week later as rectal bleeding or sepsis. The surgeon must have a high index of suspicion for these severely morbid and potentially life-threatening injuries when the patient presents with illness in the early postoperative course. In these cases, emergency resuscitation, immediate diversion with drainage of abscess, and proper supportive care are crucial.

Presentation

RUF may manifest with pneumaturia, fecaluria, rectal bleeding, rectal voiding, leakage or watery diarrhea, and

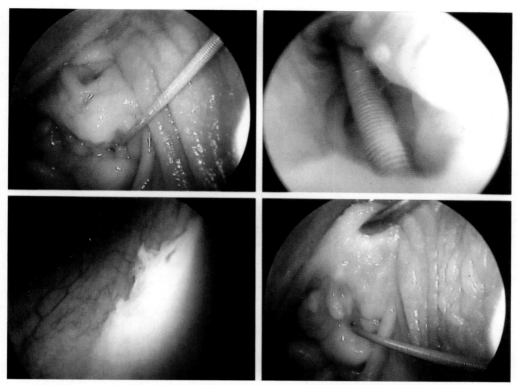

Figure 23-7 Systematic treatment strategy for ureteroarterial fistulas proposed by Krambeck and associates.[77]

often severe rectal and pelvic pain. Patients may also present with life-threatening bleeding, intra-abdominal abscess, sepsis, and necrotizing fasciitis, particularly if the diagnosis is delayed.[122] When a fistula recurs after initial surgical repair, the patient is rarely acutely ill. Recurrent urinary tract infections are the common presenting complaints in patients with long-standing RUF.

Diagnosis

These fistulas are commonly debilitating and resistant to repeated repair procedures. Therefore, careful preoperative staging evaluation and fecal and urinary diversion are almost universally recommended. Reports of RUF have suggested algorithms for RUF treatment; however, no RUF repair procedure is clearly preferred. Because a full description of all RUF repair options is beyond the scope of this chapter, the critical aspects of patient evaluation and preparation before repair are highlighted instead.

Most surgeons who treat RUF agree that fecal and urinary diversion should be performed in most cases before any definitive repair. Diversion of fecal and urinary streams from the fistula allows inflammation to improve or resolve before repair. Diversion alone is sufficient therapy to allow a small, nonradiated fistula to heal in approximately 20% to 25% of cases.[123]

Evaluation before repair includes imaging by retrograde urethrogram and VCUG and possibly CT of the abdomen and pelvis in cases of sepsis and suspected abscess. Diagnostic studies should be postponed in the presence of fever or sepsis and undertaken only after proximal urinary diversion, administration of intravenous antibiotics, and resolution of the acute process. Cystoscopy, proctoscopy, and manual examination with the patient under anesthesia are necessary to determine the extent of radiation damage or tissue necrosis surrounding the fistula, the fistula size and location, the rectal sphincter condition, and evidence of associated urethral or bladder neck stricture. It is also important to gauge bladder capacity and compliance, which both may be impaired by radiation.

VUDS is excellent for assessment of storage abnormalities; however, in some cases the fistula may large enough to preclude the accumulation of fluid in the bladder. In these situations, the surgeon must rely on the visual assessment of bladder distensibility at the time of cystoscopy. When the bladder is extremely contracted or fibrotic, preservation of the bladder is not likely to provide a functional outcome. Consideration of the rectal sphincter should also be made by anal manometry if any doubt about its competence exists.

Management

After diagnosis of RUF and initial control with fecal diversion by colostomy or ileostomy and urinary diversion by suprapubic tube or rarely ileal conduit, a waiting period of 3 to 9 months is common. During this time, inflammation and infection may heal, and in a small percentage of iatrogenic cases the fistula may resolve spontaneously.[123] Once the inflammation has settled and stabilized and the patient is deemed fit for surgery, several surgical approaches may be used.

The optimal approach is based on the surgeon's experience and the state of the patient's urinary and bowel function. Standard surgical principles of RUF repair are similar to those of other urinary fistula repairs such as careful operative planning because the first attempt at closure is the best attempt. Second, the judicious use of tissue interpositions in the plane between the rectum and the urethra is recommended. Omentum, gracilis muscle, sartorius muscle, and buccal mucosal grafts have been described for this use. Some surgeons also advocate that a buccal mucosal graft be placed over the prostatic urethral defect at the time of repair to decrease the incidence of urinary extravasation and to provide a healthy epithelialized layer of tissue on the urethral side.[122] The disadvantage of the buccal mucosal graft is the need to reposition the patient from prone to supine during the operation. Complications associated with the surgical repair of RUF by any means include bleeding, wound infection, and early or late recurrence of the fistula. After the surgical procedure, patients are maintained on oral antibiotics, and a cystogram is performed at 3 weeks.

Various surgical techniques have been described for repair of RUFs. Some urologists favor a posterior or perineal approach. A perineal approach provides familiar exposure and easy use of dartos or gracilis tissue flaps. Disadvantages associated with this approach include a theoretical risk of impotence, limited exposure, and the possible presence of significantly scarred tissues. An anterior transanorectal approach provides good exposure and also easily allows use of dartos, gracilis, or rectal tissue flaps for interposition.[124] Although rectal sphincter muscles may be divided, some studies support that an anatomic repair maintains fecal continence.[125,126]

CONCLUSION

Urinary fistula can be a devastating complication of abdominal and pelvic surgery or radiation therapy. The desire for prompt correction must be tempered by an understanding of the need for careful preoperative staging and planning, which are vital to the success of repairs and to the reduction of recurrence rates. Preoperative concerns include resuscitation of septic patients, correction of metabolic derangements if present, control of infection, and proper drainage of urine and any infected fluid collection. In staging stable patients, the surgeon should perform all necessary imaging and endoscopy to confirm the diagnosis, exclude associated injuries, and evaluate the size and location of the fistula. Only after obtaining all this information can the surgeon create a "roadmap" for repair. It is also necessary for the

surgeon to discuss this plan with the patient preoperatively as part of informed consent. Finally, meticulous attention to the surgical principles highlighted in the chapter and listed in Box 23-1 help ensure successful fistula repair. Surgeons must have great respect for fistula surgery because recurrence of the disorder is always a possibility.

KEY POINTS

1. IVP, or retrograde pyelogram if IVP is equivocal, is of paramount importance in excluding a ureterovaginal fistula (present concurrently with 10% of VVFs).

2. VUDS is a useful adjunct preoperatively to identify patients with SUI who would benefit from concomitant anti-incontinence surgery at the time of VVF repair. Additionally, bladder capacity and compliance should be assessed in patients who have received radiation prior to fistula repair.

3. The incidence of incontinence following urethrovaginal fistula repairs is 20% to 70%. A synthetic sling is never appropriate as an anti-incontinence option in this setting. Autologous fascial sling is the preferred and ideal method of anti-incontinence repair during urethrovaginal fistula repair.

4. If a patient does not present within 2 weeks of symptoms (when inflammation is minimal), formal repair of urinary fistulas should be delayed for a minimum of 2 to 3 months to allow inflammation to resolve and the fistula tract to mature. When the fistula tract is a result of radiation, repair is usually delayed for a minimum of 8 months to 1 year to allow the ischemic injury to stabilize.

5. Essential technical points in the repair of urinary fistulas include optimal exposure, wide mobilization of tissues, tension-free approximation, watertight closure, multi-layer repair, lack of overlapping suture lines, and interposition of vascularized graft.

6. The ureterovaginal fistula is the most common ureteral fistula, and most are caused by hysterectomy. Ureteroaortic fistulas are uncommon and have a 100% mortality if undiagnosed or left untreated.

7. Rectourethral fistulas are almost exclusively reported in men following prostatectomy. Increasing numbers have been reported with the rising prevalence of brachytherapy and external beam radiation use.

REFERENCES

Please see www.expertconsult.com

COMPLICATIONS OF ENDOUROLOGIC PROCEDURES

Chapter 24

COMPLICATIONS OF TRANSURETHRAL RESECTION OF THE PROSTATE

Mitchell H. Sokoloff MD
Professor of Surgery and Chief, Section of Urology, University of Arizona College of Medicine, Tucson, Arizona

Kiarash Michel MD
Urologist, Cedars-Sinai Medical Center, Los Angeles, California

Robert B. Smith MD
Professor of Urology, David Geffen School of Medicine, University of California–Los Angeles, Los Angeles, California

During the 1990s, we witnessed an increase in the average size of prostate glands we treat by transurethral resection (TUR). This is primarily a consequence of the widespread acceptance and use by both urologists and internists of pharmacologic agents as frontline therapy for benign prostatic hypertrophy (BPH).[1] Although the mechanisms and effects of these compounds (which include α-adrenoceptor antagonists, 5α-reductase inhibitors, antiandrogens, and other hormonal treatments) are rather disparate, we group them together for simplicity. The symptomatic relief in men treated with these agents can be substantial, but the effect on prostatic volume is variable.[2,3] Therefore, during the period between the appearance of a man's symptoms (which, we assume, coincides with the initiation of medical therapy) and the need for surgical therapy, the prostate can often increase in size. Correspondingly, the timing of surgery is delayed, and the men we take to the operating room for TUR are, on average, older than were patients in the late 1990s. The aging of our patient population is reflected in an increased prevalence of comorbidities, which can increase the risks of perioperative complications.

Several innovative technologies (discussed elsewhere in this textbook) have been introduced with the goal of diminishing potential side effects of surgical intervention. Despite a plethora of these minimally invasive and alternative procedures, transurethral resection of the prostate (TURP) remains the gold standard for the treatment of men with BPH.[4,5] When done correctly and methodically, TURP not only is an effective and durable therapy for BPH but also can be performed safely with minimal complications. Since the last edition of *Complications of Urologic Surgery,* the morbidity and mortality associated with TURP have been reevaluated. The reevaluation was initiated because of shortcomings in data used in comparison studies between TURP and newly introduced minimally invasive techniques. These earlier reports used data derived from large retrospective studies conducted in the 1980s.[6,7] Several groups since updated their results with patients treated during the 1990s and noted a much lower incidence of morbidity and mortality.[5,8] Clearly, improvements in surgical technique, better perioperative monitoring of fluids and electrolytes, refinements in anesthetic care, and the availability of video endoscopy have diminished intraoperative and postoperative morbidity and mortality.

Following the successes of pharmacologic therapies, as well as the introduction and initial enthusiasm for the minimally invasive procedures, the number of TURP procedures performed annually in the United States has diminished. This change is unfortunate for the urologist in training because the technical aspects of transurethral surgery are among the most difficult operative techniques for the neophyte surgeon to perfect. With the advent of lightweight cameras and high-resolution television monitors, teaching the mechanics of TUR has been made easier. These improvements alone, which enhance the ability of a mentor to direct and supervise a student while improving visualization of the prostatic bed during TURP, may account for decreased resection time and a subsequent reduction in intraoperative bleeding and fluid absorption.

Nonetheless, the subtleties of TURP can be mastered only with experience. The incidence of complications of transurethral surgery is inversely proportional to the experience of the surgeon. Therefore, at our institution, it is policy that a resident physician must be highly proficient with endoscopic procedures before advancing to TURP. This chapter is intended not only to help the urologist manage TURP-related complications but also, more importantly, to help obviate unnecessary complications by stressing fundamental techniques that should be used in all endoscopic cases. Too often, complications arise when these basic concepts are circumvented to conserve that all-important commodity, time.

GENERAL CONSIDERATIONS

No absolute size limit exists for TURP. Rather, a time constraint of 1 hour for resection should be the surgeon's guide. TURPs requiring >1 hour to complete are associated with a higher incidence of complications, including water intoxication syndrome (*TUR syndrome* [TURS]), urethral strictures, sepsis, and excessive blood loss. If greater duration is anticipated, open prostatectomy should be considered.

Absolute indications for TURP include acute urinary retention, recurrent infections, recurrent hematuria, and renal insufficiency or failure.[9] Most commonly, TURP is performed on men with moderate to severe bladder outlet symptoms that are refractory to pharmacologic therapy. The role of preoperative diagnostic tests is controversial. The American Urological Association Symptom Index and uroflowmetry are useful both to detect severity of symptoms and to assist with monitoring patients after resection.[1] Unfortunately, these measurements often do not correlate with the degree of mechanical obstruction.[10] Furthermore, these determinations do not always accurately differentiate neurologic causes from obstructing lesions. In questionable cases, a complete urodynamic evaluation with pressure-flow studies may be necessary.

The surgeon must accurately estimate prostatic size preoperatively. This can be done through a combination of approaches, including digital rectal examination, cystoscopy, and transrectal ultrasound. Prostatic size may be misjudged if a digital rectal examination is performed when large amounts of residual urine are present because the base of the bladder may be palpated, thus obscuring the prostate but possibly being mistaken for the prostate. Any question of prostatic malignant disease, as suggested by the presence of suspicious lesions or abnormalities in prostate-specific antigen (PSA) serology, must be resolved in patients who are candidates to receive primary therapy for prostate cancer.

We prefer to resect in two stages when the gland is too large to manage in a single 1-hour session. Although this technique is appropriate when the gland is found during resection to be larger than anticipated, it is questionable, in our opinion, whether a planned two-stage resection is ever justified. The necessary second anesthesia and possible septic sequelae in such cases favor one-stage open prostatectomy. Conversely, it is possible to resect one lateral lobe or the middle lobe and one lateral lobe and still obtain an excellent functional result. This approach is preferable to an incomplete resection of all lobes because the incidence of postoperative slough, hemorrhage, and obstruction is increased with incomplete resection of all lobes. Therefore, if it is impossible to complete the full resection in 1 hour, if the surgeon has concerns over water intoxication through open venous sinuses, or if the surgeon has undermined the trigone, stopping TURP after half-complete resection often results in a good outcome.

Small, fibrotic glands should almost invariably be removed by the transurethral route. Transurethral incision of the prostate at the 4- and 8-o'clock positions may work well to relieve obstructive symptoms in such patients.[11] Resection may not be necessary. Carcinoma of the prostate that causes lower urinary tract symptoms should also be managed transurethrally if a patient has persistent symptoms after androgen ablative therapy. Associated lesions, such as vesicoureteral reflux, vesical calculi, diverticula, vesical neoplasms, and stones, may alter the decision with regard to the route of prostatectomy.

SURGICAL INSTRUMENTATION

When the urologic surgeon begins an endoscopic procedure, it is essential that an appropriate array of instruments be immediately available. Many complications encountered in transurethral surgery are attributable to shortcuts employed because the surgeon did not have appropriate instruments on hand. Moreover, a dedicated operating room should contain all the endoscopic and associated equipment necessary for routine, as well as complicated, cases. The nursing staff should be well versed in the unique setup of the endoscopic suite and equipment and should be familiar with the mechanics, proper functioning, and configuration of each instrument. In addition, the operating table should be freely adjustable by the surgeon and should have radiologic capabilities in case emergencies arise in which cystography or urethrography becomes necessary.

The instrumentation for standard adult endoscopic procedures should include a full set of van Buren sounds up to 30 Fr. All sizes should be available because overly rapid dilation of a stricture is a major cause of false passages. Similarly, a filiform and followers of woven silk or LeFort sounds and a urethrotome should be included.

A full selection of insulated resectoscope sheaths in calibers to accommodate all loop sizes is mandatory. Sheaths with short beaks are preferable because they are less likely to cause injury to the urethra or trigone than are long-beaked sheaths. For similar reasons, the beaks should be inspected for smoothness before each use. Appropriate obturators are necessary for each sheath. It is sometimes helpful to have on hand an obturator with a screw tip that can accommodate a filiform thread. Copious amounts of water-soluble jelly for proper lubrication of sounds and sheaths are required for any endoscopic procedure.

Whereas the 30- and 70-degree lenses are essential for cystoscopic evaluations of the bladder, the 12-degree lens is optimal for TURP. Because fiberoptic light sources are fundamental components of an endoscopic suite, extra bulbs or an alternative light source should be available. Two resectoscopes should be available, the design of which should be the choice of the individual surgeon. The one-handed instrument of the Iglesias design that frees the opposite hand for rectal or suprapubic manipulation has become the standard. When a one-handed instrument is chosen, an O'Connor rectal shield can be used to enable the physician to perform periodic rectal manipulation without causing contamination. The rectal portion of the shield should be well lubricated to prevent irritation and possible rectal injury.

Continuous flow resectoscopes are customary in most endoscopic suites. These instruments allow for uninterrupted resection as well as improved visualization. Because the resection is not interrupted every few minutes to empty the bladder, operative time can be decreased. However, the constant pressure of the continuous flow sheath often compresses veins in the prostatic bed, thus obscuring potential sources of water absorption (resulting in TURS) as well as masking the actual amount of potential blood loss. If a continuous flow resectoscope is unavailable, a percutaneous suprapubic cystotomy can be placed immediately before resection. This approach is advantageous if heavy postoperative bleeding is expected because the volume of irrigant entering through a cystotomy and exiting out a single-lumen urethral catheter is greater than that through a three-way urethral catheter.

A full selection of appropriate resectoscope loops with regard to both size and wire caliber should also be available. The thinner the wire, the better the cutting capability is and the poorer the coagulating capacity of the loop. Several loops of each size should be available in the event of breakage.

A lithotrite, an electrohydraulic lithotriptor, or a laser filament of the surgeon's choice should be available to handle unsuspected vesical or urethral calculi. These calculi should be removed before resection of the prostatic adenoma. Similarly, flexible and rigid grasping forceps are useful in the event that material cannot be removed from the bladder by manipulation of the resectoscope loop. Often, frequent levering of the resectoscope sheath successfully evacuates fragments of tissue from the bladder. A Toomey syringe or an Ellik evacuator is also helpful for rapid elimination of vesical debris. The connecting hose should be of large caliber, rigid, and short, with an airtight seal between the syringe or evacuator and the nozzle that adapts to the resectoscope sheath. To facilitate filling of the syringe or evacuator, a deep bowl of sterile irrigating solution should be prepared. The Ellik evacuator should be inspected for bulb strength and integrity.

Surgical instruments for performing meatotomy, vasectomy, and perineal urethrotomy should be available. For such procedures, the minimal requirements include two towel clips, four straight hemostats, one Adson thumb forceps, one scalpel, and one needle holder. The type of suture material depends on the preference of the surgeon.

Two electrosurgical units should be available in case the primary unit malfunctions. Desirable features include a weighted foot pedal that will remain relatively stationary during the procedure and a sound mechanism with which cutting and coagulating currents can be differentiated by ear to help prevent the wrong pedal from being pressed inadvertently. To avoid thermal burns to the patient, a warning light or buzzer is imperative for detecting short circuits or improper patient grounding. In addition, no contact should occur between the patient and the metallic part of the operating table.

The operating table should be freely adjustable by the surgeon, and the tray should be large enough to facilitate collection of irrigating fluid and resected tissue. The ideal table should have radiologic capabilities in case emergencies arise in which cystography or urethrography is necessary. Semiadjustable or completely adjustable chairs should be available to the surgeon. Operating time may be decreased if the surgeon can adjust the patient's or his or her own relative position.

IRRIGATING SOLUTION

Generous stores of suitable irrigating fluid are imperative. Distilled water should not be used, given its tendency to hemolysis and increased risk of TURS. The ideal irrigating solution should be nonelectrolyte (so as not to interfere with electrical current) and iso-osmotic; solutions composed of 3.3% sorbitol, 5% mannitol, and 1.5% glycine readily satisfy these criteria. Glycine should not be used in patients with hepatic dysfunction because ammonia is a metabolic byproduct in the breakdown of glycine, and hyperammonemia may result. Sorbitol is metabolized to glucose, and its use can cause hyperglycemia. This condition may be a threat to diabetic patients, especially when large amounts of fluid are absorbed or extravasated. Mannitol has the advantage of being an osmotic diuretic, and it potentially helps to unload the patient of increased volume expansion. However, mannitol is not evenly distributed throughout the total body space, and hypervolemic changes may be temporarily compounded and may further contribute to manifestations of TURS.

PATIENT PREPARATION

The identification and preoperative correction of potential medical problems are of primary importance in decreasing morbidity and mortality associated with TURP. The surgeon must ensure that each urologic patient has undergone a thorough medical evaluation.

Cardiac Function

The patient's cardiac status is especially important because he may be challenged by massive shifts in fluid volume and serum electrolyte composition. Cardiac disease has always accounted for a significant proportion of mortality associated with TURP and is becoming more prominent, corresponding to the aging of our patient population. In addition to proper preoperative evaluation, adequate intraoperative monitoring is essential.

In high-risk patients, central venous pressure and pulmonary wedge pressure measurements may be necessary. Patients who are receiving anticoagulation medications present an additional dilemma to the transurethral surgeon. Discontinuing these medications may increase the likelihood of a thrombotic cardiac event; continuing the medication increases the probability of significant postoperative hemorrhage. These patients may be candidates for resection using one of the minimally invasive techniques.[12] When TURP is compulsory, consultation with the patient's cardiologist or cardiac surgeon is mandatory before any decision regarding discontinuation of any cardiac medication is made.

Renal Function

It is important to know the renal reserve of the patient to determine his capacity to handle the extra fluid volume. Serum creatinine and creatinine clearance tests are adequate for this purpose. If compromised renal reserve is detected, an attempt should be made to identify the cause and to correct it before the surgical procedure (e.g., catheter drainage for long-standing obstructive uropathy). Bladder drainage should be instituted in patients with upper urinary tract obstruction and the creatinine level should be allowed to stabilize before TURP.

Patients with compromised renal function have deficient clotting mechanisms because of abnormal platelet function.[13] Evidence also indicates that uremic patients have compromised resistance to infection.[13] Most large transurethral series indicated a significantly higher mortality rate among patients with compromised renal function. Patients with uremia secondary to upper urinary tract obstruction and prostatism must be watched carefully for postobstructive diuresis after a catheter has been passed. The diuresis is caused by the inability of the obstructed kidney to concentrate urine, the abnormal handling of sodium by the obstructed kidney, and the hyperosmolar effect of the elevated urea.[14] In addition, most of these patients start out with fluid overload.

Postobstructive Diuresis

In the case of postobstructive diuresis, daily weights should be monitored and urine output replaced on a milliliter per milliliter basis with 5% dextrose in half normal saline until the load of urea has been stabilized. Potassium is replaced as it is excreted; frequent urine and serum electrolyte measurements are essential to manage these patients properly. Moreover, calcium and magnesium can also be excreted and their levels must be monitored and replaced as needed. When serum urea nitrogen levels have stabilized, one can begin to reduce fluid replacement so as not to perpetuate this diuresis. Rarely should fluid replacement be <1500 mL of the total urine output per 24-hour period. When urine output is <250 mL/hour, fluid replacement less 50 mL of the urine output per hour is given. For outputs >250 mL, generally 100 mL/hour is subtracted from the replacement until the diuresis slows.

Infection

Urine culture and sensitivity determinations are mandatory in preparation for transurethral procedures, especially for patients with an indwelling catheter. Patients with significant urinary bacterial growth should be given appropriate parenteral antibiotic agents preoperatively, intraoperatively, and postoperatively to decrease the risk of bacteremia. Bacteremia has been noted in as many as 50% of patients undergoing transurethral surgery.[15] Patients with valvular heart disease or prosthetic devices must receive broad-spectrum antibacterial coverage. These protocols are well established in the medical literature.[16]

Prophylactic coverage with preoperative antibiotics of patients with sterile urine has been a controversial topic.[17] All patients should have a urine culture performed several days before the anticipated procedure. For those men with negative cultures, it is our procedure to administer ciprofloxacin 400 mg intravenous (IV) 1 hour before beginning resection. Most studies indicate that some prophylactic antibacterial coverage before resection is indicated in these patients.[18] Active urinary tract infections must be treated and eradicated, as demonstrated by a follow-up negative culture. Men with indwelling catheters should be treated as if they were infected. Traditionally, these patients were admitted to the hospital the day before the surgical procedure for IV antibiotics. In today's cost-conscious environment, however, such antibacterial coverage can be accomplished with a several-day course of oral agents with a broad gram-negative spectrum (e.g., as ciprofloxacin). In all patients, we continue antibiotic coverage after resection until 24 hours after the catheter has been removed.

Coagulation Issues

Because hemostasis in transurethral surgery is sometimes a problem, a coagulation profile should be obtained before any major procedure, and specific deficiencies should be corrected. This profile should include prothrombin time, partial thromboplastin time, platelet count, and bleeding time for patients with suspected platelet dysfunction. As mentioned earlier, the decision to continue administration of anticoagulant agents (e.g., aspirin, dipyridamole [Persantine]) is made by the surgeon and medical consultants. Men receiving warfarin (Coumadin) who require the maintenance of anticoagulation for prosthetic devices (e.g., artificial heart valves) should be treated with heparin preoperatively to refine coagulation parameters.[19] Warfarin can be discontinued several days preoperatively and resumed in the postoperative period after the major risk of postoperative hemorrhage has abated. If severe coagulopathy exists and is refractory or unreasonably costly to correct, alternative surgical plans may be necessary. Several of the currently available minimally invasive procedures mentioned earlier, as well as total prostatectomy, can be employed.

Other Medical Issues

Diabetic patients should have their disease under the tightest control possible to help minimize their risk of developing hyperosmolar syndrome. Patients with a high serum glucose level have increased serum osmolarity, which can cause an increased water shift from the intracellular and extracellular spaces. Thus, extravasated fluid absorbed during resection may move to the intravascular space at an accelerated rate and exacerbate the hyponatremia associated with TURS. Control of serum glucose levels helps to alleviate this problem. Patients in whom this is not possible may be treated with the early use of a loop diuretic. Patients with other medical conditions, such as obstructive pulmonary or peptic ulcer disease, should undergo appropriate preoperative management. Vigorous pulmonary toilet prevents many of the pulmonary complications associated with TUR. The use of conventional acid pump inhibitors, histamine antagonists, and oral slurries reduces the incidence of stress gastrointestinal bleeding in the postoperative period. In brief, improvements in preoperative patient evaluation and management, enhanced perioperative monitoring of fluids and electrolytes, and refinements in anesthetic care have diminished the incidence of intraoperative and postoperative morbidity and mortality.

SURGICAL APPROACH

Anesthesia

The decision regarding choice of anesthetic agents should be made after consultation with the patient, the surgeon, and the anesthesiologist. Regional (spinal or epidural) anesthesia, as opposed to general anesthesia, is our preference. With regional anesthesia, in the immediate postoperative period the patient is not as restless and coughs less, thus reducing the risks of increased Valsalva pressures and postoperative hemorrhage. With the additional infusion of a long-acting intrathecal narcotic (e.g., morphine sulfate [Duramorph]), the incidence of bladder discomfort and spasms in response to the catheter is reduced. Several reports have advocated using local anesthesia with sedation (especially for smaller glands).[20]

Regional anesthesia allows the patient to respond to pain in the event of complications such as intraperitoneal extravasation. It also permits better assessment of possible TURS. The anesthetic should be of sufficient duration to allow for unplanned occurrences. It should be given at the level of at least T9 to prevent discomfort from bladder distention during the procedure.

Blood loss should be monitored by both the surgeon and the anesthesiologist, although estimation is often difficult. The amount of blood lost during TURP is related to the size of the prostate as well as the time of resection. The anesthesiologist must watch for signs and symptoms of TURS and be prepared to treat it. If the venous sinuses are opened early in the procedure, the anesthesiologist should be notified to be alert for suspicious signs and symptoms. The serum sodium concentration should be assessed in the recovery room in such patients. If the operating time is prolonged, intraoperative determinations should be made as well. Should the sodium level be decreasing, IV fluids should be changed so that no free water is given, and furosemide (Lasix) should be administered.

Toward the end of the procedure, when hemostasis is being achieved, the anesthesiologist should ensure that the patient's blood pressure is in the preoperative range. Hypotension occurring at the end of the procedure may mask significant arterial bleeding, which may be the source of troublesome hemorrhage in the postoperative period. Should hypotension exist, ephedrine or similar agents should be administered to normalize the blood pressure.

Patient Positioning

When positioning the patient for an endoscopic procedure, the legs should be well padded at the knee brace to protect against peroneal nerve injury. For more extensive procedures, the legs should be wrapped to guard against venous stasis and possible subsequent embolic events. Approximately 5% of patients undergoing TURP develop deep vein thrombosis, which is related to the duration of resection and to the positioning of the patient.[17] Resection should be kept to <1 hour. For patients with a history of venous disease or conditions predisposing to a hypercoagulable state, pulsatile stockings should be employed.

Technique for Benign Adenomatous Hypertrophy

Although several different techniques of TURP have been described, it is most important for the neophyte surgeon to select a method with which he or she is most comfortable and to perform each resection in a methodical, step-by-step manner. It is mandatory that thorough cystoscopic evaluation be performed before resection of obstructive adenomatous tissue. The bladder should be the first area examined because cystoscopic manipulation of the prostatic urethra may cause troublesome and obscuring hemorrhage. The 12- or 30-degree lenses are used for resection, but the 70-degree lens allows for more complete inspection of the bladder wall. The presence of coexistent bladder tumors, diverticula, or vesical calculi must be excluded. If found, they should be dealt with before the prostatic resection.

Bladder tumor resection sites must be meticulously examined for possible perforation because the bladder may become extremely distended during TURP. Bladder diverticula of small capacity with an open neck need no therapy when the preoperative cystogram reveals complete emptying of the diverticulum. By contrast, if the neck is small and residual urine is present in the diverticulum, transurethral incision of the diverticulum is advisable. Vesical calculi, when present, should be handled by litholapaxy or by electrohydraulic or laser lithotripsy. If the stone is too large for endoscopic treatment, open cystolithotomy and open prostatectomy should be considered.

After concomitant vesical disease has been excluded or treated, careful evaluation of the obstructing adenoma should be made with regard to its anatomic relationship with the trigone, bladder neck, verumontanum, and external urinary sphincter. These relationships must be indelibly fixed in the surgeon's mind before resection is performed.

The distance from the adenoma to the trigone is an important determination. As the trigone hypertrophies and the prostatic fossa lengthens, this distance decreases, thus increasing the chance of a trigonal injury. The bladder neck and trigone should be inspected to determine the amount of middle lobe tissue present; the appropriate resection is then planned. The length of the prostatic urethra proximal to the verumontanum should be measured with respect to the length of the loop excursion. When the fossa is shorter than the loop excursion, care must be taken during the resection to avoid encroaching on the trigone and ureteral orifices.

The amount of prostatic tissue distal to the verumontanum should also be determined to help protect against injury to the external sphincter. The bulk of the adenoma should be judged by palpating the cystoscope with the rectal finger. It is especially important to gauge the thickness of the adenoma at the posterior vesical neck, one of the common potential sites of perforation. The external sphincter should then be visualized in relation to the verumontanum at the apex of the prostate during resection; the surgeon must be able to differentiate between the cut surface of adenoma and that of muscle tissue because the spatial relationship of the external sphincter, verumontanum, and adenoma is constantly changing.

A 24-Fr sheath will suffice for most resections and should be used in preference to larger sheaths, except when large adenomas exist. A 28-Fr loop can be accommodated in a 26-Fr sheath. Thus, it is never necessary to use a 28-Fr sheath. If, after satisfactory dilation and lubrication, the sheath is noted to drag, an internal urethrotomy or perineal urethrostomy should be substituted whenever possible (see later). If instrument drag should occur midprocedure, a smaller sheath should be substituted. When a 24-Fr sheath is already in use, an internal urethrotomy or a perineal urethrostomy in the middle of the procedure may be wise.

A detailed anatomic discussion of all techniques of TURP is beyond the scope of this chapter. The order in which lobes of the prostate are resected is largely one of personal preference. Ideally, the neophyte operator should employ various methods during the initial phases of training to choose the method that best suits his or her talents. Variant adenomatous configuration may require that the surgeon deviate from a routine pattern, but a uniform method should be followed whenever possible.

By initially resecting the posterior bladder neck area and middle lobes, one improves the flow of irrigating fluid from the prostatic fossa into the bladder. Resected chips of adenomatous tissue may then flow more readily into the bladder and not hamper the surgeon. Another advantage of beginning in this area is that resection of the middle lobe and posterior bladder neck can be done when the operator is fresh and when visualization is optimal. This technique reduces the risk of trigonal injury or perforation of the posterior bladder neck.

When circular muscle fibers of the posterior bladder neck are seen, resection in this area should be terminated. One should be especially careful not to use widespread coagulation in the area of the bladder neck; otherwise, bladder neck contracture may occur. Only pinpoint fulguration of arterial bleeders should be employed. The posterior bladder neck is a very common site of perforation. Careful attention to detail without resecting through the circular muscles of the bladder neck will help obviate this complication. Moreover, when evacuating chips with the resectoscope, the beak of the resectoscope should be placed underneath the bladder neck because leverage on the resectoscope sheath emptying the bladder may cause a perforation.

The adenoma is thinnest in the anterior portion of the prostatic fossa, and care must be taken to avoid perforation. Multiple venous sinuses may be encountered in this area. Early entrance into venous sinuses may lead to TURS. During resection, the resectoscope beak should be positioned so that the verumontanum is often in view, thus protecting the external sphincter from injury. Whenever possible, full use of the loop's sweep should be made, and the entire length of the prostatic adenoma should be resected with each excursion.

Patients with small prostates, in which a loop excursion may exceed the length of the prostatic fossa, must be handled so as not to encroach on the trigone. When the prostatic fossa is markedly elongated, two loop excursions may be necessary, or the sheath should be moved to the apex while the loop is still extended. The latter method is quicker and facilitates a smooth resection. If the lateral lobes appear so bulky that three loop widths will not complete the resection laterally into the area of the surgical capsule, it is preferable to employ an encirclement technique rather than the side-to-side, step-down method.

In patients with large prostates, resection time may be greatly reduced by using continuous flow resectoscopes that make it unnecessary to stop resection periodically to empty the bladder. Alternatively, punch suprapubic cystotomy can be performed before the procedure; this cystotomy also allows for continuous runoff of irrigating fluid. Postoperative bladder irrigation can then be run through the suprapubic tube and out a single-lumen Foley catheter, thereby increasing the volume and rate of irrigation.

In the final stage of the procedure, the apical adenomatous tissue lying distal to the verumontanum is resected. The external urinary sphincter should be visualized to guard against injuries, and the beak of the resectoscope should be placed just proximal to the sphincter. Any apical tissue that protrudes into the lumen of the prostatic fossa, as viewed from the area of the membranous urethra, should be resected. In patients who have considerable adenomatous tissue distal to the verumontanum, pushing the loop forward to resect in a proximal direction may help decrease the chance of injury to the sphincter.

After resection, the bladder is freed of prostatic chips with a Toomey syringe or an Ellik evacuator, and final hemostasis is achieved. If open venous sinuses cause excessive bleeding, catheter traction should be employed in the initial postoperative period. It is rare, in our experience, not to enter a venous sinus in the terminal phases of prostatic resection. Before removing the resectoscope, the surgeon should ensure that the patient's blood pressure during the final stages of the procedure

is nearly normal. Hypotension at the end of the procedure may mask significant bleeding arteries that may open up when the blood level returns to normal in the recovery room, thus causing postoperative hemorrhage.

A 22- or 24-Fr Foley catheter is then inserted and is connected to straight drainage. If clots form and obstruct the catheter lumen, intermittent hand irrigation usually suffices to clear them. Alternatively, three-way catheters with continuous saline irrigation can be used to prevent clots from forming. With careful observation and skilled nursing care, these three-way catheters can be used with minimal risk.

Catheter traction is often employed, and ≥30 mL of fluid should be placed in the catheter balloon to ensure that the balloon remains outside the prostatic fossa. When a balloon distends the prostatic fossa, contraction of the prostatic capsule is prevented. Such contraction is a major hemostatic mechanism. To prevent this contraction, a correspondingly larger volume should be placed in balloons when larger adenomas are resected. Up to 90 mL may be placed in a 30-mL catheter balloon chamber. Traction necessary to control venous sinus bleeding can be applied initially with meatal pressure by tying a moist sponge around the catheter or by weighted traction (<1 lb over the end of the bed; e.g., a 500-mL bag of saline). Traction using meatal pressure should never be employed for longer than a few minutes because necrosis of the meatus can result. Weighted traction over the end of the bed can be left for longer periods, as necessary. If bleeding persists, traction should be intermittently released to prevent pressure necrosis of the bladder neck. This complication has never occurred in our experience and may be more of a theoretical concern than a true potential problem.

Technique for Carcinoma of the Prostate

The same indications for operative intervention for hyperplasia apply to carcinoma of the prostate. With the widespread use of luteinizing hormone–releasing hormone agonists and antiandrogens, however, we perform fewer palliative resections of neoplastic prostate tissue. In fact, controversy exists about whether hormone therapy is justified for obstructive disease or whether its use should be withheld until the patient becomes symptomatic from metastatic disease. Nonetheless, when massive neoplastic involvement of the prostate occurs and causes obstruction, many urologists favor transrectal needle biopsy to confirm the diagnosis of carcinoma, followed by chemical or surgical castration.

Although castration often ameliorates obstructive symptoms resulting from locally advanced cancer, TURP is still an important treatment for obstruction in men with hormone-refractory disease and for intractable bleeding. Furthermore, when benign adenomatous hyperplasia exists in conjunction with carcinoma and is the prime lesion responsible for outlet obstruction, TURP should be performed in preference to hormone manipulation.

Cystoscopic evaluation is helpful in distinguishing between obstruction caused by adenomatous hyperplasia and that caused by massive infiltrative carcinoma. Some debate exists regarding the traditional role of TURP in the management of such patients with urinary retention and locally advanced carcinoma of the prostate. Many patients with complete or nearly complete urinary retention may be well managed by catheter drainage and radiation therapy, with or without adjunctive hormone treatment. It is essential, however, that those patients experiencing urinary retention do not undergo irradiation with a urethral Foley catheter in place. Such patients should be drained of urine through a suprapubic tube during the course of radiation therapy. Severe urethral stricture can result if radiation therapy is given with a Foley catheter in the urethra. Seven weeks, however, are often required for sufficient shrinkage of the prostate and a decrease in the radiation reaction to occur before the catheter can be removed and the patient is allowed to void.

Although it is thus possible to obtain significant shrinkage of enlarged neoplastic glands with radiation therapy, we prefer TUR for this group of patients. It is our belief that TURP obviates the need for long-term suprapubic catheter drainage during the period of radiation therapy and reduces the possibility that the procedure may be necessary following radiation therapy. In our experience, patients who undergo TUR after definitive radiation therapy often have a higher incidence of incontinence, bleeding, and infection because of compromise of the sphincter by fibrosis secondary to the therapy and the inability of the prostatic fossa to heal following irradiation. The onset of incontinence may be delayed because progressive fibrosis of the sphincter does occur following radiation therapy (administered by either external beam or interstitial seeds).

When TUR of prostate carcinoma has been performed and subsequent radiation therapy is contemplated, it is best to delay radiation therapy for 8 weeks to allow reepithelialization of the prostatic fossa. Fewer irritative symptoms result. If the patient has already received the full course of radiation therapy and later develops lower urinary tract obstruction, TUR should be performed. However, these patients have a greater risk of delayed healing of the prostatic fossa, bleeding, urinary incontinence, and urethral stricture formation, and they should be informed accordingly.

Special care must be taken when performing resection in cases of carcinoma of the prostate because the incidence of postoperative bleeding is higher in these patients than in those who have benign disease. Prothrombin time, platelet count, and examination of the urine for fibrinolysis should be part of the preoperative evaluation. If troublesome postoperative hemorrhage ensues, primary fibrinolysis and primary intravascular coagulation must be considered potential causes.

When carcinoma exists in conjunction with hyperplasia, the surgical technique remains essentially the same as in benign adenomatous obstruction. If the prostate is extensively involved with carcinoma, however, some modification in the technique may be necessary. Often, anatomic features are distorted; the bladder neck and membranous urethra may be the only remaining landmarks. In patients with extensive carcinoma, the urethra is often rigid, and maneuverability of the sheath is limited. In such cases, perineal urethrostomy may allow improved manipulation of the sheath and facilitate the resection. In patients with prostatic obstruction secondary to scirrhous carcinoma, a channel cut often suffices for relief of obstruction because tissue will not fall into the fossa as with adenomatous tissue. Exceptional care must be taken in the region of the apex in men with carcinoma, especially those who have been irradiated. If the carcinoma appears to be infiltrating the prostatic apex, incontinence is a common sequela of resection, no matter how careful the surgical technique may be. The patient with such apical extension should be apprised preoperatively of this potentiality.

It is our approach to perform a limited resection of the apex of such patients and to consider postoperative hormone manipulation to cause enough softening and regression of the local lesion to allow satisfactory voiding. One can always resect persistent apical tissue at a later date should obstruction remain. It is difficult to put apical tissue back in a patient whom you have made incontinent.

Technique for Prostatic Abscess

Modern antibiotic treatment has made prostatic abscess a rare lesion. During the course of TURP, however, it is not uncommon to encounter small pockets of purulent material that persist following acute or chronic episodes of infection. These pockets, however, usually are sterile.

Occasionally, a patient presents with acute obstructive symptoms secondary to a prostatic abscess. The abscess areas are often fluctuant but occasionally may be so firm that they resemble carcinoma. Before the use of modern antibacterial chemotherapy, incision and drainage by perineal exposure were the procedures of choice. Today, appropriate parenteral or broad-spectrum antibiotics alone often suffice. If the patient presents with acute urinary retention, however, a small urethral catheter or punch suprapubic cystostomy may be necessary until the appropriate antibiotic therapy has been administered and has had a chance to resolve the problem. If clinical resolution of the abscess is not achieved with parenteral antibiotics or if the patient's condition deteriorates during antibiotic therapy, prostatic imaging (e.g., computed tomography scan) and drainage of the abscess should be performed. The initial approach to drainage of the prostatic abscess is to place a computed tomography–guided percutaneous or transrectal drain into the abscess cavity. If the approach proves futile, TURP may be entertained for a more definitive drainage procedure. In most cases, the abscess is seen bulging into the lumen of the prostatic urethra. Simple unroofing of the most prominent portion of the bulge is usually all that is necessary. If significant hyperplasia is also present, it can be resected then or later, depending on the general status of the patient.

Technique for Prostatitis

TURP should be employed only rarely in patients with prostatitis, and patients should be properly forewarned that their symptoms may persist. Irritative symptoms must not be confused with obstructive symptoms; the former are often worsened by an ill-advised resection. When prostatitis is associated with adenomatous obstruction or prostatic calculi and if the patient has severe, debilitating symptoms, a properly performed resection may be of benefit. Radical TURP offers the best chance for symptomatic relief in these patients.[21] All tissue surrounding the prostatic calculi should be resected. If prostatic calculi are present between the adenoma and the surgical capsule, resection should extend well into the surgical capsule in an attempt to remove most of the inflamed tissue. In patients with inflamed prostates, coagulation should be used sparingly to decrease subsequent fibrosis in the prostatic fossa. When severe symptoms persist, total prostatectomy may be the only means of benefiting such patients.

POSTOPERATIVE MANAGEMENT

It is imperative that catheter drainage be employed well into the postoperative period. An obstructed catheter can cause distention of the prostatic capsule with resultant hemorrhage. A three-way catheter with continuous irrigation lessens the likelihood of clot formation. This catheter must be carefully monitored, however. Should a clot occlude the lumen, bleeding could be worsened by the continuous infusion of irrigating fluid, which further distends the bladder and prostatic capsule, perhaps opening venous sinuses.

We recommend the use of postoperative prophylactic antibiotics until the catheter is removed, although the choice to do so, of course, is up to the surgeon. Bladder spasms may indicate an obstructed catheter. If clots in the bladder are ruled out as a cause of the spasms, appropriate anticholinergic agents may be administered. If a large amount of solution is left in the balloon at the time the catheter is placed, reduction in the size of the balloon to 30 mL will lessen bladder spasms. Discontinuation of traction, if used, also diminishes the incidence of bladder spasms.

Patients should be kept at bed rest in the initial 24 hours following TURP. Full ambulation is allowed during the first postoperative day, but the patient should be discouraged from sitting for prolonged periods. Bowel movements should be kept soft to prevent excessive strain during this period. We routinely prescribe stool softeners for our patients. If an enema is necessary, it should be given with extreme caution to avoid possible rectal perforation or manipulation of the prostate, which may result in bleeding. Heavy lifting should be avoided for 4 to 6 weeks postoperatively.

COMPLICATIONS

Mechanical Difficulties

It is beyond the scope of this chapter to describe all possible mechanical malfunctions that can occur during TUR. The best way to prevent problems is to require that the technicians who maintain the instruments routinely check all equipment after each use. If the surgeon closely inspects the instruments while assembling them, he or she may also discover potential sources of difficulty.

Problems of Instrument Introduction

Phimosis

In the postoperative period, phimosis may trap secretions and cause periurethral drainage around the catheter, possibly leading to severe urethritis and subsequent stricture formation. Phimosis may be severe enough to cause difficulty in passing instruments. In such cases, circumcision should be performed to facilitate instrument introduction and better antiseptic preparation. It should be possible to determine whether phimosis is likely to be a problem and to obtain proper preoperative patient consent. In the absence of consent for circumcision, a limited dorsal slit suffices to allow instrument introduction.

Meatal Stenosis

Meatal stenosis of congenital, inflammatory, traumatic, or iatrogenic origin may also be present. This condition not only can prevent passage of a resectoscope but also may cause instrument drag, which hampers the sheath's maneuverability and interferes with the tactile sensation of the surgeon. Meatal stenosis in the postoperative period is also a cause of purulent urethral drainage with all its potential sequelae. Meatotomy should be adequate to resolve problematic stenosis. Incomplete incision fails to prevent subsequent damage and possibly leads to worse postoperative meatal stenosis, more symptomatic than the original condition. Urethral calibration of the area may determine the proximal extent of the stenosis. If the stenotic area is long, it may be wise to perform an internal urethrostomy with a straight urethrotome or with the direct vision Winter-Ivy instrument. Severe long strictures may be bypassed with this use of a perineal urethrostomy (see later).

It is controversial whether the meatotomy incision should be made dorsally or ventrally. A dorsal meatotomy incision causes less subsequent splaying of the urinary stream but limits the extent of the incision; bleeding is often a consequent problem. The ventral meatotomy is usually satisfactory. If it becomes necessary to perform a radical meatotomy to ensure proper instrument mobility, reconstruction of the meatus, using a frenular flap, may be performed at a later time.

Intraoperative Priapism

Erection during TUR is another possible cause of difficulty. It is not uncommon for a patient to develop priapism during TURP. It may occur with any mode of anesthesia and often persists stubbornly despite all therapeutic attempts. A trial of hypotensive anesthesia is of occasional benefit. When a patient is under spinal anesthesia, judicious administration of amyl nitrite may be helpful, as well as intracavernosal injection of an α-adrenergic agent (e.g., ephedrine). Temporary cessation of manipulation may allow the phallus to detumesce. Under no circumstances should the procedure simply continue. Forcing the instruments through an erect penis may result in meatal and urethral injury. If erection persists, perineal urethrostomy can bypass the problem (see later), but troublesome hemorrhage may occur if the incision veers from the midline. On occasion, a procedure must be terminated because of a patient's erection.

Urethral Stricture

Urethral strictures and the formation of false passages often present problems for the surgeon. Mild strictures may be dilated with van Buren sounds. False passage formation is a common hazard when dilating anesthetized patients with these instruments. Sounds should never be forcibly introduced; the curve of the instrument should allow for smooth passage using only pressure of the fingers. It is often helpful to place a free hand in the patient's rectum to guide the sound, thus helping to prevent the formation of a false passage.

Should a false passage be encountered, a filiform may be passed through the urethra, by using a urethroscope with a 0- or 30-degree lens. Dilation with woven silk followers is then performed. Timberlake obturators with a screw tip to accommodate the filiform threads are useful in ensuring proper passage of the resectoscope sheath. If the surgeon cannot satisfactorily negotiate the true urethral passage, the procedure is best terminated and attempted at a later date. Approximately 90% of patients can accept a 26-Fr resectoscope without difficulty. If the resectoscope does not move freely in and out of the urethra after apparent satisfactory dilation and lubrication, an internal urethrotomy or perineal

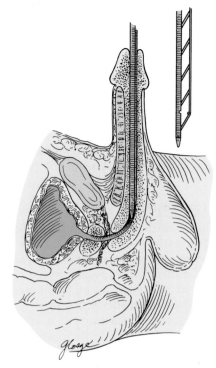

Figure 24-1 Technique for internal urethrotomy. A straight urethrotome is the preferred instrument. The penis is held perpendicular to the pubis to avoid injury to the membranous urethra.

urethrostomy should be considered. It is *never* necessary to use a 28-Fr sheath.

Internal Urethrotomy

When an internal urethrotomy is performed for individual strictures, we prefer to use the Winter-Ivy instrument and cut the stricture under direct vision. If the urethra is too tight in general to allow the resectoscope to move freely, we prefer to perform the internal urethrotomy with an Otis urethrotome. The urethrotome need only be set at 36 Fr, with one cut made in the 12-o'clock position. If the penis is held perpendicular to the pubis during internal urethrotomy, injury to the membranous urethra is avoided (**Fig. 24-1**). Catheterization is necessary for only 48 to 72 hours postoperatively. Some surgeons routinely perform internal urethrotomy before TURP. We do not agree with this approach because of associated complications including sepsis, hemorrhage, subsequent stricture formation, and development of chordee.

Perineal Urethrostomy

Many urologists advocate perineal urethrostomy to bypass distal urethral strictures. Perineal urethrostomy is also invaluable in facilitating maneuverability of the resectoscope in patients with short suspensory ligaments of the penis or a long phallus. Some urologists routinely perform the procedure in TURP when resectable tissue is expected to exceed 40 g. In addition, should a patient develop an erection at the beginning of a procedure, it is one way to proceed with the operation, thus obviating potential urethral injury while maintaining the ability to maneuver the resectoscope with ease. Perineal urethrostomy, however, is considered by many surgeons to be a cumbersome, difficult, and often time-consuming procedure. Brisk hemorrhage can result if the incision is not kept in the midline.

A simple and successful method of performing perineal urethrostomy employs resectoscope sheaths of different sizes. With this technique, the distal urethra must be dilated to a sufficient caliber to accommodate a 24-Fr resectoscope sheath. The sheath is passed into the bulbous urethra to the point at which the urethra turns upward toward the urogenital diaphragm. The fenestra of the resectoscope beak is then readily palpable in the perineum (**Fig. 24-2A**). After ensuring that the fenestra is in the midline, the surgeon makes an incision (using a scalpel) just large enough to allow the smaller sheath to be passed through the urethral wall and to exit through the perineum (see Fig. 24-2B). Then, using a 26-Fr sheath with the 24-Fr Timberlake obturator fitted snugly into the proximal end of the 24-Fr sheath, the larger sheath is passed into the distal urethra as the smaller sheath is withdrawn from the meatus (see Fig. 24-2C). The 24-Fr obturator is replaced in the larger sheath by its appropriate obturator. The surgeon then passes a larger sheath into the proximal urethra and bladder while taking care to hug the anterior wall of the bulbous urethra when negotiating the turn toward the urogenital diaphragm (see Fig. 24-2D). This is the crucial part of the procedure. If the surgeon is not successful in accomplishing this maneuver, the 24-Fr sheath is reinserted into the distal urethra and is advanced through the existing skin incision in the perineum, and the entire procedure is repeated until it is successful.

Sutures are not necessary with this technique; the larger sheath tamponades the perineal urethrostomy site during the procedure and hemorrhage is rarely a problem. If the resectoscope is inadvertently extracted from the perineal urethrostomy site during the course of the procedure, the entire maneuver is repeated. *One should never attempt simply to push the sheath back through the perineal urethrostomy because severe urethral injury and hemorrhage may result.*

During the postoperative period, the catheter should not exit through the perineal urethrostomy site; delayed wound healing and prolonged urinary leakage occur from this site. A catheter guide is helpful in passing the catheter from the meatus and distal urethra into the bladder to avoid the urethrostomy site. When a Foley catheter is left indwelling for 72 hours after the TURP, coursing the entire urethra, complete healing is accomplished and it would be unlikely for perineal leakage to occur when the catheter is removed. Urethral strictures at the site of the perineal urethrostomy have not been seen.

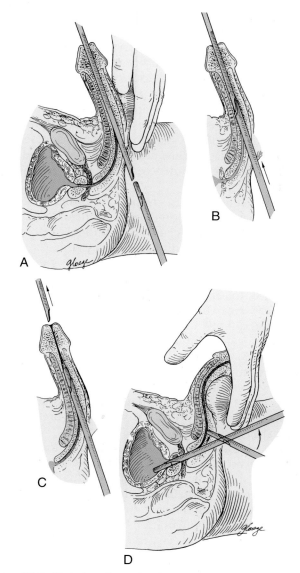

Figure 24-2 Technique for perineal urethrostomy. **A,** The fenestra of a 24-Fr resectoscope sheath palpated in the perineum. **B,** A small incision over the 24-Fr resectoscope beak has been made in the perineal urethra. A 28-Fr sheath with a 24-Fr obturator has been inserted into the fenestra of the 24-Fr sheath. **C,** Both sheaths are advanced into the urethra distal to the perineal urethrostomy. The 24-Fr sheath has been withdrawn. The 28-Fr obturator is now placed in the appropriate sheath. **D,** The 28-Fr sheath is advanced into the bladder, with care taken to hug the anterior wall of the bulbous urethra during introduction.

Bleeding

The amount of perioperative bleeding is primarily determined by prostatic size and resection time. As such, surgical technique is a significant factor, and it is paramount that the surgeon select a method with which he or she is most comfortable and perform each resection in a methodical, step-by-step manner. Preoperative evaluation of the patient's coagulation profile is an essential prophylactic measure in preventing excessive hemorrhage. Transfusion rates should be <1%.[5] Careful electrofulguration of bleeding arteries decreases the chance of delayed hemorrhage that can result from the sloughing of tissue secondary to massive fulguration of the prostatic fossa. Blood pressure levels must be normal at the termination of the procedure to ensure that significant bleeding points are not masked by hypotension. When venous sinuses are opened during the procedure, it is not necessary to terminate the resection. The level of irrigating fluid should be lowered and furosemide should be administered. Free water should not be given (see later).

Bleeding venous sinuses respond to catheter traction; indiscriminate fulguration does not control this type of bleeding and may even cause an additional hemorrhage. Unroofing of venous sinus bleeding vessels is a common occurrence if a truly complete resection is performed. Postoperatively, a continuous three-way irrigation catheter is used, to lessen the chance of a blood clot occluding the catheter. One must be careful, however, because should the catheter occlude, continuous inflow of fluid may cause overdistention of the bladder and dilation of the prostatic urethra, thus causing further bleeding. Bladder rupture can also occur. Attentive nursing care is necessary if continuous irrigation is used. It is our contention that a closed continuous irrigation system with intermittent hand irrigation as necessary is preferable to a standard two-way catheter.

If it is necessary to reoperate to control hemorrhage, thorough evacuation of clots from the bladder and prostatic fossa should be performed. Systematic examination of the entire prostatic fossa for bleeding sites should be conducted, using the irrigating fluid under low pressure. Appropriate fulguration may then be accomplished. It may be necessary to remove clots that adhere to the prostatic fossa with a resectoscope loop to visualize sites of hemorrhage. In our experience, a common area in which undetected postoperative hemorrhage occurs is the anterior bladder neck where pieces of prostate tissue often can be pulled in during resection, flip up, and reside just inside the bladder neck. Careful observation of this area is essential if an obvious bleeding site is not found on reexploration elsewhere in the prostatic fossa. Rarely, open surgical exploration may be necessary, with direct fulguration or suture ligation of bleeding sites. A circumferential bladder neck suture may be of benefit in stubborn cases; only rarely should it be necessary to leave a pack in the prostatic fossa.

If troublesome postoperative hemorrhage ensues, primary fibrinolysis and primary intravascular coagulation must be considered potential causes, especially in patients with adenocarcinoma of the prostate. Fibrinolysis may occur in conjunction with disseminated intravascular coagulation.[22] Fibrinolysis secondary to urokinase is easily detected by incubating the blood clot in a urine sample. If clot lysis occurs, IV ε-aminocaproic acid (Amicar) should be administered immediately, and the patient should be given oral therapy later. Five grams are given at once, followed by 1 g/hour until the bleeding stops.

The administration of Amicar to patients who have both fibrinolysis and disseminated intravascular coagulation, however, is hazardous, and intravascular coagulation must be ruled out before Amicar is used. The diagnosis of disseminated intravascular coagulation is made when the patient is found to be thrombocytopenic and hypofibrinogenemic, with an associated increase in the prothrombin time secondary to a decrease in the concentration of accelerator globulin. Decreased levels of prothrombin in factor VIII (antihemophilic factor) further substantiate the diagnosis. In such clinical situations, the threshold to consult a hematologist should be low.

Disseminated intravascular coagulation is managed with heparin dosed at 80 to 100 U/kg subcutaneously (SC) every 4 to 6 hours or 20,000 to 30,000 U/day IV continuous infusion. Continuous IV infusion is preferable to the intermittent IV or subcutaneous method. If associated urokinase activity is present, Amicar may be added to heparin after the clotting factors (platelet count, fibrinogen, and prothrombin) have begun to return to normal. Transfusion with appropriate blood components, such as platelet packs and fresh frozen plasma, is an important adjuvant in stubborn cases. The use of Amicar routinely in TURP for benign disease is not warranted. In a randomized, double-blind controlled study using Amicar in patients undergoing TURP for benign disease, we were unable to find any benefit in the Amicar-treated group.[23] Use of Amicar is appropriate only if fibrinolysins are detected and only after disseminated intravascular coagulation has been excluded.

In cases of stubborn hemorrhage, some surgeons advocate the placement of a Foley balloon catheter within the prostatic fossa. A 24-Fr Foley catheter with a 30-mL balloon is inserted into the bladder and the balloon is inflated to 15 mL. The catheter is withdrawn until resistance is felt. The balloon then resides within the prostatic fossa. An additional 15 mL of fluid is then added and the amount increased in 10 to 15 mL increments until hemostasis is achieved. Prolonged traction with the balloon in the prostatic fossa is not recommended, given the risk of traumatic injury. Although numerous surgeons favor prolonged catheter traction for stubborn bleeding vessels, we favor compression of the prostatic urethra with the balloon inflated within the bladder, as just described; compression of the prostatic fossa then allows the capsule to contract.

Undermining of the Trigone

Undermining of the trigone occurs because of overzealous resection of the bladder neck and proximal prostatic urethra. If such a situation occurs, a urethral catheter should not simply be advanced, using feel, into the bladder at the termination of the resection and the balloon inflated. Not too uncommonly, the catheter does not make the bend at the proximal prostatic urethra and instead directly enters the false passage below the bladder neck. In this case, inflating the balloon only exaggerates the false passage and worsens the bladder neck–prostatic urethral dissociation. Instead, the catheter should be inserted into the urethra and advanced into the bladder under control. A 21-Fr cystoscope with a 30-degree lens should be advanced under direct vision into the bladder. Once in the bladder, a 0.038 wire or a whistle tip ureteral catheter should be placed into the working channel of the cystoscope and advanced into the bladder. The cystoscope and lens should then be removed over the safety wire or ureteral catheter. With the wire or ureteral catheter in place, a council-tip three-way catheter can be advanced over wire into the bladder. If a council-tip catheter is not available, a makeshift catheter can be made simply by cutting the very tip of the three-way catheter and keeping clear of the balloon. The catheter should be well lubricated.

Once the catheter has been fully advanced, the indwelling safety wire or ureteral catheter is removed. Hand irrigation should be performed before inflating the balloon to ensure proper positioning of the urethral catheter. Resistance to complete insertion of the catheter in the urethra, or ease of irrigating the catheter coupled with difficulty aspirating through the catheter after having instilled an adequate volume into the bladder, should warn the surgeon of improper placement of the urethral catheter. In such a situation, a repeated trial of catheter placement under wire or ureteral catheter guidance should be attempted. Otherwise, a cystogram in the operating room can be performed to evaluate the catheter placement.

Resection of the Intravesical Ureter

Resection of the ureter or ureteral orifice is often the result of carelessness. To minimize the chance of inadvertently resecting the ureteral orifices, both ureteral orifices should be carefully visualized before resection of the bladder neck or middle lobe. Resection should not be performed until the orifices are clearly seen. If the surgeon believes that the resection will be too close to the ureteral orifices, a pure cutting electrical current setting should be employed for the bladder neck resection. Avoiding a coagulating current minimizes the chance of stricturing should the orifices be inadvertently resected. If the ureteral orifice is resected with a pure cutting current, simple drainage of the bladder with a urethral catheter should suffice. An IV pyelogram and voiding cystogram should be performed postoperatively. If the ureteral resection is more pronounced, a cystogram should be performed in the operating

room to exclude the possibility of an intraperitoneal perforation.

If a coagulating current was used during the resection of the ureteral orifice, an attempt should be made to stent the ureter at the termination of the TURP. The ureteral catheter should be left in place for 4 to 6 weeks. An IV pyelogram should be performed 1 to 2 weeks after removing the ureteral catheter. Repeat imaging should be performed 2 to 3 months later to evaluate for the development of a delayed ureteral stricture. A cystogram should also be performed to evaluate for vesicoureteral reflux.

Extravasation of Fluid

Symptomatic perforation of the bladder neck and prostatic capsule should occur only rarely. It is not uncommon, however, in performing complete TURP to have small, insignificant perforations. If a major perforation occurs early during the resection, large amounts of fluid may extravasate into the retroperitoneal space and cause significant discomfort or delayed resorption and exacerbation of TURS (see later). Spinal anesthesia allows the symptomatic extravasation to be discovered while the patient is still in the cystoscopic room, where appropriate therapeutic measures may be immediately initiated. General anesthesia often delays the diagnosis and requires the patient to be returned to the operating suite for possible treatment. General anesthesia further complicates the situation by masking many of the early symptoms of TURS.

Another sign of significant perforation extravasation is distortion of the prostatic urethra in which the lumen is narrowed and the length of the prostatic urethra is elongated. The bladder neck and trigone may appear distant. Perforations posteriorly in the prostatic capsule usually occur at the bladder neck area. If the perforations are in this position or if the prostatic urethra is severely distorted, a cystogram should be performed. A cystogram is also indicated if abdominal distention is noted and if the patient complains of abdominal discomfort. In the event that an intraperitoneal perforation has occurred, the patient should undergo exploration and the site of the perforation should be closed through a cystotomy incision. A careful search to rule out injury to a hollow viscus should be performed.

Rarely are lateral or anterior perforations associated with intraperitoneal extravasation. Expectant therapy with catheter drainage and diuretics may suffice for small and moderate perforations and even large perforations in the lateral and anterior area. Close observation of the patient is imperative. Careful monitoring of serum electrolytes for the initial 12 hours following surgery is mandatory to decrease the risk of undiagnosed TURS.

Retroperitoneal perforations are routinely managed with catheter drainage. These perforations occur commonly and usually remain undiagnosed. Large retroperitoneal perforations are associated with severe discomfort. If the patient is symptomatic, a small suprapubic incision should be made and a Penrose drain should be placed in the retropubic space. If the patient is infected preoperatively and if parenteral antibiotic coverage has not already been administered, a Penrose drain should be placed immediately. Prophylactic antibacterial coverage is not mandatory in patients with sterile urine preoperatively.

Transurethral Resection Syndrome

TURS may develop when venous sinus or capsular perforation occurs early in the course of resection or when resection time is prolonged. The syndrome is characterized by confusion, hypertension, bradycardia, nausea, vomiting, and visual disturbances.[24,25] Dilutional hyponatremia is the accepted cause, and symptoms usually do not manifest until the serum sodium concentration drops to <125 mEq. Hypertension and mental confusion are the predominant symptoms. Hypotension, bradycardia, or restlessness secondary to hyponatremia may follow. When general anesthesia has been employed, restlessness, disorientation, and nausea may not be present. The only manifestations of delusional hyponatremia in such patients may be increasing hypertension and increasing pulse or venous pressure. For these reasons, spinal anesthesia is the preferred method of anesthesia. In a patient with a large prostate that requires resection under general anesthesia, it is wise either to place an arterial line or to perform repeated intraoperative blood draws to evaluate the patient's plasma sodium concentrations during the procedure.

If perforation occurs of if venous sinuses are open during the resection, a loop diuretic (furosemide, 40 to 120 mg) should be administered. In addition, IV fluids should be changed to normal saline so that no free water is given. In patients with severe hyponatremia, the judicious administration of hypertonic saline (3%) may be necessary. The amount of sodium deficit can be easily calculated using established formulas.[26] For TUR-induced hyponatremia, sodium can be replaced quickly without fear of cerebral edema, because the loss of sodium occurs over such a short period.

In patients who have had perforation with large amounts of extravasation, the intraoperative sodium value may be misleading because significant absorption may occur in the first few postoperative hours. Frequent electrolyte determinations are necessary during this time, with the continued restrictions of free water and the liberal use of loop diuretics. The use of 5% mannitol solution as an irrigating medium in patients helps to obviate TURS because of its osmotic diuretic effect. Because of its hyperosmolar nature, however, mannitol may cause faster intravascular volume expansion that allows the extravasated fluid to be absorbed more easily and thus perhaps increases the amount of hyponatre-

mia. Of the other traditionally used solutions, glycine should not be used in patients with hepatic dysfunction because of concerns about hyperammonemia, and sorbitol can cause hyperglycemia, a worry in patients with diabetes.

During the procedure, if perforations have occurred, it is essential to reduce the height of the irrigating fluid to <60 cm to minimize the amount of fluid extravasated. Rarely, in our experience, has percutaneous drainage of this extravasated fluid been indicated.

Infection

Infected urine in the postoperative period is common and is difficult to remedy completely until the prostatic fossa reepithelializes. Eradication of preoperative urinary tract infections is mandatory before TURP. Patients without evidence of bacteruria also should be given prophylactic antibiotic coverage. Nonetheless, the incidence of postoperative infections is not inconsequential.[5,6] Preoperative infection and prolonged postresection catheterization are the most likely causes. In men with postoperative urinary tract infections, appropriate antibacterial coverage should be given followed by antibacterial suppression for 2 weeks postoperatively. During the healing phase, the presence of pyuria is expected. It does not necessarily indicate infection and should not be treated without a positive culture to justify the administration of antibiotic agents. Even then, antimicrobial therapy may lead to drug resistance or superinfection.

Incontinence

Incontinence is a feared complication of any form of prostatectomy, and the patient must be forewarned of this possibility. The incidence of permanent urinary incontinence after TURP should approximate 0.5% and can be the result of both sphincteric injury and detrusor instability.[6,27] Temporary incontinence is most common and usually resolves in a few days or weeks. Some degree of incontinence can be seen ≤1 year postoperatively and rarely is an incontinence procedure indicated without observing the patient for signs of improvement during a minimum of several months to 1 year. Irritative symptoms such as urgency and urge incontinence are generally the result of irritability from the resected prostatic fossa as well as from detrusor instability. If this occurs, treatment with an anticholinergic agent is usually effective. Patients with continued incontinence of the urgency variety should undergo urodynamic evaluation, especially if they are unresponsive to anticholinergic agents.

Urinary Obstruction and Retention

Approximately 6% of men are unable to void after TURP.[6] Many more have a less than optimal urine stream following prostatectomy. Patients at increased risk of having weak streams or inability to void spontaneously postoperatively, such as patients with poorly controlled diabetes mellitus, patients with chronic urinary retention, and patients with a potential neurogenic cause of urinary retention, should undergo preoperative urodynamic evaluations to delineate the origin of their urinary retention more accurately and to assess the contractility of their detrusor muscle.

Urethral stricture, bladder neck contracture, inadequate tissue resection, and atonic bladder dysfunction all need to be considered in the differential diagnosis of patients who have a weak urinary stream or who are unable to void spontaneously postoperatively. Usually, patients with an atonic bladder or inadequate resection never have a good urine stream postoperatively. Conversely, patients who develop urethral strictures or bladder neck contractures initially have an excellent urine stream, only to experience a diminution in caliber and force during the first few weeks following surgery. In such patients, a cystoscopic evaluation is essential. If no obstruction is noted, urodynamic evaluation of the bladder should be performed. In addition, urine flow rate should be documented and urethral resistance calculated. These can easily determine whether an obstructive lesion truly exists.

Urethral strictures occur in <5% of patients following TURP.[6] The membranous urethra, penoscrotal junction, and fossa navicularis are the most common sites for such strictures. Because trauma from the resectoscope is the most common cause, gentle technique, including proper preliminary urethral dilation and instrument lubrication, is an important prophylactic measure. By using the smallest available instrument and limiting the resection time to <1 hour, the incidence of stricture formation can be decreased further. If a preexisting stricture is found or if the urethra is simply too small to accept the smallest resectoscope sheath comfortably, an internal urethrotomy or perineal urethrostomy should be performed (as described earlier). Assessment of the entire urethra by panendoscopy before attempting to insert the resectoscope blindly lessens the incidence of false passage formation and permits more accurate assessment of the urethral channel. Use of a small-caliber Silastic catheter in the postoperative period also reduces the incidence of stricture formation. However, the caliber of the catheter should be sufficient to allow easy irrigation of clots. Rarely should a catheter <22 Fr be used.

If catheter traction is necessary postoperatively, the catheter should be removed as soon as possible to lessen the likelihood of trauma or ischemia to the penoscrotal junction and thereby decrease the possibility of subsequent stricture formation. The passage of a 22-Fr sound 8 weeks postoperatively will allow a stricture to be detected before it becomes severe enough to cause a management problem. Periodic dilation usually prevents the development of this complication.

Bladder neck contractures following TURP can be troublesome. Contractures can occur in ≤5% of patients following the procedure.[28] These complications seem to occur more commonly in patients with small, fibrotic prostates. Although the cause of bladder neck contractures is unknown, indiscriminate fulguration of the bladder neck and excessive catheter traction of the bladder neck have been implicated.

Initially, patients with a circumferential contracture of the bladder neck should be treated transurethrally with an incision of the bladder neck. If this does not allow the bladder neck to open, a "Mercedes Benz–type" incision or a four-quadrant, cross-like incision of the bladder neck should be performed. If this maneuver proves unsuccessful, circumferential resection of the bladder neck should be performed. Patients who demonstrate the tendency for bladder neck contracture have a high risk of recurrence once the initial contracture has been surgically corrected. Among patients who develop postoperative bladder neck contracture, 40% to 50% will experience some degree of recurrence after resection.[29] Those patients who have had two resections of bladder neck contractures have a ≤75% chance of developing a third contracture. We believe that if a patient has a third bladder neck contracture, it is warranted to consider open surgical repair with a Y-V plasty.

Continued obstructive symptoms secondary to inadequate tissue resection should be relatively rare. If a patient has significant apical tissue distal to the verumontanum, extreme caution should be used when resecting this tissue. This is clearly the focus of most obstruction when inadequate tissue has been resected. This condition is not a serious complication of surgery because it is far better to perform a repeat resection in a patient for minor apical obstruction than to make a patient incontinent with an excessive resection during the first procedure.

The problem area of inadequate resection is the anterior prostatic tissue. Often, during the course of the resection, anterior tissue will fall into the prostatic lumen after the supporting lateral lobe tissue has been removed. Paying attention to this possible cause of inadequate resection and reevaluating the anterior area at the terminal phases of the procedure will lessen the likelihood of this occurrence. Additionally, the surgeon must carefully check for flaps of prostatic tissue that may act as a ball valve in the postoperative period.

Most patients with poor bladder tone who void inadequately following TURP have to be managed with intermittent self-catheterization. Such bladder dysfunction generally occurs in patients with long-standing chronic obstruction and, perhaps, with associated diabetes mellitus. Many times, patients with poor detrusor tone can be placed in reasonable balance by TURP, and even if a relatively atonic bladder and a mild increased voiding resistance are diagnosed preoperatively, it is worth an attempt at TURP.

Sexual Function

Retrograde ejaculation is an expected sequela of TURP. Patients should be made aware that this condition will occur in the postoperative period. When patients have normal antegrade ejaculation following TURP, the occurrence of a bladder neck contracture should be suspected. Preserving the bladder neck during TURP to preserve antegrade ejaculation is rarely indicated. Continued obstruction is the most likely sequela of this maneuver. If the patient desires children following prostatectomy, he should be referred to a fertility specialist. Sperm can be collected by catheterization, pooled, and artificially inseminated, if desired. If so, a solution of sodium bicarbonate should be instilled into the bladder before ejaculation.

TURP should rarely affect potency, although most series estimate an impotence rate of 4%.[30] Four percent of men undergoing nonurologic surgical procedures allege a 4.3% incidence of postoperative impotence.[1] Many men may confuse retrograde ejaculation with impotence. Finally, patients who had good erections before TURP may have potency problems for psychological reasons. Diagnostic studies for evaluation of patients with erectile dysfunction after TURP are occasionally required.

CONCLUSION

TURP remains the gold standard for the treatment of men with BPH. When done correctly and methodically, TURP not only is an effective and durable therapy for BPH but also can be performed safely with minimal complications. Improvements in surgical technique, perioperative monitoring of fluids and electrolytes, anesthetic care, and the availability of video endoscopy have diminished intraoperative and postoperative morbidity and mortality. Nonetheless, the subtleties of TURP can be mastered only with time and practice, and the incidence of complications of transurethral surgery is inversely proportional to the experience of the surgeon.

KEY POINTS

1. Due to the widespread use and success of medical therapies, the average size of prostates in men needing TURP has increased. Consequently, the difficulty of the operation has increased.
2. Despite the introduction of new technologies, TURP remains the gold standard for endoscopic management of enlarged prostates.
3. Before undergoing TURP, men need first to be evaluated for the presence of prostate cancer as TURP can complicate the management of prostate cancer if it is diagnosed at the time of resection.
4. Proper preoperative planning, including familiarity with and assurances of availability of a wide range of endoscopic instruments, is paramount to patient safety during TURP.
5. Communication among the urologist, anesthesiologist, and operating room staff is important in order to recognize and quickly address complications that might arise during TURP.

REFERENCES

Please see www.expertconsult.com

Chapter 25

COMPLICATIONS OF TRANSURETHRAL RESECTION OF BLADDER TUMORS

Eric A. Singer MD, MA
Chief Resident in Urology, University of Rochester School of Medicine, Rochester, New York

Ganesh S. Palapattu MD
Assistant Professor of Urology, Pathology, and Oncology, University of Rochester School of Medicine, Rochester, New York

Transurethral resection (TUR) not only is the initial treatment for superficial bladder tumors but also provides tissue for the pathologic evaluation of tumor stage and grade. These features make the procedure both therapeutic and diagnostic.[1] This chapter discusses strategies to reduce perioperative complications and to maximize patient outcomes. Because TUR of bladder tumors (TURBT) shares many techniques and hazards with TUR of the prostate (TURP), we refer to the excellent discussion in Chapter 24 at several points.

GENERAL CONSIDERATIONS

Most patients who undergo TURBT have already had office-based cystoscopy. This office procedure gives the surgeon an opportunity to note the location, number, and appearance of bladder lesions and also to look for possible barriers to successful resection such as problems with mobility (hip or knee range of motion) and urethral or bladder access (phimosis, stenosis, stricture). These findings should be relayed to the operating room scheduling staff in a timely fashion to ensure that the appropriate personnel, equipment, and operating room time are available.

SURGICAL INSTRUMENTATION

The equipment used for TURBT is nearly identical to that used for TURP. Various endoscopic sheaths (e.g., 20-Fr, 24-Fr, 27-Fr, and deflecting sheaths) with their respective obturators, resecting loops (24-Fr and 27-Fr loop, rolling ball, and right-angle electrodes), Marberger cold-cup biopsy forceps, a generator with grounding pad (with easy access to a backup generator), lenses (30-degree and 70-degree lenses with spares), irrigation tubing and irrigant, water-soluble lubricant, urethral sounds, light source with camera and printer (and replacement components for each readily available), evacuators (Toomey, Ellik, or Creevy) with specimen cups and labels are needed. Additionally, retrograde pyelograms or cystography may be necessary so fluoroscopy with protective shielding, catheters (ureteral and urethral), and contrast material should be immediately available. A dedicated cystoscopy suite is an excellent way to centralize all the necessary equipment and to ensure that the operating table is both maneuverable and compatible with lithotomy stirrups and C-arm fluoroscopy. Numerous urethral catheters should be on hand for postprocedure bladder drainage including conventional Foley and coudé catheters as well as three-way catheters for continuous bladder irrigation (CBI or Murphy drip).

All instrumentation should be maintained regularly so that worn or ill-fitting parts can be serviced. The nursing staff and surgeon should inspect the setup before starting the case to confirm that the necessary equipment has been picked and that any contingency items are immediately available. This step may seem to add time to the procedure, but it is far riskier to proceed only to need an item urgently and find out that it is broken or was mislabeled during processing and is therefore not on hand. It is the surgeon's ultimate responsibility to confirm the good working order of the equipment, and a preprocedure check should become as much a habit as is "right patient/right site" preoperative verification for patient safety.

IRRIGATING SOLUTIONS

Copious amounts of the surgeon's irrigant of choice must be readily available. An experienced team of nurses who understand that any loss of visibility not only prolongs the procedure but also increases the likelihood of an adverse event is invaluable.

Because the bladder does not readily absorb its contents, the use of sterile water is safe, is unlikely to result in hemolysis or hyponatremia (TUR syndrome [TURS]), and yields outstanding endoscopic visualization. In a comparison of glycine and sterile water use for the resection superficial bladder tumors, the two solutions were found equally effective and sterile water was less expensive.[1] However, for long resections of large hypervascular tumors, changing to an iso-osmotic fluid should be considered. Advances in bipolar technology allow the use of normal saline solution as the irrigant, thus lessening the risk of hyponatremia.[2]

Sorbitol, mannitol, and glycine are all suitable options, but their metabolic profiles must be considered (see Chapter 24). Sorbitol is metabolized to glucose and can result in hyperglycemia; this possibility makes sorbitol a less desirable choice for diabetic patients. Mannitol, an osmotic diuretic, can cause intravascular fluid shifts if it is absorbed, thus further exacerbating hyponatremia. Finally, ammonia is a metabolic breakdown product of glycine, which can increase the risk of hyperammonemia and resultant encephalopathy in patients with poor hepatic function. Bladder perforation, which is addressed later in this chapter, is an absolute contraindication to continued resection regardless of irrigant.

PATIENT PREPARATION

The National Surgical Quality Improvement Program (NSQIP) laid an important foundation for the development surgical risk reduction strategies. McLaughlin and colleagues[3] reported on a pilot study that examined the risk factors associated with 30-day morbidity in a non–Veterans Affairs urology setting (including open, laparoscopic, and endoscopic procedures). Not surprisingly, these investigators found that patients with comorbidities such as heart disease (hypertension, angioplasty, myocardial infarction, congestive heart failure), lung disease (dyspnea, asthma, chronic obstructive pulmonary disease), diabetes (with or without end-organ damage), cancer (second nonmetastatic solid tumor initially treated within 5 years, prior chemotherapy), laboratory abnormalities (anemia, elevated blood urea nitrogen), or poor operative risk scores (Charlson comorbidity index score, American Society of Anesthesiologists physical status class 3 to 5) or patients who underwent longer procedures or required intraoperative blood transfusion were much more likely to suffer a complication within the first 30 days of surgery.[3] Hollenbeck and colleagues[4] also used NSQIP data specifically to identify risk factors for adverse outcomes following TURBT. These investigators found that the presence of disseminated bladder cancer, weight loss (≥10%), low serum albumin, elevated serum creatinine, dependent functional status, and emergency status were significant preoperative predictors of adverse outcomes. Perioperative predictors included postoperative hyponatremia and the need for intraoperative blood transfusion. Because of the epidemiology of bladder cancer, patients undergoing TURBT are likely to have one, if not several, of the risk factors identified in the two foregoing studies.

Preoperative Evaluation

Maximizing patient health status preoperatively is always beneficial. Attention to cardiopulmonary status and renal function and identification of issues with coagulation are of specific concern. Following a detailed history and physical examination, correspondence with a patient's primary care provider and consultation with an anesthesiologist can help identify areas for optimization before TURBT. Preoperative electrocardiogram, chest radiograph, and laboratory studies (complete blood count, prothrombin time/partial thromboplastin time/international normalized ratio [PT/PTT/INR], chemistry-14, or comprehensive metabolic panel) allow the patient to be referred for evaluation by a specialist if needed. Blood bank crossmatching may need to be considered in selected cases.

Medication Counseling

Patients need to be counseled about which medications (prescription, over the counter, and supplements) they should discontinue, how long they must abstain preoperatively, and when it is safe to resume their usual regimen. Preoperative planning for patients taking anticoagulants (warfarin) and antiplatelet agents (clopidogrel, aspirin and other nonsteroidal anti-inflammatory drugs) requires careful coordination with the prescribing provider. Some patients, such as those with artificial heart valves, cardiac stents, or hypercoagulable states, may need to be admitted and heparinized to mitigate the risk of clot formation. Postoperatively, determining when patients should resume their usual medication regimen will require weighing the risks of bleeding against those of thrombus formation.

Patients with diabetes and hypertension pose different challenges. Diabetic patients will need to modify their insulin regimen to account for not eating or drinking after midnight before the surgical procedure. The blood glucose concentrations of diabetic patients must be checked on arrival to the hospital/surgical center and monitored closely throughout their stay. A patient with type 2 diabetes who takes an oral hypoglycemic agent can withhold the medication until it is clear that he or she can resume the usual diet postoperatively. If needed, insulin can be given to manage high blood glucose concentrations. Patients who take angiotensin-converting enzyme inhibitors or angiotensin receptor blockers should not take these agents because they can result in significant hypotension on induction of general anesthesia.[5,6]

Infection

A documented negative urine culture is mandatory before transurethral surgery. Any suspicion of infection should result in immediate culture, appropriate antibiotic therapy, and rescheduling of the procedure until the urine has been documented to be sterile on repeat culture. Preoperative antibiotic prophylaxis, usually with a quinolone, is my practice unless allergy or another aspect of the patient's medical history (e.g., documented urinary tract infection with resistance to that agent, artificial heart valve, joint replacement) necessitates a change. The patient is similarly discharged home on a short course (i.e., 1-3 days) of oral antibiotics.

ANESTHESIA AND POSITIONING

Anesthesia

Selecting the appropriate anesthetic regimen is a collaborative process involving the patient, the anesthesiologist, and the surgeon. For TURBT, the choice is between regional (spinal or epidural) and general (laryngeal mask or endotracheal tube) anesthesia. If a regional approach is chosen, the anesthesiologist should be prepared to deepen the patient's sedation, and even intubate if needed, to prevent the patient from coughing or bucking during the procedure. Sudden movement can result in significant complications such as imprecise resection, hemorrhage, and bladder perforation. If the tumor is located laterally in the bladder, general anesthesia is appropriate because a paralytic agent can be given to eliminate leg adduction should current from the resecting loop stimulate the underlying obturator nerve.[7-9] Similarly, injection of 30 mL of local anesthetic (e.g., 1% lidocaine) as an obturator block can significantly decrease nerve sensitivity and adductor strength.[10-19]

Patient Positioning

Proper positioning is a fundamental aspect of any procedure performed in the lithotomy position. The surgeon, the anesthesiologist, and the nursing team should concur that all bony prominences are adequately padded and that the patient's legs are secured within the stirrups with minimal risk of nerve injury (Table 25-1). The patient should be appropriately covered to prevent hypothermia and its sequelae (impaired drug metabolism, prolonged emergence from anesthesia, coagulopathy, postoperative discomfort)[20] because a significant amount of body heat can be lost ambiently and through the irrigating fluid used intraoperatively. Warming the irrigant or using a warming blanket or forced air device can be beneficial in longer cases. Because patients with malignant disease have an increased risk of venous thromboembolism, sequential compression devices are applied to the lower extremities for all cases that may last >1 hour.[21] It is critical to have the sequential compression devices in place and functioning before anesthetic induction, when the risk of deep vein thrombosis increases.

TABLE 25-1	Nerve Injury Due to Lithotomy Positioning	
Nerve Injured	**Physical Deficit**	**Caused by**
Sciatic	Inability to flex knee	Excessive external hip rotation
Femoral	Inability to flex hip or extend knee	Excessive external hip rotation
Common peroneal	Foot drop (loss of dorsiflexion)	Compression of lateral knee at proximal fibula

From Gonzalgo M. (2006). Bladder cancer: superficial. In: Parsons J, Wright E, eds. *The Brady Urology Manual*. London: Informa Healthcare; 2006.

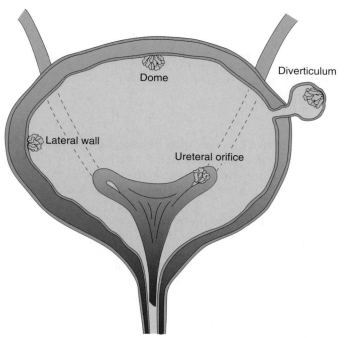

Figure 25-1 Office-based flexible cystoscopy allows the surgeon to map out the location of tumors and plan an appropriate resection. High-risk or challenging resection areas include the dome (perforation), lateral walls (obturator reflex), and ureteral orifice (obstruction).

SURGICAL APPROACH

Resection

As mentioned earlier, the information gathered during office-based flexible cystoscopy can aid in the planning of TURBT. Adjustments in equipment selection and technique may need to be made based on the size, location, and number of tumors seen (**Figs. 25-1 and 25-2**).

Diffuse Carcinoma In Situ

The initial standard therapy for carcinoma in situ is intravesical therapy with attenuated mycobacterial bacille Calmette-Guérin (BCG).[22] If carcinoma in situ is believed to involve extensive segments of the bladder,

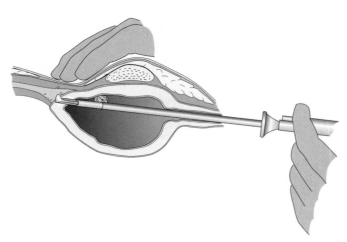

Figure 25-2 Resecting a tumor on the anterior wall of the bladder can be facilitated by using one's nonoperative hand to apply downward suprapubic pressure (anterior to posterior) to bring the area of interest into view. Care must be taken to control the end of the resectoscope at all times; the dome of the bladder can be perforated resulting in potential bowel injury.

representative biopsies with hemostatic fulguration are preferable to cauterizing large swaths of the bladder mucosa. Extensive use of electrocautery over a large surface area can result in bladder contracture.[23]

Tumor Involving the Ureteral Orifice

Tumor near or involving the ureteral orifice poses the challenge of obtaining complete resection and adequate hemostasis while preserving the caliber of the intramural ureter. Resecting with a pure cutting current and the judicious use of pinpoint cautery (with a right-angle cautery electrode) at the lowest effective setting for hemostasis make ureteral stricture unlikely.[24-28] If postoperative flank pain develops, a renal ultrasound scan can be performed to evaluate for hydroureteronephrosis. If this condition is present, a percutaneous nephrostomy tube can be placed. Tumor location at the ureteral orifice should not deter appropriate endoscopic management.

Reflux of urine into the upper tracts, which may occur with ureteral stenting (either anterograde or retrograde) or through vesicoureteral reflux following resection of the ureteral orifice, was shown to increase the risk of seeding and tumor occurrence in the ureter and renal pelvis in some retrospective studies.[29-32] Conversely, Solsona and colleagues[33] found no significant difference in upper urinary tract recurrence patterns when refluxing and nonrefluxing patients were studied after TURBT. Regardless, close follow-up and monitoring for bladder as well as upper tract tumor recurrence are advisable. Patients who symptomatically reflux after TURBT have been successfully managed with the endoscopic injection of bulking agents.[34] Surgical reimplantation of the refluxing ureter is also possible.

Tumor on the Anterior Surface

Resecting a lesion on the anterior surface of the bladder can be facilitated by using one's nonoperative hand to apply downward suprapubic pressure (compressing the anterior wall toward the posterior wall) on a bladder only partially filled with irrigant to allow better visualization of the tumor.[7,24]

Tumor at the Dome

Resection at the bladder dome is challenging because of its anatomic relationships. That the bladder dome is the furthest point from the trigone makes visualization difficult; the more irrigant is used to clear away blood, the further the point of interest travels from the resectoscope. A continuous flow resectoscope sheath can be especially useful in this situation. Additionally, bowel can overly the dome and be injured by transmural current from aggressive electrocautery. Finally, elderly patients in general and postmenopausal women in particular have significantly thinner bladder walls; therefore, perforation is an even greater concern in these patients. Taking care not to overdistend the bladder and paying meticulous attention to resection technique and depth are important when working at the bladder dome.

Tumor at the Lateral Wall

In addition to the anesthetic options discussed earlier, the surgeon can use several techniques to lessen the likelihood of a complication stemming from the inadvertent stimulation of the obturator nerve during resection of a laterally located tumor. Preventing overdistention, decreasing the cutting or coagulation current settings, and using intermittent cautery can lessen the incidence of adductor contraction.[7,11,35] The endoscopic injection of local anesthetic into the tumor base can also deliver an obturator nerve block if a percutaneous attempt was not made preoperatively.[35] Finally, use of a bipolar resecting system restricts the flow of current to between the two electrodes of the resecting loop and thus decreases stimulation of the obturator nerve.[36,37]

Tumor in Bladder Diverticula

The anatomic differences of bladder diverticula are critical to remember. By definition, they lack the muscularis propria layer, a feature that renders them thinner and much easier to perforate. This characteristic can also complicate the pathologic staging of lesions within diverticula. Golijanin and colleagues from Memorial Sloan-Kettering Cancer Center in New York[38] put forth post-TURBT staging and treatment recommendations based on their experience. These investigators suggested that conservative treatment is appropriate when the tumor is confined to the diverticula, it can be resected in its endoscopic entirety, and the patient is agreeable to close follow-up. For large or high-grade tumors, transurethral biopsy followed by partial cystectomy may be more prudent than attempting complete TUR.[39]

Reducing Cautery Artifact

Although typically not considered a complication, excessive cautery artifact is both counterproductive and preventable. Cold-cup biopsies can be obtained before resection or fulguration. Adjustment of the resectoscope's power to the lowest effective setting and the preferential use of pure cutting current also aid the pathologist in the grading and staging evaluation.[23] Alternatively, obtaining hemostasis by fulguration after adequate specimens have been obtained helps to preserve the microscopic appearance of the samples. Use of bipolar energy has not been shown to decrease the degree of cautery artifact when compared with monopolar resection.[40] Based on the principles of electrosurgery, contact surface and time between the loop and tumor tissue predict the degree of cautery injury to the tissue. Excessively slow movement of the cautery loop can char the tissue and prevent clean cutting. As such, initiation of the cautery pedal before tissue contact, and swift, controlled movement of the loop through the tissue will maximize specimen presentation.

Use of Lasers

Several different types of lasers have been used to treat bladder cancer, including neodymium:yttrium-aluminum-garnet (Nd:YAG), argon, potassium titanyl phosphate (KTP), and holmium:YAG.[41-44] The Nd:YAG laser was found to be equally effective as conventional TURBT in a prospective randomized trial, and it is therefore the laser of choice for some surgeons. Because laser energy vaporizes or coagulates the tissue it contacts, cold-cup biopsies should be performed before the laser is used to resect a suspicious lesion. Similarly, determining tumor depth or muscular invasion is not readily possible with this type of resection; for this reason, patients with papillary low-grade tumors are the most appropriate population for this technology.[45] The most significant complication of laser use is the transmural passage of energy resulting in the perforation of an adjacent structure such as an overlying loop of bowel, but this risk is low.[1,46,47]

Complications of Transurethral Resection of Bladder Tumors

Because nearly all patients with bladder cancer undergo TURBT at least once, TURBT is the most common surgical therapy for this disease.[48] In studies of postoperative resource use, patients who have had TURBT often need additional medical services and readmission at higher rates than do similar patients receiving other ambulatory procedures.[49,50] It is incumbent on all urologists to review their practice patterns to lessen the complications associated with this procedure.

Overall Morbidity and Mortality

Although TURBT is typically a safe and well-tolerated procedure, urologists must be mindful of the morbidity (5.1%[35]-43.3%[51]) and mortality rates (0.8%[52]-1.3%[51]) reported in the literature.

Mechanical Difficulties

The list of possible mechanical failures or difficulties than can occur during TURBT is myriad. The surest way to minimize this frustrating event is by carefully examining the selected equipment before initiating the procedure. Clear, timely communication between the surgeon and the operative team (anesthesia and nursing) regarding unexpected findings and the need for replacement, additional, or specialized equipment or any adjustments in the estimated operative time can help increase efficiency and patient safety.

Problems of Instrument Introduction

Barriers to effective transurethral surgery such as phimosis, meatal stenosis, or urethral stricture should be noted during flexible office cystoscopy. If an operative intervention is needed to correct one of these conditions before TURBT, the surgical consent form should be amended and the necessary additional equipment should be selected. The techniques for circumcision, meatal dilation or meatoplasty, and optical internal urethrotomy are described in greater detail in Chapter 24 and in other surgical texts.[53] If for some reason office cystoscopy has not been performed before TURBT, the surgical consent form should reflect the possible need for additional interventions.

Postoperative Bleeding

Postoperative bleeding is the most frequently reported complication of TURBT; rates range from 2% to 13%.[35,51,54] Intraoperative or postoperative bleeding is typically associated with large tumors and extensive or complex resections.[35,55] Careful examination of all resected areas under little to moderate distention is important to avoid missing small vessels temporarily tamponaded by a distended bladder. Unfortunately, coughing or bucking by the patient on emergence from general anesthesia can cause a significant increase in blood pressure that results in a loss of hemostasis. Prompt management (removal of stimulus, sedation, or antihypertensives) can decrease systemic blood pressure and allow clot formation. If symptomatic hypotension or tachycardia ensues that does not respond to a fluid bolus, transfusion of packed red blood cells, laboratory tests (complete blood count, PT/PTT/INR, basic metabolic panel), and resuscitative measures are indicated.

Insertion of a transurethral catheter is common after TURBT. Choosing a three-way (20-24 Fr) catheter enables the use of CBI (or Murphy drip) in the recovery room, if needed. One should be extremely cautious in using CBI following bladder wall resection because of the risk of bladder perforation, and CBI should be used only when oozing from the tumor bed is noted despite hemostatic measures. It is critical to include orders for scheduled and as needed (PRN) manual irrigation with 60 to 120 mL of normal saline through a 60-mL catheter-tipped syringe to remove any sediment or small blood clots that may have formed. The relatively small lumina of the inflow and outflow tracts in a three-way catheter, even in a large 24-Fr catheter, can become clotted shut easily and can lead to iatrogenic bladder perforation if the bladder continues to fill but is unable to drain. CBI should be gravity fed only; it must never be attached to an intravenous pump. Additionally, CBI is contraindicated in patients with bladder perforation. Titrating the flow for pink urine is usually adequate to limit clot formation. All nursing staff caring for a patient on CBI must be oriented to the apparatus, must strictly monitor and record the amount of irrigant instilled and returned, and must understand how to calculate urine output (total output − irrigant instilled = urine output).

Sudden observation of significant hematuria in the early postoperative period likely suggests arterial bleeding in the resection bed. In these cases, early return to the operating room for endoscopic inspection or fulguration is advisable because it will result in prompt resolution of bleeding in the stable patient. If, on rare occasions, the degree of postoperative hemorrhage is significant and results in physiologic changes (hypotension, tachycardia) despite fluid resuscitation or repeated transfusions, returning the patient to the operating room for clot evacuation and fulguration after resuscitation is also advisable. If hemorrhage is still uncontrollable, conversion to open cystectomy or embolization of the internal iliac artery by interventional radiology or vascular surgery may be necessary.[56-59] Selective and superselective embolization techniques have been developed in the attempt to minimize potential morbidity.[60-62] In summary, the surgeon should first consider taking the patient back to the operating room for hemostasis. After determining that this is not advisable, other measures may be used.

Bleeding From Unresectable Disease, Radiation, or Chemotherapy

Significant hematuria in an oncology patient, regardless of cause, often results in urologic consultation. The urologist should also be familiar with intravesical agents that are commonly used to manage hemorrhagic cystitis resulting from unresectable tumor, prior external beam radiation, or chemotherapy. Some of these patients may be poor operative candidates, thus making intravesical treatments valuable temporizing measures.

Use of a 1% alum solution (50 g of aluminum ammonium sulfate or aluminum potassium sulfate dissolved in 5 L sterile water)[63] functions as an astringent by causing protein precipitation and vasoconstriction.[64] This can be delivered in the same manner as saline CBI. The alum will cause a precipitate to form, so manual irrigation through a piston syringe (60-mL catheter-tipped syringe) is required to ensure adequate outflow. Aluminum absorption is possible, especially if large portions of the bladder have been resected. Signs of aluminum toxicity, which is more likely in patients with renal dysfunction and can be fatal, include lethargy, confusion, seizures, and metabolic acidosis.[63,65] Alum irrigation should be stopped immediately and blood should be sent for serum aluminum level testing.

Chapter 24 discusses the use of intravenous and oral ε-aminocaproic acid (Amicar; an inhibitor of plasminogen activators that interferes with fibrinolysis) in the management of post-TURP bleeding. The same regimen can be employed after TURBT, or the agent can be mixed as a solution for use with CBI. It is important to rule out disseminated intravascular coagulation as the source of bleeding by evaluating the patient's platelet count and fibrinogen level before initiating ε-aminocaproic acid therapy.[66] Instillation of intravesical formalin has been used to manage refractory hematuria resulting from advanced bladder cancer and hemorrhagic cystitis secondary to external beam radiation or cyclophosphamide chemotherapy.[67] Formalin causes protein denaturation and precipitation in the bladder mucosa that result in blood vessel occlusion.[68] This treatment should not be considered first-line therapy, and it is not advisable to use it in the immediate postoperative period because absorption is possible. Pretreatment cystography is recommended to evaluate for reflux and bladder integrity.[63] Complications, both local and systemic, include bladder contracture, urinary incontinence, vesicoureteral reflux, ureteral stricture and obstruction, acute tubular necrosis, vesicovaginal or enterovesical fistula formation, myocardial injury, and bladder rupture.[69-77] Bladder fibrosis with reduced capacity and resultant urinary frequency is a common side effect.[63]

Bladder Perforation

Bladder perforation is one of the most significant complications associated with TURBT. It can result in numerous sequelae including hemorrhage, TURS, infection, the need for urgent open surgery, tumor spillage, peritonitis, and death.[51,78] Bladder perforation typically occurs extraperitoneally. This complication can usually be managed with drainage through a urethral catheter, although intraperitoneal rupture is possible and often requires surgical repair (open or laparoscopic). At the time of suspected rupture, the location of bladder wall perforation can aid in determining the necessity for on-table cystography. Injuries in the anterior bladder wall, dome, or high posterior wall necessitate a cystogram to rule out intraperitoneal extravasation. Distention of the abdomen during resection may warrant a cystogram or immediate laparotomy, based on the index of suspicion. If small exposed areas of perivesical fat are observed during resection, without an obvious extravesical pocket or plane, prompt completion of the procedure and placement of a large bore catheter may be sufficient without a cystogram.

The incidence of post-TURBT perforation may be underestimated. In a prospective study, Balbay and colleagues[79] performed cystography after TURBT in a series of 36 patients with suspected bladder cancer. These investigators found contrast extravasation in 58.3% of their patients, compared with other series reporting perforation in only 1% to 5% of cases.[35,80,81] The significance of subclinical perforations detected by cystography is unclear. In an editorial accompanying the Balbay report,[79] Soloway raised concerns about the oncologic efficacy of radical TUR, meaning that resecting to the point of perforation, even if done deliberately, poses a risk to the patient from tumor spillage. Regardless, one must be cognizant of possible bladder perforation during aggressive resections.

Skolarikos and colleagues[80] attempted to determine the impact of bladder perforation during TURBT on extravesical tumor recurrence by examining the records of >3400 patients. These investigators found the incidence of perforation to be only 1% and identified several risk factors associated with extravesical tumor recurrence. The most significant risk factor was the need for an open surgical repair of the perforation, followed by intraperitoneal location of the bladder defect and tumor size >3 cm.[80] These investigators also noted that patients with extravesical disease after perforation repair fared far worse than did the rest of the cohort. In contrast, other studies examining outcomes after TURBT-associated perforation did not detect an increase in extravesical disease frequency or poorer outcomes.[35,82] Mindful assessment of inflow and outflow irrigant volumes during extensive resection may prompt recognition of serious occult bladder perforations.

Although rare, it seems plausible that perforation during TURBT can lead to extravesical disease, which carries a dismal prognosis. It is unclear whether perforation should prompt consideration of systemic treatment in an attempt to mitigate any increased risk of soft tissue seeding.[80] Additionally, the use of perioperative intravesical chemotherapy is contraindicated in the presence of bladder perforation. The loss of the demonstrated risk-reduction benefit of postoperative intravesical chemotherapy combined with a theoretical increase in disease progression resulting from perforation reinforces the severity of this complication.

Transurethral Resection Syndrome

Although TURS is covered in depth in Chapter 24, several differences in its origin and presentation should be considered when this complication arises after TURBT. Post-TURBT hyponatremia is usually the result of bladder perforation and the extravasation or extravesical absorption of irrigant fluid, in contrast to absorption across open prostatic venous sinuses during TURP. Because the irrigant is not directly introduced into the patient's circulatory system and must be absorbed across the peritoneum, the initial presentation may be delayed. Dorotta and colleagues[78] reported a case series of four such events and noted that the time to serum sodium nadir was 2 to 9 hours,[78] compared with of 1 to 6 hours[83-86] following prostatic resection. Hyponatremia, intravascular hypovolemia with an increase in total body water, hypotension, oliguria, acute renal failure, metabolic acidosis, and mental status changes are all described in TURBT syndrome.[78]

Early detection, rapid assessment, and immediate treatment are critical when a surgeon is faced with this complication. Management is nearly identical to that for TURS described in Chapter 24. The procedure should be halted, a bladder catheter should be left in place, blood should be sent immediately for serum chemistry testing, and resuscitation with normal saline should be started. The patient's sodium deficit should be calculated and serial measurements made to ensure the proper rate of correction. Use of hypertonic saline poses the risk of central pontine myelinolysis caused by rapid electrolyte and fluid shifts in the brain, and one should consult with specialists in, for example, nephrology or critical care medicine. Diuretics (e.g., furosemide) can facilitate hemoconcentration but should be used only in a euvolemic patient. Drainage of the peritoneum or retroperitoneum can be accomplished through an open surgical procedure with simultaneous repair of the bladder perforation or by placement of a percutaneous drain under ultrasonic guidance by interventional radiology; surgical repair of the bladder can be performed later, once the patient's condition has been stabilized. Transferring the patient to a monitored setting such as an intensive care unit is advisable.

Infection

Dysuria is common after transurethral bladder surgery, thus patients may have difficulty differentiating the expected symptoms from infection. Similarly, a dipstick urine analysis is difficult to interpret. A short course of postoperative prophylaxis with oral antibiotics is reasonable until the bladder mucosa has had an opportunity to heal. A suspected infection should be cultured immediately. Empiric antibiotics can be started and tailored to microbial sensitivities once results become available.

Urinary Retention

Instrumentation, anesthesia (general, spinal, or epidural), and postoperative narcotics can all lead to acute urinary retention, especially in men. Although many patients are discharged from the hospital or surgical center with a catheter in place, most patients who undergo resection of superficial or small to medium lesions may not require an indwelling Foley catheter. Recovery room orders should clearly indicate that patients must void adequately before discharge (specify both a volume and the time in which it must be passed); otherwise, a urethral catheter should be inserted and an office voiding trial performed. Men who take α_1-antagonists or 5α-reductase inhibitors should continue receiving their medications at the usual prescribed dose. Urinary retention that occurs weeks to months after TURBT should be investigated with cystoscopy to evaluate for urethral stricture, bladder neck contracture, or tumor recurrence and should be managed appropriately.

COMPLICATIONS OF PERIOPERATIVE INTRAVESICAL CHEMOTHERAPY

Several series showed that intravesical chemotherapy (e.g., mitomycin C) administered in the immediate postoperative period provides a significant reduction in cancer recurrence (50% at 2 years) for patients with superficial disease.[87-90] It is recommended that patients receive such treatment within 6 hours of resection unless bladder perforation is suspected or the patient has an allergy to the chemotherapeutic agent of choice.[91]

The common side effects of intravesical chemotherapy include irritative voiding symptoms consistent with cystitis (dysuria, frequency, and hematuria).[92] All the agents currently used can result in fibrosis and contracture of the bladder, usually as a result of long-term exposure, and thiotepa has been shown to cause bone marrow suppression if it is absorbed.[93] Operating room and postanesthesia care unit staff must also be educated regarding the safe administration, monitoring, and disposal of intravesical chemotherapy agents and supplies. Intravesical BCG is absolutely contraindicated in the postoperative setting; use of this agent can result in systemic sepsis (BCG-osis) and death. BCG should not be given until the bladder epithelium has been allowed to heal for at least 14 days and gross hematuria has resolved.[94]

CONCLUSION

TURBT continues to play an integral role in the management of bladder cancer. Careful preoperative preparation, attention to operative technique, and diligent postoperative monitoring and follow-up will help decrease the risk of morbidity and mortality while maximizing the benefit to the patient.

KEY POINTS

1. Equipment should be inspected by the surgeon and nursing team before its use to ensure proper selection and good working order.
2. Depending on the type of diathermy selected, all irrigant solutions are suitable for use with TURBT, each with its unique advantages and limitations.
3. A thorough preoperative evaluation, including anesthesia and subspecialty referral when indicated, optimizes the health of the patient and lessens the likelihood of complication.
4. Documentation of a negative urine culture is a requirement before TURBT.
5. Careful patient positioning and padding can prevent severe lower extremity nerve injury and lasting disability.
6. Office-based, flexible cystoscopy can assist in planning a successful procedure by providing a resection map. Tumor located on the anterior wall, on the lateral walls, at the dome, in a diverticulum, or involving the ureteral orifice may require special equipment or additional anesthetic considerations.
7. Bleeding is the most common complication associated with TURBT. Depending on its severity, it can be managed with CBI through a three-way catheter (using saline, alum, or ε-aminocaproic acid), repeat endoscopic fulguration, open surgery, or arterial embolization.
8. Perforation increases the risk of numerous other complications including bleeding, infection, TURS, and possible disease spread. Careful planning, appropriate equipment selection, diligent attention to operative technique, and effective communication among the surgical, anesthesia, and nursing teams lessen the likelihood of perforation occurring.
9. TURS can be a lethal complication. Prompt identification and management are critical. Transferring the patient to a monitored setting (intensive care unit) is often appropriate.
10. Post-TURBT intravesical chemotherapy is contraindicated in patients with known bladder perforation. Intravesical BCG is absolutely contraindicated in the immediate postoperative setting.
11. Staff members who are responsible for administering, monitoring, and disposing of intravesical chemotherapeutics must understand how to maintain a safe working environment for themselves and for their patients.

REFERENCES

Please see www.expertconsult.com

Chapter 26

COMPLICATIONS OF URETEROSCOPIC SURGERY

Eric L. Kau MD
Fellow in Endourology, Minimally Invasive Urology Institute, Cedars-Sinai Medical Center, Los Angeles, California

Christopher S. Ng MD
Attending, Minimally Invasive Urology Institute, Cedars-Sinai Medical Center, Los Angeles, California

Gerhard J. Fuchs MD
Medallion Chair in Minimally Invasive Urology; Director, Minimally Invasive Urology Institute; Vice Chairman, Department of Surgery, Cedars-Sinai Medical Center, Los Angeles, California

Endoscopic surgery for diagnosis and treatment of disorders of the upper urinary tract is an important minimally invasive tool in the urologists' armamentarium. Since 1929, when Young and McKay[1] documented first the use of a cystoscope to perform a ureteropyeloscopy in a child, and with Marshall's first use of a flexible passively deflecting fiberoptic ureteropyeloscope in 1964,[2] ureteropyeloscopy has progressed significantly.

Even with the greatly increased range of indications for ureteroscopic surgery (URS) and retrograde intrarenal surgery (RIRS), the rate of complications has steadily decreased. This change is partly the result of technologic advances such as the development of smaller ureteroscopes and ureteropyeloscopes as well as advances in energy sources (holmium and neodymium:yttrium-aluminum-garnet lasers, thulium laser) and the use of smaller endoscopic equipment such as guidewires, access sheaths, graspers, and baskets.[3-5] In addition, the skill level of urologists has improved significantly because URS and RIRS are index cases for resident education in the United States. Furthermore, the American Urological Association (AUA) and academic endourologists have conducted frequent didactic and hands-on courses to instruct the urologic workforce in the safe and efficient use of this technique and to promote technologic advances. Routine indications for URS and RIRS now include the evaluation and treatment of many conditions of the upper urinary tract including ureteral and renal stone disease, strictures of the ureter, ureteropelvic junction (UPJ) obstruction, or intrarenal strictures, as well as upper urinary tract (low-grade) transitional cell carcinoma (TCC) management and treatment of intrarenal bleeding (e.g., arteriovenous malformation).[3-6]

In 1988, Flam and colleagues[7] presented 180 patients treated with URS for ureteral stones and noted treatment success rates for proximal, distal, and overall stones of 68%, 82%, and 78%, respectively.[7] The accompanying complication rates were 17% for access and manipulation failures, 4% for perioperative ureteral injuries, and 9% for postoperative complications.[7] In contrast, a multisurgeon study from 2006 reported treatment success rates of 87.3% for proximal stones, 94.2% for distal stones, and 91.7% overall, with an overall complication rate as low as 1.9%.[8]

Prevention is still the best management of complications. Adherence to proper protocol (e.g., patient selection criteria, preparation, technique, knowledge of technology, and postoperative care) should make complications of URS and RIRS rare occurrences for both the subspecialist and the general urologist. In this chapter, we discuss the indications for URS and RIRS, describe the techniques used to perform URS and RIRS to ensure a minimum of complications, describe both the intraoperative and postoperative complications of upper urinary tract endoscopic surgery, and detail the treatment options for successful management of these complications.

PATIENT SELECTION

URS is routinely employed for management of a wide variety of upper urinary tract disorders, such as stones, strictures, and selected TCCs. Most stones in the ureter are amenable to URS with rigid and flexible instrumentation. With very few exceptions, regardless of size and composition, laser lithotripsy successfully fragments and vaporizes ureteral stones at any level, and the resultant stone fragments are readily removed with stone baskets to render the ureter completely free of stones. In the kidney, stones up to an aggregate size of 1.5 cm have become routine indications for RIRS in many institutions; however, larger stones in the renal collecting system, depending on the patient's preference or the surgeon's comfort and experience, may be better suited for percutaneous nephrostolithotomy.[3-5] Another alternative for larger stone burden is the combination of simultaneous RIRS and extracorporeal shockwave lithotripsy. This approach can be used for a stone burden larger than for RIRS monotherapy but deemed not quite large enough for the more invasive percutaneous approach.[9]

Strictures in the ureter, at the UPJ, and intrarenal strictures are also amenable to URS in selected cases. In the ureter, URS of short strictures (<0.5-1.0 cm) generally yields good results, and the UPJ stricture without crossing vessel and without massive hydronephrosis is also well suited for the ureteroscopic approach. Intrarenal strictures including the management of caliceal diverticula can also be managed using the RIRS technique in many cases.

Papillary transitional cell tumors of low grade can be treated with URS in the ureter and kidney in an organ-preserving fashion. Higher-grade lesions can be addressed in this way as a palliative measure in the patient with poor global renal function.[10]

CONTRAINDICATIONS

The only absolute contraindication is active, untreated infection. In such circumstance, the infection would need to be treated appropriately with antibiotics. In the patient with infection and obstruction, the upper urinary tract needs to be drained with an indwelling stent or percutaneous nephrostomy first and antibiotic treatment started. After eradication of the infection, the procedure can then be performed under antibiotic cover.

Uncorrected bleeding diatheses or ongoing anticoagulation therapy are relative contraindications. Careful instrumentation and use of direct contact energy sources (laser) can avoid bleeding problems. If treatment needs to be performed under such conditions referral to a subspecialty endourology center is advisable.

PREPARATION

Routine examinations before upper urinary tract endoscopy include imaging studies (computed tomography [CT] or intravenous [IV] pyelography) to assess the upper tract anatomy and pathology so that appropriate treatment can be selected. A complete patient history and physical examination as well as clearance for anesthesia are also routine.

An important step for prevention of septic complications is to confirm a negative urine culture by obtaining a preoperative urine sample. Further, the use of broad-spectrum antibiotics in the operating room, forced diuresis (10-20 mg of IV furosemide), and performance of upper urinary tract endoscopic surgery under low-pressure conditions (no pressure bags or other means of "power" irrigation) are equally important.[5]

Usually, URS is performed with the patient under anesthesia, although in some cases of distal ureteral disorders or endoscopic surveillance for upper tract TCC, local anesthesia is sufficient. Most cases of higher complexity are treated using general anesthesia; spinal or epidural anesthesia is rarely used. Especially in patients with kidney disorders, general anesthesia with control of respiratory excursions decreases renal movement and thereby improves the precision of laser application, increases treatment efficiency, and reduces the risk of injury.

TECHNIQUE OF UPPER URINARY TRACT ENDOSCOPY

Before upper urinary tract endoscopy, cystoscopy with complete examination of the bladder should be performed. The patient is placed in low lithotomy position and is prepared in a sterile fashion. A rigid cystoscope, usually 21 Fr, is the endoscope of choice because it easily allows the passage of guidewires and an open-ended ureteral catheter. After inspection of the bladder floor, posterior wall, lateral walls, and dome, the ureteral orifices along the trigone are identified.

Using a 0.035 guidewire through a 5-Fr open-ended ureteral catheter and with the aid of fluoroscopy, the guidewire is advanced into the distal ureter. The ureteral catheter can then be advanced over the wire. By placing the open-ended catheter over the wire, improper placement and potential damage of the intramural ureter are prevented (especially in the male patient with an enlarged prostate or the female patient with a large cystocele). A retrograde pyelogram using contrast is then obtained to visualize the collecting system and to assess the potential technical difficulties of guidewire and instrument advancement. The 0.035 guidewire is once again placed through the open-ended catheter and is advanced up the ureter and into the renal pelvis under intermittent fluoroscopic control. This wire becomes the safety wire once the angiocatheter is removed and is not usually used until the treatment is finished; then the ureteral stent is safely placed over this wire.

If ureteral or UPJ obstruction is encountered, the open-ended catheter is advanced over the safety wire above the level of obstruction to obtain a urine sample for culture from the renal pelvis. This maneuver allows observation of a hydronephrotic drip and inspection of the gross appearance. If urine appears putrid, the treatment should be abandoned, a stent should be placed, and treatment should be performed after appropriate antibiotic therapy has eradicated the infection.

Once access to the renal pelvis is obtained, a 10- to 20-mg dose of furosemide is given. This induces diuresis and helps to prevent pyelovenous reflux, thereby reducing subsequent risk for infection (**Fig. 26-1**). If passage of the guidewire is difficult secondary to altered anatomic features (e.g., a tight ureteral orifice, a tortuous ureter, a strictured ureteral segment, or an obstructed stone), this increases the risk of damage to the ureter. Frequently, a hydrophilic Glidewire can be successfully used to negotiate the obstacle. Because the Glidewire may once successfully negotiated past the obstacle may slip out of the ureter easily (easy in–easy out), it is advisable to exchange this wire immediately for a regular 0.035 wire once the obstacle has been bypassed. To accomplish the exchange, the angiographic catheter is advanced over the Glidewire above the obstacle and then the wire is exchanged, to establish a safety wire securely in the kidney. In complicated cases, ureteroscopic placement of a guidewire may be necessary to negotiate a difficult ureteral passage (obstruction or tortuosity) safely (**Fig. 26-2**).

If Glidewire placement is unsuccessful or if safety wire access is lost and is unable to be replaced, drainage of the kidney with a percutaneous nephrostomy should be performed. Depending on the situation (obstruction

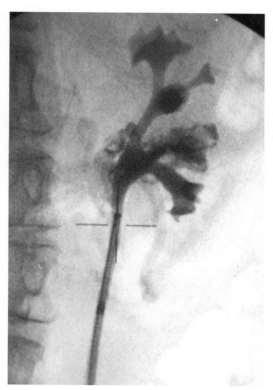

Figure 26-1 Injection of contrast shows pyelovenous reflux as well as possible forniceal rupture secondary to increased intrarenal pressure with possible complications of infection and extravasation.

with infection or ureteral injury versus absence of obstruction and complications), percutaneous drainage should be performed immediately or postponed until dictated by clinical necessity. In experienced hands, careful access with an ureteroscope to the level of obstruction may allow safe placement of a safety wire in most instances, but generally, the risk of injury is too high to recommend this maneuver as a regular step (**Fig. 26-3**; see also Fig. 26-2).

After placement of the safety wire, the next step is advancement of an ureteroscope. Usually, a 9.5-Fr rigid ureteroscope is used first for optical dilation of the intramural and distal ureter. A second guidewire (working wire) is placed through the work channel into the ureteral orifice and up into the renal pelvis. The semirigid ureteroscope is then advanced over the working guidewire, and the tip of the scope is negotiated between the two wires into the distal ureter. This maneuver allows for safe advancement of the ureteroscope in 95% of patients.

Optical dilation allows the intramural ureter and distal ureter to be visualized. Dilation is performed under direct vision, to minimize the risk of ureteral injury. To facilitate this move, the bladder should be emptied first (forced diuresis will fill the bladder quickly), and the scope is turned clockwise and counterclockwise until the two wires are arranged in an inverted-V fashion with the working wire on the bottom of the intramural ureter and the safety wire on top. Usually, the scope is advanced to the level of the pathologic process or as far as it reaches in case of renal disease (typically, up to the midproximal ureter in male patients and to the proximal ureter or renal pelvis in female patients). In the rare case in which the ureter cannot be sufficiently dilated to allow passage of the ureteroscope, it is prudent to place an indwelling double-J ureteral stent and avoid causing any potential ureteral trauma through overly aggressive dilation. The indwelling stent passively dilates (paralyzes) the ureter and the patient can return for a second look in 1 to 2 weeks with an easily accessible ureter.

Alternative options for dilation of the ureteral orifice include coaxial dilators, serial dilators, and balloon dilation. However, because these techniques are performed under fluoroscopic and tactile control only and do not allow for direct visualization of the ureter, the risk of ureteral damage is increased. In addition, these auxiliary one-time-use devices add to the cost of the procedure. If blind dilation was performed, one should then inspect the ureter before blind passage of guidewires to make sure that no mucosal tears have occurred, with their subsequent risk of false passage or ureteral perforation.

If the pathologic process is within the reach of the rigid ureteroscope, the ensuing surgical procedure is performed mostly with a rigid instrument; otherwise, a flexible instrument is used (upper third of ureter and kidney). After successful optical dilation, a 7.5-Fr flexi-

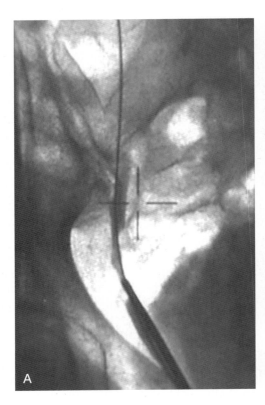

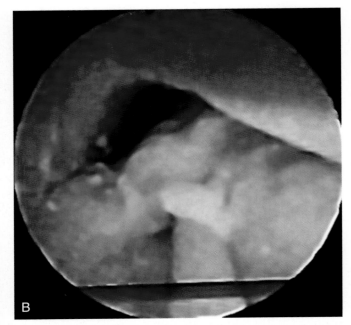

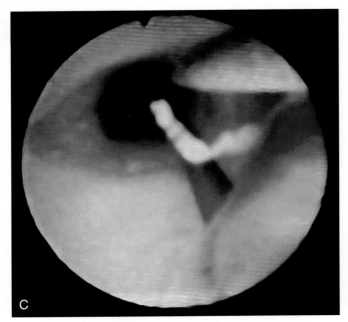

Figure 26-2 **A,** Tight ureter with stone after previous pelvic surgery with false guidewire passage. On the retrograde pyelogram, the guidewire appears to be in the "correct" position. The false passage was suspected because the 5-Fr angiographic catheter was difficult to advance. The next step then is endoscopic inspection of the ureter. **B,** Endoscopic appearance of the false passage. The blue wire passes submucosally (false passage), whereas under direct visual control the green wire negotiated the true lumen. **C,** After successful removal of the stone, the ureter above the false passage confirms the correct position of the green guidewire. The blue wire can now be removed and an indwelling stent placed over the green (safety) wire. After an indwelling time of 2 weeks, the false passage will have healed.

ble ureteropyeloscope is placed over the second guidewire and can be advanced to the level of interest. If the area of interest (i.e., stone, tumor, or stricture) is within the ureter, the ureteropyeloscope (rigid or flexible) is advanced to that level. At this point, an energy source such as a holmium laser fiber can be introduced through the work cannel of the flexible endoscope and treatment can begin. During URS and RIRS, saline irrigation is used to ensure adequate visualization of the field. Our preference is placing large 3-L saline irrigant bags to gravity drainage (60 cm above patient level). This technique does not unduly increase the pressure within the renal collecting system and thereby greatly reduces pyelovenous and pyelolymphatic reflux with the risk of infectious complications.

Power irrigation through handheld spring-loading syringes, pressure bags, or pump systems should be not used because of the increased risk of forniceal rupture, extravasation, and infectious complications. Cautious hand irrigation can occasionally be helpful to dislodge a stone (e.g., from lower calyx) into a location better suited for treatment. The use of a ureteral access sheath, usually reserved for larger renal stone burdens, can also help to keep intrarenal pressured low (especially when infection-induced struvite stones are treated) while at the same time improve irrigant flow and visibility.

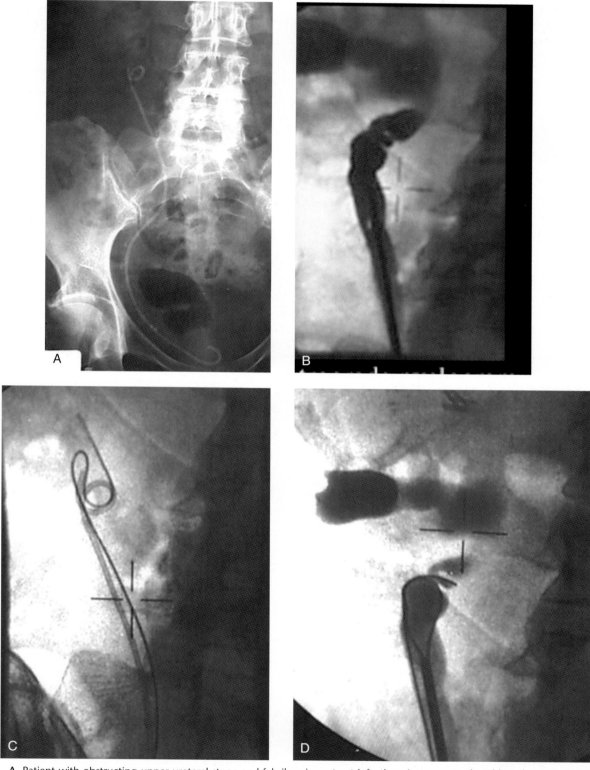

Figure 26-3   A, Patient with obstructing upper ureteral stone and febrile urinary tract infection. A stent was placed but the patient did not defervesce and ultrasound still showed high-grade hydronephrosis. The patient is receiving warfarin (Coumadin) therapy. **B,** Retrograde pyelogram shows that the stent was not placed correctly up into the kidney secondary to ureteral kinking caused by an obstructing radiolucent stone (compare with **C**); the proximal end of the stent is coiled in the ureter and the fluoroscopically placed guidewire similarly cannot negotiate the obstructed tortuous ureter. **C,** Comparison with the retrograde pyelogram in **B** reveals that the proximal end of the stent is coiled in the ureter. Therefore, the kidney remained obstructed. As the fluoroscopically placed guidewire similarly cannot negotiate the obstructed tortuous ureter, further direct endoscopic evaluation and manipulation of the obstructed ureter are required. **D,** Under endoscopic control, the ureteral obstruction and the tortuous ureter can be negotiated safely with a hydrophilic Glidewire.

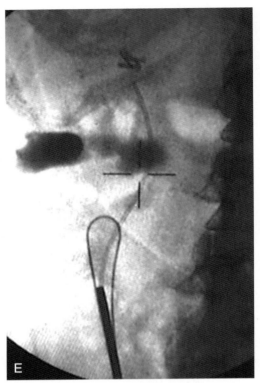

Figure 26-3, cont'd **E,** After successful negotiation of the tortuous ureter with the hydrophilic Glidewire, an angiographic catheter is placed over the wire into the kidney, and a urine sample for culture and sensitivity testing is obtained. Then the Glidewire is exchanged for a regular 0.038 guidewire, and a ureteral stent is placed for renal decompression and management of the infection.

TABLE 26-1	Early (Intraoperative) Technical Complications of Ureteroscopic Surgery and Management
Early Complications (Technical)	**Management**
Ureteral injury Mucosal tear with or without extravasation	Ureteral injury Drainage ([1] stent; [2] stent + Foley; [3] stent + Foley + PCN)
False passage (guidewire)	Endoscopically correct guidewire placement and stent for 2 wk
Perforation (with extravasation), false passage	Drainage with stent (safety-wire), check with ultrasound/CT, PCN drainage of urinoma or hematoma
Ureteral bleeding (from scope or energy source)	Observe; most will cease unless perforation or damage of large, adjacent vessel
Ureteral intussusception or avulsion	Laparoscopic or open surgery required
Damage to adjacent structures (vessels, bowel)	Open surgery likely required

CT, computed tomography; PCN, percutaneous nephrostomy.

INTRAOPERATIVE COMPLICATIONS

Ureteral Injury

Ureteral injury can manifest through bleeding, mucosal tears, false passage and perforation, intussusception, and avulsion, as well as occasional damage to adjacent structures (Table 26-1).

Ureteral Bleeding

Bleeding in the ureter should very rarely become an issue. Minimal bleeding is typically encountered from instrumentation of the tight ureteral orifice, from an edematous or tight ureter, or from contact with renal mucosa as precipitating factors. Mild oozing with the use of energy sources or when copious edema is present (impacted stone, previous instrumentation, and stenting), especially in the anticoagulated patient, is a minor complication during ureteropyeloscopy. The decreased visualization that results can make the case at hand more difficult but usually should allow safe and successful completion of the procedure. Although the bleeding is usually minimal and self-limiting, more severe or prolonged bleeding may necessitate the termination of the procedure (e.g., ureteral TCC, extensive edema, anti-coagulated patient). Too aggressive of an approach in stone fragmentation, in fulgurating upper tract TCC or performing an endopyelotomy for ureteral stricture or UPJ obstruction can lead to more severe bleeding (**Fig. 26-4**). Depending on the severity, treatment may range from termination of the procedure and placement of an indwelling double-J stent (usually sufficient) to superselective angioembolization or laparoscopic or open repair of the injury (extremely rare, highest risk at crossing of ureter with iliac vessels and at UPJ).[11,12]

In the literature, minor bleeding complications have been noted to range from 0% to 2.1%, whereas prolonged bleeding complications have ranged from 0% to 1.0%.[3,13-16] During URS and RIRS, the need for blood transfusion is extremely rare.

Mucosal Tear of Ureter

A mucosal tear is a minor complication that can be caused by instrument trauma, stone manipulation, or inadvertent use of energy sources. Treatment can usually be completed, and for management of this injury a double-J ureteral stent is placed. This injury may weaken the ureteral wall, and stone fragments may migrate and exit the ureter through the tear. Once healed, the stone fragments may remain submucosally. This may lead to a ureteral stricture or formation of a stone granuloma.[3] Therefore, all stone gravel from above the level of the

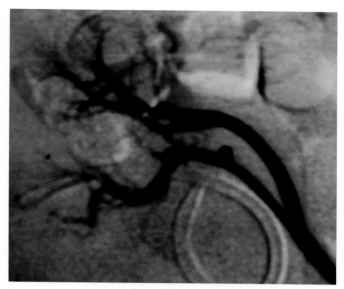

Figure 26-4 Four weeks after uneventful ureteroscopic electroincision of a right UPJ obstruction, the patient presented with intermittent gross hematuria and a falling hematocrit. Renal ultrasound showed no significant obstruction and no perirenal fluid collection. Ureteroscopic evaluation revealed brisk intermittent bleeding from the area of the previous incision. Selective angiography confirmed a pseudoaneurysm of the lower pole segmental artery crossing over the UPJ. Superselective angioembolization was successfully performed.

tear should be completely removed. Continued aggressive instrumentation of the area also could potentially lead to a false passage or perforation of the ureter, so utmost care needs to be exercised. Usually, it is best to reposition the stone remnants to a higher location, fragment them there, and cautiously remove the stone fragments across the injured area without increasing the injury further.

Ureteral False Passage

A false passage can occur during instrumentation when the ureteral wall mucosa is perforated but the ureteral wall itself remains intact. This complication typically occurs during attempted passage of a guidewire above a tightly obstructing, embedded stone or when negotiating a tortuous or strictured ureter (see Fig. 26-2). It also can happen while using too much force during passage of the ureteropyeloscope. Blute and associates[13] and Grasso and Bagley[16] cited the incidence of false passage as 0.9% and 0.4%, respectively.

To treat this injury, it first must be recognized. Using direct vision or contrast to confirm guidewire placement in the renal pelvis, a double-J stent is placed to allow the false passage to heal. If the safety wire is already in place and is not the cause of the false passage, placement of the double-J stent should not be difficult and usually is sufficient to allow the defect to heal in a matter of 2 weeks.

Ureteral Perforation

Perforation of the ureteral wall typically occurs when too much force is applied during access or instrumentation or fragmentation of a tightly impacted ureteral stone (**Fig. 26-5**). Kramolowsky[17] noted a 17% (24 of 142 procedures) perforation rate in 1987, and Stoller and colleagues[18] cited a 15.4% rate of perforation in 1992; 79.2% (19 of 24) of the perforations occurred using a larger 12.5-Fr ureteroscope, unlike the commonly used smaller-caliber scopes of today.

Grasso's[3] multistudy review from 1988 to 1998 noted that the rate of perforation ranged from 0% to 4.6%, with the highest rate occurring in the earliest study. Khambrick and associates[8] added their institutional data in addition to 9 studies published from 2000 to 2002. For the 4274 patients, the perforation rate was 1.2% (51 of 4274). Using 27 studies with ≥100 procedures each, Johnson and Pearle[19] noted a perforation rate of ≤2% with the use of smaller-caliber ureteropyeloscopes.

Treatment, as in other ureteral injuries, requires providing adequate drainage of the collecting system. This drainage is ideally accomplished with a double-J ureteral stent. If the perforation is large, stenting may not be adequate, and the patient may additionally need a percutaneous nephrostomy tube placed to avoid significant extravasation and formation of a urinoma (**Fig. 26-6**). In many cases, successful endoscopic treatment can be performed in an antegrade or retrograde fashion after a 2-week cool-down period with appropriate drainage and antibiotic coverage. However, in cases with more severe damage and formation of urinoma, eventually laparoscopic or open surgical repair of the injury may be necessary if healing occurs with stricture formation.

Ureteral Intussusception

Ureteral intussusception is a rare complication of URS. It is described as the "invagination of the mucosal sleeve resulting from partial-thickness circumferential injury to the ureter with subsequent traction of the mucosa within the ureteral lumen."[19] Like in ureteral avulsion, it is most often seen when basketed stones are forcefully and sometimes blindly removed from the ureter. Although few cases are documented in the literature, intussusception has been shown to occur in both an antegrade and a retrograde fashion.[20] In 1994 Park and associates[21] described an intussusception after retrograde pyelography, and in 1996 Bernhard and Reddy[22] described it after dilation of a previously ureteroscopied ureter with a 12-Fr peel-away sheath. Visualization of the second injury noted that the ureter was white and impassable.

This injury should be suspected when ureteral obstruction occurs after instrumentation. In intussusception, unlike in edema, obstruction by blood clots or stone fragments, or partial ureteral injury, a safety wire

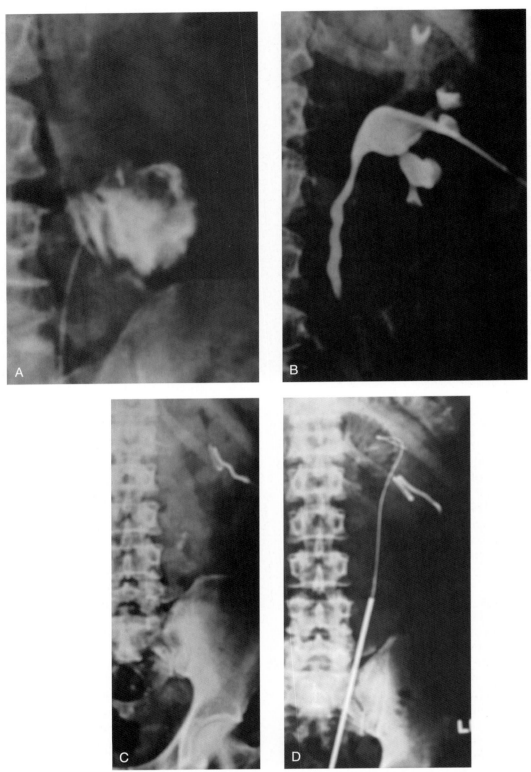

Figure 26-5 **A,** After attempted guidewire and Glidewire manipulation of impacted upper ureteral stone, the retrograde pyelogram shows extravasation suggesting perforation below the level of the stone. **B,** PCN is placed. A nephrostogram shows no contrast passing by the completely obstructing stone. After 2 weeks of PCN drainage, the stone can be approached in a retrograde fashion or, if it is still not accessible, in an antegrade fashion using the established PCN access. **C,** After 2 weeks of PCN drainage, a plain abdominal radiograph shows the two upper ureteral stones in an unchanged location. **D,** After successful placement of a safety wire (correct position in kidney confirmed by placing the angiocatheter over wire and contrast injected to outline renal collecting system), the stones can be treated in a retrograde fashion. As the kidney-ureter-bladder study shows, the stones have been successfully removed; a more invasive antegrade approach was not needed.

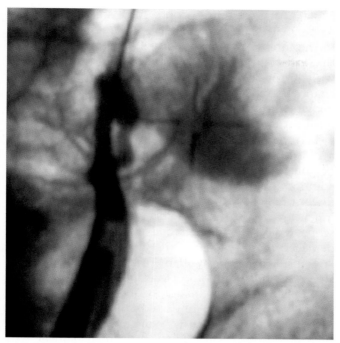

Figure 26-6 Patient presenting with macrohematuria and anemia. Previous history included aortofemoral bypass surgery 10 years earlier and ureteral stone removal 3 years earlier. On cystoscopy, brisk bleeding from the left orifice is noted. Ureteroscopically, no intraureteral bleeding source can be seen, but on injection of contrast material a fistula tract to the iliac artery and contrast runoff through the artery are confirmed. Immediate open surgery was initiated.

typically is unable to bypass this injury.[22] If the injury is identified, a percutaneous nephrostomy tube will need to be placed. As in avulsion, subsequent laparoscopic or open surgery will be needed to repair the damaged segment. Prevention with avoidance of forceful advancement of a rigid ureteroscope or access sheath or pulling against resistance at stone removal is paramount in avoiding ureteral intussusception.

Ureteral Avulsion

Ureteral avulsion is one of the most severe but very rare complications to be encountered in URS. It also should be easily preventable. The most common location for ureteral avulsion has been noted to be at the proximal third of the ureter when basketed stones too large for the caliber of the ureter are forcefully and sometimes blindly removed from the ureter. This maneuver may cause the distal segment of ureter to be pulled out from the urethra along with the stone. This severe complication should be avoided by always visualizing the ureteral wall slide by as the stone is pulled. Any resistance the stone encounters as it is being pulled through the smaller-caliber ureter should signal the stoppage of further risky downward manipulation and the need for additional stone fragmentation. After encountering resistance and stopping further basket manipulation, it

may be impossible to disengage the basket from the stone.

If the basket with the trapped stone is still mobile upward in the ureter, disengagement may be easy by just advancing the fully opened basket. The basket may then separate from the stone and thus allow further fragmentation before smaller debris is removed with multiple passages of the basket. If the trapped stone basket is wedged in the ureter and cannot be moved upward into the more dilated ureteral segment, this situation is remedied by breaking down (disassembling) the basket and removing the sleeve of the basket from the ureter. This maneuver leaves the "naked" basket in place, and the ureteroscope (rigid in the distal two thirds of the ureter, flexible in the proximal third) is then advanced along the stem of the basket up to the trapped stone. The trapped stone is then fragmented very cautiously. The surgeon must try to avoid damaging both the ureter and the wires of the basket. Once the stone is completely fragmented to pieces of 2 to 3 mm, the basket can be cautiously withdrawn. If fragmentation leaves the wires of the basket intact, it may be possible to reassemble the basket and use it further until completion of the case.

When avulsion is suspected, a retrograde pyelogram should be immediately performed. The presence of complete extravasation from the distal ureter and the absence of contrast in the proximal ureter confirm this diagnosis. Unfortunately, laparoscopic or open surgery will be necessary at this point to repair the avulsed ureter. A percutaneous nephrostomy tube should be placed at the time of injury because a ureteral stent will be difficult to place and will not allow adequate drainage. If the proximal ureter is injured, primary repair may be an option; however, if the ureter is devascularized at the area of injury, creation of an ileal ureter or autotransplantation may be required. Injuries to the midureter can be fixed primarily or with ureteroneocystostomy and an accompanying Boari flap or psoas hitch.

For avulsion distal to the iliac vessel crossing, a ureteroneocystostomy is the recommended repair. Occasionally, a transureteroureterostomy is performed, but especially for patients with a history of stone disease or upper urinary tract TCC, transureteroureterostomy is contraindicated. Rarely, the defect may be so severe or the renal function so compromised through prolonged conservative management of the condition that nephrectomy may be more prudent than an attempted repair.

From 1988 to 2001, 4 studies that included 1751 procedures showed an incidence of ureteral avulsion ranging from 0% to 0.6%.[13-16,23] A review of 10 studies published in 2006 noted an avulsion rate of 0.14% (6 in 4274 patients).[8] Motola and colleagues[24] reported avulsion during placement of a 16- to 14-Fr peel-away sheath. As data show, ureteral avulsion should rarely if ever be encountered during URS.

Damage to Adjacent Structure

Vascular injury during URS is a serious complication. In the literature, it has been reported during retrograde endopyelotomy during incision for UPJ obstruction.[25-27] Brooks and colleagues[26] reported one patient ($n = 9$) that experienced significant bleeding after retrograde endopyelotomy requiring 4 U of packed red blood cells and eventual superselective angioembolization. In a series of salvage endopyelotomies, Ng and associates[27] also reported one patient ($n = 22$) that encountered significant bleeding postprocedurally that required selective angioembolization. With 77 patients, Kim and colleagues[25] reported a 4% (3 patients) rate of significant hemorrhage that required blood transfusion and eventual angioembolization in 2 patients after fluoroscopically controlled Acucise endopyelotomy (see Fig. 26-4).

As shown in the literature, treatment of vascular injury during URS procedures will frequently resolve conservatively but may in rare instances require blood transfusion. In cases of more serious, prolonged bleeding, angiography and selective angioembolization of the bleeding vessel may be necessary. Laparoscopic or open surgery would appear to be the treatment of choice should these fail.

Stackl and Marberger[28] noted in their experience that ureters which have been scarred by previous surgeries (e.g., aortofemoral bypass, radical hysterectomy) and radiation are more vulnerable to perforation at the crossing with the iliac vessels and damage to adjacent vascular structures. Similarly, it makes sense that extra caution is used when instrumenting ureters in these patients as to avoid concomitant perforation, intussusception or avulsion.

Instrument Failure

Malfunction or Breakage

Actively deflectable flexible ureteropyeloscopes are technologically complex instruments that have made significant advances since their initial use in the 1970s and 1980s.[4,5,29] They are an invaluable part of a urologists' armamentarium and currently can cost from $12,000 to $20,000 (digital technology) each. The unfortunate reality is that flexible ureteropyeloscopes are relatively fragile. In 2006, Monga and associates[30] performed a prospective randomized study comparing 7 different flexible ureteropyeloscopes. The average number of cases before repair ranged from 3.25 to 14.4, and the average operating time before repair ranged from 105 to 494 minutes.[30] In contrast, one study showed that newer-generation ureteropyeloscopes may be more durable because a single scope was used for 50 cases and >76 hours elapsed before repair was needed.[31]

About half of the damage described may be caused by urologists themselves; the other main causes of damage occur during the cleaning and sterilizing process. Sung and colleagues[32] evaluated the cause of damage for ureteropyeloscopes. In flexible ureteropyeloscopes, >50% of total repairs were the result of damage to the internal working channel. Laser perforations of the work channel were the primary cause of this damage, with 90% located in the distal 3 to 4 mm of the working channel. For semirigid ureteroscopes, damage to the body of the shaft secondary to excessive force was the most common cause, implicated at 35% of all repairs.[32]

Fortunately, most user-related scope damage can be avoided, and with proper precautions the life span of a flexible ureteroscope can be significantly prolonged. In addition, by prompt recognition of scope damage and discontinuation of use, the damage can be repaired at much lower cost than would be incurred by complete scope replacement if a scope were further used and damaged more severely. Particularly, activation of the laser inside the working channel, lasering a target (stone, stricture, and tumor) too close to the scope lens, and improper and extreme handling of a scope against resistance (narrow ureter, impacted stone, narrow infundibulum) should be easily avoidable. Failure to heed such precautions will lead to instrument damage that reduces visibility or will make the scope nonfunctional. This failure necessitates removing and replacing the ureteropyeloscope or even terminating the procedure if no backup scope is available.

Certainly, although backup instruments represent a considerable expense that not all urologists and institutions can afford, they are necessary in the best interest of successful treatment completion. Catastrophic failure with breakage of the ureteropyeloscope in the ureter has been documented.[7,33] In one case, open surgical intervention was needed to remove the ureteropyeloscope that was in locked deflection.[33]

In our own experience, bringing in manufacturers' representatives for training sessions to teach proper handling, cleaning, and sterilization of ureteropyeloscopes to the technical staff as well as training the surgeon on the proper and safe use of ureteropyeloscopes, auxiliary equipment, and energy sources has greatly extended the time intervals between repairs. Moreover, all our instrument breakages are analyzed, and the mechanism of disuse is tracked to allow further education of all staff members potentially involved in the damage. Another preventive measure, especially useful for inexperienced users, is the use of ureteral access sheaths to facilitate manipulation in and out of the ureter and to protect the flexible scopes from undue stress.[30]

EARLY POSTOPERATIVE COMPLICATIONS

Infection

Urinary Tract Infection, Bacteremia, and Sepsis

The documentation of urinary tract infection (UTI), bacteremia, and sepsis after endoscopic surgery of the upper urinary tract has not been consistent in the urologic

TABLE 26-2 Early (Postoperative) Medical Complications: Prevention and Management

Early Complications (Medical)	Prevention and Management
Acute urinary retention	Avoid overdistention of bladder intraoperatively Voiding trial for male patients with large prostates
Infection	
Bacteremia, sepsis	Preoperative sterile urine, perioperative IV antibiotics Sterile technique, drainage (stent or PCN)
Urethritis, prostatitis, cystitis	Antibiotics and symptomatic (antispasmodic)
Periureteral Fluid Collection (Extravasation)	
Hematoma (sterile/ infected)	Observe (sterile); PCN: drain (infected)
Irrigation fluid	Observe (sterile); PCN: drain (infected)
Positional	
Nerve damage	Proper positioning and cushioning Evaluate, physical therapy
DVT	Proper positioning and cushioning, pulsatile stockings Medical treatment

DVT, deep vein thrombosis; PCN, percutaneous nephrostomy.

literature (Table 26-2). Studies have defined infection complications as low-grade fever, culture-proven UTI, pyelonephritis, and urosepsis. The terms *bacteremia* and *sepsis* especially elicit many opinions in the infectious disease community.[34] *Bacteremia* is defined as the culture-proven presence of bacteria in the circulating blood, usually associated with fever, whereas *sepsis* is defined as clinical evidence of bacteremia in addition to evidence of a severe systemic response or shock syndrome.

In terms of UTIs after ureteropyeloscopy, the more current literature is fairly consistent in showing the postoperative incidence to be <2%.[14,16,23,24] Additional data have shown that low-grade fevers (<38.5°C) occur in 1.4% to 6.9% of patients after treatment.[13-16,23] The clinical relevance of that data is undetermined. Grasso and Bagley[16] documented a 0.5% incidence of pyelonephritis in their series of 584 patients. Undoubtedly, the most serious infectious complication is septic shock syndrome, which has a reported mortality rate of 28.6% even in otherwise healthy patients.[36] In these large studies, the rate of sepsis after URS ranged from 0% to 0.3%.[13-16,23] No deaths were reported.

To minimize infectious complications during ureteroscopic and intrarenal surgery, a documented negative urine culture is mandatory. This can be obtained on routine preoperative workup or after treating a patient with appropriate antibiotics for a positive urine culture. Additionally, perioperative IV antibiotics are also recommended.[37] Jeromin and Sosnowski[38] reported in 1998 that their patients were not routinely given perioperative antibiotics. Their results showed a 21.9% (345 of 1575) rate of low-grade fevers and a 4.6% (74 of 1575) rate of active or recurrent UTIs.[38] Both rates were significantly higher than were those in the earlier studies mentioned in association with antibiotic prophylaxis. If infection is encountered before instrumentation with the ureteropyeloscope, adequate drainage with a double-J stent or percutaneous nephrostomy as well as appropriate antibiotics is mandatory. Sterile technique throughout the procedure is standard of care.

In >3000 procedures at our institution, we did not experience any incidents of urosepsis. In few cases, temporary temperature elevations up to 38.5°C postoperatively were noted, but these usually resolved within 24 to 36 hours. In addition to the measures mentioned earlier (negative urine culture, perioperative antibiotic cover), we attribute the absence of more severe infectious complications to the use of forced diuresis, which is started with 20 mg of IV furosemide (children, 5-10 mg) once access to the kidney with a safety guidewire has been obtained. Forced diuresis (IV fluids and furosemide) helps prevent pyelovenous and pyelolymphatic reflux and thereby reduces the risk of bacteremia or fluid overload.

Another precaution against pyelovenous and pyelolymphatic reflux and infectious complications is the use of gravity irrigation only (≤60 cm of water above patient level). In addition, we maintain a low-pressure environment in the kidney through frequent aspiration (inflow ≤2 minutes before aspiration). Intermittent aspiration is facilitated by using a three-way connector for irrigant and suction (suction connected to suction pump). Additional benefits of intermittent aspiration are the improved visualization and reduced risk of energy-related damage of the kidney. We strongly believe that strict adherence to these measures is the reason that our infectious complication rates are so low compared with those of other groups that use pressurized irrigant (syringe irrigation, pressure bags or pumps), with the risk of increasing pyelovenous and pyelolymphatic reflux and thereby causing infectious as well as overhydration complications. If a patient has a history of infection-induced stone or intraoperatively a struvite stone is encountered, it is advisable to culture the stone and continue antibiotic coverage at least until a negative culture from the stone is confirmed.

Extravasation

Periureteral Fluid Collection (Irrigation Fluid, Urinoma, or Hematoma, Sterile or Infected)

During ureteroscopic and intrarenal surgery, perforation of the ureter (direct instrument damage) or forniceal rupture (instrument damage or increased fluid pressure) can lead to extravasation of irrigation fluid, urine, and blood. This extravasation can lead to flank pain, fever, and ileus.[39] Further complication eventually can result in formation of an infected urinoma or hematoma. Saline irrigation is necessary because a large amount of extravasation of hypotonic fluid into the retroperitoneum can lead to hyponatremia. If the perforation is large enough, stone fragments can migrate into the perirenal space or the retroperitoneum.[7,11,28,39] In four studies the rates of stone extrusion were 0.5%, 1.2%, 1.6%, and 2.3%. Fortunately, in most instances these stones may be left outside the collecting system without any need for further intervention.

Extravasation may be underreported in the literature because many urologists do not routinely perform a retrograde pyelogram at the conclusion of the procedure. When perforation and extravasation are encountered, it is safest to terminate the procedure promptly. Usually, sufficient drainage is provided by an indwelling double-J ureteral stent, which can be readily placed over the safety guidewire. Typically, the stent should be left indwelling for ≥2 to 4 weeks to allow the injury to heal.[28] Further manipulation in the presence of documented perforation can lead to increasing the size of the defect and subsequently increasing the amount of extravasation and subsequent complications. The extent of fluid collections is best documented on CT and then followed with ultrasound examination. If the patient remains asymptomatic, stent drainage and continued outpatient observation are management techniques of choice. If the patient has clinical signs of infection, percutaneous drainage of the fluid collection is indicated with appropriate antibiotic coverage. If at that time the leak from the ureter or kidney persists, percutaneous nephrostomy tube drainage of the kidney is needed to reduce the risk of fistula formation.

Complications From Positioning During Ureteroscopic Surgery

Neuropathy through prolonged compression of nerves and deep vein thrombosis after prolonged procedures have been occasionally described. Moreover, a rare complication is overextension of lower body limbs under anesthesia, especially in patients with previous surgery (e.g., hip or knee replacement). It is important to inquire about reduction of range of motion beforehand, to prevent these rare complications.

Neuropathy through compression of exposed nerves can be avoided by careful positioning, avoiding overextension, and cushioning all pressure points. Lasting nerve damage after URS has not been described in the literature.

Deep Vein Thrombosis

Deep vein thrombosis after RIRS is a rarely reported complication.[16,27] Grasso and Bagley[16] reported a single case after 584 procedures (0.2%). Pulmonary embolism was reported in a single patient after retrograde endopyelotomy.[40] To avoid these complications, prophylactic measures are recommended such as sequential compression device boots for patients at high risk for developing thromboembolic complications or when a procedure is expected to last >3 hours.

LATE POSTOPERATIVE COMPLICATIONS

Ureteral Injury

Stricture Formation

A ureteral stricture has been defined as the "narrowing of the ureter causing a functional obstruction."[41] Review of the literature from 1988 to 2006 showed that the incidence of post-URS/RIRS stricture ranges from 0.2% to 1.4%.[8,13-16,23]

Stricture formation is a major postoperative complication that can lead to permanent renal dysfunction and even possible nephrectomy (Table 26-3). Ureteral trauma during URS is the primary cause. This complication can arise in the form of mechanical injury from the ureteropyeloscope or other accessory instrument, thermal injury from a laser fiber, perforation, or the presence of an impacted stone.[42] Ureteral perforation has been implicated in increasing the likelihood of ureteral stricture formation. In a retrospective review from 1983 to 1986, Kramolowsky[17] documented a 17% perforation rate in 142 procedures. Subsequently, strictures developed in 7 of the 24 patients with perforations.[17] Stoller and colleagues[18] noted a stricture rate of 5.9% for

TABLE 26-3	Late Technical Complications: Prevention and Management
Late Complications (Technical)	**Prevention and Management**
Stricture Formation (Extremely Rare)	Maintain observation of the following types of patients: • Difficult to treat (i.e., impacted stones, especially Steinstrasse) • Long-standing hydronephrosis • Ureteral injury • Previous pelvic or retroperitoneal surgery • Previous radiation therapy Primarily, treatment of strictures is endoscopic (ureteroscopic or laparoscopic); open repair is used for more complex strictures. Keep log and re-call patients with the listed difficulties.
Retained Stents	Treat encrusted stents by fragmenting encrustations before removing stent to avoid intussusception or avulsion.

patients with intraoperative ureteral perforations, whereas only a 3.5% overall stricture rate for the 85 patients studied. Lytton and colleagues[39] followed 16 patients (12 minor, 4 major) with ureteral perforations from 1982 to 1985 and noted a single case of "intramural ureteral stenosis." This complication was thought to result in part from the patient's previous pelvic radiation for Hodgkin's disease. In data from 1983, Stackl and Marberger noted no stricture formation in a study of 19 patients, 3 of whom required open surgery, after ureteral perforation.[28]

In the setting of an impacted stone, Roberts and associates[43] noted a 24% (5 of 21 patients) development rate of ureteral stricture. Four of the patients were noted to have a perforation at the stone site and subsequently were discovered to have a stricture at the same location. The mean time of detection was at 2.6 months.[43] In a large series of 165 patients, Mugiya and colleagues[44] noted a 17% (28 of 165) rate of stricture formation at stone impaction site and found that a longer impaction time correlated with a statistically significant increased likelihood of developing a stricture.

The increasingly common use of flexible hydrophilic access sheaths has raised concern for potential for stricture formation. Two studies from the same institution examined this issue. Kourambas and associates[45] noted no stricture formation in 23 patients who had access sheaths placed without dilation, whereas Delvecchio and colleagues[46] identified 1 stricture in 71 patients on follow-up. The stricture was not attributed to access sheath use.[45,46]

Johnson and Pearle[19] reviewed five studies published from 1996 to 2001 relating to ureteropyeloscopy, upper tract TCC, and stricture formation. In the endoscopic management of upper tract TCC, continued surveillance with fulguration of the tumor lining the mucosa is necessary. Not surprisingly, an increased stricture rate of 9.3% was noted in the combined series of 161 renoureteral units. The mean follow-up was 44.5 months. Both intraureteral bacille Calmette-Guérin and radiation therapy, which have been documented to cause stricture or ureteric obstruction on their own, may have contributed to this outcome.[47,48]

Treatment of ureteral strictures involves obtaining imaging such as a retrograde or antegrade pyelogram to visualize the length of the strictured segment. Endoscopic management with a holmium laser incision, cold knife incision, or balloon dilation has shown to be more suitable for shorter strictures (usually <1 cm long), whereas open or laparoscopic intervention is needed for denser or longer strictures.

As with other complications of URS, attention to detail and safe technique can avoid ureteral injury and subsequent stricture formation in almost all cases. It is of utmost importance to learn when a ureter is too tight to accommodate the instrument, rigid or flexible, and to avoid undue force when advancing the instrument.

TABLE 26-4	Management of Late Medical Complications of Ureteroscopic Surgery and Retrograde Intrarenal Surgery
Late Complications (Medical)	**Management**
Infection secondary to retained stone/stent/extravasation (rare)	Treat with antibiotics and remove cause of complication

Similarly, when segments of the ureter are dilated to accommodate an instrument, a cautious approach is necessary to avoid ureteral perforation, avulsion, or intussusception. When the ureter is too tight for immediate passage of an instrument or dilating device, placement of an indwelling ureteral stent is advisable. The indwelling stent almost invariably allows passive dilation of the ureter over time and facilitates a successful staged procedure after about 2 weeks of indwelling time.

Retained Stents

Retained ureteral stents after a urologic procedure can lead to encrustation and can necessitate additional and frequently complex procedures for their removal. With meticulous use of a postoperative stent book, urologists can keep a rolling log of patients who need their stents removed (Table 26-4; see also Table 26-3). Unfortunately, as Aravantinos and colleagues[49] noted, poor compliance by patients with follow-up may be the main reason for this problem.[9]

Stent encrustation has been noted to be most dense at the upper and lower curl, but it can include the entire stent.[50] A study of 299 stents by El-Faqih and colleagues[51] noted that ureteral encrustation occurred in 9.2% of indwelling ureteral stents retrieved at <6 weeks, 47.5% of stents from 6 to 12 weeks, and 76.3% of stents at >12 weeks. For those stents that remained for ≤3 months, a 30% rate of luminal occlusion was cited; however, the incidence of clinical obstruction was noted to be only 4%.[51] This finding is consistent with the concept that the persistent-to-intraluminal flow ratio of 60 to 40 provides more than adequate extraluminal flow.[50,51]

Treatment of encrusted retained stents may need a multimodal approach with the use of percutaneous nephrolithotomy, extracorporeal shockwave lithotripsy, ureteropyeloscopy, and cystolitholopaxy.[49-52] In the case of complete stent encrustation, at our institution we start with cystolitholapaxy for the distal curl with subsequent ureteroscopic treatment of the encrustations of the ureteral portion of the stent, followed by treatment of the proximal curl. If the encrustation of the proximal curl is >2 cm, we employ the percutaneous approach for the renal and proximal ureteral portions of the treatment while a second team simultaneously treats the bladder and distal ureteral portions.

KEY POINTS

1. Complications of URS and RIRS should be extremely rare.
2. Prevention of complications is the best management.
3. Adherence to proper protocol (e.g., selection criteria, preparation, technique, and postoperative care) will avoid complications of URS in almost all cases.
4. Always establish a safety wire bypassing the ureteral disorder and into the kidney.
5. Always visualize the actions of your instruments and energy sources.
6. When unsure or when encountering complications, use fluoroscopic imaging for orientation and assessment of possible complicating factors or complication.
7. When still unsure or when encountering complications, consider early placement of a double-J stent over the safety wire and return another day for a second session. It is always better to be safe than sorry.

REFERENCES

Please see www.expertconsult.com

Chapter 27

COMPLICATIONS OF PERCUTANEOUS RENAL SURGERY

Michael Lipkin MD
Resident, Department of Urology, New York University Langone Medical Center, New York, New York

Ojas Shah MD
Assistant Professor of Urology and Director of Endourology and Stone Disease, Department of Urology, New York University Langone Medical Center, New York, New York

Percutaneous renal surgery (PRS) is commonly employed to treat a variety of urologic conditions, from stone disease to upper tract urothelial carcinoma. Despite increasing surgical experience and advances in technology, complications can still occur. Prompt recognition of complications along with timely treatment can minimize the impact of these complications. This chapter reviews the spectrum of complications that can occur during and after PRS. Diagnosis, treatment, and preventive measures are presented.

HEMORRHAGE

Intraoperative Hemorrhage

Patients undergoing PRS are at risk for significant intraoperative bleeding and subsequent blood transfusion. The transfusion rates from various series have ranged from 1% to 34%.[1-7] Several factors have been shown to be associated with an increased risk for transfusion. These include surgical technique, surgeon experience, preoperative anemia, advanced patient age, increased stone surface area, and the need for multiple tracts.[4,6,8] Intraoperative complications such as infundibular tear or pelvic wall tear have been shown to significantly increase blood loss. Other factors that have been shown to predict increased blood loss during PRS include diabetes, longer operating time, and increased parenchymal thickness.[6,8]

Operative technique is a modifiable risk factor, and certain principles, if followed, can help reduce the risk of significant blood loss. The collecting system should be accessed through a posterior calyx along the direction of the infundibulum. This technique avoids the blood vessels that course adjacent to the infundibulum.[9] The posterior calyx that provides the most direct access to the targeted stone should be chosen. Once access is established, the tract should be dilated only up to the peripheral aspect of the collecting system. Care should be taken not to dilate the tract too far medially because this increases the risk of pelvic wall tear and injury to the hilar vessels. Stoller and colleagues[4] reported that renal pelvic perforation is a risk factor for excessive blood loss.

The impact on blood loss by the method of tract dilation is controversial. Davidoff and Bellman[10] found that the use of balloon dilators was associated with significantly less blood loss and lower transfusion rates when compared with the Amplatz serial dilators. Another series demonstrated that Alken serial dilators were associated with significantly greater blood loss than were either balloon dilators or Amplatz dilators.[6] Turna and colleagues[8] reported that Amplatz serial dilators were associated with significantly greater blood loss compared with balloon dilation. However, Osman an associates[11] reported on 300 patients who had tracts dilated with Alken dilators, none of whom required a transfusion. Other investigators have found no difference in blood loss among methods of dilation.[4,12]

Once access is obtained and the tract is dilated, a working sheath is often placed. Care must be taken to keep the working sheath in the collecting system to limit parenchymal bleeding. Excessive torquing of rigid instruments through the working sheath may injure renal parenchyma and vasculature and therefore should be avoided. Flexible nephroscopy or placement of additional nephrostomy tracts should be performed instead, as demonstrated by Lam and colleagues.[13] These investigators reported that the use of multiple tracts and flexible instruments decreased transfusion rates for their patients undergoing percutaneous nephrolithotomy (PCNL) in the treatment of staghorn calculi. Accessing the appropriate calyx, or using multiple access tracts when appropriate, can reduce the amount of blood loss and the number of complications.[14] Care must also be taken when removing stone fragments through an access sheath because sharp fragments can tear the sheath. Further manipulation of the fragments and sheath can lead to significant bleeding.[15]

Once access is obtained and the working sheath is in place, it is not unusual for some bleeding to continue. However, if bleeding is such that visibility is compromised, certain measures should be taken. First, the surgeon should assess the position of the working sheath. If the end of the sheath has withdrawn into the parenchyma, simply repositioning the sheath back into the collecting system may correct the problem. If this maneuver does not correct the problem, or if the sheath is not malpositioned to begin with, then other interventions need to be undertaken. Inflation of a 30-Fr dilating balloon in the tract for 10 to 20 minutes with subsequent placement of a large nephrostomy tube (24-28 Fr) usually controls the bleeding. If bleeding persists, the nephrostomy tube should be clamped for 2 to 3 hours to allow the blood to clot and tamponade the injured vessel or vessels. Administration of mannitol may hasten this process by causing renal swelling within the capsule that may help tamponade vessels along the nephrostomy tract.[4,16] The nephrostomy tube is left to straight drainage when unclamped if the patient has no signs of continued bleeding.

If these maneuvers are unsuccessful, a specialized nephrostomy tamponade catheter can be inserted (Kaye, Cook Medical, Spencer, Indiana).[17] This catheter has a peripherally located balloon that is inflated in the nephrostomy tract while urine drains through the inner core. The catheter is typically left inflated for 2 to 4 days. The foregoing measures are usually successful at controlling bleeding from peripheral vessels along the nephrostomy tract. Significant bleeding can also arise from injury to the main renal vein, and this bleeding can be controlled using a tamponade approach. Gupta and colleagues[18] reported successful management of this complication in four patients by inflating a Council balloon catheter adjacent to the point of venous injury. When the foregoing measures fail, or when significant arterial injury is suspected, then one should proceed to renal angiography with selective embolization.

Antegrade Endopyelotomy

Percutaneous endopyelotomy has the additional risk of bleeding when the ureteropelvic junction (UPJ) is incised. DiMarco and colleagues[19] reported a transfusion rate of 1.3% in their series of antegrade endopyelotomy. In cases involving secondary UPJ obstruction or ectopic kidneys, preoperative imaging with computed tomography (CT) or magnetic resonance angiography is recommended to delineate vascular anatomy. Some investigators advocate the use of endoluminal ultrasonography (US) for this purpose.[20,21] Hendrikx and associates[21] reported the use of endoluminal US, which detected 15% more crossing vessels than CT angiography and concluded that its use better prevents bleeding

complications. When significant hemorrhage arises from the incised UPJ, a 24-Fr balloon should be inflated across the area and left in place for 10 minutes. If bleeding persists once the balloon is deflated or the patient becomes hemodynamically unstable, the balloon is reinflated, and renal angiography should be performed with embolization if possible. Rarely, open surgical exploration with possible nephrectomy may be necessary if the foregoing measures fail.

Tubeless Percutaneous Renal Surgery

Nephrostomy tube–free, or tubeless PRS, has been reported. The reported advantages of tubeless PRS are decreased pain and speedier recovery leading to decreased length of stay.[22] The transfusion rates for tubeless PRS have been reported to be approximately 5%.[23,24]

Certain techniques have been applied to tubeless PRS to minimize blood loss and the risk for transfusion. Jou and associates[25] performed electrocauterization of bleeding points along the nephrostomy tract and inside the collecting system. These investigators found that this method leads to a significantly lower transfusion rate. They were able to obtain a bloodless tract in 33.7% of patients, and these patients were left without a nephrostomy tube. When bleeding persists, these investigators advocate leaving a nephrostomy tube in place. Hemostatic fibrin glue can be placed in the nephrostomy tract to aid in hemostasis. Shah and associates[26] reported on the use of Tisseel Vapor Heated Sealant (Baxter AG, Vienna). They prospectively compared patients who underwent tubeless PRS with Tisseel sealant placed in the tract at the end of the case to those without Tisseel sealant. These investigators found no significant difference in the change in hematocrit between the two groups.

Care must be taken to avoid injecting the Tisseel sealant into the collecting system because it can form a solid clot that could possibly obstruct the collecting system.[27] Patients with continued bleeding at the end of the procedure should have a nephrostomy tube left in place to control bleeding. Tubeless PRS is not recommended for patients requiring more than two tracts or patients with residual stone who need a staged procedure. Success has been shown in cases with supracostal access and for larger stone burdens, although these situations require further investigation to prove safety.[22,24,26] The rate of stone clearance with tubeless PRS has been reported to range from 83% to 93%.[22,24,26]

Postoperative Hemorrhage

Patients continue to be at risk for significant bleeding for the first several weeks postoperatively.[5,7,28] Most patients who bleed postoperatively can be managed conservatively, but approximately 1% will require invasive treatments.[5,7,10,28] If bleeding occurs with the nephrostomy tube in place, the measures discussed earlier may be employed. If significant bleeding from the tract is encountered after removal of the tube, digital tamponade should be performed with subsequent placement of a tamponade catheter or large nephrostomy tube under fluoroscopic guidance. If a nephrostomy tube is placed, it should be clamped. The patient should then be placed on bed rest and transfused as needed. Renal angiography with selective angioembolization should be performed on patients who continue to require blood transfusions or who become hemodynamically unstable.

Delayed bleeding often occurs approximately 1 to 3 weeks postoperatively.[5,7,28] When angiography is performed on these patients, the most common causes of bleeding are laceration of a segmental artery, arteriovenous malformation, pseudoaneurysm, and arteriovenous fistula.[1-3,5,7,29] Renal angiography with selective embolization is highly effective in treating these lesions (**Fig. 27-1**).[5,7,28] The nephrostomy tube must sometimes be removed so that the bleeding site may be localized during these procedures. When renal angiography and embolization are unsuccessful, open surgical exploration with vascular repair or nephrectomy may be necessary. El-Nahas and colleagues[7] reported 39 (1.3%) of 2909 patients (3878 PCNL procedures) over a 10-year period who had severe perioperative bleeding requiring renal angiography and embolization. Twenty-nine of these patients had severe bleeding before discharge, where the other 10 patients developed bleeding after discharge at a mean of 6.3 days. Renal angiography with selective embolization was successful in treating 36 of the 39 patients. The other 3 patients required exploration, and 1 required nephrectomy. These investigators identified upper calyx puncture, solitary kidney, staghorn stone, multiple punctures, and operator inexperience as significant risk factors for severe bleeding.[7] In another large series, Srivastava and colleagues[5] identified stone size as the only significant risk factor predicting these serious vascular complications.

Kessaris and colleagues[28] reported that 17 of 2200 patients (0.8%) who underwent PRS over a 10-year period required angiography and embolization for uncontrolled significant bleeding. Twenty-four percent of these patients presented in the immediate postoperative period (<24 hours), 41% in the early postoperative period (2-7 days), and 35% in the late postoperative period (>7 days). Superselective or selective angiographic embolization of such lesions, using Gianturco coils, absorbable gelatin sponges, or platinum microcoils, is generally quite successful. This study reported success in 15 of 17 such cases with selective or superselective embolization.[28,29]

Another cause of perioperative bleeding after PRS is perinephric hemorrhage (**Fig. 27-2**). This complication should be suspected in patients who have decreasing hemoglobin with clear urine draining from both the nephrostomy tube and the bladder. Perinephric hemorrhage can occur in cases with difficult access. Malpositioning of the working sheath outside the renal parenchyma is another possible cause.

"Sandwich therapy" with shock wave lithotripsy and subsequent second-look PCNL is another potential risk factor. In these situations, subcapsular or perinephric hemorrhage caused by shock wave lithotripsy may be exacerbated by further tract and collecting system manipulation. Patients in whom this is suspected should be evaluated with CT scan. This situation can typically be treated conservatively with monitoring of hemoglobin, serial physical examinations, hemodynamic parameters, and imaging as needed because the bleeding is usually confined to the retroperitoneal space. Affected patients should be treated with blood transfusions as needed, and rarely exploration may be required if hemodynamic instability cannot be controlled or if bleeding is persistent.

COLLECTING SYSTEM INJURIES

Perforation and Extravasation

Perforation of the collecting system can occur any time during PRS (**Fig. 27-3**). When the working sheath is located outside the collecting system secondary to perforation, large amounts of fluid can extravasate. Lee and associates[30] reported that perforation with extravasation occurred in 7% of 582 cases of PCNL. Perforation should be suspected if perirenal or renal sinus fat is visualized, if other perirenal structures are visualized, or if the patient's abdomen or flank becomes distended. Large amounts of fluid can quickly accumulate in the retroperitoneal space or, less commonly, the abdominal cavity. This fluid can cause difficulties in ventilating the patient during the procedure, electrolyte abnormalities secondary to fluid absorption, and ileus postoperatively.[31]

CT- or US-guided percutaneous drainage of the fluid is sometimes necessary if the patient is having serious respiratory distress, if prolonged ileus does not resolve spontaneously, or if infection of the fluid is suspected. Once perforation is recognized, serious consideration should be given to terminating the procedure. If the procedure is nearly completed, it may be possible to complete it with low-flow irrigation, provided the patient remains stable. Concerns that arise when the procedure is continued are stone migration outside the collecting system and tumor cell spillage during percutaneous resection of urothelial carcinoma. Once the procedure is terminated, a nephrostomy tube should be left in place. Most perforations heal in 72 hours, but it may be prudent to wait 7 days and perform a nephrostogram to confirm closure of the perforation before going back to complete the stone extraction or tumor removal. On rare occasions, open surgical repair may be

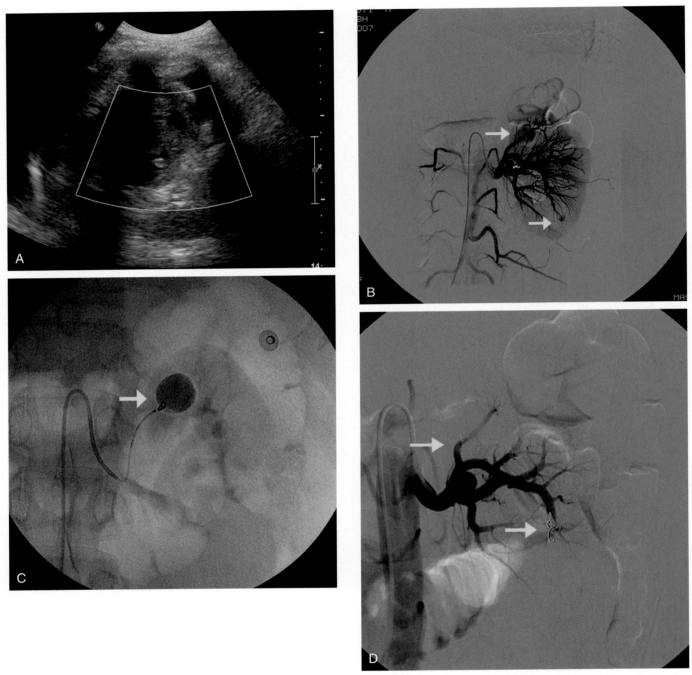

Figure 27-1 Pseudoaneurysm and vascular injury requiring selective angioembolization. **A,** Renal US scan demonstrating the "yin-yang" sign of vascular disease. **B,** Renal angiogram demonstrating a pseudoaneurysm of an upper pole vessel and blush seen from an injured lower pole artery (*arrows*). **C,** Selective embolization of the upper pole pseudoaneurysm (*arrow*). **D,** Coils seen occluding upper pole and lower pole vascular injuries (*arrows*). *(Courtesy of Dr. Timothy Clark.)*

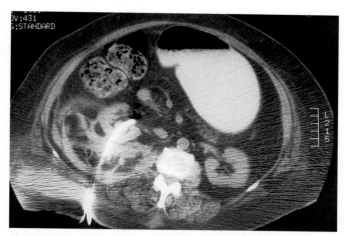

Figure 27-2 Perinephric hemorrhage and hematoma displacing the right kidney anteriorly and medially. *(Courtesy of Dr. Dean Assimos.)*

necessary.[30] This complication can be limited by paying close attention to proper access and dilation techniques, by taking care to keep the working sheath in the collecting system, by judicious stone fragmentation, and by fluoroscopic monitoring of nephrostomy tube insertion and removal.

Ureteral Avulsion

Ureteral avulsion is an extremely rare complication of PRS. It is most commonly caused by attempts at antegrade basketing of large, impacted ureteral stones, but it can also occur with dilation or incision of the UPJ and tumor resection.[30,32] This complication mandates prompt open surgical exploration, although when necessary, nephrostomy tube drainage may be used as a temporizing measure to allow stabilization of the patient. This complication can be avoided by making sure stones are fragmented into pieces small enough to be removed in the basket, as well as by adhering to proper endopyelotomy, endoureterotomy, and resection techniques.

Extrarenal and Extraureteral Stone Fragment Migration

Extrarenal and extraureteral stone fragments are generally not of any clinical consequence, provided the urine and stone are not infected and the stone is far enough from the collecting system and ureter not to cause periureteral inflammation with subsequent stricture formation (**Fig. 27-4**).[33,34] Retrieval should not be attempted in most cases because this may enlarge the perforation. The occurrence of this complication can be minimized by avoiding collecting system perforation or, if one has occurred, recognizing it and stopping the procedure, as well as applying proper stone removal techniques.

Stricture

The development of a stricture following PRS occurs rarely, with a reported incidence of <1%. The most commonly affected segments are the proximal ureter and the UPJ.[1,2] Strictures can form as a result of inflammation secondary to stone impaction or from procedural trauma including intracorporeal lithotripsy. Patients who have undergone cutaneous urinary diversion with proximal ureteral calculi may be at increased risk for stricture formation because of an intense inflammatory response (obliterative pyeloureteritis) that may be secondary to infection and other local factors.[35] Ureteral strictures can be asymptomatic, and patients undergoing PRS should be routinely evaluated for this complication with postoperative imaging.[36] Most ureteral strictures that develop after PRS can be managed with endourologic techniques, provided the stricture is <1.5 cm and is not in a radiated field. However, open or laparoscopic reconstruction may be required in patients with more extensive strictures or in patients in whom an endoscopic approach has failed.

Infundibular Stenosis

Infundibular stenosis is a rare complication that can occur after PRS.[2,37,38] Parsons and colleagues[39] reported a 2% incidence following PCNL. They identified prolonged operative time, large stone burden requiring multiple procedures, and extended postoperative nephrostomy tube drainage as independent risk factors for this occurrence. These investigators postulated that factors that increase local inflammation could include prolonged instrumentation or the use of large amounts of energy to break up stones. This complication is usually detected in the first year after PRS. Infundibular stenosis should be managed endourologically, with open surgery reserved for those in whom this approach fails. For patients who are asymptomatic without evidence of impaired renal function, close observation is an option.

Retained Foreign Bodies

On occasion, a piece of equipment used in a percutaneous procedure can break off in the renal collecting system. This can occur during any stage of the procedure. Lynch and associates[40] reported on a piece of plastic drape that was translocated into the collecting system during tract dilation. Instruments should be inspected periodically during and at the end of procedures to ensure that nothing is broken or missing. Every effort should be made to find the foreign body and remove it because it can act as a nidus for stone formation or infection or cause a granulomatous reaction within the kidney.

The foreign body can usually be extracted with a rigid or flexible nephroscope and graspers or a basket. Fluo-

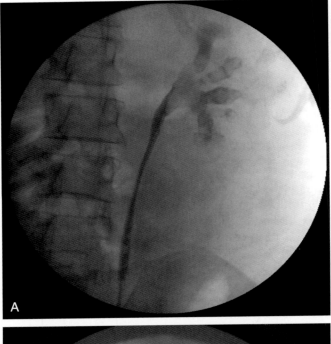

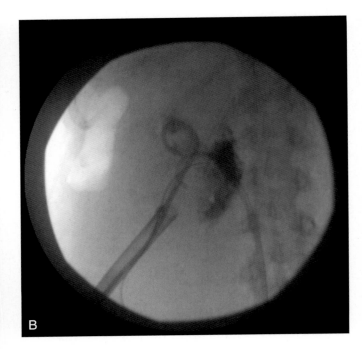

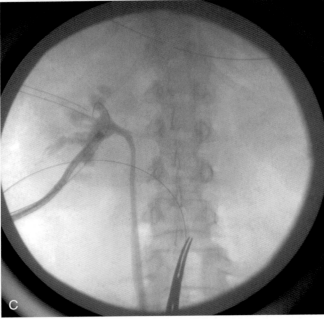

Figure 27-3 Renal pelvis injury/perforation with extravasation. **A,** Initial left retrograde pyelogram demonstrates kidney with multiple filling defects consistent with a large stone burden. **B,** Perforation noted intraoperatively under direct visualization when perirenal fat is seen near the end of the case. Left nephrostogram demonstrates extravasation. **C,** Postoperative nephrostogram after 7 days confirms healing of the renal pelvis with resolution of extravasation and clearance of stone burden with no evidence of filling defects and no stones seen with flexible nephroscope. *(Courtesy of Dr. Brian Matlaga.)*

roscopy can aid in removal of the foreign body if it is opaque. If the foreign body is discovered after nephrostomy tube removal, a retrograde ureteroscopic approach can be performed. If this fails, percutaneous extraction may be necessary. This complication can be limited by replacing instruments before instrument fatigue develops. Careful manipulation of wires, laser fibers, other lithotripter devices, baskets, and tubes can also minimize the incidence of this complication. Postoperatively, the tips of nephrostomy tubes, such as Malecot catheters, may become entrapped in the collecting system as a result of ingrowth of fibrous and inflamma-

tory tissue. If this occurs, it can be managed by a ureteroscopic approach or the creation of a new nephrostomy tract and endoscopic removal of this tissue.[41]

Tumor Seeding

Tumor seeding of the nephrostomy tube tract is a potential but rare complication of percutaneous resection of urothelial carcinoma. It has been reported after resection of poorly differentiated, locally invasive disease.[42] More commonly, it has been noted in association with percutaneous drainage of an obstructed system in

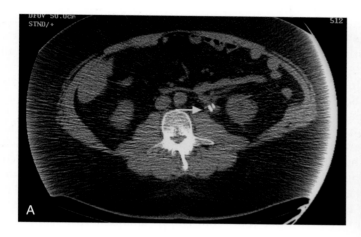

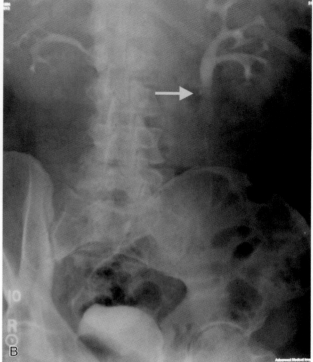

Figure 27-4   Left extraureteral stone. **A,** CT scan postoperatively demonstrates a stone fragment (*arrow*) adjacent to the ureteral stent in the region of the proximal ureter. **B,** Postoperative intravenous pyelogram reveals that the stone fragment lies adjacent to the left proximal ureter causing mild extrinsic compression (*arrow*) but no significant hydronephrosis and drainage of contrast material distally. *(Courtesy of Dr. Joshua Wein and Dr. Rupa Patel.)*

patients with transitional cell carcinoma.[43-45] Numerous series have performed percutaneous resection without evidence of tract seeding with long-term follow-up.[46-49] This complication can be minimized by proper selection of patients with low-grade, noninvasive tumors. Special care should be taken to maintain proper position of the working sheath, to perform the procedure with low-pressure irrigation, and to have low-pressure postoperative drainage with properly sized nephrostomy tubes.

Nephrocutaneous Fistula

Nephrocutaneous fistula formation is a rare occurrence after PRS.[50] It is usually caused by distal obstruction secondary to ureteral edema, obstructing stone, blood clot, or stricture. Delayed development of nephrocutaneous fistulas has been reported to occur in patients with genitourinary tuberculosis.[51] Relief of the obstruction by either placement of a ureteral stent or removal of stone usually allows the fistula to close.

Injury Resulting From Energy Sources

The performance of PRS has been aided by the continued advances in design of lithotripsy and ablative energy sources. Although these advances have improved efficacy and safety, the potential for energy-related complications should not be underestimated. Intracorporeal damage from these sources can range from minor to extensive. To avoid these complications, the surgeon should have a thorough knowledge of each energy source before it is used.

Ultrasonic lithotripsy is a commonly used energy-source technique for PCNL.[32] Collecting system or ureteral perforation can occur with this device, especially if excessive pressure is applied to these tissues. The probe can become clogged with debris, thus causing overheating that could result in thermal injury. As mentioned earlier, a piece of the lithotripter can break off. One case report noted that the tip of an ultrasonic lithotripter broke off and migrated to the left pulmonary artery.[52]

As a result of the development of newer devices with better safety profiles, electrohydraulic lithotripsy is used less frequently for PCNL.[53] The most common complications associated with electrohydraulic lithotripsy are perforation of the collecting system and bleeding, which are managed as previously described.

The holmium:yttrium-aluminum-garnet laser is commonly used for lithotripsy, for incision of strictures, and for the ablation of upper tract tumors. Although the laser has been shown to have an excellent safety profile, complications can still occur.[54] These include hemorrhage, perforation of the collecting system, and thermal injury. Investigators have also reported that heat generated from the laser can interact with hydrogen gas and can generate an explosion in the collecting system that leads to perforation and hemorrhage.[55] These complications can be minimized with careful technique and use of appropriate energy settings.

Pneumatic lithotripters and hybrid devices (pneumatic and US) are also used during PCNL.[56-58] A small risk of perforation and hemorrhage also exists with these devices.

Electrocautery and electroresection are used during PRS for resection of tumors and to control bleeding. The patient should be properly grounded to prevent thermal burns. Only nonconductive materials should be in contact with the collecting system and ureter to prevent current dispersal that could lead to thermal injury. The risk of hemorrhage can be minimized by maintaining proper orientation with respect to adjacent vascular structures. When electrocautery or electroresection is performed, sterile glycine is typically used as irrigant, with an associated risk of fluid absorption and secondary hyponatremia. This risk can be minimized by maintaining the lowest possible irrigation pressures and limiting resection time. Bipolar electrocautery devices have been created that can be used with sterile saline irrigation. These newer devices reduce the risk of hyponatremia from fluid absorption.

INJURY TO ADJACENT STRUCTURES

Lung and Pleura

The lung and the pleura are the perirenal structures most at risk of injury during PRS.[1,2] The incidence of intrathoracic complications has been reported to be between 0.3% and 15.3%.[59-63] These complications include pneumothorax, hydrothorax, hemothorax, and nephropleural fistulas (**Fig. 27-5**). They occur more commonly with supracostal access when compared with infracostal access.[59,61,62,64] Hopper and Yakes[65] studied 43 randomly selected patients with CT imaging during maximal inspiration and expiration and predicted that during maximal expiration the pleura and lung would be traversed 86% of the time on the right and 79% of the time on the left with a supra–11th rib approach. These investigators also predicted that the pleura and lung would be traversed 29% of the time on the right and 14% on the left with a supra–12th rib approach. These rates are higher than those noted clinically, with reported rates ranging from 3.3% to 15.3% for supracostal approaches, although one series did report hydrothorax in three of four cases performed with supra–11th rib access.[59-61]

Munver and colleagues[62] analyzed their experience with supracostal access for PRS. Of 300 total access tracts, 98 (32.6%) were supracostal, and of these 73.5% were supra–12th rib and 26.5% were supra–11th rib. The overall complication rate for supracostal access was 16.3% (supra–11th rib, 34.6%; supra–12th rib, 9.7%), significantly higher than the rate of 4.5% for subcostal approach in the same series. Seven of the 8 intrathoracic complications in this report occurred during supracostal access, including 6 complications during supra–11th rib access.

In a more recent series, Lojanapiwat and Prasopsuk[61] reported a significantly greater incidence of hydrothorax with supra–12th rib access than with subcostal access (15.3% versus 1.4%). A working sheath should be used with a supracostal approach to provide a barrier to the influx of fluid and air into the pleural cavity if the parietal pleura is violated. Routine intraoperative chest fluoroscopy is recommended at the termination of PRS to evaluate for obvious hydrothorax or pneumothorax, and routine postoperative chest radiography is not required if results of fluoroscopy are normal and the

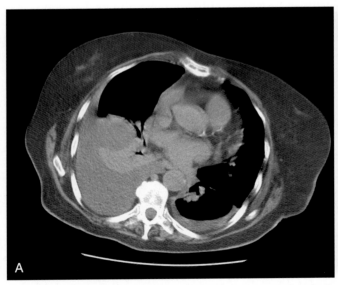
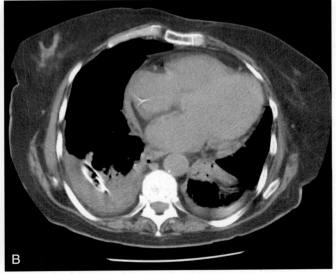

Figure 27-5 Hydrothorax. **A,** Chest CT scan demonstrates right hydrothorax. **B,** Hydrothorax was managed with tube thoracostomy. *(Courtesy of Dr. Dean Assimos.)*

patient has no signs of pulmonary compromise.[66] Preoperative CT imaging during expiratory and inspiratory phases with coronal, sagittal and three-dimensional reformats may be used in preoperative planning of access tracts to avoid intrathoracic complications.[67]

Patients with small-volume, asymptomatic hydrothorax or pneumothorax can be observed. When patients exhibit signs of pulmonary compromise or become unstable, aspiration or tube thoracostomy may be required. In cases of PRS for struvite stones, if hydrothorax occurs, it is prudent to place a chest tube to prevent development of empyema from potentially infected irrigation fluid and urine. Rarely, thoracoscopy or formal thoracotomy may be required if the foregoing interventions fail or if complex pleural effusion or empyema develops.

Nephropleural fistula can manifest intraoperatively, immediately postoperatively, or ≤1 to 2 weeks postoperatively. In the immediate postoperative period, this complication should be suspected if thoracic fluid persists despite tube thoracostomy drainage. Delayed nephropleural fistula should be suspected in patients who have undergone PRS and who present with shortness of breath with or without flank pain. The diagnosis is best made with retrograde pyelography. Treatment consists of draining the pleural fluid with tube thoracostomy and decompressing the collecting system with a ureteral stent.[64]

The intercostal vessels can be lacerated during supracostal access, with resulting hemothorax. Tube thoracostomy and open surgical thoracotomy may be necessary if this complication occurs. To minimize the risk, access should be obtained directly above the rib to avoid the intercostal vessels.

Colon

Colonic perforation is a rare complication of PRS, reported in <1% of cases.[30,32,68-70] The likely reason for this low incidence is that the colon is rarely retrorenal. Hadar and Gadoth[71] and Sherman and colleagues[72] analyzed the relationship of the kidney and colon on CT scan and found that the colon was retrorenal in approximately 0.6% of individuals. Patients at higher risk for colonic injury include those with congenital anomalies such as horseshoe kidney and other forms of renal fusion and ectopia, as well as those with colonic distention resulting from jejunoileal bypass, partial ileal bypass, neurologic impairment, and "institutional" bowel. Other proposed risk factors are lower pole puncture, left-sided procedure, previous colonic surgery, older age, and female sex.[68,73] El-Nahas and associates[69] reviewed their experience with 5039 PCNL procedures to try and identify risk factors for colonic perforation. These investigators reported 15 colonic perforations (0.3%). The only significant risk factors identified on multivariate analysis were older patient age and the presence of horseshoe kidney. Preoperative CT scan should be considered in patients at high risk, to detect the presence of a retrorenal colon, and CT guidance can be used to direct percutaneous access in these patients.[74]

Early recognition and diagnosis of colonic perforation are of critical importance. Serious infectious complications can occur when diagnosis or management is delayed. Signs of colonic perforation include passage of gas or feculent material through or around the nephrostomy tube, intraoperative diarrhea or hematochezia, and peritonitis.[68,69,73,75] These patients usually present with fever. Patients can present after the nephrostomy tube is removed with feculent material draining from the nephrostomy site.[76] Some investigators recommend antegrade nephrostogram at the end of the procedure to evaluate for colonic perforation.[69]

In the majority of cases, colon injuries can be managed conservatively if the perforation is retroperitoneal and the patient does not have signs of sepsis or peritonitis (**Fig. 27-6**).[69,77] An indwelling ureteral stent and Foley catheter should be placed and the nephrostomy tube should be pulled back into the colon. The patient should be administered broad-spectrum antibiotics and placed on a low-residue diet. A contrast study should be performed through the colostomy tube in 7 to 10 days, and the tube should be removed if no evidence of nephrocolic fistula is noted.[78,79] Open surgical management is required in patients with transperitoneal perforation, peritonitis, or sepsis and in those in whom conservative management has failed. Delay in diagnosis may increase the need for open surgical management.[69]

Small Intestine

The second and third portions of the duodenum are adjacent to the lower pole and pelvis of the right kidney and may be injured during PRS, although this complication is very uncommon.[80] Such an injury may occur if the renal pelvis is perforated during dilation, during placement of the working sheath, or during stone removal or tumor excision. This complication should be suspected if intestinal mucosa and contents are visualized, and it is usually diagnosed when contrast material is seen in the duodenum during intraoperative or postoperative nephrostogram. Surgical exploration is required in cases of large perforations or in patients with signs of sepsis or peritonitis. Patients with small injuries who are clinically stable can be managed conservatively. Conservative management includes antibiotics, nasogastric suction, and parenteral hyperalimentation. The nephrostomy tube should be positioned correctly in the collecting system to ensure adequate drainage. A nephrostogram and an upper gastrointestinal radiograph study are performed 10 to 14 days following the injury to assess for closure of the fistula.

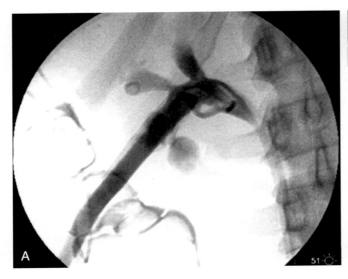

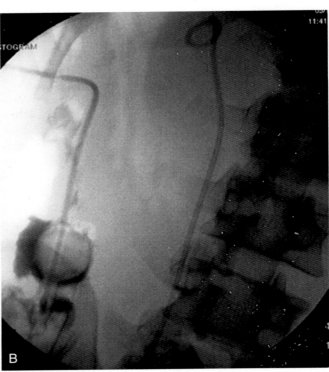

Figure 27-6 Colon injury. **A,** Postoperative nephrostogram demonstrates contrast within the large intestine. **B,** The nephrostomy tube was removed, and colon tube was placed in addition to an indwelling ureteral stent and Foley catheter. The patient healed without complications, and the colon tube was removed 7 days later, when a cologram confirmed no evidence of fistula.

Liver, Gallbladder, and Spleen

The liver is rarely injured during PRS. Hopper and Yakes[65] studied the relationship between the liver and kidney and reported on the risk of liver injury with different access approaches. These investigators reported that the risk of injury with an 11th-12th rib intercostal approach was minimal. The risk increased to 14% for a 10th-11th rib approach during inspiration. Hepatomegaly increases the risk of injury to the liver, and for these patients preoperative CT imaging should be obtained and CT-guided access should be considered to minimize this risk. If injury to the liver is diagnosed postoperatively, the nephrostomy tube should be left in place for 7 to 10 days to allow for maturation of the tract. After this time, the tube can be carefully removed, but if high-volume bleeding is noted, the tube should be reinserted immediately. Retrograde placement of an internalized ureteral stent at the time of nephrostomy tube removal may aid in preventing the development of a renobiliary fistula. Injury to the gallbladder can also occur during access. Patients may present with signs of peritonitis, and treatment consists of cholecystectomy.[81]

Splenic injury is very uncommon during PRS, likely because of the spleen's cephalad position.[82,83] Hopper and Yakes[65] also analyzed the relationship between the kidney and spleen and noted that the spleen should not be at risk of being traversed with an 11th-12th rib supracostal approach during expiration, but the risk during inspiration was 13%. This risk increased to 33% when a 10th-11th rib approach was used. In patients with splenomegaly, the risk is even higher, and CT imaging should be performed preoperatively to aid in the planning and obtaining of safe access. Injury to the spleen can cause significant internal bleeding and in some cases hypovolemic shock. The diagnosis is established with CT or US. Although some patients with splenic laceration can be managed nonoperatively, most patients require splenectomy.[1,2,83]

Lymphatics

Perforation of the collecting system during PRS may cause disruption of adjacent lymphatics that could lead to chyluria.[84] Management of this complication consists of optimizing urinary drainage and maintaining the patient with total parental hyperalimentation until the chyluria resolves. Somatostatin may aid in the treatment of these cases.[85] For refractory cases, renal pedicle lymphatic ligation can be performed.[86,87]

MEDICAL COMPLICATIONS

Infection and Sepsis

It is mandatory for all patients with urinary tract infections to be treated with the appropriate antibiotic therapy before they undergo PRS because of the risk of bacteremia and sepsis from the extravasation of bacteria into the pyelovenous or pyelolymphatic channels. Antibiotic therapy for patients with urinary tract infections should be initiated at least 1 week before the procedure. The use of prophylactic antibiotics in patients with sterile urine culture is controversial. Mariappan and associates[88] reported on the use of prophylactic antibiotics in patients with stones >2 cm or pelvicalyceal dilation with negative urine cultures. These investigators found that in these patients, prophylaxis with 1 week of ciprofloxacin significantly decreased the risk of urosepsis after PRS. Another study comparing patients with negative preoperative urine culture who received either single-dose antibiotics in the operating room or continuation of antibiotics until the nephrostomy tube was removed found no difference in rates of postoperative fever, bacteriuria, or bacteremia.[89]

Negative preoperative urine cultures do not preclude patients from developing bacteremia or urosepsis. Rao and colleagues[90] demonstrated that patients without bacteriuria may still develop bacteremia and endotoxemia. This is likely because negative urine culture results do not predict negative pelvic urine or stone culture results. Margel and colleagues[91] found that 25% of patients with a negative urine culture result had a positive stone culture result. In these patients, the most common organisms found in the stone culture were gram-positive organisms; *Enterococcus* was reported in 42% of the cultures. In another study, Mariappan and colleagues[92] found that bladder urine culture results were positive in only 5.6% of patients, whereas 42.6% of patients had positive results of pelvic urine or stone cultures. These investigators also found that positive results of pelvic urine and stone cultures were associated with a significantly greater risk for urosepsis than were positive results of bladder urine cultures. It is important to send renal pelvis urine and stone for culture during PCNL, to help predict and guide therapy in the event of urosepsis.

Purulent urine may be unexpectedly encountered at the time of accessing the collecting system. When this occurs, it is sensible to delay treatment, leave a nephrostomy tube in place to drain the collecting system, culture the fluid, and give the patient appropriate antibiotic therapy. Even with these precautions, patients can still develop urosepsis when the stone is eventually treated.[93]

Sepsis has been reported in 0.6% to 1.5% of patients undergoing percutaneous stone removal.[1,2,32] These patients should be aggressively managed with antibiotic therapy and fluid resuscitation, as well as with other supportive measures such as steroids and pressors. If the patient does not respond to these measures, CT imaging is recommended to assess for injury to adjacent structures or other complications that could be contributing to the sepsis. Fungal urosepsis should be considered in patients who are at risk, such as those who are immunocompromised or diabetic or who have had prolonged ureteral stenting.[94]

Fluid Overload

Irrigating fluid can be absorbed during PRS. Collecting system perforation and bleeding have been shown to increase the amount of fluid absorbed significantly.[95] Careful intraoperative monitoring of the input and output of irrigating fluid can help detect this problem. Signs of fluid absorption and subsequent fluid overload include unexpected hypertension and hypoxemia. Fluid absorption can be minimized by maintaining the lowest irrigation pressure that permits visibility. The use of a working sheath can reduce pressure in the pelvicaliceal system and thereby can reduce fluid absorption.[95] Limiting the duration of the procedure and discontinuing the procedure in the setting of significant collecting system perforation also reduce this complication. Normal saline solution should be used as an irrigant whenever possible to limit the development of hyponatremia. The administration of diuretics may be required for managing the hypervolemic patient with signs of fluid overload.

Hypothermia

Core body temperature has been shown to decrease during PRS. *Hypothermia,* defined as core body temperature <36°C, may occur. Decrease in core body temperature is multifactorial, and causes include vasodilation secondary to anesthesia, length of the procedure, exposed body surface, low room temperature, and the use of room temperature or cold irrigant. The consequences of hypothermia include impaired platelet function, altered enzymatic drug clearance, and shivering leading to significantly increased oxygen consumption. Increased oxygen consumption combined with decreased oxygen delivery can lead to cardiac ischemia or arrhythmias. Measures such as the use of warmed irrigant, proper patient coverage, use of heat-preserving drapes, and keeping patients as dry as possible can help reduce the risk of hypothermia.[96]

Positioning-related Injuries

Proper positioning of patients undergoing PRS is essential. Patients are typically placed in the prone position, and injuries to the brachial plexus and other peripheral nerves, shoulder dislocation, and cutaneous skin trauma can occur. All pressure points should be padded and patients should be positioned to avoid strain on joints. If neurapraxia is suspected, prompt neurologic evaluation is warranted. Most of these injuries resolve over time with conservative treatment such as physical therapy.

Some groups have advocated that PCNL should be performed with patients in the supine position.[97,98] One concern of performing PRS in the supine position is the potential increased risk of damaging adjacent organs, particularly the colon. Ng and colleagues[97] reported on 62 patients who had PCNL in the supine position and found no complications related to positioning. Manohar and colleagues[98] demonstrated that the supine position can be used safely and effectively in obese and high-risk patients for PCNL. US proved to be useful in aiding in and obtaining access in these reports.

Air Embolism

Air embolism has been reported during PRS.[99,100] This complication can occur after air is injected into the collecting system to help delineate the anatomy or as a result of airflow reversal in an ultrasonic lithotripter. Intraoperative signs of air embolism include hypoxemia, bradycardia, and even cardiopulmonary arrest. Other causes should be excluded. Management includes placing the patient in the left lateral decubitus position with the head and thorax tilted downward. A central venous access line can be placed to attempt to aspirate the air. Postoperatively, one case of complete blindness and symptoms consistent with stroke was reported. This patient was managed successfully with hyperbaric oxygen treatment with complete resolution of his symptoms.[100]

Deep Vein Thrombosis and Pulmonary Embolism

Deep vein thrombosis has been reported to occur in 1% to 3% of patients undergoing PRS.[32,101] Thromboembolic disease prevention stockings and sequential compression devices help to minimize the risk of deep vein thrombosis. Early postoperative ambulation should be encouraged to help decrease the risk as well. If postoperative deep vein thrombosis does occur, treatment is aimed at preventing propagation of the thrombus and embolic events.[102] Treatment usually consists of anticoagulation, although in the immediate postoperative period bleeding is often a concern. In these patients, an inferior vena cava filter may need to be placed. However, in patients with a mature nephrostomy tract, anticoagulation is usually well tolerated.

Mortality

Postoperative death is extremely rare in association of PRS. The mortality rate is reported to be 0.2%.[103] Most reported deaths were caused by myocardial infarction or pulmonary embolism, and this complication occurred in high-risk patients. Careful preoperative evaluation and patient preparation are critical to preventing mortality. In patients who are at high risk, intraoperative invasive monitoring and postoperative cardiac monitoring can help prevent mortality.

Loss of Renal Function

The effects on renal function from PRS are believed to be minimal. Reports of imaging studies before and after PRS have demonstrated small parenchymal scars at the tract site.[104,105] Chatham and colleagues[106] evaluated patients before and after PCNL with technetium-99m mercaptoacetyltriglycine nuclear renography. These investigators demonstrated stable or improved renal function in 84% of patients and deterioration of function in 16%. Handa and associates[107] found a significant increase in serum creatinine of 0.14 mg/dL 1 day after PRS. However, Yaycioglu and colleagues[108] demonstrated no significant change in creatinine concentration at a mean follow-up of 15.6 months after PNL in patients with normal and impaired renal function. Using nuclear renography, Dawaba and colleagues[109] evaluated renal function in children undergoing PCNL and found a stable selective glomerular filtration rate in 52.8% of renal units, an increase in glomerular filtration rate in 41.7% of renal units, and a decrease in glomerular filtration rate in 5.6% of renal units. Urivetsky and colleagues[105] demonstrated that no change in urinary enzyme activity before and after PCNL.

Patients with staghorn calculi are unique in their increased risk of renal function deterioration. Teichman and colleagues[110] reported that 25% of patients with staghorn calculi treated with PCNL had a decrease in renal function. These investigators cited solitary kidney, recurrent calculi, hypertension, complete staghorn calculus, urinary diversion, and neurogenic bladders as further risk factors for functional deterioration in this group. These findings support the idea that the functional deterioration in this group of patients is not likely to be procedurally related, but rather the result of their stone disease and comorbidities.

Acute renal loss is very uncommon following PRS. It is usually secondary to uncontrollable hemorrhage. The incidence has been reported to be between 0.1% and 0.3%.[32,111] The long-term risk of renal loss has been estimated to be 1.6% in patients who have had staghorn calculus treated with PCNL.[112]

CONCLUSION

PRS is associated with a variety of complications. These include, but are not limited to, hemorrhage, injury to the collecting system and kidney, injury to adjacent organs, infection or sepsis, and even death. Proper patient selection and appropriate preoperative workup can help minimize these complications. Surgical technique plays a large role in preventing complications, and care must be taken during each step of the procedure. Prompt recognition of complications when they occur is critical, and most complications can be managed conservatively.

KEY POINTS

1. Hemorrhage, the most common complication of PRS, can occur intraoperatively or postoperatively. It is usually managed conservatively.

2. In patients with delayed postoperative bleeding, one should have a high index of suspicion for an arteriovenous fistula or pseudoaneurysm. This complication can be managed conservatively in most cases, although patients in whom conservative management fails should be treated with angiography and selective embolization.

3. Perforation of the collecting system should be suspected if perirenal or renal sinus fat is visualized. When perforation is recognized, the procedure should be terminated, and a nephrostomy tube should be left in place.

4. Tumor seeding is a potential but rare complication of percutaneous resection of urothelial carcinoma. It can be minimized by proper selection of patients with low-grade, noninvasive tumors.

5. The lung and pleura are the perirenal structures at greatest risk of injury. Intraoperative fluoroscopy of the chest is recommended at the end of PRS to rule out obvious hydrothorax or pneumothorax. Postoperative chest radiography is not required unless patients develop signs of pulmonary compromise.

6. Patients at higher risk for colonic injury include older patients with congenital anomalies such as horseshoe kidneys, colon distention, or previous colon surgery. Preoperative CT imaging should be considered in these patients to detect the presence of retrorenal colon.

7. Colonic perforation is managed by retraction of the nephrostomy tube into the colon, placement of an indwelling ureteral stent and Foley catheter, use of broad-spectrum antibiotics, and institution of a low-residue diet. This approach allows healing in the majority of cases.

8. Negative preoperative urine culture results do not predict negative stone or pelvic urine culture results. Therefore, it is recommended to start patients on broad-spectrum antibiotics (i.e., fluoroquinolones) 1 week preoperatively.

9. The effects of PRS on renal function appear minimal. Many patients undergoing PCNL, particularly for staghorn calculi, have deterioration of their renal function over time, although this is likely the result of their stone disease.

REFERENCES

Please see www.expertconsult.com

COMPLICATIONS OF LAPAROSCOPIC PROCEDURES

Chapter 28

SPECIAL CONSIDERATIONS IN LAPAROSCOPY

Lee Ponsky MD
Assistant Professor, Case Western Reserve University, Cleveland, Ohio

Surena F. Matin MD
Associate Professor, University of Texas M. D. Anderson Cancer Center, Houston, Texas

Since the first laparoscopic nephrectomy was performed in 1991, the laparoscopic approach has been described for almost every urologic procedure, and in many cases it has become the standard of care.[1] In 1999, Fahlenkamp and colleagues[2] reported their review of >2400 laparoscopic cases and specifically evaluated the complications associated with these procedures. They identified a complication rate of 4.4%. The reintervention rate was 0.8%, and the mortality rate was 0.08%. These investigators also found that the complication rate increased in parallel with the difficulty of the procedure but was inversely related to the surgeon's experience.

Permpongkosol and associates[3] assessed complications associated with urologic laparoscopic surgery during a 12-year period in 2775 patients. These investigators confirmed an overall intraoperative complication rate of 4.7% and a postoperative complication rate of 17.5%. Operative reintervention occurs in <1% of patients undergoing laparoscopy, but clinical findings may be blunted and insufficient for a prompt diagnosis.[4] Imaging in patients who are acutely ill postoperatively may be necessary to determine whether exploration is required.[4] Although all surgical procedures carry their own risks and benefits, it is imperative that urologists be aware of the potential complications and considerations specific to laparoscopy.

ANESTHETIC CONSIDERATIONS

Several anesthetic considerations are specific to laparoscopy. As with most operations, complications correlate with a higher American Society of Anesthesiologists score.[3] Age alone does not seem to predict a higher risk.[3,5] Rather, the associated medical comorbidities usually define the risk, and as it happens, older patients have higher numbers of comorbidities. Permpongkosol and colleagues[3] showed that the incidence of complications at their high-volume institution plateaued in the year 2000 and remained steady thereafter. Vascular injuries were the most common type of intraoperative complications, and the overall incidence varied from 15% (laparoscopic simple nephrectomy and prostatectomy) to 41% (laparoscopic nephroureterectomy).

Pneumothorax, acidosis resulting from hypercapnia, and oliguria are among the main causes of anesthetic complications during laparoscopic surgery.[6,7] Subcutaneous emphysema is a minor complication that can often be seen with protracted procedures. This results when the insufflating gas dissects the subcutaneous tissues and causes distention and crepitus from the eyelids down to the scrotum. As long as carbon dioxide (CO_2) is the insufflating gas, and CO_2 is currently the insufflating gas of choice in nearly all cases, this subcutaneous emphysema usually resolves in ≤24 hours without sequelae.[8] No difference in CO_2 absorption appears to exist between the transperitoneal and retroperitoneal approaches, based on a prospective nonrandomization study.[9] In the absence of pneumothorax, pneumoperitoneum itself decreases the thoracic cavity space, with a resulting decrease in tidal volume and an increase in peak airway pressure. To maintain adequate minute ventilation, tidal volume or respiratory rate must be increased to compensate.[7]

Pneumoperitoneum with CO_2 can result in respiratory acidosis, particularly in patients with underlying pulmonary disease.[10,11] Several precautions are taken by the anesthesia team to prevent or at least minimize respiratory acidosis, including increasing minute ventilation and using intravenous rather than inhaled anesthetics. Intraoperative end-tidal CO_2 and arterial blood gasses are monitored closely. If necessary, minimizing insufflation pressure is another step the surgical team can take to minimize acidosis.

Oliguria is seen regularly during laparoscopic surgery, but this condition reverses soon after desufflation.[12-14] The cause appears to be multifactorial, with increased parenchymal, vascular, and intra-abdominal pressure producing a measurable decrease in renal blood flow and venous return to the heart. These changes are temporary and do not cause renal tubular damage.[14-16] Probably the most serious problem with laparoscopy-associated oliguria in a stable patient is failure of recognition and overtreatment with fluids that leads to fluid overload.

Laparoscopy and associated pneumoperitoneum can result in pneumothorax and pneumomediastinum.[17] These complications can be life-threatening in cases of tension pneumothorax or pericardial tamponade. If either of these situations is suspected, immediate desufflation of the pneumoperitoneum is indicated. Because of the rapid solubility of CO_2, the condition usually resolves promptly. If symptoms persist or if the patient is clinically unstable, thoracostomy or pericardiocentesis may be required.

Occasionally, intentional pneumothorax is created such as during resection of locally invasive renal tumors or when a severe desmoplastic reaction is present.[18] In these cases, as long as the patient remains clinically stable, it is reasonable to complete the procedure laparoscopically. Communication with the anesthetic team is paramount so if any sudden changes are detected, the pneumoperitoneum can be decreased immediately. Repair of the diaphragmatic defect can then be performed, and the CO_2 can be evacuated. Because of the rapid absorption of CO_2, any chest tubes that are placed can usually be removed soon, as long as no air leak is detected.

Venous gas embolism is a rare but potentially fatal complication of laparoscopy that can occur even during initial access before any instruments are inserted.[19] The positive pressure of the CO_2 pneumoperitoneum results in gas entry into the venous system. Clinically, the patient can develop rapid-onset hypotension followed by cardiovascular collapse. This condition may result in the auscultation of the characteristic "mill-wheel" murmur, which is one of those complications requiring rapid coordination and communication with the entire team to recognize promptly and manage appropriately. The surgical team should immediately desufflate the pneumoperitoneum, and both teams should help place the patient in the Trendelenburg, left lateral decubitus position. This positioning will help mobilize the gas embolism into the right ventricle. A central venous catheter can then be placed and used to attempt aspiration of the embolus. Because CO_2 is very soluble in blood, rapid absorption usually occurs.

POSITIONING AND NEUROMUSCULAR INJURIES

Neuromuscular injuries are not specific to laparoscopy. However, the laparoscopic surgeon must be aware of the potential for injuries to occur as a result of patient positioning required for certain laparoscopic approaches. The use of copious padding should go without saying,

but these injuries can occur despite the use of proper padding. Neuromuscular injuries are among the most commonly reported complications after laparoscopic urologic surgery.[20] The brachial plexus and ulnar and median nerves are the upper extremity nerves most commonly at risk. The femoral, obturator, and peroneal nerves are the most common lower extremity nerves at risk of injury resulting from positioning. The patient may complain of pain, numbness, tingling, or decreased strength as a result of the injured nerve.[21-23] Appropriate padding and avoidance of stretching or compression of nerves can help to minimize injuries. The surgeon must know which positions may place the patient's limbs on stretch or at increased pressure points. For example, patients placed in the lithotomy position with abduction of the lower limbs should have concomitant hip flexion to decrease the risk for perioperative neuropathy of the obturator nerve.[21]

Extreme body habitus, either thinness or obesity, and smoking during the perioperative period seem to promote neuropathy despite adequate positioning.[22] Moreover, as the operative time increases, so does the risk of neuromuscular injury.[23] Early recognition of the injury and of initiation of physical therapy are important in the recovery of patients with these neuromuscular injuries. Both the patient and the physician need to be aware of the potentially prolonged course of recovery in these cases.

Of all the possible neuromuscular injuries, rhabdomyolysis is the most serious because it can lead to renal failure.[24] *Rhabdomyolysis* results from prolonged pressure to skeletal muscles leading to muscle ischemia, edema, compartment syndrome, and subsequent muscle necrosis. The tissue necrosis causes metabolic acidosis, and myoglobin is released from the necrotic muscle. The high levels of myoglobinemia can cause renal tubular obstruction with subsequent acute renal failure requiring temporary or even long-term dialysis. Rapid diagnosis is essential for the prompt treatment of this potentially serious complication. The patient may complain of severe pain immediately postoperatively in the area of ischemia, such as the legs, or in the dependent flank and gluteal area for patients in the lateral decubitus position.[25] The patient's urine may be dark and may look like hematuria, which is usually the first sign of rhabdomyolysis. If this condition is suspected clinically, the urine should be tested for myoglobin, the serum should be tested for creatine phosphokinase, and the arterial blood gas should be evaluated for metabolic acidosis.

As soon as rhabdomyolysis is suspected, aggressive hydration, diuresis, and urinary alkalization should be initiated. It is critical to monitor the patient's serum electrolytes actively, including creatinine and potassium, to ensure adequate renal function because hemodialysis may be indicated. Patient-related factors often associated with rhabdomyolysis are a high body mass index and a thick muscular build. Associated technical factors include prolonged operative time, the lateral decubitus position, and use of the kidney rest.[24-27]

Wolf and colleagues[24] published results of a multi-institutional survey evaluating neuromuscular injuries during laparoscopy. The study identified neuromuscular injuries in 2.7% of cases. Patients who developed rhabdomyolysis were significantly heavier (91 versus 80 kg) and underwent longer procedures (379 versus 300 minutes). The investigators concluded that abdominal wall neuralgias, peripheral nerve injuries, and joint or back injuries occur no more frequently during laparoscopy than during open surgery; however, the risk of rhabdomyolysis may be increased during laparoscopy. These investigators recommended positioning patients in a partial rather than a full flank position to reduce the risk of some of the associated injuries. Other surgeons have also suggested eliminating or minimizing the use of the kidney bridge altogether.[26,28] Use of the kidney bridge results in significant hemodynamic changes independent of table flexion, as well as causing undue pressure to the dependent paraspinal and gluteal musculature.[27] Surgeons themselves are not immune from neuromuscular symptoms as a result of their own body positioning during laparoscopic surgery.[24]

ACCESS INJURIES

Achieving access to the target area for laparoscopic procedures can be a source of both minor and life-threatening injuries. With Veress needle access, the access needle is inserted blindly, and this maneuver can result in injury to any of the abdominal structures. In one study, this procedure accounted for ≤18% of the reported injuries.[29] Most access-related injuries involve either the visceral or vascular organs or a combination. With the Veress needle, appropriate use and placement are imperative to help minimize access injuries. The Veress needle should be checked to ensure that the spring-loaded blunt center of the needle retracts as intended. The surgeon should brace his or her hand on the patient while advancing the needle to avoid inadvertently advancing the needle too far. Once the Veress needle is advanced and is felt to be in an appropriate position, safety checks should be done routinely to assess appropriate positioning before proceeding to the next step. If a safety check fails, one should not proceed to the next step. The access needle should be aspirated first to ensure absence of blood or succus. A small amount (≈1-2 mL) of sterile fluid can be injected through the access needle and should flow freely into the abdomen. When the syringe is removed, the fluid in the needle should immediately drop down to confirm good placement.

Alternatively, a "drop-test" is used to help confirm intraperitoneal placement. This test is done with a small amount of saline solution or water placed in the access needle. If appropriate intraperitoneal placement has been achieved, the fluid should quickly drop into the abdominal cavity. Insufflation can then begin. Immediate insufflation pressure should not generally exceed 7 to 8 mm Hg at a low flow. This is a higher than normal peritoneal pressure resulting from the resistance created by the thin Veress needle. Because of the high-capacity, low-pressure nature of the peritoneal cavity, the intra-abdominal pressure should remain low as gas insufflates. In addition, visual evaluation of gas distribution is important to ensure proper placement, as well as percussion of the abdomen in all quadrants to confirm symmetric tympani. Uneven distribution of gas indicates preperitoneal placement. Access obtained in the midline or just off midline poses risk of injury to the great vessels, which in a thin patient may be <1 inch below the umbilicus.[30]

Umbilical access risks placement of the needle or trocar into the aorta, right common iliac artery, or left common iliac vein (**Fig. 28-1**). In this location, the needle or port is angled 45 degrees craniocaudally to avoid these structures and to aim into the pelvis. Using imaging-based positional anatomy, investigators have shown that the anterior superior iliac spine (ASIS) may be a more reliable indicator than the umbilicus for the aortic bifurcation, which is located 4.8 ± 1.6 cm above the ASIS plane.[31] Thus, access done at the level of the ASIS with an angle of insertion of approximately 45 degrees in the sagittal plane should avoid the aortic and vena caval bifurcation. In obese patients, this angle may need to be reduced slightly to avoid the more

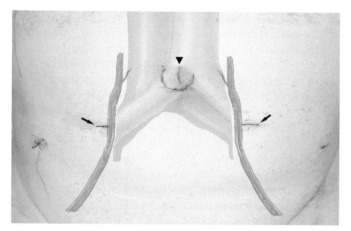

Figure 28-1 The location of the major abdominal vessels and of the inferior epigastric vessels in relation to surface landmarks is shown in a photograph of a patient with the superimposed course of vessels. The umbilicus (*arrowhead*) acts as a superficial landmark for the aortic and vena caval bifurcation. Direct entry at 0 to 30 degrees in the sagittal plane by a needle or trocar creates a high risk of puncturing the aorta, right common iliac artery, or the left common iliac vein. The inferior epigastric vessels take an ascending course medially and eventually travel in the substance of the rectus muscle. A port placed at or just below the umbilicus at the paramedian location (*arrows*), such as is frequently done during pelvic cases (e.g., laparoscopic prostatectomy), poses a higher risk of causing injury to these vessels. (*Copyright S. F. Matin, 2007.*)

copious preperitoneal fat. Based on the same measurements, the ideal location of paramedian ports is also at the level of the ASIS, but >6 cm from the midline to avoid the epigastric vessels.[31]

If blood or succus material is evident from the initial aspiration, the Veress needle should be held in place. The anesthesia team should be notified if major vascular injury is suspected. If the patient is stable and no evidence of active bleeding is present, an alternate site can be used to obtain access to the abdomen. The initial needle is not removed because it can help control any potential bleeding and will help the surgeon identify the site of and degree of injury. When an alternate site is used to obtain access, care should be taken to not overinsufflate the abdomen because this maneuver can raise the abdominal wall and thus lift the initial access needle away from the area of injury, which can often be extremely difficult to identify later.

Deciding to convert to an open approach is not considered a complication, whereas not converting to an open approach in a timely fashion can exacerbate complications. In most cases, except with major vascular injuries, Veress needle injuries usually heal with conservative management, whereas trocar injuries generally require formal repair. Any gross spillage of bowel content requires repair. Vascular and visceral injuries may be worse than initially appreciated laparoscopically. Through-and-through injuries may occur that include the back wall of the vessel or bowel and that may not be appreciated laparoscopically.[29] Bowel and retroperitoneal vascular injuries comprise 76% of all injuries sustained during primary access.[29] The retroperitoneal approach is associated with less visceral injury than is the transabdominal approach, but it does not eliminate this possibility.[2] Not all visceral injuries are identified or suspected at the time of injury, as a result of peristalsis, retraction, and failure to appreciate the possibility of an injury.[29] Postoperatively, if the patient has persistent pain, drainage from a trocar site, fever, or peritoneal signs, or a combination of these, a high index of suspicion for visceral injury should be considered. Rapid radiographic evaluation and surgical exploration are essential because delay in diagnosis is a significant independent predictor of mortality.[29]

In addition to the steps outlined in Box 28-1, several other precautions can be taken to minimize the risk of injury during initial access. These include inspection and palpation of the abdomen before placing ports, with avoidance of prior scars or palpable masses (including aneurysms). Placement of a nasal or oral gastric tube and Foley catheter before obtaining access may help to minimize hollow organ injuries. Consider the Hasson technique whenever concern exists about injury, particularly vascular access injury, as well as in very thin patients or if prior scars are present. Access should be obtained away from the quadrant with scars. Once the first port is placed and the abdomen is insufflated, addi-

---

BOX 28-1 | **Factors Facilitating Safe Placement of Trocars During Laparoscopic Surgery**

Surgeon experience
Low table height
Noting of anatomic landmarks and abdominal scars
Adequate skin incision size for trocar
Application of appropriate axial force during trocar insertion
Use of the Trendelenburg position (for umbilical access)
Elevation or stabilization of abdominal wall
Transillumination of abdominal wall vessels
Avoidance of lateral deviation of needle or trocar
Avoidance of angling of needle or trocar toward the midline

Data from Chandler JG, Corson SL, Way LW. Three spectra of laparoscopic entry access injuries. *J Am Coll Surg.* 2001;192(4):478-490; and Philips PA, Amaral JF. Abdominal access complications in laparoscopic surgery. *J Am Coll Surg.* 2001;192(4):525-536.

---

tional ports should be placed under direct vision. Transillumination of the abdominal wall by the laparoscope can help avoid injury to abdominal wall vessels.[30] Vascular injuries are sometimes noted after insertion of the laparoscope with the finding of intraperitoneal blood or a retroperitoneal hematoma. Specific injuries to vascular and organ structures are discussed later in this chapter.

The current availability of optical, blunt-tip, and radially dilating trocars has lowered the incidence of vascular and bowel injuries during access as well as port site hernias.[32,33] Some surgeons find optical access trocars to be very safe and even use them without establishing pneumoperitoneum, whereas others continue to insufflate the abdomen before trocar insertion.[34,35] However, uninsufflated midline optical access should not be done, as the visual landmarks are not reliably seen in the midline. Uninsufflated optical access, if done, should be performed laterally such that the individual abdominal muscular layers can be identified during placement, thus ensuring safety. Adequate knowledge of prevention factors remains critical; these tools are only as safe as the person holding them. No absolutely safe method for laparoscopic access exists because all forms (e.g., Veress, Hasson, optical, blunt, with pneumoperitoneum, without pneumoperitoneum) have been associated with complications.[29,30] Each method requires knowledge of its limitations and possible pitfalls, particularly when great vessels are at risk, such as with midline or just off–midline insertion, in thin or very obese patients, or in patients with prior abdominal sepsis.[29,36] Prompt recognition of vascular injury during access is obviously critical. Rapid identification of bowel injury is likely important because delayed diagnosis is associated with a significantly higher rate of mortality.[29,36]

VASCULAR INJURIES

Vascular injuries are the most common injuries occurring during urologic laparoscopy. These complications are most often related to either access injuries (discussed earlier) or dissection injuries. Bleeding resulting from injury to an abdominal wall vessel is not an uncommon cause of bleeding during laparoscopy. This injury is often noticed when blood drips into the abdomen from a trocar site or from around the trocar at the skin level. It may not be noted until after the trocar is removed, hence the rationale for removing ports under direct vision during laparoscopic exit. This type of injury typically occurs to the inferior epigastric vessels (see Fig. 28-1) during pelvic surgery.[31,37,38]

Our practice is to look laparoscopically before these ports are placed to try to identify pulsations of the epigastric vessels, which are sometimes visible intracorporeally, even in obese patients. We then use a finder needle through the proposed port tract. If the vessels happen to become punctured, this becomes evident, and bleeding will be limited and minimal once the needle is withdrawn. That location is then identified as a poor site for trocar placement. If no bleeding occurs during passage of the needle, a local anesthetic is infiltrated and the port is placed in the exact location and angle. If the epigastric arteries are injured, electrocautery is usually not successful in controlling the bleeding. Suture ligation, with a Keith, Stamey, or Carter-Thomasson needle, is often needed to control this type of bleeding. Temporary control can be obtained by tamponading the bleeding by torquing the trocar against the abdominal wall.[30]

A balloon port or Foley catheter can also be used temporarily to tamponade the bleeding until the completion of the procedure and subsequent formal control with suture ligation.[29,30] Delayed hemorrhage from the epigastric vessels can result from vasospasm or temporary occlusion from the port. In these cases, management may consist of direct cut-down, exploratory laparoscopy employing the maneuvers detailed earlier, or exploratory laparotomy. In the case of a delayed presentation consistent with a large rectus sheath hematoma, cross-sectional imaging should be used before repeat exploration to assess the size and extension of the hematoma. Angiographic embolization can be considered in cases of large rectus sheath hematoma because the bleeding site may be difficult to identify by direct cut-down or laparoscopy.

Injury to the superior mesenteric artery (SMA) is a dire complication of left-sided nephrectomy with open or laparoscopic surgery.[39-44] This complication commonly occurs if the anatomic features are distorted by prior surgery, adenopathy, or particularly large tumors that push medially or have an anterior shelf obstructing the renal vein such that the SMA is mistaken for the left renal artery.[43,44] The SMA sometimes has its origin off midline or takes a sharp turn toward the left, thus putting it in closer proximity to the kidney and renal hilum than is expected (**Fig. 28-2**).

The most common complaint from acute occlusion of the mesenteric artery is extreme epigastric abdominal

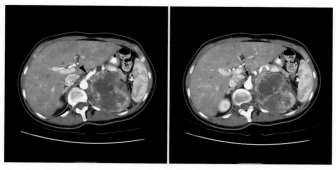

Figure 28-2 Abdominal CT of a patient showing a large left renal mass demonstrating the proximity of the celiac axis (*arrowhead*) as well as the superior mesenteric artery (*arrow*) to the renal mass. (*Copyright S. F. Matin, 2007; used with permission.*)

pain, but this could be blunted in the postoperative patient.[45] Other clinical signs include tachycardia and a low urine output resulting from hypovolemia from fluid sequestration into bowel and peritoneum. Fever may not be present until late into the course.[45] Laboratory studies include a blood gas determination for metabolic acidosis, which is nearly always present, and serum amylase and creatine phosphokinase concentrations, which are elevated late in the course.[45] Plain radiographs are nondiagnostic but with careful inspection may reveal so-called thumb-printing of bowel from mucosal edema.[45] Duplex ultrasound is suboptimal in these cases because residual pneumoperitoneum and subcutaneous emphysema degrade the ultrasound image.

Complete laceration or ligation of the SMA requires surgical correction with primary suture repair or graft interposition. The treatment of choice is primary anastomosis.[43,45,46] In cases of an incomplete ligation or incomplete injury such as can occur with an intimal tear resulting from aggressive traction, exploratory surgery may not readily identify the injury if no damage is visible. Immediate arteriography may be more helpful because it can show whether the anatomic features are intact and the SMA is patent.[45] If the patient has an incomplete injury with some continuity of the SMA, then angiographic stenting may be done. The patient may still require exploration with resection of any nonviable bowel.

Injury of the SMA is associated with a very high mortality rate and can be fatal, even with a timely diagnosis. One should always contemplate this potential complication before and during left nephrectomy.[41,42]

Challenges with controlling intraoperative bleeding as a result of laparoscopic dissection are unique to laparoscopy because the ability to apply pressure and pack the area may be difficult. As soon as vascular injury is recognized, the surgeon must determine whether an attempt at controlling the injury laparoscopically should be made.

If a grasper is being used for retraction in the non-dominant hand, rapid application of this instrument may provide the quickest response. If so, this instrument must be firmly anchored with the nondominant hand to avoid worsening the situation as a result of surgeon distraction. Again, communication between the surgeon and the anesthesiology team is imperative. The insufflating pneumoperitoneum pressure may be temporarily increased to 20 mm Hg to help tamponade any bleeding, but this technique also risks a gas embolus if a large opening in a vein such as the renal vein or vena cava is present. Pressure can be applied gently to the bleeding area with laparoscopic instruments, and smaller surgical sponges (4 × 18 cm) can be placed into the abdomen through 12-mm trocars to help control the hemorrhage. Using atraumatic instruments, the site of bleeding can be grasped or pressure applied to control the bleeding, and the area may need to be dissected to identify the exact source more accurately. Once the source of bleeding is identified, it can be controlled with suture ligation, clip placement, or a stapling device, depending on the location, type, and extent of injury and the surgeon's comfort with laparoscopic intracorporeal suturing. Additional trocars can be placed if more instruments may be helpful. Some surgeons place a hand-assist port in these cases to provide manual compression.

If the surgeon believes that the bleeding cannot be controlled expeditiously and appropriately by laparoscopic means, the option is to convert to an open approach. If bleeding is controlled temporarily with pressure from laparoscopic instruments and open conversion is being contemplated and the patient is stable, it is beneficial to call for any instruments that may be needed before making the incision. Pneumoperitoneum should be maintained during open conversion, and the laparoscope can remain in the abdomen to expose the abdominal wall as the incision is being made. Once the abdomen is opened and the pneumoperitoneum is lost, hemorrhage may worsen. It is essential that an open surgery set be available in the operating room in case urgent or emergency conversion is necessary. In difficult cases, it is also helpful to plan the site of incision at the beginning of the case and to prepare all areas into the sterile field should open conversion become necessary. With regard to the location of the incision for open conversion, we make it wherever the best exposure is obtained, rather than creating the most convenient incision by connecting the port sites. The priorities in this case are expediency and optimal exposure, not cosmesis.

Finally, at the end of every laparoscopic procedure, the pneumoperitoneum should be lowered for several minutes to evaluate for bleeding that may have been tamponaded by the pneumoperitoneum. We routinely eliminate the pneumoperitoneum, perform specimen extraction, close the incision, and then reinsufflate and evaluate for any fresh clots. Either method is acceptable as laparoscopic exit.

ABDOMINAL ORGAN INJURIES

Injury to any of the solid organs can occur during initial access or during laparoscopic dissection. If solid organ injury is suspected, the site should be thoroughly inspected and evaluated for the ability to manage the injury laparoscopically. The back wall of a viscous organ should be evaluated to ensure that it is not a through-and-through injury. It is not considered wrong to convert to an open surgical procedure, and depending on the surgeon's comfort with laparoscopic suturing, it may be reasonable to perform a laparoscopic repair. However, waiting too long to decide can lead to catastrophic consequences.

Puncture or minor injuries to solid organs such as the liver and spleen can often be managed with pressure and hemostatic agents. Laparoscopic argon-beam coagulation is also often helpful. Care must be taken when using the argon beam because it infuses gas very quickly (≈10 L/minute) into the peritoneum, and if the surgeon is not aware of this possibility, the insufflation pressures can reach dangerous levels and possibly result in tension pneumothorax. The pneumoperitoneum is thus vented through one of the trocars while the surgeon uses the argon beam laparoscopically.

If a splenic injury cannot be controlled through conservative measures, splenectomy may be required and can be done laparoscopically if the patient is stable and if the surgeon is comfortable with this approach. Our personal experience using thrombin-activated hemostatic agents such as gelatin matrix and oxidized cellulose has been favorable in patients with splenic injuries, given that splenectomy is rarely, if ever, necessary following the trend seen with blunt trauma.[47] The pancreas is at risk of injury when approaching the left kidney (**Fig. 28-3**). If injury to the tail of the pancreas is suspected, a drain should be placed near the area of the suspected injury, and amylase and lipase levels in the drain fluid can be followed postoperatively. Patients may require a prolonged course with bowel rest in many cases of pancreatic injury.[48]

Injury to the small or large bowel can also occur during dissection. Small punctures and lacerations can be closed primarily using intracorporeal laparoscopic suturing if the bowel has been prepared. More substantial injury may require formal resection and anastomosis. In cases of gross fecal spillage, temporary diversion is usually necessary. The posterior wall should be evaluated for a through-and-through injury. A more problematic solution may be encountered with electrosurgical injury, in which the extent of damage may not be readily apparent. Judgment should be exercised to

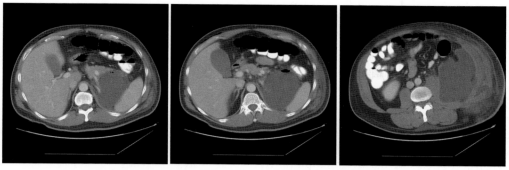

Figure 28-3 Abdominal CT of a patient presenting with abdominal pain and nausea after undergoing a difficult retroperitoneal left laparoscopic nephrectomy 1 week earlier. A large fluid collection is seen in the retroperitoneal space consistent with pancreatic fluid. (*Copyright S. F. Matin, 2007.*)

incorporate a larger area into the repair than is visually apparent. Prompt recognition of bowel injury is very important because a delay in diagnosis is associated with a higher rate of mortality.[29,36] With any major abdominal organ injury, it may be advisable to consult a general surgeon to ensure appropriate evaluation and management.

Bladder injuries should be suspected with the development of intraoperative hematuria or sudden development of gas distending the Foley drainage bag. Injuries to the bladder typically occur at midline suprapubic access locations in patients with a distended bladder or in those with a history of prior surgery.[30] If the site of injury in the bladder is not easily identified, the use of intravesical methylene blue can help to localize the site of injury. Small Veress needle injuries can often be managed conservatively with catheter drainage only, whereas larger intraperitoneal bladder injuries require formal repair in addition to bladder drainage. If any concern for ureteral injury exists, intravenous methylene blue injection or cystoscopy with stent placement can be performed. It may be necessary to place additional trocars for appropriate suture repair, and extended postoperative Foley catheter drainage may be indicated.

ELECTROSURGICAL COMPLICATIONS

Electrosurgery is arguably the single most-used surgical technique, yet it is perhaps the least understood and least appreciated by surgeons. A comprehensive review is not possible in this chapter because of space limitations, but general concepts and common types of injury are discussed.

Electrical current for medical purposes operates at frequencies of 240 kHz to 3.3 MHz, above the range where neuromuscular stimulation or electrocution occurs.[49] Electrical current can be *monopolar*, whereby the current travels from a generator, through the active electrode (i.e., handheld unit) into tissue, and out through the return electrode (i.e., grounding pad). This

BOX 28-2	Types of Electrosurgical Injury With Which the Laparoscopic Surgeon Must Be Intimately Familiar

Poor grounding pad contact
Direct organ injury
Insulation failure
Capacitative coupling

is the most common form of electrosurgery used and results in the most frequent types of electrosurgical injury. Not surprisingly, electrosurgery is one of the most common causes of litigation.[50,51] A *bipolar* circuit functions with the circuit traveling between two electrodes placed close together and the current traveling in the tissue between the electrodes. In this case, a grounding pad is not necessary. Thus, it is a potentially safer form of electrosurgery because current does not travel throughout the body, and it eliminates the risk of burns resulting from capacitative coupling or injury at the site of a poorly placed grounding pad.[49,52]

Electrosurgical injuries are listed in Box 28-2 and can result from poor grounding pad contact, direct organ contact injury, insulation failure, or capacitative coupling.[49,53] *Direct injury* occurs when an exposed metal part of the electrode unintentionally contacts tissue. This can occur if a metal portion of the active electrode is out of the field of view when the current is activated. This also occurs if the electrode tip contacts a second metal instrument and this instrument is in contact with tissue outside the field of view. It is the duty of both the surgeon and the camera operator to ensure that all active electrode surfaces are in view during the procedure and that these surfaces do not come in contact with another metal instrument during activation.

Injury caused by *insulation failure* occurs when the insulating coat of the instrument has been breached as a result of age or forceful handling or when a very high voltage of electricity is used. If the breached insulated portion is in contact with an organ when the current is activated (and frequently this portion is out of laparoscopic view), then unintended and unrecognized injury occurs. Probably the best demonstration that insulation is not an absolute barrier is capacitative coupling. *Capacitative coupling* occurs when insulation is placed between two conductors and, with enough applied voltage, a charge builds up on one conductor then travels across the insulation to the other conductor.[54] This was a greater risk when metal cannulas with plastic collars were used. Rather than the capacitatively coupled current being dispersed by the large diameter metal contact through the body wall, the plastic collar reduced the surface area, increased the current density, and resulted in a burn.

Tissue itself can become the second conductor when it comes in contact with a plastic insulator covering the electrode. Insulation failure and capacitative coupling can lead to unrecognized injury that manifests postoperatively and, particularly with bowel injury, can be life-threatening.[53,55,56] Grounding pad burns can be a particularly serious problem during radiofrequency ablation procedures, which use very high current and power settings.[57]

An important phenomenon that some surgeons and many trainees do not readily grasp is *current density*. The size of tissue or any other conductor determines the amount of heat generated. The smaller the size of the conduit, the greater is the resistance and thus the higher the heat generated. Current density is the reason tissue is heated at the electrode tip but not at the grounding pad or why serious skin burns occur when the grounding pad is not placed properly, thus resulting in less surface contact and higher current density at the grounding pad level (**Fig. 28-4**). Witness the phenomenon of current density the next time a vessel is held by forceps and a monopolar current is applied. Coagulation may not occur where the vessel is being held by the forceps but rather some distance away where the vessel diameter may be just a little smaller.

The same rationale applies when electrosurgery is used during tissue dissection. The smaller the surface contact of the electrode to the tissue, the more quickly the tissue is dissected with minimal thermal spread and dessication. Conversely, the larger the surface contact between the electrode tip and the tissue, the more slowly the tissue is dissected and the greater is the dessication. The knowledgeable surgeon dynamically manipulates these factors during surgery for safe and effective dissection. Another factor that predisposes to injury is simply the overzealous use of electrosurgery. For example, the retropubic space is a largely avascular plane requiring little to no electrosurgery, yet during robotic prostatectomy, one can frequently witness exuberant use of electrosurgery during mobilization of the bladder.

Various devices are now available to help minimize the risk of electrosurgical complications from insulation failure, including systems that detect insulation defects

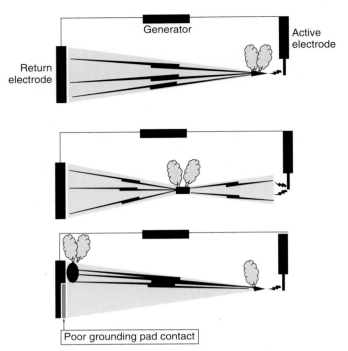

Figure 28-4 These diagrams illustrate the concept of current density, an important phenomenon to understand for both patient safety and effective electrosurgery. The tissue temperature generated is based on the following equation: Temp = $(I^2 / r^4) \times R \times t$, where I = current, r = radius of tissue, R = tissue resistance, and t = time. As can be seen from the equation, the most important determinant of where and how much heat is generated is the radius of tissue in which the current is traveling. Small changes in tissue diameter lead to large changes in the heat generated. A skilled surgeon maintains maximal current density during electrosurgery by controlling the amount of electrode contact with tissue (= radius) and, secondarily, by time. The *top panel* in this figure illustrates the ideal situation, with maximal current density at the point of active electrode contact with a minimal amount of tissue. The *middle panel* illustrates a situation in which contact is made with a larger radius of tissue, but the tissue radius becomes smaller at a point away from the intended site, thereby significantly increasing current density at that location. The same phenomenon can occur if the radius of tissue is the same but the resistance changes. Thus, tissue effects are unintentionally seen at a different location rather than at the point of electrode contact. The *bottom panel* illustrates how grounding pad burns occur when contact of the pad with tissue is poor. *(Copyright S. F. Matin, 2007.)*

and capacitative coupling.[58] Newer forms of tissue dissection hold the promise of reducing such adverse events. The ultrasonic or harmonic scalpel uses no electricity but rather depends on high-frequency mechanical friction resulting in heat and tissue dissection. Tissue sealants and hemostatic agents can also be used to aid with hemostasis. These products were reviewed by Klingler and colleagues.[56] Box 28-3 lists steps taken to minimize electrosurgical complications during laparoscopy.

MECHANICAL MALFUNCTION

Nearly all mechanical appliances can malfunction and cause a complication.[59] Clips and staplers have been the

BOX 28-3	Steps to Take to Minimize Electrosurgical Complications During Laparoscopy

1. Carefully inspect insulation covering the electrosurgical device.
2. Use the lowest possible power setting.
3. Use low-voltage, continuous ("cut") current whenever possible.
4. Use brief intermittent activation as opposed to continuous prolonged activation.
5. To dissect efficiently, make minimal contact with tissue to maximize current density and to minimize surrounding tissue damage.
6. Do not activate the electrode when it is not in contact with the intended tissue (this causes an open circuit).
7. Do not activate the electrode near or directly with another metal object.
8. Do not use hybrid metal-plastic cannula systems.
9. Use active monitoring devices to eliminate the risk of insulation failure or capacitive coupling.

Adapted from Ulmer BC. *Electrosurgical Self-Study Guide.* Boulder, CO: Clinical Education Department, Valleylab, Inc; 1997.

most notorious and obvious, because their failure is immediately recognized by the absence of hemostasis. In a survey of living donor nephrectomy, the most common hemorrhagic complication was caused by arterial bleeding, and in most of these cases, clips had a statistically worse complication of all hemorrhagic events. Nonlocking clips were the most likely to be associated with severe complications.[59] The deaths of two kidney donors were associated with the use of multiple nonlocking clips. Metal nonlocking clips are not indicated for ligation of the renal artery.[60,61] Use of the plastic locking Hem-o-Lok clips (Teleflex Medical, Markham, Ontario, Canada) has become standard for most urologists performing laparoscopic nephrectomy. Unfortunately, even this product has caused complications, although in many cases these complications were the result of poor application rather than primary mechanical dysfunction.

In 2006, Teleflex voluntarily issued a contraindication for the use of these clips specifically during laparoscopic donor nephrectomy. Because the U.S. Federal Drug Administration labeled this notification as a "recall," a short-lived panic was induced among laparoscopic surgeons.[62] This contraindication does not affect open donor nephrectomy or laparoscopic radical nephrectomy. Correct use of these locking clips includes placement of at least two clips proximally and cutting tissue to leave at least a 2- to 3-mm cuff of tissue. The locking tip should extend beyond the edge of the artery and should not pinch tissue because this can negate the locking efficacy.

Endovascular stapler failure has been reported to occur in 1% to 1.7% of cases.[63,64] What is most notable, however, is that endovascular complications are usually preventable. That all phases of instrument use are prone to problems underlies how important it is for the surgical team as well as the surgeon to understand the use of these instruments before clinical application. One of the most common preventable causes of stapler failure is application of the stapler over a previously placed clip or staple. This can cause misfiring of the staples, improper staple formation, or poor cutting of tissue.[63,64] Prompt recognition is critical to initiating steps for alternative hemostasis in these cases.

PATIENT SELECTION

The list of contraindications for laparoscopic surgery has been modified significantly over the years. Obesity, for example, used to be considered a relative contraindication to laparoscopy as these patients were found to have a higher risk of adverse events compared with nonobese patients.[65] Obese patients may in fact be at higher risk of complications because their risk is higher with open or laparoscopic surgery, but it is certainly not worsened as a result of the laparoscopic approach.[66] Certain factors, however, remain significant contraindications for surgery generally and for laparoscopic surgery specifically. These factors include uncontrolled bleeding diathesis, active infection, and bowel obstruction. A past history of peritonitis should at the least be a cause for pause and contemplation. If the peritonitis was localized (e.g., with an appendiceal abscess), then a laparoscopic approach may still be reasonable (e.g., for a left nephrectomy). If the peritonitis was generalized and diffuse, however, a laparoscopic approach may not be in the patient's best interest because of the likelihood of extensive dense adhesions. Surgery in an earlier radiated field should likewise be a cause for contemplation with regard to access and type of surgery.

CONCLUSION

Although complications can occur with any surgical procedure, awareness of laparoscopy-specific complications is imperative. Clinical findings may have a delayed presentation and in the acute setting may be insufficient for a prompt diagnosis. Specific anesthetic complications relative to laparoscopy require a surgeon's knowledge, such as pneumothorax, gas embolus, and oliguria.

Neuromuscular and positioning complications can occur as in any operation, with particular body habitus and other patient-related factors as contributors. Access complications leading to vascular, solid organ, or viscus organ injury are well recognized and require knowledge of the proper application of access instruments. No access technique is fully safe, but when appropriate precautions are implemented, these complications can be minimized.

Any organ injury requires timely management. Rapid identification of any injury with expeditious and appropriate management is essential. Failure to recognize a bowel injury can lead to potentially morbid and fatal consequences.

The knowledge of the surgeon and surgical team with regard to instruments and equipment can help to minimize endomechanical injuries. Familiarity with the principles of electrosurgery is imperative for the surgeon, but it is even more important for those surgeons working in a laparoscopic environment. The laparoscopic surgeon must be aware of patient-related factors influencing a laparoscopic approach, as well as his or her own limitations and skill level when considering an advanced procedure.

KEY POINTS

1. Careful positioning and awareness of specific neuromuscular vulnerabilities is critical to minimizing the risk of neuromuscular injuries.

2. All forms of access are associated with potential complications. The laparoscopic surgeon should be keenly aware of the limitations of whichever technique he or she routinely uses and be prepared to resort to an alternative method.

3. Always consider the potential for injury to the SMA during left-sided nephrectomy, particularly when the anatomy is distorted by tumor, lymph nodes, or prior surgery.

4. Bowel injuries require prompt diagnosis and management to minimize the risk of mortality.

5. The laparoscopic surgeon should have a good understanding of the concepts of electrosurgery, including the dynamic use of current density and the hazards of direct injury, insulation failure, and capacitative coupling.

6. All phases of instrument use are prone to problems, particularly as a result of misapplication. Knowledge of the proper use of endomechanical instruments minimizes this risk.

REFERENCES

Please see www.expertconsult.com

Chapter 29

COMPLICATIONS OF LAPAROSCOPIC RENAL SURGERY

Alon Z. Weizer MD
Assistant Professor, Department of Urology, University of Michigan, Ann Arbor, Michigan

J. Stuart Wolf Jr MD
David A. Bloom Professor of Urology, Department of Urology, University of Michigan, Ann Arbor, Michigan

Since the first report of laparoscopic radical nephrectomy in 1991 by Clayman and colleagues,[1] the indications for laparoscopic renal surgery have expanded tremendously. Although laparoscopic radical nephrectomy was initially thought to be most appropriate for benign renal disease, several series demonstrated equivalent oncologic control and safety when it and other laparoscopic procedures were compared with open radical nephrectomy with long-term follow-up.[2-4] This success, combined with improvements in surgical techniques, hemostatic agents,[5] and new devices, has prepared the way for other procedures including laparoscopic partial nephrectomy.[6,7]

Despite the benefit of reduced duration and intensity of convalescence to patients,[8] adoption of laparoscopic nephrectomy has been slow compared to adoption of laparoscopic procedures in other specialties such as laparoscopic cholecystectomy.[9] One reason cited for the slow diffusion of laparoscopic renal surgery is the lack of a common and straightforward procedure through which urologists can master basic laparoscopic skills. In addition, a burgeoning literature suggests that a large number of cases are required to achieve competence for certain laparoscopic procedures; this surgical volume may not be available to many practicing urologists.[10] Finally, several studies demonstrate that complications are significantly higher during a surgeon's early experience with laparoscopy.[11] When these factors are combined, the opportunity cost for implementing laparoscopic renal surgery for many practicing urologists appears to be too high.

The inclusion of laparoscopic experience in urology residency combined with postgraduate courses or "mini" fellowships to train practicing urologists in laparoscopic skills is likely to increase the use of laparoscopic techniques for renal surgery.[12,13] In the absence of improved hands-on training, and given that concern about complications is a major impediment to the

adoption of renal laparoscopy by practicing urologists, a greater understanding of the complications associated with laparoscopic renal surgery would be of benefit.

In this chapter, we discuss the general complications of laparoscopic renal surgery related to patient positioning, laparoscopic access, kidney mobilization, surgical closure, and postoperative recovery. In addition, we describe complications related to specific benign and malignant indications for laparoscopic renal surgery. We hope that an understanding of the identification, prevention, and management of these complications will improve the ability of practicing urologists to provide laparoscopic renal surgical procedures to their patients.

GENERAL COMPLICATIONS

Complications Related to Patient Positioning

The first reports of laparoscopic renal surgery by a transperitoneal approach described patient positioning in a full flank position with the table flexed. Subsequently, surgeons realized that such extreme positioning was not necessary for exposure, and it increased the risk of neuromuscular injuries.[14] More common now is a modified lateral decubitus position (45 rather than 90 degrees), without table flexion or elevation of the kidney rest. When a retroperitoneoscopic approach is chosen, however, a full lateral decubitus position with the kidney rest fully elevated and the operating room table maximally flexed is necessary to open up the space between the ribs and the iliac crest. The lateral decubitus position is associated with several complications.

Rhabdomyolysis

In a review of 6 case reports and 2 case series, 13 patients were reported to have developed rhabdomyolysis in association with laparoscopic nephrectomy.[15] In the setting of a solitary kidney (after laparoscopic nephrectomy), the impact of rhabdomyolysis can be profound; hemodialysis was required in 4 patients and 1 developed permanent renal insufficiency.

Rhabdomyolysis is suspected when skin changes and unusual pain of the dependent hip or thigh are noted. In severe cases, the urine may be discolored. Urine myoglobin testing is confirmatory, but early treatment is recommended based on clinical findings. Aggressive intravenous hydration and urine alkalinization can attenuate the impact of rhabdomyolysis on renal function. Orthopedic consultation to measure tissue pressures, to detect the exceptionally severe case that develops into compartment syndrome, should be considered. Preventative measures to reduce the risk of rhabdomyolysis include avoiding table flexion and ensuring that all pressure points are appropriately padded. Risk factors include male gender, muscularity or obesity, and prolonged operative times.[14,15] Given that risks appear to be additive, it may be best to avoid heavy patients early in a urologist's experience, when operative times may be prolonged.

Nerve Injuries

Other nerve injuries, including motor or sensory neuropathies, are reported in 1% to 3% of patients undergoing renal laparoscopy.[11,14,16] Brachial plexus injuries can occur if significant pressure is placed on the axilla in the full lateral decubitus position. This complication can be avoided by preventing compression of the axilla with an axillary roll placed under the upper rib cage (but not compressing the axilla). This measure is not necessary in the modified flank position (partial flank position, 45 degrees). Wrist drop and foot drop can occur when the superior hand or foot are not adequately padded. A rigid arm support attached to the operating room table is more secure than a stack of pillows in terms of supporting the wrist. Foam and pillows are adequate for padding the feet. Careful attention by all members of the operative team to proper fixation of the patient to the operating room table and to padding pressure points before initiating the surgical procedure can help prevent neuromuscular complications.

Neuropathies, usually motor, related to positioning should prompt immediate consultation with a neurologist. Sensory neuropathies are more likely related to the incisions for surgery (even the small ones for laparoscopic ports) or surgical dissection trauma to nerves coursing along the quadratus lumborum and psoas muscles (ilioinguinal, iliohypogastric, and genitofemoral nerves). Incision-related injuries may be unavoidable, but surgical dissection trauma to nerves can be reduced by attention to anatomic features. In most cases, the sensory deficits are transient. Symptomatic improvement while awaiting resolution can be provided by oral gabapentin or amitriptyline.

Other Complications

Testicular or scrotal injuries can result from positioning between the thighs. Scleral edema can develop in the dependent eye. Back or joint pain is not uncommon after a prolonged surgical procedure. Patients with preexisting musculoskeletal pain appear to be more prone to notable postoperative pain in the same locations. Finally, the dependent lung can become atelectatic during a prolonged procedure. In general, many of these complications can be avoided by reducing operative times.

Complications Related to Access and Surgical Approach

Three approaches with unique complications are commonly used to perform laparoscopic renal surgery: hand-assisted transperitoneal, standard transperitoneal, and retroperitoneal. Most studies have not shown a significant advantage of one approach over another and we use each type of access based on the anatomic features of the patient and the planned surgical procedure.[17,18]

Hand-assisted Laparoscopy

Gas Leakage Several commercially available devices can be used to allow a surgeon to use one hand to assist with laparoscopic renal surgery.[19] These devices are fixed into a 6- to 9-cm incision and create a seal around the hand by various methods that prevent loss of carbon dioxide (CO_2) to maintain insufflation. These devices can fail to seal adequately, with resulting CO_2 leak and loss of insufflation pressure and working space. Although any devices can leak as a result of physical tearing or other damage, several factors associated with surgical technique can cause persistent hand-port CO_2 leakage during the procedure.[19] Of these factors, incision size is probably the most important. Most of these devices come with a template to mark the incision, and typically the incision is made as long in centimeters as is the surgeon's glove size. This incision length needs to include both the skin and the fascial layer beneath. Ideally, the incision needs to be large enough to accommodate the surgeon's hand but small enough to prevent both dislodgment of the device during hand exchanges and gas leakage around the edges.[20] When the incision is too small, the surgeon risks neuromuscular injuries and fatigue.[21]

Vessel and Viscus Injury The midline placement of the hand-assistance device does not risk injury to abdominal wall vessels, but with a paramedian incision (as used in obese patients) or Gibson incision,[22] the risk of injury to the inferior epigastric or circumflex iliac vessels exists. Incision for the hand-assistance device (or for intact extraction) should be planned carefully if the patient has other incisions from previous procedures because ischemia to segments of the anterior abdominal wall must be considered. Another issue with placement of these devices is related to the portion that secures them to the incision. During placement of these devices, the potential exists for inadvertent entrapment of bowel or omentum. On placement of the device, check to make sure bowel has not become entrapped between the device and the abdominal wall.

Wound Complications Because of the larger incision made to accommodate a surgeon's hand, hand-assisted laparoscopy carries risks of wound complications greater than does standard laparoscopy, but these risks are still lower than with open surgery.[22-24] This risk depends somewhat on where the incision is placed. In patients with a normal body habitus, we usually make a periumbilical midline incision. We typically enter the peritoneum at the base of the umbilicus. It is easy to deviate from the midline when the patient is in the flank position, and we mark the midline using a permanent marker when the patient is in the supine position before positioning for the procedure. In patients with previous intra-abdominal surgery, this incision can allow the surgeon to perform lysis of adhesions before initiating the laparoscopic portion of the procedure. We estimate incision placement by determining where the ipsilateral wrist touches the skin when the distal interphalangeal joint touches the costal margin.

For obese patients, a paramedian incision provides easier access to the ipsilateral renal unit than does a midline incision. However, in obese patients, it is easy to angle between the skin and fascial incisions. As a result, the device may be placed farther away or closer than anticipated. If the device is too far from the kidney, the need to push the hand farther into the abdomen may injure the surgeon and may place pressure on the patient's abdominal wall that generates ischemia to the skin edges and compromises the skin and fascial closures. If the device is too close, the intra-abdominal hand may be hindered in movement.

Hernia, wound dehiscence, and wound infection can complicate any incision for laparoscopy, but these complications appear to be more common with hand-assistance procedures.[23] The incidence of herniation of the incision for the hand-assistance device ranges from 3% to 5%.[22-24] Although this rate is less than that described for intraperitoneal incisions for open surgery, this complication degrades some of the benefit of laparoscopic renal surgery. These incisions can be difficult to close because of their small size relative to the thickness of the subcutaneous fat in some patients, the positioning of the patient, and the irregularity between the skin incision and the fascial defect. We typically grasp the edge of the fascia with a Kocher clamp, run a long-lasting absorbable suture from both ends of the fascial incision, and intermittently place an interrupted suture with another absorbable suture to support the closure.

Dehiscence, which is rare, can be recognized by leakage of peritoneal fluid and ileus. Drainage of other fluid should alert the surgeon to a potential of bowel injury (i.e., fistula).

Hand-assistance wound complications, including infections, are more prevalent among obese patients.[24] Appropriately sized incisions may reduce pressure on the skin edges. Although hand-port incisions carry the greatest risk of these complications, the need to enlarge trocar incisions for specimen extraction or in situ morcellation creates increased potential for similar complications. Preoperative antibiotics along with careful attention to closure at the end of a long procedure, with irrigation of the subcutaneous tissue, can reduce the incidence of these complications.

Transperitoneal Laparoscopy: Needle and Trocar Injuries

Two approaches are commonly used to obtain access to the peritoneal cavity for standard transperitoneal laparoscopy. The commonly used Veress needle is passed into the peritoneal cavity through a small skin incision. These guarded needles are activated when engaging resistance (i.e., fascia) but become sheathed when they enter a cavity. After passing the needle firmly until resistance is lost, a 10-mL syringe containing 5 mL of sterile saline is attached to the syringe and is first withdrawn to ensure that succus or blood does not return, followed by injection of the fluid and attempted withdrawal once again. Fluid should not return, and after the syringe is removed, the fluid in the needle should flow inward. These maneuvers verify that the tip of the needle does not reside in a hollow viscus, but they do not confirm correct intraperitoneal placement. This is assessed by the *opening pressure*. The CO_2 insufflation line is connected to the Veress needle, and flow is initiated. If the pressure registered on the insufflator remains <8 mm Hg during the first few hundred milliliters of gas insufflation, then correct Veress needle placement is confirmed. If the pressure rises to >8 mm Hg, withdraw the needle a few millimeters, twist it axially, and tilt the distal tip upward slightly. When the pressure reading is elevated because the Veress needle tip was in omentum, this maneuver often lifts the tip out of the omentum and causes pressure to fall. If the pressure remains elevated, then immediately cease insufflation and try again at a different angle or a different location.

Some texts recommend avoiding high insufflation flow rates during initial insufflation through the Veress needle, but changing the flow setting on the insufflator is unnecessary because the caliber of the Veress needle limits the gas flow to 2 L per minute. Signs of inappropriate needle placement include asymmetrical abdominal expansion, subcutaneous emphysema, passage of flatus, and withdrawal of blood or succus. In addition, it is important to communicate with the anesthesiologist during this portion of the procedure because peritoneal stretch with insufflation can cause bradycardia, and the time of greatest risk of venous gas embolism is during initial insufflation.

Our practice is to attempt Veress needle placement a maximum of three times; if correct placement is not confirmed after the third attempt, then a different entry method should be used. Many urologists prefer to avoid the Veress needle altogether and use one of the alternatives in all cases. A common method is placement of a self-retaining Hasson trocar through a directly visualized small incision through the abdominal fascia into the peritoneum.

Another alternative to the Veress needle is use of a nonbladed visualizing trocar (Optiview, Ethicon Endo-Surgery, Cincinnati, Ohio). Some surgeons advocated use of this device for initial abdominal access, without prior insufflation. Further experience revealed that initial access with these and similar devices can result in bowel or great vessel injury.[25-27] When access is difficult and a laparoscopic approach is preferred, a hand-assisted approach provides the potential for open lysis of adhesions or conversion to an open surgical procedure if the adhesions are too dense.

Once pneumoperitoneum has been attained with a Veress needle, the primary port is placed. Here a non-bladed visualizing trocar has a distinct advantage by allowing direct viewing of the structures in front of the trocar. Nonbladed trocars for placement of secondary ports also likely reduce the risk of injury.

Injuries related to access include damage to visceral organs, intestine, and blood vessels. Injuries from the small-caliber Veress needle usually can be addressed laparoscopically. When these structures are injured with a trocar, however, repair may be more difficult. Abdominal wall vessel injuries are discussed later. Intra-abdominal injuries may require conversion to open surgery or hand-assistance procedures. Overall, access-related injuries account for 0.2% to 0.6% of complications associated with laparoscopic renal surgery, and knowledge of these complications and of their management is important for any surgeon commonly performing laparoscopic surgery.

Retroperitoneal Laparoscopy

Inadequate Exposure   A critical issue related to the retroperitoneal approach is limited working space. This situation can be further compromised by failure to place the ports in the appropriate locations. After the previously described patient positioning, we make a 2- to 3-cm incision over the tip of the 12th rib and the tip is exposed under direct vision. A Tonsil clamp is then used to puncture the lumbodorsal fascia to enter the retroperitoneum. We find this primary port site to provide a good view of the operative area. After using a finger to create a space posterior to the kidney, the balloon dilator is placed and inflated. If the device is placed in the correct location, the retroperitoneal contents can be seen sliding off medially to expose the posterior abdominal wall musculature. When dilation is performed anterior to the kidney, access to the renal hilum is compromised, although an additional port placed in front of the 11th rib can be used to elevate the kidney again. The initial two secondary ports are placed, in our practice along a subcostal line with one at the base of the 12th rib and one above the iliac crest, with care taken not to violate the peritoneal cavity.

Entry into the peritoneal cavity further limits the already small working space of the retroperitoneum. Entry can occur during balloon dissection (especially if scarring limits balloon expansion), during port placement (particularly the medial ports), or during perirenal dissection (most commonly at the upper pole or anteriorly). If the rent in the peritoneal membrane is small, a Veress needle or a 5-mm trocar can be placed on the intraperitoneal side and left open to vent gas from the peritoneal cavity, thus maintaining a pressure gradient favoring expansion of the retroperitoneal space. If the opening is large, however, it may be necessary to convert the procedure to an intraperitoneal approach.

Vascular Injury   Balloon dilation has been reported to cause avulsion of the renal hilum.[28,29] As the balloon is inflated, visualization of bleeding should be noted with concern. If brisk bleeding is encountered on deflating the balloon, rapid conversion to an open surgical procedure through a subcostal incision should be considered because renal vein injury can be life-threatening. Lesser bleeding, typically from the gonadal vein or tributaries of the renal vein, can be managed with various laparoscopic techniques.

Complications Related to Kidney Exposure

Bowel Injury

To gain access to the kidney on the left side, it is necessary to mobilize the descending colon off the entire surface of the kidney. On the right side, the colon is already placed medially, and it is often necessary only to incise the peritoneum overlying the right kidney. Colon injuries related to access and thermal injury can occur in ≤1.5% of patients.[30] To reduce the risk of thermal injury, we use cold scissor dissection for the initial portions of colon mobilization. If a thermal injury to the colon occurs, the extent of the injury can be underestimated at the time of initial inspection; this injury may become more apparent as the surgical procedure progresses. The duodenum needs to be reflected off the renal hilum on the right side, and injury can occur easily to this fragile structure. Additionally, both small bowel and large bowel are at risk during any medial dissection and during the passage of instruments into the abdomen.

For a clearly minor serosal injury, place one or more Lembert sutures to buttress the site. For full-thickness injury, consultation with a general surgeon should be considered,[31] although the current trend is to manage many of these injuries, even of the colon, with primary closure. Depending on the skill of the surgeon, nonabsorbable suture can be used to close a full-thickness injury in two layers. Alternatively, the procedure can be converted to a hand-assisted approach and the segment of bowel can be resected or repaired through the incision.[32,33] Avoidance of electrocautery near the bowel, minimized traction on the bowel, and careful instrument passage can prevent bowel injuries.

Spleen Injury

Injury to the spleen during laparoscopic left renal surgery has been reported to occur in ≤1.3% of cases.[30] Small thermal injuries or tears can often be managed by hemostatic agents and gentle pressure alone.[34,35] Splenic injuries can be very difficult to control, however, and splenectomy may be required. Moreover, delayed hemorrhage can occur from even small splenic injuries that appeared well controlled intraoperatively.[36] Blood transfusion and supportive care may be adequate care in some such patients,[36] but in others splenic embolization or splenectomy may be required. Patients undergoing splenic embolization or splenectomy should be provided appropriate vaccination postoperatively.

Pleural Injury

During medial rotation of the spleen to expose the upper pole of the left kidney, the diaphragm and pleura can be injured through either cautery or sharp dissection. On the right side, injury can occur when a large liver is being reflected. Small injuries can be managed by placement of a 14-gauge angiocatheter through the chest wall connected to sterile intravenous tubing and placed in a basin of water to provide a water seal. The defect is closed using absorbable suture with intracorporeal suturing. At the conclusion of the procedure, forceful ventilation by the anesthesiologist evacuates the CO_2 from the chest cavity prior to angiocatheter removal. If the injury is large or cannot be closed adequately with sutures alone, then placement of a chest tube at the conclusion of the procedure may be warranted. If the surgeon is not comfortable with intracorporeal suturing, conversion to an open procedure may be necessary to close the defect in the pleura.[37,38]

Pancreatic Injury

The tail of the pancreas is reflected medially to expose the left renal hilum. Avoiding overly aggressive retraction or electrocautery in this area can prevent injury. Injury to the pancreas typically manifests as abdominal pain, nausea, vomiting, fever, and abnormal laboratory values.[39] Minor injuries typically can be managed conservatively with bowel rest, total parenteral nutrition, and percutaneous drainage of pancreatic fluid collections. In severe cases, consultation with a general surgeon may be necessary. Prolonged but eventual recovery is the expected outcome for this complication.

Hepatobiliary Injury

Thermal burns to the liver typically do not require any intraoperative management, nor do minor tears, but larger tears in the liver capsule or incision into hepatic parenchyma may require coagulation with the argon beam coagulator or placement of hemostatic agents.[36] Occasionally, the gallbladder may be injured during removal of adhesions. If this occurs, consultation with a general surgeon to remove the gallbladder is recommended.[40]

Chylous Ascites

An uncommon complication is lymphatic leakage (with formation of chylous ascites) following left-sided laparoscopic renal surgery, owing to lymphatic disruption during mobilization and dissection of vascular structures.[41-43] The use of bipolar devices may reduce the risk of lymphatic leakage, and large lymphatic channels can be directly cauterized or clipped. Although chylous ascites can often be managed conservatively with total parenteral nutrition or medium-chain triglyceride diets and somatostatin, surgical intervention to ligate the source of lymphatic leakage is sometimes required. Biologic adhesives have been used successfully in this setting.[43]

Vascular Injury

Left Side On the left side, the gonadal vein typically drains into the renal vein. This vessel can usually be ligated if necessary with clips or bipolar electrocautery. In multiparous women, this vessel can be quite large and a stapler may be required. Undue traction on surrounding tissue without adequate mobilization can tear the vein. The gonadal artery may also be visualized and controlled with clips or bipolar electrocautery, although this vessel is small and typically is managed effectively even with monopolar electrocautery. The iliac vessels are at risk during dissection of the ureter or distal dissection of the descending colon.

Less common vascular injuries include trauma to the inferior mesenteric artery (most commonly in the setting of a large lower pole mass that displaces the dissection medially), the superior mesenteric artery (most commonly in the setting of a large upper pole mass that displaces the dissection medially), and the inferior mesenteric vein (when inadvertent dissection into the colonic mesentery occurs). Suspected injury to the superior mesenteric artery necessitates vascular surgery consultation because the bowel may be rendered ischemic. Inferior mesenteric artery and vein injuries can be managed by ligating the bleeding vessel. Aortic injuries are rare, usually occurring during dissection of the base of an atherosclerotic renal artery, and they may require conversion to an open surgical or hand-assistance procedure because aortic bleeding is difficult to control with laparoscopic instruments.

Any vascular injury may be increased in likelihood by poor visualization or loss of normal anatomic features. In addition, failure to keep the camera "true" with regard to the viewing angle can cause misidentification of vessels. Conversion to a hand-assisted approach or an open surgical procedure may be warranted to provide the surgeon more direct tactile feedback when other anatomic cues are lost.

Right Side On the right side the gonadal vein drains directly into the inferior vena cava. Therefore, injury of the gonadal vein on the right side is more problematic than on the left side. To avoid injury, the gonadal vein should be identified inferiorly and dissection should occur lateral to the vein. Traction on the vein can easily create a pseudoaneurysm close to the insertion of the gonadal vein into the vena cava, or it can frankly tear the inferior vena cava. Unlike the adrenal vein on the left, which drains into the renal vein and is usually straightforward to manage, the short right adrenal vein drains directly into the vena cava. Especially during radical nephrectomy for a large tumor, this vessel is at risk for avulsion if it is not identified and ligated purposely. Because of the more fragile nature of venous structures, the inferior vena cava is more prone to injury than is the aorta. Predominantly sharp dissection, or only very gentle blunt dissection, should be used around the inferior vena cava. When the inferior vena cava is torn, pressure can be applied and, depending on the skill level of the surgeon, this vessel can be sutured or the procedure can be converted to an open operation. Conversion to an open procedure is recommended if the inferior vena cava is stapled as a result of misidentification.[44] If a decision is made to convert to an open surgical procedure, pressure should be maintained on the injury and all open instruments should be prepared because the loss of insufflation will uncover venous bleeding that was held in check by the pneumoperitoneum.

Retroperitoneal Approach A critical issue during retroperitoneoscopic renal mobilization is continuous awareness of anatomic landmarks because this the approach may not be intuitive to surgeons early in their experience.[45] Once the anatomic features are learned, however, this approach typically allows immediate access to the renal hilum. When approaching the hilum, however, it is easy to keep following the psoas muscle medially and to be in too posterior a location and thus dissect under the great vessels. If this situation is not recognized, it can lead to injuries of the lumbar vessels that are very difficult to control.[18,29] To aid in maintaining landmarks,

we keep the psoas muscle as our horizon at all times. Misorienting the camera can lead to disastrous complications such as stapling across the inferior vena cava after mistaking it for the renal vein.[44] The gonadal vein and the ureter, which are often readily apparent if balloon dissection is performed in the correct plane, are useful landmarks. Once identified, these landmarks can be traced to the renal hilum. During dissection toward the hilum, ureteral, vascular, and even visceral injuries can occur during the retroperitoneal approach. Injuries are managed in a manner similar to that described with other approaches to the kidney, but the limited working space may make laparoscopic management more challenging. In some circumstances, the extraction site for the kidney can be used to manage complications with an open approach if the kidney is removed intact.[29]

Complications Related to Exiting

Vessel Injury

Complications related to completing laparoscopic renal surgical procedures are associated with the ports. Removal of ports should occur under direct vision to determine whether injury to an abdominal wall vessel has occurred.[46] Vascular injuries can be managed using the Carter-Thomason device by placing a figure-of-eight suture around the injured vessel. Alternatively, a cutdown procedure can be performed and the vessel can be directly ligated. If this complication is recognized postoperatively, the patient may require angiographic embolization to control bleeding, or a return to the operating room may be required. The incidence of problematic abdominal wall vessel injury appears to be lower with nonbladed trocars.

Port Site Bowel Complications

The fascia of all ports ≥10 mm should be closed to prevent bowel entrapment. In pediatric patients, all ports ≥5 mm should be closed. Closure can be accomplished with a variety of devices, including the Carter-Thomason device, which is our preferred method.[47] The sharp tip of this device can cause bowel or visceral injury, however, so closure should be performed under direct vision. Ports that have been enlarged to facilitate extraction can be closed using a variety of methods. The Carter-Thomason device can be used to place a figure-of-eight suture to close 2- to 2.5-cm incisions (as at the primary retroperitoneal access site), but for larger incisions external suturing with running or interrupted suture is required. As with closure of other abdominal incisions, the risk of inclusion of bowel exists, and the incision should be closed carefully under direct vision to avoid this complication. Although proper closure of a port site markedly reduces the risk, it does not guarantee against herniation or bowel entrapment.

Other Postoperative Complications

Hemorrhage

A review of our experience demonstrated that 3.7% of patients undergoing renal or adrenal laparoscopy had postoperative hemorrhage.[36] We found that hemorrhage typically occurred at ≤24 hours of the surgical procedure and was associated with abdominal pain, tenderness, and hypoactive bowel sounds. Increasing age, medical comorbidities, operative time, and intraoperative blood loss (especially related to splenic or liver injury) increased the risk of postoperative hemorrhage. We also found that unless an imperative surgical indication was present, these patients could be managed conservatively. Although hemorrhage increased the hospital stay and the risk of ileus and possibly prolonged early recovery, most patients achieved recovery similar to those without hemorrhage by 2 weeks. A low hematocrit value on the first postoperative day associated with hemodynamic instability can alert the surgeon to this problem. If necessary, ultrasonography or computed tomography (CT) can be used to confirm the diagnosis.

Unrecognized Bowel Injury

Unrecognized bowel injury is a serious complication associated with any laparoscopic surgical procedure. The signs and symptoms should be familiar to the urologist performing laparoscopic renal surgery because these findings differ in presentation from those of open surgical complications. Patients often complain of disproportionate abdominal pain. In cases of bowel entrapment at a port site, the patient may report localized pain. Initially, the patient may not appear toxic and often has leukopenia rather than an elevated white blood cell count. A high fever and hemodynamic instability may not occur until the patient is septic. An abdominal CT scan should be considered in those patients who are not following the normal postoperative course. If a bowel injury is identified, consultation with a general surgeon for exploratory laparotomy and fecal diversion may be warranted.[16]

SPECIFIC COMPLICATIONS

Benign Disease Indications

Donor Nephrectomy

Laparoscopy is the preferred management for donor nephrectomy and may be responsible in large part for the increase in the number of living related donors for renal transplantation.[48] Although these renal units are anatomically normal, the need to remove a functional organ with adequate ureteral and vascular length for anastomosis in the recipient, while maintaining safety for the donor, leaves a small margin for complications

in this procedure. In several large series, major complications were reported in 3.4% to 17.1% of patients.[49-52]

Complications most likely to affect the quality of the graft relate to vascular injury. The left kidney is the most frequently removed from the donor in most institutions. We prefer to ligate the tributaries of the renal vein (lumbar, adrenal, and gonadal) with bipolar energy. When these branches are large, we place a single clip on the portion remaining in the patient. By avoiding clips on the renal vein, we obviate the risk of stapler malfunction when the device is fired over a surgical clip. In a series of 8 stapler malfunctions involving the renal vein during laparoscopic nephrectomy, the most common cause was stapling over a clip.[53] In a reported donor nephrectomy series, 6 of 738 cases resulted in vascular injury caused by staple misfiring or malfunction and necessitating conversion to an open surgical procedure.[51]

Other vascular injuries reported during laparoscopic donor nephrectomy include laceration of the renal vessels during dissection, clip dislodgment from the renal artery stump, and vascular tears at the junction of the renal vessels and the aorta or inferior vena cava.[52] A significant number of reports of slippage of Hem-o-lok clips off the renal artery during laparoscopic donor nephrectomy caused the U.S. Food and Drug Administration to prohibit the use of these clips to control the renal artery during this procedure.[54] This prohibition is limited to laparoscopic donor nephrectomy, and these clips can still be used at the surgeon's discretion during simple or radical nephrectomy. This decision should be based on the length of remaining arterial stump for secure clip placement.

Several aspects of laparoscopic donor nephrectomy can compromise the function of the graft in the recipient. Ureteral injury can result in inadequate length for ureteroneocystotomy. To ensure adequate distal ureteral blood supply to prevent anastomotic strictures, many urologists preserve the gonadal vein along with the ureter during harvesting.[55] Delayed graft function is likely related to many factors, including prolonged warm ischemia time and vasospasm in the graft. Moreover, delayed graft function is related to overall graft survival.[55] Hand-assistance procedures may minimize warm ischemia time,[56] and these procedures may be safer than bag entrapment as for intact extraction after standard laparoscopy. Several reported cases of renal laceration and hematoma were related to injury from specimen entrapment.[57] "Resting" of the kidney and the use of diuretics and papaverine minimize vasospasm in the kidney and reduce the incidence of delayed graft function.[55] Up to 2% of patients report testicular pain, leg numbness, or other scrotal problems following laparoscopic donor nephrectomy related to gonadal vein ligation (in young patients) and possible injury to the ilioinguinal or genitofemoral nerves.[51]

Simple Nephrectomy

The term *simple nephrectomy* encompasses a large number of benign indications. Laparoscopic nephrectomy has been reported for xanthogranulomatous pyelonephritis, other infectious causes (tuberculosis), polycystic renal disease, and nonfunctioning (chronic hydronephrosis, failed pyeloplasty, reflux nephropathy) or atrophic kidneys. In a meta-analysis of laparoscopic renal complications, simple nephrectomy had the highest incidence of conversion to an open procedure, at 3.7%.[30] The predominant causes of complications associated with this procedure are inflammation distorting normal tissue planes and the lack of working space resulting from enlarged and distorted renal units.

The colon may be at more risk of injury than in other laparoscopic renal surgical procedures because inflammation makes mobilization difficult. A complete mechanical bowel preparation is indicated in this population, in whom the risk of injury approaches 1%.[58-62] A common pitfall during colon mobilization in laparoscopic simple nephrectomy is dissection into the colonic mesentery. A through-and-through dissection can occur easily without recognition. This dissection increases the likelihood of vascular injury, including injury to the mesenteric and contralateral renal vessels.[44] A clue to this incorrect dissection is the finding of vessels directed toward the colon. A large mesenteric opening does not require closure. Small openings may require closure to prevent the possibility of internal hernia.

If colon injury does occur, the extent of the injury should guide management. Treatment can range from reinspection of the area at the conclusion of the procedure for serosal injuries to laparoscopic repair or resection of full-thickness tears. Depending on experience and access to intraoperative consultation, laparoscopic management may be possible, or this injury may require conversion to an open procedure for repair and completion of the operation.

A second potential problem encountered with simple nephrectomy caused by lack of tissue planes is difficulty with renal hilar dissection and management. Inflammatory processes such as xanthogranulomatous pyelonephritis or chronic hydronephrosis resulting from nephrolithiasis may create significant perihilar inflammation or adenopathy that prevents successful isolation of the renal artery and vein. Although we prefer to ligate the renal artery and vein separately, in this circumstance it is often best to place a single clip on the renal artery (to stop blood flow) and then use a vascular laparoscopic stapler to control the hilum distal to the clip. Although not recommended as a routine measure, a stapler can be used to ligate the entire hilum en bloc with little risk of arteriovenous fistula.[63,64]

The real risk in using a stapler to ligate the entire hilum en bloc is not arteriovenous fistula formation, but rather the possibility that the stapler will misfire because too much tissue remains around the hilum for the device to close adequately. Enough dissection needs to be performed to thin the tissue bundle. If that is not possible, consideration of conversion to a hand-assistance procedure or an open operation is warranted, given that failure to control the hilum can be life-threatening. If the stapler does fail, the hilum en bloc can often be clamped again for temporary hemostasis. If feasible, a second trocar can be placed adjacent to the one with the stapler and a second stapler can be introduced more proximally on the vessels. The risk here is injury to a great vessel if the surgeon is disoriented.[60]

Because simple nephrectomy is not an oncologic procedure, the tendency exists to dissect close to the kidney. Although the space within Gerota's fascia or a subcapsular plane may provide the best mobilization and dissection of the kidney, this often places the surgeon very close to the renal sinus, where multiple arterial and venous branches may be encountered and vascular control may be more difficult. Identification of the gonadal vein with dissection of this vessel toward the renal hilum typically places the surgeon proximal enough on the renal artery and vein to avoid managing multiple branches.

A common problem encountered intraoperatively is failure to progress. Although this is not a complication, awareness of lack of progression during the case and conversion to hand-assistance procedures or an open operation can prevent the risks associated with prolonged operative time. Failure to progress often results from difficulty with mobilization of the kidney, owing to chronic infection, previous nephrostomy tube, and prior operation on the kidney or ureter, for example.[60-62]

The major risks in patients following laparoscopic simple nephrectomy are infection and abscess formation, especially in patients with xanthogranulomatous pyelonephritis. Before the procedure, obtain a urine culture from the patient and treat any infection appropriately. In such cases, it may be advantageous to leave a drain in place following the procedure. In cases of infection caused by chronic reflux nephropathy, ligate the ureteral stump with a clip. Despite preventive measures, many patients managed by simple nephrectomy have an infectious complication. Medical comorbidities such as diabetes can increase this risk.

Renal Cyst Decortication

Renal cyst decortication is often performed in patients with autosomal dominant polycystic kidney disease to alleviate the discomfort associated with enlarged kidneys.[65] Additionally, patients with sporadic simple cysts associated with pain or obstruction of the renal unit can be managed with renal cyst decortication.[66]

In general, this procedure requires mobilization of the colon and surrounding structures to gain access to the cyst. In patients with autosomal dominant polycystic kidney disease, extensive mobilization of the kidney may be required to address all the accessible cysts. For solitary cysts, the kidney is mobilized only as needed to provide access to the cyst based on approach and the surgeon's preference. After opening the cyst and draining the fluid, the cyst wall is excised. The base of the cyst is fulgurated with argon beam coagulation.

The most common reported complication of cyst decortication is ileus.[64,65] This complication can occur in patients with autosomal dominant polycystic kidney disease as a result of the irritating nature of the cystic fluid. Cauterization of the base of the cysts, copious irrigation with saline solution at the conclusion of the surgical procedure, and use of a closed drain may prevent this complication.[67]

Inadvertent entry into the collecting system with urine leak has been reported with cyst decortication. The use of intravenous indigo carmine at the conclusion of the procedure helps to identify violations of the collecting system. If leakage is present, the opening can be closed with laparoscopic suturing and a ureteral stent is placed. If this complication is recognized postoperatively, a ureteral stent followed by percutaneous drainage for persistent leak is appropriate.[68]

Retroperitoneal hematoma has been associated with this procedure. This complication can occur during excision of the cyst wall with inadvertent incision into surrounding normal renal parenchyma. Care to avoid normal kidney and careful fulguration with argon beam coagulation can decrease the risk of postoperative hematoma.[67]

Nephropexy

The most common complication of laparoscopic nephropexy for the management of symptomatic nephroptosis is recurrence of symptoms resulting from failure of the pexing suture or material.[69] We use three-point fixation with suture to position the kidney and place all sutures before we tie them down, with an additional flap of posterior peritoneum fixed to the anterior upper pole. Mesh can also be used to fix the kidney in place. A particular complication associated with this procedure is nerve entrapment or injury during suture placement. Because the sutures are placed in the psoas fascia to anchor the kidney in place, a risk of injury to the genitofemoral, iliohypogastric, and ilioinguinal nerves exists. Entrapment can result in neuroma and pain, whereas ligation can cause loss of sensation. Care to identify the nerves (which may resemble the psoas tendon) can avoid this complication.

Oncologic Indications

The need to adhere to oncologic surgical principles makes laparoscopic radical nephrectomy, partial nephrectomy, and nephroureterectomy quite different from renal laparoscopy for benign indications. Inade-quate resection or mishandling of the specimens can result in tumor recurrence or metastasis. Although these procedures share many complications of the benign indications for laparoscopic renal surgery, several additional complications are reviewed here.

Radical Nephrectomy

Local recurrences and port site metastases have been reported following laparoscopic radical nephrectomy. Both tumor biology and technical factors are important in the development of these complications. Although port site metastases following laparoscopic radical nephrectomy for renal cell carcinoma were initially attributed to morcellation, with three cases reported to date,[70,71] the subsequent three cases reported in the literature occurred after intact extraction.[72-74] The experience at our institution includes two port site metastases from renal cell carcinoma, one associated with morcellation and one with intact extraction. As such, morcellation (if performed correctly) does not appear to be the causative factor. One of the best arguments for intact extraction is that, with the advent of targeted therapies for renal cell carcinoma, tumor size and staging nuances may affect the eligibility of patients for clinical trials, and morcellation may exclude patients who otherwise would benefit from these trials.[75]

Renal cell carcinoma does not seem to share the same high tendency of urothelial carcinoma to implant into wounds; the historical rate of wound implantation in open surgical radical nephrectomy series was approximately 0.5%. Nonetheless, care should be taken to avoid violating the specimen when mobilizing and removing the kidney regardless of the approach elected (morcellation or intact extraction). If radical nephrectomy is performed using a hand-assisted approach, the kidney can simply be removed through the hand-assistance incision if it comes out easily; if the fit is tight, then the specimen should be placed into an entrapment sac first to avoid tearing or rupturing the specimen in situ. If a hand-assisted approach was not used, then the urologist can use intact extraction or morcellation. Morcellation is classically performed with a double-layered impermeable nylon sac, although one report suggested that the thinner self-opening sacs can be used safely as long as the incision at the morcellation site is opened enough to allow morcellation under vision.[76] If the specimen is violated, copious irrigation with sterile water is recommended. We irrigate the morcellation port site with sterile water in all cases.

Partial Nephrectomy

Laparoscopic partial nephrectomy continues to evolve as a more surgeons adopt this approach and new devices, techniques, and products permit improved hemostasis.[5,77] The spectrum of complications of laparoscopic partial nephrectomy does not significantly differ from that of open partial nephrectomy, but rates of urologic complications appear to be slightly increased with laparoscopic partial nephrectomy.[78]

Hemorrhage is the most frequent procedure-specific complication of partial nephrectomy (as well as open partial nephrectomy). In our first 100 cases, postoperative hemorrhage occurred in 9% of patients.[79] The rate of hemorrhage in our second 100 patients is 5% (unpublished data). As discussed earlier, the majority of patients can be managed conservatively.[36] Blood transfusion requirements ranged from 0% to 25% in reported series.[7,77-80]

The risk of hemorrhage is related to depth of the resection. With superficial lesions penetrating <5 mm into the renal parenchyma, we find that intraoperative hemostasis can be obtained easily with argon beam coagulation and biologic adhesives, even without clamping of the renal hilum. Postoperative hemorrhage is rare. For deeper lesions not requiring resection into the renal sinus, vascular clamping is used but hemostasis can still be obtained with only argon beam coagulation and biologic adhesives. The hemorrhage rate in such cases, with this technique, is approximately 5%. For resections that enter the renal sinus, a cellulose bolster is sutured into the defect, along with argon beam coagulation and biologic adhesives to assist in hemostasis. The risk of hemorrhage can be held to approximately 5% in this manner.

Another issue related to hemostasis involves the use of tissue sealants. Although a full discussion is beyond the scope of this chapter, the surgeon should be aware of potential allergic reactions related to the use of bovine thrombin especially in patients who have been previously exposed to this product during other surgical procedures (commonly cardiac surgery). An allergic reaction can produce coagulopathy that can be life-threatening to the patient. The surgeon must have the patient's complete surgical history before these products are used and, if necessary, must review prior operative reports to determine whether the use of the hemostatic agents could place the patient at risk.[81,82]

Most laparoscopic partial nephrectomies should reasonably be completed with a clamp time of ≤30 to 45 minutes. Although a warm ischemia time of ≤60 minutes has been reported to be safe, if a longer ischemia time is anticipated because of the complexity of the procedure, several maneuvers may assist in limiting ischemic injury. We routinely give 12.5 g of mannitol before clamping the renal hilum, followed by an additional 12.5 g when the hilum is unclamped. In addition, we have begun to cool the kidney with iced saline solution immediately after clamping. Preliminary evidence suggests that this technique can reduce ischemic injury and is not as complicated as other methods described in the literature.[77,80]

Prolonged renal ischemia can result in postoperative acute tubular necrosis and acute failure of the kidney. These complications are especially problematic if the partial nephrectomy is performed for absolute indications (solitary kidney, poor renal function). Because suturing is required for deeper resections, the likelihood of prolonged ischemia times during laparoscopic partial nephrectomy is greater in the setting of deep tumors. Given the considerable learning curve of sutured bolster application for laparoscopic partial nephrectomy, it is recommended that early in a surgeon's experience the procedure should be limited to small exophytic tumors, to allow the surgeon to gain comfort with the steps of the procedure.[83]

The argon beam coagulator that is used to obtain hemostasis around the parenchymal edges of the tumor has been reported to cause pneumothorax if the argon gas is not evacuated.[84] The gas can be evacuated with the suction irrigator or by opening the stopcock on a 5-mm port.

Although rare, patients may present postoperatively with sudden gross hematuria. This finding should prompt consideration of arteriovenous fistula. The risk of arteriovenous fistula may be higher with larger tumor resections and the need to place a running suture to control the renal sinus. Although CT may identify the fistula, angiography (interventional radiology) can identify the fistula and allow for management in the same setting.[85]

Urine leak has been reported in 3% to 5% of patients undergoing laparoscopic partial nephrectomy.[7,25,80] If the collecting system is entered, the surgeon should leave a closed drain near the tumor resection bed and a Foley catheter in the bladder. If no drainage is noted from the drain, the catheter is removed 1 to 2 days postoperatively, and the drain is monitored before removal. For those patients with urine output from the drain, the drain can be left in place for several weeks to allow healing of the fistula. If this fistula persists, a Foley catheter and an indwelling ureteral stent can be placed to promote healing. Occasionally, persistent urinomas require percutaneous drainage under ultrasound or CT guidance.[77,80]

Intraoperative alteration of the surgical procedure can be considered a complication. The percentage of patients undergoing unplanned nephrectomy in several large series was 14% and that of open conversion was 2%.[86] The factors most associated with conversion and completion nephrectomy in one study were age and tumor size.[86] Early in their experience, surgeons should select appropriate patients to avoid this potential complication. Even in the best of circumstances, conversion to open surgery or nephrectomy may occur, and patients should be counseled regarding this risk.

Nephroureterectomy

Complications peculiar to laparoscopic nephroureterectomy pertain to the management of the distal ureter. Various techniques have been described for managing the distal ureter during laparoscopic nephroureterectomy.[87-91] Complete excision of the ureter with a cuff of bladder is a mandatory part of the procedure. A retained distal ureteral stump continues to be at risk for tumor recurrence, and surveillance of a retained ureteral stump can be difficult.

Leakage of urine from the bladder is a potential complication of laparoscopic nephroureterectomy. Depending on the manner of managing the distal ureter, a drain may be placed in the pelvis adjacent to the bladder, or a large-caliber urethral catheter may be all that is needed. Again depending on the distal ureteral resection method, a cystogram may be considered at the time of urethral catheter removal, 5 to 14 days postoperatively. Persistent bladder leak can typically be managed with prolonged Foley catheter drainage. Occasionally, persistent urinoma requires percutaneous drainage.

Several reports of tumor seeding have been reported with laparoscopic nephroureterectomy.[92,93] Up to 50% of patients develop vesical or extravesical recurrence following nephroureterectomy.[87,91,94] As opposed to renal cell carcinoma, urothelial cell carcinoma readily implants locally (which is why morcellation is not considered for this procedure). Although the major technical imperatives are avoidance of tumor violation and prevention of tumor spillage, tumor biology is critical as well; high-grade tumors are more likely to implant than is low-grade disease. Careful attention to surgical technique and location of the tumor in the collecting system can reduce the potential for tumor violation and spillage. If tumor is spilled, copious irrigation with water may reduce implantation. Prevention is the best way to prevent this dreaded complication.

CONCLUSION

Laparoscopic approaches to the kidney are the standards of care for many benign and malignant conditions. An adequate technical skill set and an understanding of the expected anatomic features and of the stages of each procedure are the first steps in avoiding potential complications. For laparoscopic oncologic surgery, adherence to oncologic principles is an additional imperative. Surgeons adopting laparoscopic approaches should select appropriate cases initially because experience level is significantly associated with complications.

KEY POINTS

1. Increased patient weight and prolonged operative time place patients undergoing laparoscopic renal surgery at increased risk of rhabdomyolysis. Attention to patient positioning may help avoid this complication, and early identification may limit the impact of this complication on renal function.

2. Hand-assisted laparoscopic renal surgery carries a wound complication rate somewhat higher than that of standard laparoscopic renal surgery, although it is still less than that of open surgery.

3. If difficulty is encountered with Veress needle placement for transperitoneal laparoscopy, alternative approaches include placement of the needle in a different location, the use of optical trocars or a Hasson cannula, and conversion to hand-assisted laparoscopy.

4. Failure to place the retroperitoneal balloon dilator posterior to the kidney for retroperitoneoscopic renal surgery can compromise the procedure and increase the risk of peritoneal entry, which can further decrease the ability to perform the procedure.

5. Injuries to the liver and spleen during kidney mobilization can often be managed with hemostatic agents, argon beam coagulation, and pressure, but these injuries increase the likelihood of postoperative hemorrhage.

6. Consider CT imaging for patients with disproportionate pain and leukopenia because these findings may be early warning signs of an unrecognized visceral injury.

7. Stapler misfire during laparoscopic nephrectomy is a life-threatening complication and often results from application of the stapler over clips.

8. Port site metastases from renal cell carcinoma and urothelial cell carcinoma are related to biologic aggressiveness and specimen handling. Gentle specimen handling, including the use of specimen entrapment bags when indicated, can reduce the risk of metastases.

9. The major complication associated with laparoscopic partial nephrectomy is hemorrhage, and it appears to be more common than after open surgical partial nephrectomy.

10. Various approaches are available for the management of the distal ureter for laparoscopic nephroureterectomy. Regardless of approach, complete removal without tumor spillage is important to prevent recurrence of disease.

REFERENCES

Please see www.expertconsult.com

Chapter 30

COMPLICATIONS FOLLOWING LAPAROSCOPIC ROBOT-ASSISTED RADICAL PROSTATECTOMY

Scott M. Gilbert MD, MS
Assistant Professor, Urologic Oncology, Department of Urology, University of Florida College of Medicine, Gainesville, Florida

David P. Wood MD
Professor of Urology, Division of Urologic Oncology, Department of Urology, University of Michigan, Ann Arbor, Michigan

The surgical management of prostate cancer has undergone significant changes over the past several years. Although laparoscopy has been relatively underused in the treatment of many urologic malignant diseases,[1] the approach has gained popularity among patients with prostate cancer, hospitals, and surgeons. Consequently, the proportion of prostate cancer operations performed laparoscopically has increased dramatically. Much of this increase has been driven by the development of robotic systems, the implementation of dedicated clinical programs at centers of innovation, and the rapid adoption of robotic technology nationwide. Although reliable rates robotic technology use are difficult to estimate at this time, the significance of the increase is underscored by market forecasts, which suggest that laparoscopic robot-assisted prostatectomy is now more common than is the standard open approach.[2]

Although early evidence showed that laparoscopic robot-assisted prostatectomy was associated with reduced blood loss, decreased transfusion rates, and lower narcotic requirements postoperatively,[3] data regarding more durable—and arguably more clinically meaningful—outcomes, such as long-term cancer control, functional recovery, and health-related quality of life, are lacking.[4] As the approach has become more common, assessing complications associated with laparoscopic robot-assisted prostatectomy has become increasingly relevant and important. In this chapter, we review several of the most common and concerning complications associated with laparoscopic robot-assisted prostatectomy, including those related to the approach (access, anesthetic and physiologic considerations), as well as the potential intraoperative and postoperative complications related to the surgical procedure itself.

PREOPERATIVE CONSIDERATIONS AND COMPLICATIONS

Patient Selection

As with open radical prostatectomy, determining surgical candidacy is an important element of the preoperative evaluation before recommending laparoscopic robot-assisted prostatectomy for a particular patient. In general, candidates for a laparoscopic approach include patients with clinically organ-confined, biopsy-proven prostate cancer at relatively low risk for adverse cardiopulmonary and anesthetic complications associated with the surgical procedure. In some circumstances, anesthetic considerations related to pulmonary disease and the ability or inability to compensate for the hemodynamic, cardiovascular, and metabolic changes associated with laparoscopy may serve as relative contraindications.

Surgical considerations may also influence the appropriateness of a laparoscopic robot-assisted approach. Prior intra-abdominal and pelvic surgical procedures or disease processes and previous radiation therapy may increase the technical difficulty of laparoscopy, and these factors should be assessed carefully on a case-by-case basis as potential contraindications. Although no clear guidelines are available regarding antecedent conditions and treatments, prior surgical procedures and intra-abdominal and pelvic inflammatory processes likely increase the degree of difficulty and may result in relatively higher complication rates.

Similarly, salvage laparoscopic robot-assisted prostatectomy following radiation therapy may be particularly challenging. In complex cases characterized by anticipated fibrosis, adhesions, and altered anatomic features, the decision to proceed with a laparoscopic approach should be based on risk assessment, the surgeon's experience, and consideration of alternative approaches. As in open radical prostatectomy, patients undergoing laparoscopic robot-assisted prostatectomy should receive appropriate perioperative antibiotic and deep vein thrombosis prophylaxis.

System Considerations

System Setup and Patient Positioning

To facilitate optimal system setup, a modified low lithotomy position with Trendelenburg decline is typically used for laparoscopic robot-assisted prostatectomy. This position allows the operating component of the robotic system to come into close proximity to the patient, with the operating arms and camera oriented toward pelvic targets, including the prostate, bladder, seminal vesicles, urethra, and genitourinary diaphragm. Trendelenburg positioning is used to minimize interference of the peritoneal contents in the surgical field and may vary in degree depending on whether a transperitoneal approach or an extraperitoneal approach is used.

Close attention to positioning is important to prevent pressure- or traction-associated injuries. Accordingly, all pressure points should be padded adequately, and the surgical team, including the anesthesiologist and nursing staff, should ensure that areas of potential injury are addressed before sterile skin preparation and draping. The weight of the patient's legs should be transmitted through the heel and foot, minimal pressure should be present on the lateral aspect of the calves and thighs, the extension of the hip and thigh should be anatomic to minimize the risk of femoral nerve injury, and the lower back should be contoured with lumbar support if necessary. If the arms are positioned by the patient's side, the wrists and elbows should be well padded, and care should be taken to protect the patient's hands and fingers from injury secondary to positioning of the table, robotic equipment, or the assisting surgical team. When the patient's arms are not tucked, a natural anatomic position of the arm and shoulder should be achieved to prevent brachial plexus injury.

Once the patient has been correctly positioned, he should be secured to the surgical table to prevent shifting during the surgical procedure. This goal can be achieved relatively easily by using padded straps across the patient's chest. A crossing configuration, using two straps running from above the ipsilateral shoulder across the chest to the contralateral chest side wall, secures the patient to the table while providing additional support to the patient's shoulders and arms.

Access and Approach

Laparoscopic robot-assisted radical prostatectomy may be performed through either a transperitoneal or an extraperitoneal approach. Although the transperitoneal approach is more commonly used, the extraperitoneal approach is preferred by some surgeons because the peritoneal contents can be avoided. Both approaches have advantages and disadvantages and present different potential challenges in access. Regardless of which approach is used, initial access to the peritoneal or prevesical space is typically achieved through a small periumbilical or infraumbilical skin incision. Unless the surgeon has chosen to use a Hasson technique, which is relatively uncommon, blind access is achieved for the placement of the first port, and subsequent working ports are then established under direct vision.

Transperitoneal Approach The transperitoneal approach uses intraperitoneal access with secondary entry and development of the extraperitoneal perivesical space. Access to the peritoneal cavity may be gained either using insufflation through a Veress needle followed by blind placement of the initial camera port or using a Hasson technique when direct visualization is preferable. Following standard laparoscopic principles, confirmation of an intraperitoneal position is necessary before insufflation. Abnormally high initial intra-abdominal pressures indicate probable malpositioning, and insufflation should not be initiated in this setting. Repositioning, removal, and replacement of the device are options to establish correct placement before insufflating the abdomen. Nonvisualized passage of the Veress needle and the initial trocar following insufflation is associated with potential injury to gastrointestinal and vascular structures. If an injury is suspected after placement of the Veress needle, insufflation should be delayed and the needle should be carefully removed in the trajectory of entry to avoid converting a penetrating injury to a potentially more severe laceration.

Once safe access has been established in a different location, the area of initial entry and potential injury should be examined closely. In cases of small penetrating injuries, no additional management is required for bowel or bladder entry.[5] However, the surgeon must use his or her discretion regarding the need for repair or conversion to an open procedure. In the presence of a significant injury, such as larger visceral lacerations or an expanding mesenteric hematoma, open repair may be prudent.

Injuries associated with trocars are generally more severe than are those associated with Veress and spinal needles. These injuries require stabilization of the trocar, open conversion, and repair of the injury. Perforation of the small bowel or large intestine is the most common injury associated with initial blind trocar placement. The extent of this type of injury usually requires open repair, although in selected cases of less severe injury, skilled laparoscopic surgeons have elected to perform laparoscopic repair. Early, if not immediate, recognition and repair are essential avoid the development of peritonitis, sepsis, and related cardiovascular collapse and to ensure the safety of the patient. Significant bladder injuries may also occur during the establishment of access, as well as during the initial dissection and development of the perivesical space. Occult bladder injuries can be detected with intravesical instillation of dilute methylene blue. As with bowel injuries, small penetrating injuries associated with narrow-gauge needles can be managed conservatively, whereas large defects require laparoscopic or open repair and prolonged catheter decompression.[5] Urinary decompression with a Foley catheter reduces the risk of injury and should be routine practice before laparoscopic access is gained.

Previous abdominal surgical procedures may alter the approach in gaining initial access to the peritoneal space. Omental and small bowel adhesions to the anterior abdominal wall increase the risk of bowel injury when access is obtained blindly, and some surgeons prefer to use a direct visualization technique (Hasson) with a cut-down approach to place the first trocar under vision through a small skin incision and fasciotomy. Although this technique is conservative and reduces the chances for potential bowel injury, it increases the chance of troublesome air leak throughout the case, given the relatively large fascia opening required. A figure-of-eight fascial stitch can be used to reinforce the point of trocar entry, reduce the tendency of air leak, and ensure maintenance of intercavity pressure for the duration of the surgical procedure.

Major vascular injuries are rare and have been reported in 0.11% to 2.0% of laparoscopic cases.[6,7] The aorta and common iliac vessels are the most commonly injured vascular structures. Mesenteric vessels may also be injured, resulting in mesenteric hematoma followed by possible vascular compromise and bowel ischemia. Clinical signs of significant bleeding are hypotension followed by compensatory tachycardia. After trocar entry into a major vessel, injury is readily apparent on removal of the obturator. If the trocar has not been withdrawn or manipulated, a blunt obturator should be replaced through the lumen and the trocar should be left in place while preparations are made for open conversion and repair. An emergency laparotomy should proceed rapidly with vascular control and repair.

The inferior epigastric artery and veins are additional sources of vascular injury, particularly during placement of subsequent lateral working ports. Sharp trocars may lacerate the inferior epigastric vessels on passage through the anterior abdominal wall and may result in troublesome bleeding throughout the case and potentially significant hemorrhage in the postoperative period if the injury is not recognized and addressed intraoperatively. Less commonly, blunt dilating trocars may cause laceration or avulsion secondary to the additional force required for port placement. The risk of injury can be minimized when the vessels are directly visualized and ports are placed >6 cm from the midline.[8] Consequently,

lateral working ports should always be placed under direct vision. Use of a spinal needle to map the transabdominal course of the trocar may also help prevent injury to the inferior epigastric vasculature, in addition to other internal structures such as small bowel, by serving as a guide and directing the subsequent placement of the larger trocar.

Recognized inferior epigastric injuries should be managed promptly either laparoscopically or with a cut-down technique. When laparoscopic ligation or electrocautery is possible, additional skin incisions or port placements may be avoided. In some instances, the location of the injury may prevent adequate control without additional port placement. These cases may be managed effectively with additional port placement and subsequent internal ligation. When access to the site of bleeding is difficult, an externally placed (on the skin level) hemostatic occluding figure-of-eight stitch can be placed in the quadrant of identified bleeding to provide occlusion and control. The Carter-Thomason fascia suturing device is useful in this application because it allows full-thickness transabdominal suturing. Unrecognized or inadequately managed, hemorrhage from the inferior epigastric vessels may progress to a significant rectus sheath hematoma resulting in clinically significant pain, acute blood loss, anemia, and possible hemorrhagic shock.

The consequences of vascular injury are not limited to hemorrhage. Although uncommon, the risks of gas embolism and resulting cardiopulmonary collapse are elevated during laparoscopy. Embolism is less common when one uses carbon dioxide (CO_2) compared with other insufflants, given the dissolvability of CO_2 in blood.[8] In cases of unrecognized intravascular entry, injury, and insufflation, a CO_2 embolus may precipitate rapidly and may result in catastrophic consequences such as acute cardiovascular collapse. This is the most common cause of a gas embolism in the setting of CO_2 insufflant. Classic signs include an abrupt increase in end-tidal CO_2 accompanied by a sudden decline in oxygen saturation and a subsequent decrease in end-tidal CO_2.[8] Such cases should be managed on an emergency basis with immediate cessation of insufflation and repositioning of the patient in the left lateral decubitus position to minimize right ventricular outflow. The patient should then be ventilated with 100% oxygen, and in extreme circumstances, aspiration of the air embolism may be required.

During prolonged cases, and in settings associated with persistent CO_2 leak, subcutaneous emphysema may develop during the course of the surgical procedure. Scrotal emphysema is common with the extraperitoneal approach, and in prolonged cases, emphysema may tract up the abdominal wall and involve the subcutaneous tissues of the neck and face. This problem is directly related to the extent of CO_2 leakage around the port, which may be exacerbated by prolonged surgical time, use of high insufflation pressures, and insufflant leak around the fascia opening. Palpable crepitus is the principal clinical sign. When subcutaneous emphysema is associated with high CO_2 blood levels, delayed extubation may be required to allow the partial pressures of CO_2 and of oxygen to normalize. Maintaining intraperitoneal pressures of ≤15 mm Hg assists in minimizing this complication.

Extraperitoneal Approach The extraperitoneal approach requires port placement slightly lower than in the transperitoneal approach but in the same configuration. Potential benefits of the approach include reduced anesthetic problems associated with increase intraperitoneal pressures, avoidance of the peritoneal contents and all associated intraoperative and postoperative consequences (ileus), and decreased need to retract the bowels during the surgical procedure. The working space is smaller, however, and care must be taken in developing the extraperitoneal space before port placement, particularly in the cranial and lateral areas where the robot working ports are placed. A balloon dilator is used to develop the prevesical space bluntly and may result in laceration or avulsion of pelvic vessels when the device is not placed correctly or in cases associated with fused tissue planes. Initial port placement to gain proper access to the space is essential because improper placement may result in occult or obvious intraperitoneal entry and bothersome intraperitoneal leak throughout the procedure. In cases of suboptimal development of the prevesical space, the working space can be limited, resulting in a relatively reduced ability to manipulate the working elements and translating to more difficult surgical dissection. In the event of an intraperitoneal communication, a 5-mm port can be placed into the peritoneal space for decompression. Conversion to an intraperitoneal approach should be done if a large intraperitoneal CO_2 leak occurs.

Injury to intraperitoneal structures is less common with an extraperitoneal approach because the peritoneal contents are avoided. Nonetheless, small bowel and large intestine injuries are possible secondary to unintentional peritoneal entry during establishment of access. Vascular and bladder injuries are the most common injuries when establishing the extraperitoneal space. These injuries may occur either during initial port placement into the prevesical space or during subsequent balloon dilation of the space, particularly when the initial port is not positioned correctly. In these cases, avulsion injuries to pelvic veins and blunt pressure–associated trauma to the bladder may occur.

Venous bleeding should be controlled through a combination of insufflation pressure tamponade and focal ligation. If the inferior epigastric vessels have been injured with initial dilation of the space, additional ports should be placed to facilitate achievement of hemostasis. In placing the additional lateral working ports during the extraperitoneal approach, care must be taken to dissect the peritoneum bluntly and superiorly, to allow for adequate cranial working port placement. This maneuver is most commonly performed through the initially placed camera port, with the camera used as the blunt dissector as well as for visualization during this portion of the procedure. Following adequate peritoneal reflection, the inferior epigastric vessels are generally well visualized and can be avoided during the placement of lateral trocars.

Ergonomic and work space considerations are particularly important during the extraperitoneal approach, given the reduced working space available. In particular, proper port placement is important in robot-assisted prostatectomy to ensure that instruments do not interfere with one another during the procedure. The consequences of suboptimal port placement range from troublesome access of assistant instruments to interference among the various robotic working elements, either internally or externally. These issues are preventable given careful preoperative consideration and port placement tailored to the patient's anatomic features and the surgical approach. In general, suboptimal port placement is more problematic in the extraperitoneal approach because the working space is somewhat more confined relative to a transperitoneal approach. Secondary port placement may also be troublesome for the duration of the surgical procedure if careful planning is not taken into account. Such suboptimal situations result in conflicting working elements in delivery of instruments and needles, limited assistant access to the surgical area, and displacement of the working arms as the camera is moved closer to the surgical field.

Positioning the Robot Working-Element
In positioning the operating element of the robotic system, care must be taken to ensure that unintentional contact between the robot and the patient does not occur. The only contact between the robot and the patient occurs through the working ports, and at no time should any other moving or static element of the robot place pressure on the patient's core or extremities. The most common area of potential contact is between the working elements (arms) and the patient's thighs. This contact can be avoided by pivoting the arms of the robot up and away from the patient when the robotic arms are attached to the working ports. One practical concern that may go unrecognized but is potentially serious is the placement of equipment (cables, light source, camera, suction tubing) in the vicinity of the patient's face and the endotracheal tube. Care should be taken when considering placement of these laparoscopic accessories, and if at all avoidable, they should be routed away from the area of the patient's head. In laparoscopic robot-assisted prostatectomy, however, these accessories are often placed in that area out of necessity. In these cases, a protective foam barrier may

be placed over the patient's face after the endotracheal tube has been secured. This measure may prevent facial injuries such as corneal abrasion and may also reduce the risk of unintentional dislodgment of the endotracheal tube during the surgical procedure.

Critical system failures, although uncommon, may occur, requiring abortion of the robot-assisted approach and conversion to either a straight laparoscopic procedure or open prostatectomy. Early field experience with the robot system indicated technical or system failures in 0.4% to 2.6% of cases.[9,10] In some cases, system errors may prevent initiating the surgical procedure, whereas in others, these errors occur intraoperatively and result in suboptimal system performance. Although information on estimates of system failure is limited, the impact of this system-specific complication on patient- and cancer-related health outcomes has not been measured to date.

Physiologic Consequences and Anesthetic Considerations

Laparoscopy is associated with several well-described physiologic changes that affect respiratory workload, cardiopulmonary functioning, and acid-base equilibrium. Although these changes may not universally lead to adverse consequences, in certain settings and in some cases, complications may result. CO_2 absorption and hypercapnia alter acid-base status and result in respiratory acidosis.[11] However, patients with significant pulmonary problems, such as chronic obstructive pulmonary disease, may be unable to compensate for excess CO_2 through respiratory exchange, and they may develop exaggerated acid-base disturbances and associated cardiac arrhythmias. Prolonged or marked acidosis may have serious consequences at the cellular level that interfere with normal cellular processes across systems. Exposure to increased levels of CO_2 may also increase heart rate, cardiac contractility, and vascular resistance through sympathetic stimulation that increases the cardiac workload and may thus precipitate cardiac stress and reversible ischemic disease or cardiac arrhythmia.[12] Cardiac abnormalities other than tachycardia and ventricular extrasystoles, such as bradycardia secondary to peritoneal irritation and vagal stimulation, may also become apparent during laparoscopy.[13]

Beyond consequences related to altered acid-base status and the direct effect of hypercapnia, laparoscopy may also impair cardiopulmonary functioning through a pressure effect. Diaphragm motion may be limited, thereby decreasing functional reserve space as intra-abdominal pressure increases[5] and necessitating compensatory peak airway pressure support to maintain a constant tidal volume. In patients with significant pulmonary disease, positive end-expiratory pressure may be required to maintain adequate ventilation.[5] Trendelenburg positioning may further exacerbate these

problems because the diaphragm has even more limited motion, and functional reserve is decreased further.

Venous return may also be affected by pneumoperitoneum. In euvolemic and hypovolemic patients with relatively low atrial pressures, venous return is reduced secondary to the pneumoperitoneal pressure transmitted to the vena cava. Conversely, in hypervolemic states characterized by high atrial pressures, venous return is increased through vena cava resistance to the pneumoperitoneum. Additional pressure-related hemodynamic consequences may be seen. Low levels of insufflation in the range of 5 to 20 mm Hg cause a stimulatory effect on the cardiovascular system characterized by decreased peripheral vascular resistance, increased heart rate, and enhanced contractility of the myocardium. Higher pressures, however, particularly those approaching or exceeding 40 mm Hg, are associated with decreased venous return and decreased cardiac output. In cases of significantly increased pneumoperitoneal pressure (>40 mm Hg), capacitance vessels collapse, arterial resistance increases, and venous return decreases.[14] Accordingly, intra-abdominal pressure should be maintained at levels ≤20 mm Hg.[15,16]

Oliguria resulting from the pressure effects of increased intra-abdominal pressure may lead to low urine output and may increase the potential for postoperative azotemia. This complication effectively results from an intraperitoneal compartment syndrome leading to decreased renal vein blood flow and compression of the renal parenchyma.[17,18] Higher pressures are associated with an increasing probability of oliguria. Although the effect may be directly mediated by the pneumoperitoneal pressure, modulation of antidiuretic hormone and vasopressin levels may also contribute to it.[19] In cases of extended surgical time and insufflation, CO_2 may be stored in tissue and may require a significant period to clear postoperatively.

INTRAOPERATIVE SURGICAL COMPLICATIONS

Although open and laparoscopic robot-assisted prostatectomy techniques share many of the same operative risks, some potential surgical complications are unique to the laparoscopic approach. Accordingly, surgical complications can be broadly classified as those related to surgical intervention (radical prostatectomy) and those related to surgical approach (open versus laparoscopic robot-assisted procedures). The surgical intervention group consists of intraoperative and postoperative complications common to both types of surgical procedures, such as hemorrhage, wound infection, and rectal injury, as well as longer-term functional impairments, such as bladder neck contracture, postprostatectomy urinary incontinence, and sexual dysfunction. In addition to this group of well-defined complications, the potential for other types of intraoperative complication exists with the laparoscopic robot-assisted approach. In this section, various types of surgical complications associated with prostatectomy and the laparoscopic approach are reviewed.

Hemorrhage

Although surgical bleeding can be problematic during prostatectomy, the pressure effect associated with laparoscopy results in relatively low levels of blood loss, and significant hemorrhage during laparoscopic robot-assisted prostatectomy is relatively uncommon.[20,21] The hemorrhagic advantage of laparoscopic prostatectomy over the open counterpart is underscored by the differential blood loss between the two approaches: blood loss of <200 mL is common following laparoscopic robot-assisted prostatectomy and translates to a reduced incidence of postoperative transfusion (1%-2%) and a higher average postoperative hematocrit for most patients.[22,23] Nonetheless, in some cases, bleeding may be problematic either during the operation or in the postoperative period when areas of inadequate hemostasis were not identified during the surgical procedure.

Sources of bleeding are the same as those described for the open procedure: the dorsal venous complex and Santorini's complex overlying the anterior and lateral surfaces of the prostate and bladder, the inferior vesicle and proximal prostatic vascular pedicles, the neurovascular bundles coursing posterolateral to the prostate, the apical prostatic vessels, and the bladder neck. Venous bleeding, such as that encountered with division of the dorsal venous complex, is less troublesome during laparoscopic robotic prostatectomy compared with the open approach secondary to the pneumatic pressure of the working space. Nevertheless, venous bleeding may still be a potential source of hemorrhage, particularly in the delayed setting when the hemostatic effect of laparoscopic insufflation is no longer operational.

Hemostatic techniques available to control venous and arterial bleeding range from standard suturing and electrocautery to more device-based methods, such as vascular staples and laparoscopic hemostatic clips. Bleeding of large veins and venous complexes may be controlled effectively using suture ligatures or vascular staples. The dorsal venous complex, for example, has been controlled in several ways, including predivision placement of a hemostatic figure-of-eight suture ligature, control with suture oversewing after division, and use of a laparoscopic vascular stapler. If problematic dorsal venous complex bleeding is encountered, temporary increase of the insufflation pressure may improve visualization to allow accurate hemostatic control.

Unnecessary bleeding from small arteries may be encountered during sharp dissection and when hemostatic control is not complete. During seminal vesicle dissection, for example, vasal and seminal arteries may

retract posteriorly following division, with resulting bleeding that is subsequently difficult to expose and control. Control of the proximal pedicles generally relies on hemostatic staples, hemoclips, or electrocautery; however, in cases characterized by misapplication or dislodgment, pedicle bleeding may be significant.

Additionally, in nerve-sparing procedures, antegrade dissection of the periprostatic fascia may result in bleeding in exchange for avoidance of thermal or mechanical injury to the neurovascular bundles. In general, this bleeding does not cause significant hemorrhage postoperatively, and it can be controlled with either discrete bipolar electrocautery or application of hemostatic agents. Minimizing bleeding in laparoscopy is important because blood loss generally correlates with efficiency, not only in the time saved not spent searching for sources of bleeding and subsequent control but also in maintaining optimal visualization of the surgical field. When the operative field becomes contaminated with blood, the visual benefits of laparoscopy diminish slightly.

Visceral (Bladder and Bowel) Injury

During laparoscopic robot-assisted prostatectomy, visceral injury may be mechanical, electrical, or thermal and may involve the bladder, ureters, bowel, or rectum. Bladder injury, although uncommon, has been reported with a laparoscopic approach. Typically, injury occurs during the transperitoneal approach with division of the urachus and development of the retropubic space. The incidence is <2% during laparoscopic prostatectomy, and this complication can be effectively managed with two-layer closure and bladder decompression.[24] In cases of multiple cystotomies or when the integrity of the anterior bladder has been compromised secondary to misguided surgical dissection, additional repair may be necessary.

Inadvertent bladder injury can be prevented by maintaining visualization of the fibrous tissue separating the adventitia of the anterior bladder and the posterior abdominal wall. This plane ultimately leads to pubic symphysis, at which point the anterior prostate can be identified and defined by removing excess investing periprostatic adipose tissue. Partial bladder distention has been advocated by some surgeons to assist in identification of the bladder during this surgical step, although bladder decompression and maintenance of correct surgical orientation may be safer. Excessive bleeding may indicate incorrect surgical dissecting through the serosa and detrusor of the bladder and should prompt corrective measures.

Bowel injury, like bladder injury, is uncommon following laparoscopic robot-assisted prostatectomy, but it can be devastating if it is not recognized and repaired expediently. Most commonly, insult to the small or large bowel results from retraction during the surgical procedure. This injury may result from either assisting elements, such as graspers, laparoscopic suction, and needle delivery devices, or the active working elements of the robotic system. Recognized injuries should be repaired immediately, either laparoscopically or through an open conversion when a laparoscopic repair is not possible or safe. During operative repair, the peritoneal contents should be irrigated thoroughly, and broad-spectrum antibiotic coverage should be included in the postoperative care. Unrecognized bowel injuries may manifest with symptoms including significant fever, nausea, abdominal distention and ileus, and signs consistent with peritonitis. Less clinically acute symptoms, but as concerning, include diffuse abdominal pain and low-grade fever in the absence of leukocytosis and should alert the surgical team of a possible intra-abdominal process.[8]

Visceral injury may result from misdirected electrocautery through several mechanisms. Unintended activation can result in direct injury to unintentionally targeted structures, such as the bladder and bowel, in cases of accidental electrocautery activation during visceral contact. Although injury may be minor, thermal injury and the resulting tissue necrosis may lead to significant injury following direct activation. Injury may also occur through direct coupling, resulting in unintended transmission of electrocautery current to adjacent structures. If the coupling occurs outside of the field of vision, the resulting injury may go unrecognized. Capacitive coupling may also occur in tissues and areas surrounding metal laparoscopic ports. In these cases, insulation failure allows current to escape along the shaft of an instrument and results in potential injury to tissue outside of the field of vision. In contrast to mechanical injury, thermal injury is more likely associated with delayed presentation, and injuries to the bowel, such as bowel necrosis and leak, may not develop for several days.

Rectal Injury

Rectal injury, a rare but significant complication during radical prostatectomy, has been reported in 1% of 3% of open surgical procedures.[25-27] Risks for injury include previous pelvic radiation and periprostatic inflammation. Although rectal injury has not been commonly reported during laparoscopic robot-assisted prostatectomy, it is an important potential complication that may lead to subsequent events including pelvic abscess formation, rectourethral fistula, and sepsis. Although the impact of direct visualization and antegrade dissection used for the laparoscopic approach on the risk of rectal injury has not been firmly established, these features of the laparoscopic approach may facilitate improved identification and dissection of Denonvilliers' fascia and thus allow the surgeon to establish the correct posterior plane. However, for inexperienced surgeons,

and in cases of distorted anatomic features resulting from previous inflammation or treatment effect, poorly defined surgical planes or suboptimal visualization may be disorienting. In such cases, the posterior plane should be established with sharp dissection from the base toward the genitourinary diaphragm. Avoiding electrocautery during this portion of the dissection decreases the chance of thermal injury to the anterior rectum.

In the event of a recognized rectal injury, the defect can be closed primarily using two-layer closure (running internal mucosal closure reinforced by a layer of interrupted imbricating Lembert sutures) followed by conservative observation in cases characterized by healthy, nonirradiated tissue with a high probability of healing. In cases of significant spillage or contamination following rectal injury or if the tissue has been previously irradiated, a temporary diverting colostomy should be considered. Unrecognized injuries present a significant management problem and may result in a rectourethral fistula requiring a delayed posterior sagittal repair (York-Masson).

Ureteral Injury

Ureteral injury is an uncommon complication, although the ureteral orifices are at risk during the development and division of the bladder neck during laparoscopic prostatectomy. In the event that they are close to the vesicle neck, they may also be at risk for obstruction during urethral anastomosis. Direct injury may occur during division of the posterior bladder neck or dissection of an intravesical median lobe by transection of the urethral orifices or thermal injury secondary to cautery effect. Indirect injury may occur during retraction of the bladder following division of the bladder neck by a number of mechanisms, including mechanical injury or electrothermal coupling insult. During bladder neck reconstruction, the ureteral orifices may be at risk of suture ligation if they are in close proximity to the bladder neck and suture line. In extremely uncommon but problematic cases, the ureteral orifices may be everted to an extravesical position following reconstruction and may result in complete urine leak postoperatively. Open conversion, reconstruction of the bladder neck, stent placement, or ureteral reimplantation may be required to manage clinically significant ureteral injuries.

Port Hernias and Wound Dehiscence

On completion of the case, port sites >10 mm should be closed to prevent postoperative small bowel entrapment and herniation during a transperitoneal approach. Herniation can also be prevented by visual inspection of the port entry site and fascia closure before removal of the final camera port. Typically, the Carter-Thomason suturing device is useful for placing simple and figure-of-eight fascial sutures. If bowel does become entrapped in a port site, laparoscopy should be performed with concomitant external manual reduction of the bowel loop. The portion of bowel in question should then be examined, and if it is not viable, bowel resection may be required. When an extraperitoneal approach is used, ports generally do not require fascial closure because intraperitoneal contents are contained within the peritoneum and are therefore not able to herniate through the port sites. The central incision, which is typically extended for retrieval of the specimen, should be closed with care, to ensure adequate suture strength and fascial apposition to prevent fascial dehiscence.

EARLY POSTOPERATIVE COMPLICATIONS

Urethral-vesical Anastomotic Leak

The rate of urethral-vesical anastomotic leak varies according to surgical technique, the surgeon's experience, and the patient's anatomic features. In laparoscopic radical prostatectomy, urine leak ranges from 1% to 10% depending on definition.[22,24,28]

Laparoscopic robot-assisted prostatectomy offers several advantages in reducing the risk of anastomotic leak, including direct visualization and the ability to perform a running anastomosis. Nonetheless, apposing the bladder neck and the proximal urethra may be a challenging step in the surgical procedure given the constant tension that must be applied throughout the reconstruction to counteract the separating effect of insufflation. Several competing factors must be considered when performing the anastomosis during laparoscopy. Although vision is greatly aided, during this portion of the procedure the CO_2 insufflation may actually be counterproductive because it tends to pull the anastomosis apart while the surgeon is attempting to deliver the initial posterior stitches distally to the urethra for proper apposition. This problem can be partially resolved by reducing the insufflation flow rate and pressure setting, in addition to maintaining suture tension throughout the anastomosis. Undue tension or carelessly applied tension on the first several anastomotic stitches may result in urethral tears that further compromise the integrity of the anastomosis and may predispose to anastomotic stricture. In cases of suboptimal anastomosis, the urine leak is most often located posteriorly as a result of a lack of complete apposition of the bladder neck and urethra in this location when the initial sutures are placed.

Urine leak may be more difficult to diagnosis following an intraperitoneal approach secondary to a tendency to peritoneal fluid drainage. If a leak is suspected, however, additional diagnostic tests should be performed, including drain fluid creatinine determinations or a cystogram to visualize the leak. Management is generally conservative and consists of continued extra-vesical drainage and bladder decompression with a Foley catheter. A cystogram can be performed before catheter removal to ensure resolution of the leak, although this is not required in all cases. In cases characterized by persistent urine leak, a ureteral injury or fistula should be considered as a potential source other than anastomotic leak. In cases of transperitoneal prostatectomy, anastomotic urine leak may contribute to prolonged ileus, which has been reported in approximately 3% of cases.[22]

Femoral and Obturator Nerve Injury

Nerve injury may result from patient positioning, inadequate padding, and prolonged surgical duration. Femoral nerve injury is relatively more common during laparoscopic prostatectomy given the low lithotomy positioning typically used. Lower leg weakness, inability to ambulate, and paresthesias are usually observed and should alert the surgical team of potential femoral nerve palsy. Management is conservative, and most injuries resolve with physical therapy and time. Other nerves may be injured during surgery as well. Direct surgical injury to the obturator nerve may result either from mechanical or electrical current insult, similar to the risk in open prostatectomy.

Novice laparoscopic surgeons should be aware that the pneumoperitoneal and pneumoretroperitoneum used for the transperitoneal and extraperitoneal approaches, respectively, distort the anatomic appearance of the external iliac vein and cause the obturator nerve to appear more medially than in the open surgical approach. Such visual disorientation may contribute to injury to the pelvic side wall structures, particularly during concurrent laparoscopic lymph node dissection. If transected, the nerve should be repaired immediately. Nerve palsy resulting from a traction injury secondary to surgical positioning manifests postoperatively and may require formal neurologic evaluation and nerve conduction studies to quantify the extent of injury. These injuries are most often managed conservatively with physical therapy; however, the course of recovery may be prolonged, and it may take months before strength and sensation return to preinjury levels.

Urinary Tract Infection and Wound Infection

Although urinary colonization is common following prostatectomy and the associated prolonged catheterization, symptomatic urinary tract infection is, in general, not a significant or prevalent problem. The risk of perioperative urinary tract infection can be minimized through numerous measures, including the use of appropriate antibiotics preoperatively, early cessation of therapy postoperatively to reduce the risk of selective resistance and *Clostridium difficile* infection, the use of silver-lined antibacterial catheters, and appropriate catheter care during the early postoperative period. Some physicians also prescribe a single or short antibiotic course at the time of catheter removal, although this practice is of unclear benefit.

Postoperative wound infection is another uncommon infectious complication of laparoscopic robot-assisted prostatectomy. Contributing factors include suboptimal skin preparation, inadequate sterile surgical technique, prolonged length of operation, suboptimal timing of preoperative antibiotic administration, incorrect selection of antibiotic coverage, surgical treatment in the setting of active infection or colonization, rectal or bowel injury, and lack of wound irrigation before skin closure. Cellulitis may be treated with antibiotics and observation. Deeper wound infections require drainage through wound opening and initiation of wound care. Deeper infections, such as pelvic abscesses, should be drained percutaneously if possible, and cultures should be obtained during drainage to determine the most effective antibiotic therapy.

Thromboembolic Complications

The rate of clinically evident deep vein thrombosis has been low in relatively large laparoscopic series. For example, in one large laparoscopic series, the rate of thromboembolic complications was only 0.3%.[24] Despite the associated risks of pelvic surgery and relative venous stasis secondary to laparoscopic insufflation and intracavitary pressure, deep vein thrombosis does not appear to be more common than in the open approach. The suspicion of deep vein thrombosis or pulmonary embolus should be high in the presence of leg tenderness, respiratory distress, or decreased oxygen saturation. Use of continuous sequential compression devices or subcutaneous heparin reduces the risk of this complication, although some surgeons are hesitant to use heparin in the postoperative period routinely secondary to the risk of pelvic hematoma and potential adverse consequences such as anastomotic compromise. If deep vein thrombosis or pulmonary embolus is detected, however, prompt management with anticoagulation to prevent thrombus propagation is warranted.

INTERMEDIATE AND LATE POSTOPERATIVE COMPLICATIONS AND CONSEQUENCES

Given the relatively recent implementation of laparoscopic robot-assisted prostatectomy, most early clinical reports focused on intraoperative and early postoperative complications. Although reports regarding early functional treatment-related consequences are emerging, the extent of treatment-related impairments and functional recovery following laparoscopic robot-assisted prostatectomy has not been fully characterized. Nonetheless, clinical results reported to date indicate that during and beyond the learning curve, the laparo-

scopic approach is safe, and complications are relatively uncommon.

Overall, complications vary and are likely modified by case complexity, the surgeon's experience, and other still unidentified clinical factors. Intraoperative complications have been reported to be as low as 2.3% and range fairly narrowly to approximately 5% in currently reported case series.[29,30] Major complications and the need for repeat exploration following laparoscopic robot-assisted prostatectomy also appear to be rare, occurring in 1.7% and 1% of cases, respectively.[30]

Factors resulting in deviation from the anticipated postoperative course, such as treatment-specific complications, delay in discharge, or unplanned medical care for unexpected problems occur in ≤10% reported cases. Transient urinary retention following early catheter removal appears to be a significant contributor to this proportion and has been reported in ≤13% of cases following laparoscopic robot-assisted prostatectomy, whereas hematuria occurs in only 1% of cases.[30] Although reports may underestimate the true incidence of adverse events following laparoscopic robot-assisted prostatectomy given the common limitations of capturing and attributing surgical complications comprehensively and systematically, the type and frequency of complications reported thus far appear to support the safety of the robotic approach.

Functional complications and recovery following laparoscopic robot-assisted prostatectomy are of particular interest to most surgeons and patients, but they are more difficult to interpret, largely because assessment varies from surgeon to surgeon and from case series to case series. Most series have reported favorable recovery of urinary continence. Experience groups report 12-month incontinence in 1% of cases,[31] whereas others report return to baseline urinary function in >70% of cases and subjective continence in 90% of cases using more standard assessment methods.[29] Continence rates also appeared to be relatively favorable during the initial case experience with laparoscopic robot-assisted prostatectomy; one group reported that 90% of surgical patients did not require urinary control pads following the surgeon's initial 72 cases.[32]

Recovery of sexual function appears to be more variable and, as reported after the open procedure, more problematic. In one series, only 53% of patients achieved a baseline sexual function score following prostatectomy, although subjective potency was observed in 80%.[29] The impact of sexual problems is common even among the most experienced groups; despite a 93% probability of achieving an erection sufficient for intercourse, only slightly more than half of patients returned to baseline functioning following bilateral nerve-sparing procedures.[31] These results should be considered in the context of transparent reports of functional outcomes following laparoscopic robot-assisted prostatectomy, such as one case series reporting that only 19%

of patients reached baseline sexual function 12 months postoperatively.[33] Nonetheless, laparoscopic robot-assisted prostatectomy appears to have equaled the open approach in at least preliminary outcomes.[34,35]

Cancer control following laparoscopic robot-assisted prostatectomy, measured by proportion of positive margin, prostate-specific antigen failure, and disease progression, is one element of effectiveness for which adequate information is not yet available on which to draw reliable conclusions. Positive margins of 21% have been reported by some investigators,[29] whereas others have experienced 5-year biochemical recurrence in 8.4% cases.[31] As with other surgical interventions, surgical experience (measured by volume) has an important effect on outcomes and consequences following laparoscopic robot-assisted prostatectomy whether the procedure is performed in referral centers or in nonacademic community settings.[36]

Perhaps intuitively, surgeon-related factors appear to be more important than are patient-related factors. Although complications may or may not vary according to approach (transperitoneal versus extraperitoneal)[37] or other important clinical factors, such as body mass index,[38,39] the experience of the surgeon appears to be a principal determinant of the likelihood of postoperative complications.[40] Nevertheless, much of the information regarding the important consequences of treatment is incomplete, and additional study and assessment are necessary to determine the frequency and severity of treatment failure following laparoscopic robot-assisted prostatectomy.

CONCLUSION

Laparoscopic robot-assisted prostatectomy has become a common surgical approach in the management of early-stage prostate cancer. Complications may be related to the surgical procedure (prostatectomy), the approach (laparoscopy), or both. Overall, major and minor complications are relatively uncommon following laparoscopic robot-assisted prostatectomy and are consistent in type and frequency (other than hemorrhage) with the complications observed following open radical prostatectomy. Surgical experience appears to be an important mediator of complications. This finding indicates a learning curve and is a major influence on outcome. Nonetheless, despite the rapid diffusion of the laparoscopic approach and the growing experience with robot-assisted prostatectomy, a comprehensive understanding of the complications, consequences, and outcomes is currently in the early phase of development.

KEY POINTS

1. Proper patient selection and positioning will limit risk of complication.
2. Extraperitoneal approach eliminates risk of small bowel or major vascular injury.
3. Pneumoperitoneum limits bleeding.
4. Rectal injuries can be closed robotically.
5. Urethral vesicoanastomotic problems occur infrequently and usually are managed with catheter drainage rather than re-exploration.

REFERENCES

Please see www.expertconsult.com

Chapter 31

COMPLICATIONS OF MINIMALLY INVASIVE RECONSTRUCTION OF THE UPPER URINARY TRACT

Elias S. Hyams MD
Resident Physician, Department of Urology, New York University School of Medicine, New York, New York

Michael D. Stifelman MD
Director of Robotic Surgery and Minimally Invasive Urology, Department of Urology, New York University School of Medicine, New York, New York

The role of minimally invasive techniques in urologic surgery has burgeoned since the late 1990s. Although laparoscopy has become the standard of care for certain ablative urologic procedures (e.g., radical nephrectomy and adrenalectomy), its techniques have been increasingly employed for urologic reconstruction (e.g., radical prostatectomy and pyeloplasty). Intracorporeal suturing has been the most challenging aspect of laparoscopic reconstruction, although emphasis on laparoscopic suturing in training and more widespread use of robotic techniques have made this aspect of treatment less daunting.

Reconstruction of the upper urinary tract includes but is not limited to the following procedures: pyeloplasty, ureteroureterostomy, retrocaval ureter repair, ureteral reimplantation, psoas hitch or Boari flap, ileal ureter, and ureterolysis. All these procedures have been performed laparoscopically,[1-5] and many have been performed robotically.[6-9] Laparoscopic reconstruction with or without robotic assistance requires advanced skills; complications may result from both technical and patient factors, although meticulous technique can help to minimize morbidity. Comfort with open surgical techniques is essential for any laparoscopic surgeon to ensure competent intervention when conversion to an open procedure or open reoperation is required.

This chapter briefly reviews preoperative considerations for patients having minimally invasive urologic reconstruction. It then reviews the epidemiology of intraoperative and postoperative complications associated with these procedures and ways to address these complications should they occur.

PREOPERATIVE CONSIDERATIONS

General Considerations

See Chapter 28.

Operative Planning

Reconstruction of the upper urinary tract relies on a thorough understanding of a patient's anatomy related to both disease and anatomic variation. Planning for pyeloplasty should include computed tomography (CT) or magnetic resonance angiography to assess for crossing vessels and delineate hilar anatomy. For pyeloplasty or ureteral reconstruction, CT and magnetic resonance urography can be used to characterize the lesion of interest, for instance the length and location of stricture. Diuretic renal scans are useful to assess relative renal function and extent of obstruction. Additionally, if minimally invasive ureterolysis is planned, biopsy of retroperitoneal tissue should be considered before ureteral manipulation to exclude malignancy.

Patients should have a mechanical bowel preparation before reconstructive urologic surgery to increase working space and improve exposure. If a secondary repair is being performed or if the patient has had prior abdominal surgery, bowel adhesions may be present and bowel decompression may facilitate suturing and decrease the risk of injury. A bowel preparation is also useful for upper urinary tract reconstruction because it may be necessary to harvest bowel for ureteral interposition.

The decision to use minimally invasive techniques in lieu of open surgical methods depends primarily on the surgeon's preference and experience. Regarding the use of pure laparoscopy versus robotics, both have theoretical advantages, but few data suggest that one technique is superior to the other for reconstruction. For example, data are conflicting regarding the superiority of robotic to laparoscopic pyeloplasty, and long-term comparative data are lacking.[10-12] In sum, most reconstructive procedures have been safely and effectively performed laparoscopically with or without robotic assistance, or with pure robotics, and a surgeon should select the technique with which he or she is most familiar. Robotic techniques may have greatest advantage for surgeons without considerable laparoscopic suturing experience and thus permit better technical results than with pure laparoscopy.

Selection of transperitoneal versus retroperitoneal approaches for reconstruction depends primarily on the surgeon's preference. Both approaches are safe and effective for upper urinary tract surgery.[13-15] Retroperitoneal access may be safer in patients with extensive prior abdominal surgery, although disadvantages include limited working space and a potentially steeper learning curve.[16]

Intraoperative Complications

General principles of perioperative care apply to patients having urologic reconstruction and include the use of bilateral sequential compression boots, prophylactic antibiotics, and generous padding to all pressure points. Neuromuscular pain secondary to operative positioning is a frequently reported complication in large series of urologic laparoscopy.[17]

Complications related to access and pneumoperitoneum are discussed in Chapter 28. Management of visceral and vascular injuries is also discussed at length in that chapter. This section describes complications specific to minimally invasive reconstructive procedures and recommendations regarding their management.

Minimally Invasive Pyeloplasty

Laparoscopic pyeloplasty was first described in 1993 and has become standard of care at centers where advanced laparoscopy is performed.[18,19] This procedure has been shown to be safe and effective for primary and secondary ureteropelvic junction (UPJ) obstruction and for transperitoneal and retroperitoneal approaches.[20,21] Different types of reconstruction are performed including Anderson-Hynes dismembered pyeloplasty (typically with crossing vessels or a redundant renal pelvis) and Y-V plasty (typically with no crossing vessels or a high insertion), among others.[22] Robotic assistance was first reported by Sung and colleagues in 1999,[23] and numerous series have been published demonstrating the equivalence or superiority of this technique with the specific advantage of facilitated intracorporeal suturing.[24-26] In published reports of robotic pyeloplasty, intraoperative complications have been negligible and no conversions to an open procedure have been noted.[6,9,11,12,24-28]

Numerous series have demonstrated a low intraoperative complication rate for laparoscopic pyeloplasty.[20,22] In a series of 147 patients who underwent laparoscopic transperitoneal pyeloplasty, 2 cases of bowel injury were reported, including a serosal injury to the small bowel and an inadvertently clipped colonic diverticulum.[22] Both injuries were repaired laparoscopically during the same surgical procedure with no sequelae. Clipping of a colonic diverticulum can be repaired laparoscopically by excising the diverticulum with a laparoscopic gastrointestinal anastomosis (GIA) stapler.[29] No intraoperative complications were reported in a large series of patients who underwent extraperitoneal laparoscopic pyeloplasty.[15] Other large series of laparoscopic pyeloplasty have reported no intraoperative complications.[30,31] In the largest multi-institutional series to date of robotic pyeloplasty, a single minor intraoperative complication was noted among 140 patients; the patient had a minor intraoperative splenic laceration that was successfully managed with pressure and topical hemostatic agents.[9]

Both pure laparoscopic and robotic techniques have been used safely to perform secondary pyeloplasty including procedures after endopyelotomy and primary pyeloplasty.[6,19,20] Because dissection for secondary pyeloplasty can be hindered by fibrosis around the renal pelvis and proximal ureter, it is generally helpful to remove excess fibrosis from around the ureter before anastomosis is performed. One intraoperative complication occurred in a series of 36 patients who underwent laparoscopic transperitoneal repair of secondary UPJ obstruction; this patient had bleeding requiring conversion to an open procedure.[20] In a large multi-institutional study, no intraoperative complications were noted in 23 patients who underwent secondary robotic pyeloplasty. Minimally invasive pyeloplasty has also been safely performed in patients with upper urinary tract anomalies.[6,9,32]

The reported rate of conversion from laparoscopic to open pyeloplasty is ≤1.6%.[13-15,21] Rassweiler and associates[33] reported a single conversion in their large series of retroperitoneal laparoscopic pyeloplasty based on significant anastomotic tension and the requirement for open dissection and fixation of the kidney during suturing. The risk of conversion to an open procedure is higher during the early portion of the learning curve for laparoscopic pyeloplasty and decreases significantly as experience improves.[21] Conversion to an open approach may be necessary early in the learning curve based on failure to progress as well as more urgent indications.[34] Mufarrij and associates[9] reported no open conversions in a series of 140 robotic pyeloplasties. Facilitated intracorporeal suturing with robotic techniques may limit the rate of conversion to open procedures based on failure to progress, particularly early in a surgeon's laparoscopic experience.

The risk of significant bleeding from laparoscopic or robotic pyeloplasty is low. Inadvertent injury to major vessels may be minimized with good operative planning including CT angiography to identify crossing vessels or anomalous vascular anatomy. However, in our experience, imaging may not be completely reliable; both false-positive and false-negative results of imaging for relevant vessels may occur. Therefore, a laparoscopic Doppler probe (Vascular Technology, Nashua, New Hampshire) can be used to confirm the presence or absence of crossing vessels and can potentially further decrease the risk of vascular injury.

Laparoscopic suturing is the most challenging aspect of laparoscopic pyeloplasty. Technical complications of suturing (e.g., stricture, urinary extravasation) may be minimized by meticulous technique, but patient-related factors (e.g., history of diabetes, secondary repair) may influence the incidence of these complications. Technologic advances such as Lapra-Ty clips (Ethicon, San Angelo, Texas) may be used to minimize tissue trauma during suturing.[35] Moreover, robotic assistance has decreased the learning curve for anastomotic suturing and is likely to reduce complications related to the suture line early in a surgeon's experience.

Creating a tension-free anastomosis requires careful intraoperative planning and may decrease the risk of complications related to ureteral ischemia and suture line breakdown. Too much ureter or pelvis may be inadvertently removed, thus leading to difficulty in creating a tension-free suture line. It is generally helpful not to remove redundant pelvis until the anastomosis is complete. Creating a relaxed suture line may be particularly difficult during secondary repair in a patient with a small renal pelvis or ischemic proximal or distal tissue. Intraoperative techniques for safely creating more length include nephropexy, reverse psoas hitch, and creation of a "handle" in the renal pelvis to decrease the manipulation of healthy tissue. Traction sutures can also be placed in the ureter or pelvis to decrease manipulation of tissue and decrease the risk of ischemia.

Ureteral stent placement across the anastomosis is essential to minimize the risk of urinary leakage. Complications of stent placement include submucosal tunneling and incomplete advancement into the bladder or kidney, depending on the direction of placement. Retrograde stenting requires a second surgeon to place the stent cystoscopically while the laparoscopic surgeon confirms placement in the renal pelvis. If anterograde placement is performed, the bladder can be filled with 300 mL of methylene blue; refluxed dye confirms correct distal positioning of the stent. Initial evidence indicates that stentless laparoscopic pyeloplasty in patients having primary repairs is safe; however, the data are preliminary.[36]

Minimally Invasive Ureteral Reconstruction

Laparoscopic ureteral reconstruction has been performed in all portions of the ureter for diverse indications including trauma, stricture, neoplasm, and anatomic abnormalities.[4,37-40] Procedures have included laparoscopic ureteroureterostomy, psoas hitch, Boari flap, ileal ureter, neovesicoureterostomy, ureterolysis, and retrocaval ureter repair. Only case reports and small series of these procedures exist because of limited indications and technical complexity. Reports have noted successful robotic ureteral reconstruction including ureteroureterostomy, retrocaval ureter repair, ureteral reimplantation with and without psoas hitch, and ureterolysis with omental wrap.[8]

Laparoscopic ureteroureterostomy was first reported for treatment of infiltrative endometriosis and has been performed without significant intraoperative complications or need for conversion to an open procedure.[41] This technique has been successfully performed for treatment of midureteral stricture and iatrogenic ureteral injury.[2,38,40] Skill with intracorporeal suturing is required to perform the ureteral anastomosis safely and expeditiously. A unique consideration for ureteroureterostomy relates to the "watershed" blood supply of the midureter and the potentially increased risk of ischemia during manipulation and suturing. Techniques for reducing the risk of ischemia include minimizing the manipulation of tissues (e.g., using traction sutures), using a Doppler probe to avoid disrupting arterial flow, minimizing medial dissection of the ureter and potential disruption of the vascular supply, and ensuring that the ureteral edges appear pink and healthy before anastomosis. Robotic techniques have been used safely and successfully for ureteroureterostomy in a patient with an obstructed upper pole system and crossed renal ectopia with fusion.[7,42]

Ureteral stent placement is recommended in all patients having ureteral repair and can be placed in retrograde fashion either preoperatively or intraoperatively. If the stent cannot traverse the obstruction, it can be placed in retrograde fashion to the distal end of the stricture and can help to identify both the ureter and level of obstruction. If the ureteral length is insufficient for primary anastomosis, techniques such as psoas hitch or Boari flap can be performed to gain length distally. These techniques have been performed laparoscopically,[4,43] but urologists without advanced laparoscopic skills may require conversion to an open procedure. Bowel interposition or autotransplantation may be necessary if more conservative techniques are unsuccessful. Understanding the patient's anatomy and extent of disease is essential to ensure appropriate operative planning and management of the patient's expectations preoperatively.

Despite limited data, evidence indicates that the intraoperative complication risk of ureteral reconstruction is low. No significant intraoperative complications were noted in small series of laparoscopic ureteral reimplantation (for indications including reflux, distal ureter injury, and low-grade distal ureteral transitional cell carcinoma [TCC]),[4,37,44] laparoscopic Boari flap,[43,45] and laparoscopic ureterocalicostomy[46] or in case reports of laparoscopic ileal ureter,[3] robotic ureterocalicostomy,[47] retrocaval ureter repair,[39,48] and laparoscopic transureteroureterostomy in pediatric patients.[49] In addition, no complications were observed in another report of robotic reconstruction procedures including ureteroureterostomy, ureterocalicostomy, and ureteral reimplantation.[8]

Minimally Invasive Ureterolysis

Laparoscopic ureterolysis was first reported by Kavoussi and associates in 1992.[50] Laparoscopic dissection within a fibrotic retroperitoneum can be challenging given diminished tactile feedback. However, low morbidity was reported in several series of laparoscopic ureterolysis.[51,52] Intraoperative ultrasound can help to identify the ureter if fibrosis obscures retroperitoneal anatomy.[53]

Ureteral injury is one potential complication of laparoscopic ureterolysis. Ureteral injuries should be repaired either laparoscopically or with an open procedure, based on the extent and location of injury. Omental wrapping or intraperitonealization can be performed to protect the ureteral anastomosis. Vascular injury can occur; Fugita and associates[54] reported one iliac vein injury in their series from 2002. Pneumothorax and subcutaneous emphysema have also been reported during laparoscopic ureterolysis.[55,56]

Reported conversion rates to open procedures have been ≤15% in series of laparoscopic ureterolysis.[51,54] Conversion has been required secondary to technical difficulty with periureteral fibrosis, vascular injury, and other emergency indications.

Hand-assisted techniques can be used to shorten operative time and reduce technical difficulty. One series of hand-assisted laparoscopic ureterolysis reported a small ureteral injury that was repaired with simple absorbable suture.[51]

Robotic ureterolysis has been safely performed without intraoperative complications.[53] Improved visualization from robotic technology may facilitate identification of the ureter, and the precision of robotic Pott scissors and greater degrees of freedom may facilitate the dissection and potentially decrease the risk of injury.

POSTOPERATIVE COMPLICATIONS

Most complications of laparoscopic or robotic surgery are postoperative.[13-15] In addition, intraoperative injuries may not be recognized until the postoperative period. Symptoms that cannot be explained by physical examination or routine studies should prompt further evaluation. CT can lead to diagnosis in most patients with unexplained pain, fever, leukocytosis, or decreasing hematocrit following urologic laparoscopy.[57] See Chapter 28 for a thorough discussion of general postoperative complications of urologic laparoscopy, including trocar site hernia or infection, ileus or bowel injury, bleeding, and medical complications. This section discusses postoperative complications specific to minimally invasive upper urinary tract reconstruction.

Minimally Invasive Pyeloplasty

See Tables 31-1 and 31-2 for summaries of postoperative complications from major series of laparoscopic and robotic pyeloplasty. These studies did not use standardized definitions of complications and thus may not be directly comparable. Minor and major complications were often grouped together in determining the total complication rate in these studies.

The reported postoperative complication rate for laparoscopic pyeloplasty is 2% to 22%.[33,58,59] A meta-analysis of laparoscopic pyeloplasty series revealed an 8% postoperative complication rate including hematoma, urinoma, pyelonephritis, bowel serosal injury, transient ileus, thrombophlebitis, and UPJ anastomotic stricture.[60] Increasing experience with laparoscopic pyeloplasty within series revealed decreasing rates of postoperative complications.[58] Extraperitoneal laparoscopic pyeloplasty has published complication rates of ≤13%.[13-15]

Postoperative complication rates for robotic pyeloplasty have also been low. In the largest series to date of robotic pyeloplasty, a 7.1% major and 2.9% minor complication rate was reported.[9] The most common major complication in this series (7 of 10) was stent migration, with no difference noted between the use of retrograde and anterograde techniques for stent placement. The investigators admitted erring on the side of longer stent placement and relying on reflux of methylene blue dye through the proximal end of the stent to confirm anterograde placement. One patient in this series, with body mass index of 42, had gluteal necrosis that occurred during a 5-hour procedure and required subsequent fasciotomy. The investigators mentioned that their operative times have decreased and that they do not flex the operating table during surgical procedures in obese patients, to allow for more even distribution of weight. Additionally, one patient in this series developed an obstructing blood clot in the renal pelvis that necessitated a percutaneous nephrostomy tube that was left in place until stent removal. The investigators noted that irrigation of the renal pelvis before closure can help to minimize likelihood of this complication. Finally, a single patient had worsening hydronephrosis and pyelonephritis postoperatively that required stent exchange.

In another series of 92 patients undergoing robotic-assisted laparoscopic pyeloplasty, 3 patients (3%) had early complications requiring reintervention.[24] The first patient required stent exchange and percutaneous nephrostomy tube placement for clot-related obstruction of the renal pelvis and colic with urine extravasation; the second patient bled into the collecting system 2 days postoperatively and despite conservative treatment required open secondary pyeloplasty; and the third patient, who had excessive urine extravasation after inadequate closure of the renal pelvis, required

TABLE 31-1	Postoperative Complications of Laparoscopic Pyeloplasty			
Reference	**No. Cases**	**Approach**	**Postoperative Complication Rate (No. Patients)**	**Postoperative Complications (No. Patients)**
Soulie et al[15] (2001)	55	Retroperitoneal	12.7% (7)	Hematoma (3), urinoma, severe pyelonephritis, anastomotic stricture (2) requiring open pyeloplasty at 3 wk and delayed balloon incision at 13 mo
Inagaki et al[22] (2005)	147	Transperitoneal	7.5% (11)	Laparoscopic repositioning of drainage tube for urinary leakage (2), retroperitoneal hematoma, diagnostic laparoscopy (negative) for suspected bowel injury, blood transfusion (2), CHF, superficial antecubital thrombophlebitis, transient ileus, persistent urinoma
Moon et al[1] (2006)	170	Transperitoneal (3) Retroperitoneal (167)	7% (12)	Colon injury requiring right hemicolectomy POD 6; reexploration for port site bleeding 12 hr postoperatively, myocardial infarction, perinephric urinoma treated conservatively, heavy hematuria, port site infection, uncomplicated UTI, unexplained postoperative fever or rigor, ipsilateral renal pelvic stones (3)
Zhang[73] (2005)	50	Retroperitoneal	4% (2)	Prolonged duration of retroperitoneal drain for urine leak (2)
Mandhani et al[30] (2005)	92	Transperitoneal	18.4%	Paralytic ileus (6), blood transfusion, prolonged drain output (6), pyelonephritis, meatoplasty, SWL, ureteroscopy for stent migration, percutaneous stenting, repair of port site hernia
Eden et al[21] (2004)	124	Retroperitoneal	4.1% (5)	Myocardial infarction 6 hr postoperatively, bleeding from a subcostal artery lacerated during port insertion requiring return to operating room 10 hr postoperatively, superficial port site infection, renal calculus formation (2)
Jarrett et al[29] (2002)	100	Transperitoneal	11% (11)	Urinary ascites secondary to drain migration requiring laparoscopic exploration and drain repositioning (2), retroperitoneal bleeding requiring PCN, blood transfusion (3), CHF, pneumonia, superficial antecubital thrombophlebitis, transient ileus; persistent urinoma requiring percutaneous drainage
Turk et al[31] (2002)	49	Transperitoneal	2% (1)	Anastomotic leakage POD 1 requiring laparoscopic repair
Hemal[74] (2003)	24	Transperitoneal (12) Retroperitoneal (12)	12.5% (3)	Prolonged ileus (3) (all transperitoneal)
Sundaram et al[20] (2003)	36	Transperitoneal (all secondary)	22.2% (8 cases)	Anastomotic leakage at postoperative cystogram POD 2 (4) (3 managed with continued Foley catheter and retroperitoneal drain, 1 required PCN), UTI, pneumonia, atelectasis, fever, bilateral upper extremity weakness although related to patient positioning, renal calculus formation at 2 mo
Klingler et al[75] (2003)	40	Transperitoneal	17.5% (7 cases)	Anastomotic stricture, reoperation (2) (nephrectomy in 1 patient for recurrent stricture/urosepsis/deteriorated renal function, open ureterocalicostomy in 1 patient for ischemic anastomosis/recurrent stricture); renal pelvic clot retention (2) requiring PCN in 1 patient; urinoma, urosepsis from recurrent UTI (2) requiring PCN in 1 patient

CHF, congestive heart failure; PCN, percutaneous nephrostomy; POD, postoperative day; SWL, shock wave lithotripsy; UTI, urinary tract infection.

TABLE 31-2 **Postoperative Complications of Robotic-assisted Laparoscopic Pyeloplasty**

Reference	No. Procedures	Postoperative Complication Rate (No. Patients)	Postoperative Complications (No. Patients)
Mufarrij[9] (2008)	140	7.1% (10) (major) 2.9% (4) (minor)	*Major:* stent migration (7), clot obstruction, gluteal compartment syndrome requiring fasciotomy, pyelonephritis/obstruction *Minor:* febrile UTI, urine leak (2), splenic laceration (intraoperative)
Palese et al[6] (2005)	35	11.4% (4)	UTI requiring oral antibiotics, pyelonephritis requiring IV antibiotics (2), gluteal compartment syndrome
Patel[28] (2005)	50	2% (1)	Renal colic after stent removal at 21 days requiring restenting (retrograde pyelogram showed widely patent anastomosis)
Schwentner et al[24] (2007)	92	3.3% (3)	Bleeding into renal pelvis/colic with urine extravasation requiring stent exchange and PCN, bleeding into collecting system 2 days postoperatively initially managed conservatively then requiring open pyeloplasty 3 mo later, insufficient closure of resected renal pelvis and excessive urine extravasation requiring transperitoneal exploration and primary closure of renal pelvis
Weise and Winfield[27] (2006)	31	6.5% (2)	Afebrile UTI, urine leak with ileus treated nonoperatively
Gettman et al[26] (2002)	9	11% (1)	Urinary leakage requiring open exploration and repair of incompletely closed renal pelvis
Bernie et al[12] (2005)	7	28.6%	Febrile UTI requiring IV antibiotics, gross hematuria from bleeding at anastomotic site requiring readmission and conservative treatment

IV, intravenous; PCN, percutaneous nephrostomy; UTI, urinary tract infection.

open repair of the renal pelvis. This last patient had prior treatment of UPJ obstruction but the exact treatment was not mentioned. Two other patients in this series had prior pyeloplasty, and 9 had prior endopyelotomy or ureteroscopy, none of whom had significant complications. In a series of 31 patients with robotic-assisted laparoscopic pyeloplasty, 1 patient had nonfebrile urinary tract infection and 1 had a urine leak with ileus that was treated nonoperatively.[27]

Bleeding or hematoma formation can occur following minimally invasive pyeloplasty. Soulie and colleagues[13] reported that 2 of 61 patients developed hematoma in the lumbar fossa following laparoscopic pyeloplasty. Rassweiler and associates[33] reported 5 cases of postoperative hematoma in 143 patients undergoing laparoscopic pyeloplasty. Hematoma can generally be managed conservatively by following serial hematocrit levels and transfusing as necessary. Hemodynamic instability or a precipitous drop in hematocrit may necessitate urgent reoperation. One may need to drain a hematoma percutaneously at a later point based on persistent symptoms or infection.[13-15] CT scan is generally the best modality for diagnosing postoperative hematoma.[57] Delayed bleeding can occur as well; in one series, a patient required hospitalization for retroperitoneal bleeding 1 month after laparoscopic pyeloplasty.[22]

Urinoma is another important complication following minimally invasive pyeloplasty. Urine leakage occurs in ≤2.3% of patients undergoing laparoscopic pyeloplasty,[22,59] and this complication can occur despite meticulous suturing and ureteral stent placement. Urinoma may be indicated by flank or abdominal pain, fever, or elevated liver function tests on the right side.[57] Soulie and colleagues[13] reported that 2 of 61 patients developed postoperative urinoma. Rassweiler and colleagues[33] reported urinary extravasation in 2 of 143 patients after laparoscopic pyeloplasty. Secondary pyeloplasty and congenital abnormalities may be risk factors for urinary leak.[25,26]

In the early postoperative period, leakage can be detected by persistently elevated drain output and can be confirmed by checking fluid creatinine levels. Drains may be required for a prolonged period if leakage persists. Within a urinoma, drains can be repositioned if necessary, including laparoscopically.[22,29] If one suspects urinoma after the acute postoperative period, CT with intravenous contrast is the diagnostic modality of choice. Delayed images may be needed to reveal active urine leak. Urinomas can generally be managed conservatively by leaving stents in place to optimize drainage or by replacing stents for ≥2 weeks and then assessing drainage of the upper urinary tract. Placement of a Foley catheter, or leaving the catheter in place, may also decrease pressure on the upper urinary tracts and maximize healing if leakage is noted. Percutaneous drainage of urinoma may be required if conservative measures fail.[17] Percutaneous drains may be gradually devanced and serial imaging done to ensure resolution of the collection. Reactive pleural effusions can result from urinary leakage abutting the diaphragm; these effusions may require drainage if symptoms develop or if infection is a consideration. The risk of urinary leakage may be reduced by control of suture tension during collecting system closure (e.g., with Lapra-Tys).[35] Generally, urinary leakage has no significant sequelae, but periureteral scarring can occur. Repeat laparoscopy to suture an insufficiently closed site is rarely necessary but may be performed.[31]

Stent obstruction can occur after minimally invasive pyeloplasty. Rassweiler and colleagues[33] reported that 1 of 143 patients developed stent obstruction after laparoscopic pyeloplasty. A second stent can be placed, the stent can be changed, or percutaneous nephrostomy tube placement with or without anterograde stenting may be necessary. Stent migration can also occur requiring repositioning through ureteroscopy or removal depending on timing relative to surgery.[30] If stent migration below the anastomosis is identified late, stenosis may require reoperation. Proper positioning of the double-J stent should be carefully confirmed before leaving the operating room,[30] and erring on the side of longer versus shorter ureteral stents may be helpful. Acute obstruction after stent removal may require repeat stenting or nephrostomy tube placement. If a patient presents with ipsilateral flank pain before stent removal, imaging (e.g., kidneys, ureters, bladder) should be performed to ensure the stent is in proper position.

Stricturing at the UPJ following stent removal causes obstruction 2.5% to 3.6% of the time.[61] Stenting or nephrostomy tube placement may be required to relieve obstruction in these patients depending on symptoms, the presence of infection, and serum creatinine concentrations.[17,58] Conservative treatment of stricture can be attempted, such as with balloon dilation or endopyelotomy. However, secondary pyeloplasty may ultimately be required, and alternative techniques such as ureterocalicostomy may be necessary depending on the patient's anatomy (e.g., insufficient renal pelvis for anastomosis). Stents are typically removed 4 to 6 weeks after repair and the anastomosis evaluated at 6 to 8 weeks by renal scan or intravenous pyelogram. Depending on the timing of restricturing, this process may be considered a treatment failure or a complication. Success rates for both laparoscopic and robotic pyeloplasty are high and early restricturing is uncommon.[24,62] Mufarrij and colleagues[9] reported that 3 of 140 patients required treatment of recurrent stricture after robotic pyeloplasty; 2 patients required endopyelotomy and 1 required repeat pyeloplasty. These investigators

attributed these failures most likely to ischemia or technical factors.

Minimally Invasive Ureterolysis

Reported postoperative complications of laparoscopic ureterolysis have been mild and have included prolonged ileus, epididymitis, urinary retention, and port site erythema.[54] No postoperative complications were reported in one series of hand-assisted laparoscopic ureterolysis.[51] In a series of five laparoscopic ureterolysis procedures, one patient had a small perioperative ureteral leak that was managed with prolonged Foley catheter drainage and ureteral stent placement.[53] No postoperative complications occurred after five robotic ureterolysis procedures reported in the same article.[53]

Postoperative complications of ureterolysis are similar to those listed earlier for pyeloplasty and may include urinary extravasation and ureteral obstruction secondary to recurrent fibrosis or ischemic changes in the ureter. Intraperitonealization and omental wrapping can help to decrease the risk of recurrent obstruction, although these procedures may be technically challenging. Efforts should be made to diagnose and treat the underlying cause of fibrosis if possible. Ureteral stent placement may be helpful to minimize the risk of postoperative urinary leak and obstruction.

Unusual complications of ureteral manipulation can occur during ureterolysis. One of our patients developed a midureteral leak after robotic ureterolysis with omental wrapping. Stent placement was performed but the patient had recurrent flank pain and a renal scan demonstrated partial mechanical obstruction. Ureteroscopy revealed a mild midureteral stricture as well as a ureteral diverticulum with a Weck clip within the lumen of the diverticulum. Balloon dilation and stenting were performed and subsequent ureteroscopy revealed sealing of the diverticulum; however, the patient required subsequent laser endoureterotomy and balloon dilation for recurrent stricture.

Minimally Invasive Ureteral Reimplantation

Laparoscopic ureteral reimplantation has been shown to be safe, with a low postoperative complication rate. No postoperative complications were reported in one small series of patients who underwent laparoscopic reimplantation for distal ureteral stricture refractory to endoscopic management.[44] No major postoperative complications were noted in a small series of patients who underwent distal ureterectomy and reimplantation for low-risk ureteral TCC.[37]

Stricture can occur at the site of anastomosis following minimally invasive reimplantation. The diagnosis can be made initially with renal ultrasound and then confirmed by excretory urography. Confirmation of drainage at the time of stent removal can minimize the risk of patients who present again with obstruction. Ureteral stent placement is generally indicated to drain the obstructed system, although percutaneous nephrostomy tube placement may be necessary. Stricture can be managed conservatively with dilation, but it may ultimately require anastomotic revision. Obstruction secondary to edema can occur postoperatively and is generally minimized by stenting for 4 to 6 weeks postoperatively; however, transient obstruction can also occur after stent removal and may require stent replacement for several weeks.[37] One method of minimizing the risk of technical complications is to determine the location of the new ureteral orifice cystoscopically and then assess tissue apposition during the suturing process.[63]

Urinary leak can occur following ureteral reimplantation and can be managed as discussed earlier with maximal drainage and consideration of percutaneous drain placement. A cystogram should be performed at the time of stent removal to confirm the absence of leak. Reflux into the ureter through the repair confirms patency of the anastomosis, provided a refluxing anastomosis was performed. If a nonrefluxing anastomosis was performed, diuretic renal scan or an intravenous pyelogram can be performed to confirm the absence of obstruction at the ureterovesical anastomosis.

Minimally Invasive Ureteroureterostomy

The primary postoperative complications of laparoscopic ureteroureterostomy include anastomotic stricture and urinary leakage. However, published rates of postoperative complications for laparoscopic ureteroureterostomy have been low. In a small series of ureteroureterostomy for iatrogenic injury of the pelvic ureter, no postoperative complications were noted ≤13 months after surgery.[2] Midureteral strictures have also been repaired laparoscopically with good drainage and without complications.[38]

Obstructed retrocaval ureter has been repaired by laparoscopic resection of diseased retrocaval ureter and ureteroureterostomy without postoperative complications.[39,64,65] This procedure has been safely performed both transperitoneally and retroperitoneally.[66]

Laparoscopic ureteral surgery has been reported for upper urinary tract TCC and has been shown to be safe. Proximal ureteral segmentectomy and ureteropelvic anastomosis have been performed for low-risk TCC in the proximal ureter without complications.[67] Laparoscopic distal ureterectomy with ureteral reimplantation has also been safely performed for low-grade TCC.[68] Oncologic outcomes at short-term follow-up have been encouraging in these patients. Patients should be carefully selected for any minimally invasive procedure for management of ureteral malignant disease, and principles of open oncologic surgery should be respected.

Minimally Invasive Boari Flap

Laparoscopic Boari flap has been described for long distal ureteral strictures and has been shown to be safe and effective.[5,43] In a small series of laparoscopic Boari flap, one patient with a history of pelvic radiation developed uroperitoneum after Foley catheter removal.[5] The urinoma did not resolve with reinsertion of the catheter, and the patient required exploratory laparoscopy during which a small vesicotomy was laparoscopically repaired. The patient had no sequelae of this complication.

The risk of urine leakage can be minimized by leaving a Foley catheter in place for 7 to 10 days postoperatively and confirming the absence of a leak with cystography. In patients with a history of pelvic radiation, the Foley catheter should be left in place for ≥2 weeks to maximize healing. Ureteral stents should be left in place for 6 weeks to allow for complete healing of the ureter.

Minimally Invasive Ileal Ureter

One case of laparoscopic ileal ureter has been reported after laparoscopic ureterectomy for ureteral TCC in a patient with a solitary kidney.[3] No complications were associated with this procedure. Complications can arise from bowel manipulation and suturing including ileus, bowel obstruction, and bowel leak. Management of these complications is discussed in Chapters 28 to 30.

Minimally Invasive Ureterocalicostomy

Laparoscopic ureterocalicostomy has been performed without complications.[46] Robotic assistance may significantly facilitate the suturing component of this operation.[47]

Minimally Invasive Transureteroureterostomy

Laparoscopic transureteroureterostomy was reported in a series of three pediatric patients without significant postoperative complications.[49] Transient urinary leak occurred in one patient that resolved in <24 hours. Leaving a drain near the anastomosis is recommended to ensure the absence of leakage before the Foley catheter is removed. The literature on open transureteroureterostomy indicates an incidence of urinary leakage of ≤6%.[68]

Obstruction of the common ureter is noted infrequently in series of open transureteroureterostomy and has not been reported for laparoscopic transureteroureterostomy.[68-70] Intraoperatively, a stent can be placed either in the recipient ureter or across the anastomosis, although some investigators argue that stenting the recipient ureter is more useful for maintaining ureteral patency during the anastomosis and for preventing placing sutures through the back wall.[49] Overall, series of open transureteroureterostomy demonstrate a low complication rate and the rare occurrence of obstruction; in skilled hands, laparoscopic transureteroureterostomy is likely to have similarly a similarly low complication rate.

CONCLUSION

In competent hands, minimally invasive urologic reconstruction is a safe and effective surrogate for open techniques. Inexperience with laparoscopic suturing is the main obstacle to the dissemination of these techniques into the community. As training programs emphasize laparoscopic suturing more, robotic techniques become more popularized, and demand from patients grows for minimally invasive reconstruction, these techniques will become more prominent in urologic practice.

Unfortunately, reports of complications for urologic reconstruction, and for much of urologic laparoscopy, do not use standardized definitions of complications. Such standardization would help to improve our understanding of the epidemiology of operative morbidity and would inform strategies to minimize the risk of these procedures.[59] Certain classification schemes for complications do exist, however, and modifying them to reflect urologic procedures specifically could increase the utility of reporting for our field.

Because of the learning curve for laparoscopy and intracorporeal suturing in particular, movement has been made toward credentialing of urologists in laparoscopic techniques to improve safety.[71] Training for laparoscopy should proceed incrementally to minimize morbidity in the early portion of the learning curve. Training modules have been implemented to improve the efficiency and safety of laparoscopic training for

urologists.[72] The benefits of robotic techniques, specifically regarding intracorporeal suturing, need to be balanced against cost issues regarding the purchase and maintenance of robotic systems.

KEY POINTS

1. All upper tract reconstructive procedures have been performed safely and effectively using minimally invasive techniques, including laparoscopy and robotic surgery.
2. Thorough preoperative planning is critical for upper tract reconstruction, including preoperative imaging geared toward the type of surgery being performed and counseling about the different types of reconstruction that may be required depending on intraoperative findings.
3. Minimizing manipulation of tissue during upper tract reconstruction is critical to reduce risk of ureteral stricture and urinoma formation.
4. Maximal drainage of the urinary tract after upper tract reconstruction (i.e., ureteral stent placement, percutaneous drainage, and bladder drainage) reduces the risk of urine leakage and urinoma formation postoperatively.
5. Robotic surgery will be used increasingly for upper tract reconstruction based on facilitation of intracorporeal suturing, and it may decrease risk of complications, particularly during surgeons' early experience.

REFERENCES

Please see www.expertconsult.com

Chapter 32

COMPLICATIONS OF ROBOTIC SURGERY

Brian H. Irwin MD
Assistant Professor of Surgery, Division of Urology, University of Vermont College of Medicine, Burlington, Vermont

Joseph R. Wagner MD
Director of Robotic Surgery, Connecticut Surgical Group/Hartford Hospital, Hartford, Connecticut

The use of robotic-assisted laparoscopic surgery in urology has increased dramatically since the first robotic prostatectomy was performed by the Frankfurt Group in 2001.[1] In 2001, approximately 250 robotic-assisted laparoscopic prostatectomies were performed worldwide, whereas >33,000 procedures were performed in 2006 (data supplied by Intuitive Surgical, Sunnydale, California). With this explosion, the need for urologic surgeons to understand the complications specific to robotic-assisted cases has increased as well. Minimizing complications related to this type of complex surgical endeavor takes a team effort including circulating and scrub nurses, anesthesiologists, technical support specialists, and surgeons and their assistants. At Hartford Hospital in Connecticut, >2000 robotic-assisted laparoscopic urologic procedures have been performed including radical prostatectomies, radical cystectomies with various urinary diversions, pyeloplasties, ureteral calicostomy, partial nephrectomies, adrenalectomies, vesicovaginal fistula repairs, bladder diverticulectomies, ileal ureteral creation, and distal ureterectomies with ureteral reimplantation. The goal of this chapter is not to cover all aspects of every possible urologic procedure performed with robotic assistance, but rather to provide an overview of possible complications related specifically to this new modality.

PREOPERATIVE PREPARATION AND PATIENT SELECTION

The roles of patient preparation and selection cannot be overemphasized in their ability to prevent and alter the outcomes of possible complications of surgery. This is especially true during the early learning curve of any newly developing surgical technique. The ideal patients for robotic surgery are relatively thin, have no surgical history of the abdominal cavity, and are otherwise physiologically healthy. A thorough cardiopulmonary evaluation is critical to avoid many possibly devastating complications. The many physiologic changes associated with pneumoperitoneum are well documented and are described elsewhere in this book. Pneumoperitoneum with the strict and exaggerated positions required for robotic-assisted surgery places these patients at risk for potential cardiopulmonary compromise intraoperatively.

The surgeon must determine and discuss the patient's expectations preoperatively. Informed consent, open communication, and presentation of realistic expectations are the hallmarks of patient satisfaction and the avoidance of malpractice suits.[2] We invite all our patients who undergo robotic prostatectomy or cystectomy, regardless of outcome, to join our patient support list, which contains each patient's name, age at surgery, date of surgery, and preferred method of contact (phone or e-mail). Surgical candidates are given this list at their preoperative consultation. The patient should be counseled regarding pain expectations as well as the need for catheters and drains in the postoperative period. It is not uncommon in our practice to see patients who initially think that the robot will provide pain-free and complication-free surgery. This is clearly not the case.

The patient should be informed of the possible need for conversion to a laparoscopic or even an open procedure in the event of unfavorable anatomic features, intraoperative complications, or mechanical failure. With proper maintenance, mechanical failures are extremely rare.[3] Mechanical problems are generally detected before the patient is brought to the operating room, and a discussion can be held whether to proceed with another approach or postpone the procedure. We have had three intraoperative failures requiring conversion to a laparoscopic approach, all of which were completed successfully.

An empty bowel at the time of operation serves two purposes: (1) it maximizes the working space within the pneumoperitoneum, and (2) it minimizes bowel spillage should a bowel injury occur. Patients are instructed to take a clear liquid diet starting the day before the procedure, followed by nothing by mouth except for sips of water with medications starting at midnight before the operation. Patients are requested to undergo a mechanical bowel preparation in the form of 8 ounces of magnesium citrate given in the afternoon before the operation followed by a Fleets enema in the evening.

Before the induction of general anesthesia and endotracheal intubation, prophylactic antibiotics are administered in a form appropriate for the procedure (most typically a first- or second-generation cephalosporin). The patient receives an injection of 5000 U of unfractionated heparin subcutaneously and pneumatic antiembolism stockings are applied. After induction, an orogastric tube is placed and a Foley catheter is inserted to ensure complete decompression of the stomach and bladder during port insertion.

Patient Positioning

Patient positioning varies dramatically depending on the specific requirements of the surgical procedure. Positioning injuries can be potentially devastating; however, in most cases, they can be avoided with proper preparation and forethought.

Renal or Adrenal Surgery

During renal or adrenal surgical procedures, the patient is typically placed in a 45-degree semilateral decubitus position with gel pads used to support the operative side (**Fig. 32-1**). A padded neurologic armrest is used to support the arm gently. In this semilateral position, an axillary roll is not required. The patient's upper leg is extended over the flexed lower leg with pillows placed in between. The table is left flat and is not flexed. It is necessary to roll the patient from a near supine position for port placement to a full flank position intraoperatively. To allow this drastic change in position, the patient is secured with 3-inch wide cloth tape passed over the patient and around the table several times to

secure the patient's head, shoulders, chest, hips, and legs. Upper and lower body warming blankets are used to maintain the patient's core body temperature. In this position the robotic device can be used to approach the renal fossa in a position over the patient's ipsilateral shoulder and can also be used to gain access to the lateral pericolic gutters and upper pelvis.

Pelvic Surgery

Positioning for pelvic surgery usually requires the use of extreme Trendelenburg positioning (often >20 degrees head down) (**Fig. 32-2**). This positioning should be minimized when possible. Options for supporting the patient's head and shoulders include straps extending across the shoulders and chest, shoulder bolsters, and vacuum bean bag devices. Straps across the chest can worsen ventilatory problems already aggravated by Trendelenburg positioning, particularly in patients with restrictive pulmonary disease, obesity, or other comorbid diseases. Shoulder bolsters must be well padded and placed with ample room for the patient to rest gently against them. These bolsters should be placed directly in line with the acromion on either side to avoid brachial plexus injuries. Vacuum bean bag devices must be well padded because they also can cause pressure injuries.

For pelvic surgical procedures, patients are placed either into a modified dorsal lithotomy position with the use of stirrups or into a split-leg position with the legs straight but supported under the knees and laterally flexed at the hips (see Fig. 32-2). Modified dorsal lithot-

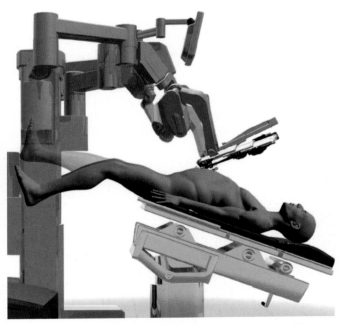

Figure 32-2 Patient positioning for robotic pelvic surgery. The patient is placed into a modified dorsal lithotomy position with the use of stirrups or split-leg supports. The robot is brought in between the patient's lower extremities. (*Courtesy of Intuitive Surgical, Sunnydale, California.*)

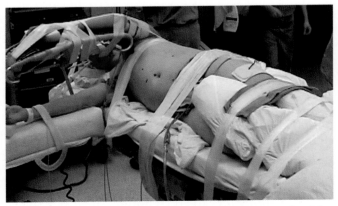

Figure 32-1 Patient positioning for robotic renal surgery. Careful attention to positioning and padding by the anesthesia, nursing, and surgical teams is critical. The robot is brought into the surgical field over the patient's ipsilateral shoulder.

omy positioning has the advantages of allowing the legs to be protected somewhat by the stirrups themselves and of lowering them out of the way of the moving robotic arms during the procedure and during robotic docking and undocking. However, stirrups may make patients more prone to pressure neuropathies and neurologic stretch injuries. To minimize the risk, it is crucial to maintain a straight line from the patient's heel, to knee, to contralateral shoulder and to ensure that the hip position is not hyperextended.

The split-leg configuration may provide support in a more anatomic position and may thus decrease the risk of neurologic compression injuries. Stretch injuries can still occur, particularly femoral neuropathies resulting from hip overextension. The split-leg configuration has the disadvantage of less room for the robotic surgical cart to approach the patient. In our experience, the creation of ample room between split legs or stirrups and the robotic arms has become less problematic with the newer-generation da Vinci S surgical system (Intuitive Surgical, Sunnyvale, California) than with the standard da Vinci system. The robot is then placed between the patient's legs (**Fig. 32-3**).

Complications directly attributable to patient positioning during pelvic and renal surgery have included rhabdomyolysis,[4-18] musculoskeletal pains, and ventilatory difficulties.[19-23] Neurologic injuries, including ulnar,[24,25] brachial,[26] femoral,[27-29] and peroneal[30,31] nerve neurapraxias, as well as cerebral edema, have also occurred. A head-down position and severe blood loss can lead to retinal blindness, and this complication is well-documented across surgical disciplines.[32] Needless to say, this situation can occur during robotic prostatectomy, particularly early in the learning curve.

Port-related Complications

Most port-related injuries can be avoided in much the same way as in standard laparoscopic surgery. Peculiar to the use of robotic assistance is an even greater necessity to position ports in exact locations. Port misplacement may render a robotic procedure impossible because the robotic arms will clash with each other or with the patient. Poor port placement could result in conversion to a laparoscopic open procedure.

Initial access into the abdominal cavity can be safely obtained using either a standard Hasson technique, a Veress needle, or a visual trocar. All subsequent ports should be placed under direct vision using standard laparoscopic techniques. Special care must be used in patients who have had prior abdominal operations because these patients are prone to adhesion formation and any port placement technique is more likely to allow inadvertent bowel injury. Transillumination and knowledge of common vascular anatomy (i.e., location of inferior epigastric arteries) can be particularly helpful in avoiding major vascular injuries within the abdominal wall as well as bothersome venous bleeding at port sites.[33-35] In our experience of >2000 robotic cases, 2 patients required reoperation for bleeding, 1 for an inferior epigastric arterial injury at a robotic arm port site.

In general, robotic ports should be spaced approximately 8 cm apart. Placing robotic ports closer than this can lead to clashing of robotic arms and poor access to the surgical field. Port sites for renal surgery are as depicted in **Figure 32-4**. Typical port placements for pelvic surgery for both the three-arm and four-arm da Vinci systems are shown in **Figure 32-5**.

Proper port removal is as important as port placement in avoiding postoperative complications. As with placement, all ports should be removed under direct vision. The pneumoperitoneum should be allowed to fall to ≤5 mm Hg to ensure that the port site shows no evidence of bleeding.

Port site hernias can be avoided by the use of sutures placed with a fascial closure device. In general, port sites >10 mm should be closed at the fascial level; however,

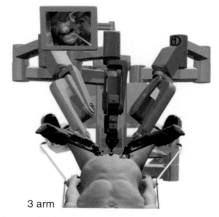
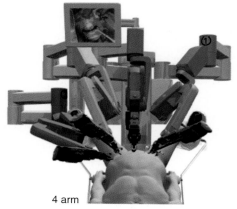

3 arm   4 arm

Figure 32-3 Robot and robotic arm positioning for both a three-arm and a four-arm system during pelvic surgery. *(Courtesy of Intuitive Surgical, Sunnydale, California.)*

ports placed with a dilating tip may not require fascial closure if ≤12 mm. Port site disease recurrences have been documented following laparoscopic nephroureterectomy[36-40] and radical robotic cystectomy.[41]

INTRAOPERATIVE COMPLICATIONS

General Considerations

Although most anesthesiologists are comfortable with short laparoscopic procedures such as cholecystectomy and hernia repair, for example, they may be less well versed in major, longer laparoscopic cases and may inappropriately treat the patient as they would for an open surgical procedure. Decreased blood loss, decreased insensible loss, and decreased urine output resulting from insufflation pressures can result in fluid overload. Nitrous inhalants should be avoided because they can cause bowel distention with decreased exposure. Insufficient ventilation can result in hypercapnia with pul-

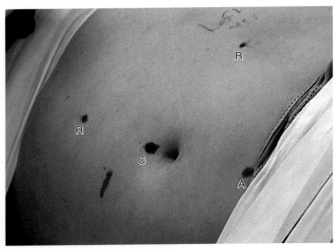

Figure 32-4 Port sites for robotic renal surgery: two 8-mm robotic trocars (R), one 12-mm robotic camera trocar (C), and one 12-mm assistant trocar (A).

monary arrest or fatal arrhythmias. A multi-institutional review by Gill and colleagues[42] revealed that 35% of complications were the result of the physiologic changes that occur during laparoscopy. Open communication with the anesthesia team before and during the surgical procedure will prevent many of these complications.

At the end of the procedure, the patient should be examined for signs of significant subcutaneous emphysema, particularly after longer procedures. The presence of diffuse crepitus is associated with mucosal absorption and resultant laryngeal obstruction in a patient in whom hyperventilation may be required to expel excess carbon dioxide. Therefore, extubation in this setting must be controlled. Lack of a cuff leak around the endotracheal tube with a deflated balloon, chest radiographic evidence of pneumomediastinum, direct visualization of laryngeal coaptation, and baseline pulmonary insufficiency are all indications for delayed extubation.

Bleeding is another more common complication of minimally invasive surgery. In a review of complications during urologic laparoscopic procedures, bleeding was the most commonly cited intraoperative complication.[43] Bleeding can result from injury of the primary organ or of an adjacent organ as well as injury to major vascular structures. These injuries can be thermal or can result from blunt trauma or stapler or clip misadventure. Depending on the situation, pressure, endoclips or staplers, fibrin sealants, Surgicel (an oxidized cellulose hemostatic agent), temporary elevation of the insufflation pressure, or free suturing techniques can generally salvage the situation. However, one should not hesitate to obtain adequate assistance when necessary from general surgical or vascular colleagues or even convert to an open procedure if necessary. All members of the surgical team need to be well versed in the steps to undock the robotic surgical cart in the event of such an emergency.

Many intraoperative complications result from injury of adjacent local organs. The keys to minimizing intraoperative complications are solid knowledge of local and intra-abdominal anatomy, a high index of suspi-

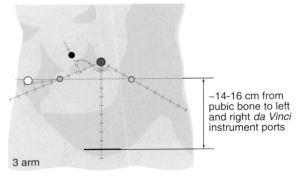

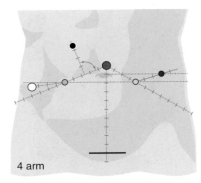

~14-16 cm from pubic bone to left and right *da Vinci* instrument ports

3 arm

4 arm

Figure 32-5 Color-coded port sites for robotic pelvic surgery: white (12-mm assistant trocar), black (5-mm assistant trocar), blue (8-mm right robotic trocar), red (12-mm robotic camera trocar), yellow (8-mm left robotic trocar), and green (8-mm robotic fourth arm trocar). *(Courtesy of Intuitive Surgical, Sunnydale, California.)*

cion for injury, and the ability to recognize and repair these injuries intraoperatively. In the robotic-assisted approach, the lack of tactile feedback may increase the possibility of injury to a local structure. For this reason, all moving instruments must be kept within the visual field at all times to avoid inadvertent injury.

Renal or Adrenal Surgery

Injuries sustained during renal and adrenal surgery are site specific. Right-sided surgical procedures predispose patients to injuries involving the duodenum, ascending colon and hepatic flexure, liver, and inferior vena cava. The adrenal veins come directly off the inferior vena cava and are very short on the right side. These veins can bleed excessively if they are not controlled carefully. Left-sided renal or adrenal surgical procedures can lead to injuries of the aorta, splenic flexure and descending colon, pancreas, and spleen. Diaphragmatic injuries can occur on either side. In our experience, the most common indication of a diaphragm laceration is loss of space around the upper pole as the diaphragm is pushed inferiorly by the insufflation pressure. At times, this laceration can be accompanied by hemodynamic or ventilatory changes. As long as no lung laceration is present and the patient is stable, the injury can be repaired, and carbon dioxide will be rapidly reabsorbed. If the pneumothorax prevents adequate exposure or if the patient is hemodynamically unstable, a small Heimlich valve tube can be placed to evacuate the pneumothorax and complete the procedure.

Pelvic Surgery

Nongenitourinary structures commonly encountered during pelvic surgery include the bowels, particularly the rectum, and neurovascular structures in the region. These structures also can be avoided in most cases with a proper knowledge of anatomic landmarks.

Injuries to the iliac veins during pelvic lymph node dissection can cause significant bleeding. Most injuries can be repaired robotically with distal control if necessary and with fine suturing technique. However, larger injuries may necessitate conversion to an open procedure for surgical correction.

During pelvic lymph node dissection, visualization of the obturator nerve is important. Because the operator in the console is physically separated from the patient, the operator will not feel any adductor activity as would be expected with dissection close to this nerve in open or laparoscopic surgery. This muscle activity, however, can usually be appreciated visually within the console.

Rectal injuries are among the more common complications described during any approach for prostatectomy. Rectal injuries in the robotic-assisted setting tend to be smaller than those created during open surgery. We suspect that the reason is the increased sharp rather than blunt dissection employed during robotic prostatectomy. This situation emphasizes the need for a high index of suspicion to avoid problems with unrecognized perforations. The rectum can be tented up beside the prostate laterally and is particularly susceptible to injury during non–nerve-sparing prostatectomy when dissection is performed lateral to the neurovascular bundles. We routinely place a 32-Fr chest tube into the patient's rectum during positioning to permit easy insufflation testing of the rectum when necessary. When recognized, rectal injuries should be closed with a two-layer technique with absorbable suture. In our experience at Hartford Hospital, we have had two rectal injuries. The first was recognized intraoperatively during salvage prostatectomy (**Fig. 32-6**). This injury was repaired in a two-layered fashion followed by interposi-

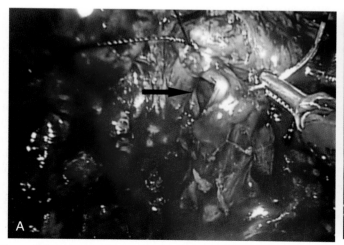
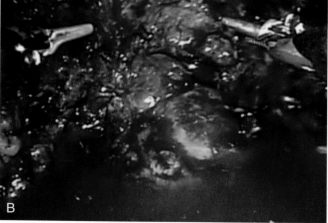

Figure 32-6   **A,** Rectal injury (*black arrow*) repaired in two layers with 2-0 absorbable suture. **B,** Air is insufflated into the rectum after repair to ensure a tight closure.

tion of a J-shaped omental flap and passed by a tunnel through the peritoneal reflection in the cul de sac of Douglas. The second injury manifested in a delayed fashion 6 weeks postoperatively in a patient with a prior history of a colonic-vesical fistula resulting from diverticulitis. The fistula resolved with 3 weeks of Foley catheter drainage, and no further intervention was required.

Ureteral injuries in the robotic-assisted laparoscopic literature have been most commonly reported in association with radical prostatectomies. These injuries most often occur during posterior dissection between the prostate and Denonvilliers' fascia while approaching the vasa differentia and seminal vesicles or while dissecting the bladder neck from the base of the prostate. In this region, the ureter is subject to potential transection or obstruction if it is incorporated into a bladder neck repair or the anastomosis. This situation can be particularly problematic if the ureteral orifices are close to the bladder neck or if a large median prostatic lobe exists. We routinely give all our patients an ampule of indigo carmine intraoperatively. Although this precaution is usually unnecessary because the orifices are well away from the bladder neck and are never seen, in difficult cases it allows us to avoid the annoying wait for blue efflux if the injection is not given until problems arise.

We have had one ureteral injury at our institution, in which the right ureter was obstructed during a posterior bladder neck repair and was incorporated into an interrupted anastomosis. This injury was treated with percutaneous nephrostomy tube placement. Attempts to pass an antegrade stent were unsuccessful. Cystoscopic transection of the obstructing suture, antegrade passage of a wire, ureteral stent placement, and prolonged Foley catheter drainage successfully addressed the issue without long-term sequelae.[44] Since that time we have favored anterior bladder neck repairs in an attempt to avoid inadvertent ureteral injury during bladder neck repair and to allow visualization of the orifices during the anastomosis. On the rare occasion when the ureteral orifices are particularly close to the cut bladder neck, bilateral double-J ureteral stents can be placed to provide visualization during the dissection and creation of the anastomosis and to ensure postoperative patency.

In 2001, early in our learning curve at another institution, a ureteral transection was recognized intraoperatively by the lack of blue efflux from the right ureteral orifice. A wire was passed into the ureteral orifice and was seen curling in the pelvis, a finding indicating ureteral transection. The prostatectomy and anastomosis were completed, the ureter was dissected from the iliac veins distally, and a standard ureteral reimplantation was performed in the dome of the bladder over a stent.[45] The urologic literature has established that a ureteral reimplant, rather than a primary ureteral repair, is the preferred approach for distal ureteral injuries. Although distal ureteral injuries during prostatectomy have been primarily repaired successfully laparoscopically,[46] we believe that this approach is more prone to anastomotic breakdown and stricture.

Reconstructive Surgery

Robotic assistance can be particularly helpful in reconstructive urologic surgery. At our institution, this technique has been applied to pyeloplasty, ureterocalicostomy, bladder diverticulectomy, ureteral reimplantation, and vesicovaginal fistula repair. Current robotic carts are capable of very fine suturing with enhanced optics and motion scaling that make them well suited to creation of the meticulous anastomoses often required in reconstructive urologic surgery. As in open or laparoscopic surgical reconstructions, several principles must be adhered to in the creation of a successful anastomosis. These principles include preserving an adequate blood supply at the cut surfaces, minimizing tension on healing edges, maintaining patency during the healing process, and apposing the mucosa to promote healing. Several articles have addressed the benefits of running[47-51] versus interrupted[52,53] anastomoses. Although no one technique is appropriate for all situations, general principles can again be applied. Running anastomoses tend to be more watertight and provide a more even distribution of tension; however, they can be more ischemic and if performed in a circumferential fashion can lead to cicatrix and stricture formation. Compared with running anastomoses, interrupted anastomoses can be more prone to leakage between sutures, but they provide less restriction of blood flow to the anastomosis.

IMMEDIATE POSTOPERATIVE COMPLICATIONS

Bleeding Complications

The exact incidence of bleeding following robotic surgery is not known. However, bleeding is rarely an indication for intervention in the immediate postoperative course in our experience. We have found that most patients with evidence of postoperative bleeding can be managed expectantly with intervention required for hemodynamic instability. We have seen several patients with an apparent postoperative hemorrhage and a subsequent fall in hematocrit who remained hemodynamically stable with adequate urine outputs. As the hematocrit approached 25%, most of these patients stopped bleeding and required no intervention. Only one patient required a 2-U transfusion for bleeding followed by successful expectant management. We traditionally obtained commuted tomography imaging in these patients to identify and localize any bleeding, but these scans were universally unhelpful because they did not lead to any change in intervention.

In >1900 prostatectomy cases to date, 2 of our patients have required reoperation for bleeding complications. One patient had an epigastric artery injury from a robotic arm 8-mm port site that required ligation. The second patient had unidentifiable pelvic ooze requiring exploration resulting from hemodynamic instability. The hematoma was evacuated, Surgicel and FloSeal hemostatic sealant were placed along the neurovascular bundles, and the patient did well.

Urinary Extravasation

Complications following reconstructive urologic procedures involving urine leakage are reported in nearly every series published within the specialty of urology. This finding underscores the frequency of these complications. At our institution, the incidence of urinary extravasation following prostatectomy has decreased with the increased experience of the surgeons. We believe that any reconstructive procedure during which the urinary tract is violated should involve placement of a drain around the urinary tract closure. This maneuver helps to avoid the devastating complications of sepsis and urinary peritonitis that can be seen in the absence of controlled leaks. Creatinine levels are checked routinely before drain removal to assess for evidence of urinary extravasation. Following prostatectomy, drains are removed on postoperative day 1 if the fluid creatinine concentration is <3 mg/dL. We have had six patients with immediate urine leaks (<1%), all of which closed in ≤1 week with continued Foley and pelvic drainage.

To date, we have had four patients with delayed urinary leaks manifesting between 3 and 6 weeks postoperatively typically with fever, lower abdominal pain, and bladder spasms uncontrolled by anticholinergic therapy. Two leaks resolved uneventfully with 2 weeks of Foley catheter drainage. A third required placement of a percutaneous transgluteal drain and 2 weeks of Foley catheter drainage. The fourth continued with persistent leakage from an abdominal drain as documented in a cystogram. This complication was managed with diversion of the urinary stream away from the anastomosis with placement of bilateral externalized single-J ureteral stents through the urethra with subsequent resolution of the leak.

Early Urinary Retention

In the literature describing both open and laparoscopic procedures, efforts have been made to attempt earlier and earlier catheter removals. Early catheter removal has been shown to have an increased incidence of early urinary retention, most likely because of edema at the anastomsis.[71,72] We generally remove the catheter on postoperative day 8, and this approach seems to limit early urinary retention.

Ileus

Ileus is reported in the literature with an incidence ranging from 1.5% to 4.2% following robotic-assisted laparoscopic prostatectomy.[54-60] In the majority of cases, these complications have been associated with urinary extravasation from the urethrovesical anastomosis.[60] This is a disadvantage of the intraperitoneal approach typically performed for robotic-assisted prostatectomy because it allows for the presence of urinary peritonitis and subsequent ileus. An extraperitoneal approach may decrease the incidence this problem.[61-64]

Deep Venous Thrombosis and Pulmonary Embolism

Patients undergoing robotic-assisted surgery often fall into a very high-risk category for the development of deep vein thrombosis and resultant pulmonary embolism. Risk factors common to these patients include pelvic surgery, oncologic surgery, Trendelenburg positioning, dorsal lithotomy positioning, and prolonged pneumoperitoneum.[65] For these reasons, all measures should be taken to minimize the risk of these potentially life-threatening complications. Patients should receive subcutaneous heparin before the induction of anesthesia. This therapy should be maintained throughout the hospital stay. Lower extremity compression devices should be applied before positioning and should be maintained at all times while the patient is in bed throughout the hospital course.

Systemic Complications

Cardiovascular and pulmonary systemic complications are relatively rare and are rarely associated specifically with a robotic approach. Although certain aspects of positioning and the procedure can exacerbate underlying conditions as outlined earlier, these issues are most commonly related to the patient's underlying disease and warrant consideration on a case-by-case basis.

Infection

Wound infections following robotic surgery are rare. They are reported with an approximate incidence of 1% in most series.[54,57,58,66-68] Postoperative fluid collections (seromas, lymphoceles, hematomas, or urinomas) are common following laparoscopic and robotic urologic procedures. When these collections become infected, they require drainage and administration of appropriate systemic antibiotics. Drainage can be accomplished in most cases by placement of percutaneous drains. Multiple drains may be placed if needed, but in rare cases open evacuation of infection fluid or tissue and drain placement may be necessary.

LONG-TERM COMPLICATIONS

Hernias

Port site hernias occur rarely if ports have been closed appropriately as described earlier. The rate of inguinal hernia following radical prostatectomy has been reported to be approximately 12%.[69,70] Investigators have hypothesized that stripping the peritoneum from the floor of Hesselbach's triangle weakens the area and makes it more prone to hernia formation. The general surgeons at our institution prefer to fix hernias secondary to robotic prostatectomy through an open approach (i.e., Lichtenstein-type repair) to avoid the possibility of mesh application directly over bowel without interposed peritoneum.

Bladder Neck Contractures

Bladder neck contractures and anastomotic obstruction can largely be avoided by abiding by the principles of reconstructive surgery discussed earlier. When these complications do occur, they can be quite frustrating for patient and surgeon alike. The bladder neck contracture rate among our patients is 2%. Initial treatment modalities include dilation, incision, and resection. Our current preference is for incision. Most patients do well with one intervention. However, we have two patients with troubling recurrences. One patient is managing well with intermittent catheterization twice a day and an insurance incontinence pad. The other required transurethral resection for a dense fibrotic stricture every 4 months despite catheterizations twice daily and eventually underwent a Mitrofanoff procedure.

Urinary Incontinence

We ask the patient with localized prostate cancer to begin Kegel exercises as soon as he makes the decision to undergo surgical treatment. Some studies have suggested that patients with increased preoperative urinary symptoms or significantly enlarged prostates are more apt to have continence issues postoperatively.[73,74] Surgeons are always searching for techniques to improve long-term continence as well as the rapidity in which continence is gained.[75,76] Although the efficacy of these techniques can be debated, it is conservative to state that preservation of the bladder neck and maintenance of urethral length are important determinants of future continence. Every effort should be made to achieve this surgical result while maintaining oncologic principles.

Patients still requiring pads at 6 months are started on biofeedback. Anecdotally, we believe that patients benefit considerably by this intervention. Patients with mild (one pad/day but more than an insurance pad) incontinence at 1 year try various combinations of α-agonists, anticholinergics, or tricyclic antidepressants in addition to Kegel exercises. If symptoms persist, urodynamic studies are performed and, if appropriate, surgical procedures such as collagen injection, bladder sling, and sphincter are considered. Patients with moderate or severe incontinence (two pads/day or more) undergo immediate urodynamic testing at 1 year with appropriate recommendations.

To date, we have had four patients undergo a surgical procedure. A bladder sling in two patients decreased incontinence from one to two pads daily to an insurance pad. Two patients went from one pad daily 6 months postoperatively to three pads daily after salvage radiation. A urinary sphincter rendered them completely continent.

Erectile Dysfunction

The patient's level of preoperative sexual function, age, and comorbidities together with the surgical technique all play large roles in determining postoperative sexual function. Again, surgeons are continuously honing their techniques to improve potency outcomes. The veil of Aphrodite technique developed by Dr. Menon has been shown to improve potency while maintaining surgical margin rates.[77,78] As with techniques to improve continence, the efficacy of all these techniques can be debated, but it is conservative to state that the more periprostatic tissue that can be left unmanipulated while maintaining oncologic principles, the better.

Data are starting to accrue in support of the early, perhaps even preoperative, use of phosphodiesterase inhibitors.[79,80] Starting the night the catheter is removed, we ask all patients interested in future potency to start a low dose of a phosphodiesterase inhibitor at bedtime; a full dose is taken before sexual encounters. Unfortunately, the lack of prescription coverage makes this approach a considerable financial burden to the patient. Patients are instructed to follow this plan as much as is financially feasible.

For men not responding adequately to phosphodiesterase inhibitors, numerous other options are available including penile injections, intraurethral suppositories, penile vacuum pumps, and penile elastic rings. In most series, potency has been shown to improve over 6 to 24 months.[81] Therefore, permanent interventions such as penile implants are delayed until we are sure that future erectile function is not going to occur.

CONCLUSION

With proper patient selection and preparation, careful positioning, and meticulous attention to the details of anatomy, the incidence and effects of many complications following robotic surgery can be minimized. More and more complex reconstructive and extirpative urologic surgical procedures involving the kidneys, adrenals, and pelvic organs will become possible with the continued development of new technologies. With these technologies comes the need for urologic surgeons to continue to anticipate and strive to avoid any accompanying potential complications.

KEY POINTS

1. Proper patient selection is important, particularly early in the robotic learning curve.
2. Obtaining informed consent and managing patients' expectations preoperatively will result in improved patient satisfaction.
3. Open communication during positioning and surgery among surgeons, anesthesiologists, and nurses will avert many complications.
4. Proper port placement is critical; poor port placement will result in robotic arms clashing with each other or the patient.
5. Most robotic surgery complications are not robot specific; they can occur with laparoscopic or with open approach. An understanding of laparoscopic port placement, the physiologic changes associated with laparoscopy, and the potential complications from the procedure itself are mandatory.

REFERENCES

Please see www.expertconsult.com

COMPLICATIONS OF RETROPERITONEAL SURGERY

Chapter 33

COMPLICATIONS OF NEPHRECTOMY

Eric C. Nelson MD
Clinical Research Fellow, Department of Urology, University of California–Davis, Sacramento, California

Christopher P. Evans MD
Professor and Chairman, Department of Urology, University of California–Davis, Sacramento, California

Surgical removal of the kidney was reported as early as 1861. However, the first planned nephrectomy was probably performed by Gustav Simon in 1869 for a ureterovaginal fistula.[1] Because early nephrectomies were associated with high mortality rates as a result of peritonitis, the flank incision became the preferred approach until the 1950s, when effective antibiotic prophylaxis was developed. In 1969, Robson and colleagues[2] published a seminal article describing their surgical management of renal tumors through the thoracoabdominal approach. Early control of the renal vessels, en bloc excision of kidney and adrenal with Gerota's fascia remaining intact, and extended lymphadenectomy allowed improved survival compared with simple nephrectomy.[2]

The principles outlined by Robson and associates still form the basis for treatment of similar tumors. Since that time, however, advances in imaging techniques have improved detection of smaller lesions and have caused a significant downward stage migration. This change may partially account for improvements in the morbidity and mortality of nephrectomy. Evolving surgical techniques, anesthesia improvements, newer antibiotics, and effective intensive care contribute as well.

PREOPERATIVE CONSIDERATIONS

Cardiopulmonary Complications

Some possible life-threatening cardiopulmonary complications common to all surgical procedures include hypovolemic shock, myocardial infarction, pneumonia, pulmonary embolism, and pulmonary insufficiency. Renal surgery may cause severe stress to the cardiopulmonary system through patient positioning effects, blood loss, and other causes. The slow-growing nature of renal neoplasms allows treatment of significant occlusive cardiovascular lesions before nephrectomy. Revascularization of the coronary arteries and carotid endarterectomy may allow safer renal surgery. However anticoagulation during cardiac surgery increases the risk of tumor bleeding.

Patients undergoing nephrectomy frequently are placed in the flank position for surgical access. This position may severely stress the cardiopulmonary system, especially if the operating table is broken or a kidney rest is extended. First, pressure on the great vessels may decrease preload and increase afterload, thereby decreasing cardiac output. Second, ventilation is severely decreased by the flank position. In addition to limiting the excursion of the dependent diaphragm, increased ventilation-perfusion mismatching may further decrease oxygen exchange and lead to hypoxia. These combined cardiopulmonary effects may make this position intolerable for some patients with limited reserve.

These issues necessitate careful preoperative screening of patients for pulmonary diseases and cardiac status. Cardiology and pulmonology consultation should be obtained if any doubt exists about the patient's condition. Preventive measures instituted preoperatively and invasive monitoring intraoperatively may increase safety for some patients. The potential for blood loss and large hemodynamic shifts should prompt preoperative blood typing. In addition, autologous blood donation should be offered to patients.

Urologic Complications

Preoperative workup of the urinary tract, in addition to imaging of the operative site, should include assessment of contralateral kidney function in addition to total kidney function by creatinine and urea nitrogen levels. Urinalysis and, if indicated, urine culture and sensitivity should be performed to ensure that the urinary tract is not infected before operation. If urinary tract infection is found, antibiotics with adequate coverage should be given.

Patient Preparation

General intraoperative preventive measures are very important in avoiding complications common to any surgical procedure. Strict adherence to evidence-based recommendations ensures best possible outcomes. Antibiotic prophylaxis should be initiated ≥30 minutes before incision. Two large-bore intravenous access ports must be in place. Subcutaneous heparin should be initiated preoperatively to decrease the risk of deep vein thrombosis. Alternatively, compression hose, or preferably sequential compression devices, should be placed on the lower extremities unless contraindications such as open ulcers exist. If this is the case, some evidence suggests that placement of these devices on the arms may still provide some antithrombotic effects. The patient must be positioned carefully with pressure points sufficiently padded. Factors pertaining to specific positions are discussed later.

General Complications

Complications particularly relevant to nephrectomy include pneumonia, hypertension, and acute renal insufficiency. The risk of pneumonia may be higher after renal surgery compared with other abdominal procedures because of a combination of factors. The pulmonary issues discussed earlier lead to atelectasis intraoperatively.

Because of the kidney's location, the patient's postoperative discomfort with deep breathing may be significant; it may decrease clearance of secretions from the nonventilated space and set up an environment conducive to bacterial growth. Prevention and treatment of postoperative pneumonia are discussed later.

Nephrectomy represents the removal of an important component of the body's mechanism for maintaining blood pressure within the normal range. The incidence of postoperative hypertension is <8%, usually mild, and it frequently resolves.[3] In the long term, hypertension develops in some kidney donors, but it is not significantly different from hypertension in matched population controls or siblings.[4] Postoperative acute renal insufficiency may be multifactorial, relating to removal of a large percentage of the body's functional nephrons, direct or indirect manipulation of the contralateral kidney that causes arterial spasm, and rhabdomyolysis related to patient positioning. Postoperative acute renal insufficiency is usually transient but may require dialysis in some cases. Long-term renal insufficiency has not been shown to be a concern in patients with normal contralateral kidneys.[4]

SURGICAL APPROACH

Many incisions have been described for nephrectomy. These may be classified into anterior, flank, and poste-

rior approaches. Indications for specific incisions include patient body habitus, size and location of the renal lesion, other concurrently planned operations, indications for lymphadenectomy, and the surgeon's experience.

Site Verification

The Joint Commission (formerly the Joint Commission on Accreditation of Healthcare Organizations) reported statistics on wrong-site surgery and showed that the incidence is increasing; 90 cases occurred in 2005 alone. Approximately 10% of cases are reported to be urologic. Rigorous adherence to policies designed to prevent these occurrences is necessary to optimize patient care (Box 33-1).

Anterior Incisions

The advantages of anterior incisions, whether midline, subcostal, or chevron (**Fig. 33-1**), include quick exposure to the renal pedicle and the great vessels. This feature may not be as important for prevention of tumor seeding as was first thought; however, ease of exposure and familiarity with anatomy are still advantages. Procedures in trauma cases are performed through anterior approaches for quick access to the renal vessels and exposure to the entire abdomen. Some patients cannot

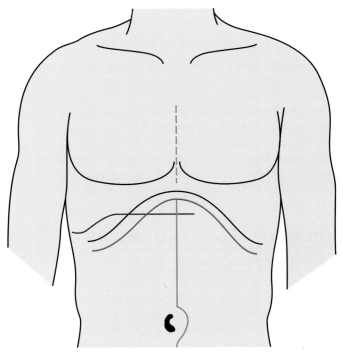

Figure 33-1 Diagram demonstrating anterior incisions. Midline incisions (*blue*) may be extended superiorly if exposure of the thoracic vena cava is necessary. The subcostal incision (*red*) may be extended across the midline if a complete chevron incision is necessary. A thoracoabdominal incision (*green*) offers excellent exposure to the superior renal pole and thoracic vena cava.

Example of Wrong-site Surgery Policy

Definition
Wrong-site surgery is a broad term encompassing all procedures performed on the wrong patient, wrong body part, wrong side of the body, or at the wrong level of the correctly identified anatomic site.

Predisposing Conditions
All patients undergoing surgery are considered at risk for wrong-site surgery. Certain situations increase the risk of wrong-site surgery, however, such as multiple surgeons or surgical procedures during a single encounter, or unusual room setup, equipment setup, or patient positioning.

Personnel
The entire surgical team must work to ensure compliance with the outlined procedures. With any change of personnel, repeat verification of procedure site shall be done.

Marking the Site
All surgical procedures involving left/right distinction, multiple sites, or anatomic levels require surgical marking by a physician member of the surgical team. An indelible marker visible after the patient has been prepared and draped shall be used to initial the surgical site. In no case will the opposing side be marked.

Patient Transfer
The anesthesia provider shall not move the patient from the preoperative holding area until the surgical site is positively identified and marked, if appropriate.

Documentation
On transfer to the operating room, the circulating registered nurse (RN) verbally confirms the patient's identity with the patient and ensures agreement among all medical records, the surgical site and marking, the surgical team, and the anesthesia provider. The circulating RN documents that this has been done. In addition, the circulating RN documents the completion of the Surgical Pause before incision.

Surgical Pause
Immediately before the skin incision, the entire team actively participates in a timeout during which the key information regarding patient, surgery, and surgical location is verified.

Conflict Resolution
In the event of any disagreement or conflict with any step of this procedure, the surgical procedure is suspended until the conflict is resolved by the attending physician.

plasms, left nephrectomy with significant thrombus extension into the vena cava, and other preoperative indications for bilateral dissection. Although rarely indicated because of the accuracy of modern imaging techniques, the anterior approach also allows exploration of the abdomen for metastatic disease. Some investigators advocate extended lymphadenectomy with nephrectomy, and this procedure is easiest through an anterior approach.

The disadvantages of anterior approaches include transection of multiple muscle groups for subcostal or chevron incisions. If the operation is performed transperitoneally, any spillage of tumor or infectious material may have greater consequences than if the material is confined to the retroperitoneum. If the operation is intended to be retroperitoneal, anterior approaches may not be best because entry into the peritoneal cavity may accidentally occur. Transperitoneal operations are associated with formation of adhesions and possible future small bowel obstruction. This complication was estimated to occur in 2% of patients in some series.[7] Obese patients may not be suitable candidates for anterior approaches because of difficulties associated with excessive extraperitoneal and intraperitoneal fat.

Flank Incisions

Flank approaches may be preferable for uncomplicated nephrectomies. This approach allows access to the retroperitoneum while avoiding entry into the peritoneum or chest. Careful attention must be given to positioning and padding of the patient. Taping the hips too tightly to the operating table can result in gluteal necrosis. The incision may be accomplished in the 10th or 11th interspaces, or the 10th, 11th, or 12th ribs may be resected. If an intercostal incision is performed, the incision should be made immediately superior to the rib to avoid damage to the intercostal nerve and to the vessels that run immediately below each rib and extend between the internal oblique and transversalis muscle layers. Up to 23% of patients have a flank sag postoperatively as a result of injury to intercostal nerves that causes laxity of flank muscles at that level (**Fig. 33-2**).[8] This condition may be difficult to distinguish from a true hernia, which is a rarer complication requiring surgical treatment to prevent incarceration. Such hernias are more commonly seen in persons with poor nutritional status, diabetes, or other risk factors for poor wound healing. Computed tomography (CT) imaging aids in establishing the diagnosis of an incisional hernia. Postoperative pain from flank incisions may be significant, especially during deep inspiration. Pain may become a long-term problem as a result of neuritis or entrapment of an intercostal nerve in the sutures or surrounding scar tissue. This complication may be prevented by careful reapproximation of the muscle layers. Fortunately, these issues usually resolve with time. Reassurance may be all that

tolerate flank approaches for cardiovascular reasons. Other indications for anterior approaches are planned bilateral nephrectomy in patients with polycystic kidney disease, large or upper pole tumors, bilateral renal neo-

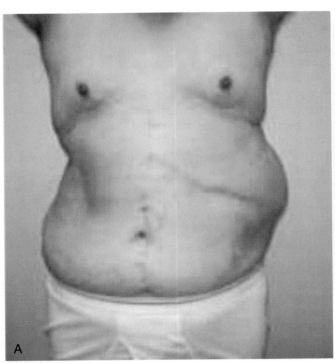
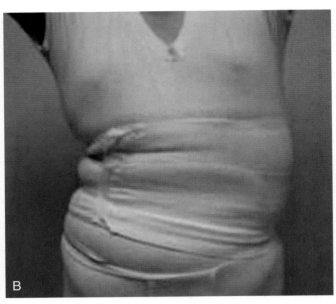

Figure 33-2 **A,** This patient is a 63-year-old man who underwent left splenectomy through a midline incision secondary to lymphoma and nephrectomy through a flank incision for T3b renal cell carcinoma (RCC). Although the surgical margins were negative, two sequential RCC recurrences of the diaphragm and renal bed were resected through a subcostal incision. Despite subsequent repair of a flank incisional hernia, the patient continues to have flank laxity, in part because of transected intercostal nerves. **B,** Photograph showing management of flank laxity with an abdominal binder.

is required, but some patients require local steroid injections for analgesia.

Thoracoabdominal Incisions

The thoracoabdominal incision is a large incision now usually reserved for large or complicated radical nephrectomies. The extensive incision allows exploration of the peritoneal, retroperitoneal, and thoracic compartments with biopsy or wedge resection of any suspicious lesions. The exposure to the upper pole of the kidney is excellent, and therefore this incision may be used when an extensive upper pole lesion is anticipated. Vena cava thrombi with known extension above the diaphragm or into the right atrium may require entry into the thoracic cavity, and a right thoracoabdominal incision provides good visualization of the thoracic vena cava and right atrium. The disadvantage of this incision is the considerable morbidity associated with it. The size of the incision predisposes it to infection. Postoperative discomfort of the patient may be considerable because of the extensive wound and the necessity for a chest tube. Spillage of tumor or infectious particles may be problematic given that both the peritoneum and the thoracic cavity are affected. Caution must be exercised when the left thoracoabdominal incision is used, to avoid injury to the spleen during incision of the diaphragm. The division of the costal cartilages anteriorly

may lead to significant postoperative pain if these cartilages are not fixed securely with nonabsorbable suture. Rare complications include postoperative hemidiaphragmatic paralysis from division of the phrenic nerve and an annoying clicking sensation from nonunion of the costal cartilages.[9]

Lumbodorsal Incisions

A distinct advantage of lumbodorsal incisions is decreased postoperative pain. This incision allows entry into the retroperitoneal space without division of any muscle groups and thereby minimizes the surgical trauma, which is one cause of postoperative discomfort of patients. Wound breakdown is uncommon with lumbodorsal incisions because the only layer to be divided, the lumbodorsal fascia, is very strong. The disadvantages of this incision center on the limited exposure it provides. Because extensive dissection of the vascular pedicle is very difficult, this incision is inadequate for renovascular surgery and radical nephrectomies with large tumors, upper pole disease, or suspected tumor extension or tumor thrombus. Division of the costovertebral ligament of the 12th rib may improve upper pole exposure. However, this maneuver risks damage to the costal neurovascular bundle. Because of the limited exposure provided by lumbodorsal incisions, they are less commonly used than are anterior or flank approaches. At present, laparoscopic surgery has widely replaced the lumbodorsal approach to minimize incision size and postoperative pain.

INTRAOPERATIVE COMPLICATIONS

Hemorrhage

Angiography is not routinely performed before nephrectomy. Thus, prevention of significant intraoperative hemorrhage requires accurate knowledge of renal anatomy and blood supply as well as the variations commonly encountered.

Arterial Anatomy

In the majority of patients, a single renal artery branches laterally off the aorta and enters the renal hilum. On the right, the renal artery usually courses posterior to the vena cava. Multiple renal arteries are not uncommon, seen in >25% of patients in some series.[10] These arteries, if present on the right, generally pass anterior to the vena cava. The renal arteries are end circulation. If the artery or any of its branches is occluded, ischemic infarction of the kidney or the respective segment will occur.

Because the gonadal artery, adrenal artery, and inferior phrenic artery also lie in close proximity to the areas of dissection, these vessels are vulnerable to injury. The inferior phrenic arteries are the first abdominal branches of the aorta and generally have branches coursing inferior to supply a portion of the adrenal circulation. The adrenal arteries branch from the aorta at the level of the celiac trunk anteriorly and course laterally to the adrenals. Additional adrenal arterial branches frequently originate from the renal artery. The gonadal arteries branch laterally off the aorta below the renal arteries. Alternatively, they may occasionally branch off the renal artery. The right gonadal artery most often passes anterior to the vena cava.

Venous Anatomy

Venous drainage of the kidney, in contrast to the arterial circulation, has many collateral vessels. The right renal vein drains directly into the vena cava, usually without being joined by other veins. The left renal vein is usually joined by the left gonadal vein, left adrenal, and a lumbar vein before it passes anterior to the aorta to join the vena cava. Both renal veins generally lie anterior to the corresponding renal artery. Multiple renal veins are less common than are multiple arteries but they do occur in approximately 1% of patients, generally on the left. The renal vein may divide, with one limb anterior and one posterior to the aorta. Alternatively, only the posterior branch may remain.[11] The extensive collateral vessels of the renal venous system prevent slowly occurring occlusive processes such as tumor thrombus formation from causing kidney damage, renal failure, or other symptoms. Because of the greater collateral circulation on the left, the left renal vein may be ligated acutely with probable survival of the renal unit. The right lacks such extensive collateral vessels.

Statistics of Hemorrhage

Radical nephrectomy has classically been considered a bloody surgical procedure. Neovascularization and additional collateral circulation to renal tumors can be extensive. In historical series, most patients required transfusions with average amount reaching 2 L.[2] More modern series report an average blood loss of 300 mL and a transfusion rate of only 15%.[12] Hemorrhage during nephrectomy for neoplastic conditions is more likely compared with benign conditions.[13] Close attention to surgical technique may minimize complications associated with hypotension, anemia, and blood transfusion. Adequate venous access must be ensured preoperatively to allow rapid resuscitation and possible blood transfusion.

Preoperative Embolization

Preoperative embolization is an attractive option when tumor extent makes extensive vascularity probable (**Fig. 33-3**). Infarction of the entire kidney should theoretically reduce blood loss, although most studies have not found this to be the case.[14] Some surgeons believe that embolization may allow easier dissection of the kidney because it forms an edematous plane immediately surrounding the infarcted tissue. Arterial embolization also allows earlier ligation of the renal vein. In cases anticipated to have a difficult hilar dissection or anterior approaches, in which the anatomic access to the artery is more difficult, angioinfarction may be helpful. Examples include patients with large hilar tumors overlying the artery, bulky nodal disease encasing the artery, or

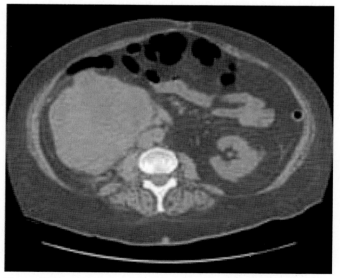

Figure 33-3   This 63-year-old woman had a T3c tumor measuring 16 × 13 cm that was managed with preoperative embolization.

bulky venous thrombus. Early ligation of the vein or mobilization of the kidney itself may allow better-visualized division of the renal artery.

In patients with tumor thrombus (discussed later), embolization may cause some regression in the extent of the thrombus.[15] More importantly, in the case of an occluded renal vein, it may allow early division of the collateral venous drainage that encircles the kidney in the perinephric fat. This technique may allow much easier surgical approach and dissection. Although it is not routinely necessary, preoperative embolization may assist in management of large, hypervascular tumors.

Common complications of embolization include the *embolization syndrome* consisting of nausea, vomiting, fever, and flank pain. Nephrectomy should be carried out ≤48 hours after embolization to minimize these symptoms. Another alternative is placement of a thoracic epidural catheter before embolization, a strategy we routinely employ. Embolization contributes to postoperative ileus. Thus, some degree of bowel preparation or a clear liquid diet preoperatively may by useful. More serious complications include acute renal failure, which may be exacerbated by accidental embolization of the contralateral kidney through reflux of the embolizing agent. Accidental embolization of other organs also occasionally occurs and causes serious complications such as heart failure and spinal cord injury. Occasionally, an associated tumor thrombus may embolize and may possibly cause sudden death.[16] The mortality rate for embolization with a variety of techniques has been reported to be ≤3.3% when embolization is used for palliation in inoperable cases.[17] However, the actual complication rate for preoperative embolization is probably lower.

Vessel Dissection

Among the principles of radical nephrectomy, as originally described by Robson and colleagues,[2] are early control and ligation of the renal vasculature to prevent hematogenous tumor spread. Regardless of the incision used, the renal artery should be ligated first to prevent renal congestion. Careful dissection is necessary to confirm the identity of the renal artery. Depending on the approach, the celiac artery, superior mesenteric artery, contralateral renal artery, and lumber vessels may all be mistaken for the renal artery. If an injury occurs to one of these vessels, immediate recognition and primary repair will minimize subsequent complications. Consultation with a vascular surgeon, if available, is suggested. When approaching the renal artery, care should be taken to prevent avulsion of any branches listed earlier. Adrenal arterial branches are particularly prone to such injury. Although they are small, they may bleed profusely.

The renal artery may be ligated but left undivided if the anatomic features dictate it. Once the renal vein is

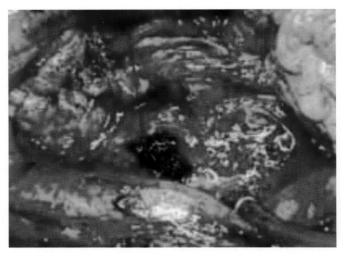

Figure 33-4 Surgicel bolster tamponading a retracted lumbar vein oversewn with figure-of-eight sutures on a UR5 needle.

ligated and divided, exposure to the renal artery may be improved. If the renal vein does not decrease in size after ligation of the renal artery, multiple renal arteries may be present.

The renal vein must be handled with care because a lumbar vein may drain posteriorly into it, especially on the left. The thinner walls of the vein make avulsion of these small veins a real possibility. The distal segment may retract into the paraspinous muscles and render hemostasis difficult. Prevention of this complicating factor begins with recognition. Preoperative imaging may be helpful in some cases.[18] If lumbar veins are visualized, some incisional approaches with more limited visibility should be avoided. If avulsion of these veins occurs, compression of the bleeding site while completing removal of the kidney will improve exposure and thereby facilitate hemostasis. Figure-of-eight sutures in the paraspinous muscle to oversew the bleeding site are usually effective. A bolster of Surgicel (an oxidized cellulose hemostatic agent; Johnson & Johnson Wound Management, Somerville, New Jersey) placed under the figure-of-eight suture will assist in tamponade of the retracted vein (**Fig. 33-4**).

Hematoma

Hematoma formation following radical nephrectomy may complicate the patient's postoperative course. In addition to the ability of the retroperitoneum to hold large amounts of fluid, the potential space left behind from bulky tumors allows significant bleeding without causing symptoms. The patient's hematocrit and blood pressure should be carefully followed, and one should realize that healthy individuals may lose ≤25% of their intravascular volume before significant symptoms occur. Even small hematomas may become infected and form abscesses. Verification of a dry surgical bed is an absolute necessity.

Drains are not routinely needed for nephrectomy. When significant intraoperative hypotension has occurred, some vessels may be in spasm, which may cause delayed postoperative bleeding. Placement of a closed drain for 24 to 48 hours postoperatively will permit early identification of bleeding.

Injury to Nearby Organs

Spleen

Splenic injury is a well-known complication of intra-abdominal surgery, and left nephrectomy is the third leading cause of iatrogenic splenic injury.[19] Wide ranges of statistics are given (from 2%-26%), but most modern series report splenic injury in approximately 5% to 10% of cases.[20]

Risk factors for splenic injury include prior abdominal surgical procedures, obesity, increasing age, large left kidney (i.e., polycystic kidney disease), and upper pole lesions.[21] Most case series show very different rates in donor nephrectomy–associated splenectomy and in splenectomy complicating radical left nephrectomy for neoplastic disease. Cooper and colleagues[21] speculated that this discrepancy reflects the different goals of surgery. Donor nephrectomies carry a risk of splenectomy of only 1% to 2%.[7,21] In addition, retroperitoneal approaches carry a much smaller risk of splenic injury.

Prevention of splenic injury begins with careful planning of the surgical approach and recognition of the importance of adequate exposure to the upper pole of the left kidney.[22] Splenic injuries occur in different ways. The most common cause is excessive traction on the splenic attachments that rips the splenic capsule. In addition, direct injury during dissection of large tumors may lacerate the splenic capsule, and retractors may damage the spleen if excessive force is placed on them or if countertraction is too great. In addition, direct injury during division of the diaphragm is a rare cause of injury from thoracoabdominal incisions.

Avoidance of splenic injury requires an understanding of the splenic attachments. The spleen is attached to all surrounding structures including the diaphragm, colon, stomach, and kidney (the lienophrenic, lieno-colic, lienogastric, and lienorenal ligaments, respectively). The most superficial attachment, a lieno-omental band, was described by Lord and Gourevitch.[23] Early division of the inferior lienocolic and lienorenal attachments allows safe retraction of the spleen, although care should be taken to pad all retractors well and to avoid excessive pulling. Some investigators advocate coloepiploic mobilization or separation of the greater omentum off the colon from the midpoint of the transverse colon to the splenic flexure. Mejean and associates[24] retrospectively demonstrated decreased rates of splenic complications ostensibly from increased splenic mobility as a result of early and more complete division of the colic attachments. These investigators further suggested that the subcostal incision is superior to the midline incision for avoiding excessive traction on the splenic ligaments.[20]

Splenic injury is easily recognized by immediate bleeding from this highly vascular organ. Traditional treatment proceeded to immediate splenectomy. Increasing experience with splenorrhaphy from trauma surgery shows that significant numbers of spleens may be salvaged. Superficial lacerations may be treated with argon beam coagulation or hemostatic products such as Avitene (Davon, Cranston, Rhode Island) or Surgicel. Packing with laparotomy sponges to promote hemostasis followed by repeat examination is recommended. Deeper lacerations may require bolsters or splenic wrapping with mesh to tamponade the bleeding. Excessive intraoperative bleeding may be controlled by manual compression of the splenic vessels as they course near the tail of the pancreas until splenorrhaphy or splenectomy is completed.

Postoperative management of splenectomy includes vaccination for pneumococcal, *Haemophilus,* and meningococcal infections. Some investigators advocate preoperative vaccine administration to patients who are undergoing left nephrectomy and who have risk factors for splenectomy because the morbidity is minimal compared with the risk of postoperative vaccine administration.[21] Sepsis in splenectomized patients is much more serious than in immunocompetent persons, and the incidence is probably ≥10 times greater. Drains in splenectomized patients, if used, should be removed as quickly as possible to decrease the risk of overwhelming infection.[21]

Pancreas

Pancreatic injuries are rare compared with injuries of other nearby organs. Historical series in open kidney donor nephrectomies gave an incidence of <1%.[7] Pancreatic injuries may occur with right nephrectomy during performance of Kocher's maneuver to mobilize the second portion of the duodenum. However, most injuries occur secondary to the close proximity of the tail of the pancreas to the hilum of the left kidney. Retraction, avulsion of surrounding structures, and direct laceration may all injure the organ. Intraoperative bruising may also cause postoperative pancreatitis or asymptomatic elevation of amylase and lipase concentrations. Risk factors probably include prior operations, inflammation surrounding the kidney, larger lesions, or any other cause of difficult dissection.

Prevention of pancreatic injury includes development of the plane between Gerota's fascia and the visceral peritoneum during dissection of the superomedial pole of the left kidney. Identification, complete mobilization, and careful retraction of the pancreas will help to avoid any avulsion injuries.

Recognition of pancreatic lacerations requires immediate repair. It is important to inspect for injury to the pancreatic duct. If no injury is noted, simple repair of the pancreatic capsule with nonabsorbable suture and an omental bolster is all that is necessary. If the duct is involved, distal resection of the pancreas is probably preferable. General surgical consultation should be obtained if available. The distal pancreas is resected and the duct is closed. The capsule of the pancreas is then closed over the stump. In these cases, placement of a surgical drain is indicated.

Postoperative management of the patient who has undergone significant pancreatic manipulation includes monitoring of amylase and lipase level, especially as the patient begins to eat. Any patients with significant injury to the pancreas require placement of a nasogastric tube. Parenteral alimentation should be considered early in the postoperative course. If clinical signs or symptoms of pancreatitis do not resolve, a CT scan should be performed. Fluid collections possibly representing a pancreatic leak, if found, require aspiration by interventional radiologic means. The fluid should be sent for measurement of amylase, lipase, pH, Gram stain, and culture. Infected liquid suggests the presence of necrotizing pancreatitis and requires emergency laparotomy for débridement and drainage. If the fluid is not infected, a percutaneous drain should be left and total bowel rest instituted. The addition of octreotide decreases pancreatic output and may be helpful in some cases. The starting dose is 50 μg subcutaneously three times daily, with titration up to 200 μg three times daily based on fistula output.[25]

Duodenum

Duodenal injuries most commonly occur during dissection anteromedial to the right kidney. The second part of the duodenum is most commonly involved. Far more uncommon is injury to the distal duodenum immediately adjacent to the ligament of Treitz. Such injuries occur on reflection of the left mesocolon medial to the inferior mesenteric vein where the mesocolon can be quite thin, or due to thermal injury or direct laceration.

Duodenal injuries are rather rare; in one series only a single injury to the duodenum occurred in 344 right nephrectomies.[20] Risk factors may include prior operations, inflammation surrounding the kidney, larger lesions, or any other cause of difficult dissection and adherence of the duodenum.

Prevention of duodenal injury includes careful dissection and the use of padded retractors. When necessary, Kocher's maneuver mobilizes the duodenum away from the operative field.

Careful inspection of the duodenum for lacerations and hematomas should be performed. Duodenal laceration should be closed with a two-layer technique and possibly reinforced with omentum or jejunum. If a duodenal hematoma is found, it should be opened and drained to prevent transient small bowel obstruction.

The duodenum can then be repaired and covered with an omental bolster or jejunal tissue. If more extensive injury occurs, general surgical consultation should be considered. With standard preoperative prophylactic antibiotic coverage only for skin organisms, consideration should be given to adding gram-negative and anaerobic coverage, especially if no bowel preparation was used. Postoperatively, nasogastric suction should be maintained until intestinal peristalsis resumes.

Liver

Liver injury during nephrectomy in general is relatively rare. Many large case series list no liver lacerations. Causes of liver injury generally include forceful retraction during right nephrectomy. Preventive measures include adequate padding of retractors and division of the triangular and coronary ligaments if necessary to achieve adequate mobilization.

On recognition of a liver injury, or during intentional resection of liver extensions of the primary tumor, the liver laceration may be managed with Bovie or argon beam coagulation. For larger defects, Surgicel bolsters with horizontal mattress sutures of 2-0 silk or 1 chromic gut on a blunt-point needle may be more appropriate. If bleeding makes repair difficult, total obstruction of hepatic vascular inflow may be obtained by Pringle's maneuver (**Fig. 33-5**). The hepatic artery and portal vein are isolated at the porta hepatis and are

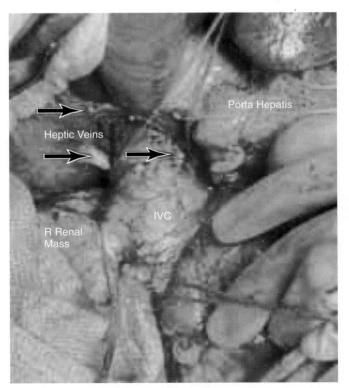

Figure 33-5 Photograph demonstrating technique for isolation of the porta hepatis for possible Pringle's maneuver. In addition, umbilical tapes isolate the right renal vein and the inferior vena cava (IVC) above and below the tumor.

cross-clamped. Studies in liver donors indicated that significant ischemic injury does not take place with intermittent total occlusion from 10 minutes progressing to 30 minutes alternating with 5-minute reperfusion intervals.[26] If the extent of liver injury is judged to present a risk of postoperative bile leakage, drain placement is indicated.

If recognized and treated appropriately, iatrogenic liver injuries typically follow an uncomplicated course postoperatively. If a significant bile leak develops, percutaneous drainage is indicated. Low-output fistulas typically close with conservative management, whereas high-output fistulas may require intervention with minimally invasive techniques.

Colon and Stomach

Injuries to the stomach, colon, and jejunum or ileum are very rare and are generally thermal injuries from accidental electrocautery arcs. Similar risk factors exist and probably include prior operations, inflammation surrounding the kidney, larger lesions, possibility of tumor extension into surrounding organs, or other causes of difficult dissection. Preventive measures include mechanical bowel preparation if the chance exists of tumor extension complicating resection or necessitating bowel resection. Closure of any hollow viscus is generally accomplished with a double-layer technique with possible omental bolstering. If unanticipated spillage of colonic content occurs, extensive irrigation with sterile water, drain placement, and postoperative antibiotic prophylaxis for gram-negative and anaerobic organisms should be initiated.

Adrenal Glands

Radical nephrectomy as outlined by Robson and associates[2] included adrenalectomy to maintain the integrity of Gerota's fascia. Improvements in imaging have allowed improved preoperative assessment of tumor volume, extension, and adrenal involvement. In addition, significant stage migration resulting from increasing numbers of incidentally found tumors at early stages mandates reassessment of the practice of routine adrenalectomy. Studies of pathology specimens showed that the incidence of adrenal invasion is directly related to the stage of the primary lesion. Stage T1/2 lesions in general have a <2% chance of adrenal involvement if no adrenal abnormalities are seen on preoperative CT. Upper pole lesions, multifocal lesions, and radiologic stage T3/4 lesions have a much greater incidence (from 7.8% for T3 to 40% for T4).[27-30] In addition, up to one third of patients with adrenal involvement show evidence of extensive nodal or metastatic disease.[31]

In light of the foregoing data, some surgeons perform adrenal-sparing radical nephrectomies in some patients to spare them from future adrenal insufficiency if metachronous contralateral disease develops that requires adrenal resection. In these patients, the chance for adrenal injury exists during renal mobilization. Usually, a well-defined plane separates the adrenal gland from the kidney. If this plane is not developed sufficiently, traction on the kidney may result in tears of the adrenal capsule, which may bleed profusely. Small injuries may be oversewn or treated with argon beam electrocautery. However, adrenal hemostasis using these methods is marginally successful and adrenalectomy is often the best solution. The vasculature of the adrenal gland, discussed earlier, is at particular risk of injury during nephrectomy, whether adrenalectomy is planned or not.

Diaphragm

Perforation of the diaphragm and parietal pleura with resulting pneumothorax is a possible complication of renal surgery regardless of the approach. The incidence probably rises with increasingly superior flank incision sites. Rates of iatrogenic pneumothorax through sub-12th rib flank incisions are negligible, whereas 11th interspace and 10th interspace incisions have a moderate risk. The overall risk of pneumothorax in modern series varies from 1% to 10%. In general, pneumothoraces requiring chest tube placement occur in approximately 1% of cases.[32-35]

Prevention involves careful attention to the anatomic features during dissection of the diaphragm off the costal attachments. For operations in which Gerota's fascia is opened, such as partial nephrectomy, this tissue can be used to buffer the upper aspect of the flank incision from the retractor. Many surgeons routinely obtain a postoperative chest radiograph to assess for pneumothorax requiring chest tube placement. Several studies examined the necessity for routine chest radiography postoperatively and concluded that it was unnecessary.[36,37] Although the incidence of pneumothorax from the variety of incisions discussed earlier is variable, this complication is usually recognized intraoperatively. The investigators found that only approximately 1% of patients undergoing nephrectomy had pneumothoraces of potential clinical significance that were missed intraoperatively. Many of these pneumothoraces resolved spontaneously with no negative consequences. The investigators concluded that routine chest radiography is unnecessary. Chest radiography should be obtained on the basis of intraoperative pleural injury or postoperative indications such as central line placement, symptoms, or physical examination findings.[37]

If a pleural injury is detected intraoperatively, it should be covered with a sponge to prevent entry of blood from the surgical field into the pleural cavity. At the end of the procedure, a 10- to 12-Fr Robinson catheter can be passed through the pleurotomy to aspirate the air. A pursestring suture is placed around it. The distal end of the catheter is placed under water while the anesthetist hyperinflates the lung to 40 mm Hg. Attention should be paid to blood pressure because cardiac preload is decreased with lung hyperinflation.

The catheter is then removed and the suture is tied to close the defect. If the pleurotomy is too large to close with this technique, chest tube placement is probably advisable. If no intrathoracic bleeding is noted, a smaller chest tube may be placed, or even a pigtail catheter can be inserted into the second intercostal space. Careful closure of the diaphragm with the sutures on the abdominal side of the repair facilitates pleural healing. Postoperatively, pneumothorax should be monitored with serial upright end-expiratory chest radiographs to verify resolution before the chest tube is removed.

INFECTION

Currently, infectious complication rates from nephrectomy excluding superficial wound infections are probably approximately 3% to 5%.[38] To minimize the risk of spreading infection, the urinary tract's normal sterile state must be verified preoperatively. Positive preoperative urine culture necessitates adequate antibiotic coverage for several days before the surgical procedure. Postoperative infections after any surgical procedure include wound infections, abscesses, pneumonia, pyelonephritis, cholecystitis, and infections caused by antibiotic treatment such as *Clostridium difficile* colitis. Our discussion focuses on those infections that may be more specifically related to nephrectomy.

Pneumonia

Postoperative pneumonia is a common nosocomial infection to which patients undergoing nephrectomy may be especially prone. Radical nephrectomy for neoplastic disease is associated with a greater incidence of pneumonia compared with nephrectomy for benign conditions.[13] Some degree of atelectasis is nearly universal in patients undergoing general anesthesia, especially if the operation is performed with the patient in the flank position. The proximity of the incision site to the diaphragm and the division of accessory muscles of inspiration make deep breathing painful during the postoperative period. This situation perpetuates the stasis of fluid in the atelectatic lung segments, fluid that serves as an ideal culture medium for nosocomial pathogens. Major surgery may also suppress the immune system and thus increase susceptibility to infections.

Prevention of postoperative pneumonia includes preoperative evaluation of respiratory reserve and pulmonary status. Consultation with a pulmonologist is indicated if any doubt exists about the patient's status or if the patient has any history of obstructive, restrictive, or severe infectious pulmonary diseases. These risk factors should be addressed and minimized by adequate treatment preoperatively. Postoperatively, adequate pain control, incentive spirometry, and early ambulation are important for quickly decreasing atelectasis and the risk of pneumonia.

Abscess

Abscess formation is a rare complication of urologic surgery (1.7% in one series for renal cell carcinoma).[20] Risk factors are similar to those for wound infection, including preoperative urinary tract infection, entry into gastrointestinal organs, entry into kidney parenchyma or collecting system, and postoperative renal hemorrhage. In addition to avoidance of these risk factors, adequate irrigation, prophylactic antibiotics, and drain placement if indicated minimize the chance of abscess formation. In the presence of risk factors for infection, unexplained postoperative fever should prompt an abdominal CT search for an abscess. If an abscess is found, treatment involves percutaneous drainage by interventional radiologic means and empirical antibiotics. Antibiotic coverage is adjusted if necessary when culture and sensitivity results become available. With increasingly precise interventional radiology techniques, open débridement of abscesses is rarely necessary.

SPECIAL POPULATIONS

Tumor Thrombus

Renal cell carcinoma frequently involves vascular structures. Four percent to 25% of tumors show thrombus.[39] Such vascular extension may manifest as lower extremity edema, varicocele, dilated superficial abdominal veins, proteinuria, pulmonary embolism, right atrial mass, or loss of function in the involved kidney. If a tumor thrombus is found, surgical preparation should probably include a magnetic resonance imaging (MRI) scan in addition to other preoperative imaging studies, to assess the proximal extent of the tumor thrombus (**Fig. 33-6**).[40,41] Preoperative MRI accurately measures the extent of tumor thrombus in approximately 98% of cases.[42] If an interval of ≥2 weeks exists between MRI and the surgical procedure, for level II and III thrombus, a follow-up study such as ultrasound, transesophageal echocardiography, or repeat MRI should be considered to ensure that significant thrombus propagation has not occurred. Invasive approaches such as venacavography are rarely indicated.

Fortunately, such tumor thrombi do not necessarily indicate metastasis, and survival of patients after complete removal is better than in patients with primary tumor invasion into Gerota's fascia. Although some centers are describing experimental techniques, tumor thrombus remains one of the main indications for open surgical management.[43] In patients with level III or IV tumor thrombus, the importance of adequate preoperative assessment of the cardiopulmonary system should be emphasized in the presence of possible cardiopulmonary bypass.

An uncommon complication of tumor thrombus extension above the hepatic veins is Budd-Chiari syn-

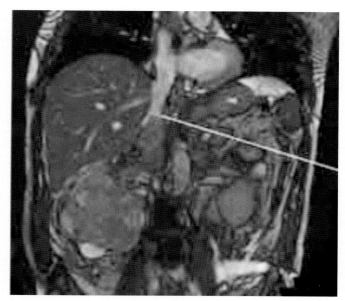

Figure 33-6   This 58-year-old man was found to have a tumor thrombus. This MRI was obtained to confirm the proximal extent of tumor thrombus.

1. Adequate exposure of the primary lesion
2. Adequate exposure to the vena cava
3. Exposure of the contralateral renal vein
4. Ability to mobilize the liver
5. Ability to extend incision if necessary to include the chest
6. Complete control of vena cava above and below the thrombus to avoid pulmonary embolism
7. Avoidance of cardiopulmonary bypass if possible
8. Protection of natural venovenous shunt pathways.

The inferior vena cava above and below the thrombus, both renal veins, and the portal vein should be isolated with umbilical tapes and Rummel tourniquets (see Fig. 33-5). Lumbar veins that will be draining into the opened area of the inferior vena cava are best ligated beforehand. If an unrecognized lumbar vein is bleeding into the open vena cava to a significant extent, it can be occluded either posterior to the vena cava with a sponge stick or within the vena cava with a Kittner device. The Rummel tourniquets can be tightened to occlude the major veins. Alternatively, Satinsky and vascular clamps can be used. Although some vascular surgeons prefer not to use clamps on the vena cava, we have not encountered problems with this method.

Ligation of the hepatic veins permits increased hepatic mobilization and isolation of an addition 4 cm of infrahepatic vena cava. This technique facilitates infrahepatic vena cava control as well as rotation of the liver to the left side of the inferior vena cava and thus gives excellent exposure to the right adrenal gland and retrohepatic inferior vena cava (**Fig. 33-7**).

When the tumor thrombus extends into the right atrium, opening the chest cavity is probably necessary. This procedure may be accomplished by midline sternotomy, thoracoabdominal incision, or xiphisternal extension of a chevron incision. A second small parasternal incision has also been described to access the thoracic cavity. The extent of tumor thrombus and whether or not it invades significant portions of the vena cava or right atrium dictate the operative time needed for complete excision. This time, in turn, dictates the need for venovenous bypass or hypothermia, cardiac arrest, and exsanguination.[47] Several groups have developed excision techniques for increasingly proximal levels of thrombi without cardiopulmonary bypass through transabdominal approaches.[48] Regardless of the approach, the complication most to be avoided is fragmentation of the thrombus leading to pulmonary embolism.

Verifying complete thrombus removal before reestablishing venous flow is critical. Various methods for removing remnant clot have been described, including manual "milking down" of the thrombus, placement of a Foley catheter past the thrombus followed by inflation and removal, and direct visual techniques employing flexible cystoscopes.[49]

drome or hepatic venous outflow obstruction. The classic acute presentation of Budd-Chiari syndrome consists of sudden-onset ascites, hepatomegaly, right upper quadrant pain, and elevated liver function test results. This syndrome is rarely seen in renal cell carcinoma–associated tumor thrombus formation, in which a more gradual onset of similar symptoms is typical.[44] Treatment involves an expeditious surgical procedure to relieve hepatic vein obstruction and thereby spare liver parenchyma if possible. In spite of surgical intervention, severe symptoms usually indicate irreversible liver injury and the onset of hepatic failure. The largest series of patients with renal tumor thrombus–induced Budd-Chiari syndrome showed no survival for >6 weeks in seven patients with severe cases. The outcome of five patients with mild cases was probably similar to that in patients with equivalent renal disease without Budd-Chiari syndrome.[44] Surgeons should carefully consider patient selection for surgery in the presence of Budd-Chiari syndrome in light of probable poor outcomes.

Surgical technique for vena cava thrombectomy has undergone many changes. Because all investigators agree that the proximal level of tumor thrombus dictates the surgical approach, accurate assessment with preoperative imaging is important. At least six systems to categorize thrombi have been proposed.[45] Probably the most widely used is the Mayo Foundation (Rochester, Minnesota) classification, which divides thrombi into four groups based on their relationship to the renal vein ostia, hepatic veins, and diaphragm.[46] Various surgical approaches have been advocated for every level.

Basic principles guiding the choice of surgical approach are as follows:

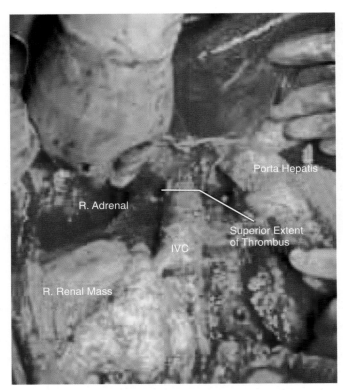

Figure 33-7 Photograph of liver rotated to the left to allow exposure of the retrohepatic vena cava. Note the ligated hepatic veins. IVC, inferior vena cava.

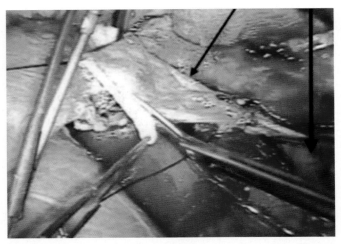

Figure 33-8 Reconstruction of the inferior vena cava with defatted pericardium. The *thin arrow* indicates the medial border of the graft sewn to the vena cava. The *thick arrow* indicates the vena cava inferior to graft.

Some complications of nephrectomy with thrombus removal are secondary to inadequate reconstruction of the inferior vena cava. Decreased cardiac preload may cause heart failure in some individuals with limited reserve. Decreased renal drainage of the contralateral kidney may cause acute renal insufficiency requiring dialysis. This condition may be reversible with the development of venous collateral vessels. It is always advisable to perform reconstruction of the inferior vena cava with graft material if inadequate vein remains following resection of adherent tumor thrombus. If the chest cavity is open, defatted pericardium may be used as autologous graft material (**Fig. 33-8**).

Cardiopulmonary bypass may be associated with small increases in morbidity and mortality. Most morbidity related to the bypass itself is from two different mechanisms. First, cardiopulmonary bypass results in a systemic inflammatory response through multiple biochemical mechanisms. These mechanisms are generally brought about by contact of the blood with the extracorporeal gaseous interface and biocompatible surfaces of the cardiopulmonary bypass machine. The inflammatory mediators (complement, cytokines) activate leukocytes, vascular endothelial cells, and platelets and generate a systemic response that damages organs.[50] Second, cardiopulmonary bypass generates multiple small emboli from lipoprotein aggregates, gaseous emboli, and other particulate matter. These affect end-organ capillary beds, particularly in the heart, brain, lungs, and kidneys. Healthy individuals with adequate reserve usually have no problems, but patients with significant comorbidities of any of these organs may be significantly affected.[50] Ongoing research is focused on overcoming these difficulties.[51]

Other postoperative complications of cardiopulmonary bypass are usually manageable. Bleeding from heparinization and inadequate reversal with protamine may be extensive. Patients may also experience continuing temperature dysregulation following bypass. In addition to complications of cardiopulmonary bypass, hypothermic circulatory arrest leads to ischemic damage to body structures, some of which may be irreversible. Neural tissue is especially susceptible to such injury, and temporary neurologic dysfunction, stroke, and death may result. These complications are generally rare in radical nephrectomy.[52] Prevention includes shortening operative time to decrease the risk of ischemia. Despite these added risks, hypothermic circulatory arrest may decrease the risk of warm ischemia to the liver and contralateral kidney. Increased visualization and operative time may reduce the risk of tumor thrombus embolization.[52]

Cytoreductive Nephrectomy

Two prospective studies from the Southwest Oncology Group and the European Organisation for Research and Treatment of Cancer demonstrated a modest survival advantage for cytoreductive nephrectomy before immunotherapy.[53,54] Morbidity from the renal neoplasm itself, such as pain and hematuria, may require palliative nephrectomy even in patients with extensive metastatic disease. However, in patients with lower performance status, it is advisable to attempt more conservative measures such as improved pain control and renal angioinfarction.

One article compared morbidity and mortality of cytoreductive nephrectomy in patients with tumor thrombus with radical nephrectomy in patients who did not have metastatic disease. Zisman and colleagues[39] found no increase in complications of surgery compared with patients undergoing similar radical nephrectomies without metastatic disease.

Locally Recurrent Disease

Clinical series have reported an incidence of isolated local disease recurrence in the absence of other metastatic disease of <2%.[55-57] Any T stage primary tumor may be affected. It is controversial whether local recurrence represents remnant disease from positive margins, residual lymph node disease, recurrence in residual adrenal gland (**Fig. 33-9**), or a form of metastasis. Positive margin status during open nephrectomy should be rare in the absence of grossly evident disease. Careful dissection with the avoidance of tumor spillage should minimize this possible risk factor. Obviously, patients with positive margin status and patients with gross tumor spillage in the incision require close follow-up because surgical extirpation is the only efficacious treatment available for renal cancer.

In patients with no evidence of metastatic disease in whom resection of local disease recurrence is complete, long-term survival may be achieved in ≤30%.[57] Some investigators have suggested adjuvant immunotherapy in these patients to enhance outcomes.[58] Longer recurrence-free intervals may correlate with improved survival after repeat resection.[56,59]

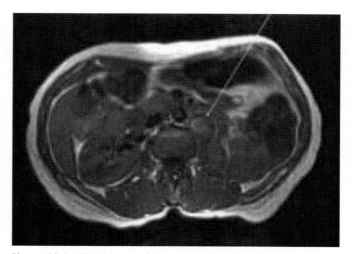

Figure 33-9 This 51-year-old woman had undergone left simple nephrectomy 6 years earlier. The pathology report showed Fuhrman grade 4/4 renal cell carcinoma, chromophobe type. This MRI demonstrated the indicated recurrence, which was found to be Fuhrman grade 2/4 chromophobe type within the residual adrenal gland.

Complications of repeat resection may be significant. Wide resection of the possible neoplastic recurrence may require en bloc resection of adjacent organs and may thus increase the risk of complications, infection, and perioperative mortality. Older series showed several mortalities.[58,60] More recent series, although reporting no deaths, showed a complication rate of 13% to 42%.[57,59] Because of the significant complication rate and the small chance of a survival benefit in patients with local recurrence and metastatic disease, these patients should not be considered for repeat resection.[57] No efficacy was shown for any adjuvant or adjunctive therapies including chemotherapy, immunotherapy, external beam radiation therapy, or intraoperative radiation therapy. As systemic therapy for renal neoplasms develops, recommendations regarding proper treatment of metastatic disease will undoubtedly undergo significant change.

Donor Nephrectomy

The ethical issues surrounding living donor nephrectomy depend in part on the actual morbidity and mortality of the operation. At this time, most living donor nephrectomies in the United States are performed with minimally invasive techniques including laparoscopy and hand-assisted laparoscopy. In some other countries, miniaturization of the incision is practiced. Because the operation carries no direct medical benefit to the patient, optimization of outcomes is imperative. Investigators have estimated that the perioperative mortality rate is approximately 0.03% and that rate of major complications of donor nephrectomy is approximately 1.8%.[4] These rates, much lower than in nephrectomy performed for renal cancer, reflect the elective nature of the procedure, the extensive preoperative workup, and the ability to abandon the operation or resect the contralateral kidney.

Postoperatively, contralateral renal hypertrophy maintains glomerular filtration rate between two thirds and three fourths of preoperative levels. Long-term sequelae of donor nephrectomy include increased blood pressure, especially systolic, although most patients have blood pressure remaining in the normal range or easily managed mild hypertension. Rates of hypertension in kidney donors mirrors national rates, but this finding may reflect selection bias favoring healthy donors. In addition, proteinuria compared with preoperative values develops in 13% to 22% of patients.[4,61] To our knowledge, no studies have shown any clinically significant effects from these complications of donor nephrectomy.[61]

The surgical technique for open donor nephrectomy is similar to that for simple nephrectomy. Different centers use a variety of incisions for the approach. Extraperitoneal approaches may minimize the risk of subsequent adhesions and possible small bowel obstruction requiring reoperation. Rates of small bowel obstruction were ≤2% in older series.[7] However, meticulous dissection of the renal pedicle with sparing of all renal vessels may be easier through an anterior transperitoneal incision, particularly if any aberrant vessels exist. Care must be taken when dissecting the ureter to avoid damaging the collateral vessels from the renal hilum to the proximal ureter. These vessels maintain blood supply in the transplanted organ and damage to them may cause ureteral necrosis. Complete mobilization of the kidney is performed before the renal vessels are clamped, to minimize warm ischemia time. In the transplanted kidney, application of papaverine may be indicated to avoid possible renal artery spasm.

Elderly Patients

Definitions of *elderly* have been changing as the population ages. Case series have moved from 60 to 65 years as age cutoffs to 70 to 75 years. Historically, elderly patients were thought to benefit very little from surgical extirpation of neoplasms because the morbidity and mortality associated with surgery were thought to exceed the benefit possible over the remaining life span. These concepts have changed significantly for many neoplasms including renal cancer. Studies have shown nonsignificantly higher rates of morbidity and mortality for nephrectomy in elderly patients.[62] Indeed, most of the increased problems are probably the result of the greater number and incidence of comorbidities commonly associated with increasing age. These comorbidities can usually be managed preoperatively to optimize outcomes.

Perioperative strategies to decrease complication rates include minimizing of operative time, earlier consideration of blood transfusions, and possible gastric tube placement to decrease pneumonia rates. Extraperitoneal approaches may decrease ileus and allow sooner return to normal diet, a factor that may be more important in elderly patients. Postoperative intensive care for 24 to 48 hours may allow earlier recognition of possible complications.

Transitional Cell Carcinoma

The current treatment standard for most cases of upper urinary tract transitional cell carcinoma is nephroureterectomy with a cuff of bladder. Low-grade, low-stage lesions may be managed more conservatively.[63] Increasing numbers of nephroureterectomies are performed laparoscopically in some centers. However, open nephroureterectomy still offers unparalleled exposure for difficult cases. It may be performed through many different incisions. Single incisions include midline or a combination of midline and subcostal. Alternatively, two incisions may be used such as a flank or subcostal combined incision with a Gibson or lower midline incision for distal ureteral dissection. In some cases, the distal ureter may be resected endoscopically or laparoscopically. Ideally, en bloc resection of the whole specimen is accomplished, although some institutions divide the ureter to make subsequent resection easier. Surgical dissection of the kidney is identical to that performed in radical nephrectomy. The adrenal gland may be spared in most cases. The cuff of bladder should be resected because this technique decreased the disease recurrence rate in one study.[64]

Complications of nephroureterectomy are similar to those of radical nephrectomy. Other complications associated with cystotomies such as urinoma or fistula formation are rare. In addition, the contralateral ureteral orifice may be damaged by the dissection of bladder cuff. This complication may result in anuria secondary to obstruction of the remaining ureter at the ureteral orifice. Gentle dissection prevents this complication. Management includes retrograde stent placement if possible or nephrostomy if stent placement fails.

KEY POINTS

1. Advantages of anterior incisions, whether midline, subcostal or chevron, include quick exposure to the renal pedicle and the great vessels.
2. Up to 23% of patients will have a flank sag postoperatively as a result of injury to intercostal nerves that causes laxity of flank muscles at that level.
3. In cases anticipated to have a difficult hilar dissection or anterior approaches, in which anatomic access to the artery is more difficult, preoperative renal artery embolization may be helpful.
4. The most common cause of splenic injury is excessive traction on the splenic attachments that rips the splenic capsule.
5. In cases of pancreatic injury, if injury of the duct is noted, distal pancreatectomy is the preferred method of management.
6. If bleeding makes repair of liver injury difficult, total obstruction of hepatic vascular inflow may be obtained by Pringle's maneuver.
7. Perioperative strategies to decrease complication rates in elderly patients include minimal operative time, earlier consideration of blood transfusions, and possible gastric tube placement to decrease pneumonia rates.

REFERENCES

Please see www.expertconsult.com

Chapter 34

COMPLICATIONS OF PARTIAL NEPHRECTOMY

Guilherme Godoy MD

Fellow in Urologic Oncology, Bruce and Cynthia Sherman Fellowship in Urologic Oncology, Division of Urologic Oncology, Department of Urology, New York University Langone Medical Center, New York, New York

Rebecca L. O'Malley MD

Resident in Urology, Division of Urologic Oncology, Department of Urology, New York University Langone Medical Center, New York, New York

Samir S. Taneja MD

The James M. Neissa and Janet Riha Neissa Associate Professor of Urologic Oncology; Director, Division of Urologic Oncology, Department of Urology and New York University Cancer Institute, New York University Langone Medical Center, New York, New York

Since first reports in 1869 to 1870 by Simon[1] and in 1887 by Czerny,[2] partial nephrectomy has been used to manage many different urologic diseases. The major application of partial nephrectomy since the early 1990s has been as an alternative to radical nephrectomy in the treatment of small renal tumors.[3-15] This technique has proven oncologically safe for early tumors confined to the kidney. More recent efforts have been made to duplicate open partial nephrectomy techniques in laparoscopic tumor resection and thereby shorten recovery time and reduce postoperative morbidity. The significant downward stage migration of renal tumors resulting from increase in the incidental diagnosis has prompted investigators to expand indications and increase the use of partial nephrectomy.[16-18] Despite this change, the use of the partial nephrectomy remains low nationally, even for small renal tumors, likely a reflection of the perception of increased morbidity relative to radical nephrectomy.

PREOPERATIVE CONSIDERATIONS

The absolute indications for partial nephrectomy include tumor in a solitary renal moiety, bilateral renal tumors, or preexisting azotemia that would preclude the ability to perform nephrectomy without requiring that the patient undergo dialysis. Despite these indications, in selected patients of this type, nephrectomy followed by dialysis may be indicated for maximal oncologic efficacy. Relative indications include medical illnesses predisposing to renal disease, preexisting medical renal disease, renal stones, recurrent renal infection, mild azotemia, and multifocal tumors associated with a genetic syndrome. *Elective partial nephrectomy* is defined as that in which the patient has none of the foregoing risk factors, normal renal function, and a radiologically normal contralateral renal moiety. Studies have suggested a greater overall reduction in glomerular filtration rate (GFR) in patients undergoing radical nephrectomy as compared with partial nephrectomy (discussed later).[19] Because this finding may correlate with higher likelihood of morbidity and mortality not related to oncologic factors, the impetus for consideration of elective partial nephrectomy may be greater in the future.

In considering patients for partial nephrectomy, host factors to be considered include overall health and the ability to tolerate surgery, the presence of comorbidities predisposing to renal disease, bleeding diathesis or a need for anticoagulation, and baseline renal function. Although the need for perioperative anticoagulation does not preclude partial nephrectomy, it certainly does increase the risk of postoperative bleeding, and as such it may be a reason for considering nephrectomy in an otherwise fragile patient. Renal anatomic variants including duplication, anomalous location, and anomalous vasculature are important to be aware of in operative planning, but they do not preclude partial nephrectomy. Previous renal surgery for any indication must be evaluated carefully to ensure that partial nephrectomy will be feasible. Finally, body habitus may influence the operative approach and the decision for surgical intervention.

Retrospective studies demonstrated that patients undergoing partial nephrectomy have better long-term renal function than do patients undergoing radical nephrectomy.[20,21] More recently, investigators demonstrated that the likelihood of having a GFR >45 mL/minute or >60 mL/minute was greater among patients having a partial nephrectomy.[19] The inherent implication of these findings is that individuals undergoing partial nephrectomy may indirectly reduce their risk of nononcologic morbidity and mortality as a result of preserved renal function. A significant positive correlation exists between reduced GFR and cardiovascular mortality or other medical illnesses. Some investigators have suggested that the risk of cardiovascular or nononcologic mortality is greater among patients undergoing radical nephrectomy as compared with partial nephrectomy.[22] Whether this finding is ultimately related to selection bias remains to be determined in prospective evaluation. Nonetheless, the findings are provocative in suggesting that elective partial nephrectomy should be considered in most patients in whom the procedure is technically feasible, and broadening of the indications may be of value.

Consideration of the tumor is essential in selecting candidates for partial nephrectomy and in planning the surgical procedure. Tumor size and location should be considered within the framework of surgeon's technical experience and comfort level when deciding whether partial nephrectomy is appropriate. In these tumors, ample margin can be obtained with limited concern of damaging the remaining renal blood supply. Historically, elective partial nephrectomy was considered appropriate for exophytic tumors <4 cm. In retrospective evaluation of early series, central tumors and larger tumors had worse oncologic outcomes. Admittedly, the majority of patients in those categories may not have had elective indications for partial nephrectomy. As surgeons have become comfortable with the technique, indications for elective partial nephrectomy have been expanded to include central tumors, and those in the T1b (4-7 cm) category. Thus far, no apparent decline in cancer control has been reported among those series.[4]

OPERATIVE PLANNING

Operative planning of partial nephrectomy requires rigorous understanding of arterial anatomy and the relationship of blood supply and collecting system (**Fig. 34-1**). This knowledge allows planning of the necessity for renal ischemia, the line of resection for margin control, and the likelihood of necessary venous and collecting system repair. Several groups demonstrated the utility of preoperative three-dimensional image reconstruction using computed tomography (CT) or magnetic resonance imaging (MRI).[23] These modalities are extremely useful in identifying multifocality, anomalous vasculature, and venous tumor thrombus in segmental renal veins.

Planning of the incision is important. Partial nephrectomy can be performed through a variety of incisions including a traditional flank, subcostal (intraperitoneal), thoracoabdominal, or the more recently described "mini-flank" (subcostal extraperitoneal).[24] We prefer perform open partial nephrectomy through an extraperitoneal approach, using a supracostal 11th rib incision. The advantages of such an approach include the ability to tamponade postoperative bleeding and contain urine leaks in the retroperitoneum, to reduce postoperative ileus, and to allow proper exposure for elongation of the renal hilum and "stretch" of the kidney. Disadvantages include increased pain limiting postoperative inspiratory effort, risk of pleural injury, and flank denervation bulge, which often arises from stretch of the intercostal nerve during rib distraction. The subcostal approach is feasible, but we have found it difficult to bring the kidney up to the level of the skin as we can easily do with hilar mobilization through a flank incision. The "mini-flank" incision may represent a compromise between these two approaches, by taking advantage of the benefits of each.

A decision to be made in operative planning is that of open versus laparoscopic partial nephrectomy. Various laparoscopic techniques for partial nephrectomy exist including hand-assisted, robot-assisted, and pure laparoscopic partial nephrectomy. A discussion of the reported benefits and weaknesses of each is beyond the scope of this chapter, but the decision of technique must be made by each surgeon based on his or her own operative comfort level. Given the faster general convalescence with laparoscopic partial nephrectomy (see later), in our center we prefer this technique whenever feasible and reserve open partial nephrectomy for those patients with solitary kidney, significant multifocality, or very centrally located tumor.

A good benchmark is for the surgeon to determine, within his or her own skill set, an estimated ischemia time for renal reconstruction based on tumor size and position. Although the optimal time for tolerable ischemia is not clearly defined, we use a benchmark of 30 minutes by estimate. If it appears that >30 minutes would clearly be required, we would consider open partial nephrectomy. When using a transperitoneal approach, the most difficult tumors for exposure and resection are those located in the medial posterior segment. Increased morbidity for partial nephrectomy in a solitary kidney has been reported for laparoscopic as compared with open partial nephrectomy even in centers of excellence, a finding suggesting that these procedures are best performed by open partial nephrectomy in most cases.[25]

GENERAL COMPLICATIONS

The general complications related to the renal surgery, incision, and medical comorbidity are discussed else-

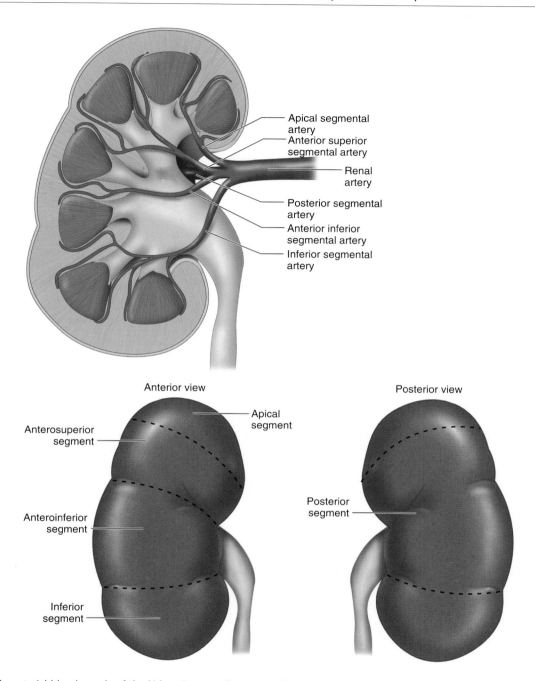

Figure 34-1 The arterial blood supply of the kidney is generally reproducible with five major segmental branches. On occasion, when a tumor is localized to a single arterial segment, selective segmental arterial occlusion may be feasible, thereby reducing the risk of renal ischemia. In resecting, the line of resection should not cross the direction of segmental flow, to avoid peripheral infarct. Similarly, on reconstruction, knowledge of the direction of blood supply relative to the defect is essential.

where in this book. This chapter focuses attention on complications specifically related to partial nephrectomy. The main technical complications of partial nephrectomy include bleeding, urine leak, renal dysfunction, vascular fistula or malformation, positive margin, renal infarct, and on rare occasions renal loss.

The learning curve of partial nephrectomy remains a major challenge for the urologic community, but in more recent series morbidity is improving. In fact, some

series comparing morbidity, length of stay, and cost differential associated with partial and radical nephrectomy reported no significant differences and concluded that the nephron-sparing approach can offer the benefit of maximal parenchymal preservation while adding little additional morbidity.[5,8,15] Analyzing >1800 nephrectomies performed between 1991 and 1998 in 123 of the Department of Veterans Affairs Medical Centers (VAMC), Corman and colleagues[8] compared the complication rates of radical nephrectomy and partial nephrectomy within a 30-day period following the operation. These investigators observed no statistically significant difference in the mortality and morbidity rates between the radical and the nephron-sparing approach. These observations were also seen in a referral practice, rather than in a population-based practice such as the VAMC. Comparing complications and also the associated costs of radical and partial nephrectomy for localized renal cell carcinoma during a 7-year period (1991-1997), Shekarriz and colleagues[5] did not observe significant differences between these two modalities. Observations such as these are clearly based on institutional experience, and training of community urologists to perform partial nephrectomy with low risk of morbidity remains a challenge.

Open Partial Nephrectomy: Incidence

Classically, the critical technical challenge of partial nephrectomy has been balancing vascular control to reduce the risk of significant intraoperative hemorrhage against the risk of ischemic injury resulting from prolonged clamping. In most open series, hemorrhage has been the most common intraoperative complication.[26-28] The reported incidences of other significant postoperative complications include those of urinary fistula (0%-17.4%), acute renal failure (0%-26%), and postoperative bleeding (0%-4.5%).[26-31]

In the early experience with open partial nephrectomy, reported complications were high, ranging ≤30.1% in one series. In that series, hemorrhage was the fourth most common complication, whereas acute renal failure was more common, occurring in 42.3% of patients.[7] In preventing bleeding and renal dysfunction, the surgeon's challenge is to balance efficient reconstruction with as minimal an ischemic injury as possible. Recognizing the deleterious effect of prolonged arterial clamping on renal function, surgeons have adopted a more permissive bleeding strategy and improved reconstructive techniques. Thompson and colleagues,[32] when comparing two groups of patients operated before and after 1995, reported an incidence of hemorrhage of 1.5% and 1.2%, respectively. The incidence of acute renal failure was also much lower (3.8% and 1%, respectively); dialysis was required in only 2% of those operated before 1995 and in 0.6% of those treated thereafter.[32] Urinary fistula or leak has also been historically frequent complication in some early series (57.6%),[7] whereas in comparative series reported by Thompson and associates, urine leak was noted in 2.6% and 0.6% of cases before and after 1995, respectively.[32] Clearly, the learning curve of partial nephrectomy has reduced morbidity.

Van Poppel and colleagues[26] prospectively compared the complications of nephron-sparing surgery and radical nephrectomy in a phase III multicenter trial. These investigators found in the nephron-sparing group a rate of severe hemorrhage (defined as blood loss >1 L) of 3.1% and urinary fistula of 4.4%, whereas in the radical nephrectomy group severe hemorrhage was seen in only 1.2%.[26] Reoperation for complications was necessary in 4.4% of the nephron-sparing group and in 2.4% of the radical nephrectomy group.[26] As such, partial nephrectomy has been considered safe and desirable, despite a higher rate of perioperative and early postoperative complications, given the potential benefit of preserving the renal function.[26] We have experienced an extremely low rate of complications with contemporary partial nephrectomy by adhering to the specific technical concepts outlined later in this chapter. With careful attention to detail, partial nephrectomy can be very safely performed for the most patients with early-stage renal tumors.

Laparoscopic Partial Nephrectomy: Incidence

Link and associates[33] reported their experience with 217 laparoscopic partial nephrectomies. Despite a slightly increased blood loss, these investigators showed a complication rate of only 10.6% overall, including urine leakage in 1.4% and delayed renal hemorrhage in 1.8%.

Permpongkosol and colleagues[34] reported on a 12-year experience with complications seen at a single high-volume center involving 2775 urologic laparoscopic procedures. Regarding the 345 patients who underwent laparoscopic partial nephrectomy, these investigators showed a 28% rate of overall complications and a 5.8% rate of major complications.[34] The transfusion rate was noted to be 6%, whereas open conversions were required in 3.5%.[34] Similarly, another report on the 5-year outcomes of laparoscopic partial nephrectomy in an experienced laparoscopic center showed an incidence of intraoperative complications of 6% (mostly hemorrhage) and a postoperative complication rate of 13%.[35] Of the patients with postoperative complications, only 2% had urine leakage and 2% had retroperitoneal bleeding from the tumor bed that required repeat exploration with subsequent completion nephrectomy.[35]

Finally in another series, when comparing laparoscopic with open partial nephrectomy, a higher rate of major intraoperative and postoperative complications (5% versus 0% and 11% versus 2%, respectively) and more prolonged ischemia time (27.8 versus 17.5 minutes, respectively) were noted in the laparoscopic cohort, although overall complication rates were acceptable for both procedures.[35] In more contemporary series, the rates of complication have declined, and with operator experience, these rates should be similar to those noted with open partial nephrectomy.

One patient in the series reported by Link and colleagues[33] required angioembolization 2 weeks postoperatively as a result of pseudoaneurysm development.

This complication had been rare, and only two other cases of pseudoaneurysm after laparoscopic partial nephrectomy had been reported before in the literature.[36] Subsequently, several investigators reported pseudoaneurysm, arteriovenous fistula, and delayed bleeding requiring angioembolization on a more frequent basis than that observed with open partial nephrectomy. This finding may be related to the technique of suture repair employed.

SPECIFIC COMPLICATIONS

Positive Margin

Oncologic efficacy in renal cancer relies on a negative tumor margin during partial resection. Although investigators have demonstrated that the thickness of margin does not appear to be important in predicting recurrence-free survival, a negative margin remains essential.[37] Simple enucleation of the tumor is certainly technically the simplest approach, but in our opinion it increases the likelihood of microscopic residual disease.

Planning the line of renal incision is heavily dependent on the tumor position and the extent of subcortical tumor. Tumors that are predominantly exophytic can be incised in a shallow incision around the circumferential base of the tumor. Tumors that are predominantly endophytic require true resection of a segment of the kidney to ensure adequate margin. We have found the technique of intraoperative ultrasound most useful for mapping the line of renal incision during both open and laparoscopic partial nephrectomy (**Fig. 34-2**). The ultrasound probe is passed over the kidney from normal cortex toward the center of the tumor. Radial passes of the ultrasound probe allow mapping of the subcortical extent of the tumor. The line of renal incision is then planned on this basis.

During excision, arterial ischemia is useful in allowing direct visualization of the renal incision as it progresses. This feature is perhaps most important in laparoscopic partial nephrectomy because tactile feedback is less available to assess the surgeon's position in the kidney relative to the tumor. Incision into the tumor, or too close to it, can be redirected by a repeat incision at a greater depth starting 1 to 2 cm proximal to the leading edge of the incision. We have used visual landmarks in the kidney to guide the adequacy of our renal incision during laparoscopic partial nephrectomy. For example, if a tumor is radiologically positioned within 10 mm of the renal sinus or collecting system (**Fig. 34-3A**), then visual entry of these structures confirms the adequacy of margin (see Fig. 34-3B).

During laparoscopic partial nephrectomy, we have found ischemia essential to guide the renal incision visually. Because no tactile feedback is available, the incision is guided visually, and if it appears too close,

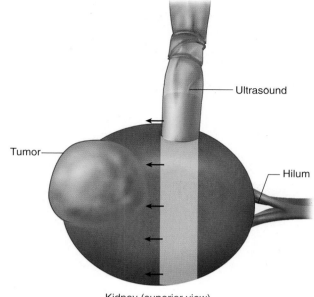

Kidney (superior view)

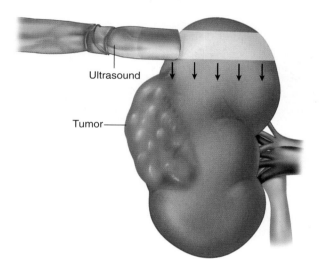

Kidney (anterior view)

Figure 34-2 In mapping a tumor by ultrasound scan, the probe is passed across the tumor in each direction to determine the extent of subcortical tumor and to ascertain the optimal line of incision. Tumor can often extent tangential or lateral to the visible exophytic component of the tumor. The probe can be passed across the tumor in radial or perpendicular lines (like the spokes of a wheel) to assess the extent of tumor fully.

or the tumor is exposed in the incision, then reestablishing the cut 2 to 3 cm proximal to the leading edge of the incision with a deeper angle will allow recovery of the margin.

Frozen section analysis of shaved margins is widely used to confirm the adequacy of the incision, and although this analysis may reassure the surgeon and patient, it is likely inaccurate in predicting oncologic efficacy. Sampling error and artifactual expansion of the

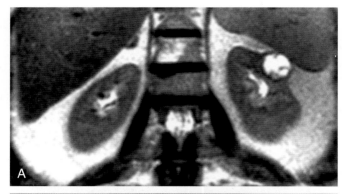

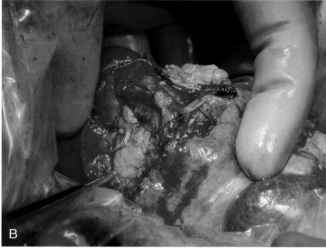

Figure 34-3 On observing the position of a tumor to be within 10 mm of the renal sinus (**A**), exposure of the sinus during resection (**B**) is essential to ensure adequacy of margin.

defect during incision render this technique of margin analysis of little value.

Bleeding

Because partial nephrectomy requires transection of multiple blood vessels during renal incision, it is perhaps intuitive that bleeding is a potential consequence. Bleeding can occur intraoperatively, immediately post-operatively, and at a delayed interval up to several days or weeks after the surgical procedure. Intraoperative bleeding usually occurs from the cut parenchyma, but it can occur from the hilum if the vessels are not carefully dissected during exposure. Preoperative knowledge of the individual renal vascular anatomy is essential in this regard. Bleeding has generally been feared in partial nephrectomy. For large and central tumors, selective embolization or extracorporeal resection of the tumor followed by autotransplantation has been performed, in an attempt to provide clean margins with limited blood loss. In the contemporary era, such techniques are generally not necessary if one adheres to basic tenets of vascular control and renal reconstruction.

The fundamental tenets of renal reconstruction are as follows:

1. Closure of the collecting system
2. Suture or coagulation control of small transected intraparenchymal vessels
3. Prevention of retraction within cut large central blood vessels
4. Compression of the defect to aid in venous tamponade

A variety of tools and techniques can be employed for each tenet, but with attention to each, good outcomes can be achieved.

Parenchymal bleeding during resection is usually handled by clamping of the renal artery or vein. In most open partial nephrectomies, arterial clamping is adequate because venous tamponade through hilar stretch and manual compression is easily achieved. Brisk bleeding on renal incision despite clamping can indicate a missed renal artery, and if it is not easily identified, a hilar cross-clamp can be placed during both open and laparoscopic procedures. When performing this maneuver on the left side, the position of the aorta, adrenal, pancreas, and superior mesenteric artery should be known before the clamp is placed. On the right, avoidance of the duodenum and porta hepatic is essential. If brisk bleeding is noted with the venous clamp in place, then venous hypertension resulting from continued arterial inflow should be suspected. Removal of the venous clamp can reduce bleeding in these cases.

Numerous techniques exist for repair of cut renal vessels. Direct suture ligature with 4-0 absorbable sutures is generally preferred. We find it most effective to identify vessels during renal parenchymal incision and suture ligate them before division. The renal parenchyma is separated with a small Freer instrument, and on identification of the vessel, a direct suture ligature is placed and the vessel is divided with tenotomy scissors (**Fig. 34-4**). In this fashion, the line of resection can be controlled and redirected. During laparoscopic partial nephrectomy, coagulative techniques are more practical for sealing small transected blood vessels. Insufflation pressure generally provides adequate slowing of venous ooze to allow effective coagulation. We prefer the use of a wet electrode, but various tools could be used.

In laparoscopic partial nephrectomy, we have described a technique of single-pass suturing that meets all the basic tenets of reconstruction. In this technique, a suture is passed into the defect through the renal capsule (**Fig. 34-5**) and is fixed to the surrounding capsule with a locking clip. The suture is passed in a running fashion through the central portion of the defect to incorporate the collecting system and larger cut vascular channels (**Fig. 34-6**) and then is advanced out of the defect through the contralateral capsular

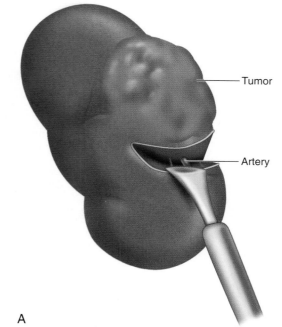

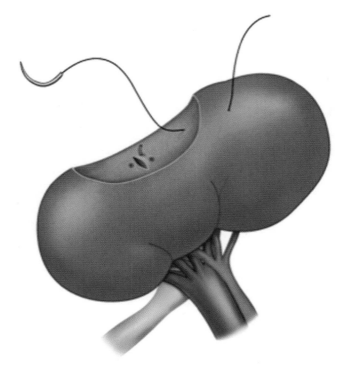

Figure 34-5 A 2-0 Vicryl suture on an SH (small half-circle) needle is passed through the outer renal capsule approximately 2 cm from the cut edge of the resection bed into the base of the renal defect. The end of the suture is knotted and preloaded with a 5-mm locking hemoclip (Hem-o-Lok, Pilling Weck Canada LP, Markham, Ontario, Canada) to anchor the suture at the outer capsule. *(Courtesy of Division of Urologic Oncology, Department of Urology, New York University Langone Medical Center, New York, 2009.)*

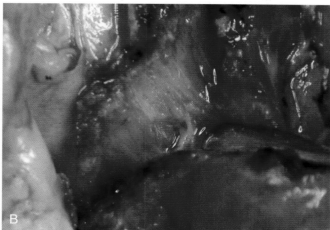

Figure 34-4 Separation of the renal parenchyma with a Freer instrument (**A**) allows visualization of arterial branches as they enter the specimen (**B**). On recognition of the vessel, it is directly suture ligated, thereby avoiding placement of deep sutures that may inadvertently injure or ligate a more proximal branch point of the vessel or adjacent vessels. *(B, From Nieder A, Taneja SS. The role of partial nephrectomy for renal cell carcinoma in contemporary practice. Urol Clin North Am. 2003;30:536.)*

edge. In doing so, the free end of the suture is secured with a clip while cinching down against the capsule (**Fig. 34-7**). The radial tension of the stitch pulls the central vessels into the defect rather than allowing them to retract. To date, the technique has resulted in no cases of delayed bleeding or vascular malformation.

If brisk bleeding occurs after removal of the arterial clamp, one should again consider the possibility of venous compression or twisting of the renal pedicle, thus impairing venous outflow. If the vein is not compromised, then suture repair of bleeding should be performed while one manually compresses the defect. Reclamping of the artery should be avoided because of the increased risk of ischemic injury following reperfusion.

In cases of immediate postoperative bleeding, initial management should be conservative with transfusion, bed rest, and serial monitoring of hematocrit. Expanding retroperitoneal hematoma can worsen bleeding through stretch of the renal defect. Therefore, if multiple transfusions are required, hemodynamic instability is noted, or the hematocrit is not responsive to transfusion, then one should give early consideration to angiography and selective embolization. In these patients, unlike in renal trauma, attention must be focused on the resection bed in which any visible vessels can be embolized, even if they are not actively bleeding. Intermittent hemorrhage is common, and bleeding may not actually be seen on angiography.

In patients with delayed bleeding (hematuria or flank hematoma) following discharge from the hospital, early angiography should be performed given the high likelihood of arteriovenous fistula or pseudoaneurysm. If the index of suspicion is low, or if the bleeding is minimal and the patient is hemodynamically stable, then one

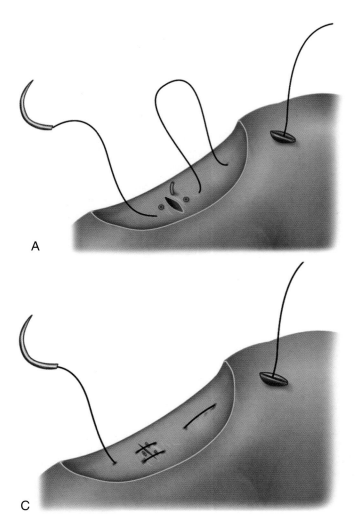

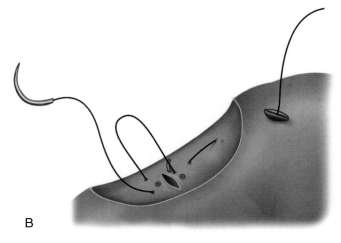

Figure 34-6 A to **C,** The suture is passed in a running fashion along the collecting system opening until closure is complete. Adjacent muscular arterial branches or central venotomies are included in the suture to provide central compression. In those cases in which the collecting system is not entered, the central, deepest portion of the defect is closed with a similar running suture. *(Courtesy of Division of Urologic Oncology, Department of Urology, New York University Langone Medical Center, New York, 2009.)*

could first perform a duplex ultrasound scan or magnetic resonance angiography (MRA) because these techniques are less invasive (**Fig. 34-8**). If an abnormality is not noted and bleeding persists, then angiography would be required anyway. Selective angioembolization is extremely effective in the management of these complications.[36] We have on occasion seen delayed hematuria resulting from decompression of an extrarenal hematoma through the collecting system. In these cases, a small, fluid-filled defect (closed urinoma) is noted at the resection bed on an MRI urogram.

Infarct

In performing partial nephrectomy, preservation of the vascular supply of the retained segments of kidney is essential to avoid renal infarction. Although the functional significance of infarct is not known, certainly infarcted tissue likely decreases the preserved renal reserve over time. Large infarcted segments can result in renin-mediated hypertension, and if a large portion

of the repaired collecting system loses blood supply, this situation can promote leak.

Avoiding infarct again relies on knowledge of renal arterial anatomy. Given the end-arterial nature of renal blood flow, maximizing proximal vascular preservation should be the goal of resection. In approaching polar lesions, straight rather than tangential amputation is desirable, but if the lesion is primarily located within the anterior or posterior segmental vasculature, then a significant amount of parenchyma can be preserved through a tangential cut. Within the anterior and posterior segment, we find that starting the parenchymal incision away from the hilum and cutting toward the center of the kidney will allow identification of arterial branches as they enter the specimen, thereby avoiding radial infarct. We find that starting the incision from the hilum and working outward results in a higher likelihood of injury to main branches and thereby promotes additionally infarcted kidney (**Fig. 34-9**).

On separation of renal parenchyma along the planned line of incision, individual vessels are identified as they

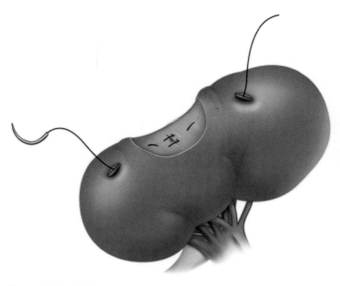

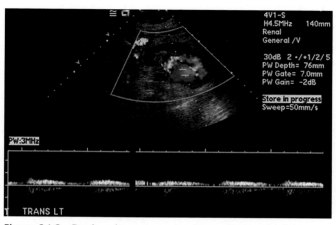

Figure 34-8 Duplex ultrasonography demonstrating the "yin-yang" sign of turbulent mixing of arterial and venous blood following laparoscopic partial nephrectomy. *(Courtesy of Michael Stifelman, MD.)*

Figure 34-7 While the surgeon holds the leading edge of the suture on tension, the needle is passed out of the resection bed through the outer renal capsule opposite the site of entry. A locking hemoclip (Hem-o-Lok, Pilling Weck Canada LP, Markham, Ontario, Canada) is used to cinch the suture, compress the defect, and lock the suture in place. Compression of the resection defect is provided by cinching the suture ends in the direction of the central portion of the defect. *(Courtesy of Division of Urologic Oncology, Department of Urology, New York University Langone Medical Center, New York, 2009.)*

enter the specimen, are suture ligated, and are transected sharply to avoid the necessity for deep suture placement for retracted blood vessels (see Fig. 34-4). This technique is more difficult to recapitulate in laparoscopic surgery, and as such, the likelihood of radial infarct is higher in laparoscopic partial nephrectomy owing to the suturing techniques typically used in the laparoscopic procedure. We have adapted a modified suturing technique (described earlier) to reduce the likelihood of major infarct or vascular complication.

The general management of infarct is observation. In patients with severe hypertension resulting from infarcted kidney, nephrectomy should be performed.

Urine Leak

Urine leak rates reported in the urologic literature depend on the operator's definition. This definition has varied widely from leakage for >72 hours to leakage persisting for >3 months postoperatively. We generally define urinary fistula following partial nephrectomy as urine leakage persisting for >4 weeks after the surgical procedure. Nonetheless, any duration of postoperative urine leak must be appropriately managed by the surgeon. Simple principles of drainage, prevention of infection, and avoidance of ureteral obstruction generally allow resolution of the leak.

Careful closure of the collecting system generally prevents urine leak. In cases of large resection bed, or in

tumors resected from the anterior or posterior segment with tangential renal incision, small caliceal injuries may not be identified, and these are often the site of persistent leak. In general, meticulous closure of the collecting system is performed with a layer of interrupted absorbable 4-0 braided sutures. This stage is followed by a second layer of imbricated sutures that attempt to pull the parenchyma together around the defect and thereby reduce tension on the primary closure (**Fig. 34-10**). In the laparoscopic setting, the collecting system is closed with a running absorbable 2-0 suture, and tension is removed from the closure by anchoring the suture to the surrounding renal capsule. Serial sutures are placed more widely to allow an imbricating effect.

Two modifications of technique have greatly reduced our leak rate with open partial nephrectomy: (1) retrograde instillation of methylene blue through the renal pelvis and (2) the use of a layer of tissue adhesive over the closure. The use of tissue adhesive is most important in laparoscopic partial nephrectomy because small caliceal injuries are often difficult to identify. We have adopted a standardized technique of infiltrating Gelfoam (Pfizer Inc., New York) with fibrin sealant (Tisseal, Baxter International Inc., Deerfield, Illinois), molding it to the resection defect, and then activating it through infiltration of thrombin. Additional hemostatic materials are packed into the defect, and then the kidney is folded over the materials using horizontal mattress sutures of 3-0 absorbable non-braided suture anchored to the surrounding renal capsule. In the laparoscopic technique, this latter maneuver is not performed.

Urine leak presents in one of two ways. Early leaks often become evident in the recovery room and persist, whereas delayed leaks manifest 5 to 14 days postoperatively and may become symptomatic. It is not clear whether most delayed leaks were simply unrecognized early because of inadequate drainage and lack of symp-

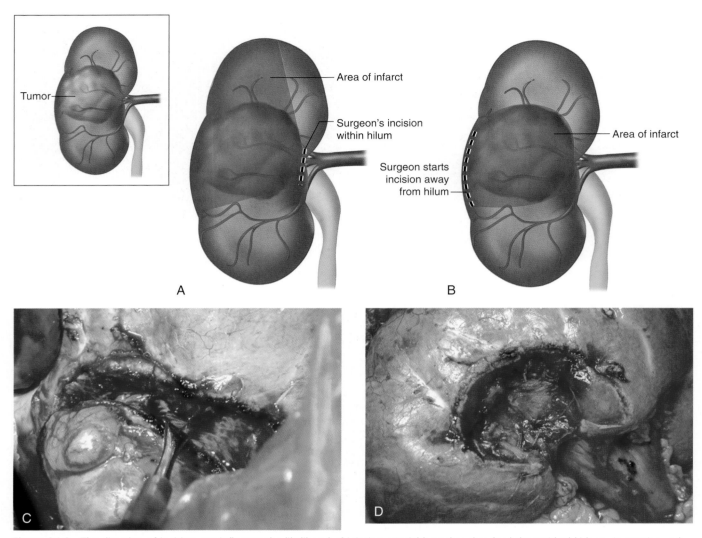

Figure 34-9 The direction of incision can influence the likelihood of injuring arterial branches that feed the residual kidney. As arteries and more proximal branch points are present in the hilar region, we generally prefer to start resection on the side of the tumor opposite the hilum. This is particularly relevant when operating in the anterior or posterior segment. **A,** If the incision is carried out from the hilum, infarct radial to the defect can often be seen. **B to D,** When starting the resection away from the hilum, larger central vessels are preserved and the surrounding kidney remains well perfused.

toms. The old tenet that urine leakage frequently occurs in the first 24 to 72 hours but then resolves is not entirely true. In fact, most renal reconstruction for elective partial nephrectomy should be watertight. Early leakage generally indicates poor collecting system closure or unrecognized collecting system injury, and in our experience this leakage rarely stops within the first few days.

Early leak is suspected if drainage of >30 to 40 mL per shift is noted >48 hours after the surgical procedure. Large-volume drain outputs within the first 24 hours may lead one to suspect leak, but intervention is not required unless infection is noted, serum creatinine becomes markedly elevated because of reabsorption, or the patient has no urine output (solitary kidney). In these cases, renal obstruction may be suspected and

early imaging is advised. Urine leak beyond 48 hours is confirmed by measurement of drainage creatinine level relative to serum. If the drainage is pure urine, creatinine levels will generally be >30 mg/dL. When the drainage creatinine is even moderately higher that of the serum, then at least part of the draining fluid is urine and a urine leak is likely present. Minimal creatinine elevation may suggest a resolved urine leak with some dilute urine still in the retroperitoneum. After leak confirmation, we generally perform an immediate ultrasound scan or noncontrast CT study for assurance that the drain is properly positioned, that no undrained urinoma is present, and that the kidney is well drained.

If all these tenets are met, the patient is discharged home with prophylactic antibiotics and a drain in place.

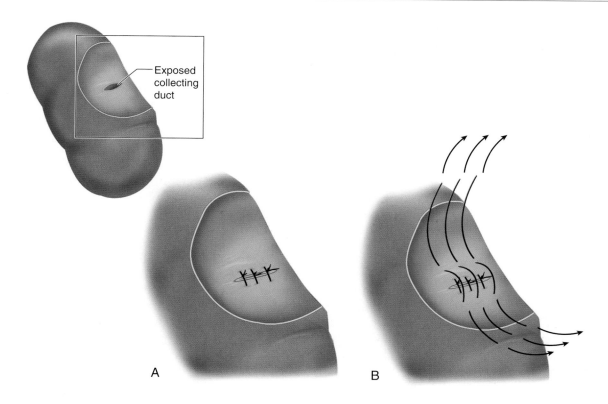

Figure 34-10   Two-layer collecting system closure involves two interrupted layers of absorbable suture. The first layer (**A**) incorporates the edges of the collecting system, whereas the second layer (**B**) attempts to imbricate normal renal parenchyma to remove tension from the first line. The use of interrupted rather than running suture reduces the likelihood of tearing the collecting system with the suture.

Patients are monitored weekly with electrolytes and renal ultrasound studies to rule out worsening urinoma or drain migration. In cases of undrained fluid, the drain is repositioned to sit immediately adjacent to the leak point. This maneuver can be facilitated by contrast CT with delayed cuts. Ideal drain placement is immediately adjacent to the kidney to allow a drain tract to form. In cases of high-output leak, the drain can be converted from suction to gravity, but a follow-up ultrasound scan within a few days is warranted to rule out a secondary fluid collection.

Presentation of delayed leak is usually the result of flank pain, fever, or drainage from a port site or incision. In a patient with fever, evaluation should include a complete blood count with manual differential, blood and urine cultures, and a chest radiograph to identify other potential sources of infection. CT with intravenous contrast should include delayed images to identify urinary extravasation, provided renal function is acceptable for receiving iodinated contrast. Ultrasound can alternatively be used to identify a perirenal fluid collection. Before percutaneous drainage, broad-spectrum antibiotics should be administered. The drain is best positioned immediately adjacent to kidney, but in cases of infection, maximal drainage is paramount to allow defervescence, and this may be best achieved with the patient in the most dependent position.

In the absence of infection, similar evaluation of renal function and imaging to identify fluid collections should be performed. On percutaneous drainage, the fistula output may be quite high initially because of the presence of a large potential space outside the kidney. Maximal kidney drainage is necessary to promote antegrade drainage over time. In general, a ureteral stent is not necessary unless evidence indicates ureteral obstruction, blood clots or debris within the collecting system, or a very large collecting system opening. In our experience, stents often worsen the leak initially, possibly as a result of reflux. It is essential to have a concomitant urethral catheter in place while the leak is perpetuated, particularly in a man with high-pressure voiding. We have generally avoided stent placement unless absolutely necessary because most leaks will close with prolonged drainage.

Resolution of urine leak generally requires scarring in of the potential space around the kidney. This occurs as scar tissue fills in around the drain forming a drain tract. We generally prefer to leave the drain on gravity drainage to promote antegrade urine flow within the collecting system. On converting to gravity drainage, a follow-up ultrasound scan within 36 to 48 hours will confirm that no urine collection has formed around the kidney or drain tract. If it has, then the drain should be returned to suction. Urine collections prevent the formation of a drain tract and delay leak closure. Over a period of 2 to 4 weeks, if properly drained, a drain tract should have formed, and on confirmation of the absence of urinoma, the drain can be advanced back 2 to 3 cm to allow the tract to close between the tip of the drain and the kidney. Every 48 to 72 hours, the drain can be pulled back another 2 to 3 cm until it is removed. During this time of drain advancement, one should monitor for urinoma formation and fever, a finding suggesting recurrence of the urinoma within the drain tract. In cases of high drain outputs (>300 mL/24 hours) more prolonged observation (≤12 weeks) may be necessary before attempting drain advancement. Low-output leaks require minimal observation before closure can be achieved. In this regard, closure of a leak is an active process initiated by the surgeon rather than a passive physiologic process.

Urine leak can also result from ureteral injury. Excessive dissection of the renal pelvis, the lower pole of the kidney, and the proximal ureter should be avoided because it can cause devascularization, ischemia, and necrosis with subsequent fistula formation in the dissected segment. On completion of the procedure, fat should be interposed between the lower pole of the kidney and the upper ureter to avoid adherence, scarring, and subsequent stricture of the ureter.

Renal Function

Measuring renal functional outcomes after elective partial nephrectomy is most difficult given the compensatory ability of the remaining kidney. Conventional beliefs have been that renal dysfunction following partial nephrectomy is related to the length of renal arterial clamping and the amount of parenchyma resected. In truth, many factors may influence the function of the operated kidney including intraoperative blood pressure variations, fluid resuscitation during the case, and aggressive handling of the kidney. Intraoperative blood loss may result in a higher risk of renal dysfunction because of the possibility of hypotension and reduced tissue oxygenation. When operating on an individual with two kidneys, the risk of postoperative azotemia and the necessity for dialysis depend on the functional reserve of the remaining kidney. Patients with diabetes, hypertension, and known vascular disease are more likely to have transient azotemia postoperatively. Individuals with a solitary kidney are also affected by these factors, but clearly, the risk of azotemia is more strongly affected by renal arterial clamping than in patients with two kidneys and normal renal function.

In patients with bilateral functioning kidneys, the reported rate of acute kidney injury after open surgery has been 4%,[35] whereas chronic kidney disease has been reported to occur in 2% to 8% of patients.[32,35] Similar patients in laparoscopic series were shown to have negligible rates of renal dysfunction.[38-40] In patients with solitary kidneys, the rates of acute kidney injury after open procedures are more evident, ranging between 13% and 38%, with chronic kidney disease occurring from 3% to 30% of these patients.[31,41,42] In laparoscopy series, these data have not been consistently reported. Analyzing an initial cohort of 430 patients who underwent laparoscopic partial nephrectomy at the Cleveland Clinic, Gill and colleagues[43] observed that in 22 cases with solitary kidneys and 2 of which electively converted to an open procedure, a single patient (4.5%) required temporary dialysis and the chronic kidney disease incidence rate was 13%.

Several maneuvers to reduce renal ischemia have been proposed. The use of an osmotic diuretic, such as mannitol, immediately before and shortly after clamping of the renal artery is thought to reduce the accumulation of free oxygen radicals in the tissues. Similarly, cooling of the kidney during ischemia is believed to reduce the likelihood of tissue injury. During open partial nephrectomy, we have used both these maneuvers. The kidney is placed within an intestinal bag with the opening loosely cinched around the renal pedicle. On ice slush packing, the bag serves to hold the ice to the renal surface. After clamping, a period of 5 to 10 minutes is necessary to reach the nadir core temperature within the kidney. We generally begin to operate on the kidney during this period to reduce total ischemia time, but other surgeons advocate waiting a full 5 minutes before renal incision.

In general, we do not clamp the renal vein because stretch of the pedicle usually sufficiently reduces venous backflow. Investigators have suggested that retrograde circulation of venous blood may allow low level tissue oxygenation in the setting of arterial clamping. This possibility has been suggested for laparoscopic partial nephrectomy as well.[44]

In the setting of laparoscopic partial nephrectomy, several investigators have attempted to use various methods of intracorporeal kidney cooling.[45-47] We have not found these methods to be practical, and it is questionable how effectively the kidney is cooled. Instead, we use a technique of renal arterial clamping, venous clamping during deep resection in which large venous channels are exposed, and early clamp removal, to allow shorter warm ischemia time. Clearly, this technique is related to operator comfort in reconstruction in the presence of bleeding.

An alternative to the use of vascular clamping is manual compression of the renal parenchyma. This technique is quite effective in open partial nephrectomy, particularly for polar lesions. In laparoscopic surgery, the technique can be applied through hand assistance, but this approach is more cumbersome because one-hand suturing is required. Even if the renal vessels are not clamped, they should be fully dissected in case of the need for urgent clamping. Surgery can then be performed by squeezing the renal parenchyma with the hands and using only enough pressure to control the bleeding.

Because of the increased risk of azotemia in the setting of a solitary kidney, we generally avoid arterial clamping in these patients whenever possible.[25] In most cases, this situation requires open surgery, but in the case of small exophytic tumors, a laparoscopic approach with no arterial clamping can be considered.

Postoperatively, attention should be given to avoiding or minimizing nephrotoxic or harmful medications such as angiotensin-converting enzyme inhibitors, nonsteroidal anti-inflammatory drugs, and aminoglycosides. Individuals at high risk, including those with solitary kidney, large (>50%) renal resections, prolonged ischemia times, preexisting renal insufficiency, and severe vascular disease, should be prepared mentally for the possibility of temporary or even permanent hemodialysis.

Reoperation

Urine leak rarely requires reoperation, but in cases of persistent ureteral obstruction perpetuating the leak, recurrent abscess, or severe intraperitoneal leak (laparoscopic), a repeat operation may be necessary. Reoperation for bleeding is required when angiographic techniques fail to control postoperative bleeding. In most cases, reoperation for leak or bleeding results in nephrectomy.

CONCLUSION

Partial nephrectomy for tumor resection is an increasingly important technique for practicing urologists to master. The long-term benefits may be greater than initially perceived. Careful preoperative imaging, knowledge of renal anatomy, attention to patient- and tumor-related risk factors, and meticulous surgical technique are essential for achieving good surgical outcomes. Complication rates should be acceptably low if following fundamental tenets of surgical technique.

KEY POINTS

1. Knowledge of renal arterial anatomy is essential for performing partial nephrectomy.
2. Complication rates with both open and laparoscopic partial nephrectomy vary with operator experience, but both can be acceptable with careful attention to detail.
3. The risk of bleeding and urine leak should be balanced against the risk of renal dysfunction from prolonged arterial clamping.
4. Renal incision should be planned by ultrasound study according to arterial anatomy and should be started away from the hilum to minimize the risk of infarct.
5. Identification and direct suture ligature of retracted blood vessels within the line of incision avoid retracted sutures deep in the incision bed.
6. At the time of urine leak, the drain should be positioned to remove any extrarenal urine collections completely. A stent is rarely required unless ureteral obstruction is present.

REFERENCES

Please see www.expertconsult.com

Chapter 35

COMPLICATIONS OF RENOVASCULAR SURGERY

David Canes MD
Assistant Professor of Urology, Tufts University Medical School, Boston, Massachusetts

John A. Libertino MD
Chairman, Institute of Urology, Lahey Clinic, Burlington; Professor of Urology, Tufts University Medical School, Boston, Massachusetts

Lesions of the renal artery, including stenoses and occlusions, have a final common pathway of renal ischemia with two clinically relevant findings: hypertension and renal insufficiency. The endocrine effects, mediated through the renin-angiotensin-aldosterone axis, result in hypertension. The cumulative effects of decreased blood flow on the end organ lead to progressive renal impairment. Diagnosis during a window of time before massive parenchymal loss ensues affords the opportunity to intervene and change the natural history of renal disease.

Of intrinsic renal artery lesions, the most common cause is atherosclerosis, accounting for two thirds of all cases. It is most often part of generalized vascular disease in a given patient and can be expected to progress in 40%. The remaining two thirds of stenotic renovascular disease cases result from mural dysplasia, most commonly in young women as a result of medial fibroplasia. Other renovascular diseases include aneurysms, emboli, and traumatic injuries. Less commonly, Takayasu's disease with periarteritis and the endothelial nodules of neurofibromatosis may affect the renal arteries.

Few fields demonstrate the ebb and flow of surgical trends quite like renovascular surgery. In 1954, Freeman[1] reported the first case of renal thromboendarterectomy and noted "prompt and persistent reduction in the patient's blood pressure that followed this procedure." Over the next half-century, various anatomic and extra-anatomic reconstructive procedures were developed. Renal revascularization was subsequently almost exclusively the therapy of choice for renovascular hypertension. With the advent of diagnostic-value angiotensin-converting enzyme inhibitors, as well as the therapeutic value of other medical antihypertensives, fewer patients were surgical candidates. Catheter-based treatment with percutaneous transluminal renal angioplasty (PTRA) was first reported in 1964 by Dotter and Judkins.[2] Renal angioplasty was performed for renovascular hypertension in 1978,[3] and was carried out concomitant with stenting in 1987.[4] As a result, younger, healthy patients with less advanced disease are now favored for this approach.

In an analysis of hospital discharges in the United States between 1988 and 2001, combined aortic and renal revascularizations decreased by 73%, isolated renal revascularizations decreased by 56%, and endoluminal procedures increased 173%.[5] Management to this day remains controversial, and although PTRA has come into favor, urologists must understand the complications of all procedures, including historical ones. As is sometimes the case, exuberance for specific procedures continues until the pendulum swings.

The complications of renovascular surgery are grouped in a useful paradigm in Table 35-1. This chapter systematically reviews pertinent complications of common surgical and endoluminal treatments for this disease complex.

PATIENT SELECTION

As with any surgical procedure, careful patient selection is the first step to avoid complications. Patients with functionally significant renovascular lesion are candidates for surgery if the following is true: poor control of hypertension after appropriate medical therapy, poor patient compliance with medical treatment, total renal artery occlusion or dissection, deterioration of renal function as manifested by elevated blood urea nitrogen or creatinine level, cross-sectional imaging demonstrating parenchymal loss, angiographic evidence of progressive renal arterial disease, anuria from arterial occlusion in a solitary kidney, or a combination of the foregoing.[6]

Renal artery stenosis can be corrected by numerous surgical techniques, the details of which are described elsewhere (Box 35-1).[7] In general, aortorenal bypass with autologous saphenous vein graft is preferred.[8] In cases of severe atherosclerosis of the aorta, splenorenal

TABLE 35-1	Complications of Interventions for Renal Artery Stenosis*		

Blood Pressure Response
  Hypertensive crisis
  Rebound hypertension
  Persistent hypertension
Renal Function Response
  Acute renal failure
  Infarction of renal unit
  Worsening renal function
	A	**Cardiovascular**
		  Myocardial infarction
		  Cerebrovascular accident
		  Emboli (atheromatous, cholesterol)
			B

Surgical
Technical
  Hemorrhage
  Renal artery/graft thrombosis
  Intimal dissection
  Anastomotic disruption
  Anastomotic stenosis
Conduit related
  Saphenous vein aneurysm
  Synthetic graft delayed bleeding
  Synthetic graft–enteric fistula
	C	**Procedure or Site Specific**
		Saphenous vein donor site
		  Skin flap necrosis
		  Bleeding, hematoma
		Splenorenal
		  Pancreatitis
		  Postsplenectomy immunocompromise
		Hepatorenal
		  Gangrenous cholecystitis
		  Bile duct injury
		PTRA ± stent
		  Hematoma, AV fistula, hemorrhage,
		  dissection, perforation, emboli,
		  stent restenosis, stent thrombosis
			D

*Complications are grouped in categories: (A) related to physiologic perturbances, overall success; (B) related to cardiovascular comorbidity, diffuse atheromatous plaque; (C) related to technical factors, and (D) site-specific surgical complications.
AV, arteriovenous; PTRA, percutaneous transluminal renal angioplasty.

BOX 35-1	**Spectrum of Nonmedical Interventions for Renal Artery Stenosis**

Endoluminal Repair
PTRA
PTRA with stent

Reconstructive Surgery
Aortorenal bypass
Renal artery reimplantation
Thromboendarterectomy
Excision and primary reanastomosis
Extra-anatomic bypass
• Splenorenal
• Hepatorenal
• Gastroduodenal-renal
• Iliorenal
• Mesentorenal
• Thoracic aortorenal
Ex vivo reconstruction and autotransplantation

Ablative Surgery
Partial nephrectomy
Nephrectomy

PTRA, percutaneous transluminal renal angioplasty.

(left-sided renal artery stenosis) or hepatorenal (right-sided renal artery stenosis) bypass is preferred, to reduce the troublesome complications associated with atheroemboli from clamping a diseased aorta.[9-13] Alternative inflow may be employed in appropriate circumstances from the iliac artery, superior mesenteric artery, gastroduodenal artery, and thoracic aorta. Patients with mural dysplasia extending into segmental vessels or associated with aneurysms are better served by ex vivo repair with autotransplantation.[14-16] Indications for autotransplantation should not be overzealously extended when acceptable forms of in situ repair could be accomplished.[6] Thromboendarterectomy has been largely abandoned but is occasionally performed for ostial stenosis of accessory arteries or bilateral renal artery stenosis.

Nephrectomy is of course reserved for patients who are poor surgical risks and in whom medical therapy has failed and for patients with extensive unreconstructable branch vessel disease, extensive unsalvageable unilateral parenchymal damage, or complete occlusion and infarction following arterial reconstruction. Nephrectomy is also indicated for total renal artery occlusion unless the following are true:

1. Angiography, isotope renography, or intravenous pyelography demonstrates a nephrogram.
2. Angiography detects retrograde filling of distal circulation by perihilar collateral vessels.
3. Intraoperative backbleeding from a renal arteriotomy occurs.
4. An intraoperative or preoperative biopsy demonstrates intact glomerular architecture.[17,18]

PTRA is most successful in young women with fibromuscular dysplasia, in whom little controversy exists over its use for this indication. In patients with atherosclerosis, nonostial lesions respond best to PTRA.[19,20] Outcomes for ostial lesions secondary to atherosclerosis are improved with PTRA and stenting.[21]

CARDIOVASCULAR COMPLICATIONS AND OVERALL MORTALITY

Renal artery stenosis in patients with atherosclerosis is often a manifestation of global vascular atheromatous disease. Technical advances in surgical procedures, anesthetic care, and perioperative monitoring have made this high-risk patient population appropriate surgical candidates. It is paramount that the urologist understand that medical comorbidity is the rule rather than the exception in this group. Cherr and colleagues[22] reviewed their series of 500 hypertensive patients undergoing surgical intervention for atherosclerotic renovascular disease. Cardiac comorbidity was present in 70% of patients, including angina, prior myocardial infarction, left ventricular hypertrophy, congestive heart failure, or prior revascularization (coronary artery bypass grafting, percutaneous transluminal coronary angioplasty). Cerebrovascular comorbidity was present in 32%, including prior transient ischemic attack, stroke, or endarterectomy. During early experience with surgical revascularization of the renal artery, excluding the fibrodysplastic group, coronary artery disease was the leading cause of operative mortality.[23]

Thus, after documenting the need for PTRA or open surgical reconstruction of renovascular disease, the patient must be extensively evaluated for extrarenal atherosclerosis with particular attention to coronary and carotid circulations. In addition to a carefully obtained history and physical examination, all patients should undergo electrocardiography, cardiac stress testing, noninvasive carotid studies, and directed angiography where indicated.[24] Obviously, correctable coronary or carotid artery disease should be addressed before operative intervention for renovascular disease, to reduce associated perioperative morbidity and mortality.[13]

Perioperative mortality rates from contemporary surgical series are acceptably low. More useful data predictive of early mortality arise from subgroup and multivariate analysis. Cherr and colleagues[22] reported a 4.6% 30-day overall mortality rate. However, mortality was 0.8% for isolated renal artery repair and 6.9% for combined aortic or bilateral repair.[22] On multivariate analysis, only advanced age and clinical congestive heart failure were significant predictors of mortality. The extent of the surgical procedure was not significant, probably because increased morbidity may be more a reflection of diffuse vascular disease in patients requiring more extensive surgical intervention. Darling and colleagues,[25] in a report of 568 patients, had a 5.5% mortality rate, 4% for unilateral and 10.5% for bilateral repair, and 22.3% for emergency repair. In this series, bilaterality was a significant predictor of mortality ($P < .05$).

Over the period from 1988 to 2001, the Nationwide Inpatient Sample database was used to analyze treatment trends, and mortality figures were comparable to these reports. The in-hospital mortality rate was 5.2% for combined aortic and renal revascularization, 2.2% for isolated renal revascularization, and 0.8% for angioplasty and stenting.[5] Significant predictors included advanced age (>75 years), emergency admission, and nonwhite race. The finding on multivariate analysis that emergency repair predicts increased perioperative mortality is important because approximately 3% of our patients require an emergency operation for repair of renal artery rupture or dissection with complete occlusion after PTRA.[20] In the case of young, otherwise healthy women with fibrous dysplasia, as expected, the opposite is true, with 0% operative mortality reported in one series for this subgroup.[26]

To summarize, preoperative cardiovascular screening, risk stratification, and preoperative targeted extrarenal revascularization are paramount. The overall early mortality rate for surgical repair of renovascular stenosis is in the 5% range, and it is even lower in patients with unilateral or fibrodysplastic disease. Bilateral or concomitant aortic repair should be approached with caution. Emergency procedures are associated with significantly increased mortality. The mortality rate for PTRA is approximately 1%.

PHYSIOLOGIC COMPLICATIONS

Hypertensive Crisis

Even with patent inflow after successful revascularization, hypertensive crisis may occur in the early postoperative period. The following may potentiate hypertension in this setting:

1. Intraoperative fluid overload
2. Vasoconstriction from hypothermia
3. Sympathetic overdrive from poor incisional analgesia

Once these correctable factors have been addressed, calcium channel blockade or sodium nitroprusside is appropriate. Dramatic hypertension should also initiate radiographic imaging to exclude graft thrombosis. In any of the foregoing situations, continuous hemodynamic monitoring in an intensive care setting may be appropriate.

Rebound hypertension intraoperatively or immediately postoperatively may also result from abrupt withdrawal of antihypertensive medications.[22] Patients receiving high doses of single-agent therapy with β-blockers and angiotensin-converting enzyme inhibitors should instead receive low doses by initiating combination therapy with vasodilators or calcium channel blockers. Furthermore, constitutive activation of the renin-angiotensin-aldosterone axis with or without concomitant diuretic therapy results in volume contraction. This poses a delicate situation to our anesthesia colleagues, who must replete volume at the very least with central venous monitoring and preferably with a pulmonary artery catheter. Too little volume correction results in hypovolemia and graft thrombosis, whereas hypervolemia potentiates hypertension, as discussed.

Persistent Hypertension

The end point of blood pressure response is important. Failure of blood pressure to respond can be considered a late complication of treatment, even when a technical error may not be apparent. The ultimate response depends on the clinical subgroup. In the atherosclerotic group, approximately 5% to 20% of patients have a failed hypertension response to revascularization.[22,24,26,27] In the fibromuscular dysplasia group, whereas the overall cure rate is higher, failures are comparable, in the range of 10%. The natural history of hypertension in patients whose condition is eventually improved or cured after revascularization is frequently that of a slow, gradual decline over several weeks.

Renal Failure: Acute and Chronic

Acute renal failure is reviewed in Chapter 34. The same considerations apply here with regard to warm ischemia time and its influence on postoperative acute renal failure. Proper preclamping renal protection with intravenous hydration, mannitol, and heparinization is applicable. Warm ischemia time is best kept to <30 minutes when possible.

When surgical revascularization is indicated in the setting of atherosclerotic ischemic nephropathy, how often can deteriorating renal function be expected? Cherr and colleagues[22] reported that 10% of their cohort were worsened after surgical repair. In general, this complication falls within the range of 10% to 25% across various series in the literature.[24,27,28] In a series reported by Marone and colleagues[29] in a cohort of patients with atherosclerotic renovascular disease and a mean serum creatinine level of 2.6 mg/dL, renal functional decline occurred in 17%, with progression to end-stage renal disease requiring dialysis. Predictors of progression to dialysis on multivariate analysis in the study by Marone and associates were twofold: (1) completely occluded renal artery (odds ratio, 4.63), and (2) baseline creatinine concentration, with each 1 mg/dL increase conferring a 1.8-fold increased progression to dialysis. Unfortunately, successful rescue of renal function may be difficult to predict. Other studies failed to substantiate reliable predictive factors.[30] Therefore, generalizations regarding patient selection are lacking. As a rule of thumb, we would not consider for revascularization a patient with a serum creatinine ≥4 mg/dL, unless the patient had a solitary kidney, normal renal size, and a tight stenosis or total occlusion.

TECHNICAL SURGICAL COMPLICATIONS

Renal Artery or Graft Thrombosis

Renal artery thrombosis is the most common complication of renal vascular reconstruction and is most common after either placement of a Dacron graft or endarterectomy. Predisposing factors include small Dacron grafts, renal atrophy associated with thin-walled diseased arteries and high intrarenal vascular resistance, hypotension, and hypovolemia. Thrombosis of both venous and synthetic grafts is partially strongly affected by the adequacy of peripheral runoff and the adequacy of resection of the endothelial plaques in atherosclerotic vessels.[20] Routine postoperative imaging is essential to assess graft patency. At the Lahey Clinic in Burlington, Massachusetts, this imaging is performed either with Doppler ultrasonography or nuclear scintigraphy (diethylenetriamine pentaacetic acid or mercaptotriglycylglycine) in the first 24 hours postoperatively.

Hemorrhage

Postoperative hemorrhage requiring reoperation is in some measure a technical failure, but it may also be a function of the structural integrity of the arterial wall in diseased segments. In the presence of systemic heparinization, minor bleeding from suture holes in renal and aortic anastomoses has been helped by the use of Prolene suture material.[20] Otherwise, thrombogenic mesh is usually sufficient to control needle hole bleeding. Bleeding may also occur during the first 24 hours from poorly controlled perihilar collateral vessels, which may grow to considerable size in the presence of high-grade renal artery stenosis.

Unrecognized venous bleeding may occur from the adrenal vessels during and after difficult dissection of the left renal artery. In some patients, the adrenal gland is adherent to the anterior portion of the renal artery, vein, and perihilar tissue. The adrenal gland must be handled gently for this reason, and intraoperative hemostasis must be compulsively maintained. Other technical aspects of the vascular anastomotic technique may account for bleeding, including gaps in the placement of adjacent sutures or the apposition of diseased vessels. Late hemorrhage may rarely result from infected graft suture lines.

Intimal Dissection

In severely atherosclerotic vessels, intimal plaques can be dislodged, resulting in intimal dissection or emboli. Suture needles should always be placed from intima to adventitia to avoid this complication. Double-armed sutures permit this maneuver on both the arterial and venous portions of the anastomosis.

Anastomotic Disruption

Fortunately, serious bleeding from a disrupted anastomosis is rare. When it occurs, it is usually associated with approximation of diseased vessels or errors in technique.

Anastomotic Stenosis

As a general rule, the single most important factor responsible for long-term patency is a wide, flawless anastomosis with the renal artery. Loupe optical magnification and fiberoptic head lamps are helpful to permit precise placement of sutures. For other complications specific to the choice of certain grafts, see later.

Saphenous Vein Complications: Stenosis and Aneurysms

In the case of the saphenous vein graft, procurement is critical to short- and long-term success. Meticulous technique in exposure and excision prevents mural trauma and ischemia. The graft must be handled gently and without stretching, tributaries should be carefully tied in continuity with fine silk, and areolar tissue should be kept on the specimen. Fibrotic stenosis may develop at the site of venous valves; therefore, a valveless segment of vein should be used when possible.[31] In addition, transmural ischemia of the graft may lead to subendothelial fibroblastic proliferation and late stenosis.[31] Prolonged ischemia of the saphenous vein should also be avoided at all costs. The graft should remain in situ until the renal vessels are mobilized and it is ready for use. If the graft must be removed prematurely, it should be placed in cold Ringer's lactate solution or autologous blood.

A small risk of aneurysmal dilatation of the saphenous vein graft exists, as first indicated by Ernst and colleagues in 1972.[32] This risk is particularly increased in children.[31] The true cause of saphenous vein graft aneurysms is not known; however, the incidence is <1%.[33] Late rupture of a saphenous vein graft has also been reported.[34]

Synthetic Grafts: Thrombosis, Delayed Bleeding, and Fistula Formation

Dacron grafts and silk sutures have been abandoned because of delayed complications of late bleeding from arterial-enteric fistulas and a high rate of thrombosis.[35] Only if autogenous graft is not available should polytetrafluoroethylene (PTFE) be used exclusively. Although concerns prevail about graft occlusion, infection, and enteric fistulas with synthetic grafts, one series suggested that these concerns may be unfounded.[36] Early and late occlusion occurred in 1.4% and 4.8%, respectively. We still maintain that synthetic material be used only when autogenous graft is not available.

Embolic Complications

Placement and release of vascular clamps on a diseased aorta may result in atheroemboli distally. As the section on patient selection suggests, this complication is best avoided by choosing an extra-anatomic bypass for the patient with extensive aortic atheroma. Even with the most judicious preoperative evaluation, however, some component of aortic disease may be encountered. Therefore, it is crucial to determine the proper anastomotic site based on imaging and confirmed with palpation of the aorta to determine the softest location for an intended anastomosis. Systemic heparinization also aids in preventing catastrophic emboli but does not reduce the risk entirely. In addition, the lower extremities should be routinely prepared and draped in the sterile surgical field so that the immediate femoral or distal pulse may be palpated and thrombectomy performed if necessary.

PROCEDURE OR SITE-SPECIFIC COMPLICATIONS

Saphenous Vein Donor Site

Improper harvesting of the saphenous vein, aside from the stenotic and aneurysmal complications discussed earlier, may lead to donor site complications. The saphenous vein should be obtained from the thigh opposite the renal lesion to permit two surgeons to operate simultaneously. The incision should be made directly over the vein to avoid the complication of devascularized skin flaps, which can result in necrotic wound edges and wound sepsis. Accuracy in this task is facilitated by two maneuvers: (1) preoperative skin marking overlying the course of the vein with the patient standing and (2) finger dissection between the trunk of the vein and the skin. The thigh incision should not be closed until the bypass procedure has been completed. This technique ensures that any delayed bleeding caused by systemic heparinization can be recognized and controlled appropriately.

Aortorenal Bypass

Particular complications to be avoided in this setting are autologous graft kinking, twisting, or and misalignment, as well as atheroemboli. The saphenous vein graft must be oriented properly to avoid misalignment during implantation. In addition, although it is preferable to leave the vein too long rather than too short, it should not be so long as to bend into an acute angle at any point. Such acute bends or kinks are certain to result in graft thrombosis. Excision of the aortic wall is not necessary because intraluminal aortic pressure spreads the edge of a linear aortotomy. In addition, localized endarterectomy should not be performed because intimal plaque fragments may dislodge and embolize to the lower extremities on removal of the clamp.

Splenorenal Artery Bypass

Careful oblique and lateral angiography of the celiac axis preoperatively is essential to establish the patency of this artery when splenorenal artery bypass is entertained. Whereas most reconstructive surgical procedures of the renal artery are accomplished transperitoneally, we prefer a retroperitoneal flank approach for left-sided repairs. Complications specific to this technique are predictable by proximity. Pancreatitis and pancreatic pseudocyst may be prevented by delicate handling of the pancreas because several small pancreatic branches must be ligated and divided from the splenic artery.

Splenectomy is a possible complication of this technique, usually in response to inadvertent splenic laceration. As routine practice, removal of the spleen is not necessary because the spleen continues to receive adequate collateral blood flow from the short gastric arteries. Inadequate length of splenic artery is occasionally encountered and can be overcome with a saphenous vein interposition graft. This maneuver enables tension-free anastomotic bypass.

Hepatorenal Artery Bypass

The same admonition to image the celiac axis as a prerequisite applies similarly here. Careful dissection of the porta hepatis is essential to avoid common bile duct injury. When the right hepatic artery has an anomalous origin and is used for an inflow source, concomitant cholecystectomy is routinely performed. Failure to do so may result in gangrenous cholecystitis.

Percutaneous Transluminal Renal Artery Angioplasty With or Without Stenting

Since its introduction in 1964, PTRA has been used widely to treat patients with renovascular hypertension and ischemic nephropathy secondary to renal artery stenosis. Nonostial unilateral lesions and those secondary to medial fibroplasia without branch involvement are most amenable to treatment with PTRA. Ramsay and Waller[37] reviewed the literature including 691 PTRA procedures, in which 9.1% of patients experienced complications, including 3 fatalities (cholesterol embolism, bowel infarction, cerebral hemorrhage). Puncture-related complications not inherent to PTRA but inclusive of all endovascular interventional procedures are of course possible, including femoral artery puncture site bleeding, arteriovenous fistula, groin hematoma, and retroperitoneal hematoma. Arterial complications include renal artery dissection, thrombosis or occlusion, segmental infarction, and hematoma. Renal artery perforation is a rare complication requiring emergency surgical exploration.

Endoluminal stents provide better results than does angioplasty alone,[21] particularly for ostial lesions. Complications include those of PTRA listed earlier with the addition of stent restenosis, thrombosis, and technical failure. Technical factors listed by Lederman and colleagues[21] that promote decreased complication rates include use of soft guidewires, careful device sizing using quantitative angiography, low-pressure predilation before stent deployment, stent deployment with the guiding catheter as a delivery sheath, and high-pressure stent postdilation. Nevertheless, rates of restenosis after PTRA with stent for atherosclerotic renal artery stenosis range from 13% to 65%.[38] In general, published results of PTRA with or without stenting in atherosclerotic disease do not report functional improvement comparable to that seen after primary surgical repair.

The lack of correlation between immediate angiographic technical success and durable outcome from the standpoint of blood pressure or renal function may relate to atheroemboli. Hiramoto and colleagues[39] elegantly performed ex vivo angioplasty and stenting on endarterectomy specimens fitted into PTFE and showed that thousands of microscopic atheromatous fragments are released. Unlike contrast nephropathy, an acute event that resolves within 2 to 3 weeks, these atheroemboli may contribute to a slow decline in renal function as they occlude afferent arterioles. Whereas these purely experimental results may not mimic the in vivo situation, they are intriguing.

SPECIAL CONSIDERATIONS

Pediatric Population

Renovascular disease is a significant cause of hypertension in children, and it comprises 10% of pediatric referrals for hypertension evaluation.[40] In contrast to the adult population, arterial dysplasia accounts for most cases. Although rare, special postsurgical late complications from growth spurts have been reported, one in which an autologous graft avulsed from the aorta requiring emergency reoperation. Pursestring suture contracture is also possible with arterial growth, and interrupted sutures may be preferable.

Stanley and colleagues[41] reviewed their experience in 57 children with renovascular hypertension over a 30-year period and highlighted several notable differences in complications seen with childhood renovascular surgery. In this population, autogenous internal iliac artery grafts are favored over vein grafts for bypass.

Aneurysmal dilation of vein grafts is clearly more common in children (≤20%), attributed to differences in the intrinsic blood supply in the wall that predispose these patients to mural ischemia. Another important difference between the adult and pediatric population relates to aortic reimplantation, a procedure often avoided in adults because of early thrombosis. In children, reimplantation is a more durable means of revascularization. Splenorenal bypass is to be avoided because the celiac artery fails to grow in some children, with resulting functionally significant stenosis with advancing age.

Stanley and colleagues[41] also downplayed the role of percutaneous renal angioplasty (PRA) and explained that neither proximal ostial lesions nor more distal segmental stenoses are well managed. In children, narrowings may represent true hypoplasia, and PTA would result in vascular disruption. In these cases, operative repair is more appropriate.

Laparoscopic or Robotic Surgery

Case reports of minimally invasive approaches to renovascular surgery are sporadic. Laparoscopic aortorenal bypass was performed successfully in a porcine model.[42] In humans, both laparoscopic and robotic-assisted repairs of renal artery aneurysms have been reported.[43,44] Of course, potential complications of these approaches include all the complications associated with the minimally invasive surgical milieu. The reader is referred to Chapters 29 and 32.

Transplant Renal Artery Stenosis

PTRA should be the initial treatment of choice for transplant renal artery stenosis. Lohr and colleagues[45] reviewed the literature on this subject. Of 90 patients undergoing PTRA for this indication, graft loss occurred in only 1 patient, and recurrent stenosis in 2. Vascular surgical repair, however, was associated with an 11% rate of graft loss and a 6% restenosis rate.

Surgery After Failed Percutaneous Transluminal Renal Angioplasty

This category is increasingly relevant to urologists. Wong and colleagues[38] reviewed their experience of 51 patients undergoing surgical management for failed PTRA. The surgeon must be aware that PTRA will generate emergency cases, as in this series in which operation was required in 4 patients for acute thrombosis, renal artery rupture, and infected pseudoaneurysm. In the long term, failed PTRA was associated with either emergency repair or nephrectomy in 16% of patients in the foregoing series. In addition, the success of operative repair depends on the underlying cause. In general, revascularization for failed PTRA was more beneficial to blood pressure with underlying fibromuscular dysplasia as opposed to atherosclerosis. In these patients, surgery is generally associated with more extensive renal artery exposure and complex operative management as a result of perivascular fibrosis and inflammation.

The presence of stents is also important. In the foregoing series, three patients had endoluminal stents, which the investigators correctly pointed out excluded thromboendarterectomy and reimplantation as options. Landing sites for bypass may also be compromised.

Surgery for Renal Artery Aneurysms

For this rare entity, surgical repair is subject to the overall list of complications already discussed. Investigators from Dusseldorf, Germany[46] reported their extensive experience with operative reconstruction of renal artery aneurysms in 94 patients. Mortality rates are generally low, and in this series no mortality occurred in elective (nonruptured) cases. The overall morbidity rate was 17%, including transient dialysis in 3 patients, bleeding in 3, and graft occlusion in 1. Long-term patency was 83% at 4 years.

Surgery for Renal Artery Dissection

In this acute process, surgical results are generally poor, with renal loss the most common complication. In a report by Muller and colleagues,[47] surgical revascularization was aggressively pursued, favoring resection with vein interposition graft in 25 of 28 reported patients. Early complications occurred in 5 patients (20%), including thrombosis and bleeding. Even with this aggressive approach in which primary nephrectomy was not performed, 8 of 25 (32%) of kidneys were lost on late follow-up. Only 38% benefited permanently from revascularization.

Perhaps the most relevant aspect of these cases with regard to complications of surgical intervention is strict adherence to rational surgical indication. In general, consideration of a combination of aneurysm size and associated symptoms is appropriate. English and associates[48] reported on their experience in their series of 62 aneurysm repairs. Most investigators would agree that whereas the risk of rupture is theoretical in most patients, women of childbearing age should certainly be considered for prophylactic repair. Patients with aneurysms of significant size (exact cutoff debated, 2.0 cm accepted), associated hypertension, or embolism are also candidates for repair. In the series reported by English and colleagues[48] and using such selection criteria, rates of morbidity and mortality were low and acceptable at 1.6% and 12%, respectively.

KEY POINTS

1. Fewer patients with renal artery stenosis are surgical candidates, with interventional radiology procedures accounting for the majority of treatments.
2. Careful patient selection in remaining cases is the key to avoiding complications.
3. In this population, coexistent global vascular disease often exists, and cardiovascular complications dominate. Coronary and carotid circulations require attentive preoperative evaluation.
4. Renal artery thrombosis is the most common complication of renal vascular reconstruction.
5. Achieving a wide, flawless anastomosis is the most important factor responsible for long-term patency of surgical revascularization.

REFERENCES

Please see www.expertconsult.com

Chapter 36

COMPLICATIONS OF RENAL STONE SURGERY

Bruce I. Carlin MD
Former Assistant Professor of Urology, Washington University School of Medicine, St. Louis, Missouri

Michael Paik MD
Urologist, Private Practice, Northwest Community Hospital, Arlington Heights, Illinois

Donald R. Bodner MD
Professor and Interim Chair, Department of Urology, Case Western Reserve University School of Medicine, Cleveland, Ohio

Martin I. Resnick MD
Former Chair, Department of Urology, Case Western Reserve University School of Medicine, Cleveland, Ohio

Most complex renal stones are treated with minimally invasive or noninvasive measures. Percutaneous nephrolithotomy, retrograde ureteroscopy, and extracorporeal shock wave lithotripsy (ESWL) have almost eliminated the need for open renal stone surgery. Although the role of open renal stone surgery is not as prominent as it once was, urologists must maintain proficiency and knowledge of a variety of open renal techniques. Many complete staghorn calculi associated with intrarenal scarring or infundibular and caliceal stenosis are still treated with open renal techniques, especially if intrarenal reconstruction of the collecting system is required.

We reviewed our experience with open renal stone surgery. From 1991 to 1995, 780 stone procedures were performed at the Case Western Reserve School of Medicine Affiliated Hospitals in Cleveland, Ohio, including 42 open stone cases (5.4%). The distribution of our procedures is listed in Table 36-1.

The clinical urologist must be adept not only in the performance of these procedures but also in appropriate preoperative and postoperative management of patients. Of our 42 patients who underwent open stone procedures, 5 (12%) of our patients experienced complications. Three occurred in patients who underwent anatrophic nephrolithotomy. One patient sustained a pneumothorax, another developed postoperative pneumonia, and a third experienced bladder outlet obstruction secondary to clot retention. One patient who underwent pyelolithotomy developed *Clostridium difficile* colitis. Finally, a patient who underwent pyelolithotomy and ureterolithotomy developed a retained large stone fragment that caused ureteral obstruction and sepsis. This patient was managed initially with percutaneous nephrostomy tube placement followed by ureteroscopy and ESWL.

The complications that occur secondary to open renal surgery are directly related to the particular procedure. The goals of any procedure for stone removal—open, minimally invasive, or noninvasive—are to remove all stone fragments and to preserve maximal renal function. In this chapter, we review the techniques of the various open renal stone procedures and discuss their specific complications.

HISTORY OF OPEN RENAL SURGERY

Hippocrates is credited with performing the first operation on the kidney. In his time, it was common practice to drain renal and perirenal abscesses; on occasion, the collecting system of the kidney was entered and the stone was extruded either at the time of surgery or during the postoperative period. Celsus, Galen, and other early physicians mentioned kidney stones in their writings, but none believed extraction to be safe or feasible. In 1501, Cardan of Milan described removing 18 stones when a renal abscess was drained. Hevin,[1] in 1778, is credited with first using the term *nephrolithotomy*.

European surgeons, in the 1700s and early 1800s, limited use of nephrotomies to obstructed, infected kidneys; if the stone could not be readily removed, it was left to pass through the fistulous tract. Before the late 1800s, nephrolithotomy remained an imprecise

TABLE 36-1	Management of Renal Stones at Case Western Reserve School of Medicine From 1991 to 1995	
Type of Operation (n)		**Percentage of Total (%)**
Extracorporeal shock wave lithotripsy		68
Retrograde ureteroscopy		22
Percutaneous nephrolithotomy		5
Open cases (42):		5
Pyelolithotomy (15)		
Simple pyelolithotomy (5)		
Extended pyelolithotomy (7)		
Pyelolithotomy with pyeloplasty (3)		
Anatrophic nephrolithotomy (14)		
Ureterolithotomy (7)		
Radial nephrolithotomy (6)		

operation usually performed inadvertently in association with drainage of renal and perirenal abscesses. Intrarenal hemorrhage was a major problem when the procedure was specifically performed for removal of intrarenal stones because knowledge of intrarenal anatomy was limited. The gradual evolution of modern nephrolithotomy in the 1960s closely followed research on intrarenal anatomy, physiology, renal preservation, and perioperative techniques.

Dr. William Ingalls[2] is credited with performing the first deliberate nephrolithotomy in the United States at the Boston City Hospital in 1872 in a patient whose perinephric abscess he had previously drained. In 1880, Henry Morris,[3] an English surgeon, performed the first nephrolithotomy on an apparently healthy kidney with no associated abscess. He subsequently described his initial experience with 34 nephrolithotomies with 33 recoveries and 1 death. His results established that nephrolithotomy is a safe surgical procedure and refuted the previous teachings that renal stones should be removed only from an abscess cavity.[4]

Surgeons practicing in the early 1900s had an excellent understanding of gross renal anatomy, but it was not until the studies of Jozsef Hyrtl,[5] a 19th-century Viennese anatomist, that the intrarenal vasculature was defined. He described a relatively avascular plane between the anterior and posterior segments of the renal artery. "The Intrinsic Blood Vessels of the Kidney and Their Significance in Nephrotomy" was then published in the *Bulletin of the Johns Hopkins Hospital* by Max Brödel,[6] a medical artist at the Johns Hopkins Medical School. In this classic report, Brödel accurately described the branching of the main renal artery and its lack of free anastomosis between segmental branches. The relatively avascular plane between the anterior and poste-

rior arterial segments, known as *Brödel's white line*, was also noted.

Cullen and Derge,[7] in 1909, suggested that the nephrotomy incision be made with a thin silver wire passed between arterial branches from within outward. These investigators recommended an L-shaped nephrotomy incision to avoid ischemic infarction of the papillary tips. In the late 1920s, after studying the effect on the kidney of different incisions, Deming[8,9] concluded that the best nephrotomy incision was longitudinal through the avascular plane described by Hyrtl and Brödel. Smith and Boyce[10] then combined this incision with intrarenal reconstruction of the collecting system to remove staghorn calculi and improve renal drainage.

Improvements in intraoperative stone localization with radiography and the use of hypothermia to preserve renal function deserve special mention. Robson[11] was the first to suggest the use of intraoperative radiographs to localize renal stones. Refinements in radiography and the development of ultrasonography (US) helped to diagnose renal stones more accurately not only preoperatively but also intraoperatively. Subsequently, the use of intraoperative radiographs and US, along with direct palpation and needles for localization, helped to define the exact location of the stone further.

A significant advance in open renal surgery occurred when investigators learned that the adverse effects of ischemia could be prevented by hypothermia. It was known as early as 1880 that ischemia resulted in kidney damage. Litten[12] noted histologic damage to the epithelium of the proximal tubule when the kidney was made ischemic. Other investigators[13-15] also noted ischemic changes when the total clamp time was 30 minutes, and they found that these changes were reversible only when the time elapsed was <1 hour.

Renal cooling reduces cellular metabolic activity and consequently protects the proximal tubule from ischemic damage. The optimal temperature to which the kidney must be cooled is controversial, but temperatures of 15°C to 20°C appear to be most effective. Numerous methods are available to cool the kidney, and little practical difference appears to exist among them.[16-22] Hypothermia, by whatever method, is an important adjunct to open renal surgery and should be considered when the renal artery is clamped for any prolonged period of time.

RENAL ANATOMY

To understand the principles of open renal surgery better, the intrarenal arterial anatomy and associated collecting structures are first reviewed. In 70% to 80% of kidneys, the main renal artery branches in the distal third of the vessel before it enters the renal hilum into the anterior and posterior segmental arteries, each of which is an end artery with no collateral circulation

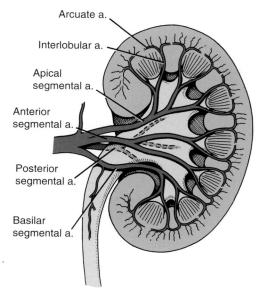

Figure 36-1   Anatomy of the renal artery.

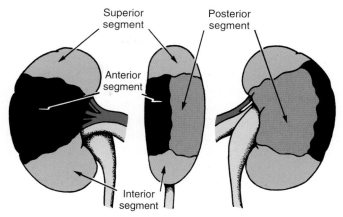

Figure 36-2   Vascular segments as determined by distribution of the renal artery.

(**Fig. 36-1**). Further branching continues in an orderly manner, with 8 to 12 interlobar arteries coursing along opposite sides of the infundibulum toward the papilla. The interlobar arteries then branch into the transmedullary arteries, which form near the renal parenchyma and enter at the caliceal cup. They are paired and pass into the medulla through the interpapillary spaces to reach the cortex, and some continue as the arcuate arteries.

The kidney is divided into four surgical segments by division of the renal artery: superior, inferior, anterior, and posterior segments (**Fig. 36-2**). In approximately 50% of patients, the first division of the main renal artery is the posterior segment, which supplies the posterior portion of the kidney; however, in one third of patients, the first branch supplies the inferior pole. The posterior branch continues without division to supply the posterior segment of the kidney. The anterior segmental artery is the larger division and divides into three or four branches because it is the continuation of the main renal artery. The anterior division typically supplies the superior, inferior, and anterior segments. The artery to the inferior segment enters the renal hilum, descends obliquely to its lower border, and then crosses the renal pelvis and divides into the anterior and posterior divisions.

The exact number and distribution of the calices constitute the most variable components of renal anatomy. The ureter generally is a direct continuation of the renal pelvis. In most kidneys, the pelvis divides within the substance of the kidney into two or three main sections known as *infundibula,* or *major calices.* These structures divide into secondary or tertiary sections known as the *minor calices.* The calices are well-defined units that can be simple and drain a single

papilla or can be complex and drain multiple papillae. The total number of calices averages 8 but ranges from 4 to 12. Polar calices are the most variable and are frequently complex, the superior division often being the most complex. The remainder of the calices are paired anteriorly and posteriorly along an imaginary line that divides the kidney longitudinally. The anterior calices are irregularly arranged at an angle 70 to 75 degrees from the frontal plane, whereas the posterior calices are more regularly arranged at a 20-degree angle from the frontal plane.

PREOPERATIVE CONSIDERATIONS

Approximately 15% to 20% of all urinary calculi are struvite or "infection" stones. They occur more frequently in females than in males (2:1) and often form a staghorn or branched configuration in the kidney. Infection stones occur most frequently in patients with neurogenic bladders and recurrent urinary tract infections (UTIs) as well as in patients with long-term indwelling catheters and external urinary diversions. Typically, the infections associated with struvite stone formation are caused by urease-producing bacteria, which include *Proteus mirabilis, Providencia, Klebsiella,* and occasionally, *Pseudomonas.* Strains of *Pseudomonas* appear to be the most difficult to eradicate and are consequently associated with the highest incidence of stone recurrence.[23] *Escherichia coli* is not a urea splitter, and infections associated with *E. coli* should be suspected of being superinfections and not associated with the formation or growth of the stone.

All UTIs must be treated adequately before open renal surgery to prevent the postoperative complications of sepsis, abscess formation, and wound infection. It is often difficult to eliminate the bacteria totally in the presence of an infection stone, in an infundibular or intracaliceal scar, or in a kidney with areas of patchy pyelonephritis.[24] The presence of retained bacteria is likely in these kidneys despite negative results of bladder urine cultures.

Preoperative infections should be treated for a minimum of 24 to 48 hours with an appropriate antibiotic, the selection of which is based on results of in vitro culture and sensitivity studies. Aminoglycosides and other nephrotoxic agents should be reserved for patients with resistant infections with tested sensitivities. It is advisable to repeat urine cultures once the antibiotics have been discontinued to ensure that the infection is completely resolved. At the time of operation, cultures of any mucinous material in an obstructed calix and of stone fragments removed from the kidney should be obtained. These cultures are helpful in the selection of postoperative antibiotics, because the bacteriologic features of the stone may differ greatly from the preoperative urine cultures.[25] The exact duration of postoperative antibiotics is controversial, but a 2- to 4-week course of antibiotic suppression is usually reasonable. Urine cultures should be repeated after the antibiotics have been discontinued.

If the infection stone is removed completely during the surgical procedure, if urine cultures are monitored closely postoperatively, and if all recurrent infections are promptly treated, the risk of recurrent stone formation can be markedly diminished.[26] The main cause of recurrent stone formation is the presence of residual stone fragments left at the time of surgery. It is well recognized that systemic antibiotics sterilize only the surface of the stone and bacteria remain harbored deep within the interstices.[27] Removing all the stone fragments therefore is most important.

INTRAOPERATIVE AND POSTOPERATIVE COMPLICATIONS

Pulmonary Dysfunction

Pulmonary dysfunction is the most common complication and it occurs in 5% to 10% of all patients undergoing open renal surgery.[27] Birch and Mims[16] reviewed their experience with patients undergoing anatrophic nephrolithotomy and found a 37% incidence of pulmonary complications, especially atelectasis. The lateral, or flank, position is most frequently used to enter the kidney, especially when hypothermia is considered.

A substantial incidence of pulmonary complications occurs with this approach. The patient is positioned in such a way that lateral flexion on the table and additional use of the kidney rest will maximally separate the iliac crest from the costal margin. The patient's head is in the Trendelenburg position, and the feet are down. This position creates such stress on the respiratory and skeletal systems that most unanesthetized patients cannot tolerate it. A 14.5% decrease in vital capacity in the unanesthetized patient and a 14% decrease in the tidal volume in the anesthetized patient have been reported when this position has been used.[28,29] These reductions in respiratory capacity are the result of direct restriction of the chest wall in all directions, with excursion most limited laterally.[30]

Concern has been expressed that the downward lung may be at increased risk for pulmonary complications secondary to venous congestion and the inability to expand fully; however, clinical experience has shown that these complications occur with equal frequency in both lung fields.[16] Postoperative pulmonary problems also are complicated by the position of the patient's wound. Deep breathing and coughing are extremely important but painful. Pulmonary physical therapy and incentive spirometry should be instituted in the postoperative period. Ultrasonic aerosols may also help, but whether they should be used routinely is debatable. Early ambulation is of great importance to minimize postoperative complications.

Pneumothorax

Pneumothorax occurs in <5% of patients undergoing open surgical removal of renal stones. Patients with a history of prior renal surgery or pyelonephritis are at increased risk for developing a pneumothorax. These patients often have adherence of the upper pole of the kidney to the diaphragm and the attached pleura, thus making inadvertent entry into the chest more common. Because of the attachment of the pleura to the ribs, pleural injury is also more frequent when the 11th or 12th interspace is used for the incision than when a 12th rib or subcostal incision is used.

When a small pleural entry is recognized, it can be closed with a running or pursestring chromic suture. The anesthesiologist is instructed to inflate the lung fully before completing closure of the pleura to ensure that no air remains. If concern exists that the pleural incision is not adequately closed, use of a small chest tube is appropriate. The tube can be removed 48 hours postoperatively. A portable chest radiograph should be obtained in the recovery room if pleural repair has been performed or if pneumothorax is suspected. If pneumothorax is confirmed on this film, a chest tube should be considered and follow-up chest radiographs are essential.

Pulmonary Emboli

Pulmonary emboli can occur after any surgical procedure, and specific techniques to prevent them are controversial. Early ambulation is important, and perhaps thigh-high elastic stockings or sequential venous compression stockings should be considered in the high-risk patient. Boyce[31] reported 3 fatal (0.3%) and 9 nonfatal (0.9%) pulmonary emboli in his series of 951 patients undergoing anatrophic nephrolithotomy, for a total incidence slightly higher than 1%.

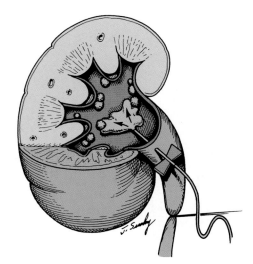

Figure 36-3 In coagulum pyelolithotomy, the ureter is occluded and the coagulum injected.

TABLE 36-2	Anatrophic Nephrolithotomy From 1963 to 1982: Mortality*	
Cause of Death		**No. Patients**
Myocardial infarction		1
Pulmonary embolus		3

*Mortality = 0.42% in <3 months.
Modified from Boyce WH. Surgery of urinary calculi in perspective. *Urol Clin North Am.* 1983;10:585-594.

A fatal pulmonary embolism was also reported in association with coagulum pyelolithotomy (**Fig. 36-3**).[32] Figure 36-3 illustrates a coagulum pyelolithotomy in which a mixture of thrombin, calcium chloride, and cryoprecipitate is injected into the renal pelvis to form a coagulum to remove all the stones. It is believed in this instance that the embolus occurred secondary to over-filling of the renal pelvis and subsequent pyelovenous backflow with intravascular leakage of the coagulum.

Cardiovascular Complications

In addition to pulmonary complications from open renal surgical procedures, cardiovascular changes should be considered. In the flank position, decreased venous return is the rule and hypotension may be encountered. It is important to add flexion and raise the kidney rest gradually while continually monitoring blood pressure. Mediastinal shifting and displacement of the liver have been implicated in the hypotension, and the use of elastic stockings may improve venous return.[33] In his series of 951 patients undergoing anatrophic nephrolithotomy, Boyce[31] reported 1 myocardial infarction for an incidence of slightly higher than 0.1% and accounting for 1 death (Table 36-2).

Hemorrhage

Significant postoperative renal hemorrhage occurs in <10% of open renal surgical procedures.[34] A urologist's ability to operate on the kidney with minimal blood loss and preservation of renal function is directly related to his or her knowledge of the intrarenal arterial anatomy and the various vascular segments (see Figs. 36-1 and 36-3). The avascular plane between the anterior and posterior branches of the renal artery must be identified to make intersegmental nephrostomy inci-

sions without causing massive hemorrhage. The kidney should be completely mobilized and the main renal artery fully dissected. The posterior segment is clamped, and methylene blue injected intravenously if anatrophic nephrolithotomy is considered. The avascular plane can be easily differentiated from Brödel's white line (**Fig. 36-4**).

To minimize hemorrhage during the procedure, the kidney can be cooled and the renal artery clamped. Precise closure of the collecting system with repair of the intrarenal vessels and careful closure of the renal capsule minimize subsequent postoperative hemorrhage. When postoperative bleeding is encountered, it is frequently intrapelvic and occurs spontaneously 1 to 2 weeks after the procedure. The bleeding often results from inadequately closed intrarenal vessels, and expectant treatment is usually sufficient. Blood transfusions, intravenous fluids, and bed rest often stabilize the patient.

The administration of aminocaproic acid (Amicar) may also be of benefit when hemorrhage does not immediately subside.[35] Aminocaproic acid is an antifibrinolytic agent and is helpful because of the high levels of urokinase in the urinary system. It is administered intravenously for approximately 24 hours, and the bleeding is often controlled within the first day. Aminocaproic acid can be continued orally and gradually discontinued.

If bleeding persists and hypotension develops despite conservative management, arteriography should be performed to identify open vessels and the presence of arteriovenous shunts. When recognized, bleeding and hypotension should be treated with embolization by an experienced angiographer. Exploration with direct repair is required only when all other measures fail. Boyce[31] reported an average blood loss of 778 mL and considered it excessive when the blood loss was >1000 mL (Table 36-3). He reported hemorrhage by this definition in 6.8% of his patients undergoing anatrophic nephrolithotomy.

Complications Associated With Vascular Manipulation

When extensive nephrotomies are required, it is often advantageous to clamp the main renal artery. This helps

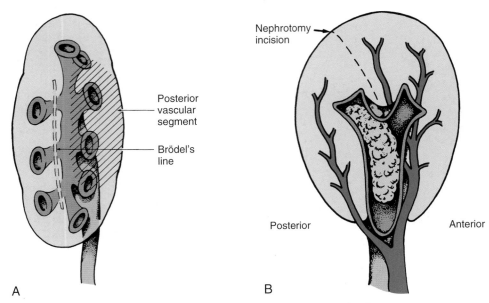

Figure 36-4 **A** and **B,** The nephrotomy incision will be made after the avascular plane is defined.

TABLE 36-3	Anatrophic Nephrolithotomy From 1963 to 1982: Morbidity (Complications With Recovery In 951 Patients)
Cause of Death	**No. Patients (%)**
Hemorrhage >1000 mL (reoperation, 3 patients)	65 (6.8)
Arteriovenous fistulas reoperated	4 (0.4)
Atelectasis, any degree, by radiograph	232 (24.4)
Pneumothorax	36 (3.8)
Pulmonary embolus	9 (0.9)
All others, including temperature >100°F, gastrointestinal bleeding	153 (16.1)

Modified from Boyce WH. Surgery of urinary calculi in perspective. *Urol Clin North Am.* 1983;10:585-594.

not only in reducing intraoperative blood loss but also in diminishing kidney turgor, to permit easier localization of stone fragments and entry into the collecting system. Clamps can damage the vessel to which they are applied; therefore, atraumatic clamps should be used and placed meticulously. Care should be exercised in dissection of the renal artery before placement of the clamp; to reduce injury to the vessel, the adventitia and small vessels around the artery should be preserved. In Boyce's[31] large series of anatrophic nephrolithotomies, he reported no instance of either acute or delayed injury to the renal artery. Once the vascular clamp is removed, the vessel should be inspected for injury to the renal artery or one of its segments; this injury can be easily recognized, and, if present, it can be repaired.

Renal vein injuries are extremely rare because the renal vein is not clamped during periods of hypother-

mia. It is also important not to clamp the renal vein during the hilar dissection because this can lead to venous thrombosis and subsequent renal infarction.

Once the renal artery is carefully dissected, it is important to be sure that the patient is well hydrated with increased amounts of intravenous fluids and that no hypotensive episodes occur. Mannitol should be administered 5 to 10 minutes before clamping of the renal artery.[36,37] The administration of mannitol is beneficial because it increases renal plasma flow, decreases intrarenal vascular resistance, prevents cellular swelling, and flushes renal tubules of cellular debris. Mannitol also increases the osmolarity of the tubular fluid and thus helps protect the kidney from hypothermic injury during periods of surface cooling. Additionally, mannitol protects the kidney from reperfusion injury by acting as a free radical scavenger and by arresting mitochondrial calcium accumulation.[38]

The kidney can be cooled by a multitude of techniques, all of which are effective in preventing postischemic renal failure.[16-22] Direct surface cooling with ice is as effective as other methods. The kidney is surrounded by a rubber dam, and the main renal artery is occluded. An ice slush is then placed in direct contact with the kidney (**Fig. 36-5**) and is kept in contact with the kidney until the procedure is completed and the vascular clamp is removed. The kidney suffers ischemic injury when the warm ischemia time is >30 minutes.[16-22]

Stone Migration

Migration of the stone during intraoperative manipulation of the kidney with the resultant inability to localize it is a serious problem. When pyelolithotomy is performed, the renal pelvis should be opened directly over

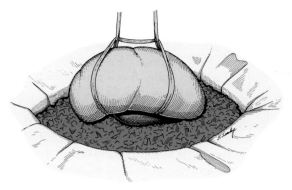

Figure 36-5 An ice slush solution is placed in direct contact with the kidney after the renal artery is first clamped. A rubber dam keeps the ice in contact with the kidney.

TABLE 36-4	Anatrophic Nephrolithotomy From 1963 to 1982
Radiograph	**Final Intraoperative Outcome (%)**
No calculi or calcification	79.5
Papillary calcification	5.0
Parenchymal calcification	15.5

Modified from Boyce WH. Surgery of urinary calculi in perspective. *Urol Clin North Am.* 1983;10:585.

the stone after the ureter distal to the stone is secured with a vascular loop. The incision should be made in a transverse direction as far away from the ureteropelvic junction as possible. An incision at this location is least likely to tear into the ureteropelvic junction. Extension is also possible along each calix, when needed. Securing the ureter distal to the stone prevents the stone from passing into the ureter. If, however, this occurs and is not recognized, it can cause acute urinary obstruction resulting in postoperative flank pain and urosepsis. These complications necessitate the performance of an emergency secondary procedure: either the placement of a percutaneous nephrostomy or the passage of a ureteral stent. When anatrophic nephrolithotomy is performed, a double-J ureteral stent should be passed down the ureter from the renal pelvis into the bladder because it protects the kidney from obstruction secondary to passage of small stone fragments. The stent can be removed cystoscopically on the seventh postoperative day.

For branched calculi that are difficult to remove with simple pyelolithotomy, extended pyelolithotomy should be considered. The renal pelvis is dissected free of peripelvic fat, and the posterior edge of the renal sinus is completely exposed. A pyeloinfundibular incision is made to conform with the location of the calculi, and the stone is then delivered.

Radial nephrotomy is also of benefit in removing renal stones. Following clamping of the main renal artery and application of hypothermia, parenchymal incisions can be made that parallel the course of the intrarenal vessels. This approach prevents transection of these vessels, lessens bleeding, and minimizes parenchymal destruction. Stone localization is facilitated by intraoperative radiographs obtained before making the incision. Whenever possible, radial nephrotomies should be made on the posterior convexity of the kidney to avoid large venous branches on the anterior surface of the kidney.

Retained Stone Fragments

Retained stones represent a major concern in terms of a nidus for further calculus formation and are reported to have an incidence of 5% to 30% (Table 36-4).[30,39-41] This complication is less problematic than in the past; the availability of less invasive measures such as ESWL and percutaneous procedures can be employed to remove small residual stone fragments. Residual stone fragments are probably of less concern for calcium oxalate, cystine, and uric acid stones than for struvite stones. Struvite stones grow faster than do the other types of stones in the presence of an associated UTI.[42] Sleight and Wickham[43] reported that 70% of retained infected stones increased in size as compared with 30% of stones without infection.

Intersegmental nephrotomy is indicated for full staghorn calculi and branched calculi with infundibular stenosis. This technique provides maximal exposure to the renal collecting system. Before making the nephrotomy incision, intraoperative radiographs should be obtained to define the extent of the stone (**Fig. 36-6**). Once the bulk is removed, further films are obtained to help localize the fragments, and final films should confirm the absence of residual fragments. If stone fragments cannot be localized, intraoperative nephroscopy may be helpful. Intraoperative US can also be employed to localize remaining fragments 2 to 3 mm in diameter.[44] US offers a distinct advantage in identifying radiolucent calculi and also in quantitating the depth and angle of the stone from the surface of the kidney. For this imaging modality, personnel must be trained in the use of this technique.

Hypertension

The potential of developing or aggravating preexisting hypertension would seem to be a concern with any surgical procedure that involves the kidney. This complication, however, appears to be unusual. Boyce and Elkins[39] reviewed 100 patients with nephrolithotomy and noted that only 2 became mildly hypertensive postoperatively. Both these patients were managed with low doses of antihypertensive medications and did well. Whether the hypertension was directly related to the

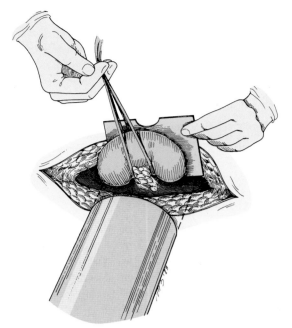

Figure 36-6 Sterilized radiographic films can be placed in direct contact with the kidney and can accurately assess residual fragments.

surgical procedure or was a natural occurrence was unclear. By careful dissection of the renal artery, accurate mapping of the avascular plane, and use of hypothermia, ischemic injuries to the kidney can be minimized.

Decreased Renal Function

Despite following all the techniques to preserve renal function as previously described, trauma to the renal parenchyma can still occur, and some patients demonstrate diminished renal function postoperatively. Boyce and Elkins[39] noted that of 100 patients undergoing nephrolithotomy, only 2 showed a decrease in renal function postoperatively and 1 of the patients required a nephrectomy. Experience with anatrophic nephrolithotomy in patients with a solitary kidney also revealed that the average preoperative renal function equals postoperative function. Although diminution in function was noted in some patients, marked improvement was noted in others. In the patients who improved, relief of obstruction and resolution of infection associated with stone removal likely contributed to the result.[45,46] The general principles of careful dissection of the renal artery, atraumatic clamping of the renal artery, use of methylene blue to help identify the avascular plane between the anterior and posterior renal segments, and use of hypothermia enable one to emulate the excellent results reported by Boyce and Elkins.

Stone Recurrence

After the eradication of all stone fragments, subsequent stone recurrence is a potential problem for all patients. The stone recurrence rate has been reported to be between 20% and 30% over 6 to 10 years.[47,48] Russell and colleagues[48] noted that the recurrence rate was only 9% in female patients but was 43% in male patients. Better control of UTIs, particularly those caused by the *Pseudomonas* strains, is helpful in lowering the recurrent stone rate. Appropriate use of suppressive antibiotics in patients with recurrent UTIs may also be of benefit in reducing recurrent infections. Acetohydroxamic acid, a urease inhibitor, may also help to slow the rate of infection stone enlargement and recurrence.

Probably the most important aspect of reducing the recurrence rate relates to identifying and treating metabolic problems as they predispose to stone formation. In Boyce's experience,[31] many of the patients who developed recurrent stones had unrecognized metabolic problems, and with a better understanding of the pathogenesis of the disease as exists now, this recurrence rate should be markedly reduced.

Chemolysis

Because a retained stone fragment can be a nidus for further infection stone formation, every effort should be made to remove all stone fragments at the time of the surgical procedure. However, when this goal is impossible, a nephrostomy tube and a ureteral stent can be left in place.

Approximately 5 to 7 days into the postoperative period, direct irrigation with hemiacidrin (Renacidin Irrigation) is started. Hemiacidrin is a 10% solution of citric acid, D-gluconic acid, magnesium acid citrate, calcium carbonate, and water at a pH of 4. Because struvite stones are soluble in acid, 73% to 100% of struvite stones can be effectively dissolved with this approach.[49-52] When irrigation is performed with hemiacidrin, the urine must first be sterile, and during irrigation, the intrapelvic pressure must be maintained at <20 to 25 cm H_2O.[50] A manometer with a pop-off valve is required to prevent introduction of the agent at a high pressure. Because the solution contains large amounts of magnesium, hypermagnesemia may result if the intrapelvic pressure is high; therefore, serial magnesium levels must be obtained. When the urine is sterile, irrigation is begun with sterile saline solution for 24 to 48 hours. The rate of the hemiacidrin irrigation can then slowly be increased but should not exceed 120 mL per hour.

The intact nature of the collecting system free of extravasation should be established by nephrostogram before the irrigation is begun. The treatment should be discontinued if the patient experiences severe flank pain or fever or if results of a urine culture become positive during the treatment period.

Urinary Leakage

Pyelocutaneous fistula producing prolonged urinary leakage represents another complication associated with renal surgery. Distal ureteral obstruction, UTI, and the presence of foreign bodies are the main causes of prolonged urinary leakage and generally resolve spontaneously within 2 to 3 weeks of the surgical procedure.

Intervention is rarely required; however, when necessary, placement of an indwelling ureteral stent is suggested, especially following anatrophic nephrolithotomy, procedures requiring extensive dissection of the renal collecting system, or procedures complicated by the presence of infection.

Urinoma formation is a rare complication resulting from premature removal of operative drains. In the presence of UTI, sepsis can result. Placement of a ureteral stent is helpful in managing this problem, and percutaneous or formal drainage may be required.

KEY POINTS

1. In order to understand the principles of open renal surgery, the intrarenal arterial anatomy and associated collecting structures must be understood.
2. All UTIs must be treated adequately before open renal surgery to prevent the postoperative complications of sepsis, abscess formation, and wound infection.
3. Preoperative infections should be treated with appropriate antibiotics for at least 24 to 48 hours before surgery.
4. Pulmonary dysfunction is the most common complication in this type of surgery and occurs in 5% to 10% of patients.
5. Migration of the stone during intraoperative manipulation of the kidney with the resultant inability to localize it is a serious problem.
6. Retained stones represent a major concern because they act as a nidus for further calculus formation. ESWL and percutaneous procedures can be used to remove small residual stone fragments.
7. After the eradication of all stone fragments, subsequent stone recurrence is a potential problem for all patients. Probably the most important aspect of reducing the recurrence rate relates to identifying and treating metabolic problems as they predispose to stone formation.

REFERENCES

Please see www.expertconsult.com

Chapter 37

COMPLICATIONS OF RENAL TRANSPLANTATION

Jeffrey L. Veale MD
Assistant Professor, Department of Urology, David Geffen School of Medicine, University of California–Los Angeles, Los Angeles, California

H. Albin Gritsch MD
Surgical Director, Renal Transplantation, Kidney and Kidney-Pancreas Transplantation Program, Department of Surgery, University of California–Los Angeles Medical Center; Associate Professor of Urology, David Geffen School of Medicine, University of California–Los Angeles, Los Angeles, California

Minor complications can quickly become life-threatening for immunosuppressed patients after renal transplantation. More than 70,000 patients are currently on the national kidney transplantation waiting list, and 520,000 patients are projected to be undergoing dialysis by the year 2010.[1] Thus the demand for kidney transplantation will continue to rise. In 2006, approximately 10,300 deceased donor and 6500 living donor kidney transplants were performed, where 30,000 new patients were added to the waiting list in the United States. Community urologists and general surgeons will increasingly be called on to participate in donor and recipient care. Early recognition of renal transplant complications can prevent serious morbidity and mortality. This chapter focuses on how to prevent and treat the complications of renal transplantation.

BASIC OPERATIVE PROCEDURE

To avoid renal transplant complications, patients should be carefully screened for cardiac disease and severe peripheral vascular disease. However, because the most common causes of end-stage renal disease are diabetes and hypertension, many patients already have these problems. Communication with the anesthesia team to avoid hypotension, hypoxia, and tachycardia will reduce the risk of post-transplant complications.

A retroperitoneal lower abdominal incision is used to expose the iliac vessels. The donor kidney is prepared by removal of the perinephric adipose tissue and ligation of small braches off the renal vessels. The donor kidney is kept ice cold until the time of reperfusion by wrapping a gauze pad with crushed ice saline around it. The renal vein or vena caval extension graft is anastomosed to the external iliac vein and the renal artery is anastomosed to the iliac artery. If possible, a patch of the donor aorta is used to facilitate the arterial anastomosis. Intravenous furosemide and mannitol are administered to reduce ischemia reperfusion injury. The ice pad and the vascular clamps are removed. Once hemostasis is achieved, the graft is carefully positioned to avoid kinking of the vessels. The ureter is passed beneath the spermatic cord and is anastomosed to the bladder mucosa with a stented extravesical approach. A submucosal tunnel is created to prevent reflux.

SURGICAL CHALLENGES

Multiple Vessels

In cadaveric donor transplants, multiple arteries can be kept on a Carrel aortic patch; occasionally when the arteries are far apart, a section of the Carrel patch can be excised and reapproximated. However, when a living donor kidney has multiple arteries, these need to be anastomosed individually to the recipient or to one another so that one accommodating donor artery can be anastomosed to the recipient. If two arteries are approximately the same size, we prefer to use the "pair of pants" technique before anastomosing to the recipient vessel. When the vessels are of different caliber or length, an end-to-side technique may be the most appropriate option. Other options for multiple arteries include (1) using the recipient's inferior epigastric artery in an end-to-end fashion with a donor artery and (2) harvesting the recipient's internal iliac artery and using it to accommodate multiple donor arteries. If the surgeon has exhausted these options, most transplant centers have a bank of vessels from deceased donors that can aid in the vascular reconstruction. In any event, a lower pole branch should always be preserved to avoid ureteral necrosis.

If multiple donor renal veins are available, the largest should be used and the others can be ligated because of internal venous collateralization. If two veins are approximately the same size, they can be sewn together with the "pair of pants" technique or individually anastomosed to the recipient's iliac vein. For right deceased donor kidneys, it is helpful to include the vena cava to extend the venous length.

Perioperative Anticoagulation

Anticoagulation is required for patients with mechanical cardiac valves, atrial fibrillation, and other diseases that increase the risk of venous thrombosis and pulmonary embolus. For patients admitted for deceased donor renal transplantation who are receiving warfarin, the international normalized ratio (INR) should be corrected to <2.0 at the time of the operation. Patients with a history of a coagulopathy or an increased risk of anastomotic thrombosis (peripheral vascular disease or multiple small vessels requiring vascular reconstruction) are anticoagulated with heparin. To limit the risk of postoperative bleeding a small bolus of 1000 U followed by a continuous infusion of 100 U per hour has been successful in preventing graft thrombosis.

Severe Recipient Peripheral Vascular Disease

Even after computed tomography (CT) and magnetic resonance imaging studies, as well as a thorough history and physical examination, a transplant surgeon may discover severe peripheral vascular disease affecting the pelvic vasculature at the time of the surgical procedure. Most calcified vessels have a soft spot along the external or common iliac artery that can accommodate the donor artery. Noncrushing Fogarty shodden vascular clamps can occlude areas with plaque with less risk of intimal injury. In rare cases the artery can be occluded internally with two Fogarty embolectomy catheters, and the balloons are deflated and removed when the assistant throws and ties down the last suture.

Poor Graft Perfusion

On release of the vascular clamps the renal parenchyma should be pink and have appropriate turgor. Arterial signals should be detectable by Doppler probe in the hilar branches of the renal artery and major sections of the parenchyma. With deceased donor allografts, perfusion is frequently patchy but this resolves in approximately 10 minutes. The pulse in the renal artery should be palpably similar to that of the external iliac artery. The allograft must be positioned to avoid kinking of the vessels. If the hilum is positioned medially, the risk of vascular injury during percutaneous biopsy is reduced. Planning the final renal position and determining the best location before vascular anastomosis reduce any

difficulty with graft positioning. Rarely, the graft may need to be placed low in the pelvis or intraperitoneally. This positioning makes renal allograft imaging and biopsy significantly more complicated, and revision of the vascular anastomosis should be considered. Arterial spasm can be relieved by topical or intra-arterial injection of papaverine or verapamil; however, this must be done with caution because of the risk of hypotension and heart block.

Bleeding

Loss of <250 mL of blood is usually possible by careful hemostasis during exposure of the iliac vessels, ligation of small branches off the allograft vessels, and meticulous placement of the anastomotic sutures. Blood loss can be diminished by flushing the donor vessels with heparinized saline solution, following the preparation of the allograft and ligating the sites of extravasation. If blood loss is significant at the time of reperfusion, the vascular clamps should be reapplied and the graft carefully inspected.

Anastomotic bleeding can usually be controlled with fine suture ligatures. If the vessels have torn, it may be necessary to take down the vascular anastomoses and reconstruct the vessels on the back table. For this reason, the nursing staff should be instructed to leave the back table set up until the operation has been completed. In addition, do not infuse Collin's or UW (University of Wisconsin) solution into the transplant renal artery when the allograft is in situ and the venous anastomosis is complete. Otherwise the patient may develop heart block and cardiac arrest because of the high potassium content of these solutions. Oozing from the anastomosis usually stops with gentle pressure and the application of cellulose gauze.

Immunosuppression Toxicity

The immunosuppressive medications used in renal transplantation may exacerbate or induce complications such as malignant disease, infections, diabetes mellitus, hematologic disorders, neurotoxicity, and metabolic disorders. Surgeons involved in the care of renal transplant patients must be aware of these complicating factors because they may impact on the optimum surgical management. Unlike heart or liver transplantation, dialysis provides an alternative renal replacement therapy. If severe complications occur, the recipient's life may need to be saved by discontinuation of immunosuppression.

Cardiovascular Disease

Patients with end-stage renal disease have a substantial risk for cardiovascular disease. Diabetes is the most common disease leading to renal transplantation, and almost all patients with renal failure develop hypertension. Additional cardiovascular risk factors associated with end-stage renal disease include increased extracellular fluid volume, anemia, high plasma levels of homocysteine, and thrombogenic factors. Additionally, uremia may accelerate atherogenesis and proteinuria is associated with hyperlipidemia. Patients who are undergoing dialysis and who are taking calcium salts as phosphate binding agents develop vascular calcifications, which can complicate the technical aspects of the transplant operation.[2] Cardiovascular risk factors are exacerbated by immunosuppression that can cause glucose intolerance (corticosteroids and calcineurin inhibitors) and hyperlipidemia (sirolimus and calcineurin inhibitors). Cardiovascular disease is the leading cause of allograft loss and death after transplantation. Prevention and careful preoperative evaluation rather than treatment are the best ways to avoid cardiovascular complications.

UROLOGIC COMPLICATIONS

Urinary Extravasation

Ischemia of the distal ureter, the most common cause of urinary extravasation, results in leakage at the ureterovesical anastomosis. The allograft ureter receives blood supply solely from the renal artery; therefore, preservation of all the arterial branches (especially lower pole arteries) is essential to ensure viability of the ureter. Careful procurement of kidneys and the practice of leaving the shortest length of ureter that allows for a tension-free ureterovesical anastomosis also help to ensure an adequate blood supply to the distal ureter. A stented Lich-Gregoir ureteroneocystostomy has the lowest incidence of urinary extravasation and other urologic complications.[3,4] It is helpful to distend the bladder with antibiotic solution before ureteral implantation. The bladder mucosa should be mobilized sufficiently to allow the ureter to swell in the antireflux tunnel. The anastomosis can also be tested for leakage by gently refilling the bladder. This brief procedure also ensures that the ureter has been anastomosed to the bladder because anastomosis to an ovarian cyst and thickened folds of peritoneum have been reported.[5]

In general, most cases of urinary extravasation occur soon after transplantation and manifest with allograft tenderness and decreased urinary output. Increasing wound drainage is also a frequent finding. The diagnosis can sometimes be made by ultrasound examination but is confirmed by creatinine analysis of the draining fluid, by nuclear medicine scan, or by cystogram (**Fig. 37-1**). Occasionally, upper urinary tract extravasation from a calyx, the renal pelvis, or ureteral injury is best diagnosed by an antegrade nephrostogram. Small leaks in the bladder may be treated with Foley catheter drainage. Antegrade stent and nephrostomy tube placement may

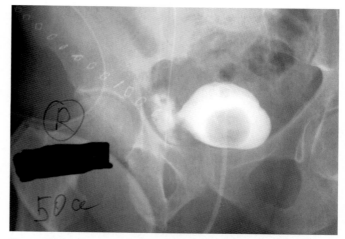

Figure 37-1   Cystogram demonstrating a bladder leak. Note the small-capacity bladder in a patient who was anuric for approximately 10 years.

also provide sufficient drainage to allow closure of a very small leak. If the leak is caused by an ischemic sloughed ureter, endoscopic management merely delays definitive treatment. Therefore, early surgical exploration and repair are usually the best solutions. The type of repair depends on the level of the leak and the vasculature of the tissues. A bladder leak can be closed primarily, with a Foley catheter left in place for ≥1 week and confirmation of closure by repeat cystogram. Ureteral leaks are best treated by resection of the distal ischemic segment and reimplantation into the bladder over a stent. If the length of ureter is inadequate, then cystopyelostomy (sometimes requiring a psoas hitch) and ureteroureterostomy to the recipient's native ureter are both viable options.

Obstruction

Common causes of allograft ureteral obstruction include Foley catheter blockage, blood clots, ureteral edema, ischemic ureteral fibrosis (stricture), kinked ureter or extrinsic compression from a lymphocele, urinoma, and hematoma. Other less common causes of obstruction include stones, prostatic hyperplasia, neurogenic bladder, abscess, rejection (which includes the ureter), and urethral strictures. Obstruction may be painless because of the absence of innervation to the renal allograft. However, obstruction should be suspected in any patient with an unexplained decrease in urine output, enlargement or tenderness of the allograft, and a rising serum creatinine level. Increasing hydronephrosis on ultrasonography is suggestive of obstruction, but this sign is not always present (**Fig. 37-2**). Low-grade dilation of the collecting system in the early postoperative ultrasound scan may occur with vigorous diuresis or edema and resolves. A mercaptotriglycylglycine diuretic renal scan is useful to determine whether physiologic obstruction is present.

Rapid reduction of obstruction can be achieved by placement of a percutaneous nephrostomy tube and antegrade stenting. If obstruction is present, the serum creatinine concentration should decrease following this procedure. Some minor obstructive processes may resolve over time with proximal diversion and stenting. Stones, blood clots, and strictures <2 cm can often be treated endoscopically. More complex obstructions require open repair. Strictures >2 cm require excision and reimplantation of the remaining healthy ureter into the bladder or native ureter as described in the previous discussion of urinary extravasation (**Fig. 37-3**).

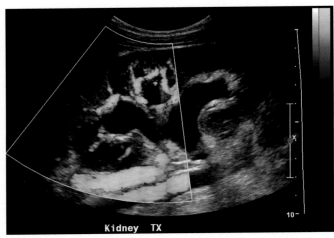

Figure 37-2 Hydronephrosis on renal ultrasound. This image suggests obstruction of the renal allograft. Note the decreased flow to the cortex of the kidney, and the prominent iliac vessels on the power Doppler image.

Extrinsic ureteral obstruction from a lymphocele, hematoma, urinoma can generally be successfully treated with external drainage.

Often obstruction can be avoided. Elderly men who have been anuric while undergoing dialysis may have unnoticed benign prostatic hypertrophy. Following transplantation, this population of patients may benefit from an α-blocker or a 5α-reductase inhibitor. If one clinically suspects a voiding abnormality, a postvoid residual determination should be obtained to detect urinary retention. Transurethral resection of the prostate (TURP) should not be performed unless the recipient has adequate urine output, because a "dry TURP" can lead to bladder neck contracture or urethral strictures. The complications of endoscopic surgery can be reduced by waiting until the renal allograft has recovered and the patient is receiving a reduced dose of immunosuppression.

Reflux

Avoiding reflux into the allograft is theoretically desirable to reduce the pressure effects and pyelonephritis that may lead to impaired graft function. Some investigators have supported this theoretical advantage.[6-8] However, this finding has not been confirmed by others.[9-14] Urinary reflux into the renal allograft is usually identified during evaluation of recurrent urinary tract infections and is usually painless. A detrusor tunnel that is five times the diameter of the ureter should be attempted when possible. Most renal transplant surgeons prefer to use the stented Lich-Gregoir extravesical

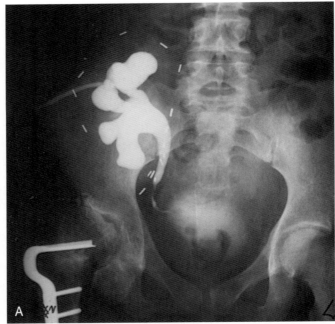
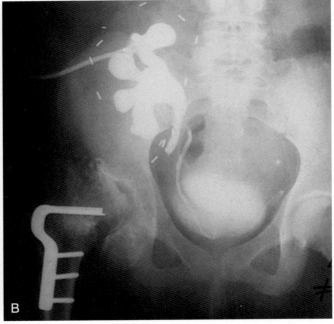

Figure 37-3 **A,** Anterograde nephrostogram of a distal ureteral stricture that manifested with urinary tract infection 11 years after living-related renal transplant. Also note avascular necrosis of the right femoral head, a complication of prolonged high-dose corticosteroids. **B,** Anterograde nephrostogram after urinary reconstruction. *(Courtesy of T. R. Hakala.)*

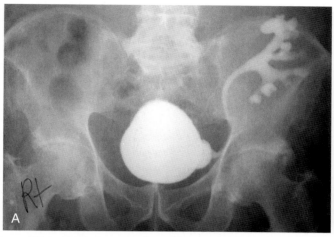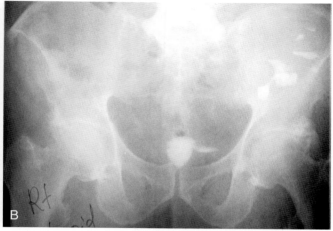

Figure 37-4 Voiding cystourethrogram. **A,** Reflux into the transplanted collecting system, with a diverticulum at the site of the ureteral anastomosis. **B,** Note some retained contrast after voiding.

technique.[15,16] When ureteral length is compromised or when the patient has a nonaccommodating bladder, a refluxing anastomosis is an acceptable option. Recipients who develop recurrent pyelonephritis after transplantation with confirmed reflux on imaging studies (**Fig. 37-4**) should initially be treated with long-term antibiotic prophylaxis. If this approach is not effective, then an endoscopic or open reconstructive procedure may be indicated.

Hematuria

In general, most renal transplant recipients develop some form of hematuria in the early postoperative period. Mild hematuria tends to resolve spontaneously over a couple of days. Moderate hematuria may develop into clots that can block the Foley catheter and occasionally require gentle manual irrigation or continuous bladder irrigation to resolve. If continuous bladder irrigation is not enough to clear the hematuria, then cystoscopy with fulguration is required.

The source of the bleeding is usually the ureteric stump. Vessels of the ureteric stump should be ligated with absorbable suture before creation of the ureteroneocystostomy. Urokinase with its natural anticoagulation properties may be responsible for some persistent hematuria.

VASCULAR COMPLICATIONS

Hematomas

Perioperative bleeding is usually caused by small vessels in the renal hilum that may not have been identified intraoperatively because of vasospasm. Close observation of vital signs and serial hematocrit determinations are necessary in the early postoperative period to detect bleeding. Most small perirenal hematomas are asymp-tomatic, although larger hematomas can produce significant flank pain, lower extremity edema, and venous or ureteral obstruction. Hematomas in the retroperitoneum often tamponade and can be treated conservatively; however, expanding hematomas require exploration.

Massive bleeding may occur with graft rupture or anastomotic leaks. Graft rupture may result from swelling from ischemia reperfusion injury or severe rejection.[17] An intraoperative biopsy specimen of the ruptured allograft should be obtained. If the renal parenchyma appears viable, the graft should be wrapped with polyglactin mesh; if hemostasis can be achieved, allograft nephrectomy may not be necessary.[18] Anastomotic bleeding is rare unless the anastomosis is infected. In this case, allograft nephrectomy is almost always required. If necessary, the iliac artery may be ligated without loss of limb, and the resultant claudication may be relieved by a surgical bypass procedure.[19] During surgical exploration of hematomas, one should resist the temptation to remove blood clots that have dissected into the retroperitoneal fat, unless active bleeding is noted in the area, because it becomes increasingly difficult to achieve hemostasis in this region. Ultrasound examination reliably detects perinephric fluid collections, but CT provides a much better assessment of the extent of blood dissection into adjacent tissues (**Fig. 37-5**).

If one elects to manage the bleeding conservatively, then aspirin and anticoagulant medications should be discontinued if possible. Blood transfusions are administered to maintain a hematocrit of ≥30%. Uremia inhibits platelet function, and most patients undergoing dialysis have abnormal bleeding times.[20] The intravenous administration of 0.3 μg/kg of 1-desamino-8-D-arginine vasopressin (DDAVP) causes the release of factor VIII from endothelial storage sites and may promote coagulation, although the effect is largely

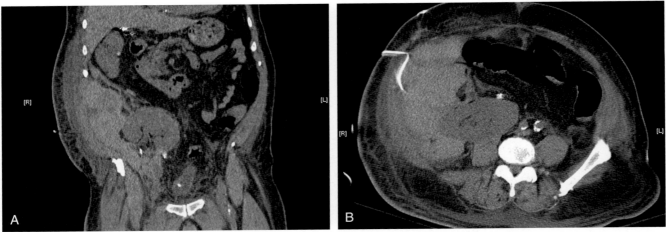

Figure 37-5 **A,** Coronal noncontrast CT scan of a large hematoma lateral to the renal allograft. **B,** Transverse noncontrast CT scan demonstrating that even a well-positioned drain does little to prevent hematoma formation.

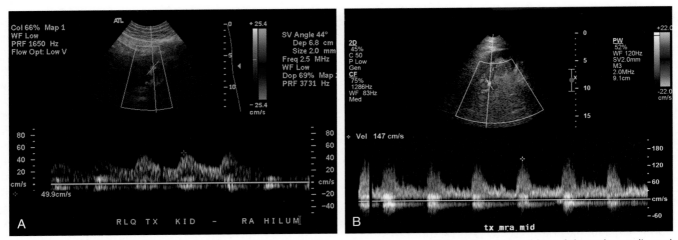

Figure 37-6 **A,** Doppler ultrasound scan of the renal hilum showing decreased velocity (49.9 cm/second) and loss of the early systolic peak tardus-parvus waveform. **B,** Normal velocity and waveform.

absent after 8 hours and DDAVP may induce tachyphylaxis. Daily intravenous conjugated estrogen (Premarin) infusion of 0.6 mg/kg for 5 days also reduces the bleeding time in uremic patients.[21] Vitamin K deficiency is fairly common in patients with renal failure and a poor nutritional state, and other coagulation parameters should be evaluated and corrected.

Renal Artery Stenosis

One of the most common vascular complications is transplant renal artery stenosis (TRAS), with a reported incidence of 1.6% to 12%.[22-25] Most cases of TRAS occur within 3 years after transplantation. The presenting signs suggestive of TRAS include poorly controlled renin-mediated hypertension, increasing peripheral edema, decreased allograft function with or without the use of angiotensin-converting enzyme inhibitors, and the presence of a bruit over the allograft. Renal artery stenosis is suspected on ultrasonography when the peak

systolic velocity is >250 cm per second with turbulence. A tardus-parvus Doppler arterial waveform is also highly suggestive of TRAS (**Fig. 37-6**).[26]

Angiography remains the gold standard, although CT angiography and magnetic resonance angiography (**Fig. 37-7A**) are helpful in making the diagnosis. The risk of contrast administration needs to be considered in patients with marginal renal function. In some cases, carbon dioxide angiography can be used to minimize the load of nephrotoxic contrast material. Evidence has linked gadolinium contrast to the development of nephrogenic systemic fibrosis in patients undergoing dialysis.[27]

Any factor that leads to intimal injury or turbulent blood flow can result in stenosis, and clinicians should try to avoid the potential causes of TRAS listed in Box 37-1. If stenosis is diagnosed in the first postoperative month, then surgical revision of the anastomosis is usually the best option. Beyond this time period, percutaneous transluminal angioplasty (PTA) (see Fig.

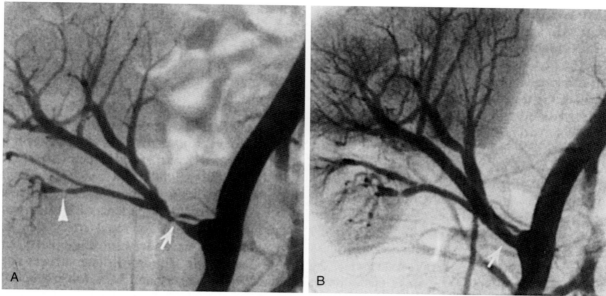

Figure 37-7 Percutaneous transluminal angioplasty of transplant renal artery stenosis. **A,** Severe stenosis of the proximal allograft renal artery (*arrow*) demonstrated on an external iliac arteriogram. The end-to-side Carrel patch anastomosis with the external iliac artery is widely patent. Also note the marked stenosis in the lower pole intrarenal branch artery (*arrowhead*). **B,** After balloon angioplasty, the proximal renal artery is widely patent (*arrow*). *(From Jordan ML, Holley JL, Zajko AB. Renal vascular hypertension in the transplant patient. In: Novick A, Scoble J, Hamilton G, eds.* Renal Vascular Disease. *London: WB Saunders; 1996:279.)*

BOX 37-1	Causes of Transplant Renal Artery Stenosis

Recipient artery atherosclerosis
Donor artery atherosclerosis
Anastomotic stricture resulting from faulty suture
 technique
Arterial injury during donor nephrectomy
Kinking of the renal artery
Disparity in donor-recipient vessel size
Rejection of the donor artery
Vascular clamp injury
Perfusion pump cannulation injury

37-7B) is usually the preferred treatment, with a durable success rate of ≤84%.[28,29] Surgical correction may be necessary after failed PTA or for lesions that are not approachable by angioplasty. An intraperitoneal approach to the vessels provides the best exposure. The surgical techniques for revascularization of TRAS include the following:

1. Resection of the stenotic segment and direct arterial reanastomosis
2. Transection of the transplant artery distal to the anastomosis and end-to-side reimplantation
3. Bypass with autologous saphenous vein or Gore-Tex graft
4. Open dilation
5. Vein patch angioplasty

The immediate technical success rate of surgical correction is between 55% and 92%, with graft loss in ≤20% and a mortality rate of ≤5.5%.[30]

Renal Artery Thrombosis

Renal artery thrombosis is most often seen in pediatric recipients. The incidence is increased in transplant recipients with thrombotic tendencies (anticardiolipin antibodies, protein C or S deficiency, or thrombocytosis). This complication can also occur in kidneys that have donor vascular disease or kidneys with multiple small arteries requiring complex bench surgical intervention before implantation (horseshoe donor kidneys, pediatric en bloc donor kidneys). Renal artery thrombosis typically occurs within the first 72 hours after transplantation.

The renal allograft vessels must be carefully inspected for intimal integrity. Fine vascular suture material should be used to create an intimal approximating anastomosis. If the allograft does not perfuse properly, the vascular clamps are reapplied to the recipient vessels, the anastomosis is taken down, the kidney is flushed with chilled Ringer's lactate solution containing 1000 U/L of heparin, and the anastomosis is carefully redone. If extensive reconstruction of the recipient vessel is required, the allograft should be removed and placed back in the ice-cold preservation solution on the back table. In transplants that have an increased risk of arterial thrombosis it may be helpful to give 1000 U of heparin before suturing the arterial anastomosis. Continuing the heparin at 100 U per hour for the duration of the hospitalization with daily acetylsalicylic acid on discharge may also help to prevent this complication in those patients with significant risk factors.

If delayed arterial thrombosis occurs, it is rarely possible to make the diagnosis in time to salvage the graft, and this complication is usually associated with severe acute rejection. The patient may experience a sudden cessation of urine flow without any discomfort. Thrombocytopenia and hyperkalemia may occur as platelets are consumed in the graft with a sudden elevation in creatinine. The diagnosis of renal thrombosis is confirmed by ultrasonography or renal scan with no blood flow to the allograft. If the diagnosis is made immediately, then the patient is rushed to the operating room for emergency open arteriotomy and thrombectomy. Unfortunately, most grafts that sustain arterial thrombosis are lost and require allograft nephrectomy.

Renal Vein Thrombosis

Renal vein thrombosis generally occurs in the early postoperative period. Some causes of renal vein thrombosis that should be avoided include kinking or angulation of the renal vein, stenosis of the venous anastomosis, intraoperative or postoperative hypotension, hypercoagulable state, acute rejection, deep vein thrombosis with extension into the allograft, and renal vein compression by a perinephric fluid collection. Prophylactic heparinization as discussed in the previous section on arterial thrombosis may also be beneficial for transplant recipients who have an increased risk for renal vein thrombosis. If venous thrombosis occurs intraoperatively, the allograft will appear cyanotic and swollen. A clot may be palpable in the renal vein.

Thrombectomy and revision of the anastomosis should be attempted as in arterial thrombosis. The vascular clamps should be carefully reapplied so that a segment of the thrombus is not dislodged into the systemic circulation. Delayed renal vein thrombosis is usually diagnosed by Doppler ultrasonography and may be confirmed by renal scan or venography. Late renal vein thrombosis (occurring >4 weeks after transplantation) is usually a result of propagation of deep vein thrombosis into the renal vein. Thrombolytic therapy with intravenous streptokinase or anticoagulation may occasionally be useful. The diagnosis of late venous thrombosis is usually made after a period of prolonged allograft ischemia, and nephrectomy is indicated.

Deep Vein Thrombosis and Pulmonary Embolism

Pulmonary embolism is the most common preventable cause of death among hospital patients in the United States.[31] A review of 4724 kidney transplantations found this procedure to have the highest risk of venous thromboembolism (1%) of any urologic procedure.[32] Possible reasons for this risk include stasis from clamping of the vein, endothelial injury from creation of the vascular anastomosis, pelvic dissection, diabetes, calcineurin inhibitors, immobility, elevated homocysteine level, and decreased venous emptying secondary to urinoma, hematoma, lymphocele, or positioning of the kidney. We recommend placement of pulsatile compression stockings before the induction of anesthesia and removal of these stockings when the patient is ready to ambulate. Anticoagulation with heparin should also be considered for high-risk recipients. Low-molecular-weight heparin should be avoided because the degree of anticoagulation is unpredictable in patients with marginal renal function and is difficult to monitor.

Lymphocele

Lymphatic collections are usually found medial to the renal allograft and may occur in 36% of transplants, although most lymphoceles are too small to require treatment.[33] The lymphatic collection arises from the lymphatics surrounding the iliac vessels that are divided during mobilization or renal hilar lymphatics of the donor kidney. Some lymphoceles may produce pain, ureteral obstruction voiding symptoms, and renal or iliac vein compression leading to deep vein thrombosis or leg swelling. The diagnosis is confirmed by ultrasound examination (**Fig. 37-8**) and aspiration of the fluid using sterile technique. Lymphatic fluid is usually clear with a high lymphocyte count, high protein content, and creatinine concentration similar to that of serum.

Small, asymptomatic lymphoceles do not require treatment. Aspiration alone may resolve the problem, but repeated aspiration is discouraged because it may lead to infection and rarely results in permanent decompression. Percutaneous closed-system catheter drainage with instillation of sclerosing agents, such as povidone-iodine (Betadine)[34] or fibrin glue,[35] has been successful. Loculated lymphoceles, collections adjacent to the renal hilum, and those that are inaccessible for safe puncture are best treated by marsupialization into the peritoneal cavity. This procedure may be accomplished by a laparoscopic or open surgical approach.[33,36] The transplant ureter, which is often incorporated into the wall of the lymphocele, must be identified and carefully preserved. A cystoscopically placed ureteral stent or intraoperative ultrasound scan may be beneficial. The peritoneal opening must be large enough to prevent bowel herniation. Omentum is usually placed in the opening to prevent closure.

The incidence of lymphoceles can be reduced by minimizing the pelvic dissection and ligating lymphatics. Avoiding the immunosuppressant agent sirolimus in the early postoperative period may also help to reduce the incidence of this complication. Additionally, placing a drain at the end of the procedure and leaving it for the initial postoperative course have been shown to reduce lymphatic collections.[37]

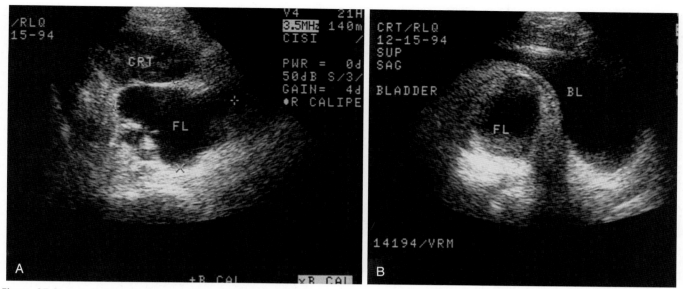

Figure 37-8 Renal allograft ultrasound with a lymphocele. **A,** The lymphocele (FL) is medial to the renal transplant (CRT). **B,** The lymphocele extends into the pelvis and displaces the bladder (BL). Attempted sclerosis of this lymphocele with povidone-iodine (Betadine) initially failed, but treatment was successful with an open peritoneal window procedure.

Arteriovenous Fistula

In renal allografts, arteriovenous fistula formation most commonly follows renal transplant biopsy. Other causes of arteriovenous fistula include trauma, infection, rupture of an aneurysm, and injury to segmental renal vessels before organ recovery. In these latter cases, segmental renal infarction of the parenchyma subtended by the injured vessel may also lead to urine leak from the underlying calyx. An arteriovenous fistula may manifest with hypertension, hematuria, or a bruit over the allograft. The diagnosis is confirmed by color duplex ultrasound examination (**Fig. 37-9**) or angiography (**Fig. 37-10**). Most postbiopsy fistulas are small and resolve spontaneously. Localized pressure with the ultrasound probe may diminish flow enough to allow localized thrombosis. Angiography with selective embolization of the feeding vessel is the treatment of choice for persistent clinically significant fistulas.[38] The incidence of arteriovenous fistula may be reduced by correcting the bleeding time and platelet count before performance of ultrasound-guided biopsy of the renal allograft cortical tissue.[39]

GRAFT REJECTION

Only kidneys from identical twin donors have no risk of rejection, require no immunosuppressive medication, and may continue to function for >40 years. Almost all other donor kidneys eventually succumb to rejection and require immunosuppression. Allograft rejection is classified into three major categories: hyperacute, acute, and chronic.

Hyperacute rejection usually begins immediately after perfusion. The transplanted kidney, after initially perfusing well, may become cyanotic, soft, and edematous.

One must exclude other causes of insufficient arterial blood supply including positional kinking of the vessels, intimal flap, or hypotension. The diagnosis is confirmed by an intraoperative biopsy of the kidney that shows polymorphonuclear leukocytes in the glomeruli and peritubular capillaries with widespread vascular thrombosis. This type of rejection results from preformed cytotoxic antibodies reactive to endothelial cells of the graft.

Hyperacute rejection can be prevented by testing the recipient serum for antibodies reactive to donor lymphocytes with a cross-match test. This test is usually performed before each renal transplantation. Recipients with a positive cross-match test result or blood type incompatibility have undergone successful transplantation with plasmapheresis, intravenous immunoglobulin, and potent immunosuppression. However, a negative cross-match test result should be obtained before every renal transplant procedure. Treatment of hyperacute rejection is disappointing and is generally associated with graft loss.

Acute rejection occurs in 10% to 40% of allografts within the first year after transplantation.[40,41] With current immunosuppression, the only presenting sign is usually a rise in the serum creatinine level. The diagnosis is confirmed by allograft biopsy. The differential diagnosis includes dehydration, ischemia reperfusion injury, drug nephrotoxicity, obstruction, and pyelonephritis. Acute rejection is often the result of an insufficient immunosuppression regimen or poor patient compliance. New methods of monitoring the immune response may allow the clinician time to increase immunosuppression and reverse the process before significant damage to the allograft occurs.[42] Approximately 90% of acute rejections are cell mediated and are characterized

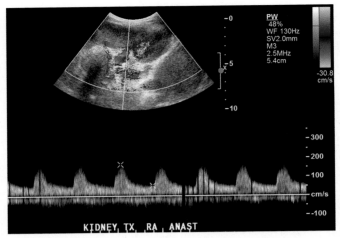

Figure 37-9 Doppler ultrasound scan of renal allograft after biopsy. Note the speckling of colors within the upper region, a finding suggestive of a fistula because blood is flowing in various directions.

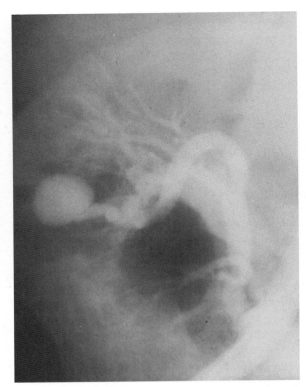

Figure 37-10 Angiogram of an arteriovenous fistula after renal allograft. Note visualization of the renal vein before the nephrogram phase. This fistula was treated with selective embolization.

by lymphocytic invasion of the interstitium and tubular epithelium. Ten percent of acute rejections show evidence of antibody-mediated rejection, characterized by complement deposition (C4d) in the peritubular capillaries. Vascular rejection signifies arterial inflammation and can result from either cell-mediated or antibody-mediated rejection. Standardized criteria for grading renal allograft biopsies have been developed and are used to guide additional immunosuppressive therapy.[43]

Acute rejection within the first year after transplantation can be successfully reversed approximately 80% of the time.[2] Acute cellular rejection is treated by high-dose methylprednisolone, by antilymphocytic antibodies, or increasing the dosage of calcineurin inhibitor medications. For antibody-mediated acute rejection, most clinicians favor rapid removal of the circulating antibodies by plasmapheresis and the neutralization of the remaining antibodies with intravenous immunoglobulin.

Chronic rejection is identified in most renal transplants after a few years. Renal allograft biopsies show evidence of accelerated atherosclerosis, interstitial fibrosis, and tubular atrophy. The pathogenesis is not fully understood but both antigen-dependent and antigen-independent mechanisms of vascular injury are implicated. The serum creatinine concentration slowly increases until the allograft fails. Although immune factors including acute rejection play a role in the development of chronic rejection, the newer term *chronic allograft nephropathy* more accurately describes the multifactorial nature of this disease. Hypercholesterolemia, hypertension, immunosuppression nephrotoxicity, ischemia reperfusion injury, and infection have all been associated with the same pathologic findings. Many clinical trials are now being designed to determine whether this process can be stopped or prevented. Increasing immunosuppressive treatment is usually not advised.

KEY POINTS

1. As the demand for kidney transplantation continues to rise, urologists will increasingly be called on to participate in donor and recipient care.
2. The allograft ureter receives blood supply solely from the renal artery; therefore, preservation of all the arterial branches (especially lower pole arteries) is essential to ensure viability of the ureter.
3. A stented ureteroneocystostomy has six times fewer urologic complications than a nonstented ureteroneocystostomy.
4. If a urine leak is caused by an ischemic sloughed ureter, endoscopic management merely delays definitive treatment. Therefore, early surgical exploration and repair is usually the best solution.
5. Recipient who develop recurrent pyelonephritis after transplantation with confirmed reflux on imaging studies initially should be treated with long-term antibiotic prophylaxis. If this approach is not effective, then an endoscopic or open procedure may be indicated.

REFERENCES

Please see www.expertconsult.com

Chapter 38

COMPLICATIONS OF URETERAL SURGERY

William J. Aronson MD

Clinical Professor, Department of Urology, David Geffen School of Medicine, University of California– Los Angeles, Los Angeles, California

The goals of ureteral surgery are to reestablish ureteral continuity, to eliminate obstruction, and ultimately to preserve renal function at the highest achievable level with minimal morbidity. Complications of open ureteral surgery are not infrequent given that these operations are often performed in the setting of prior endoscopic or open surgery or in patients with complicating factors such as prior radiotherapy, multiple prior procedures, or complex disease entities such as retroperitoneal fibrosis.

Complications of ureteral surgery are, however, often preventable with careful attention to surgical technique as well as proper preoperative and postoperative care. This chapter examines complications arising from the following procedures: ureteroureterostomy, transureteroureterostomy (TUU), ureterolysis, psoas hitch, Boari bladder flap, ileal ureter, and renal autotransplantation. The preoperative, intraoperative, and postoperative errors that lead to complications of these procedures, as well as their prevention and management, are discussed.

SURGICAL ANATOMY

To prevent surgical complications, it is vital to understand the anatomy of the ureters and neighboring structures. The upper ureters descend in the retroperitoneum anterior to the psoas muscle and adhere to the overlying parietal peritoneum. At approximately the level of the third lumbar vertebra, the ureters are crossed ventrally by the gonadal vessels coursing medially to laterally. The lower third portions of the ureters begin at the pelvic inlet where they cross anterior to the bifurcation of the common iliac artery. Here the left ureter is crossed ventrally by sigmoid branches of the inferior mesenteric vessels, and it is here that the ureter may be injured during left hemicolectomy.

As the ureters descend into the pelvis, first posterolaterally and then anteromedially to insert into the bladder, they become more difficult to identify as they become entangled in the anterior branches of the hypogastric vessels coursing medially to supply the pelvic viscera. In male patients, just before the ureters enter the bladder, they are crossed ventrally by the vas deferens. In female patients, the distal ureters enter the base of the broad ligament 1 to 2 cm lateral to the uterocervical junction and are crossed anteriorly by the uterine vessels, thus making this portion a common site of injury during radical hysterectomy.

The ureter receives its blood supply from almost all vessels near it (**Fig. 38-1**). Ureteral branches of these vessels enter the ureteral sheath and form a freely anastomotic plexus within the adventitia, which in turn sends off small branches to the ureteral mucosa.[1] Many of the perforating branches to the ureter run in close proximity to the peritoneum; therefore, great care should be taken when incising the peritoneum to avoid these branches. The greater the length of ureter mobilized during an operation, the more these perforating branches are sacrificed, thus making the ureteral blood supply more reliant on distant perforating branches feeding the adventitial plexus. To spare the ureteral blood supply, the length of ureter mobilized must be minimized and the paraureteral tissue and adventitial sheath must be preserved.

PREOPERATIVE PLANNING

Careful preoperative planning and evaluation are paramount to the success of ureteral surgery. Before ureteral surgical procedures are undertaken, factors in the patient's history that may adversely affect ureteral viability must be considered. Previous abdominal or retroperitoneal surgery may distort the ureteral anatomy and compromise the ureteral blood supply. Any history of pelvic or abdominal radiation therapy must also be elucidated inasmuch as a resultant ureteral stricture rate of 2.4% has been reported, with higher rates of injury when radiation is combined with a surgical procedure.[2,3] Previous radiation therapy to the pelvis may

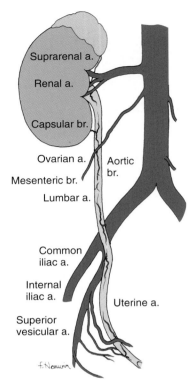

Figure 38-1 Blood supply of the ureter. Perforating arterial branches to the upper ureter emanate medial to the ureter, whereas those to the lower ureter emanate laterally. *(From Smith RB, Skinner DG, eds.* Complications of Urologic Disorders. *Philadelphia: WB Saunders; 1976:131.)*

also cause fibrosis and contracture of the bladder, thus preventing the use of a psoas hitch or Boari bladder flap reconstruction. In cases of ureteral trauma caused by ballistic weaponry, it is important to know the caliber of the weapon used because higher-velocity missiles may cause significant ureteral injury beyond the path of the bullet.[4] Failure to evaluate these issues before ureteral surgery is performed may result in serious complications owing to the use of nonviable ureter for surgical repair.

Before embarking on an open ureteral surgical procedure, the functional status of both kidneys must be established by appropriate studies. The entire anatomy of both ureters should also be evaluated preoperatively with an intravenous urogram (IVU) or a retrograde ureterogram or both, when indicated, to elucidate any distortion of the ureteral anatomy and to rule out any unforeseen obstruction or abnormality of the ipsilateral or contralateral ureter. The incidence of ureteral anomalies may be as high as 10% in urologic patients, and these anomalies need to be identified preoperatively.[5] In addition, it is critically important that any history of bladder outlet obstruction, dysfunctional voiding, or neurogenic bladder be elucidated because these condi-

tions may impede urinary outflow and compromise the ureteral repair.

When planning ureteral surgical procedures, preoperative radiographic studies such as an IVU or retrograde ureterogram may underestimate the actual extent of ureteral injury. Surgical exploration may reveal less viable ureter for reconstruction than was expected. This potential discrepancy must be anticipated and planned for accordingly. If interposition with bowel is under consideration, preoperative bowel preparation is mandatory. If renal autotransplantation is considered, then preoperative renal artery angiography should be performed, a vascular or transplant surgeon should be available if needed, and an ice machine should be available. The patient should fully consent to all potential operative procedures and complications.

INTRAOPERATIVE TECHNICAL ERRORS

General Principles

The most common cause of complications of ureteral surgery is intraoperative technical error. Regardless of the indication for ureteral surgery (i.e., an intrinsic problem such as a stricture or malignancy or an extrinsic process such as retroperitoneal fibrosis, trauma, or surgical misadventure), several basic principles must be followed.

First and foremost, do not underestimate the exposure required to mobilize the ureter. Extensive ureteral strictures may require significant bladder and kidney mobilization to minimize tension of the anastomosis. Generally speaking, for repairs of complicated ureteral strictures, I perform a full-length midline incision. The ureter must first be identified without damaging it or its blood supply. Pinching the ureter will not always cause peristalsis when the ureter is involved in a pathologic process, and therefore pinching the ureter will not always reliably identify the ureter in these complex surgical situations. It is often necessary first to identify the ureter at an uninvolved, anatomically reliable site (e.g., anterior to the iliac bifurcation) and trace it back toward the diseased segment. To preserve ureteral blood supply, handling of the adventitia should be minimal and paraureteral tissue should be spared. Gentle traction can be obtained with a fine stitch placed at the cut end of the ureter or by a vessel loop surrounding the ureter.

Technical errors such as crushing of the ureter or excessive mobilization can cause ureteral ischemia and necrosis and can thus predisposing the patient to stricture. Only viable ureter must be used for the anastomosis. Operative signs of devitalization include dense periureteral scarring, friability of tissues, and lack of bleeding from cut edges. In some instances, I use intravenous fluorescein (1 ampule) followed by inspection with Wood's lamp (ultraviolet light) to determine viability, with fluorescence visible only in the viable ureter. All nonviable ureter must be completely débrided to prevent subsequent necrosis and complications.

It is critically important to create ureteral anastomoses without tension. When ureteral injury and débridement result in lengthy ureteral gaps that prevent a tension-free anastomosis, other mobilization techniques must be considered. These include the vesicopsoas hitch, the Boari bladder flap, and downward renal mobilization. When the bladder has an adequate capacity, the vesicopsoas hitch combined with ureteral reimplantation is a highly successful and relatively simple technique to gain at least 3 to 5 cm of additional length while preserving functional bladder capacity.[6,7] In my opinion, the Boari bladder flap technique is second to the psoas hitch as the method of choice to bridge lower ureteral gaps. Although this is a highly effective technique to provide significant additional length, it has a greater risk of complications when a pedicled flap is used.[8]

Up to 8 cm of length can also be obtained through downward renal mobilization, which is accomplished by dissecting the kidney free from its perinephric attachments, displacing it downward, and affixing it to the iliac fossa. To achieve effective mobilization, the upper ureter must also be dissected from its paraureteral attachments; this approach requires division of the perforating vessels. Great care must be taken to preserve the basilar branch of the renal artery because the dissected ureter relies on this branch for its blood supply. The blood supply to the upper ureter can generally be preserved by sparing the perinephric-perihilar fat in the triangle formed by the upper ureter and renal artery. The critical arterial branches from the renal vasculature to the ureter generally course through this region.

Every effort must be made to create a watertight ureteral anastomosis.[9] Leakage of urine through the anastomosis can delay healing and cause fibrosis with subsequent stricture formation.[10] The anastomosis should also be created to allow for a maximal luminal diameter because some contraction of the anastomosis occurs postoperatively (**Fig. 38-2**). I prefer to use interrupted fine chromic sutures to avoid a pursestring effect that may result from a running closure.

The use of appropriate internal and external drainage is also essential to avoid complications. After creating a ureteral anastomosis, placement of external drains to dependent areas is mandatory. Issues concerning the need for an internal stent as well as the appropriate type of stent have not been resolved.[11] When any question exists regarding the ureteral blood supply and viability and the degree of tension and adequacy of an anastomosis, a self-retaining ureteral stent should be placed. I frequently place ureteral stents even for flawless anastomoses and have never regretted this maneuver.

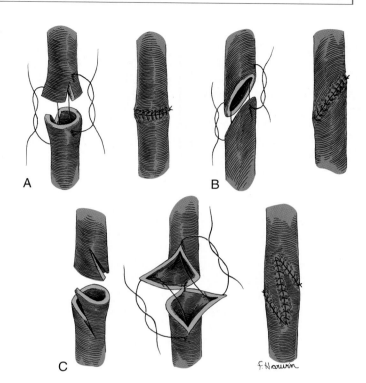

Figure 38-2 Ureteroureterostomy: techniques to maximize luminal diameter. **A,** Spatulation of ureteral margins. **B,** Oblique anastomosis. **C,** Z-plasty technique. *(From Smith RB, Skinner DG, eds.* Complications of Urologic Disorders. *Philadelphia: WB Saunders; 1976:137.)*

Open Ureteral Surgery

Ureterolithotomy

Ureterolithotomy is rarely used at present given the effectiveness of retrograde and antegrade ureteroscopy with laser lithotripsy for treating ureteral stones. Ureterolithotomy does warrant mention here, however, because of the significant risk of ureteral stricture following this procedure. In several reports evaluating management of ureteral strictures, the percentage of patients with strictures caused by ureterolithotomy ranged from 8% to 19%.[12-14]

Ureteroureterostomy

Ureteroureterostomy is frequently used to bridge short defects of the upper two thirds of the ureter resulting from traumatic or intraoperative injuries. When the basic principles of ureteral surgery are strictly followed, complications from this procedure are rare.[9,15] However, when ureteral viability is not properly assessed, the incidence of urinary fistula and stricture is higher, especially when ureteroureterostomy is performed for blast injuries to the ureter.

Transureteroureterostomy

TUU has proved highly successful for pediatric patients in several instances (e.g., when the bladder is not suitable for reimplantation of more than one ureter, for undiversion procedures, and as a salvage procedure for failed ureteral reimplantation).[16-17] TUU has also been used successfully in adults to manage defects in the lower third and occasionally the middle third of the ureter.[18,19] This procedure is especially useful when the pelvis must be avoided and when the bladder cannot be mobilized to create a psoas hitch or a Boari flap. Alternatively, TUU has been successfully employed in cases of pelvic malignant disease that is not of genitourinary origin (i.e., rectal and ovarian cancer, sarcoma) involving a distal ureter.[20] TUU is absolutely contraindicated in the presence of transitional cell carcinoma of the ureter or renal pelvis and in the presence of recurrent urolithiasis. To avoid complications, the preoperative evaluation should rule out any history of tuberculosis or recurrent pyelonephritis in either kidney as well as reflux or obstruction in the recipient ureter.

The inherent problem of performing TUU is that both kidneys are at risk if any complications with the ureteral anastomosis occur such as stricture or urine leak.[21] To avoid these complications, one should strictly adhere to the following technical principles. A generous midline incision is needed to give wide transabdominal exposure. Mobilization of the donor ureter should include paraureteral tissue as well as en bloc transfer of the gonadal vessels with the donor ureter if possible. The donor ureter should follow a gentle curve and approach the recipient ureter at approximately a 45-degree angle. It also should course above the level of the inferior mesenteric artery to avoid impingement between the cleft of the aorta and inferior mesenteric artery.[18]

In addition, the anastomosis should be tension free and watertight and must be accomplished without significant angulation or mobilization of the recipient ureter. With their experience of TUU in 253 patients, Noble and colleagues[22] recommended stenting the anastomosis until radiographic evidence of healing is present. Given that both renal units are at risk following TUU, long-term follow-up is mandatory.

Ureterolysis

As a treatment for idiopathic retroperitoneal fibrosis, ureterolysis consists of peeling the fibrous tissue off the length of the ureter, mobilizing the abdominal and pelvic ureter, and then either placing the ureter intraperitoneally, with or without an omental wrap, or displacing the ureter laterally. With mobilization of the entire ureter, as demanded by this operation, the ureter becomes completely dependent on blood supplied from the most proximal and distal perforating vessels. With the already tenuous ureteral blood supply, intraoperative nephrostomy tube placement should be strongly considered if injury to the adventitia or inadvertent ureterotomy occurs during the ureterolysis procedure. Moreover, stent placement should always be attempted

before the procedure to aid with identification and mobilization of the ureter.

The complication of recurrent ureteral obstruction after ureterolysis occurs more frequently when a clean plane of dissection has not been obtained between the fibrous tissue and the ureter. These patients usually have histologic invasion of the ureteral muscle layer by the fibrotic process.[23] Another complication of ureterolysis, late intestinal obstruction, appears to occur more frequently when an omental wrap of the ureter has been performed. In one report, this complication occurred in 14% of the procedures that incorporated omental wrapping after ureterolysis.[24]

Vesicopsoas Hitch

The vesicopsoas hitch is my first choice for managing injuries or strictures of the lower third to lower half of the ureter that are not correctable by ureteroneocystostomy alone. Prerequisites include a normal bladder capacity, no prior pelvic irradiation, and no evidence of bladder outlet obstruction or neurogenic bladder disease. Maximal length can be obtained through the use of a horizontal cystotomy, fixation of the bladder to the psoas tendon above the iliac bifurcation, and closure of the cystotomy longitudinally. Division of the peritoneal attachments and contralateral superior vesical pedicle may also increase the upward mobility of the bladder.

Great care should be taken to suture only the superficial aspect of the psoas tendon (using three interrupted nonabsorbable sutures) to avoid genitofemoral and femoral nerve injuries, which can lead to painful neuropathies.[25] Three cases of femoral neuropathy were described in detail by Kowalcyzk and colleagues.[25] In two of these patients the neuropathy resolved with conservative management that included early mobilization and physical therapy, whereas one patient required exploration and removal of the tacking suture.[25] Although a nonrefluxing anastomosis is preferred in children, Ahn and Loughlin[26] used a freely refluxing anastomosis in 17 of 24 adults undergoing a psoas hitch procedure and reported no long-term complications. In adults, a freely refluxing anastomosis is preferred if a tunneled anastomosis will leave the ureter under tension.

Boari Bladder Flap

The Boari flap is my second choice after the psoas hitch for bridging lower ureteral defects because of the inherent complications associated with a pedicled flap. However, if the bladder has adequate capacity and compliance, the Boari flap remains an effective option for bridging defects up to the level of the midureter. The flap itself is generously spiraled from the contralateral anterior bladder wall to the ipsilateral posterior wall and the base of the flap is fashioned between the dome and the trigone (**Fig. 38-3**). The base should be ≥4 cm in

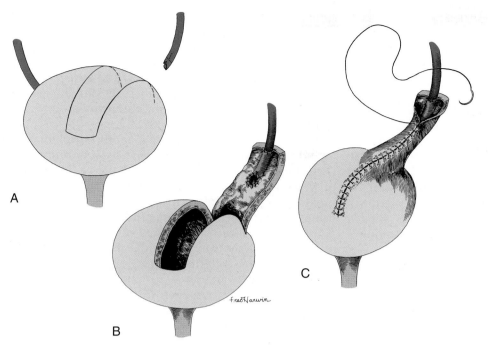

Figure 38-3 Bladder flap procedure. **A,** Creation of a tapered bladder flap, based posteriorly. **B,** Submucosal ureteral reimplantation. **C,** Closure of the bladder flap. *(From Smith RB, Skinner DG, eds. Complications of Urologic Disorders. Philadelphia: WB Saunders; 1976:142.)*

width, and great care should be taken not to injure the branches of the middle and inferior vesical arteries that supply blood to the flap. The flap is first fixed to the psoas muscle, then closed in two layers, thus incorporating larger amounts of the seromuscular layer than the mucosa to prevent excessive narrowing of the tube. Extra suture material should be used for closure at the junction of the bladder and base of the flap to prevent leakage.

The need for an antirefluxing procedure is unclear. In a series of 23 patients who underwent a Boari flap procedure with a freely refluxing anastomosis, 21 of these patients had stabilization or improvement of creatinine clearance; 22 patients also achieved complete resolution or improvement of hydronephrosis. Follow-up in this series was 5 to 14 years.[27] Complications of the bladder flap technique include decreased bladder capacity, stenosis of the bladder tube, and urine leakage at the apex of the flap or at the junction of the bladder and the base of the flap.

For more extensive ureteral strictures extending as high as the lower pole of the kidney, Olsson and associates[28] described using a psoas hitch combined with a Boari bladder flap with excellent results. These investigators described making the transverse bladder incision for the psoas hitch on the contralateral side to the ureteral stricture. After tacking the bladder to the psoas muscle (using chromic suture), this incision becomes the lateral border of the bladder flap.[28] Similarly, Sutherland and colleagues[29] described bridging a 14-cm defect with a combined Boari bladder flap and psoas hitch.

Ileal Ureter

Ileal interposition is a safe and effective technique for repairing extensive ureteral defects that cannot be repaired by the previously discussed reconstructive procedures. It is also frequently used when previous attempts at ureteral reconstruction have failed. Proper patient selection is essential to avoid complications. Patients should have a preoperative serum creatinine concentration <2 mg/dL (with good ipsilateral renal function) to avoid progressive renal impairment and electrolyte abnormalities.[30] In addition, bladder emptying must be adequate to avoid bladder outlet obstruction from mucus produced by the ileal segment.

Because the interposed ileum retains its absorptive capacity, the length of ileum used should be minimized. This can be accomplished by use of a vesicopsoas hitch distally, and if viable ureter exists proximally, it can be anastomosed to the ileum in an end-to-side fashion. Obtaining a tension-free anastomosis of the proximal ileum to the renal pelvis using adequate ileal mesentery may result in redundant ileal length, in which case the excess ileum from the midportion of the ileal ureter should be resected to minimize ileal length. I also advocate creating a freely refluxing ileal vesical anastomosis because this has not been associated with deterioration of renal function or adverse pyelographic changes.[30] If urine leakage is noted at the anastomosis, a nephrostomy tube should be inserted intraoperatively. An additional maneuver I find extremely useful is placement of a 22- or 24-Fr red rubber catheter in the interposed ileum, with the tip of the catheter in the renal pelvis and the opposite end brought through the bladder and out a suprapubic stab wound. The catheter is secured to the ileum with several chromic sutures and should remain in place for approximately 6 weeks. I believe that this maneuver prevents kinking of the ileal ureter and allows it to heal in a straight fashion. It also facilitates internal drainage during healing.

Complications of ileal interposition include urinary fistula, elongation of the ileal ureter with kinking and obstruction, mucus plug obstruction, anastomotic strictures, chronic infection with pyelonephritis, and bowel obstruction. Electrolyte abnormalities and progressive renal failure are also important complications in patients with a preoperative creatinine concentration ≥2.0 mg/dL. Chung and associates[31] reviewed their experience performing ileal ureter in 52 patients. Among 6 patients with a baseline creatinine level >2 ng/mL, 3 maintained stable renal function whereas 3 had worsening azotemia. Subjects undergoing ileal ureter with baseline renal deficiency should be consented for the high risk of worsening renal failure and metabolic abnormalities, and consideration should be given to renal autotransplantation.

Alternatives to ileal ureter replacement include reconfiguring short tubes of ileum or colon with the Yang-Monti principle or, in the case of right ureteral defects, using the vermiform appendix.[32,33] Series incorporating these alternatives are relatively small with few reports of complications, yet these approaches are based on sound reasoning. Given the urologists' increasing use and expertise with intestinal segments for reconstruction, I anticipate that these alternative forms of ureteral replacement will be used to a greater extent in the future.

Renal Autotransplantation

The majority of ureteral defects can be managed by conservative means or by reconstructive procedures such as ureteral reimplantation with or without a psoas hitch, Boari flap, ureteroureterostomy, TUU, downward renal mobilization, or a combination of these techniques. When such procedures are not possible or have failed, creation of an ileal ureter and renal autotransplantation are the only two remaining options to preserve the affected renal unit. Renal autotransplantation has proved to be safe and effective, primarily because of increasing surgical experience with renal transplantation and methods of renal preservation. Although autotransplantation is most commonly used for the surgical treatment of renal arterial lesions, it has proved extremely effective for managing long ureteral defects.[34]

Preoperative evaluation includes renal artery angiography to delineate the anatomic features of the renal artery. If peripheral vascular disease is suspected, iliac artery angiography should be performed to rule out severe atherosclerosis of the recipient iliac vessels. In patients with long ureteral defects resulting from idiopathic retroperitoneal fibrosis, Rose and colleagues[35]

recommended two additional preoperative studies: pelvic computed tomography to assess the extent of fibrosis in the pelvis and femoral venography with inferior venacavography to document adequate pelvic venous drainage. These investigators and others showed that autotransplantation is highly successful in patients with retroperitoneal fibrosis in whom ureterolysis has failed.[35-39]

The complications of renal autotransplantation include urine leakage, bleeding, and renal nonfunction. Dissection in the renal hilum should be minimized to prevent devascularization of the renal pelvis and proximal ureter, which may produce necrosis and urine leakage. Bleeding is a significant complication of autotransplantation and resulted in nephrectomy in 2 of 23 (8.6%) patients in one series.[35] Both these patients had undergone multiple prior operations on the involved kidney, and in 1 patient, bleeding resulted from nephrostomy tube erosion into an intrarenal vessel. The complication of renal nonfunction may result from inadequate renal flushing secondary to severe parenchymal disease or from excess perivascular fibrosis in the renal hilum causing vascular spasm.[35] Therefore, severe parenchymal disease and extensive fibrosis in the renal hilum appear to be contraindications to autotransplantation. An additional contraindication is the presence of any active infection, which may seed the vascular anastomoses and result in subsequent rupture.

Renal autotransplantation offers several advantages over ileal interposition for managing long ureteral defects. Autotransplantation avoids the complications of electrolyte disturbances and progressive renal deterioration frequently present in patients with a creatinine concentration >2.0 mg/dL who undergo ileal interposition. Moreover, problems associated with excess mucus secretion and chronic bacteriuria are also avoided. Alternatively, with proper patient selection, ileal interposition continues to be a highly successful technique for managing long ureteral defects.

POSTOPERATIVE ERRORS

Postoperative errors leading to complications include premature removal of surgical drains and inadequate follow-up. No set amount of time has been established for ureteral stents to remain indwelling after ureteral surgical procedures. This decision is based on clinical judgment, with the understanding that healing of the mucosa and muscle takes approximately 6 days and 6 weeks, respectively.[40-41] I generally remove stents 4 to 6 weeks after a ureteral anastomosis. A cystogram can be used to ensure that no extravasation is present after bladder reconstruction. Additionally, if a ureteral stent is in place, the cystogram before stent removal can be used to study the healing of ureteral anastomosis through reflux of contrast from the bladder.

Before removing percutaneous nephrostomy tubes, low-pressure anterograde nephrostograms should be performed to verify patency. In addition, these tubes should be capped for ≥24 to 48 hours before removal to confirm that the patient is able to tolerate the absence of percutaneous drainage.

Of critical importance is adequate follow-up, both by functional studies such as IVU and by serial renal ultrasound studies. For patients with factors predisposing them to stricture formation, such as urine leakage or borderline ureteral viability, follow-up is indicated for at least several years to rule out late ureteral obstruction.

GENERAL COMPLICATIONS AND MANAGEMENT

Urine Leakage

Urine leakage is best managed by appropriately placed drains and a urethral catheter at the time of the surgical procedure. In the absence of urine leakage postoperatively, drains should remain in place for 3 to 6 days before their advancement to allow the initial mucosal healing to occur and to protect against delayed urine leakage.

If persistent urine leakage occurs for >7 to 10 days postoperatively and a ureteral stent was not inserted intraoperatively, then a stent should be placed. Frequently, when a stent cannot be passed in retrograde fashion, anterograde placement is more successful. If a stent cannot be placed in either fashion, percutaneous drainage through a nephrostomy tube alone will allow ureteral edema to resolve and may permit resorption of previously extravasated urine that is distorting the ureter and preventing stent passage. With both percutaneous nephrostomy tube drainage and a stent in place, the fistula will heal without stricture development, and normal renal function can be expected in 63% to 95% of cases.[42-45]

In my experience, in the presence of properly placed drains and a functioning ureteral stent, urine leakage usually resolves without requiring percutaneous nephrostomy drainage. In some cases, placement of a stent may increase urinary extravasation through reflux of urine. This is particularly true in cases of bladder outlet obstruction or significant bladder instability. In these patients, a urethral catheter may be required until the leak seals.

The use of drains at the site of ureteral repair is imperative. The choice of suction drain or flat Penrose drain is based on the preference of the surgeon. When prolonged urinary drainage is anticipated, use of a non-suction drain may be preferable to avoid perpetuation of the leak. In cases of prolonged anastomotic drainage, if a suction drain was used, removing suction from the drain may allow the leak to seal. In rare instances, persistent urine leakage from abdominal drains may resolve by advancing the drain away from the operative site. Before advancing the drain, or removing suction, it may be advisable to image the retroperitoneum to rule out an undrained urine collection.

If leakage persists, distal ureteral obstruction must be ruled out and treated accordingly. This obstruction may result from either a distal stone fragment after ureterolithotomy or a previously unrecognized distal ureteral abnormality. The timing of ureteral leakage can influence management. Persistent urinary extravasation from the time of reconstruction is likely caused by technical error and usually heals with prolonged drainage. Significant extravasation in these cases can increase the risk of extraureteral scarring or anastomotic stricture.

In cases of delayed leakage, beginning >10 to 14 days postoperatively, ischemic necrosis should be suspected. In such patients, drainage remains the mainstay of management. Healing may require proximal urinary diversion through nephrostomy, and a high likelihood of stricture formation at the ischemic site exists. When healing does not occur through drainage or when leakage results in significant infection or azotemia, early repair may be warranted.

Urine leakage that fails to resolve with conservative management can be managed by either open repair or nephrectomy. In such cases, reconstruction can be extremely difficult and temporizing ureteral ligation with delayed repair may be necessary. With a normally functioning contralateral kidney, nephrectomy should be strongly considered in chronically ill or elderly, debilitated patients, especially in the presence of vascular grafts or known infection.

Ureteral Stricture

Another important complication of ureteral surgery is ureteral stricture. Before recommending therapy, one must prove, by IVU, furosemide (diethylene triamine penta-acetic acid or mercaptotriglycylglycine) renal scan, or Whitaker testing, that the stricture is causing significant renal obstruction. When a wire can be advanced beyond the stricture, endourologic management remains a viable therapeutic option. It offers the advantage of decreased postoperative pain, shorter hospitalization, and less time for convalescence compared with open surgical repair.[46] Techniques now used in endourologic management include balloon dilation, hot- or cold-knife incision, laser incision, or hot-knife incision using an Acucise catheter. These procedures can be performed either in an anterograde or a retrograde fashion.

Balloon dilation of ureteral strictures (excluding strictures of the ureteropelvic junction or ureterointestinal anastomosis) has had a varying success rate ranging from 50% to 76%, although in my experience the success rate is substantially lower.[47] Hot- or cold-knife incision of strictures appears to be more effective than balloon dilation, with success rates ranging from 43% to 100%.[48-50] Success rates with balloon dilation and incision can be expected to be much lower with strictures longer than 1.5 to 2 cm and when the stricture tissue is devascularized secondary to surgical intervention or radiation therapy.[43,46]

ACKNOWLEDGMENT

I greatly appreciate the input and contribution of Dr. Robert B. Smith.

KEY POINTS

1. In female patients, the distal ureters enter the base of the broad ligament 1 to 2 cm lateral to the uterocervical junction and are crossed anteriorly by the uterine vessels, thus making this portion a common site of injury during radical hysterectomy.

2. Surgical exploration may reveal less viable ureter for reconstruction than was expected preoperatively. This potential discrepancy must be anticipated and planned for accordingly. If interposition with bowel is under consideration, preoperative bowel preparation is mandatory.

3. When attempting to identify the strictured segment of a ureter intraoperatively, it is often necessary first to identify the ureter at an uninvolved, anatomically reliable site (e.g., anterior to the iliac bifurcation) and trace it back toward the diseased segment.

4. When ureteral injury and débridement result in lengthy ureteral gaps that prevent a tension-free anastomosis, other mobilization techniques must be considered. These include the vesicopsoas hitch, the Boari bladder flap, and downward renal mobilization.

5. TUU is absolutely contraindicated in the presence of transitional cell carcinoma of the ureter or renal pelvis and in the presence of recurrent urolithiasis. The donor ureter should course above the level of the inferior mesenteric artery to avoid impingement between the cleft of the aorta and the inferior mesenteric artery.

6. When one performs ureterolysis, stent placement should always be attempted before the procedure to aid with identification and mobilization of the ureter.

7. When one performs a psoas hitch or Boari bladder flap, prerequisites include a normal bladder capacity, no evidence of a neurogenic bladder, and no prior pelvic irradiation. Bladder outlet obstruction should be treated preoperatively.

8. In considering ileal ureter placement, patients should have a preoperative serum creatinine concentration <2 mg/dL (with adequate ipsilateral renal function) to avoid progressive renal impairment and electrolyte abnormalities.

REFERENCES

Please see www.expertconsult.com

Chapter 39

COMPLICATIONS OF ADRENAL SURGERY

Aaron P. Bayne MD
Pediatric Urology Fellow, Scott Department of Urology, Baylor College of Medicine; Urology Service, Texas Children's Hospital, Houston, Texas

Mitchell H. Sokoloff MD
Professor of Surgery and Chief, Section of Urology, University of Arizona College of Medicine, Tucson, Arizona

The landscape of adrenal surgery has changed since the late 1990s. Significantly greater numbers of adrenal operations are being performed with the use of laparoscopy. This change has led to a reduction in the overall number of complications but has also introduced new issues and complications not previously seen with conventional open surgery.[1] Moreover, advances have been made in the diagnostic methodology used for evaluating adrenal lesions and the applicability of surgery has changed. Consequently, the indications for adrenalectomy have been refined. Box 39-1 lists current clinical indications for adrenalectomy.

In this chapter, we review the major areas of complications associated with adrenal surgery. Complications of adrenal surgery are often unique to the specific underlying pathologic process and disease being treated. Thus, we separately discuss each disease and the complications associated with that treatment. These complications can be considered to occur preoperatively, intraoperatively, and postoperatively, and each is addressed. In this chapter, we try to identify pitfalls in the diagnosis of adrenal lesions, ways to avoid, recognize, and manage complications during adrenal surgery, and ways to minimize postoperative complications.

DIAGNOSTIC PROCEDURES AND PATIENT PREPARATION

Hyperaldosteronism

Primary aldosteronism is an important cause of hypertension. Classically, patients with primary aldosteronism present with hypertension and hypokalemia resulting from excess aldosterone production. However, as diagnostic criteria are refined, the actual incidence of primary aldosteronism in the hypertensive population may be 5- to 15-fold more common than previously believed.[2,3] In addition, most patients with primary aldosteronism do not have hypokalemia.[3]

The diagnosis of primary aldosteronism is usually based on a two-step evaluation involving screening and confirmatory testing (**Fig. 39-1**). Screening tests usually consist of plasma aldosterone concentration, plasma renin activity, and calculation of the ratio of plasma aldosterone concentration to plasma renin activity. Because screening can produce normal results in patients with primary aldosteronism, it is imperative to repeat screening tests in high-risk patients.[4] False-positive screenings can also occur, especially in patients with renal failure. Because no study is 100% accurate in diagnosing primary aldosteronism, it is important to confirm the preliminary screening test results with a saline load test or a fludrocortisone suppression test.

Secondary aldosteronism can be seen in patients with renal artery stenosis, malignant hypertension, cirrhosis, pregnancy, and heart failure. This form of aldosteronism is usually secondary to elevated plasma renin and angiotensin levels. Spironolactone, estrogen, angiotensin-converting enzyme inhibitors, and angiotensin receptor blockers may affect serum aldosterone concentration and must be stopped 6 weeks before screening. When evaluating patients with possible primary aldosteronism, it is important to correct hypokalemia before screening because this condition may affect plasma aldosterone concentrations.[5] Given that hypokalemia is less severe when dietary sodium is limited, patients may purposely decrease their salt intake to avoid feeling the effects of low potassium. Therefore, sodium loading is required during diagnostic evaluation.[6]

When the diagnosis of primary aldosteronism is made, the search for a surgically treatable cause requires imaging of the adrenal glands to assess for masses. Computed tomography (CT) and magnetic resonance imaging (MRI) are both accepted imaging modalities for the adrenal glands. MRI is a good alternative in pregnant women to avoid radiation exposure. Adrenal scintigraphy can show a lateralizing adrenal lesion. Adrenal vein sampling has been shown to increase the specific-

BOX 39-1	Clinical Indications for Adrenalectomy

Primary aldosteronism (solitary adenoma versus bilateral adrenal hyperplasia)
Cushing's syndrome
Pheochromocytoma
Adrenal adenoma
Myelolipoma
Adrenal cyst
Metastatic tumor
Adrenocortical carcinoma
Neuroblastoma (pediatric)
Incidentally discovered adrenal mass or "incidentaloma"

From George, K, Chow, MLB. Surgery of the adrenal glands. In: Wein AJ, Novick A, Partin A, Peters C, eds. *Campbell-Walsh Urology,* 9th ed. Philadelphia: WB Saunders; 2007:1868-1889.

TABLE 39-1 Etiology of Hypercortisolism

Type of Hypercortisolism	Proportion (%)	Female-to-Male Ratio
Corticotropin-dependent		
Cushing's disease	70	3.5:1.0
Ectopic corticotropin syndrome	10	1:1
Unknown source of corticotropin*	5	5:1
Corticotropin-independent		
Adrenal adenoma	10	4:1
Adrenal carcinoma	5	1:1
Macronodular hyperplasia	<2	1:1
Primary pigmented nodular adrenal disease	<2	1:1
McCune-Albright syndrome	<2	1:1

*Patients might ultimately prove to have Cushing's disease.
From Newell-Price J, Bertagna X, Grossman A, Nieman L. Cushing's syndrome. *Lancet.* 2006;367(9522):1605-1617.

ity of the diagnosis of surgically treatable primary aldosteronism when no lateralizing lesion was seen on imaging.[2,3] Cortisol levels should be checked during adrenal vein sampling to ensure proper catheter placement.[7] Only a highly trained radiologist should perform adrenal vein sampling because adrenal vein rupture has been reported.[8]

Once a correctable source for primary aldosteronism is found, surgical preparation should include correction of hypokalemia and control of hypertension. Spironolactone for 3 to 6 weeks preoperatively allows for resolution of hypokalemia, blood pressure control, and return of function to the contralateral adrenal gland (which may be suppressed for the primary lesion).[5] This regimen helps to minimize the operative risk of stroke, myocardial infarction, and arrhythmia. Amiloride, a potassium-sparing diuretic, and calcium channel blockers can be used to help control blood pressure. The adrenalectomy can then be performed.

Cushing's Syndrome

Cushing's syndrome is the result of glucocorticoid excess. The most common cause of glucocorticoid excess is exogenous administration. Exogenous steroid administration can occur concomitantly with endogenous hypercortisolism. Therefore, it is imperative to identify all potential sources of cortisol excess in patients. Careful history, medication review, and physical examination are needed to identify all causes of corticosteroid excess.

The endogenous causes of hypercortisolism are divided into adrenocorticotropic hormone (ACTH)–dependent causes in 85% and ACTH-independent causes in 15% (Table 39-1).[9] When screening for Cushing's syndrome, 24-hour urinary free cortisol is the preferred test. This test should be repeated three times before the diagnosis of hypercortisolism can be safely

excluded.[10] Measuring urinary creatinine helps ensure adequate urine collection.[10] Pseudo-Cushing states such as anxiety, depression, alcoholism, diabetes, pregnancy, and polycystic ovary syndrome can cause elevation of plasma cortisol.[9,11] Because urinary free cortisol testing will miss some patients with subclinical Cushing's syndrome and for the reasons listed earlier, it is recommended to confirm the diagnosis with low-dose dexamethasone suppression testing, nocturnal plasma cortisol tests, and late-night salivary cortisol testing.

The next step, once the diagnosis of Cushing's syndrome is made, is differentiating between ACTH-dependent and ACTH-independent Cushing's syndrome. Serum measurement of ACTH usually differentiates between these two. When in doubt, this finding can be confirmed with a corticotropin-releasing hormone stimulation test.

Imaging of the adrenal is warranted in all cases of ACTH-independent Cushing's syndrome. CT and MRI scans offer good anatomic detail. Typically the contralateral adrenal gland is atrophied. Adrenal adenoma and adrenocortical carcinoma are the two most likely encountered lesions.[9] Adrenal adenomas are typically >2 and <6 cm.

Many of these patients have hypertension, diabetes, and obesity and require adequate blood pressure, electrolyte, and glucose control preoperatively. These patients need steroid administration at the time of the surgical procedure that will be continued postoperatively. For patients with significant preoperative symptoms, adrenal enzyme inhibitors such as metyrapone, aminoglutethimide, and ketoconazole can also be used. Because these drugs provide only temporary blockage, some of these patients may also need preoperative mineralocorticoid and glucocorticoid supplementation.[12]

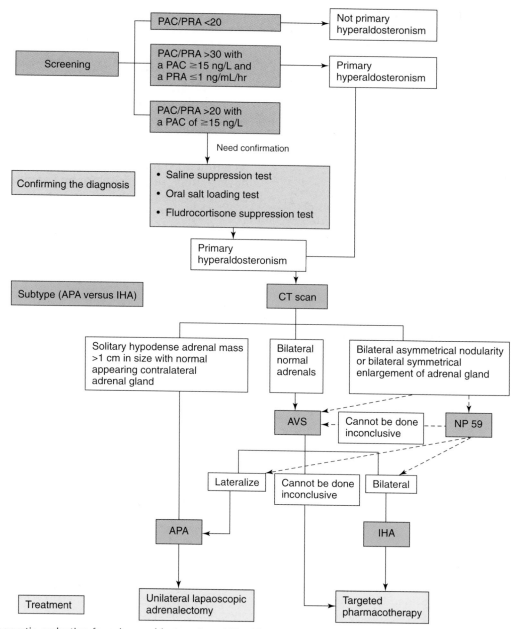

Figure 39-1 Diagnostic evaluation for primary aldosteronism. APA, aldosterone-producing adenoma; AVS, adrenal vein sampling; IHA, idiopathic hyperaldosteronism; NP, adrenal scintigraphy with ^{131}I-labeled 6-beta-iodomethyl-19-norcholesterol; PAC, plasma aldosterone concentration; PRA, plasma renin activity. *(From Al Fehaily M, Duh Q. Clinical manifestation of aldosteronoma. Surg Clin North Am. 2004;84[3]:887-905.)*

Pheochromocytoma

Any patient with unexplained, episodic hypertension or patients with recurrent episodes of tachycardia, dizziness, sweating, flushing, "spells," and headache should be screened for pheochromocytoma. These tumors tend to occur sporadically but can be seen in inherited syndromes such as multiple endocrine neoplasia types 2A and 2B and von Hippel–Lindau disease, among others. Given that some patients have only mild symptoms, thorough history and physical examination are impor-

tant especially when evaluating a patient with an incidentally discovered adrenal mass.

If the diagnosis of pheochromocytoma is not made preoperatively, this can lead to major intraoperative complications. Urinary metanephrines and catecholamines are still widely used as screening tests with good sensitivity and specificity. Plasma free metanephrines have a near 100% sensitivity with good specificity and are becoming the preferential screening test.[13,14] If the plasma free metanephrines are only slightly elevated,

BOX 39-2	Medications That May Cause False-Positive Results for Catecholamines and Metanephrines

Tricyclic antidepressants and antipsychotic agents
Levodopa
Drugs containing catecholamines
Ethanol
Withdrawal from clonidine and other drugs
Acetaminophen and phenoxybenzamine (plasma metanephrines)
Major physical stress (e.g., surgery, stroke, obstructive sleep apnea)
Labetalol and sotalol (can interfere with the spectrophotometric assay for metanephrines; measurements of catecholamines and metanephrines are not affected by most antihypertensive agents)

From Kudva YC, Sawka AM, Young WF. The laboratory diagnosis of adrenal pheochromocytoma: the Mayo Clinic experience. *J Clin Endocrinol Metab.* 2003;88(10):4533-4539.

then a clonidine suppression test can be performed to help make a diagnosis.[15] The causes of false-positive results are depicted in Box 39-2.[14]

CT and MRI of the abdomen and pelvis are both acceptable imaging modalities with high sensitivity and specificity. MRI is preferred because patients must have adequate α- and β-blockade before intravenous contrast administration for a CT scan, given that contrast can precipitate a hypertensive crisis. MRI also allows for imaging in children, in patients with allergies to contrast material, and in pregnant women.[16] Imaging should be closely inspected in patients with familial syndromes and in children. Abdominal and pelvic imaging is important because >10% of lesions occur outside the adrenal gland. Metaiodobenzylguanidine (MIBG) functional scanning may be helpful in localizing small lesions, extra-adrenal sites, and metastasis in patients with pheochromocytoma.[7] Drugs such as labetalol and tricyclic antidepressants can interfere with MIBG scans and must be discontinued well in advance of scanning.[17]

Preoperative management of patients with pheochromocytoma is essential to prevent intraoperative complications such as hypertensive crisis, cardiac ischemia, cardiac arrhythmia, and pulmonary edema.[17] Preoperative α-adrenergic blockade with phenoxybenzamine or doxazosin is highly recommended. A starting dose of 10 mg of phenoxybenzamine twice daily with increases of 10 to 20 mg daily to a total dose of 1 mg/kg is usually sufficient.[17] β-Adrenergic blockade and calcium channel blockade may also be necessary in addition to α-blockade before the surgical procedure. If blood pressure control is still not adequate, the addition of α-methyl-*para*-tyrosine may be useful.[18] Because patients have contracted blood volumes preoperatively, adequate salt and water intake is important. A thorough preoperative anesthesia evaluation should be performed as well.

Adrenal Carcinoma

Adrenal carcinomas can be hormonally active or nonfunctioning. These tumors tend to be a cause of virilization more often than do hyperfunctioning cortisol-secreting adenomas.[19] At the time of diagnosis, most adrenal carcinomas are typically >5 cm and resection is recommended for all lesions >6 cm.[20,21] Adrenal cancers have a high propensity to invade adjacent organs.[20] Invasion can be missed on preoperative imaging so the operating surgeon must have a high index of suspicion for adrenal carcinoma before surgical removal. Metastatic evaluation is also important preoperatively.

Because the preferred management of this disease is surgical removal, preparation for en bloc resection and knowledge of surrounding anatomic features are crucial. Patients must also be aware that that adjacent organ removal may be necessary because the best hope for cure is total resection. Intraoperatively, the anesthesia team should be prepared for the possibility of a long surgical procedure with significant blood loss.

Adrenal Incidentaloma

The critical determination in the evaluation of an incidentally discovered adrenal lesion is whether the lesion is hyperfunctioning. Careful history and physical examination may reveal undiagnosed signs of adrenal disease. Laboratory evaluation to rule out a hyperfunctioning adenoma and especially a pheochromocytoma should be performed in all cases.[7] Because some adrenal adenomas turn out to be pheochromocytomas, this diagnosis must be excluded before the surgical procedure (Table 39-2). Accurate diagnosis preoperatively can avoid intraoperative and postoperative complications. Imaging can be helpful as well because certain diseases have specific characteristics on CT and MRI.[19] Table 39-3 summarizes the different radiographic appearances and characteristics of adrenal tumors. Box 39-3 highlights common errors that can be made during the diagnostic evaluation of adrenal masses.

SURGICAL APPROACHES AND INTRAOPERATIVE COMPLICATIONS

Both laparoscopic and open approaches can be used for adrenalectomy. In a comparative evaluation of 50 laparoscopic adrenalectomy studies and 48 open adrenalectomy studies with >3700 patients total, Brunt[1] revealed that laparoscopic adrenal surgery was associated with a decrease in complications and a shorter duration of hospitalization. In the last few years, most adrenal surgery publications have promoted laparoscopic adrenalectomy as the treatment of choice for most

TABLE 39-2	Evaluation of Adrenal Tumors	
Hypersecretory State	**Prevalence (%)**	**Screening Test**
Hypercortisolism	5-14	Urinary free cortisol, adrenocorticotropic hormone, cortisol rhythm, 1-mg dexamethasone suppression test
Hyperaldosteronism	1.5-3.3	Potassium, aldosterone-to-plasma renin activity ratio
Congenital adrenal hyperplasia	Rare	Adrenocorticotropic hormone test
Virilization	0-11	Dehydroepiandrosterone, testosterone
Feminization	Rare	Estradiol
Pheochromocytoma	1.5-25	Urinary catecholamines/metanephrines

From Barzon L, Boscaro M. Diagnosis and management of adrenal incidentalomas. *J Urol.* 2000;163(2):398-407.

TABLE 39-3	Radiographic Appearances and Characteristics of Adrenal Tumors			
Variable	**Adrenocortical Adenoma**	**Adrenocortical Carcinoma**	**Pheochromocytoma**	**Metastasis**
Size	Small, usually ≤3 cm in diameter	Large, usually >4 cm in diameter	Large, usually >3 cm in diameter	Variable, frequently <3 cm
Shape	Round or oval, with smooth margins	Irregular, with unclear margins	Round or oval, with clear margins	Oval or irregular, with unclear margins
Texture	Homogeneous	Heterogeneous, with mixed densities	Heterogeneous, with cystic areas	Heterogeneous, with mixed densities
Laterality	Usually solitary, unilateral	Usually solitary, unilateral	Usually solitary, unilateral	Often bilateral
Attenuation (density) on enhanced CT	≤10 Hounsfield units	>10 Hounsfield units (usually >25)	>10 Hounsfield units (usually >25)	>10 Hounsfield units (usually >25)
Vascularity on contrast-enhanced CT	Not highly vascular	Usually vascular	Usually vascular	Usually vascular
Rapidity of washout of contrast medium	≥50% at 10 min	<50% at 10 min	<50% at 10 min	<50% at 10 min
Appearance on MRI[†]	Isointense in relation to liver on T_2-weighted image	Hyperintense in relation to liver on T_2-weighted image	Markedly hyperintense in relation to liver on T_2-weighted image	Hyperintense in relation to liver on T_2-weighted image
Necrosis, hemorrhage, or calcifications	Rare	Common	Hemorrhage and cystic areas common	Occasional hemorrhage and cystic areas
Growth rate	Usually stable over time or very slow (<1 cm/yr)	Usually rapid (>2 cm/yr)	Usually slow (0.5-1.0 cm/yr)	Variable, slow to rapid

*Adrenal hemorrhage and myelolipoma are usually easily characterized because of their distinctive imaging characteristics.[24,25] Myelolipomas are composed of myeloid, erythroid, and adipose tissue. On imaging, they have low attenuation on unenhanced CT, and they are hyperintense on T_1-weighted in-phase MRI. The presence of pure fat within an adrenal lesion on CT is consistent with the presence of myelolipoma. Acute adrenal hemorrhage has increased attenuation on unenhanced CT, and on T_1-weighted MRI, one sees hyperintensity secondary to methemoglobin. In chronic adrenal hemorrhage, a dark rim develops along the periphery of the mass on the T_2-weighted image because of the hemosiderin-laden macrophages.
†If the imaging characteristics are indeterminate on both unenhanced and enhanced CT, MRI may be considered to clarify the imaging phenotype.
CT, computed tomography; MRI, magnetic resonance imaging.
From Young WF. Clinical practice: the incidentally discovered adrenal mass. *N Engl J Med.* 2007;356(6):601-610.

hyperfunctioning adenomas and incidentalomas. Considerable debate exists about the management of lesions >6 cm, but a growing body of literature has demonstrated safe removal of lesions >6 cm. Although some surgeons have had some success with the removal of adrenal carcinoma laparoscopically,[22-24] the National Institutes of Health consensus is that these tumors and tumors >6 cm should be removed through an open approach.[21]

Before incision, patients should have sequential compression devices placed and should receive perioperative antibiotics. Because most laparoscopic and open procedures involve a flank approach or a modified flank approach, appropriate padding of the patient's arms,

BOX 39-3	**Common Errors That Can Be Made During the Diagnostic Evaluation of Adrenal Masses: Pitfalls in the Diagnosis of Surgical Adrenal Disorders**

Primary Aldosteronism

Challenge with sodium loading (10 g/day) before measuring plasma potassium (K+)

Repletion of K+ to normalize plasma K+ before measuring plasma or urinary aldosterone

Complete reliance on a postural aldosterone stimulation test (70% accuracy)

Failure to measure cortisol during adrenal vein sampling of aldosterone to validate correct positioning

Failure to recognize bilateral adrenal hyperplasia

Adrenal hemorrhage during adrenal vein sampling

Cushing's Syndrome Resulting From Adrenal Adenoma or Carcinoma

Failure to identify the use of exogenous steroids causing Cushing's syndrome

Inadequate physical examination essential for the diagnosis

Knowledge that alcoholism and depression can mildly elevate plasma cortisol (pseudo-Cushing's syndrome)

Inability to diagnose pituitary Cushing's syndrome by finding elevated plasma adrenocorticotropic hormone

Adrenal Carcinoma

Evaluation for metastatic disease

Incidentaloma

Metabolic evaluation to identify functional lesions

MRI to determine tissue composition

Pheochromocytoma

Careful evaluation to reveal multiple lesions

Measurement of urinary catecholes and metabolites even if plasma catecholes are normal

Evaluation for other components when multiple endocrine abnormality syndromes are suspected

From Vaughan ED. Diseases of the adrenal gland. *Med Clin North Am.* 2004;88(2):443-466.

legs, and torso is important. When patients are obese, a flank position in both the open and laparoscopic approach will allow the pannus to fall away and thus will make placement of instruments easier.[25] Patients with pheochromocytoma and some with aldosterone-producing adenomas should be well hydrated before induction of anesthesia. In patients with pheochromocytoma and adrenal cortical carcinoma, thought should also be given to pulmonary artery catheterization and arterial line placement because significant hemodynamic changes should be expected.[26] Correction of hypokalemia, control of blood pressure, and tight glycemic control should all be assessed before induction of anesthesia. Patients with Cushing's syndrome should receive glucocorticoids in the perioperative period.

The most common complications encountered during open adrenal surgery are hemorrhage, wound problems, adjacent organ injury, infections, and pulmonary problems. In the laparoscopic approach the incidence of all these problems with the exception of bleeding is significantly reduced.[1] Regardless of the approach, attention to surgical technique and knowledge of adrenal anatomy are crucial to performing successful adrenalectomy.

Port placement should be selected based on the type of laparoscopic approach used by the surgeon. Retroperitoneoscopy offers the advantages of less intra-abdominal organ manipulation. It may have some benefit for recovery but comes at the cost of a smaller working space and for some surgeons a less familiar view of the retroperitoneum compared with the transabdominal approach.[27] Retroperitoneoscopic adrenalectomy may also be favorable in the setting of previous abdominal surgery in which adhesions may complicate or limit a transabdominal open or laparoscopic approach.[28]

A transabdominal laparoscopic approach to the adrenal gland is still the most common approach. It affords a larger work space with a more familiar approach to the abdomen and may permit easier removal of large masses when compared with a retroperitoneoscopic approach.[29] In addition, during difficult dissections, a hand port can be easily placed during transperitoneal surgery to combine the benefits of tactile feedback with minimally invasive techniques.[30]

Closure of the fascia at the port sites and any incision will limit the occurrence of hernias and is particularly important in patients with Cushing's syndrome, who are prone to poor wound healing, and after transperitoneal laparoscopic adrenalectomy to limit the incidence of bowel entrapment.[31] After placing all ports it is imperative to assess for injuries from port site placement including bleeding and solid organ injury because these complications may occur during port placement.

The induction of pneumoperitoneum can cause a significant increase in circulating catecholamines in patients with pheochromocytoma. Insufflation pressures of ≤10 mm Hg have been shown to limit this catecholamine rise. This technique may help prevent cardiovascular complications before any manipulation of the adrenal gland.[26,32] Conversely, high insufflation pressures during adrenal surgery may increase the working space and tamponade bleeding vessels. Case-by-case evaluation is crucial, and high insufflation pressures should be used with caution in patients with pheochromocytoma. As always, it is important to lower the pressure at the completion of the surgical procedure to inspect for sites of bleeding.[33]

The approach for adrenalectomy should reflect the underlying pathologic process. For large tumors suggestive of adrenal cortical carcinoma, it is best to approach these cases with the possibility that multiple surrounding organs may need to be resected along with the vena cava.[34] Preparation for this is important. Accessing and obtaining vascular control are important considerations in the choice for the location of the incision. Because of high local disease recurrence rates, a laparoscopic approach is not favored for lesions that are clearly malignant.[34] Some surgeons advocate exploring large lesions laparoscopically when preoperative imaging shows no evidence of malignancy and no evidence of surrounding organ invasion (**Fig. 39-2**). Most surgeons recommend that once an adrenal carcinoma is encoun-

tered, the procedure should be converted to an open approach.[22,35]

When using a lateral flank approach, care should be taken to avoid the neurovascular bundle that runs in the bed of the 11th rib (**Fig. 39-3**). Damage can cause muscle prolapse or a flank hernia, both of which are difficult to treat. If a thoracoabdominal approach or flank approach is chosen, attention must be turned to the possibility of pleural violation and pneumothorax. A large violation is best treated with a chest tube connected to a −20-cm contained vacuum device. Smaller rents in the pleura can be easily treated and resolved intraoperatively by using a red rubber catheter to evacuate any air that is present. A pursestring suture is used to close the pleura and closure of the fascial layers occurs around the catheter, the open end of which is subsequently placed in a small container of saline solution or water. Under positive pressure, the pneumothorax is then "bubbled out" through the catheter. The catheter is removed after wound closure.

Postoperative chest radiographs should be checked in these patients. If a significant residual or expanding pneumothorax is still evident, chest tube placement may be needed.[36]

Knowledge of the relationship of the adrenal gland with other abdominal and retroperitoneal organs and the neighboring vasculature is crucial (**Fig. 39-4**). This knowledge is particularly important during mobilization of surrounding organs for exposure and when the diagnosis of adrenal cortical carcinoma is considered because en bloc organ resection may be necessary (**Fig. 39-5**).[34] During a transabdominal approach, the spleen and tail of the pancreas need to be clearly visualized and

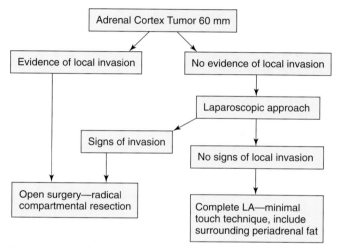

Figure 39-2 Algorithm for the surgical management of adrenal tumors ≥60 mm in diameter. LA, laparoscopic adrenalectomy. *(From Palazzo, FF, Sebag, F, Sierra, M, et al. Long-term outcome following laparoscopic adrenalectomy for large solid adrenal cortex tumors. World J Surg. 2006;30[5]:893-898.)*

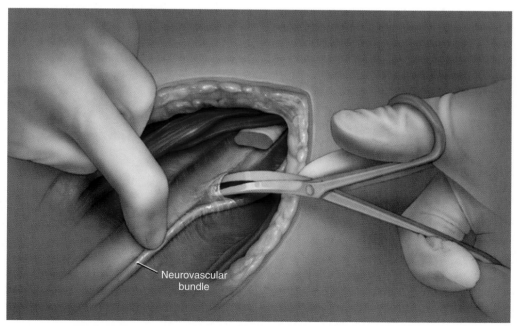

Figure 39-3 Dissection of the intercostal nerve during flank surgery. *(From George, K, Chow, MLB. Surgery of the adrenal glands. In: Wein AJ, Novick A, Partin A, Peters C, eds. Campbell-Walsh Urology, 9th ed. Philadelphia: WB Saunders; 2007:1868-1889.)*

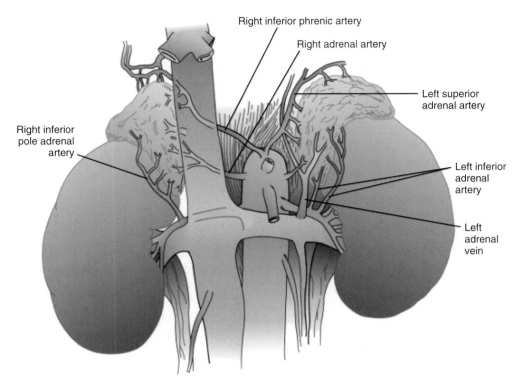

Figure 39-4   Vascular relationships. *(From Duh Q-Y, Yeh MW. The adrenal glands. In: Townsend CM, Beauchamp RD, Evers BM, Mattox KL, eds. Sabiston Textbook of Surgery, 18th ed. Philadelphia: WB Saunders; 2007.)*

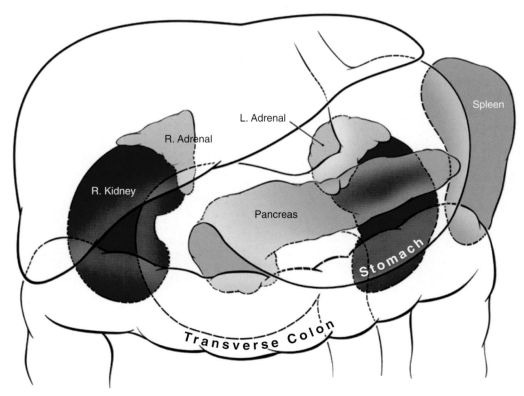

Figure 39-5   Visceral relationships. *(From George, K, Chow, MLB. Surgery of the adrenal glands. In: Wein AJ, Novick A, Partin A, Peters C, eds. Campbell-Walsh Urology, 9th ed. Philadelphia: WB Saunders; 2007:1868-1889.)*

dissected free from the adrenal gland. If a pancreatic injury is suspected drains should be left in place and care should be undertaken with dietary advancement until the type of drainage fluid is determined. If the splenic capsule has a small violation, splenorrhaphy can be performed.

For large injuries, splenectomy may be necessary. If a colon injury occurs during mobilization, repair can be attempted for serosal tears and in cases with no contamination. Spillage of enteric contents and significant bowel injury are exceedingly rare and should warrant definitive expert repair in accordance with general surgical principles.[37]

Meticulous planning and the implementation of every possible precaution will decrease the risk of complications during adrenalectomy. Preoperative bowel preparation may reduce colonic volume and make mobilization easier, especially in laparoscopic procedures, which should include placement of an orogastric or nasogastric tube. During laparoscopic adrenalectomies, once the spleen and colon are mobilized, positioning the table to elevate the left side allows these organs to fall medially and thus aid adrenal exposure.[38] When dissecting around the upper pole of the kidney it is important to limit the amount of posterior mobilization to prevent the kidney from falling medially and impairing adrenal visualization.

For right-sided lesions, liver and ascending colon are the most prominent organs requiring mobilization for visualization of the adrenal gland. These structures, as well as the inferior vena cava, duodenum, and head of the pancreas, must be clearly identified during dissection. A Kocher maneuver may be helpful to expose the inferior vena cava and any short right adrenal veins. In the laparoscopic approach an extra port may be needed to elevate the liver for adequate exposure.[39] In patients with significant retroperitoneal fat or in patients whose adrenal gland is difficult to identify, laparoscopic ultrasound examination has been successfully used not only to identify the adrenal gland but also to establish its relationship with the inferior vena cava and surrounding structures.[40-43]

Early control of the adrenal vein facilitates the surgical procedure and decreases blood loss. In the case of pheochromocytoma, early ligation of the adrenal vein is paramount because it limits catecholamine surge and helps to protect the patient from vascular compromise.[44,45] Although minimizing manipulation of the adrenal gland is important for all tumors to prevent capsular violation, it is particularly important in pheochromocytoma because this is the time of peak catecholamine levels during the operation. As mentioned earlier, preoperative management of patients with pheochromocytoma is essential, and α-adrenergic blockade with phenoxybenzamine or doxazosin is highly recommended. β-Adrenergic blockade and calcium channel blockade may also be useful, as may

the addition of α-methyl-*para*-tyrosine.[18] Adequate fluid intake and resuscitation are important. Minimizing adrenal gland manipulation is essential in patients with potentially malignant lesions to prevent tumor spillage and peritoneal contamination.[22,26,35,46,47]

Vascular injuries are common in adrenal surgery. The most frequently injured vascular structures are the inferior vena cava and the adrenal vein. Avulsion of the adrenal vein can cause significant bleeding, and special attention to the short length of the right adrenal vein is important. When a vascular injury is identified, use of compression, application of Allis clamps, intracorporeal suturing, clipping, or stapling, volume resuscitation, and communication with the anesthesiologist may all be necessary to control hemorrhage.[48,49] If the procedure is performed laparoscopically, the surgeon should not hesitate to convert it to an open operation if laparoscopic control is not possible. Having the equipment in the room to convert to an open operation is vital because bleeding may be brisk and may allow little time to wait for instruments.[49] It is also important not to staple over metal clips because this maneuver may hinder proper stapler application and lead to bleeding.[48] When using clips to ligate the adrenal vein, it is recommended to use two clips on the vena cava side to ensure vessel ligation before specimen removal.[50]

Renal artery injuries can occur and cause severe bleeding as well as revascularization and ischemia to the kidney. Identification of the end organ supplied by each artery and vein before ligation is crucial to prevent such injuries.

The surgeon must also recognize the potential for vascular anomalies and multiple adrenal vessels. Accessory adrenal veins can occur ≤10% of the time.[51] Castilho and colleagues[52] reported on converting a laparoscopic adrenalectomy in a child to an open operation when hemorrhage occurred from an unrecognized secondary adrenal vein draining to the liver. Identification and ligation of the branches off the inferior phrenic arteries should be performed when the superomedial portion of the gland is dissected.[47,53] Vascular injury can also happen during port site placement. The inferior epigastric artery as well as major mesenteric and pelvic vessels can be injured during trocar insertion.[39,49]

The role of partial adrenalectomy is debated in the literature; some investigators have reported long-term adrenal salvage rates with partial adrenalectomy particularly in patients with inherited disorders such as multiple endocrine neoplasia and von Hippel–Lindau disease.[54] Some of these patients had recurrent lesions. Many of these patients still required corticosteroid therapy postoperatively and a few had acute addisonian crisis.[54] Another series demonstrated that on pathologic examination of isolated aldosterone-producing adenomas removed by partial or total adrenalectomy, 27% of specimens had multiple adenomas in the specimen. In one series, 2 of 29 patients who underwent partial adrenalectomy had persistent hyperaldosteronism and hypertension, whereas all 63 patients who underwent total adrenalectomy had resolution of the hypertension and improvement in aldosterone levels.[55] At this time, we recommend against partial adrenalectomy in patients with no inherited syndrome and a unilateral adrenal mass. Adrenal-sparing surgery may be considered in patients with inherited syndromes, but these patients must be watched extremely closely for both recurrences and any signs of adrenal insufficiency.

POSTOPERATIVE COMPLICATIONS AND PATIENT MANAGEMENT

The postoperative management of patients undergoing adrenal surgery is dictated largely by the type of adrenal lesion removed (Box 39-4). In the postoperative period, all patients should use incentive spirometry liberally. Early ambulation is strongly encouraged. Sequential compression devices should be placed on both lower extremities. Hospital-specific guidelines on the use of routine postoperative anticoagulation are available in most medical centers. Blood counts and electrolytes should be checked in patients after the surgical procedure and again the following morning.[50] Close blood pressure monitoring is important in all patients. Any concern for bleeding should lead to appropriate and immediate imaging or intervention based on the situation.

Pheochromocytoma

Patients with pheochromocytoma should be monitored closely in either the intensive care unit or an intermediate care unit after the surgical procedure. These patients are at an increased risk for postoperative hypoglycemia, hypertension, and hypotension.[56] Hypoglycemia can occur as a result of rebound hyperinsulinemia after tumor removal.[56] Hypotension results from abrupt withdraw of catecholamines. Volume resuscitation is important in the postoperative period as is the judicious use of catecholamines.[17]

Hyperaldosteronism

After adrenalectomy for an aldosterone-producing adenoma, blood pressure should be monitored very closely and for a prolonged period. These patients are at risk for long-term hypertension, and blood pressure typically falls progressively for a few weeks after adrenalectomy.[5] During hospitalization (and perhaps after discharge), these patients should have daily potassium levels drawn because early potassium replacement may be required. Although rare, some patients may experience salt wasting and hyperkalemia from suppression of the contralateral adrenal gland, and patients must also be monitored for this complication in the postoperative

> **BOX 39-4** **Postoperative Complications of Adrenal Surgery**
>
> **Primary Aldosteronism**
> Hypokalemia: secondary to continued potassium loss immediately postoperatively
> Hyperkalemia: secondary to failure of contralateral adrenal gland to secrete aldosterone
>
> **Cushing's Syndrome**
> Inadequate steroid replacement leading to hypocortisolism
> Fracture secondary to osteoporosis
> Hyperglycemia
> Poor wound healing
> Increased risk of infection
>
> **Pheochromocytoma**
> Hypotension secondary to α-adrenergic blockade after tumor removal
>
> **Generic Complications**
> Hemorrhage
>   Inferior vena cava
>   Adrenal arteries
> Pneumothorax
> Pancreatitis
> Pneumonia
> Hiccups
>
> From Vaughan ED Jr. Complications of adrenal surgery In: Taneja SS, RM Ehrlich RM, Smith RB, eds. *Complications of Urologic Surgery*, 3rd ed. Philadelphia; WB Saunders; 2000:362-369.

period.[5] The use of potassium-sparing diuretics such as spironolactone should be stopped.

Cushing's Syndrome

Patients undergoing bilateral adrenalectomy for Cushing's disease require long-term corticosteroid replacement and are at risk of developing Nelson's syndrome.[9] These patients are also at risk of recurrent episodes of addisonian crisis. Addisonian crisis has been reported after unilateral and partial adrenalectomy; therefore, most patients require at least short-term corticosteroid and mineralocorticoid replacement in the postoperative period and some require long-term treatment.[33,37,50,54] Acute adrenal insufficiency may manifest with fever, nausea, vomiting, lethargy, and hypotension. Any patients presenting with these symptoms after adrenal surgery should be treated with dexamethasone and electrolyte correction until the diagnosis is made (Table 39-4).[50] Patients with severe manifestations of Cushing's syndrome are a higher risk for infectious and wound complications and should be watched closely. Patients with Cushing's disease have a persistent risk of fracture from osteoporosis and should be clinically monitored.[10]

Other postoperative complications can include infections such as pneumonia, urinary tract colonization,

TABLE 39-4	Symptoms and Signs in Acute Adrenocortical Insufficiency ("Adrenal Crisis")	
Symptoms and Signs (Clinical Deterioration Without Obvious Cause)		**Prevalence (%)**
Fever		70
Nausea and vomiting		64
Abdominal pain		46
Hypotension		36
Abdominal distention		32
Obtundation and lethargy		26
Hyponatremia		45
Hyperkalemia		25

Modified from May ME, Vaughan ED Jr, Carey RM. Adrenocortical insufficiency: clinical aspects. In: Vaughan ED Jr, Carey RM, eds. *Adrenal Disorders.* New York: Thieme; 1989:176; and Duh Q-Y, Yeh MW. The adrenal glands. In: Townsend CM, Beauchamp RD, Evers BM, Mattox KL, eds. *Sabiston Textbook of Surgery,* 18th ed. Philadelphia: WB Saunders; 2007.

abscess formation, and sepsis. Pancreatitis can occur from manipulation of the pancreas in addition to an overt injury. Port site complications can include hernias and hematomas. Patients may have delayed bleeding, delayed recognition of bowel injuries, and unrecognized or increasing pneumothorax. Patients should be evaluated and treated for these conditions based on their individual clinical situations. For delayed bleeding, reoperation may be necessary.[38] Local recurrences after adrenalectomy for adrenal cortical carcinoma can be seen after open and laparoscopic adrenalectomy. Patients undergoing laparoscopic adrenalectomy for malignant disease are also at risk for port site recurrences. Any patient with adrenal cortical carcinoma should be followed closely with imaging for recurrence.[34]

With a proficient knowledge of underlying adrenal disease, solid open and laparoscopic surgical technique, and a thorough awareness of the spatial relationships between the adrenal and surrounding vascular and visceral structures, surgeons can avoid or at least minimize many of the complications of adrenal surgery.

KEY POINTS

1. With the widespread use of laparoscopy, the landscape of adrenal surgery has changed dramatically over the past decade.
2. Complications associated with adrenal surgery are most often uniquely related to the underlying pathology of the disease under treatment.
3. Many adrenal surgical complications can be avoided with a rigorous diagnostic evaluation and a meticulous preoperative preparation.

REFERENCES

Please see www.expertconsult.com

Chapter 40

COMPLICATIONS OF LYMPHADENECTOMY

Ofer Yossepowitch MD
Attending Surgeon, Department of Urology, Rabin Medical Center, Petah-Tikva, Israel

Bernard H. Bochner MD
Attending Surgeon, Department of Surgery, Urology Service, Memorial Sloan-Kettering Cancer Center, New York, New York

Lymphadenectomy, the excision of the regional lymph nodes draining a tumor, is a mainstay in the surgical management of solid cancers. The procedure is essential to accurate nodal staging, which allows for uniform assessment of treatment outcomes across institutions as well as appropriate selection of candidates for additional therapies. For some cancers, lymphadenectomy has been shown to provide a therapeutic benefit. As with all surgical interventions, lymph node dissection has the potential for adverse side effects. Nevertheless, until advances in imaging and molecular markers allow for accurate assessment of nodal involvement preoperatively, lymph node dissections will continue to be of paramount importance to patients and physicians.

This chapter describes the complications associated with lymph node dissection for genitourinary malignant diseases. The intent is not only to help urologists manage these complications but also, more importantly, to help avoid these complications. Fundamental techniques and anatomic considerations that should be employed in the perioperative and operative settings are highlighted.

PELVIC LYMPH NODE DISSECTION

Removal of the pelvic lymph nodes provides diagnostic or therapeutic benefit for several major urologic malignant diseases, including bladder, prostate, and penile cancers. Although the indications and anatomic boundaries of pelvic lymph node dissection (PLND) in prostate cancer remain an area of contention, extended lymphadenectomy is now becoming a standard of care for patients undergoing radical cystectomy for muscle-invasive bladder cancer.

Radical Prostatectomy

PLND at the time of radical prostatectomy improves the accuracy of prostate cancer staging. In an era of down-ward stage migration in which many cancers harbor favorable characteristics,[1] however, a pertinent question remains whether all men newly diagnosed with low-risk, localized prostate cancer truly benefit from PLND. Opponents quote the low incidence of lymph node involvement in prostate cancer and recommend employing risk stratification models to omit PLND in men with a low risk of lymph node metastasis.[2,3] Proponents argue that currently available predictive tools are unreliable because of sampling error (i.e., models are based on limited data from inadequate dissections) and the evolution of Gleason score interpretations over time.[4]

Furthermore, an increasing body of evidence suggests that PLND improves not only staging but also recurrence-free survival.[5,6] Investigators generally agree that imaging studies, including computed tomography (CT) and magnetic resonance imaging (MRI) of the pelvis, lack the sensitivity required to supplant the reference standard of PLND. Two techniques that show promise for detection of occult lymph node metastases are positron emission tomography[7] and MRI combined with intravenous lymphotrophic superparamagnetic nanoparticles.[8] These techniques, however, require further validation before they can be incorporated into routine clinical practice.

For PLND in prostate cancer, the anatomic boundaries (i.e., extent) of dissection remain controversial. Prostate lymphatic vessels may drain by way of three major routes: ascending ducts into the external iliac lymph nodes, lateral ducts into the hypogastric and obturator lymph nodes, and posterior ducts into the sacral lymph nodes.[9] The limited PLND or node sampling for prostate cancer, as performed by many urologists, typically includes only a portion of the lymphatic tissue between the external iliac vein and obturator nerve.

Proper lymph node dissection as originally described by McCullough and associates[10] and later reiterated by Bader and colleagues[11] should include all the tissue between the external iliac vein and hypogastric vein, above and below the obturator nerve, including the obturator and hypogastric nodes. Additionally, some investigators recommend including the common iliac and presacral nodes.[5] Compared with limited PLND, appropriate dissections result in a greater node yield and a higher incidence of positive lymph node results.[12]

In one large series of PLNDs for prostate cancer, the reported incidence of lymph node metastases reached 24% in patients with a prostate-specific antigen (PSA) value of ≥10 and a Gleason score of ≥7.[11] Moreover, approximately 70% of positive lymph nodes were located along the internal iliac vessels. In approximately 20% of node-positive patients, this was the sole location of lymph node involvement and, in fact, nodal metastases were more likely to be found in the hypogastric and obturator nodes than in the external iliac nodes.

Taken together, these data provide strong support for extended PLND in patients undergoing radical prostatectomy, particularly for those with moderate- to high-risk cancers. The major concern deterring many urologists from adopting this approach is the higher incidence of morbidity.[13,14]

Radical Cystectomy

The extent of lymph node dissection required to stage and treat bladder cancer optimally at the time of radical cystectomy is equally controversial. Investigators generally agree that lymph node dissection is an important part of the surgical management of bladder cancer. In patients with invasive bladder cancer, the regional lymphatics are frequently involved and not uncommonly represent the only site of metastatic disease. Lymph node involvement, one of the strongest adverse prognostic features, is often used to determine the subsequent treatment strategy and the need for adjuvant therapy.[15] PLND not only provides valuable staging information but also enhances the rate of local disease control and survival.[16]

Despite the growing body of evidence to support the use of more extended dissection at cystectomy, no guidelines regarding the optimal boundaries of PLND have been established.[17] Mapping series indicate that the common iliac and presacral nodal regions are more frequently involved with tumor metastases than was previously recognized.[18-20]

In fact, 35% of the 599 positive lymph nodes identified in the series by Leissner and colleagues[18] were located above the bifurcation of the common iliac vessels, outside the limits of a standard lymphadenectomy template. More than half the node-positive patients had nodal metastases in the common iliac lymph nodes, and nearly one third had nodal metastases in the region of the distal aorta. These investigators concluded that had they restricted the nodal resection to the obturator fossa, >74% of all lymph node metastases would have been left behind, and 7% of patients

would have been incorrectly categorized as having lymph nodes negative for cancer. Similarly, Vazina and associates[20] demonstrated that among node-positive patients in their series, 20% with pT2 disease and 30% with pT3 disease had nodal metastases located cephalad to the bifurcation of the common iliac vessels.

Some studies support extending lymph node dissection to include all areas below the aortic bifurcation.[21,22] Several investigators reported that removal of an increased number of lymph nodes at cystectomy improved survival. This association was maintained when controlling for age and other comorbidities, features that could affect the decision to perform extensive node dissection or could influence overall and disease-specific survival.[23] Thus, based on available evidence and despite the lack of randomized trials investigating the impact of dissection boundaries on outcome, many investigators believe that the most reliable diagnostic and therapeutic approach to bladder cancer includes routine extended PLND in all patients undergoing cystectomy with curative intent. Exceptions to this recommendation include salvage radical cystectomy following definitive radiation treatment (>5000 rads). In these patients, care should be taken because extended lymphadenectomy may be associated with additional morbidity.[24]

Complications

Perioperative complications associated with PLND can be classified as local or systemic. Local complications may include deep vein thrombosis, pelvic hemorrhage, abscess formation, wound infection, and wound dehiscence. Systemic problems may include pulmonary embolism, pulmonary atelectasis, pneumonia, myocardial infarction, congestive heart failure, arrhythmias, and prolonged ileus. Additional specific complications of lymphadenectomy include pelvic neuropathies, lymphocele formation, vascular injuries, and lymphedema of the lower extremities. Nerve injures and lymphoceles are discussed in the sections that follow. Lymphedema is discussed in detail in the later section on inguinal lymphadenectomy for carcinoma of the penis.

Nerve Injuries

The spatial relationship between the pelvic lymph node chains and pelvic nerves puts pelvic nerves at risk for injury during PLND. Nerve injuries fall into three general categories,[25] as follows:

1. *Neurapraxia* is a functional injury caused by nerve compression or traction and resulting in a conduction block without overt axonal degeneration. Recovery from neurapraxia is expected to occur within a matter of weeks.
2. *Axonotmesis*, a more severe injury caused by prolonged compression or excessive traction, is charac-

terized by wallerian degeneration in which the neural elements distal to the injury site degenerate, whereas the supporting neuronal structures and envelopes (epineurium, perineurium, and endoneurium) remain intact. The supporting neuronal structures allow for nerve regeneration, and function recovers slowly over 6 months to 1 year.

3. *Neurotmesis,* the third and most severe form of injury, denotes complete division of the nerve. Recovery from neurotmesis is not expected.

Nerves that may suffer injury during major pelvic surgery for urologic malignant diseases include the obturator, femoral, and genitofemoral nerves. Injury to the sciatic nerve is extremely rare and is not addressed in this chapter.

Obturator Nerve Injury

Anatomic and Functional Considerations The obturator nerve innervates the medial adductor muscles of the thigh, namely, the gracilis, pectineus, adductor longus, adductor brevis, and adductor magnus (the most powerful adductor), as well as the obturator externus. These thigh adductors also act to a varying extent as flexors, extensors, and rotators of the leg. After arising from the L2-L4 segments of the lumbar plexus, the obturator nerve pierces the medial border of the psoas muscle and enters the pelvic cavity along the lateral pelvic wall within the obturator fossa. The nerve travels parallel to the pelvic sidewall usually above the obturator artery and vein and leaves the pelvis through the obturator foramen accompanied by the obturator vessels.

Although the obturator nerve receives sensory input from the medial aspect of the thigh, it is the only motor nerve that arises from the lumbar plexus and passes through the pelvis without innervating any of the pelvic organs. As such, this nerve can be completely dissected and mobilized within the obturator fossa without risk of denervating any of the pelvic organs. Injury to the obturator nerve itself during PLND is possible by excessive traction, crush, use of electrocautery in close proximity to the nerve, or inadvertent nerve transection.[26] Prolonged surgery associated with acute hip flexion has also been implicated in this type of injury.[27]

Clinical sequelae of obturator nerve injury can include motor deficits, sensory symptoms, or both.[26] The sensory component typically manifests as pain and diminished sensation, which extends down the medial thigh into the knee and occasionally into the hip. The pain is commonly exacerbated by extension and abduction or inward thigh rotation. When clinically apparent, weakness of the ipsilateral hip adductors may vary in severity and can be quite debilitating, particularly when the patient tries to drive an automobile.

Occasionally, electromyography is required to diagnose and isolate the motor component, particularly if symptoms are equivocal. In patients who have under-

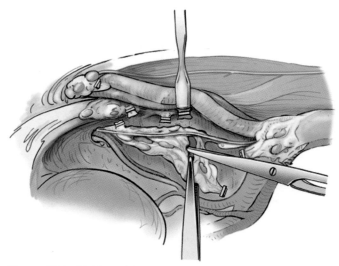

Figure 40-1 Division of the node packet, proximally and distally, should be performed only after clear visualization of the nerve throughout its entire course within the obturator fossa.

gone complete nerve resection, spontaneous recovery, when it occurs, is likely to result from a compensatory response by other thigh muscles or from the presence of an accessory obturator nerve.[28]

Technical Highlights and Intraoperative Techniques to Avoid Injury The key to avoiding damage to the obturator nerve is sound knowledge of its anatomic course and relationship to pelvic structures. Damage to the nerve typically occurs during the proximal or distal aspect of the lymph node dissection. Identifying the lymph node of Cloquet (marking the distal limit of the dissection above Cooper's ligament) is a mandatory step. Dissection above Cooper's ligament is generally safe, but any dissection below this landmark should be carried out with great attention because it may lead to inadvertent nerve damage. Proximally, the nerve can be identified lateral to the bifurcation of the common iliac vessels as it exits the psoas muscle. Complete exposure of the nerve is facilitated by its careful dissection laterally away from the accompanying obturator vessels and nodes (**Fig. 40-1**). Node packet division, proximal and distal, should be performed only after the nerve can be visualized throughout its entire course within the obturator fossa.

Traction injury or partial or complete transection of the nerve may occur while the nerve is freed from the lymph node packet within the obturator fossa. The nerve may be predisposed to injury in patients with tumor involvement of the obturator nodes, prior chemotherapy with subsequent tumor scarring, or prior pelvic irradiation because the perineural tissues may be particularly adherent to surrounding tissues. Additionally, abrupt bleeding during dissection may necessitate electrocautery in proximity to the nerve or application

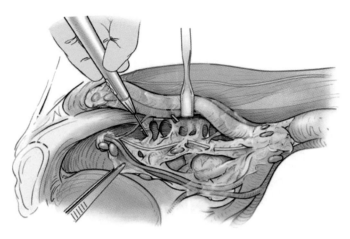

Figure 40-2   Potential sources of cumbersome bleeding during lymph node dissection in the obturator fossa: anomalous vascular tributaries emanating from the obturator vessels, vascular branches arising off the external iliac vein, and small vessels traveling between the lymph node packet and the pelvic sidewall. Prospective identification and control of these vessels permit meticulous dissection in a bloodless field.

of hemoclips in a poorly visualized field, either of which could result in inadvertent thermal injury or crush injury. Therefore, surgeons should recognize and avoid three potential sources of cumbersome bleeding during dissection in this area:

1. Anomalous vascular tributaries emanating from the obturator vessels
2. Vascular branches arising off the external iliac vein
3. Small vessels traveling between the lymph node packet and the pelvic sidewall (**Fig. 40-2**)

To avoid inadvertent damage to the nerve, the surgeon should obtain adequate visualization before sutures or hemoclips are placed deep within the obturator fossa. Any bleeding can be initially managed by packing the obturator fossa with a small sponge. Gentle pressure applied for several minutes may effectively minimize venous bleeding and allow for careful application of hemoclips to any remaining conspicuous bleeding vessels.

In general, management of obturator neuropathy should include immediate repair of intraoperative transection by epineural suture approximation using microsurgical techniques.[26,29] After repair or postoperative recognition of injury, physical therapy should be instituted promptly.

Femoral Nerve Injury

Anatomic and Functional Considerations   Arising from segments L2-L4 of the lumbar plexus, the femoral nerve emerges from the lateral border of the psoas muscle and courses along the groove between the psoas and iliacus muscles. It then enters the thigh beneath the inguinal ligament and divides into motor and sensory branches.

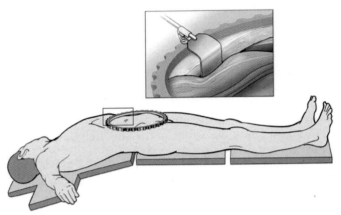

Figure 40-3   Femoral nerve injury caused by indirect compression from retracting the psoas muscle laterally while pressing on the nerve against the pelvic sidewall.

The motor divisions innervate the leg flexors, namely, the iliac, quadriceps, pectineal, and sartorius muscles, whereas the sensory branches innervate the anteromedial aspect of the thigh and leg.

Damage to the femoral nerve typically results from intraoperative nerve compression, which leads to direct nerve injury or ischemic injury secondary to reduced blood flow in the iliolumbar, lateral circumflex, or deep circumflex arteries. Causes of nerve compression include direct compression by the tips of the retractor blades and indirect compression from retracting the psoas muscle laterally while pressing on the nerve against the pelvic sidewall (**Fig. 40-3**). The severity of the injury is usually related to the duration of retraction and positioning of the patient.

Pelvic surgeons tend to place more lateral retraction on the left iliopsoas muscle to obtain better exposure near the rectosigmoid colon, a maneuver that increases the risk of injury to the left femoral nerve.[30] In addition, the paucity of vascular anastomotic branches supplying the left deep circumflex artery renders the left femoral nerve more vulnerable to ischemic injury than the right femoral nerve. Because the extrapelvic portion of the femoral nerve is angulated sharply around the inguinal ligament, excessive flexion of the thigh with abduction and external rotation of the hip in the lithotomy position carries increased risk of femoral nerve compression, particularly when "candy cane" stirrups are used.[31]

Intraoperative Techniques to Avoid Injury and Postoperative Treatment   Self-retaining retractors cause most femoral nerve injuries.[32] Therefore, urologic surgeons should become familiar with the proper placement of surgical retractors. The lateral blades should cradle the rectus muscles without compressing the psoas muscles. A folded laparotomy sponge should be used beneath each blade to cushion and protect the lateral pelvic sidewall. Proper placement of the blades should be confirmed by visualizing or palpating a clear space between the tips of the blades and the psoas muscle. Therefore, it is imperative to use the shortest available blade that can effectively retract the rectus muscle, particularly in patients with a thin abdominal wall, poorly developed rectus muscles, or a narrow pelvis.

In obese patients, surgeons tend to use a longer blade to allow retraction of the thick abdominal wall. Because the tip of a long blade may impinge excessively against the psoas muscle, obese patients are also at risk for femoral nerve injury. During lithotomy positioning, the surgeon should limit hip flexion, abduction, and external rotation to prevent postural nerve entrapment injury beneath the inguinal ligament.

Postoperatively, femoral neuropathy should prompt immediate physical therapy to prevent muscle wasting. This therapy should include early ambulation with knee stabilizers to compensate for thigh weakness and to prevent falling, as well as passive range-of-motion exercises and stretching to prevent muscle contractures. To minimize risk of thromboembolic complications, routine application of an intermittent calf compression device (e.g., Venodyne, Microtek Medical, Columbus, Mississippi) is warranted, and low-molecular-weight heparin may be used judiciously. Chronic neurogenic pain during the recovery period should be treated with non-narcotic analgesics. Drugs such as carbamazepine, which stabilizes the neuronal membrane, and amitriptyline, which blocks catecholamine reuptake at the nerve terminal, are useful adjuncts to analgesics.[31]

Femoral nerve compression almost invariably resolves spontaneously; however, the time to resolution remains quite variable. Certain neurologic deficits, particularly motor impairment, may require a prolonged recovery. As nerve function returns, motor activity will increase, not infrequently accompanied by intensified neuropathic pain. This pain, however, generally responds to the aforementioned medications. In a large series of 282 patients with femoral neuropathy following pelvic surgery, 265 patients (94%) recovered spontaneously.[32] The remainder experienced mild residual symptoms that lasted ≤4 months postoperatively.

Genitofemoral Nerve Injury

Anatomic and Functional Considerations   The genitofemoral nerve is a mixed motor and sensory nerve with a preponderance of sensory fibers. After originating from L1-L2 nerve roots, the genitofemoral nerve travels obliquely between the two bellies of the psoas muscle, perforates the psoas major, and descends along its anterior belly. It then takes a caudal course lateral to the external iliac vessels and, at a variable distance above the inguinal ligaments, divides into its terminal branches, which are the genital and the femoral branches. The genital branch receives sensory input from the skin of the scrotum in men and the mons pubis in women and innervates the cremasteric muscle.

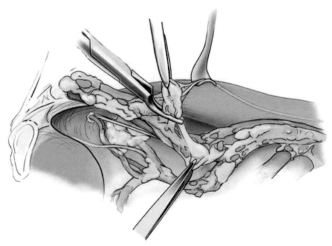

Figure 40-4   The genitofemoral nerve commonly lies in the groove between the iliac vessels and the psoas muscle, typically engulfed within nodal tissues. Complete mobilization of the artery and vein medially may facilitate identification and preservation of the nerve. Care should be taken to secure and divide all vascular tributaries from both vessels to the psoas muscle during this maneuver.

The femoral branch supplies the skin overlying the femoral triangle. Great variation of the genitofemoral sensory nerves to the inguinal region (with free communication among branches of the genitofemoral, ilioinguinal, or iliohypogastric nerves) renders the clinical sequelae of genitofemoral nerve injury inconsistent.

Intraoperative Techniques to Avoid Injury   Genitofemoral nerve injury may occur in patients undergoing standard lymphadenectomy or extended lymphadenectomy including the common and external iliac lymph nodes. The keys to avoiding inadvertent avulsion of the genitofemoral nerve are knowing its location and identifying it early. The nerve commonly lies adjacent to the common iliac vessels, in the groove between the vessels and the medial aspect of the psoas muscle (**Fig. 40-4**). Dissection of the nodal tissue should start proximally at the para-aortic or paracaval nodes in an extended template. Because the nerve is frequently engulfed within the common and external iliac lymph nodes, freeing it may require a split-and-roll technique.

Complete mobilization of the artery and vein medially may facilitate identification and preservation of the nerve. Care should be taken to secure and divide all vascular tributaries from both vessels to the psoas muscle during this maneuver. Once the nerve is identified clearly, dissecting it laterally with gentle traction away from the nodal tissue is generally straightforward and ensures that the nerve remains intact.

Lymphocele

Lymphocele is defined as a lymph collection within a thick fibrotic wall lacking an epithelial lining. The most common cause of pelvic lymphoceles is lymphadenectomy performed for staging of urologic malignant diseases. The mechanism underlying formation of pelvic lymphoceles is drainage of lymphatic fluid from transected afferent lymphatic channels into a closed space. Lack of smooth muscle cells in the wall of lymphatic vessels precludes vasoconstriction and allows lymphatic channels to remain patent >48 hours after injury. Because the peritoneum has high capacity to absorb lymph, lymphoceles typically develop after extraperitoneal surgical procedures. However, with the liberal use of abdominal imaging following radical cystectomy and laparoscopic radical prostatectomy, it became evident that lymphocele can form after intraperitoneal surgical procedures as well.

A variety of factors may contribute to the formation of lymphoceles, most commonly inadequate lymphostasis, the presence of metastatic lymph nodes, the long-term use of steroids or diuretics, prior pelvic irradiation, the extent of lymphadenectomy, and low-dose heparin administration. Of these factors, low-dose heparin has been studied most extensively.

Catalona and associates[33] and Tomic and coleagues[34] were first to suggest that subcutaneous heparin administration carries a major risk for lymphocele formation following extraperitoneal lymphadenectomy. Their observation was confirmed by Kropfl and associates,[35] who further noted that risk of lymphocele formation was considerably reduced when the heparin was injected into an upper limb as opposed to the lower abdomen or thigh. Drainage fluid from all patients who had heparin injected into the thigh was found to contain high levels of heparin, but fluid from patients who had heparin injected into the arm lacked heparin. Paucity of clotting factors and lack of platelets are believed to render the lymphatic fluid more vulnerable to the effect of anticoagulants than is blood.

Another significant risk factor for pelvic lymphoceles is extended lymphadenectomy. In one report, the rate of lymphocele formation was twofold higher in patients with prostate cancer who were undergoing extended compared with limited PLND (10.3% versus 4.6%, respectively; $P = .01$).[13] The increased risk for lymphocele formation following extended PLND in bladder cancer is less well documented.

Most lymphoceles are asymptomatic and often remain undetected. Hence, the reported incidence of pelvic lymphoceles following PLND in modern series is fairly low, ranging from 2% to 27%.[36] When symptoms do occur, they usually manifest early in the postoperative course as a sensation of pelvic fullness. As the lymphocele enlarges, symptoms related to compression of adjacent anatomic structures may become evident. Urinary frequency from bladder compression, constipation from rectosigmoid compression, pain from pressure on pelvic nerves, and edema (scrotal, labial gland, and rarely lower extremity edema) may occur as pelvic venous return is hindered. Compression of major pelvic veins may occasionally lead to thrombotic complica-

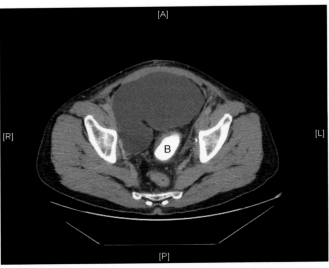

Figure 40-5 A 57-year-old man 16 days after radical prostatectomy and bilateral pelvic lymph node dissection presenting with vague abdominal pain and urinary frequency. Axial CT shows compression of the bladder (B) by a large pelvic lymphocele.

tions. Ureteral compression with subsequent hydronephrosis is rare. Associated fever is infrequent, and its presence indicates a possible superinfection, which generally requires prompt lymphocele drainage.

Physical examination is typically unremarkable. Only occasionally, in patients with very large fluid collections, is a pelvic mass just above the inguinal ligament visible or palpable. Imaging studies are required to make the diagnosis, and at the majority of centers ultrasound examination is used most commonly, particularly after prostatectomy. On ultrasound imaging, lymphoceles appear as anechoic cystic structures that may contain thin septations and debris. Occasionally, a lymphocele may be mistaken for a large postvoid residual noted on routine office evaluation. CT is more expensive but provides excellent visualization of most pelvic and retroperitoneal fluid collections. It is generally the preferred imaging modality following radical cystectomy. On CT images, lymphoceles are seen as thin-walled hypodense lesions with negative Hounsfield unit values (**Fig. 40-5**). A finding of a thickened wall with regional enhancement suggests the presence of infection.

Management Currently, no consensus exists on the optimal management of pelvic lymphoceles. In fact, only half of all pelvic lymphoceles ultimately require intervention.[36] Small, uncomplicated lymphoceles can be managed expectantly and, except for monitoring, usually require no further treatment. One should consider the relationship of the lymphocele with the iliac or femoral vein. Venous compression resulting in lower extremity venous stasis or deep vein thrombosis may be one indication for intervention in the absence of pain or infection. Large or symptomatic lymphoceles, which generally require treatment, can be managed by percutaneous techniques or surgically.

In the past, percutaneous drainage was performed by simple aspiration, but this approach was abandoned because of high (80%-90%) recurrence rates and a substantial (25%-50%) risk of infection.[37,38] This method is currently reserved for diagnostic purposes only and has been supplanted by placement of a percutaneous drainage tube. Reported success rates with the drainage tube are approaching 80%, with a mean drainage duration ranging anywhere from a few days to several months.[39] A major disadvantage of this technique, particularly when prolonged treatment is required, is the need for frequent tube exchanges as a result of clogging of the small-caliber side holes.

Sclerotherapy through a percutaneous catheter has become popular in cases of recurrent lymphoceles. Sclerosing agents offer the potential for faster resolution because these agents obliterate the lymphatic channels by a chemical effect. Instillation of sclerosing agents can be tried as an alternative when lymphoceles do not resolve after catheter drainage alone.[40] Multiple sclerosing agents have been explored over the years, including povidone-iodine, ethanol, ampicillin, tetracycline, doxycycline, bleomycin, sodium aztreonam, sodium tetradecyl sulfate, fibrin glue, and talc.[36,40] Ethanol and povidone-iodine are the two most commonly used sclerosing agents, with success rates varying between 88% to 97% and 62% to 89%, respectively.[36] Bleomycin is generally reserved for sclerotherapy of resistant lymphoceles.

The major impediment to successful resolution of pelvic lymphoceles after percutaneous drainage, either alone or in combination with sclerotherapy, is the presence of a multiloculated cavity. McDougall and Clayman[41] proposed an alternative, minimally invasive intervention for managing persistent lymphoceles: dilating the percutaneous track followed by careful endoscopic fulguration of the cavity lining. The most durable solution to refractory lymphoceles is probably internal marsupialization, which consists of creation of a peritoneal window to allow the lymphocele to drain into the peritoneal cavity. Peritoneal drainage can be performed laparoscopically or using an open technique but is contraindicated in the setting of infection because of the increased risk of peritonitis.[42] Unfortunately, complete resolution with this technique is not guaranteed, and relapse rates approach 20%.[36]

To improve outcomes, some investigators have suggested packing the cavity with omentum to prevent window closure and to facilitate transperitoneal absorption of lymphatic fluid. Other investigators have instilled diluted methylene blue solution into the drained cavity to enable precise identification of the lymphocele location and extent.[43] Open external drainage is reserved primarily for loculated, infected lymphoceles that fail to respond to percutaneous drainage and antibiotic therapy.[44]

Intraoperative Techniques to Avoid Lymphocele Formation   The key surgical tenet for avoiding or minimizing formation of pelvic lymphoceles is meticulous control of the divided lymphatic channels. Although small and innocuous lymphatic channels can be readily sealed with electrocautery, it is imperative to apply clips or suture ligatures to any major lymphatic trunks. Particular attention should be given to controlling the distal and proximal limits of the lymph node packet dissected (see Fig. 40-1). Because lymphatic vessels are frail and prone to disruption, care should be taken to avoid excessive traction on the packet before it is clipped. Whether pelvic drains actually reduce the incidence of lymphocele formation remains an area of contention. In an earlier study,[10] pelvic drains were reported to reduce the incidence of lymphocele formation, although a subsequent study of patients after radical hysterectomy failed to show any advantage.[45]

RETROPERITONEAL LYMPH NODE DISSECTION

Retroperitoneal lymph node dissection (RPLND) plays a critical role in the management of testicular cancer. Although no consensus exists on the extent and clinical benefits of lymph node dissection for renal cell carcinoma and upper urinary tract urothelial tumors, many urologists consider RPLND in these patients to be part of extirpative surgical treatment.

Germ cell tumors of the testis are both rare (accounting for only 1%-2% of all neoplasms in men) and unique because they affect almost exclusively young men <45 years old. The introduction of effective chemotherapy and improvements in surgical techniques dramatically increased overall cure rates for these tumors from approximately 25% in the mid-1970s to more than 95% today. Primary RPLND is generally indicated in patients with low-volume (clinical stage I and IIa), nonseminomatous tumors, particularly if they are poorly compliant or at high risk for retroperitoneal spread (i.e., have lymphovascular invasion, stage T2 disease or higher, or a predominance of embryonal carcinoma).

In patients who undergo primary RPLND, regardless of whether adjuvant chemotherapy is used (in those with detected micrometastases), overall cure rates approach 100%. In the absence of elevated tumor markers, RPLND is also indicated for postchemotherapy residual disease in patients with nonseminomatous tumors and occasionally seminomas. Even in patients with advanced disease, the prospects of surgical cure are excellent, largely because of the efficacy of platinum-based chemotherapy in reducing the size of the mass preoperatively, advances in surgical techniques, and the excellent cardiovascular and pulmonary capacity of younger men that allows them to withstand major surgical insults.

Overview of Complications

Perioperative morbidity of RPLND is generally related to the complexity of the surgical procedure and to prior exposure to chemotherapy, in particular bleomycin. An increased incidence of intraoperative and postoperative complications can be expected in patients with large-volume tumors and a severe desmoplastic reaction, commonly seen during postchemotherapy RPLND for metastatic seminoma. In these challenging cases, patients are best treated in tertiary referral centers by experienced surgeons who are comfortable with vascular surgical techniques. A detailed discussion of the toxicity and side effect profiles of the various chemotherapeutic agents commonly used in testicular cancer is provided in Chapter 10.

Vascular Complications

The most effective means to deal with vascular complications is to avoid them in the first place.

The split-and-roll technique with division of the lumbar arteries and veins is commonly used in RPLND for circumferential removal of the tumor and lymphatic tissues surrounding the great vessels down to the level of the anterior spinal ligament. With primary RPLND, a reported analysis of complications indicated that significant vascular morbidity is exceedingly rare.[46] With postchemotherapy RPLND, however, the chemotherapy may have caused substantial fibrosis that renders the major retroperitoneal blood vessels susceptible to injury. Therefore, it is imperative that surgeons performing RPLND in patients who have received chemotherapy have an in-depth understanding of retroperitoneal anatomy and be competent in vascular control techniques. Failure to recognize ominous preoperative signs (e.g., lower limb edema or enlarged abdominal wall collateral veins) or to appreciate the potential need for inferior vena cava (IVC) resection in patients with bulky, right-sided masses may culminate in a poor outcome or may hinder a successful resection attempt.

When operating in the retroperitoneum, surgeons should be familiar with the vascular anomalies that may be encountered, including persistence of ascending lumbar veins, a retroaortic or circumaortic left renal vein, caval duplication, and rarely a transposed left-sided vena cava. Recognizing these anomalies on preoperative imaging may minimize intraoperative blood loss and prevent unwarranted nephrectomy.[47]

Arterial Complications

Injury to critical vascular structures must be avoided. Therefore, knowledge of their typical location and anatomic course is essential.

In suprahilar dissections, the superior mesenteric artery must be identified early because inadvertent injury to this vessel may culminate in a catastrophic outcome. Securing the lymphatic trunks at the base of the superior mesenteric artery is key to avoiding excessive lymphatic leakage and possible formation of chylous ascites. Complete mobilization of the left colon mesentery, including division of the inferior mesenteric artery, is sometimes necessary to gain a better plane between the aorta and the mass. Although older patients with diffused atherosclerosis are prone to developing diarrhea and possibly ischemic colitis after inferior mesenteric artery division, this procedure is well tolerated in younger patients who have generous crossover blood supply through the arc of Riolan.

Compared with the main renal arteries, the segmental and polar renal arteries are more vulnerable to inadvertent injury and, once transected, are extremely difficult to repair. Vigilance in the area of these vessels is warranted. Bolus contrast, three-dimensional magnetic resonance angiography (MRA) can provide detailed information on renal vasculature preoperatively, but it is unclear whether routine use of this imaging technique would decrease vascular complications.[48]

As for the main renal arteries, the lymphatic drainage on the left side is immediately inferior to the renal hilum, whereas on the right side it is more remote. The proximity of lymphatic tissue to the left renal pedicle makes safe dissection of the left renal artery challenging, especially in patients with a large mass in the para-aortic region. On rare occasions, adjunctive nephrectomy may be required.[49] The right renal artery is more prone to inadvertent injury or clipping when the surgeon is dissecting a large interaortocaval mass.

In rare circumstances, en bloc aortic resection may be necessary to achieve complete tumor removal. Tumor adherence to the aorta often indicates malignant involvement, and aortic resection may be the only means to ensure surgical extirpation. In a report from Indiana University, 15 patients (1%) required aortic replacement at the time of RPLND, and all had teratoma or viable cancer on the final pathology report.[50] Peeling the tumor off the aorta in a subadventitial plane (often the most expedient cleavage plane) may permit complete tumor resection but leaves the aorta devoid of its resilient adventitial support. These rare cases are best managed by graft substitution with a tube or trouser aortoiliac graft.[50]

Venous Complications

The inferior mesenteric vein, gonadal vein, and lower lumbar veins can be safely divided after obtaining proximal and distal control. Injury to the renal veins or IVC, however, may result in substantial morbidity. The left renal vein is particularly susceptible to damage, largely because of its longer course and multiple tributaries.

Injury typically occurs during dissection of a bulky para-aortic mass that obscures the point of drainage of the left gonadal, adrenal, or ascending lumbar veins. To avoid nephrectomy, primary repair of the vein is essential. Lateral venorrhaphy in a transverse direction with 5-0 polypropylene suture can be used for small perforations in the renal vein. If a large defect is encountered, repair with a saphenous vein patch or Gore-Tex vascular graft is generally needed. Before grafting, administration of 12.5 g of intravenous mannitol, clamping of the renal artery, and concomitant cooling of the kidney are required.

Extensive injury to the renal vein mandates ligation and nephrectomy. To avoid potential injury to the left renal vein, it is often prudent to detach the mass completely at its medial border (mobilizing it off the aorta), its posterior aspect (dissecting it off the psoas muscle), and its lateral border (off the ureter and descending colon). By leaving the difficult superior dissection of the renal hilum until maximal mobilization is achieved, surgeons can more comfortably control bleeding and reconstruct the renal vein, if required.

Injury and hemorrhage involving the IVC are usually secondary to inadvertent laceration or avulsion of large fragile veins. The lumbar veins, which enter the posterolateral aspect of the vena cava and typically run with a corresponding artery at each vertebral level, are a common source of troublesome bleeding. To avoid disruption of the lumbar veins, the IVC should be retracted gently throughout the dissection, and each lumber vein should be securely controlled using sutures ligatures or hemoclips. It is particularly important to avoid tying these ligatures too tightly because inadvertent shearing through the vessel may occur.

Persistent hemorrhage from the proximal end of an avulsed lumbar vein may be difficult to control if the vein retracts into the vertebral foramen or behind the psoas muscle. Bleeding may generally be controlled by oversewing the overlying psoas aponeurosis or perivertebral soft tissues with a figure-of-eight ligature suture. Retropsoas exploration to find the origin of the lumbar vein is rarely required, and hemostatic agents often prove helpful in this setting.

En bloc resection of the infrarenal IVC during RPLND is rare but may be required if the tumor overtly invades the caval wall, if the IVC is encased by a massive retroperitoneal mass, or if extensive desmoplastic reaction impedes dissection with safe margins. It is of paramount importance to remove the tumor completely, even if a portion of the IVC is sacrificed, because incomplete tumor resection invariably compromises the patient's survival.[51]

Beck and Lalka[52] reported a 6.8% incidence of IVC involvement in 955 patients undergoing RPLND for residual bulky retroperitoneal disease following chemotherapy. In the majority of cases (67%), the final speci-men revealed carcinoma or teratoma within the vessel wall, a finding highlighting the importance of resecting the IVC to achieve complete tumor removal. When bulky, right-sided residual disease is encountered along with severe desmoplastic reaction, en bloc caval resection permits better access to the aorta and hence reduces the risk of aortic injury.

IVC resection generally triggers significant morbidity, from immediate venous congestion of the lower extremities to continued extravasation of lymphatic drainage into the peritoneal cavity and accumulation of chylous ascites.[52] Patients who undergo IVC resection in an acute setting are at particular risk. In one report of acute IVC interruption, 70% of the patients experienced significant bilateral lower extremity edema, and half of them remained edematous for >5 years.[53] In contrast, patients who have underlying IVC occlusion (complete or nearly complete) experience minimal, if any, venous congestion or third-space extravasation of lymphatic drainage.

In a study of patients with chronic IVC occlusion, 40% had no sequelae and 30% developed minimal disability following ligation of the IVC.[54] Gradual IVC occlusion, often associated with long-standing external compression from encasing tumor, allows for development of collateral veins that mitigate acute and chronic venous morbidity. Therefore, it is important for surgeons contemplating IVC resection not to sacrifice any competitive venous collaterals that have developed. When performing the lymph node dissection, one should attempt to preserve the contralateral testicular, lower lumbar, and pelvic veins to avoid compromising the venous return through the hemiazygos or azygos systems.[55] If these venous tributaries must be sacrificed to attain complete tumor resection, the intervertebral veins of Batson may provide additional means of circumventing the obstructed caval segment.

The resected IVC is best replaced by an interposition polytetrafluoroethylene graft or an autologous pericardium tube graft. Grafts in the venous system are far more likely to occlude than are arterial grafts. Slow venous flow against a hydrostatic pressure gradient, low intraluminal pressure, and the presence of competitive flow from venous collaterals all put the IVC graft at risk for occlusion.[52] Because the long-term patency of IVC reconstruction is questionable, this procedure should be reserved for patients with poor collateral circulation.

MRI and MRA can be useful in assessing the patency of the infrarenal vena cava as well as for identifying enlarged collateral vessels.[48] Normal venous pressure in the lower limbs of a patient with suspected IVC obstruction may indicate adequate collateral circulation superficially through the epigastric and axillary veins and, at a deeper level, from the hypogastric vein through the rectal plexus and portal venous system. In one reported series of patients undergoing RPLND with IVC resection, the absence or presence of preoperative venous signs and symptoms was a poor predictor of chronic venous sequelae.[52] Other early complications of IVC resection include renal insufficiency, deep vein thrombosis, and increased incidence of chylous ascites and autonomic dysfunction.

Retroperitoneal Lymphoceles and Chylous Ascites

Anatomic and Physiologic Considerations

The main lymphatic channels in the retroperitoneum are the ascending lumbar lymphatic trunks. These chains travel posterior and parallel to the aorta and IVC and are formed by the coalescence of the common iliac lymph vessels. Typically, both lymphatic trunks merge posterior and medial to the aorta to form the cisterna chyli (**Fig. 40-6**). The cisterna chyli, which is a saccular dilatation of the main lymphatic trunk, is commonly situated behind the left crus of the diaphragm. It marks the termination of the retroperitoneal lymphatic pathway and the beginning of the thoracic duct. The thoracic duct traverses the aortic hiatus into the right posterior mediastinum, courses to the left at the level of the fourth thoracic vertebra, and commonly drains into the venous system at the junction of the left jugular and subclavian veins. A distinct cisterna chyli is present in approximately half the cases; in the rest, it is replaced by a variable lymphatic plexus.[56] The cisterna chyli and thoracic duct transport lymph from the lower hemitrunk back to the circulatory system.

Anywhere from 50% to 90% of lymphatic fluid is derived from the intestine and liver. This fluid contains mostly dietary fat in the form of chylomicrons. Because intestinal lymphatic fluid is returned by the lacteals (generally into the left trunk), ingestion of a fatty meal can increase the lymph flow in the lacteals and retroperitoneal lymphatic trunks ≥200-fold compared with a fasting state. Unrecognized disruption of the cisterna chyli, the thoracic duct, or their major tributaries can lead to major lymphatic leak and development of retroperitoneal lymphoceles and, less frequently, the accumulation of chylous ascites.

Management and Intraoperative Techniques to Avoid Retroperitoneal Lymphoceles and Chylous Ascites

Small lymphoceles are fairly common after extensive RPLND and most are clinically innocuous. Symptomatic retroperitoneal lymphocele is rare. Presenting symptoms may include a sense of abdominal fullness, flank pain related to ureteral compression, and fever and chills related to lymphocele infection. CT may reveal a thin-walled cystic lesion. Any radiographic evidence of a lobulated collection containing fluid and air with wall enhancement should prompt concern of a retroperitoneal abscess (**Fig. 40-7**). Retroperitoneal abscesses are treated by CT-guided percutaneous drainage and appropriate antibiotics.

Abdominal distention, enlarging girth, and disproportionate weight gain are among the most common

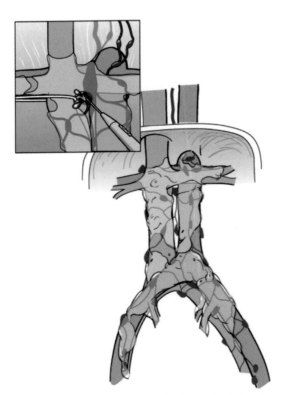

Figure 40-6 Merging of the right and left lymphatic trunks posterior and medial to the aorta to form the cisterna chyli. Inadvertent injury to this delicate structure results in marked lymph secretion into the peritoneal cavity.

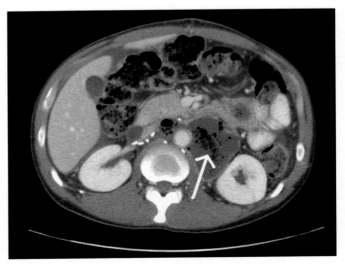

Figure 40-7 A 21-year-old man 4 weeks after postchemotherapy retroperitoneal lymph node dissection presenting with increasing left flank pain, night sweats, and elevated fever. CT shows a lobulated collection containing fluid and air with wall enhancement (*arrow*) indicating a retroperitoneal abscess.

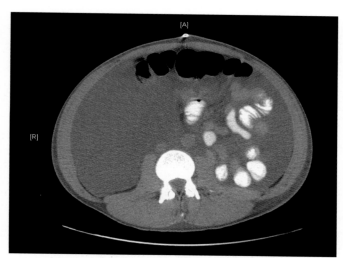

Figure 40-8 A 35-year-old man presenting with uncomfortable sensation of abdominal fullness 3 weeks following postchemotherapy retroperitoneal lymph node dissection. CT demonstrates a large amount of ascitic fluid. Paracentesis confirmed the diagnosis of chylous ascites.

signs of chylous ascites. Patients may complain of an uncomfortable sensation of abdominal fullness and dyspnea related to restriction of the diaphragm or leakage of ascitic fluid into the chest and formation of chylothorax.[56,57] The diagnosis of chylous ascites is generally made by CT scan (**Fig. 40-8**) and is confirmed by analyzing the fluid obtained by paracentesis. Typically, the fluid appears milky and odorless (provided it is sterile) and has a high content of protein (>3 g/dL) and triglycerides (twofold to eightfold higher than that of plasma).

Management of postoperative chylous ascites is primarily conservative. Treatment goals include decreasing the mesenteric lymph flow and lymph leakage into the peritoneum, alleviating mechanical symptoms related to the distended abdomen, and providing adequate replacement of nutritional losses. Common conservative measures consist of repeat therapeutic paracentesis, dietary modifications, hyperalimentation, and the administration of a somatostatin analogue. Surgical intervention is reserved as a last resort for patients for whom nonoperative management is ineffective. Diagnostic paracentesis is often required early in the evaluation of chylous ascites. Repeated attempts at therapeutic paracentesis and placement of an externalized peritoneal drain are rarely effective and may prolong the leakage of ascitic fluid, exacerbate nutritional and immunologic losses, and increase the risk of peritonitis.[58]

Dietary intervention is the mainstay of nonoperative therapy for chylous ascites. A high-protein, low-fat diet containing medium-chain triglycerides (which are transported directly into the portal circulation, thus bypassing intestinal lymphatics) yields minimal lymph flow within the major lymphatic trunks and facilitates the spontaneous closure of lymphatic fistulas. Nutritional manipulations alone or in combination with diuretics may be effective in as many as 50% of patients.[56-58] Total parenteral nutrition is generally recommended as second-line therapy when dietary manipulations fail. Hyperalimentation has the advantage of resting the bowel while restoring crucial nutritional deficits and effectively further decreases the production and leakage of lymph.

Finally, the adjunctive use of the somatostatin analogue octreotide offers additional benefit by drastically reducing the lymphatic output through the fistula within 24 to 72 hours after initiating therapy.[59] Octreotide therapy should be attempted early in the course of treatment with low-dose, subcutaneous injections of 100 μg three times daily. Close monitoring of blood glucose levels and gradual tapering of octreotide on complete resolution of the condition are prudent.

Persistent active lymphatic leakage after several weeks to months of maximal conservative management warrants a more aggressive approach. Surgical repair by direct suture ligation of a leaking lymphatic channel and peritoneovenous shunting with a LeVeen or Denver shunt have been described, although the role and timing of surgical repair remain controversial.[57] The singular difficulty with surgical ligation lies in identifying the exact locations of lymphatic leakage. Several techniques facilitate localization of large, open lymphatic channels: prescribing a heavy, fatty meal preoperatively; using lipophilic dyes; and performing lymphoscintigraphy. If a definitive fistula cannot be identified, nonselective suturing of retroaortic tissues may successfully resolve the leak.[56]

The primary means of minimizing postoperative lymphatic leakage is to secure (ligate or clip) the cut ends of lymphatic vessels throughout the procedure. Particularly vulnerable locations include the region of the right renal artery, where large tributaries to the cisternae chyli are located, and the numerous lymphatic channels overlying the left renal vein. Large lymphatic channels at the base of the pancreas and superior mesenteric artery also require meticulous control. At the completion of dissection, the surgical field must be thoroughly irrigated with warm water, and lymphostasis must be ensured.

Ejaculatory Dysfunction

Anatomy and Neurophysiology of Antegrade Ejaculation

Normal antegrade ejaculation is a coordinated, sequential process of seminal emission and ejaculation proper. During emission, the two vasa deferentia contract to propel sperm from the epididymis, mix it with fluids from the seminal vesicles, prostate, and bulbourethral glands, and deliver the ejaculate into the posterior urethra. For normal ejaculation to ensue, the bladder neck must be closed (or partially closed) at this phase. During ejaculation proper, the semen is ejected through the penile urethra. Ejaculation is prompted by the rhythmic contractions of the bulbocavernosus and ischiocavernosus muscles coupled with complete bladder neck closure and relaxation of the external urethral sphincter and urogenital diaphragm.

From a neurophysiologic standpoint, ejaculation initiates with transmission of afferent stimuli from the genital end organs through the pudendal nerve onto the cerebral cortex. Efferent impulses are transmitted through the anterolateral spinal cord columns to the thoracolumbar sympathetic outflow tract. These preganglionic fibers synapse in the ganglia of the paravertebral sympathetic trunk and exit through L1-L4 postganglionic fibers. Although individual anatomic features vary greatly, ejaculatory information is transmitted predominantly through the L3-L4 fibers and to a lesser degree through L1-L2. The efferent signals then travel through the postsympathetic fibers to the hypogastric plexus and on to the vas, ampulla, seminal vesicles, prostate, and bladder neck. Thus, whereas the ejaculatory phase is under control of a somatic spinal reflex at the S2-S4 level, seminal emission and bladder neck closure are governed by the sympathetic nervous system and are most vulnerable to damage during RPLND.

Intraoperative Techniques to Avoid Autonomic Nerve Injury

Nerve-sparing RPLND requires a sound understanding of the anatomy of the retroperitoneum. The keys to avoiding sympathetic nerve damage and ensuring preservation of normal ejaculation are prospective identification and meticulous dissection of the sympathetic trunks, the postganglionic sympathetic fibers (particularly L3 and L4), and the hypogastric plexus. The sympathetic chains run parallel to the great vessels and are located in the retroperitoneum between the medial border of the psoas muscle and the vertebral column. The right chain is typically located posterior to the IVC, whereas the left chain is located posterolateral to the aorta. The sympathetic chains and ganglia are intimately involved with lumbar vessels. Therefore, great care should be taken to avoid injury to these delicate structures during isolation and division of these vessels.

The left postganglionic sympathetic fibers emerge lateral to the aorta and then traverse anteriorly to join the hypogastric plexus near the takeoff of the inferior mesenteric artery. On the right side, postganglionic fibers emerge underneath the IVC, course medially at an oblique angle anterior to the aorta, and then converge into the hypogastric plexus. Thus, an anterior split-and-roll maneuver over the IVC can be carried out safely, whereas dissecting over the aorta may result in disruption and damage to the left postganglionic fibers

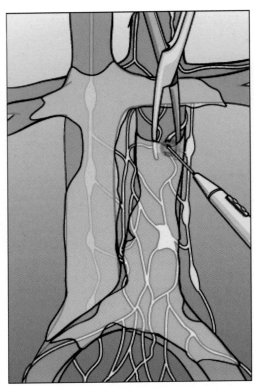

Figure 40-9 Anterior split-and-roll maneuver over the aorta may result in disruption and damage to the left postganglionic sympathetic fibers. The nodal tissue can be safely split over the inferior vena cava.

(**Fig. 40-9**).[60] The interaortocaval and para-aortic lymphatic tissue should be dissected only after the nerve fibers have been isolated and properly encircled with soft vessel loops. Isolating the subtle fibers of the hypogastric plexus, which is generally situated between the two common iliac arteries, should be done carefully.

To reduce the incidence of postoperative ejaculatory failure, two surgical approaches—nerve-sparing techniques and modified templates—have become popular. *Nerve-sparing techniques* rely on precise dissection and preservation of vital neuroanatomic structures. In patients with limited residual retroperitoneal disease, selective or unilateral nerve sparing may be contemplated if the margin of resection and oncologic safety will not be compromised. Successful nerve sparing is more difficult after chemotherapy because of nerve entrapment and fibrosis between the tumor mass and the adventitia of the great vessels.

Modified dissection templates are intended to limit the extent of dissection to anatomic regions likely to be at increased risk of metastatic disease. Prompted by the high incidence of permanent ejaculatory dysfunction in patients undergoing extensive, bilateral RPLND and driven by surgical mapping studies in testicular cancer,[61,62] modified dissection templates have been developed for low-volume disease. All minimize or avoid contralateral dissection, particularly below the level of the inferior mesenteric artery.

Combining nerve-sparing techniques with modified templates has resulted in postoperative ejaculation rates of 84% to 98%.[60,63] However, the concept of modified-template RPLND has been challenged.[64] Lack of adequate postoperative follow-up to account for surgical or pathologic sampling errors, as well as overreliance on postoperative chemotherapy, may undermine some of the conclusions drawn from these mapping studies. An analysis of >500 patients with clinical stage I to IIA nonseminomatous tumors who underwent primary RPLND, for example, found that 23% of men with retroperitoneal metastases had disease present outside the limits of the modified templates, and 20% to 30% of these tumors had chemoresistant teratomatous elements.[65]

Intraoperative use of Brindley's electrostimulation device to facilitate identification and isolation of postganglionic sympathetic fibers has been reported by several investigators. Although bladder neck closure and seminal emission can be documented endoscopically, it is unclear whether these factors affect or predict future fertility in these patients.[66] For men with retrograde ejaculation in whom emission is preserved, treatment with an α-adrenergic sympathomimetic agent may restore an intact bladder neck status and antegrade ejaculation. For patients with failure of seminal emission, transrectal electroejaculation is required to recover motile sperm for assisted reproductive techniques, with a resulting pregnancy rate of 43%.[67]

Gastrointestinal Complications

Mobilization and retraction of the duodenum may result in transient pancreatitis (manifesting as nausea and vomiting) in conjunction with elevated serum levels of amylase and lipase. Attention to proper positioning and to tension placed on the retractor blades is key to avoiding pancreatic irritation. Conservative treatment with dietary restriction is often sufficient to resolve this temporary pancreatic inflammation.

Postoperative paralytic ileus is reported in approximately 0.2% of patients undergoing primary transabdominal RPLND and in 2% of those undergoing the procedure after chemotherapy.[68] The more extensive the retroperitoneal dissection, the higher is the likelihood of protracted ileus, which usually resolves with conservative measures after an extended hospital stay. The incidence of this complication is minimized by careful mobilization of the duodenum and root of the small bowel mesentery and cautious avoidance of inadvertent pressure or serosal abrasions from retractor blades.

Direct injury to the bowel is rare and most likely occurs after chemotherapy when a large, adherent inter-aortocaval mass is dissected. This injury usually involves the third or fourth segments of the duodenum. Full-thickness injury requires primary, two-layer closure with interposition of omentum between the great vessels and the bowel to decrease the incidence of abscess formation and potentially fatal disruption of an aortoduodenal fistula. Tension-free reapproximation of the visceral peritoneum (overlying the small bowel mesentery) to the serosa (covering the duodenum) and the edge of the mesocolon minimizes the likelihood of an internal hernia. This technique also facilitates future access to the retroperitoneum (in case a salvage procedure is required) by preventing fibrous adhesions to an extensively dissected, raw retroperitoneal surface.

INGUINAL LYMPH NODE DISSECTION

Penile cancer spreads along predictable routes, following the lymphatic drainage of the penis. Initial spread to the superficial inguinal nodes is followed by extension to the deep inguinal nodes of the femoral triangle and ultimately to the ipsilateral pelvic lymph nodes. Because inguinal lymph node involvement invariably precedes the spread of distant disease, the most important prognostic indicator for patients with carcinoma of the penis remains the presence or absence of regional lymph node metastases. Metastatic penile carcinoma in the regional lymph nodes generally confers a poor prognosis; however, aggressive lymphadenectomy has been associated with improved survival and cure in 30% to 60% of patients.[69,70]

Even though the diagnostic value of groin dissection in these patients is evident and the concept of surgical curability has been confirmed in numerous studies, management of regional lymph nodes in penile cancer remains controversial. Given the inaccuracy of clinical staging (by physical examination and imaging studies) and the significant morbidity incurred with groin dissection,[71-73] many urologists are reluctant to recommend inguinal lymphadenectomy unless the lymph nodes have become overtly palpable. Because the extent of morbidity is directly related to the extent of dissection, some surgeons are now trying to limit the boundaries of dissection while relying on frozen section analysis intraoperatively for margin assessment.

Anatomic Considerations

Inguinal lymph node dissection in penile cancer can be prophylactic, therapeutic, or palliative. Prophylactic groin dissection is indicated for patients with an invasive primary tumor (TNM stage T1 at minimum) and no palpable adenopathy. In this setting, patients undergo modified superficial inguinal lymph node dissection (including the lymphatic tissue above the fascia lata) between the sartorius muscle laterally and the adductor longus muscle medially. The saphenous vein is invariably dissected from the nodal packet and is preserved. In the absence of lymph node metastases on frozen section analysis, the procedure is concluded. If metastases are detected, complete inguinal and ipsilateral pelvic dissection is performed.

Therapeutic groin dissection is indicated for men with overtly palpable adenopathy after a course of antibiotics to rule out a possible inflammatory component. In this setting, the saphenous vein has traditionally been divided at the saphenofemoral junction, the femoral vessels are skeletonized to allow for removal of deep inguinal nodes, and a sartorius muscle flap is generally rotated medially to cover the exposed femoral vessels. If a mobile nodal mass is fixed to the skin, an ellipse of involved skin should be excised en bloc with the specimen.

Palliative groin dissection is performed to remove all gross residual disease after chemotherapy. To achieve negative surgical margins, the resection often includes the inguinal ligament, the spermatic cord, and the ipsilateral testis. More rarely, the dissection also includes segments of the femoral artery and vein (with adequate reconstruction by a patch or bypass grafting) and inferior portions of the rectus abdominis and external and internal oblique muscles. Myocutaneous flaps to cover a large defect may occasionally be required and remain a necessary step to ensure adequate reconstruction.

Complications

Complications consistently reported in groin dissection series are related to disruption of the lymphatics draining the lower extremities and damage to the overlying skin flaps from devascularization. These complications include skin edge necrosis (45%-62% of dissections), wound infection (14%-17%), seroma formation (6%-16%), and lymphedema (23%-50%).[71-73] Skin flap necrosis remains a frequent complication of groin dissections.

The blood supply to the skin of the inguinal region is derived from branches of the common femoral artery. Complete groin dissection necessitates skeletonization of the femoral vessels and ligation of these branches, with potential compromise in blood supply to the raised skin flaps. Viability of the skin edges in this setting depends primarily on anastomotic vessels running along the superficial fatty layer of Camper's fascia. Because lymphatic drainage of the penis to the groin is beneath Camper's fascia, this layer can be preserved and left attached to the overlying skin when the skin flaps are fashioned.

Several surgical modifications have been developed to minimize skin flap necrosis, including avoidance of the inguinal skin crease during the initial skin incision, meticulous skin edge handling with fine hooks, creation of thicker skin flaps in which Camper's and Scarpa's fascial layers are preserved, and limitation of the extent of flap mobilization (superiorly to the inguinal ligament and inferiorly to the tip of the femoral triangle). Careful hemostasis and excision of ischemic flap margins at the end of the procedure are mandatory. Additionally, placing horizontal sutures to anchor the underlying muscle aponeurosis may reduce the tension at the flap edges. Taken together, these surgical tenets have substantially reduced the incidence of skin edge necrosis from the 50% to 60% reported historically to 8% in a study reported in 2002.[71] If skin necrosis does occur, débridement and split-skin grafting may be necessary.

Lymphedema

Lymphedema following groin dissection can be bothersome and debilitating with respect to ambulation, difficulty in standing for prolonged periods, and recurrent bouts of cellulitis induced by lymphostasis. The overall incidence of postoperative lymphedema has been reported to be ≤50%, with severe lymphedema occurring in 35% of patients.

Limiting the template of dissection, specifically by sparing the saphenous vein in these circumstances, has resulted in reduced rates of postoperative lymphedema. This concept was validated in the gynecologic literature in a study evaluating the advantages of saphenous vein preservation in lymphadenectomy for carcinoma of the vulva.[74] The study demonstrated a decrease in the incidence of chronic lower extremity edema from 32% to 3% without affecting local cancer control. Persistent lymphedema is rare but if left untreated may become progressive, chronic, and incurable.

A stepwise approach to the management of chronic lymphedema was developed and advocated by the International Society of Lymphology.[75] It consists of initial skin care, light manual massage, elevation of the affected limb, range-of-motion exercises, and intermittent compression with low-stretch elastic stockings or multilayered bandage wrapping. Failure to achieve significant improvement should prompt maintenance therapy with a 24-hour compression garment and intermittent pneumatic compression devices. Diuretics, benzopyrenes (which hydrolyze tissue proteins), and surgical intervention (e.g., resection, liposuction, and microsurgical procedures) are all of questionable efficacy. Comprehensive lymphedema therapy can produce rapid reduction in all stages of lymphedema but has the disadvantages of being labor intensive, compliance dependent, and costly.[76]

Wound infection and seroma formation are fairly uniform among contemporary reports, with incidences ranging between 10% and 15%. Impaired lymphatic drainage and the frequent occurrence of seromas render these wounds particularly susceptible to infection. Parenteral antibiotics with staphylococcal coverage and meticulous skin preparation of the genital folds by both patients (preoperatively) and the surgical team serve to reduce infective complications. Vacuum-assisted closure therapy in complex inguinal wound failures appears to be superior to conventional wound care without conferring an increased risk of local recurrence.[77]

KEY POINTS

1. Lymphadenectomy remains crucial in the surgical management of urologic malignancies, yielding both diagnostic and therapeutic benefits.
2. The split-and-roll technique should be used invariably to dissect lymphatic tissue overlying the large arteries and veins.
3. Sound knowledge of the pelvic and retroperitoneal anatomy are key to avoiding complications associated with lymph node dissections.

REFERENCES

Please see www.expertconsult.com

COMPLICATIONS OF PELVIC SURGERY

Chapter 41

COMPLICATIONS OF RADICAL CYSTECTOMY

Erik Pasin MD
Resident, Department of Urology, University of Southern California, Norris Comprehensive Cancer Center, Los Angeles, California

Maurizio Buscarini MD
Resident, Department of Urology, University of Southern California, Norris Comprehensive Cancer Center, Los Angeles, California

John P. Stein MD
Professor, Department of Urology, University of Southern California, Norris Comprehensive Cancer Center, Los Angeles, California

In the United States, bladder cancer is the fourth most common cancer in men and the eighth most common in women, with transitional cell carcinoma compromising nearly 90% of all primary bladder tumors.[1] Although most patients present with superficial bladder tumors, 20% to 40% of patients present with or ultimately develop muscle-invasive disease. Invasive bladder cancer is a lethal malignant disease. If it is untreated, >85% of patients will die of their disease within 2 years of the diagnosis.[2] Furthermore, a certain percentage of patients with high-grade bladder tumors without involvement of the lamina propria will have recurrent or progressive disease or unsuccessful intravesical management, and they may best be treated with earlier cystectomy, when survival outcomes are optimal.[3] The rationale for an aggressive treatment approach employing radical cystectomy for high-grade, invasive bladder cancer is based on several clinical observations:

1. The best long-term survival rates, coupled with the lowest local recurrence rates, are seen following definitive surgical treatment including removal of the primary bladder tumor and regional lymph nodes.[4,5]
2. The morbidity and mortality of radical cystectomy have significantly improved over the past several decades.
3. Transitional cell carcinoma tends to be resistant to radiation therapy, even at high doses.
4. Chemotherapy alone or in combination with bladder-sparing protocols has not demonstrated long-term local control and survival rates equivalent to rates reported with cystectomy.[6]
5. Radical cystectomy provides accurate pathologic staging of the primary bladder tumor (p stage) and regional lymph nodes and thus permits selective determination of the need for adjuvant therapy based on precise pathologic evaluation.

For the aforementioned reasons, radical cystectomy has become standard treatment and arguably the ideal form of therapy for high-grade, invasive bladder cancer today.

The evolution and improvements in lower urinary tract reconstruction, particularly orthotopic diversion, have been major components in enhancing the quality of life of patients requiring cystectomy. Currently, most men and women can safely undergo orthotopic lower urinary tract reconstruction to the urethra following cystectomy.[7] Orthotopic reconstruction most closely resembles the original bladder in both location and function, provides a continent means to store urine, and allows volitional voiding through the urethra. The orthotopic neobladder eliminates the need for a cutaneous stoma and a urostomy appliance, as well as the need for intermittent catheterization in most cases. These efforts have been directed to improve the quality of life of patients who must undergo bladder removal and have stimulated patients and physicians to consider radical cystectomy at an earlier, more curable stage of disease.[8]

At the University of Southern California (USC) in Los Angeles, a dedicated effort has been made to improve on the surgical technique of radical cystectomy and to provide an acceptable form of urinary diversion without compromising a sound cancer operation.[9-11] Radical cystectomy is a technically challenging operation, often performed in elderly patients with associated comorbidities that requires diligent attention to preoperative, intraoperative, and postoperative details. Despite this attention, complications do occur. Therefore, it is prudent for all surgeons to be familiar with the presentation, prevention, and treatment of the major causes of morbidity and mortality associated with this surgical procedure.

The complications of radical cystectomy can be categorized as (1) those specific to the removal of the anterior pelvic organs and associated lymphadenectomy and (2) those specific to the form of urinary diversion. This chapter focuses on the early and delayed complications associated with radical cystectomy and intestinal urinary diversion.

COMPLICATIONS OF CYSTECTOMY

Mortality

With improvements in surgical technique and perioperative anesthetic care, the early mortality rate associated with radical cystectomy has decreased from nearly 20% before 1970[12] to 1% to 5% in most contemporary series.[4,5,13-16] In a retrospective analysis of 1359 patients following radical cystectomy at USC, the most common cause of death in the perioperative period was cardiovascular, and septic complications from resulting urine and bowel leaks were the second most common (Table 41-1).[12] The USC surveillance regimen after radical cystectomy is shown in Table 41-2.

Hemorrhage

Hemorrhage is a common complication of radical cystectomy that can occur acutely intraoperatively and in

TABLE 41-1 Perioperative Mortality Rates From Radical Cystectomies, 1971 to 2001 (N = 1359 Patients)

Category	No. Perioperative Mortalities	Median Age (yr) at Surgery (Range)	Median Time (Days) to Death (Range)	Total No. Patients With Type of Complication	Complications Resulting in Perioperative Mortality (%)
Cardiovascular	8	65 (47-72)	13 (0-28)	34	24
Acute myocardial infarction	4				
Arrhythmia	2				
Cerebrovascular accident	1				
Arterial thrombosis (superior mesenteric artery)	1				
Infectious/Sepsis	8	71 (58-78)	33 (23-47)	212	4
Primary contributing factor					
Urine leak	3			72	4
Bowel leak/fistula	3			24	13
Small bowel obstruction	1				
Hematoma	1				
Pulmonary Embolus	4	69 (66-77)	20 (0-28)	25	16
Hepatic Failure	3	73 (62-78)	38 (5-48)	34*	15*
Upper Gastrointestinal Bleeding	2				
Hemorrhage, surgical site	1				
Hemorrhage	2	72 (66-77)	23 (1-44)	34*	15*
Hemophilia B	1				
Conduit-arterial fistula	1				
Unknown	2	62 (57-67)	64 (47-80)		
Total	27	67 (47-78)	28 (0-80)		

*All hemorrhagic complications regardless of primary cause are considered collectively.

the delayed setting. The bladder, prostate, uterus, and vagina are vascular organs that are drained by a rich venous supply, which necessitates careful and secure vascular control. Although several patient-related characteristics may affect intraoperative blood loss and the need for transfusion, a sound understanding of pelvic anatomy and adherence to proper surgical technique remain the cornerstones of prevention of significant bleeding in the intraoperative and delayed settings.

The blood supply to the anterior pelvic organs is derived primarily from the anterior branches of the internal iliac vessels. The anterior division of the hypogastric artery gives off seven branches supplying the pelvic viscera (superior vesical, middle rectal, inferior vesical, uterine, internal pudendal, obturator, and inferior gluteal arteries) that collectively form the lateral pedicle. At our institution, the lateral vascular pedicle is isolated, and each individual branch is clipped and divided after dissecting the obturator fossa and ligating the obturator vessels. Isolation and development of this pedicle are crucial for proper vascular control and to help minimize bleeding during radical cystectomy.

With the lateral pedicle entrapped between the surgeon's left index and middle fingers, firm traction is applied vertically and caudally (**Fig. 41-1**). This maneuver facilitates identification and allows individual branches of the anterior portion of the hypogastric artery to be isolated. The posterior trunk of the hypogastric artery, including the superior gluteal, iliolumbar, and lateral sacral arteries, is preserved to avoid gluteal claudication. All anterior branches of the hypogastric artery are isolated and divided between hemoclips down to the endopelvic fascia. The proximal aspect of each vessel is doubly clipped. We prefer right-angle hemoclips, with care ensuring that 0.5 to 1 cm of tissue projects between each clip when the pedicle is divided. This technique prevents the clips from becoming dislodged during the operation, with resulting unnecessary bleeding.

After control of the lateral pedicle, attention is directed toward the posterior pedicle. The posterior pedicle is developed after entry into Denonvilliers' space. The pouch of Douglas is incised slightly on the rectal side, and the plane between the posterior sheath of Denonvilliers' fascia and the rectum (Denonvilliers' space) is developed. A combination of sharp and blunt dissection allows the rectum to be carefully swept off the seminal vesicles, prostate, and bladder in men and the posterior vaginal wall in women. This sweeping motion, when extended laterally, helps to thin and develop the posterior pedicle, which resembles a collar emanating from the lateral aspect of the rectum (**Fig. 41-2**).

Once the posterior pedicles have been defined, they are clipped and divided down to the endopelvic fascia in the male patient. In women, the posterior pedicles, including the cardinal ligaments are divided 4 to 5 cm beyond the cervix. Again, proper hemoclip placement and technique are essential to minimize blood loss.

Although it is standard practice at USC to dissect and ligate the individual vessels of the lateral and posterior pedicles between carefully placed hemoclips, investigators have proposed that staple ligation of these pedicles contributes to significantly lower estimated blood loss and transfusion requirements compared with suture ligation alone.[17] We have not found this technique useful and in fact strongly encourage individual vessel ligation to ensure optimal vascular control.

TABLE 41-2	University of Southern California Surveillance Regimen After Radical Cystectomy			
	4 Months	**1 Year**	**2-5 Years (Annually)**	**After 5 Years (Annually)**
Orthotopic neobladder, continent cutaneous diversion*, ileal conduit†,‡	IV pyelogram (ultrasound if creatinine >1.8 mg/dL)	IV pyelogram (ultrasound if creatinine >1.8 mg/dL)	IV pyelogram (ultrasound if creatinine >1.8 mg/dL)	IV pyelogram (ultrasound if creatinine >1.8 mg/dL)
	Gravity cystogram	Gravity cystogram	Gravity cystogram	Gravity cystogram
	Comprehensive metabolic panel	Comprehensive metabolic panel	Comprehensive metabolic panel	Comprehensive metabolic panel
	Liver function tests	Liver function tests	Liver function tests	Liver function tests
	Chest radiograph	Chest radiograph	Chest radiograph	Chest radiograph
		Urine cytology	Urine cytology	Urine cytology
				Vitamin B$_{12}$ every other year

*Same as orthotopic neobladder with annual urethral washings in male patients.
†Same as orthotopic neobladder, may use loopogram to assess upper tracts.
‡Consider computed tomography of the abdomen or pelvis at 6, 12, and 24 months in pT3 or pT4 disease.
IV, intravenous.

The third major vascular structure that must be controlled before removal of the cystectomy specimen is the dorsal venous complex (DVC). Although several methods have been described, we use one of two methods of securing the DVC, both of which offer excellent vascular control. An angled clamp can be passed carefully beneath the DVC, anterior to the urethra. The venous complex can then be ligated with a 2-0 absorbable suture and divided close to the apex of the prostate. Any additional bleeding after transection of the venous complex, should it occur, can be oversewn with the previously placed absorbable 2-0 suture.

Alternatively, the DVC may be gathered at the apex of the prostate with a long Allis clamp. This technique may help to define the plane between the DVC and the anterior urethra more clearly. A figure-of-eight 2-0 absorbable suture can then be placed under direct vision anterior to the urethra and distal to the apex of the prostate around the gathered DVC. This maneuver not only affords secure vascular control but also avoids passage of instruments between the DVC and the rhabdosphincter that could potentially injure these structures and compromise the continence mechanism.

Several patient-related characteristics reported in the literature predispose to greater estimated blood loss and a higher transfusion rate. Increased body mass index was shown to correlate with a larger estimated blood loss in several retrospective analyses.[18,19] In one analysis, body mass index was the only preoperative variable on a multivariate analysis to predict increased blood loss during radical cystectomy independently.[18] Gender differences have been thought to affect transfusion requirements in patients undergoing radical cystectomy. One study found that the transfusion rate and the median number of units transfused were greater in women compared with men as a result of the rich lateral vascular pedicles unique to the female pelvis (cardinal and uterosacral ligaments).[20]

Controlled hypotensive anesthesia as a means to reduce blood loss in radical cystectomy has been studied and remains standard surgical practice in selected patients at our institution.[21] At USC, the anesthesiologist titrates intravenous (IV) nitroglycerin to lower mean arterial pressure until the cystectomy specimen is removed, at which time the blood pressure is returned to normal range. Return to normotension facilitates identification of any bleeding vessels that may not have been identified or properly secured during the hypotensive period and thus allows further pelvic hemostasis. Despite obtaining secure vascular control during the intraoperative period, postoperative bleeding may occur that requires immediate return to the operating room.

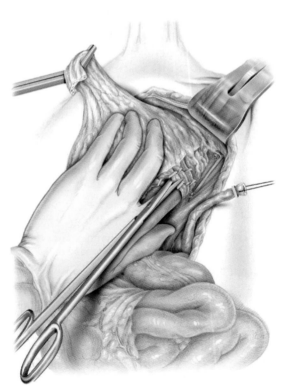

Figure 41-1 Technique for isolation and ligation of the lateral pedicle. All anterior branches of the hypogastric vessels are isolated and divided between hemoclips down to the endopelvic fascia.

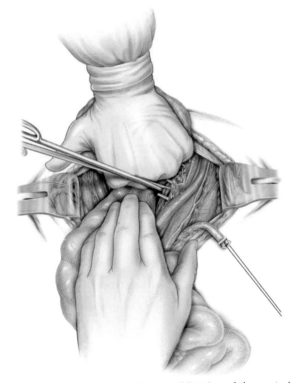

Figure 41-2 Technique for isolation and ligation of the posterior pedicle. The posterior pedicle is developed after entry into Denonvilliers' space and, with a combination of blunt and sharp dissection, resembles a collar emanating from the lateral aspect of the rectum.

In our series of 1359 patients who underwent cystectomy, 11 patients (0.8%) experienced surgically related postoperative hemorrhage, 8 of whom (72%) required return to the operating room. We routinely place a large Hemovac drain in the pelvis to drain any blood for the first 24 hours postoperatively. An undrained pelvic hematoma may predispose to abscess formation, delayed return of bowel function, or disruption of urethral-intestinal anastomoses in orthotopic neobladders.

Rectal Injury

Rectal injury as a complication of radical cystectomy has potentially grave consequences if it is not recognized intraoperatively. Contemporary cystectomy series report an incidence of rectal injury ranging from 0.3% to 9.7%.[4,5,14,15,16,22] Factors predisposing to intraoperative rectal injury include prior pelvic surgery, colonic inflammatory disease, extensive prior transurethral resection of a posterior bladder mass, direct extension of a posterior bladder mass into Denonvilliers' space, and, most importantly, prior pelvic radiation therapy.[22]

Morbidity can be minimized by prospectively identifying those patients at increased risk and employing primarily sharp dissection of the posterior bladder off the anterior rectal wall in patients with an obliterated posterior plane. Furthermore, intraoperative recognition of a rectal injury, appropriate repair, adequate decompression of the injured rectum, establishment of sufficient pelvic drainage, and aggressive nutritional and antimicrobial support are all critical to prevent significant potential sequelae.

The advent of preoperative bowel preparation in the 1970s led to numerous clinical trials that clearly demonstrated the decreased incidence of infectious postoperative complications in modern elective colorectal surgery.[23] Proper bowel preparation is also important to minimize the infectious sequelae of rectal injury. A three-tier regimen is standard practice when performing surgical procedures in which breach of the distal intestinal tract is anticipated.[23] This regimen includes the following steps:

1. Preoperative mechanical cleansing to decrease the fecal load and facilitate the efficacy of the orally administered antibiotics
2. Preoperative oral antimicrobial bactericidal therapy targeting both aerobic and anaerobic organisms
3. Perioperative parenteral antimicrobial therapy

All patients at our institution who are undergoing radical cystectomy are admitted the day before the procedure for antibacterial bowel preparation and IV hydration. A clear liquid diet may be consumed until midnight, at which time the patient is to consume nothing orally thereafter before the operation. A standard Nichols bowel preparation[23] is given, as follows:

120 mL of castor oil orally at 09.00 hours; 1 g of neomycin orally at 10.00, 11.00, 12.00, 13.00, 16.00, 20.00, and 24.00 hours; and 1 g of erythromycin base orally at 12.00, 16.00, 20.00, and 24.00 hours. We find that this regimen is generally well tolerated, it obviates the need for enemas, and it maintains nutritional and hydration support.

Key to minimizing the risk of rectal injury is a sound understanding of the fascia layers between the bladder and the rectum. The anterior and posterior peritoneal reflections converge in the cul-de-sac to form Denonvilliers' fascia, which further extends caudally to the urogenital diaphragm (**Fig. 41-3**). This important anatomic boundary in the male patient separates the prostate and seminal vesicles from the rectum posteriorly. The plane between the prostate and seminal vesicles and the anterior sheath of Denonvilliers' fascia does not develop easily. However, the plane between the rectum and the posterior sheath of Denonvilliers' fascia (Denonvilliers' space) should develop easily with sharp and blunt dissection. Therefore, the peritoneal incision in the cul-de-sac should be made slightly on the rectal side, rather than on the bladder side. This technique facilitates proper and safe entry and development of Denonvilliers' space. Occasionally, patients with an invasive posterior bladder tumor or those who have undergone

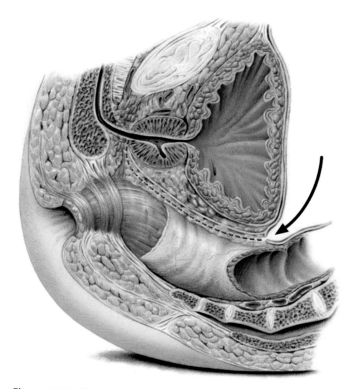

Figure 41-3 The peritoneal incision in the cul-de-sac (*arrow*) should be made slightly on the rectal side for safe entry into Denonvilliers' space and should develop easily with sharp and blunt dissection. Knowledge of the fascial layers between the bladder and rectum facilitates the posterior dissection and minimizes the risk of rectal injury.

previous pelvic radiation therapy may have this plane obliterated, thus increasing the risk of rectal injury.

Because most rectal injuries are created as a result of the shearing forces produced during blunt dissection of Denonvilliers' space, patients with obliterated posterior planes necessitate entry into this space sharply. If rectal injury does occur, it is crucial that it be identified intraoperatively. Often a small rectal laceration can be missed, and in patients at high risk for rectal injury, diligent intraoperative inspection of the anterior and lateral rectal walls is essential. When visualization is inconclusive and rectal injury is suspected, delineation of the site of injury can be accomplished by insufflating the rectum with air while the pelvis is filled with fluid.

Once rectal injury is identified, it should be closed in layers. In previous reviews, investigators had advocated that proctotomies be closed at the time of initial injury in three layers,[24] although most literature currently considers a two-layer closure sufficient.[25] A running absorbable suture is used to close the mucosa after the wound edges are débrided. Care should be taken to invert the mucosal edges into the bowel lumen when this layer is closed. The second layer of interrupted silk sutures in a Lembert fashion is used to complete the closure. If possible, the interposition of a greater omental apron is advised to discourage fistula formation,[26] particularly if rectal injury occurred in the setting of orthotopic neobladder construction, in which fresh suture lines of the neobladder and urethral anastomosis are vulnerable. Diversion of the fecal stream by means of a sigmoid loop colostomy should be performed when the rectal defect is considerable, the contamination is great, or impaired healing from previous pelvic radiation or colonic inflammatory disease is expected.[22]

Venous Thromboembolism

It lingers in the mind of every surgeon that after a dedicated intraoperative effort, acute pulmonary events developing from insidious venous clots may complicate the patient's perioperative outcome. A wealth of information has been published regarding the cause, risk factors, treatment, and prevention of venous thromboembolism since Virchow first reported on the factors that predispose to thrombosis in 1856.

Thromboembolism accounts for 1% to 4% of all perioperative complications reported in contemporary cystectomy series.[4,5,14-16] Several risk factors have been identified that predispose patients to a higher incidence of venous thromboembolism than in the general population (Box 41-1). Indisputable evidence has accumulated in the form of randomized clinical trials to demonstrate the effect of primary thromboprophylaxis in the reduction of deep vein thrombosis (DVT), nonfatal pulmonary embolism, and fatal pulmonary embolism.[27] To prevent such complications, it is common

BOX 41-1	Risk Factors for Venous Thromboembolism

Obesity
Smoking
Advanced age
Previous venous thromboembolism
Prolonged immobility/paresis
Trauma (major or lower extremity)
Central venous catheterization
Estrogen-containing oral contraceptives
Heart or respiratory failure
Myeloproliferative disorders
Acute medical illness
Inherited or acquired thrombophilia

practice for surgical patients to be prescribed some form of thromboprophylaxis during their hospital stay.

The evidence-based guidelines of the Seventh American College of Chest Physicians Conference on Antithrombotic and Thrombolytic Therapy reported that the absolute risk of DVT in hospitalized patients who undergo major urologic surgery (defined as open urologic procedures) and who receive no form of thromboprophylaxis is 15% to 40%.[27] Additionally, the conference reported that the ratio between asymptomatic DVT and symptomatic thromboembolism is approximately 5:1 to 10:1. The conference thus recommended, based on strong evidence,[28] that in patients undergoing major, open urologic procedures, routine prophylaxis with low-dose unfractionated heparin twice or three times daily is the preferred thromboprophylaxis regimen. Low-molecular-weight heparin or prophylaxis with intermittent pneumatic compressions or graduated compression stockings is an acceptable alternative.

For patients with multiple risk factors, the conference recommended combining graduated compression stockings or intermittent pneumatic compressions with either low-dose unfractionated heparin or low-molecular-weight heparin. For those patients actively bleeding or at high risk of bleeding, the conference recommended the use of mechanical thromboprophylaxis with intermittent pneumatic compressions or graduated compression stockings at least until the bleeding decreases.[27]

Because most venous thromboembolic events are diagnosed several weeks after hospital discharge, the duration of thromboprophylactic therapy necessary to prevent thromboembolism while negligibly affecting the rate of hemorrhage in postoperative patients with cancer remains unclear. One study found that enoxaparin prophylaxis for 4 weeks after surgical treatment of abdominal or pelvic cancer was safe and significantly reduced the incidence of venographically demonstrated thrombosis, as compared with enoxaparin prophylaxis for 1 week.[29] These limited data suggest that some form of thromboprophylaxis for 1 month postoperatively may be important.

At our institution, warfarin (Coumadin) and intermittent pneumatic compression devices are used as thromboprophylaxis in the postoperative hospitalization period for patients undergoing cystectomy. It has been our large experience that excellent prophylaxis of thromboembolic events with minimal effect on postoperative hemorrhage rates can be achieved with an initial warfarin load of 10 mg given through a gastrostomy tube immediately in the postanesthesia recovery unit, followed by daily administration of warfarin while monitoring the patients prothrombin time to keep within a range of 18 to 22 seconds. For patients who are particularly sensitive to warfarin, smaller doses are commonly used, and any dangerous elevation of the prothrombin time can be effectively and immediately reversed with the administration of IV vitamin K.

As seen in Table 41-1, 25 of 1359 patients (1.8%) receiving radical cystectomy in our series developed pulmonary embolism at a mean of 20 days postoperatively. Sixteen percent of these embolisms proved fatal, a finding emphasizing the potential significance of this complication after major pelvic exenterative surgical treatment of malignant disease. In our experience, the rate of hemorrhage and the need for transfusion in patients receiving low-dose unfractionated heparin or low-molecular-weight heparin are greater compared with the use of warfarin, and as such, warfarin administration in the postoperative period as a means of thromboprophylaxis for the patient after radical cystectomy has been standard practice at USC.

Ileus

Postoperative ileus is the prolonged delay in the coordinated movements of the gastrointestinal (GI) tract. This common complication of intra-abdominal surgery is often responsible for a lengthy hospital stay and significant perioperative morbidity. The following factors responsible for the pathogenesis of postoperative ileus have been elucidated: imbalances among the sympathetic, parasympathetic, and intrinsic nervous systems of the small intestine and colon; and the role of inflammatory mediators. Although a complete discussion of this extensive topic is beyond the scope of this chapter, the reader is referred to an excellent review for more detail regarding the origin and pathogenesis of postoperative ileus.[30]

Prolonged ileus after radical cystectomy is a common complication with an incidence ranging from 7% to 23% in several series.[4,5,14-16,31] In one report, ileus was the most common complication resulting in a prolonged hospital stay following radical cystectomy.[31] Chang and colleagues[31] defined ileus as a delayed return of bowel function beyond postoperative day 4. As such, larger numbers of patients from their retrospective series were

regarded as having ileus compared with other series.[31] The definition of ileus is debatable; however, the delay in recovery of coordinated intestinal movements from surgical trauma typically resolves after 3 to 4 postoperative days, with the colon the last of the intestinal segments to regain function.[30]

Because postoperative ileus prolongs hospital stay, and longer time spent in the hospital places patients at increased risk for nosocomially acquired infections and other complications, it seems prudent for physicians to tailor the standard perioperative care toward evidence-based strategies shown to help resolve postoperative ileus in the safest and most expeditious manner. Although ascertaining the best method of reducing the duration of postoperative ileus is difficult because much of the published literature is skewed by differences in study protocols, several general conclusions can be made.

Some investigators recommend placement of a thoracic epidural catheter and the use of local anesthetic to reduce the possibility of a postoperative ileus.[30] Epidural anesthesia with bupivacaine has been shown to be superior to systemic and epidural opioid with respect to reduction in postoperative ileus and without significantly affecting pain relief in patients undergoing abdominal surgical procedures.[30] Limiting the use of IV opioids and supplementing narcotics with nonsteroidal anti-inflammatory drugs may also be helpful. In addition to reducing the total amount of narcotic use, the use of nonsteroidal anti-inflammatory drugs decreases the amount of local inflammatory mediators in the intestinal wall and may minimize the duration of postoperative ileus through this alternative mechanism as well.[30]

No prospective, randomized trials have validated the use of prokinetic agents, including erythromycin or metoclopramide, in the resolution of postoperative ileus. Cisapride did show promise in previous years, although the discovery of its arrhythmogenic effect as a consequence of its prolongation of the Q-T interval led to its current unavailability in the United States.[30] Contrary to popular belief, early ambulation has no demonstrable effect in expediting the resolution of postoperative ileus. Early ambulation is to be encouraged, however, because it is beneficial primarily in the prevention of atelectasis, pneumonia, and deep vein thrombosis.[30]

Ileus that fails to resolve by the 10th to 14th postoperative day may warrant investigation into the cause. Correction of electrolyte imbalances, particularly hyponatremia, hypokalemia, and hypomagnesemia, which may occur in the perioperative period, is important to restore bowel function. A search for additional causes such as abscess from intestinal anastomotic or urine leak should also be considered.

Bowel decompression is advised to prevent the sequelae of ileus including nausea, vomiting, abdominal distention, and pain. Poorly decompressed bowel in the setting of unresolved ileus may also cause significant fluid shifts and may potentially stress enteric anastomoses and predispose the patient to anastomotic leaks. Traditionally, nasogastric decompression was the method of choice in conservative management of postoperative ileus. In addition to the general discomfort associated with nasogastric tubes, more recent literature suggested that postoperative nasogastric intubation was the single most important variable associated with the development of postoperative pulmonary complications.[32] It is therefore standard practice at USC to place an operative gastrostomy tube at the time of cystectomy in a modified Stamm fashion, in which greater omentum is interposed between the stomach and the abdominal wall, to facilitate resolution of postoperative ileus,[33] without the need for a nasogastric tube.

Bowel Leak and Enterocutaneous Fistula

The development of a bowel leak following radical cystectomy is a devastating complication associated with a significant morbidity and mortality. Up until the 1960s, the mortality rate of patients with GI fistulas was 43%.[34] Although the advent of improved methods of critical care and artificial nutrition steadily decreased the mortality rate of postoperative bowel leaks, these complications continue to pose significant anxiety, discomfort, and negative self-image for patients during the course of disease and remain a considerable source of elevated hospital cost.[34]

The finding of fever, wound infection, and elevation of white blood cell count on the fifth to seventh postoperative day or a delayed return of bowel function persisting and temporally associated with these events should raise suspicion of an intra-abdominal abscess from a potential bowel leak or an unrecognized enterotomy. Patients are often extremely ill and may display signs of sepsis, including hypotension, tachycardia, and organ system failure requiring an intensive care setting. The finding of enteric contents from a surgically placed drain confirms the diagnosis. A computed tomography (CT) scan with water-soluble oral contrast material in those patients with no external evidence of fistula is prudent and typically reveals extravasation of contrast from the bowel lumen into an intra-abdominal or pelvic fluid collection. A CT scan is also necessary to rule out any distal intestinal obstruction that may have contributed to the formation of, and will invariably prevent the closure of, the enteric fistula.

Once the complication is diagnosed, management of a bowel leak from an unrecognized enterotomy or breakdown of intestinal anastomosis is a clinical dilemma. Two schools of thought exist: emergency laparotomy and conservative management. The decision to choose one or the other is not always obvious given the lack of clear evidence-based guidelines in dealing with this complication. The decision to begin a trial of conservative management largely depends on the presence or absence of peritonitis or sepsis.[35] If drainage is adequate, or if the patient has a controlled fistula and in the absence of clinical peritonitis or multiple intra-abdominal abscesses refractory to percutaneous drainage, a trial of conservative management is warranted.[35] Maximal drainage of any intra-abdominal or pelvic fluid collections from radiographically placed drains is mandatory to treat the septic patient.

Every attempt to control intra-abdominal infection aggressively is essential because the major cause of death in this group of patients is sepsis, which is the result of a neglected or undrained intra-abdominal or pelvic abscess.[36] The abdominal incision, if displaying signs of infection, should be opened and left to heal by second intention. Cultures should be obtained and broad-spectrum antibiotic therapy should be employed and tailored to microbial sensitivity.

The patient should be made to take nothing by mouth. Proximal decompression and drainage by means of a nasogastric or gastrostomy tube should be begun, and hyperalimentation should be instituted. Total parenteral nutrition is classically indicated in patients with enterocutaneous fistulas. Total parenteral nutrition has been shown to increase the spontaneous closure rate by inducing bowel hypoactivity and to provide better nutritional preparation of the patient for reoperation after a defined period of nutritional support if the fistula fails to close spontaneously.[37]

Data regarding the use of somatostatin analogues in the conservative management of enterocutaneous fistula are debatable. Although somatostatin and its analogues have been shown to decrease fistula output thus make it easier to manage fluid, electrolytes, and protein imbalances, the therapeutic advantage with regard to reducing the time to fistula closure has not been consistently shown in clinical trials.[38-41]

Despite attention to detail and patience, with conservative treatment, only 50% of postoperative bowel fistulas close spontaneously in ≤4 to 6 weeks in the absence of distal obstruction or the loss of bowel continuity. If nutritionally anabolic and free of sepsis, the remainder of patients usually respond favorably to elective reoperation to repair the fistula and restore intestinal continuity.[35] Reoperation is best delayed for at least 3 to 4 months postoperatively.

The decision to perform acute emergency laparotomy is warranted in patients displaying peritonitis or signs of sepsis with proven or suspected intraperitoneal abscesses that are not amenable to percutaneous drainage or in which percutaneous drainage has failed.[35] The goal of laparotomy is to cleanse the abdominal cavity and pelvis of any loculated abscesses by using copious irrigation, to provide adequate drainage of the pelvis and peritoneum by means of surgically placed drains, and to control the source of contaminating infection, typically through the creation of a proximal enterostomy, irrespective of the level of injury.[35]

It may be possible to resect the affected bowel segment and primarily reanastomose it in a patient who presents with a fistula within the first 2 postoperative days. These occurrences are usually the result of technical error and may afford a cure in a minimally compromised patient with insignificant peritonitis and a normal serum albumin concentration.[35] However, intestinal diversion should be performed if the quality of bowel is suspect or if the patient has a history of radiation therapy, because primary repair often fails in these patients.

Strict attention to surgical detail during intestinal anastomosis is crucial to avoid the development of an enterocutaneous fistula. At our institution, a traditional two-layered, hand-sewn, interrupted, end-to-end anastomosis using a series of 3-0 silk sutures is performed to reestablish intestinal continuity after the appropriate segment of bowel is gathered to form the urinary reservoir. Adequate exposure to the anastomosing segments, maintenance of excellent blood supply to the severed ends, avoidance of local spillage of enteric contents that may facilitate a focal septic environment, accurate serosa-to-serosa apposition, and avoidance of tissue strangulation by sutures tied too tightly are all important details that, when methodically followed, allow for successful intestinal anastomosis.[42]

Lymphocele

Numerous studies emphasized the importance of pelvic lymph node dissection during cystectomy for invasive bladder cancer. Most of these investigators advocated lymph node dissection not only as a staging procedure but also as an integral part of the curative intent of radical surgery for invasive bladder cancer.[43-45] Although most patients undergoing radical cystectomy are elderly and have significant comorbidities, proper lymphadenectomy may still be beneficial. Studies have shown that removing more lymph nodes increased survival in patients with node-negative as well as node-positive bladder cancer.[46-48] However, opinion continues to be divided on the extent of the lymphadenectomy and the minimum number of nodes that should be removed.

The incidence of lymphocele with limited or extended lymph node dissection is 1% to 4%, according to major published series.[44,49] Most of these cases can be managed expectantly. In the USC series with extended lymphadenectomy, only two patients required percutaneous CT-guided drainage of the lymph collection, and this maneuver promptly resolved the problem in both cases.

In another study, Brossner and colleagues[45] reported the events during and after radical cystectomy in a series of 92 consecutive patients, in terms of major and minor complications, and compared minimal and extended lymphadenectomy procedures. These investigators found that extended lymphadenectomy in patients undergoing radical cystectomy did not increase morbidity within 30 days of the surgical procedure. We believe that extended lymphadenectomy causes no significant increase in complications during and after the procedure.

Wound Infection and Fascial Dehiscence

Surgical site infections and wound and tissue dehiscence are well-known postoperative complications in GI and urologic surgery. The severity of these complications ranges from mild cases needing local wound care and antibiotics to serious cases with multiple reoperations and a high mortality rate. Usually, infectious complications prolong hospitalization, with a substantial increase in cost of care.[50,51]

The incidence of wound infection and fascial dehiscence after radical cystectomy in reported series is 3% to 6% and 1% to 3%, respectively.[4,5,14-16] Several patient-related characteristics increase the risk of wound infection and fascial dehiscence in major abdominal operations. Extensive prior smoking history, diabetes mellitus, and cardiopulmonary disease are associated with increased risk of surgical site infections and abdominal wall dehiscence[52-57] by a variety of proposed mechanisms. Smoking, microvascular disease as a result of long-standing diabetes mellitus, and severe lung disease are known causes of peripheral tissue hypoxia,[58,59] which increases the risk of wound infection and dehiscence.[60] In addition, some studies suggest that hypoxia, smoking, and diabetes reduce collagen synthesis and oxidative killing mechanisms of neutrophils,[61-65] with resulting impairment of wound healing.

The association between elevated perioperative blood loss and postoperative tissue and wound complications in elective operations suggests that hypovolemia and reduction of tissue oxygenation by loss of red blood cells are also detrimental to healing and increase the risk of infection and tissue dehiscence.[66-71] Disruption of the local vascular supply, thrombosis of vessels, and tissue hypoxia are common to all tissues subject to surgical intervention.[72] Once the blood supply is restored, several factors may further complicate healing. The most important seems to be proliferation of bacteria in the wound and tissue that affects the processes involved in wound healing and increases the risk of wound infection and dehiscence. Fascial dehiscence is invariably associated with previous wound infection,[73] and it represents a serious postoperative problem that often necessitates immediate operative exploration and repair.

Occasionally, in the case of minor fascial separation, it may be possible to delay immediate repair for several months in the absence of frank evisceration or incarceration of bowel. However, immediate return to the operating room is usually mandatory in patients with evisceration or obstruction.

URETHRAL AND VAGINAL PRESERVATION IN CYSTECTOMY

As patients are living longer and with higher expectations, quality of life issues are becoming more important factors in patients undergoing radical cystectomy. These issues should not, however, override the need for providing sound oncologic surgical extirpation.

Orthotopic diversion most closely resembles the original bladder in its location and functional characteristics. Advances in surgical technique have obviated the need for external appliances and cutaneous stomas in appropriately selected patients and have made volitional voiding possible. The ideal reservoir should fulfill five criteria:

1. Maintenance of a large capacity
2. Low filling pressures
3. Protection of the upper urinary tracts
4. Relatively nonabsorptive surface area
5. Allowance for continent volitional voiding

Orthotopic diversion currently represents the procedure of choice in the properly selected patient undergoing cystectomy. Currently, >90% of male and female patients at USC undergo orthotopic lower urinary tract reconstruction.[74-76]

With the advent of orthotopic urinary diversion, preservation of the rhabdosphincteric continence mechanism has become the most important functional goal in the surgical management of the patient undergoing cystectomy; second only to the complete extirpation of the malignant disease. Based on the neuroanatomic studies of Walsh and Donker[80] and others during the early 1980s, and through steady refinement in the surgical techniques applied to radical retropubic prostatectomy,[77-80] the importance of the external striated urethral sphincteric complex in maintaining continence has become evident in those patients undergoing enterourethral anastomosis following radical cystectomy. Preservation of the rhabdosphincter and its pudendal innervation is critical in allowing the return of continence.[81]

Precise neuroanatomic and histologic studies of the pelvis and urethra have provided a better understanding of the rhabdoid sphincter and a rational basis for continence preservation in radical pelvic surgery.[81-83] Proper knowledge and preservation of the anatomic configuration of the rhabdosphincter muscle and its pudendal nerve supply[81,82] following cystectomy should provide continence and volitional voiding. Attention to anatomic details and meticulous surgical technique are of the utmost importance to optimize functional and clinical outcomes. Overall, daytime continence rates of ≥80% have been reported in most large series with orthotopic reconstruction.[9,74-76,84]

Minimal manipulation of the external striated urethral sphincteric complex (the muscle fibers of the rhabdosphincter and its fascial attachments) and of its innervation is essential in providing optimal urinary continence.[76,79,81,83] The pudendal nerve provides somatic innervation to the rhabdosphincter and enters this muscle in the perineum through the perineal nerve and from the pelvis by way of the intrapelvic branch of the pudendal nerve.[79,81] Branches of the pudendal nerve that run along the pelvic floor below the endopelvic fascia ultimately innervate the rhabdosphincter. Therefore, minimal dissection should be performed along the pelvic floor levator musculature to avoid injury to the rhabdosphincter innervation.

Our experience with the orthotopic ileal neobladder has demonstrated excellent long-term continence rates.[74-76,84] More than 85% of male patients rated their continence as good or satisfactory during the day and night. However, as with other orthotopic diversions, more patients (≈20%) achieved better continence during the day than during the night. The ultimate level of daytime and nighttime continence was achieved by 1 year postoperatively in 89% and 85% of the male patients, respectively. In general, younger patients tended to fare better than did older patients. Over an 8-year study period, only 2.7% of patients required an artificial urinary sphincter secondary to unsatisfactory continence following orthotopic bladder replacement.[75,84]

Since 1990, the USC group has also been committed to providing orthotopic lower urinary tract reconstruction in appropriately selected female patients.[9,76,85,86] In fact, many of the early neuroanatomic studies demonstrating the pudendal innervation to the rhabdosphincter complex were generated from female cadaveric dissections.[82,83] In our series of women undergoing orthotopic diversion, complete daytime continence was reported by 85% of patients, with nighttime continence rates reported by 82%. Eighty-five percent voided to completion, whereas the initial results suggested that 15% required some form of intermittent catheterization.[76] With longer follow-up, it appears that 30% to 40% of women will require some form of intermittent catheterization to empty their neobladder.

Continence-preserving Technique

Several technical issues should be considered intraoperatively to help achieve maximum continence in both men and women who require radical cystectomy and orthotopic urinary diversion. Attention to surgical detail is most important and deserves special mention.

Anterior Apical Dissection in the Male Patient

The technique of bilateral pelvic lymphadenectomy with radical cystoprostatectomy has been previously

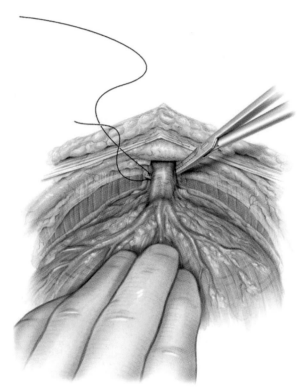

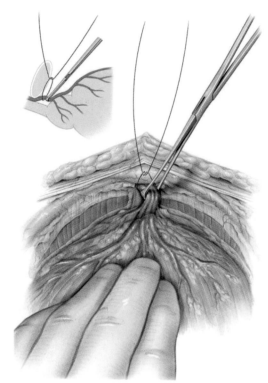

Figure 41-4 One technique for ligation of the dorsal venous complex. An angled clamp is passed beneath the dorsal venous complex, anterior to the urethra. The venous complex can then be ligated with a 2-0 absorbable suture and divided close to the apex of the prostate. If any bleeding occurs from the transected venous complex, it can be oversewn with an absorbable (2-0 polyglycolic acid) suture.

Figure 41-5 Technique of gathering the dorsal venous complex at the apex of the prostate with a long Allis clamp. A figure-of-eight 2-0 absorbable suture can then be placed under direct vision anterior to the urethra (distal to the apex of the prostate) around the gathered venous complex. This suture is best placed while the surgeon faces the head of the table and holds the needle driver perpendicular to the patient. This maneuver avoids the unnecessary passage of instruments between the dorsal venous complex and the rhabdosphincter that could potentially injure these structures and compromise the continence mechanism.

reported.[87] Urethral preparation with preservation of the continence mechanism is of critical importance when orthotopic diversion is anticipated in men.

Only after the cystectomy specimen is completely freed and mobile posteriorly is attention directed anteriorly to the urethra. All fibroareolar connections among the anterior bladder wall, the prostate, and the undersurface of the pubic symphysis are divided. The endopelvic fascia is incised adjacent to the prostate, and the levator muscles are carefully swept off the lateral and apical portions of the prostate. The superficial dorsal vein is identified, ligated, and divided. With tension placed posteriorly on the prostate, the puboprostatic ligaments are identified and are slightly divided just beneath the pubis and lateral to the DVC that courses in between these ligaments. Care should be taken to avoid any extensive dissection in this region. The puboprostatic ligaments should be incised only enough to allow for proper apical dissection of the prostate. The apex of the prostate and membranous urethra now become palpable.

Several methods can be performed to control the DVC properly, as previously described (see the earlier section on hemorrhage). A more illustrative description

follows. One may carefully pass an angled clamp beneath the DVC, anterior to the urethra (**Fig. 41-4**). The venous complex can then be ligated with a 2-0 absorbable suture and divided close to the apex of the prostate.

If any bleeding occurs from the transected venous complex, it can be oversewn with an absorbable (2-0 polyglycolic acid) suture. In a slightly different fashion, the DVC may be gathered at the apex of the prostate with a long Allis clamp. A figure-of-eight 2-0 absorbable suture can then be placed under direct vision anterior to the urethra (distal to the apex of the prostate) around the gathered venous complex (**Fig. 41-5**). This suture is best placed while the surgeon faces the head of the table and holds the needle driver perpendicular to the patient. The suture is then tagged with a hemostat. This maneuver avoids the unnecessary passage of any instruments between the DVC and the rhabdosphincter that could potentially injure these structures and compromise the continence mechanism.

After the complex has been ligated, it can be sharply divided with excellent exposure to the anterior surface

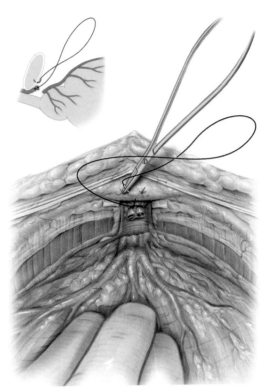

Figure 41-6 Suspending the venous complex anteriorly to the periosteum helps reestablish anterior fixation of the dorsal venous complex and puboprostatic ligaments and may enhance continence recovery.

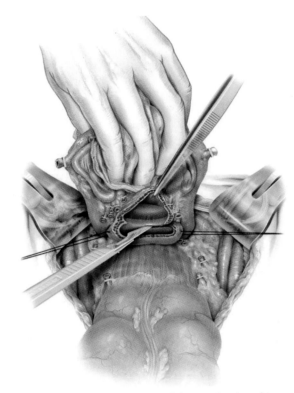

Figure 41-7 When the posterior pedicles are developed in women, the posterior vagina is incised at the apex, just distal to the cervix.

of the urethra. Once the venous complex has been severed, the suture can be used to secure the complex further. The suture is then used to suspend the DVC anteriorly to the periosteum to help reestablish anterior fixation of the DVC and puboprostatic ligaments (**Fig. 41-6**). This technique may enhance continence recovery. The anterior urethra is now exposed.

Regardless of the technique, the urethra is then incised 270 degrees just beyond the apex of the prostate. A series of 2-0 polyglycolic acid sutures is placed in the urethra circumferentially, with careful incorporation of only the mucosa and submucosa of the striated urethral sphincter muscle anteriorly. The urethral catheter is clamped and divided distally. Two sutures are placed that should incorporate the rectourethralis muscle posteriorly or the caudal extent of Denonvilliers' fascia. Next, the posterior urethra is divided and the specimen is removed. Frozen section analysis of the distal urethral margin of the cystectomy specimen is then performed to exclude tumor involvement.

Anterior Dissection in the Female Patient

When considering orthotopic diversion in female patients, several technical issues are critical to maintain the continence mechanism.

When the posterior pedicles are developed in women, the posterior vagina is incised at the apex, just distal to

the cervix (**Fig. 41-7**). This incision is carried anteriorly along the lateral and anterior vaginal wall to form a circumferential division. The anterolateral vaginal wall is then grasped with a curved Kocher clamp. This maneuver provides countertraction and facilitates dissection between the anterior vaginal wall and the bladder specimen. Careful dissection of the proper plane prevents entry into the posterior bladder and reduces the amount of bleeding in this vascular area. Development of this posterior plane and vascular pedicle is best performed sharply with the use of hemoclips and is carried just distal to the vesicourethral junction. Palpation of the Foley catheter balloon assists in identifying this region.

This dissection should effectively maintain a functional anterior vaginal wall (**Fig. 41-8**). Furthermore, an intact anterior vaginal wall helps support the proximal urethra through a complex musculofascial support system that extends from the pelvic floor, which may be an important component to the continence mechanism in these women.

Alternatively, in the case of a deeply invasive posterior bladder tumor with concern of an adequate surgical margin, the anterior vaginal wall should be removed en bloc with the cystectomy specimen. After dividing the posterior vaginal apex, the lateral vaginal wall subsequently serves as the posterior pedicle and is divided

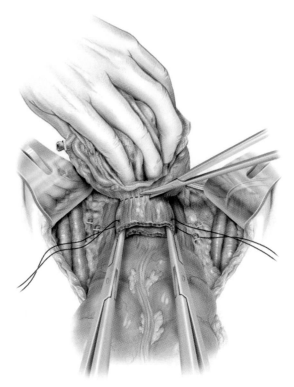

Figure 41-8 A Kocher clamp provides countertraction and facilitates dissection and preservation of a functional anterior vaginal wall.

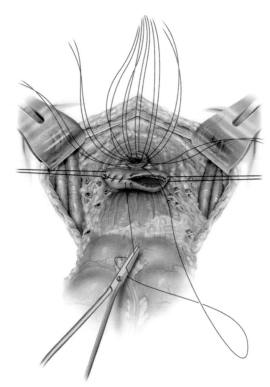

Figure 41-9 Vaginal reconstruction by a clam-shell technique and placement of urethral sutures after the cystectomy specimen is removed.

distally. This maneuver leaves the anterior vaginal wall attached to the posterior bladder specimen. Again, the Foley catheter balloon facilitates identification of the vesicourethral junction. The surgical plane between the vesicourethral junction and the anterior vaginal wall is then developed distally at this location. A 1-cm length of proximal urethra is mobilized while the remaining distal urethra is left intact with the anterior vaginal wall. Vaginal reconstruction by a clam-shell (horizontal) or side-to-side (vertical) technique is required. Other means of vaginal reconstruction may include a rectus myocutaneous flap, detubularized cylinder of ileum, a peritoneal flap, or an omental flap.

When the posterior dissection is completed (ensuring dissection just distal to the vesicourethral junction), a Satinsky vascular clamp is placed across the bladder neck to prevent any tumor spill from the bladder. With gentle traction, the proximal urethra is completely divided anteriorly, distal to the bladder neck and clamp, and the specimen is removed. The female urethra is positioned in a more anterior position than in men, and this position facilitates placement of 8 to 10 urethral sutures after the specimen is removed (**Fig. 41-9**). Frozen section analysis is performed on the distal margin of the cystectomy specimen to exclude tumor.

If the anterior vaginal wall has been preserved, the vagina is then closed at the apex in two layers. In the past, the vagina was suspended to Cooper's ligament

to prevent vaginal prolapse or the development of an enterocele postoperatively. Currently, we perform a colposacropexy incorporating Marlex mesh, which fixates the vagina to the sacrum without angulation or undue tension. Regardless of the form of vaginal reconstruction, a well-vascularized omental pedicle graft is placed between the reconstructed vagina and the neobladder and is secured to the levator ani muscles to separate the suture lines and prevent fistulization (**Fig. 41-10**).

As in men, no dissection should be performed anterior to the urethra along the pelvic floor in women considering orthotopic diversion. This technique prevents injury to the rhabdosphincter region and corresponding innervation. Some reports suggest that a sympathetic nerve-sparing cystectomy is important in maintaining continence in these women. We routinely sacrifice the autonomic nerves coursing along the lateral aspect of the uterus and vagina and rely successfully on the pudendal innervation of the rhabdosphincter region for maintenance of continence. Fluorodynamic studies in women undergoing orthotopic diversion have also identified the rhabdosphincter region as the area that provides the continence mechanism in these women. It is possible that preservation of the sympathetic nerves may contribute to the high incidence of hypercontinence and urinary retention requiring continuous intermittent catheterization reported by Hautmann and associates.[88]

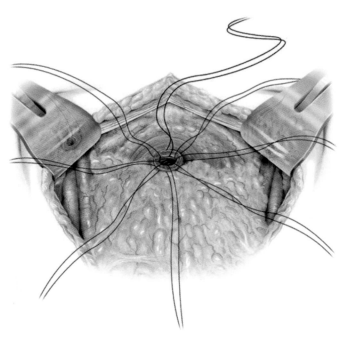

Figure 41-10 Greater omental apron interposed as a bed on which the neobladder will reside. This vascular tissue acts as a barrier to discourage fistula formation between vulnerable suture lines of the neobladder and the reconstructed vagina.

COMPLICATIONS OF CYSTECTOMY AFTER RADIATION THERAPY AND TOTAL PELVIC EXENTERATION

Total pelvic exenteration has historically been associated with a high incidence of perioperative complications, with rates ranging from 32% to 84%.[89-96] This patient population has the additional disadvantage of often having undergone high doses of preoperative radiation to the pelvic area, thus creating unique physiologic and pathologic changes to the pelvic organs and increasing the perioperative complication rate.

The complications seen with total pelvic exenteration were reviewed by Pearlman,[97] who found that complication rates varied between 30% and 70%, whereas Soper and associates[91] reported a reoperation rate of 26%. In a more recent series, overall morbidity was 28% with a reoperation rate of 18%. In this report, the incidence of bowel obstruction and fistula formation was 3% for both, significantly lower than 8% and 19%, respectively, reported by others.[99] These differences may be related to the use of omentum or pedicled muscle transposed into the pelvis required to repair the pelvic floor, to fill the dead space, and to separate suture lines. The incidence of complications appears to be lessened by the transposition of nonirradiated tissue into the pelvis.[100]

In one study,[95] 45% of patients required at least one readmission to the hospital, and 32% required addi-

tional operative procedures. The most common complications associated with exenteration in this study included wound or pelvic complications, GI or genitourinary fistulas, and small bowel obstruction. Although many complications after this surgical procedure may be considered minor, major complications are not infrequent. Specifically, serious infections of the wound or pelvis and problems with the urinary conduit are the most common major perioperative complications.[101-105]

Considerable variations have been reported in the rates for both short-term and long-term complications of the urinary conduit.[106-110] Early complications can occur in ≤10% of patients and usually involve problems with the urinary enteric anastomosis, such as leaks and obstruction. Most leaks can be managed conservatively with prolonged conduit drainage and, if needed, proximal diversion of the urine stream with percutaneous nephrostomy tubes. Late urinary complications include stenoses and fistulas, which have been reported to develop in ≤16% of patients.[111] Major complications involving the urinary and GI tracts do correlate with prior exposure to radiation therapy.[101-104] In one series,[100] 67% of patients who had undergone radiation therapy developed postoperative complications, compared with 26% of those who had not had prior irradiation.

The perioperative mortality rate for patients having undergone total pelvic exenteration ranges from 0% to 18%.[112-114] The markedly different early mortality rates may reflect surgical expertise concentrated into experienced consultant-led operative teams, careful patient selection, improved postoperative care, and antibiotic and thromboembolic prophylaxis. These reasons have been suggested to be predominantly responsible for the reduced perioperative mortality rate (from 18% to 8% over a 50-year period) and an overall complication rate in one series.[112]

Simultaneous pelvic reconstruction following surgical extirpation is increasingly popular among high-volume surgical oncology centers.[115-118] In this manner, the patient is afforded the opportunity to have these procedures done concurrent with the extirpative portion of the procedure. The creation of a neovagina, urinary diversion, and functional low colon can be performed with acceptable morbidity and gives the patient the opportunity for better organ function following this extensive extirpative surgery.[119-125]

Since the late 1980s, many surgeons have transitioned to continent urinary diversion as a means of lower urinary tract reconstruction following total pelvic exenteration without an appreciable increase in morbidity.[126-127] The rectus abdominis flap is increasingly used for vaginal reconstruction following pelvic exenteration. It is technically easy to harvest and results in an excellent neovagina with a more suitable vaginal caliber.[125] Low colon reanastomosis is routinely performed and more recently our institution has used the J-pouch to increase the likelihood of anorectal continence.[118]

Considerable morbidity may be associated with the resultant large, empty pelvic dead space left after pelvic exenteration. The pelvic dead space predisposes patients to abscesses, fistula formation, perineal wound problems, and intestinal obstruction. Thus it is prudent to fill this space with omentum or other autologous tissue. Many groups use myocutaneous flaps to fill the pelvic dead space after pelvic exenteration, especially in patients who have previously undergone irradiation. The advantages of myocutaneous flap reconstruction in the irradiated pelvis and perineal wound include reduction of dead space, interposition of well-vascularized, nonirradiated tissue, and replacement of resected skin.[125] The use of myocutaneous flaps, such as those based on the rectus abdominis, gracilis, and gluteus maximus muscles, have provided excellent results.[120,121]

In the setting of prior pelvic radiation, continent urinary reservoirs may also be predisposed to complications. Previously, sigmoid, ileum, and transverse colon were widely used for urinary diversion in the setting of prior pelvic radiation.[105,126-128] Each technique had advantages in terms of capacity and ability to avoid using radiated bowel segments; however, reported disadvantages included sustained incontinence and the incidence of ureterointestinal complications.

Wammack and associates[128] prospectively compared operative outcomes in a series of 36 irradiated patients and 385 nonradiated patients who underwent continent urinary reservoir formation with either a Mainz I pouch, using the appendix to form the continence mechanism, or an ileal intussuscepted nipple valve (Indiana pouch). Of the 36 radiated patients, 31 (86%) developed a pouch-related complication, whereas 88 (23%) of the 385 nonradiated patients developed complications. In this series, pouch-related complications were defined as failure of the continence mechanism, ureterointestinal stricture, leakage, or fistula and stomal stenosis.

Overall, a fourfold increase in complications was observed in the radiated patients. Wilson and associates[105] observed a similar increased risk of complications in radiated patients and reported a fivefold increase in complications related to the ureterointestinal anastomosis in radiated compared with nonirradiated patients undergoing Indiana pouch reconstruction.

It is apparent that complications after total pelvic exenteration are significant, particularly in patients who received prior pelvic radiation therapy. Given that urinary and bowel complications after such surgical procedures can often become demoralizing to patients with newly diagnosed malignant, if not fatal, disease, concentration is imperative on surgical detail in this patient population.

CONCLUSION

Radical cystectomy has become standard treatment and arguably the best definitive form of therapy for high-grade, invasive bladder cancer. Lower urinary tract reconstruction, particularly orthotopic diversion, has been a major component in enhancing the quality of life of patients requiring cystectomy. As with any major surgical procedure, however, complications do occur. It is important for all surgeons to be familiar with the presentation, prevention, and treatment of the major causes of morbidity and mortality associated with radical cystectomy and lower urinary tract reconstruction.

The complications discussed are among the most common associated with cystectomy. In fact, many other complications may be encountered, as the published literature testifies, and a thorough understanding of their presentation, prevention, and treatment is equally essential for a successful patient outcome. A sound understanding of surgical anatomy and adherence to proper surgical technique, familiarization with recent data regarding the most successful treatment methods, and attention to detail in the perioperative period are crucial for minimizing complications in any surgical undertaking.

ACKNOWLEDGMENT

Dr. Stein,

You will always be in my mind, my heart, and my hands. Thank you, John.

EAP

KEY POINTS

1. Cardiovascular events are the leading causes of mortality in patients immediately after cystectomy.
2. A sound understanding of pelvic anatomy and adherence to proper surgical technique remain the cornerstones in preventing significant bleeding in intraoperative and delayed settings.
3. Key to minimizing the risk of rectal injury is a sound understanding of the fascia layers between the bladder and rectum and the use of sharp dissection in the posterior plane in those patients at high risk for rectal injury. Furthermore, adequate bowel preparation, intraoperative recognition, appropriate repair, adequate decompression of the injured rectum, establishment of sufficient pelvic drainage, and aggressive nutritional and antimicrobial support are all critical to prevent possible significant sequelae from rectal injuries.
4. Routine thromboprophylaxis is imperative to prevent development of deep vein thrombosis after major open urologic surgical procedures.
5. Ileus is the most common complication resulting in a prolonged hospital stay in patients undergoing radical cystectomy. Ileus that fails to resolve by postoperative day 10 to 14 warrants investigation into its cause.
6. The decision to perform acute emergency laparotomy is warranted in the patient with a documented bowel leak who has peritonitis or signs of sepsis with proven or suspected intraperitoneal abscesses that are not amenable to percutaneous drainage or in which percutaneous drainage has failed. Conservative management with hyperalimentation may be attempted in controlled fistulous settings. Fistulas that fail to close after approximately 4 months of conservative therapy require surgical correction.
7. Lymphocele is a rare complication of radical cystectomy that usually can be managed conservatively.
8. Fascial dehiscence is invariably associated with previous wound infection and, when associated with evisceration, represents a serious postoperative problem that often necessitates immediate operative exploration and repair.
9. Preservation of the rhabdosphincter and its pudendal innervation is critical in allowing the return of continence after radical cystectomy and neobladder reconstruction.
10. Careful radiographic surveillance of the upper urinary tracts of patients with ureteroenteric anastomoses is essential to identify ureterointestinal anastomotic strictures early and to preserve kidney function.
11. Endoscopic methods of reservoir stone removal are highly effective and minimally invasive.
12. All surgeons need to be familiar with the presentation, prevention, and treatment of the major causes of morbidity and mortality associated with radical cystectomy and lower urinary tract reconstruction. A sound understanding of the surgical anatomy, adherence to proper surgical technique, familiarization with recent data regarding the most successful treatment methods, and attention to detail in the perioperative period are crucial for minimizing complications in any surgical undertaking.

REFERENCES

Please see www.expertconsult.com

Chapter 42

COMPLICATIONS OF SIMPLE PROSTATECTOMY

William J. Ellis MD
Professor, Department of Urology, University of Washington, Seattle, Washington

Jonathan L. Wright MD, MS
Assistant Professor, Department of Urology, University of Washington, Seattle, Washington

Open prostatectomy was once the primary treatment for symptomatic benign prostatic hyperplasia (BPH). However, with the advent of minimally invasive procedures and the development of medical therapies, the use of open prostatectomy significantly declined. Currently, interest is growing in the role of transurethral holmium laser enucleation of the prostate as a treatment alternative to open prostatectomy for large glands.[1] Although infrequently performed in the United States, open prostatectomy continues to be extensively performed in other countries where resources limit the medical and endoscopic options available to patients and providers.[2-4] A retrospective review in of surgical therapy for BPH performed in 1992 compared with 2002 in Spain found that although the overall rate of surgical intervention declined by 18%, the proportion of open prostatectomies performed increased.[5] Clear indications for open prostatectomy still remain, but with surgeons' decreasing familiarity with the procedure, the need to understand and recognize the complications of this procedure becomes even more important.

INDICATIONS

Open prostatectomy may be performed in prostate glands >80 to 100 g[6] when the presence of other disease requires an open surgical procedure and when the patient's anatomic features preclude appropriate positioning for endoscopic resection. Prostate glands >200 g may be efficiently enucleated with the open approach, and complication rates are low. Open prostatectomy should be considered in patients with bladder calculi or bladder diverticula that may be dealt with through an open approach. Certain anatomic factors favor open prostatectomy: severe hip or knee contractures, penile prostheses, and ureteral orifices in close proximity to the bladder neck where endoscopic visualization is limited. Patients with a penile prosthesis, particularly a semirigid prosthesis, may require perineal urethrostomy for endoscopic resection.

SURGICAL APPROACH

The suprapubic and retropubic approaches are both employed for open prostatectomy. The perineal approach is rarely used today. Surgeons are gaining increasing experience with the laparoscopic approach.[7,8] The surgical techniques are well described elsewhere, and this chapter highlights procedural details as they relate to specific complications. Briefly, the suprapubic approach involves adenoma enucleation from within the bladder by using an anterior cystotomy. This approach is often preferred when large bladder calculi or bladder diverticula must be repaired. The retropubic technique achieves enucleation through an anterior prostatic capsulotomy. The laparoscopic approach is performed extraperitoneally, and both open suprapubic and retropubic techniques described earlier can be performed.[8]

EARLY COMPLICATIONS

Hemorrhage

Widely ranging significant perioperative bleeding events have been recorded, with an incidence of 0% to 35%.[9] Much of the variability may result from transfusion thresholds, autologous blood banking, reporting, and experience of the surgeon. Large European series reported transfusion rates of 6% to 8%.[10-12] In another series of 56 patients, 36% received blood transfusions, but 80% of those patients received autologous blood for which the transfusion threshold was likely lower.[13] The second half of a Nigerian study of 240 patients showed marked decreases in clot retention and transfusion rates related to experience of the surgeon.[4]

Several surgical techniques to control intraoperative bleeding have been described. In the 1940s, Rolnick[14] advocated packing the prostatic fossa with gauze for ≥5 minutes after enucleation. Even today, this technique remains the standard for initial efforts at hemostasis.[15] After removing the packing, hemostatic sutures at the 5- and 7-o'clock positions incorporating the bladder mucosa, bladder neck, and prostatic capsule in a figure-of-eight fashion usually provide adequate hemostasis. If persistent hemorrhage is present, several additional maneuvers are available. Hemostatic agents (e.g., oxidized cellulose [Surgicel]) may be placed in the fossa along with temporary packing to assist in achieving hemostasis. To facilitate capsular contraction and tamponade, Shaikh and Malament[16] described placing an absorbable pursestring stitch at the bladder neck. The O'Conor stitch is an absorbable placating stitch placed in the posterior capsule that similarly provides capsular tamponade[17] (**Fig. 42-1**). Other investigators have described placing a nonabsorbable pursestring stitch that is brought out through the abdominal wall and is removed in 24 to 48 hours.[18,19]

Some investigators emphasize the importance of obtaining hemostasis *before* capsulotomy during the retropubic approach with ligation of the dorsal venous complex with 0-chromic ligature.[20] Exposure of the dorsal vein is accomplished by releasing the puboprostatic ligaments, incising the endopelvic fascia, and passing a right-angle clamp between the dorsal vein and the urethra. Alternatively, the dorsal vein may be ligated with figure-of-eight 2-0 chromic sutures without incision of the endopelvic fascia. Next, the lateral vascular pedicles are ligated with sutures placed at the posterolateral edges of the prostate. Studies have highlighted the importance of these lateral sutures in limiting intra-

operative hemorrhage.[21] This concept of early vascular control has been extended by some investigators to include clamping of the internal iliac arteries.[22] Once these maneuvers are complete, capsulotomy is performed in what should be a relatively bloodless field. Retropubic enucleation of small glands may result in tearing of the lateral edges of the capsulotomy with a finger and subsequent hemorrhage, which can be avoided by performing adequately sized capsulotomy.

Clot retention is prevented with continuous bladder irrigation through a 22- or 24-Fr three-way catheter or by a suprapubic tube catheter through the dome of the bladder and a two-way catheter draining the bladder through the urethra. A large-diameter outflow port is crucial to allow for clot evacuation. A 30-mL balloon is used on the Foley catheter with a general rule of 1 mL of fluid for each gram of adenoma removed. Venous bleeding can be further controlled postoperatively by placing traction on the urethral catheter to provide tamponade. Only light traction is required for adequate tamponade; tight traction increases bladder spasms. Arterial bleeding cannot be controlled well with traction and may require reoperation. Some large series reported reoperative rates for bleeding of 1% to 3.7%.[2,4,10,11] Most arterial bleeding can be endoscopically fulgurated. Selective angioembolization or hypogastric artery embolization is rarely required. Delayed bleeding (>2 weeks postoperatively) is rare and should be managed initially with bladder irrigation, Foley catheter traction, and reoperation if needed.

Infection

Infections after open prostatectomy include urinary tract infection, epididymitis, and wound infections. The rate of urinary tract infection or epididymitis following open prostatectomy is comparable to the rate after minimally invasive procedures (median, 8%; range, 3% to 17%).[6] Patients at risk include those with long-term indwelling Foley catheters, chronic urinary tract infections, or a history of epidiymitis.[23] Graham and Grayhack[23] recommended that prophylactic vasectomy be performed before open prostatectomy in high-risk patients, but this recommendation has not been critically studied and is not routinely followed. Wound infections are specific to open surgical techniques and have been reported to occur in 2.5% to 4.3%.[2,4,9,12] Preoperative urine cultures and perioperative antibiotics should be given to all patients undergoing open prostatectomy.

Incontinence

Urinary incontinence after open prostatectomy may be urge, stress, or mixed. In a survey analysis of 1804 open prostatectomies in Italy, reported rates of early and late urinary incontinence were 3.7% and 1.2%, respec-

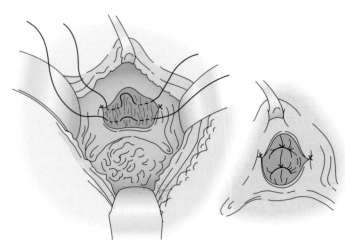

Figure 42-1 Capsule placating sutures as described by O'Conor. Two sutures are placed in the posterior fossa to aid in prostatic contraction. (*From O'Conor VJ Jr. An aid for hemostasis in open prostatectomy: capsular placation. J Urol. 1982;127[3]:448.*)

tively.[11] No distinction was made based on severity or type of incontinence. Urge incontinence, usually resulting from bladder instability, has been reported in ≤8% of cases. This complication is generally transient and resolves within 8 weeks of the surgical procedure. Stress incontinence may result from sphincteric deficiency, sphincteric injury, or neurapraxia. During apical enucleation, the urethra can often be pinched off at the apex of the adenoma. Extensive traction or tearing can disrupt the external urethral sphincter complex. Using curved Satinsky scissors for sharp dissection of the urethra at the prostatic apex can help minimize trauma to the external sphincter.

Urodynamic studies in patients before open prostatectomy and 6 months postoperatively demonstrate reversible bladder changes that can occur.[9] Whereas 22% of patients in this series had detrusor instability preoperatively, only 9% had instability postoperatively. In addition, significant changes in the maximum bladder contraction force were observed at 6 months postoperatively. In this series, 9% of patients had postoperative stress incontinence that resolved by 12 weeks. These investigators further demonstrated a reduction in bladder wall thickness present as early a 1 week postoperatively (mean, 3.3 mm versus 5.2 mm) that reached its nadir at 6 weeks (2.9 mm) and remained constant for ≤1 year. Resolution of urge incontinence may be the result of these reversible changes of bladder hypertrophy.

Neuropathy of the external sphincter after open prostatectomy has not been well described. In theory, if the capsule is not disrupted, the nerve supply should remain intact. A study of 47 men after open prostatectomy examined the electromyographic responses of the external urethral sphincter and the bulbocavernosus muscles after electrical stimulation of the bulbocavernosus reflex.[24] All men in the study had an intact reflex arc and eternal urethral sphincter with latencies within the normal range. The investigators concluded that the somatosensory components of the pudendal nerve are not compromised after open prostatectomy, but this area requires further study.

Persistent Urinary Leak

The incidence of persistent urinary leakage from the cystotomy or capsulotomy after all drains are removed is 1% to 2%.[19] In a series of 200 patients undergoing suprapubic prostatectomy, 2 patients had persistent urinary leakage.[2] Both patients were managed with Foley catheter drainage and had spontaneous resolution within 4 weeks. It is normal to have same drainage for ≤48 hours after drain removal, but failure to seal is considered persistent urinary leakage. The cause is most commonly high postvoid residuals from anatomic obstruction (e.g., urethral stricture) or poor detrusor function. Treatment is with bladder drainage until the leakage site has healed. Inadequate cystotomy or capsulotomy closure is rarely the cause of persistent leakage. A three-layer closure for cystotomies after suprapubic prostatectomies was described using perivesical fat as the third layer, with a reduction in the leakage rate from 13% to 2% ($P = .06$) in one prospective, randomized series.[25] Leakage from the capsulotomy site after retropubic prostatectomy is rarer and is usually adequately treated with bladder drainage.

Surgical drainage of the retropubic space should be performed in all open prostatectomies, either with a Penrose drain or a suction drain. Some investigators prefer Penrose drains because of the belief that a suction drain encourages leakage when the drain is placed adjacent to the suture line of the capsulotomy or cystotomy. If persistent drainage is present, the drain should be withdrawn slightly to increase the separation between the suture line and the drain. Suction drains should be taken off suction to allow a persistent tract between the suture line and the drain to collapse. Drains should remain in place until catheter removal and until drainage is <30 mL per day.

Cardiovascular and Thromboembolic Events

Cardiovascular and thromboembolic events are two of the leading causes of mortality in patients undergoing open prostatectomy. Because of limited quality data, the American Urologic Association Guidelines Panel was unable to determine mortality rates by surgical techniques.[6] However, the overall mortality from BPH has steadily declined from 7.47 deaths in 100,000 patients in the early 1950s to 0.26 deaths in 100,000 patients in the late 1990s.[6] Large open prostatectomy series reported 1 death among 1804 patients (0.06%)[11] and 2 deaths among 902 patients (0.2%).[10] Patients undergoing open prostatectomy should use graduated compression stockings and intermittent pneumatic compression devices. High-risk patients should be considered for low-dose unfractionated heparin or low-molecular-weight-heparin treatment. Patients should be encouraged to ambulate as early as the afternoon following morning operations.

Osteitis Pubis

Osteitis pubis is a rare complication of prostatectomy. Patients typically present 4 to 6 weeks postoperatively with severe pain (pubic symphysis, pelvic and lower abdomen) and low-grade fever. On examination, the patient reports pain during thigh adduction and tenderness during direct compression of the symphysis and medial compression of the pelvis.[26] Radiographic changes are usually delayed until 2 to 4 weeks after presentation. Treatment is with anti-inflammatory drugs and reassurance because the disease is self-limiting.

LATE COMPLICATIONS

Bladder Neck Contracture

The rate of bladder neck contracture is estimated to be 7.6%,[6] although some series have reported contracture rates of 3.9% to 6.25%.[2,9-13] The origin of bladder neck contracture is unclear and does not appear to be related to adenoma size. The incidence of contractures is reported to be higher following suprapubic prostatectomy than after retropubic prostatectomy.[27] The reason for the higher rate is unknown. We attempt to reduce the risk of bladder neck contracture by performing a Y-V plasty of the bladder neck after enucleation of the adenoma (**Fig. 42-2**). Bladder neck contractures may be initially treated with dilation (**Fig. 42-3**). Recurrent contractures should be treated with internal urethrotomy. Bladder neck reconstruction for refractory contractures is very rare.

Impotence and Sexual Dysfunction

Retrograde ejaculation is common after open prostatectomy. It occurs in the majority of patients at a rate similar to that seen after transurethral resection of the prostate.[6] Retrograde ejaculation is the result of resection or disruption of the internal sphincter that leads to failure of the bladder neck to close during ejaculation and thus allows the ejaculate to pass in retrograde fashion into the bladder. Erectile dysfunction after open prostatectomy is likely multifactorial, with age, comorbidities, and preexisting erectile dysfunction playing roles. In the 1994 Clinical Practice Guidelines of the Department of Health and Human Services,[28] the rate of erectile dysfunction after open prostatectomy was estimated to be 16% to 32%, depending on the approach used: retropubic (16.2%), suprapubic (17.7%), and perineal (32.3%). However, in the 2003 Guidelines on the

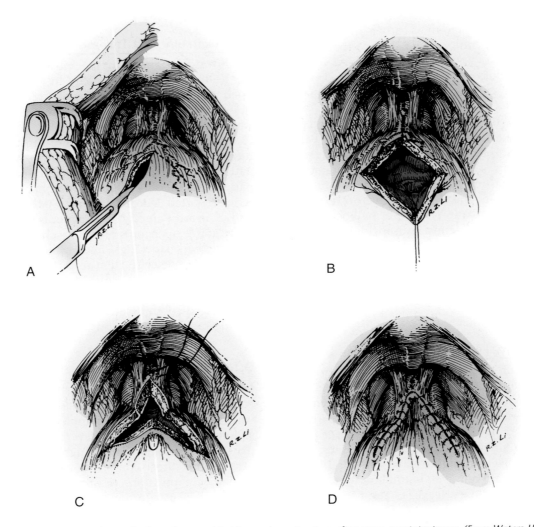

A

B

C

D

Figure 42-2 Y-V plasty of the bladder outlet for refractory bladder neck contracture after open prostatectomy. *(From Waters HB. Suprapubic and retropubic prostatectomy for benign hyperplasia. In: Fowler JE, ed.* Mastery of Surgery: Urologic Surgery. *Boston: Little, Brown; 1992:378.)*

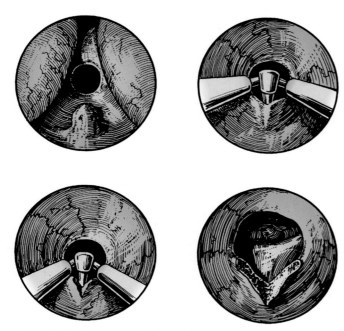

Figure 42-3 Transurethral incision of a bladder neck contracture using the Collings knife. One incision can be made at the 6-o'clock position or two incisions can be made at the 4- and 8-o'clock positions. *(From Waters HB. Suprapubic and retropubic prostatectomy for benign hyperplasia. In: Fowler JE, ed.* Mastery of Surgery: Urologic Surgery. *Boston: Little, Brown; 1992:377.)*

management of BPH by the American Urologic Association, no estimate of the risk of erectile dysfunction was given because data were lacking.[6]

A review of large series found a lack of reporting on erectile dysfunction. One of the problems in the older literature was the lack of information on preoperative sexual function such that preexisting sexual dysfunction could not be evaluated.[28] In a more recent series of 32 men in whom preoperative and postoperative sexual function was evaluated, 81.2% of men had normal sexual function preoperatively and 78.6% had normal

erections after the surgical procedure.[9] Libido was significantly decreased at 1 week postoperatively and improved over subsequent weeks, although it was still significantly lower than preoperative levels at 6 weeks postoperatively.

CONCLUSION

Open prostatectomy continues to have a role in the management of men with BPH. It is a highly successful intervention with low retreatment rates (median, 1%; range, 0%-8%).[6] Although medical therapy and minimally invasive treatments for BPH have become more common than open prostatectomy, urologists need to be aware of the complications following open prostatectomy because lack of familiarity with the procedure may increase the complication rate.

KEY POINTS

1. Patient selection is important because other treatment options exist.
2. Complication rates can decrease through meticulous surgical technique.
3. Bleeding is best controlled by ligating the prostate pedicle within the prostatic fossa at the 5- and 7-o'clock positions.
4. Damage to the sphincter mechanism during the apical dissection is a major cause of incontinence.
5. Bladder neck contracture is a late complication that can usually be managed by dilation or endoscopic incision.

REFERENCES

Please see www.expertconsult.com

Chapter 43

COMPLICATIONS OF RADICAL PERINEAL PROSTATECTOMY

Sam D. Graham Jr MD

Retired Professor and Chairman, Department of Urology, Emory University, Atlanta, Georgia

Radical perineal prostatectomy was first performed in 1868 by Kuchler and was popularized by Young in 1905 as a treatment for adenocarcinoma of the prostate. The procedure was the operation of choice for radical prostatectomy until the value of pelvic lymphadenectomy in staging prostate cancer was recognized in the 1970s. Radical perineal prostatectomy was replaced by retropubic prostatectomy because the retropubic approach allowed simultaneous pelvic node dissection. However, the perineal approach has seen a resurgence based on the lower morbidity and a reduction in the rate of positive pelvic lymph nodes in patients presenting with adenocarcinoma of the prostate. This reduction, reported to be ≤5%, has obviated the need for pelvic node dissection in patients with a favorable Gleason sum (<7) and lower prostate-specific antigen levels (<10 ng/mL), with no adverse effect on outcome.[1,2]

The complications of radical perineal prostatectomy can be divided into two types: perioperative (at the time of surgery or ≤30 days of the surgical procedure) and postoperative (>30 days after the operation). The rates of complications are functions of the age of the patient and other comorbidities that make patient selection important in avoiding unfavorable results (Table 43-1). The usual candidates are patients who are relatively young (patients >70 years old are counseled and selected based on their life expectancy), have few comorbidities and a life expectancy of >10 years, have localized disease (organ confined), and have had no radiation therapy to the prostate.

PERIOPERATIVE COMPLICATIONS

Hemorrhage

Hemorrhage during radical perineal prostatectomy usually originates from either the dorsal venous complex or the arterial branches to the prostate or seminal vesicles. In performing radical perineal prostatectomy, the surgeon is usually able to divide the endopelvic fascia at the apex and dissect along the anterior prostate and thereby avoid the large venous tributaries that make up the dorsal venous complex (**Fig. 43-1**). On occasion, however, perforating vessels are present or the surgeon is unable to avoid the venous complex, and substantial venous bleeding results. Sometimes this bleeding can be controlled by packing the wound and waiting, although active hemostasis is often required. Electrocautery is generally useless in this situation, and the surgeon is best served by suture ligating the vessels with 3-0 polyglactin 910 (Vicryl). A figure-of-eight suture placed anteriorly to the urethra is usually sufficient.

Arterial tributaries are usually easier to control. The arterial supply to the prostate originates from a branch of the pudendal artery and is located posterolaterally to the prostate and seminal vesicles. Generally, minor tributaries from the inferior vesical artery in the anterior bladder neck can be controlled with electrocautery. The posterior pedicles to the prostate consist of a superior pedicle that enters the prostate at its posterior base and is a constant anatomic finding and the more variable inferior pedicle that is found near the apex of the prostate. These pedicles can be isolated, divided, and ligated; if a nerve-sparing operation is not contemplated, they can be cauterized.

The artery to the seminal vesicle enters the seminal vesicle at its tip and should be cauterized during the dissection. If arterial bleeding persists after the prostate is removed, the surgeon can generally isolate the sites by packing 4 × 8-inch sponges in each side of the wound and removing one and then the other. To visualize the deeper aspects of the wound adequately, it is frequently very important to have optimal lighting, which can be obtained only with a halogen head lamp and adequate retraction.

Delayed bleeding is an uncommon complication and may result from either inadequate control of vessels before closing or clotting abnormalities. The vessels

TABLE 43-1	Nerve-Sparing Radical Perineal Prostatectomy: Morbidity	
Complication	**Percentage (%)**
Strictures	6.7
Incontinence	
Significant	3.1
Minor	7.1
Rectal injury	1.3
Wound infection	1.3
Deep vein thrombosis	0.4
Cerebrovascular accident	0.4
Perioperative myocardial infarction	1.3

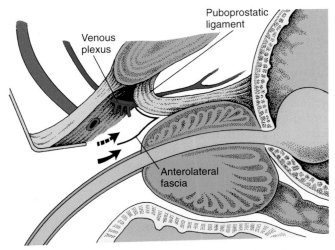

Figure 43-1 The *solid arrow* indicates the proper plane of dissection beneath the anterolateral fascia and beneath the venous plexus. Dissection above this fascia (*dotted arrow*) carries the hazard of disruption of the venous sinus and troublesome bleeding.

most easily missed during closure are on the anterior rectal surface or are retracted within the bladder neck. Vessels retracted within the bladder neck can be detected by irrigating the Foley catheter after the anastomosis is completed.

Another potential site of hemorrhage is the bulb of the penis. This bleeding usually occurs when the dissection proceeds too far anteriorly during an attempt to divide the rectourethralis. This hemorrhage will not respond to any intervention other than suture ligation.

Since 1991, average blood loss among patients in my practice has been <450 mL and the rate of transfusion approximately 5%. Among nearly 500 patients, 1 patient had clot retention resulting from arterial bleeding within the bladder and another had a bleeding diathesis resulting from abnormal clotting parameters.

Cardiovascular Complications

Cardiovascular complications include pulmonary embolus and myocardial infarction. The cardiovascular complications are a reflection of the patient population, who are generally older and have some degree of underlying cardiovascular disease. The patients are placed in a position that allows maximum drainage of the veins of the lower extremities and their legs are wrapped to the groin before positioning, measures that should prevent pulmonary embolism. I do not routinely use any preoperative anticoagulation and have seen only 4 cases of pulmonary emboli in >500 patients after radical perineal prostatectomy in the past few years.

Rectal Injury

The incidence of rectal injury in radical perineal prostatectomy is <1%. This complication can be avoided by adhering to the following principles:

1. When the central tendon is divided, the surgeon should dissect through the fat and muscle fibers until the white rectal fascia is identified distal to the rectal sphincter.
2. The surgeon should then place the index finger of the nondominant hand in the patient's rectum to aid in identifying the rectal wall, and generally an easy blunt dissection is made under the rectal sphincter and the levator ani, both of which are retracted anterolaterally.
3. The surgeon should obtain optimal exposure by retraction of both muscle groups; by placing tension on the rectum, one can easily identify the rectourethralis (**Fig. 43-2**). This should be identified, a right-angle clamp placed around the muscle bundle, and the muscle divided. Again, the index finger in the patient's rectum can be of great help in delineating the rectum.
4. After the rectourethralis is divided, the blunt dissection is directed to develop a plane between the rectum and the apex of the prostate. The index finger in the patient's rectum is most important at this stage because the relationship between the rectum and the apex is highly variable, and the plane is not as easily developed as the dissection to this point. At this point the rectum is most at risk for injury, and the surgeon should not rely strictly on visual cues to determine the plane.
5. Once the rectum is safely off the distal 1.5 to 2 cm of the apex, the posterior layer of Denonvilliers' fascia can be incised and the rectum easily dissected posteriorly between the two layers of Denonvilliers' fascia (the "pearly gates") (**Fig. 43-3**).

Another potential site of rectal injury is near the base of the prostate laterally when taking the superior pros-

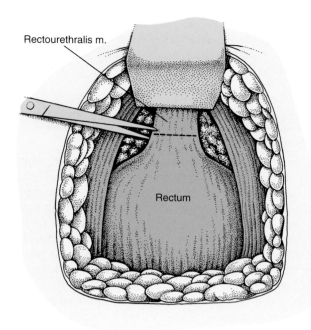

Rectourethralis m.

Rectum

Figure 43-2 Posterior view of the rectourethralis with the rectum identified. Division of this muscle drops the rectum posteriorly and permits access to the prostate.

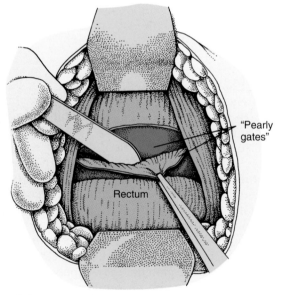

"Pearly gates"

Rectum

Figure 43-3 Incision of the overlying fascia (the "pearly gates") to expose the true capsule of the prostate.

tatic plexus. Caution should be exercised, especially when the layers of Denonvilliers' fascia do not easily separate, as seen in patients with a history of prostatitis or after multiple biopsies.

Should the rectum be injured, it can be repaired in two layers using running 3-0 polyglactin 910 and silk Lembert sutures. The wound is copiously irrigated with antibiotic-containing irrigant at the end of the procedure and a Penrose drain is placed. Colostomy is generally not needed unless the patient has had prior radiation.

Infections

Infections are uncommon and are usually associated with wound soilage during the procedure. These infections can be prevented by using preoperative antibiotics, irrigating the wound with antibiotic-containing irrigant, and avoiding wound contamination during rectal dissection.

Loss of Foley Catheter

I prefer to leave a Foley catheter in place for 12 days postoperatively. On occasion, the catheter prematurely falls out of the urethra because of either failure to inflate the Foley balloon adequately during the procedure or a defect in the balloon. I do not insert the catheter into the bladder until the anastomosis is partially completed and I do not inflate the balloon until the anastomosis is fully complete. Because the anastomosis is performed with six to eight individual polyglactin 910 sutures, the catheter can usually be reinserted by the urologist, with care taken to use adequate lubrication. If not, gentle insertion of a flexible cystoscope usually allows passage of a guidewire into the bladder. If this maneuver fails, repeat exploration in the immediate postoperative period may be indicated, or observation of the patient and exploration may be required only when the patient is unable to urinate or when a urinary fistula is suspected ≥5 days after the operation.

Oliguria and Anuria

Oliguria and anuria are infrequent complications that can have a multitude of causes, including acute tubular necrosis, edema of the trigone because of the closure of the anastomosis, obstruction by traction with the Foley catheter, displacement or blockage of the Foley catheter, or ureteral injury. The first step in this situation is to ensure that the patient is adequately hydrated and that the catheter irrigates freely inward and outward. If any tension has been placed on the catheter or drainage tube, it may be prudent to obtain a cystogram. If the patient is adequately hydrated, escalating doses of furosemide or other diuretic may be given to stimulate renal function. Edema usually resolve in time, although the diagnosis is generally one of exclusion after ruling out all other causes including renal dysfunction. If the urine output does not return within 24 hours or the patient becomes symptomatic from the renal dysfunction (i.e., becomes fluid overloaded or uremic), one or several percutaneous nephrostomies should be placed.

Persistent Fistula

Persistent fistula is infrequent and is usually the result of either a blocked Foley catheter or disruption of the anastomosis or bladder neck reconstruction. This complication usually requires no intervention other than continued catheter drainage as long as the catheter is not obstructed and the catheter tip remains in the bladder. Repeat exploration is indicated if the anastomotic disruption is complete and the diagnosis is made in the early postoperative period. If complete disruption occurs >48 to 72 hours postoperatively, however, it may be more prudent to perform a suprapubic cystostomy and repair the anastomosis later.

LATE POSTOPERATIVE COMPLICATIONS

Inability to Void

Approximately 15% of patients are unable to void after removal of their Foley catheter and require replacement of the catheter. The causes are usually edema of the anastomosis, a tissue flap in the anastomosis that will not "seat," or a hypotonic bladder. The immediate intervention is reinsertion of a Foley catheter using a smaller (16-Fr) catheter. Patients are given a repeat voiding trial 48 to 72 hours after being counseled to avoid any anticholinergic medications. Occasionally, patients require two or three catheter reinsertions before they can void spontaneously.

Anastomotic Disruption

The most common cause of anastomotic disruption after removal of the Foley catheter is either failure to insert a new catheter while the patient is in urinary retention or inability to insert a catheter with traumatic disruption of the anastomosis. This complication is perhaps the most disastrous in that the anastomotic stricture usually requires significant operative intervention. This complication can be prevented by catheterizing any patient who fails a voiding trial once he or she becomes uncomfortable or within a few hours of removal of the catheter. If the patient requires catheterization, it should be done with a 16-Fr catheter that is well lubricated and passed gently. If any resistance is encountered, the surgeon should try a coudé catheter or possibly a filiform and Councill/Graham–style catheter. Once again, careful use of a flexible cystoscope with passage of a guidewire into the bladder can obviate the need for repeat exploration. If the attempts to insert a catheter into the bladder through the urethra continue to fail, the surgeon should insert a suprapubic tube and repair the anastomosis later.

Gastrointestinal Complications

Gastrointestinal complications are generally minimal. The more common problems are diarrhea resulting from the antibiotic coverage, constipation caused by narcotics in the perioperative period, and loss of proprioception (inability to distinguish gas from solids). Occasionally, the patient may have an exacerbation of rectal hemorrhoids, which may require intervention.

LONG-TERM POSTOPERATIVE COMPLICATIONS

Impotence

The rate of erectile dysfunction is 100% in men immediately postoperatively, and erectile function may gradually return within 12 to 18 months. The mechanism of injury is the disruption of the neurovascular pathways that track along the posterolateral border of the prostate and membranous urethra. Failure to preserve the neurovascular bundles results in permanent impotence, although preservation of the bundles does not guarantee potency. Patients are more likely to regain potency if they are young (<60 years old) and were fully potent preoperatively. The rate of potency (able to achieve an erection spontaneously and maintain it sufficiently for penetration) in this group is approximately 50%. The regular use of intracorporeal or intraurethral prostaglandin in the early postoperative period has shown significant enhancement of the spontaneous potency rate. Alternatives may also include the use of the newer oral agents developed for erectile dysfunction.

Incontinence

Immediately on removal of the Foley catheter, approximately 50% to 60% of patients will exhibit some degree of incontinence, which usually resolves spontaneously within 6 to 8 weeks. If the patient does not seem to be regaining some control within 4 weeks, the urologist should rule out organic causes such as urinary tract infection or bladder neck contracture. Long-term incontinence rates have ranged from 2.8% to 3.1% at our institution when incontinence is defined as an inability to control urinary leakage that requires pads, clamps, artificial urinary sphincters, or other devices.[3] An additional 6% to 12% of patients may experience the loss of a drop or two of urine on exertion, but this is not generally a problem. Patients at highest risk for incontinence include elderly patients (>70 years old), morbidly obese patients, and patients who have had prior radiation therapy to the prostate.

Urethral Stricture and Bladder Neck Contracture

The incidence of stricture or bladder neck contracture is between 5% and 13%. The presenting symptoms are generally decreased urinary flow rates, straining, prolonged voiding times, and feeling of incomplete emptying. Resolution of the contractures follows gentle dilation ≤24 Fr of the narrowed area. Although incontinence may be a complication of this secondary procedure, it is more likely that the patient will have resolution of the overflow incontinence rather than experience incontinence because of the procedure.

KEY POINTS

1. Hemorrhage during radical perineal prostatectomy usually originates from either the dorsal venous complex or the arterial branches to the prostate or seminal vesicles.
2. The incidence of rectal injury in radical perineal prostatectomy is <1%.
3. Infections are uncommon and are usually associated with wound soilage during the procedure. They can be prevented by using preoperative antibiotics, irrigating the wound with antibiotic-containing irrigant, and avoiding wound contamination during rectal dissection.
4. Immediately on removal of the Foley catheter, approximately 50% to 60% of patients will exhibit some degree of incontinence, which usually resolves spontaneously within 6 to 8 weeks. Approximately 15% of patients are unable to void after removal of their Foley catheter and require its replacement.
5. The rate of erectile dysfunction is 100% immediately postoperatively. Erectile function may gradually return within 12 to 18 months.
6. The incidence of stricture or bladder neck contracture is between 5% and 13%. The presenting symptoms are generally decreased urinary flow rates, straining, prolonged voiding times, and feeling of incomplete emptying.

REFERENCES

Please see www.expertconsult.com

Chapter 44

COMPLICATIONS OF RADICAL RETROPUBIC PROSTATECTOMY

Basir Tareen MD

Fellow in Urologic Oncology, Bruce and Cynthia Sherman Fellowship in Urologic Oncology, Division of Urologic Oncology, Department of Urology, New York University Langone Medical Center, New York, New York

Guilherme Godoy MD

Fellow in Urologic Oncology, Bruce and Cynthia Sherman Fellowship in Urologic Oncology, Division of Urologic Oncology, Department of Urology, New York University Langone Medical Center, New York, New York

Samir S. Taneja MD

The James M. Neissa and Janet Riha Neissa Associate Professor of Urologic Oncology; Director, Division of Urologic Oncology, Department of Urology and New York University Cancer Institute, New York University Langone Medical Center, New York, New York

The description of the anatomic nerve-sparing radical retropubic prostatectomy (RRP) by Walsh[1] in 1983 revolutionized the technique, and as a result, the comfort level of urologists performing the procedure has risen to meet the increased need for radical prostatectomy in the current era of prostate-specific antigen testing. Despite numerous options for treatment of localized disease, radical prostatectomy remains the urologic gold standard of treatment.

The complication rate for radical prostatectomy appears to have declined with technical modifications to the operation and increasing experience of urologic surgeons.[2,3] Surgical morbidity following radical prostatectomy is influenced by many factors including the experience of the surgeon, the age and medical comorbidities of the patient, the size of the prostate, the anatomy of the pelvis, the volume of prostate cancer, and the use of preoperative hormonal ablation or radiation. Intraoperative complications include bleeding, rectal injury, nerve injury and, in rare circumstances, ureteral injury. Early postoperative complications include urinary leak, infection, deep vein thrombosis or pulmonary embolus, and loss of the urethral catheter. Delayed postoperative complications generally present the greatest problem to the patient. These include incontinence, impotence, voiding dysfunction, and bladder neck contracture.

PREOPERATIVE CONSIDERATIONS

Selection of a treatment modality for localized prostate cancer is multifactorial and requires extensive discussion between the surgeon and the patient. Preoperative expectations on the part of the patient are a critical determinant of postoperative satisfaction. The process of preoperative education mandates a careful and comprehensive review of the therapeutic options and their potential complications and relative outcomes.

In general, candidates for radical prostatectomy should be in good health. In contemporary prostatectomy series, the risk of myocardial infarction, pneumonia, cerebrovascular accident, and death from these causes is exceedingly low,[3-5] likely because of proper patient selection in addition to improved anesthesia techniques.[6] Selection of healthy surgical candidates is important not only from the standpoint of avoiding anesthesia-related morbidity but also because the relative advantage of surgical resection over radiation-based therapies lies in the duration of therapeutic response.

Individuals with expected longevity >10 years are ideal for the procedure and are likely to benefit the most from it. In assessing a patient's longevity, the urologist must carefully weigh the aggressiveness of the disease against the patient's health. Higher-grade cancers, which are more likely to result in disease-related morbidity in the short term, may require aggressive therapy in patients with relatively short longevity, whereas radiation-based therapies or watchful waiting may be more important in individuals with moderately differentiated disease and relatively poor health.

In this regard, Albertsen and colleagues[7] described the risk of cancer-related death in ≤15 years of diagnosis for individuals with various grades of prostate cancer. The estimated risk of death was 4% to 7% in patients with Gleason score 2 to 4, 6% to 11% in patients with Gleason score 5, 18% to 30% in patients with Gleason score 6, 42% to 70% in patients with Gleason score 7, and 60% to 87% in patients with Gleason score 8 to 10. Clearly, individuals with higher-grade disease have worse outcomes with radical prostatectomy than do patients with low-grade disease, but prediction of outcome must be balanced against disease-related risk of death.

In selecting candidates for radical prostatectomy, the presence of voiding dysfunction should be carefully elucidated. Individuals with significant preoperative obstructive voiding symptoms may actually experience relief of such symptoms following radical prostatectomy.[8] Conversely, such individuals, particularly those with large prostates, may experience a worsening of voiding symptoms or progression to urinary retention following radiation-based treatments. The improvement in quality of life resulting from the relief in voiding symptoms following radical prostatectomy may actually outweigh the detriment causes by mild degrees of stress incontinence in the view of the patient.[9]

A careful assessment of the patient's daily activities and profession may aid in determining the potential impact of stress urinary incontinence on the individual surgical candidate. Although rates of significant incontinence have drastically improved, the patient should be made well aware of the nature and potential impact of stress urinary incontinence. Similarly, the risk of impotence despite nerve-sparing procedures should be carefully delineated. Although the pharmacologic advancements in the field of erectile dysfunction have lessened the impact of postoperative impotence following radical prostatectomy, the presence of a regular sexual partner, the stability of current relationships, and cultural attitudes regarding erectile dysfunction should be carefully evaluated before the surgical procedure.

The overall impact of complications of radical prostatectomy on quality of life is a topic of intense study in many centers and is covered comprehensively in Chapter 45. Future focus will lie in preoperative identification of poor candidates for surgery on the basis of potential impact of surgical complications on quality of life.

INTRAOPERATIVE COMPLICATIONS

Bleeding

Bleeding during RRP is most commonly encountered during division of the dorsal venous complex of the penis. Before the description of the anatomic approach to radical prostatectomy by Walsh, severe hemorrhage was often encountered on uncontrolled division of the venous complex. On occasion, such bleeding was severe

enough to require cutdown onto the prepubic penile shaft and identification of the retracted, uncontrolled venous complex beneath Buck's fascia for ligation.

Despite the advances in technique, the potential for significant bleeding during division of the dorsal venous complex and the remainder of the procedure still exists. The mean intraoperative blood loss reported in large series of radical prostatectomy has varied tremendously and ranges from 579 mL to >2 L and is likely influenced by operative technique, the presence or absence of nerve sparing, time, and the experience of the surgeon.[5,10] Several surgeons have suggested various means of perioperative blood management to minimize the need for transfusion. Rates of allogeneic transfusion in contemporary series have varied from 2.4% to 21% independent of autologous blood donation.[5,11-15] Reoperation for bleeding is extremely rare, with a reported incidence as low as 0.3% in one large series.[15]

The use of autologous blood donation was previously shown to reduce the risk for allogeneic transfusion. Several investigators challenged the need for blood donation.[13,16,17] Koch and Smith[13] reported an overall transfusion rate resulting from intraoperative bleeding of 2.4% in 124 patients undergoing radical prostatectomy without preoperative autologous blood donation. Because it is unlikely that most surgeons will be fortunate enough to experience such a minimal likelihood of intraoperative and postoperative bleeding, and for this reason, it is advisable that some form of preventive management be instituted in patients undergoing radical prostatectomy.

Chun and associates[18] proposed the use of preoperative erythropoietin injections instead of autologous donation. Patients were given one to two injections of erythropoietin, provided their preoperative hematocrit was <48%.[18] On average, an increase in the hematocrit of 3% was noted when 600 U/kg was administered 7 to 14 days preoperatively. Using this method, the investigators demonstrated an identical risk of allogeneic transfusion in individuals donating autologous blood of approximately 9.6%.[18] Based on safety and efficacy from a prospective study of 283 men undergoing RRP at our institution, we currently give epoetin alfa preoperatively in two doses of 600 IU/kg.[19]

Although dorsal venous complex bleeding can occur regardless of the chosen technique of control, several anatomic points can be helpful for avoiding profuse hemorrhage. The dorsal venous complex courses beneath the pubis symphysis as a bundle of veins over the membranous urethra before it fans over the anterior surface of the prostate and bladder neck. On uncontrolled division, variable amounts of bleeding can occur. Initial descriptions of the anatomic retropubic prostatectomy included isolation of the dorsal venous complex with passage of a right-angle clamp between the membranous urethra and the complex, followed by sharp division with a knife blade. We have, in recent years, chosen to ligate the complex proximally and distally before division.

The dorsal venous complex is covered by an overlying reflection of the endopelvic fascia. To control all the veins fanning over the prostate within the complex effectively, the endopelvic fascia must be fully incised along the lateral sulcus of the anterior prostate. This incision is made in the groove between the prostate and levator musculature during gentle retraction of the prostate contralaterally (**Fig. 44-1A**). The incision must be carried to the base of the prostate and bladder neck to allow effective mobility of the proximally located veins.

A decussation of the endopelvic fascia, termed the *puboprostatic ligament,* lies at either lateral edge of the venous complex fusing its anterior surface to the posterior surface of the pubic bone. We do not routinely divide the puboprostatic ligaments, but this maneuver can be helpful in dropping the venous complex away from the pubis. This is particularly useful when operating on large glands that compress the dorsal venous complex or glands with a large anterior or retropubic component and when the puboprostatic ligaments extend onto the anterior surface of the prostate gland. In these situations, we divide only that portion of the puboprostatic ligament needed for exposure. Preservation of the puboprostatic ligament will hold the vein stump fixed, to some extent, and prevents retraction and uncontrolled bleeding.

Once the endopelvic fascia has been incised on either side of the gland and the superficial dorsal vein has been defined and fulgurated, the deep venous complex is bunched centrally for control (see Fig. 44-1B). An angled or straight long Allis clamp is inserted with one jaw in each facial incision. The venous complex is then bunched centrally at the level of the midprostate, with care taken to include all veins but avoiding prostatic capsular injury. Difficulty with bunching may be corrected with further proximal incision of the endopelvic fascia. Once the clamp is in place, the venous complex is controlled with a suture ligature of 2-0 polyglactin 910 (Vicryl) on a wide curved needle, at the level of the clamp placement. The clamp is removed during ligation of the proximal vein. Next, a suture ligature is placed around the distal venous complex as far caudad as possible (see Fig. 44-1C). This is achieved by placing the Allis clamp more apically and gently depressing the visible prostatic apex, thus exposing the distal vein as it courses over the membranous urethra. Double passage of each suture ligature will fix it in place and prevent it from slipping off on division of the vein.

Sharp incision of the dorsal venous complex is then initiated between the proximal and distal sutures (**Fig. 44-2**). A plane of dissection is developed sharply within the dorsal complex, with great care taken not to injure the anterior prostatic capsule. A sponge stick is used by

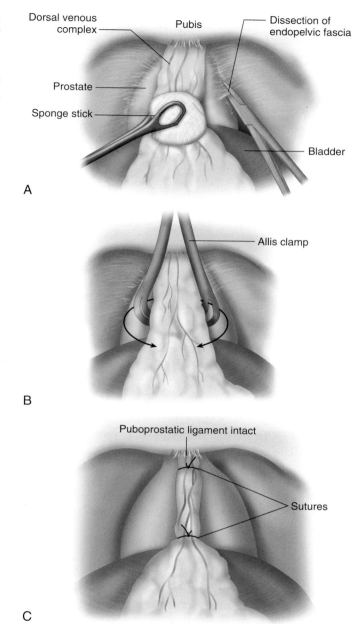

Figure 44-1 The technique of dorsal venous complex control. **A,** The endopelvic fascia is sharply incised on either side of the prostate. The incision extends from the base of the prostate to the puboprostatic ligament. **B,** An Allis clamp is used to bunch the dorsal venous complex centrally. The initial bunching is done over the midprostate, proximal to the prostatic apex. Bunching is performed by inserting the jaw of the clamp into the endopelvic fascial incision on each side and thereby incorporating all veins as they fan over the prostate. **C,** Proximal and distal bunching sutures are in place in the dorsal venous complex. The surface of the anterior prostate reveals no excluded veins coursing over the gland. The first suture is placed proximally at the level of the bunching clamp. A second suture is then placed distal to the puboprostatic ligaments, around the dorsal venous complex, as far caudad as possible without division of the puboprostatic sutures.

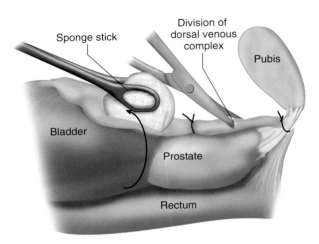

Figure 44-2 Division of the dorsal venous complex begins by incising the centrally bunched tissue between the proximally and distally placed sutures. A sponge stick is used to rotate the gland dorsally and cranially away from the pubic symphysis as the dorsal complex is divided. In doing so, the dorsal complex is rotated into the field as it is sequentially divided. Antegrade dissection is carried out within the dorsal venous complex until the membranous urethra is rotated into the field of view. Caution must be exerted to avoid anterior prostate injury.

the assistant to retract the prostate cranially and gently roll it away from the pubis as the venous tissue is divided. The surgeon should always err on the side of cutting out the distal suture rather than injuring the anterior prostate. If the distal suture is cut out, complete division of the dorsal venous complex should be completed, and then the dorsal venous complex stump can be directly suture ligated. Incision of the dorsal venous complex is sequentially carried out until the anterior urethra is exposed. An effort should be made to preserve the anterior thickness of the urethra maximally.

Bleeding can occur throughout the procedure. This bleeding often originates from the bed of the neurovascular bundle if nerve sparing is performed, from the seminal vesicular arteries, or from the bladder neck. The prostatic pedicles are usually directly ligated before division, and for this reason should not be a major source of bleeding. Bleeding from the neurovascular bundles can occasionally be controlled be clipping prostate perforating branches before division, but this is often a fruitless endeavor. In a non–nerve-sparing procedure, early ligation of the neurovascular bundle can save a great deal of trouble when one tries to suture ligate the stump once it is retracted. When steady bleeding is encountered, it is usually best to move ahead with the procedure because operative time likely predicts the cumulative blood loss. Fulguration or clipping of the neurovascular bundles may inadvertently injure the nerve and therefore should be avoided.

Some investigators have advocated an antegrade approach to radical prostatectomy to avoid early bleed-

ing,[20] but in general, if the procedure is to be performed in a timely fashion with early control of the dorsal venous complex, this should not be necessary.

Rectal Injury

Injury of the rectum occurs in <1% to 3.6% of patients undergoing radical prostatectomy.[3,4,21,22] Risk factors for rectal injury include previous radiation and periprostatic inflammation resulting from previous transurethral resection or excessive bleeding at the time of biopsy. Salvage prostatectomy carries the highest rates of intraoperative rectal injury, with reports ranging from 6% to 15%.[23,24] Immediate repair of the injury results in excellent outcome without long-term sequelae in the majority of patients.

Following division of the posterior urethra, the surgeon encounters the rectourethralis muscle along with underlying Denonvilliers' fascia. It is desirable to divide this layer in a single incision and thus enter the pararectal space and allow an adequate posterior margin of resection. If the surgeon is too timid in division, aggressive retraction of the prostatic apex can result in shearing of Denonvilliers' fascia from the posterior apex and splitting of the gland. If the surgeon is too aggressive in achieving this plane, sharp injury of the rectum can occur. In general, rectal injury results from an overzealous attempt to develop the posterior plane bluntly with the tip of the finger. If the rectourethralis is not completely divided, or if the plane does not develop easily with blunt dissection, the attached rectal wall can be torn. Sharp dissection is preferable if the apex of the gland does not lift away from the rectum easily. An obscured operative field from excessive bleeding hinders the ability to see the tissue planes clearly. Therefore, adequate hemostasis is preferable at the time of the apical dissection.

When rectal injury does occur, it is generally acceptable to repair the defect primarily in the absence of gross fecal soiling.[21,25,26] Patients should have been given a preoperative enema specifically for this reason. Débridement of devitalized tissue at the site of laceration should be followed by a two-layer closure of mucosal and muscular layers of the rectal wall. A small opening can be made in the peritoneum to pull down and interpose an omental flap between the rectal repair and the vesicourethral anastomosis. Although this maneuver is not routinely necessary, it can provide an extra safety measure if the surgeon is concerned about the viability of the rectal closure. A pedicalized flap of peritoneum or pararectal fat can serve a similar purpose. In the event of a large injury, a significantly devitalized or devascularized rectal wall, or the presence of gross soiling, serious consideration should be given to a temporary diverting colostomy along with simultaneous rectal wall repair. This procedure is certainly advisable in the setting of a previously irradiated pelvis.

The risk of rectourethral fistula following repair of rectal injury is lowered from approximately 15% to 43% to 80% by use of bowel preparation.[26] Use of prolonged bowel rest, anal dilation at the time of the surgical procedure, and the administration of broad-spectrum antibiotics have all been suggested as potential aids in lowering fistula rates. Perhaps the greatest risk of fistula formation and risk of morbidity stem from unrecognized rectal injury.[21] If a rectourinary fistula does develop and the patient is otherwise well, an initial attempt at conservative management can be attempted using bladder drainage and a low-residue diet. Complicated cases or patients with a history of radiation will likely require use of a temporary diverting colostomy.[27]

Ureteral Injury

Ureteral injury during radical prostatectomy is rare, occurring in 0.05% to 1.6% of cases.[4,28,29] When it does occur, it is usually during the bladder neck division, although with many surgeons advocating extended lymphadenectomy, the ureter may be injured above the iliac bifurcation during node dissection. In the setting of a large median lobe, care must be exercised to avoid the ureteral orifices by directly visualizing them. We prefer to use a partial bladder neck–sparing approach, and when doing so, caution must be exerted to avoid straying into the trigonal musculature.

The administration of intravenous indigo carmine on division of the bladder neck should be routinely performed to visualize ureteral efflux on both sides. This is particularly true for the surgeon inexperienced in prostatectomy, but is a good general habit for all surgeons. Occasionally, in a patient who has undergone aggressive transurethral resection of the prostate, the ureteral orifices can be cut during division of the bladder neck. Our simple solution is to perform a ureterotomy for a length of approximately 1 cm, insert an indwelling stent, and then taper the bladder neck posteriorly to relocate the orifices proximally.

On rare occasions, injury to the ureter can occur during posterior dissection of the seminal vesicles. The ureters generally enter the posterior bladder wall anterolateral to the tips of the seminal vesicles and cross toward the midline above the trigone. For this reason, blind placement of sutures should be avoided in the seminal vesical bed. If one suspects an injury, passage of a 3-Fr feeding tube can allay concerns. In rare circumstances, an on-table retrograde pyelogram can be helpful.

If ureteral injury is identified, immediate ureteroneocystostomy is indicated. The cut end of the ureter is pulled into the bladder lumen at a convenient site, spatulated, and sutured to the bladder mucosa. A long submucosal tunnel is not necessary. The vesicourethral anastomosis should be completed first to avoid tension on the ureteral anastomosis. Similarly, if tension is encountered, a Boari flap is preferable to a psoas hitch to avoid undue tension on the vesicourethral anastomosis.

Nerve Injury

Injury to the obturator nerve and femoral nerve can occur during pelvic mobilization, and these injuries are discussed in detail in Chapter 40.

EARLY POSTOPERATIVE COMPLICATIONS

Urinary Leak

Although the reported incidence of anastomotic leak is low in contemporary series, the true incidence is unknown because most small leaks are never diagnosed secondary to spontaneous resolution. In general, factors predisposing to extravasation are poorly understood. Experience at our institution suggests that the ability to achieve a watertight anastomosis does not appear to be related to the deposition of collagen because the rate of extravasation is equivalent on postoperative days 3 and 7.[30,31] Fenig and colleagues[32] did find that postoperative blood loss was associated with the degree of extravasation on postoperative cystogram. This same relationship was not true of intraoperative blood loss, a finding that left the investigators to conclude that postoperative blood loss resulted in a hematoma that may cause distraction of the vesicourethral anastomosis.

When urinary leak does occur, a combination of catheter drainage with retropubic drainage should allow closure of the leak in a short time. Pelvic suction drains can be used following radical prostatectomy, but if a leak does occur, consideration should be given to converting to gravity drainage by removing the suction bulb. Additionally, if a leak persists, gradual withdrawal of the drain can ensure that the drain tip has not migrated into the anastomosis. If the patient has significant hematuria, periodic gentle irrigation of the catheter is wise to maintain drainage. Clot retention, or catheter plugging resulting from clot, can cause leakage in the early postoperative period. Leaks persisting for >7 to 10 days are concerning to the surgeon, but a steadfast approach of maximal drainage should be maintained. Repeat exploration is hardly ever necessary.

Complete disruption of the anastomosis resulting from pelvic hematoma or seroma is a rare occurrence. Even in this setting, if the anastomosis is stented with a catheter, healing should occur. Obviously, the likelihood of bladder neck contracture is high with significant disruption of the anastomosis, and if it is relatively early in the postoperative period, consideration should be given to surgical revision of the anastomosis along with drainage of the hematoma or seroma. If significant time has elapsed since the surgical procedure, the surgeon may encounter technical difficulty with the anastomosis because of tissue friability and distortion.

In the setting of fever or pelvic pain accompanying a leak, consideration should be given to the possibility of an undrained pelvic fluid collection. Cross-sectional imaging along with percutaneous drainage can relieve the problem if it is identified.

Urinary Tract and Wound Infection

Infectious complications following radical prostatectomy are relatively unusual. The incidence in contemporary series ranges from 1% to 3%, generally consisting of wound infection.[3,22,33,34] Early recognition of wound infection is essential to minimize the need for aggressive therapy. Patients generally at risk include those with excessive abdominal pannus and those with large amounts of urinary extravasation.

The use of prophylactic antibiotics in radical prostatectomy is essentially the same as in individuals undergoing other forms of abdominal surgery. Antibiotic coverage should be broad spectrum and directed toward skin flora. We routinely use a first-generation cephalosporin administered at the time of anesthetic induction and maintained for a period of 24 hours after the procedure. Because patients have an indwelling catheter for 1 week postoperatively, the use of urinary tract prophylaxis is advocated by some surgeons following surgery. The use of antibiotics for a prolonged period postoperatively is controversial, and the benefit is not clearly demonstrated. Nonetheless, in view of the fresh incision, the risk of small amounts of urinary extravasation, and the risk of catheter-related secondary infections, we generally administer a fluoroquinolone until the catheter is removed.

Before the surgical procedure, a urine culture is advisable. Individuals with known infection should obviously be fully treated before the operation. These individuals should then have prophylactic antibiotics directed toward the offending organism.

Wound infection can result in any patient, but in general patients with significant urinary extravasation, bleeding, or excessive subcutaneous fat may be at the greatest risk. In individuals believed to be at risk because of obesity, the use of a suprafascial subcutaneous suction drain can prevent seroma formation and limit the risk of infection. Additionally, relatively loose approximation of the skin allows drainage of serous and serosanguineous fluid and thereby limits the risk of fluid collection. Subcutaneous sutures to close the "dead space" should be avoided in this situation.

When infection does occur, it is best treated by opening the incision and allowing healing by second intention. On rare occasions, periodic débridement may be required to remove devitalized tissue. The fascia underlying the infection should be carefully inspected for dehiscence, which is rare with an extraperitoneal lower midline incision. If persistent wound drainage is noted, consideration should be given to the possibility of a urine leak or a pelvic abscess.

Pulmonary Embolus and Deep Vein Thrombosis

Thromboembolic complications continue to be a major complication of pelvic cancer surgery. Although the diagnosis and management of deep vein thrombosis and pulmonary embolus are discussed in Chapters 2 and 4, routine preventive measures are an important part of radical prostatectomy. The incidence of deep vein thrombosis or pulmonary embolus in contemporary radical prostatectomy series has varied from 2% to 3.1%.[3,4,22,33,34] This rate is consistent with the 1% to 5% reported rate of patients undergoing surgical treatment of cancer of the abdomen and pelvis.[35] Much discussion has centered on the routine use of heparinoid prophylaxis for procedures that place the patient at high risk for venous thromboembolism. In a review of 1373 RRPs, Koya and Soloway and their associates[36] found only 3 instances of deep vein thrombosis with no clinical pulmonary embolus when they used only sequential compression devices and no heparinoid prophylaxis. Lepor and colleagues[15] found similarly low rates in their series of 1000 cases and as such the use of prophylaxis remains controversial.

Loss of Catheter

Occasionally, as a result of catheter malfunction or injury, the Foley catheter can fall out following radical prostatectomy. This complication is obviously of more concern 7 hours postoperatively than 7 days afterward. In the very early postoperative period (<48 hours), it is unwise to attempt blind passage of a catheter. The use of a flexible cystoscope with passage of a floppy guidewire and then a Council-tip catheter is the safest course of action. Although it is not absolutely necessary to perform this procedure while the patient is under anesthesia, it is probably most comfortable for the patient in this early postoperative period.

If one is unable to penetrate the anastomosis, or if the anastomosis is disrupted, then placement of a suprapubic cystostomy under ultrasound guidance can temporize the situation. If no urethral catheter is placed, the patient will be at high risk of bladder neck stricture with a suprapubic tube in place. On rare occasions, if nothing can be passed through the anastomosis, reoperation with replacement of the catheter and revision of the anastomosis are indicated. Although reoperation is hardly ever necessary, when it is indicated, it is best simply to perform a cystotomy and attempt antegrade passage of a catheter to establish the lumen. A wire can then be passed through the catheter for eventual retrograde catheter passage. This technique is preferable to disruption and reconstruction of the vesicourethral anastomosis.

Similarly, in the presence of unusually severe hematuria or clot retention, the surgeon should consider placement of an open or closed suprapubic cystostomy rather than catheter change. Urinary drainage can be maintained with the cystostomy while the nonfunctional urethral catheter continues to stent the vesicourethral anastomosis.

In the later postoperative period (>2-5 days), consideration should be given to leaving the catheter out as long as the patient is not in urinary retention. A retrograde urethrogram can confirm closure of the urethra. Alternatively, at this later stage, gentle passage of a catheter is usually possible at the bedside. For those patients falling in between (1-2 days), an attempt at bedside flexible cystoscopy with passage of a wire is usually acceptable, but blind passage of a catheter should be avoided. An unsuccessful attempt can be followed by one while the patient is under anesthesia.

DELAYED POSTOPERATIVE COMPLICATIONS

Impotence

Erectile dysfunction following radical prostatectomy was the primary impetus for the development of the modified anatomic approach to RRP described by Walsh. Before the anatomic description of the neurovascular bundles containing the cavernosal nerves, erectile function after radical prostatectomy was rare. Now, with the application of nerve-sparing techniques, investigators report potency in 63% to 68% of men undergoing bilateral nerve-sparing procedures and in 41% to 50% of those undergoing unilateral nerve-sparing operations.[1,3,4] Most reported series are from centers of excellence, and the reported rates of potency from community-based series are often worse, ranging from 11% to 30%.[37-39]

The assessment of postoperative potency is a critical factor in determining outcomes in prostate cancer surgery. This is described in detail in Chapter 45, but use of a validated instrument for the measurement of sexual function is critical.[40] Potency is clearly not a binary variable, and it should be treated as a graded phenomenon. Decreased preoperative erectile function is an important determinant of the likelihood of postoperative erections after nerve-sparing surgery.

Several factors influence the likelihood of retaining erectile function postoperatively. Age is a primary determinant of the success of bilateral nerve-sparing prostatectomy in preserving potency adequate for sexual intercourse. The potency rate following bilateral nerve-sparing radical prostatectomy for men <50 years old has varied from 86% to 91% compared with 75% to 80% in men in their 50s, 58% to 60% in men in their 60s, and 25% to 42% in men >70 years old.[1,3,4,41] Although it is difficult to quantitate, preoperative erectile function may be the greatest predictor of age-related return of potency. Whereas recovery of erectile function is variable, Klein and Scardino and their colleagues[42] showed that recovery of erectile function may continue even after the first postoperative year and may improve even over 2 to 3 years. The presence of risk factors for impotence such as diabetes, chronic hypertension, cardiovascular disease, and multiple medications should also be considered predictive risk factors.

In addition to patient characteristics contributing to postoperative erectile dysfunction, certain technical factors aside from cavernosal nerve preservation may contribute to this outcome as well. We believe that excessive traction, manipulation, or local cauterization of the neurovascular bundles can greatly influence the likelihood of return of function. Recognition of the nerve bundle and careful preservation of its surrounding tissues are exceedingly important in avoiding nerve injury. Neurapraxia caused by traction or thermal injury may reverse, but the increasing suggestion is that prolonged periods of postoperative erectile dysfunction may increase the likelihood of permanent impotence.

On occasion, when dividing the dorsal venous complex and or lateral periurethral tissues, the surgeon encounters bleeding in the space lateral to the urethra. This complication is most often the result of a lacerated venous branch that is partially retracted beneath the levator musculature. Care should be exercised to avoid electrocautery and or placement of deep suture ligatures during attempts to control such bleeding. The placement of sutures should limited to tacking the vessel to the surrounding levator muscle with a 3-0 or 4-0 absorbable stitch under direct vision. Deeply placed stitches in this location can cause unseen injury to the ipsilateral neurovascular bundle or continence mechanism.

To avoid traction injury to the cavernosal nerves during apical retraction of the gland, we have used a modified approach to the nerve-sparing technique of Walsh. Following division of the deep dorsal venous complex, the lateral prostatic fascia is identified on the anterolateral aspect of the prostate (**Fig. 44-3A**). The prostatourethral junction is developed by bluntly pushing the overlying levator fibers off the apex with a Kitner dissector. The fascia is incised while it is elevated from the prostate capsule with a right-angle clamp. Care should be exercised to avoid injury to the prostate capsule during this maneuver. Once incised, the lateral edge of the incised fascia is lifted away from the gland and a plane is developed between the prostate and the lateral prostatic fascial contents (inclusive of the cavernosal nerve bundle). The plane is developed with blunt and sharp dissection along the prostatic apex and the prostatourethral junction. In this fashion, the nerve is completely freed from the prostatic apex before division of the urethra or retraction of the prostatic apex (see Fig. 44-3B).

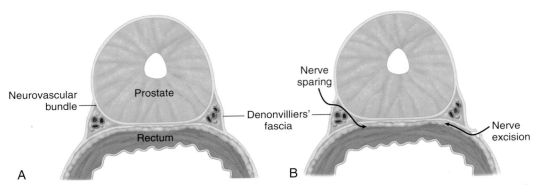

Figure 44-3 The neurovascular bundle dissection can be carried out for either preservation or wide excision. **A,** Anatomically, the neurovascular bundle is carried and is separated from the prostate by decussation of the lateral prostatic fascia and from the rectum by Denonvilliers' fascia. The lateral prostatic fascia extends over the lateral rectum dorsal to the position of the neurovascular bundles. **B,** In nerve preservation, the lateral fascia is released on the anterolateral surface of the prostate and then is rolled off the posterolateral aspect of the gland until Denonvilliers' fascia is exposed. On release of the neurovascular bundle, an incision in the posterior layer of Denonvilliers' fascia overlying the anterior rectal wall allows complete separation of the prostate from the bundle. Entry into the plane posterior to Denonvilliers' fascia allows elevation of the prostatic apex from the rectum such that no tension is placed on the nerves after division of the urethra and retraction of the prostatic apex. *(Modified from Goad JR, Scardino PT. Modifications in the technique of radical retropubic prostatectomy to minimize blood loss.* Urol Clin North Am. *1994;2:75.)*

The plane between the lateral prostatic fascia and the prostate should develop easily with a blunt sweeping motion, but occasionally sharp dissection is necessary. On lateral reflection of the fascia from the posterolateral prostate, exposure should be medial to the neurovascular bundle to allow perforation of Denonvilliers' fascia and entry into the perirectal space (see Fig. 44-3B). Carrying the plane circumferentially around the prostate can make division of the posterior urethra and rectourethralis quite simple. Occasionally, the plane is adherent, and in this circumstance consideration should be given to the possibility of extraprostatic cancer advancement or simply residual fibrosis from the prostate biopsy. In these cases, the posterior plane should be developed following division of the urethra, and one should consider intraoperative frozen sections, from the lateral and apical margin bed.[43]

Much attention has been focused on penile rehabilitation using behavioral and medical therapy to increase likelihood of potency following RRP. Numerous authors reported significantly improved potency using phosphodiesterase-5 inhibitors following radical prostatectomy both as needed for impotence and on a daily basis prophylactically immediately after the procedure and continuing during the postoperative period.[44,45] At our institution, we routinely prescribe daily sildenafil 50 mg for the first year postoperatively for these patients.

Incontinence

Incontinence remains the most feared and frustrating complication of radical prostatectomy for both patient and surgeon. Although contemporary surgical series report markedly improved rates of total continence compared with earlier series, a small percentage of cases still result in debilitating incontinence for the patient. Further underscoring the frustrating nature of the complication is the absence of any reliable preoperative or intraoperative predictors of postoperative continence.

Contemporary surgical series report rates of total continence of 80% to 95%.[1,4,3,22,46-48] The definition of *total continence* is variable, but in general, the term should apply only to those patients who have absolutely no leakage and who require no pads or devices for urine collection. Even with this definition in mind, some investigators have reported excellent continence rates. In the Baylor series, individuals undergoing surgical procedures after 1990 reported total continence rates of 95% compared with rates of <80% among individuals undergoing prostatectomy before 1990.[46] Age may also influence continence. Catalona and colleagues[3,4] reported a 96% rate of continence in men <70 years old compared with a rate of 87% among those >70 years old. Once again, the reports of incontinence rates are generally from centers of excellence in radical prostatectomy, and community-based series often report lower rates of total continence.[38-40]

In attempting to minimize the risk of incontinence in the postoperative setting, preservation of the external striated sphincter is of paramount importance. Minimizing the blind passage of clamps, periurethral dissection, and aggressive hemostatic suturing in the area of the external sphincter is critical for preservation of the sphincter. For this reason, we prefer to perform the apical dissection sharply with no passage of clamps. All suture ligatures are placed directly under vision, and no excessive efforts are made to control venous oozing in the periurethral area.

Following division of the dorsal venous complex as described, the membranous urethra is exposed. By leaving the puboprostatic ligaments largely intact, the normal suspension of the urethra to the symphysis is preserved. An effort should be made to preserve the full thickness of the "spongy" tissue of the urethra along with its surrounding sheath. This goal is accomplished by limiting anterior sharp dissection to the point at which the catheter can first be palpated. Thinning of the anterior urethra, a potential pitfall of our technique of dorsal vein division, is avoided in this fashion.

As described, we perform our nerve-sparing procedure before division of the urethra. On completion of the procedure, the nerve bundles have been released from the posterolateral aspect of the prostatourethral junction. With gentle retraction on the prostatic apex, the lateral urethra is exposed, and division of the urethra is begun 5 mm distal to the prostatourethral junction (**Fig. 44-4**). The anterior two thirds of the urethra is divided, to exposing the catheter below. The anterior and lateral anastomotic sutures are placed at this time to incorporate urethral sponge and mucosa in each suture pass. Next, once the catheter has been divided, the posterior urethra is exposed. We believe that passage of the posterior sutures is best performed at this time to facilitate inclusion of the rectourethralis and urethral mucosa in the suture passage. Because the neurovascular bundle on either side of the urethra has already been released, passage of the posterior anastomotic sutures is possible at this point.

When the surgeon assesses the patient with incontinence postoperatively, a careful historical evaluation should be performed to determine the nature of the incontinence. As discussed later, preexisting detrusor

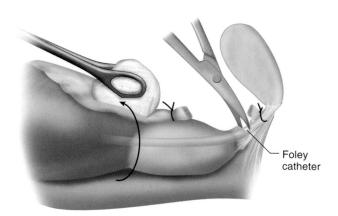

Figure 44-4 Division of the membranous urethra. The urethra is divided anteriorly following full release of the neurovascular bundles. Care is taken to preserve the full thickness of the urethra by cutting through the wall in a single stroke rather than layer by layer. In this fashion the urethral catheter is exposed.

Foley catheter

hypertrophy, instability, and decreased bladder wall compliance may contribute to postoperative voiding dysfunction. On occasion, these conditions can result in urge-related incontinence. The management of stress urinary incontinence following radical prostatectomy is discussed in Chapter 50. In general, surgical treatment of stress incontinence should be withheld until conservative treatment has failed for 10 to 12 months. In cases of severe incontinence lasting ≥6 months, complete resolution of incontinence is unlikely, and earlier intervention may be considered.

Bladder Neck Contracture

Bladder neck contracture or vesicourethral anastomotic stricture is not an uncommon complication of radical prostatectomy; it occurs in 0.5% to 17.5% of cases.[3,10,34,47,49] In most series, the risk of stricture is approximately 5% to 10%. This complication usually manifests relatively soon after catheter removal because the predisposing factors are present in the perioperative period. On occasion, late bladder neck contractures are noted, and consideration to the diagnosis should be given whenever patients complain of worsening incontinence, increased urgency or frequency, or decreased urinary stream.

Multiple factors may contribute to early contracture of the anastomosis including anastomotic urinary extravasation, poor mucosal approximation, suture reaction, and ischemia. A large review from the Cancer of the Prostate Strategic Urologic Research Endeavor (CaPSURE) database showed that men who developed stricture were older and had a higher body mass index.[49] Although these factors are self explanatory, some, such as ischemia and poor mucosal apposition may not be easily recognized postoperatively. Attention to these issues is most important intraoperatively during completion of the anastomosis. Excessive thinning or mobilization of the bladder neck, particularly when rolling an anterior bladder wall tube, can cause ischemia and should be avoided. Sutures with nonreactive characteristics such as the absorbable monofilament poliglecaprone 25 (Monocryl) should be used.

Several maneuvers can aid in ensuring mucosal apposition. Tapering of the bladder neck should be performed with a mucosal everting stitch to avoid stricture in the tapered segment of bladder neck (**Fig. 44-5**). We place anastomotic sutures in the lumen of the bladder neck for further eversion of the mucosa to maximize mucosal apposition at the anastomosis. While performing the vesicourethral anastomosis, the most difficult position at which to achieve mucosal apposition is the posterior urethra. Often, on division of the posterior urethra, the mucosa retracts, and the urethra can be thinned at this position. For this reason, when possible, we prefer to place the posterior urethral sutures before division of the posterior urethra and rectourethralis. If

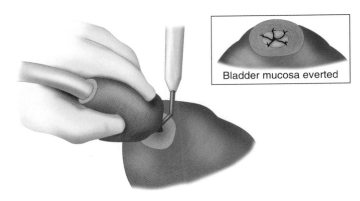

Bladder mucosa everted

Figure 44-5 The prostate is circumferentially amputated from the bladder neck by using a circumscribing cautery incision from posterior to anterior. In doing so, no blunt dissection is performed, but instead the muscle fibers are incised directly along the neck to allow the bladder to fall away from the elevated prostate. Following bladder neck division, the bladder mucosa is fully everted to maximize the likelihood of mucosa-to-mucosa apposition in the vesicourethral anastomosis.

this maneuver is not possible, sutures should be place deep into the urethral lumen to maximize mucosal capture in the suture.

Minor Complications

Inguinal hernia is another proposed complication of RRP, with a proposed incidence of 10% to 20%.[50,51] The cause has been elusive and has led many investigators to speculate that a lower midline incision in and of itself is the reason for the increased incidence of inguinal hernias. Stranne and colleagues[51] compared a survey population of various lower midline procedures versus a nonoperated group of patients and found significant differences in incidence at 24 months for development of inguinal hernia. Lepor and Robbins[52] reviewed 1300 patients undergoing RRP and showed a 13% incidence of inguinal hernias in this population, a finding suggesting that underdiagnosis of hernia on the preoperative examination was the likely reason for previously higher reported rates of postprostatectomy inguinal hernia. These investigators found the postoperative incidence of hernias to be only 8%.[52]

Urine loss during sexual intercourse or ejaculation is an often overlooked complication of RRP. Studies often focus on volume of urine loss and correlate this with greater bother and more significant lifestyle changes.[53] Abouassaly and Gill and their colleagues[54] described their experience with postprostatectomy ejaculatory urine loss in 26 patients and reported that although the amounts of urine lost were typically small, they had a major impact on quality of life and led to a great deal of embarrassment and anxiety. Koeman and associates[55] were surprised to find that 7 of 14 patients who com-

plained of "weakened orgasm" in their series also complained of involuntary urine loss.

Change in orgasm following RRP is another complication that is often not discussed with the patient or is lost when focusing on whether that patient will have potency. Other than the "dry orgasm," many patients believe that their orgasm is "weakened" or different in duration. One could hypothesize that lack of prostate and seminal vesicle contraction may contribute to this phenomenon.

The rate of *fecal incontinence* was reported to be ≤5% in men undergoing RRP who participated in a telephone survey in a study by Bishoff and colleagues.[56] Although rates of this complication are typically proposed to be higher in patients undergoing radical perineal prostatectomy, other investigators suggested that the rates of fecal incontinence noted by Bishoff and colleagues were considerably lower and that no significant differences existed between RRP and radical perineal prostatectomy in this regard.[57] A study of outcomes showed no difference between bowel symptoms in patients undergoing watchful waiting and those in patients undergoing RRP.[58]

SALVAGE PROSTATECTOMY

Selection of candidates for radical prostatectomy following radiation can be difficult. In general, the operation results in relatively low rates of cancer control, although with proper selection, some investigators have reported 10-year clinical cancer-free survival rates of 60% to 70% and biochemical recurrence-free survival rates of 30% to 43%.[42,59,60] Investigators have estimated that as many as two thirds of these patients have advanced pathologic disease (pT3a or greater).[23,42] Stephenson and Eastham[61] proposed that the 5-year progression-free rates for salvage RRP are 86%, 55%, and 28% for patients with preoperative prostate-specific antigen levels of 4 ng/mL, 4 to 10 ng/mL, and >10 ng/mL.[42,61]

A higher likelihood of rectal injury is noted in patients undergoing salvage surgery than in those patients undergoing primary radical prostatectomy, with reported rates ranging from 6% to 15%.[23,24,62] Fibrotic reaction often ablates the plane posterior to the prostate, and to avoid injury to the rectum surgeon should use sharp dissection to develop the plane. In patients with known proctitis or rectal devascularization resulting from radiation, strong consideration should be given to a diverting colostomy in the setting of rectal injury. In a properly prepared bowel, it may be acceptable to repair the injury primarily, but given the propensity for poor wound healing in the irradiated field, the surgeon should have a low threshold for proximal diversion. One option is to repair the defect primarily, but to raise a loop of sigmoid colon to a suprafascial position. If the rectum heals without difficulty, the loop can be dropped back into the abdomen and the fascia closed in a relatively minor operation. If the rectal injury does not heal, a Turnbull-style loop stoma can be matured at the bedside.

In addition to intraoperative difficulty, individuals undergoing postirradiation prostatectomy are prone to higher rates of incontinence and deep vein thrombosis than are patients undergoing primary prostatectomy.

Most groups report rates of incontinence >50%. For this reason, careful selection with regard to the possibility of cancer cure should be a fundamental tenet of salvage prostatectomy. We have not been strong advocates of the idea of palliative resection for locoregional control in this setting and believe that patient selection based on oncologic tenets is essential.

KEY POINTS

1. When performing open radical prostatectomy, the rate of bleeding varies with operator experience and technique. The use of preoperative erythropoietin or autologous blood donation can lower the likelihood of allogeneic transfusion greatly.

2. Control of the dorsal venous complex prior to division can greatly reduce blood loss during radical prostatectomy. Accurate and complete bunching of the dorsal vein hood over the base of the prostate is helped by wide incision of the endopelvic fascia back to the bladder neck.

3. Early release of the lateral prostatic fascia on the anterolateral surface of the gland facilitates release of the neurovascular bundles prior to urethral division, thereby reducing traction on the neurovascular structures.

4. In performing the urethral anastomosis, tension-free mucosal apposition is essential in avoiding bladder neck contracture.

5. Pelvic hematoma due to postoperative bleeding causes distraction of the urethral anastomosis, potentially causing urinary extravasation and eventual bladder neck contracture. In such cases prolonged catheterization is warranted.

6. Rectal injury at the time of radical prostatectomy does not require diverting colostomy in the majority of cases. Bowel preparation, antibiotics, methodical closure of the rectum, and interposition of either omental or peritoneal closure of the rectum, and interposition of either omental or peritoneal flap can all help in avoiding the need for colostomy.

REFERENCES

Please see www.expertconsult.com

Chapter 45

LONG-TERM OUTCOMES OF RADICAL PROSTATECTOMY

George J. Huang MD
Clinical Instructor, Department of Urology, Keck School of Medicine, University of Southern California, Los Angeles, Los Angeles, California

David F. Penson MD, MPH
Professor of Urology, Vanderbilt University, Nashville, Tennessee

Radical prostatectomy (RP) is a standard treatment for clinically localized prostate cancer. Furthermore, the literature indicates that RP alone may be curative in many cases of locally advanced disease.[1-4] With an estimated >100,000 cases of RP performed annually in the United States, RP is one of the most commonly performed operations in the field of urology.[5] RP provides excellent long-term cancer control and disease-specific survival, but untoward effects of surgery can negatively affect a patient's health-related quality of life (HRQOL).[6] Specifically, RP can result in urinary dysfunction in the form of stress incontinence or bladder neck contracture and sexual dysfunction in the form of anejaculation and erectile dysfunction (ED). We have a relatively good understanding of outcomes in these domains during short-term follow-up (≤2 years postoperatively), but our understanding of longer-term outcomes (after year 2) in these areas is far less complete and is still evolving.

To counsel patients properly, it is imperative that practicing urologists fully appreciate and acknowledge the side effects of RP, as well as the effects of other treatments. To date, no adequately sized randomized clinical trial has compared the long-term oncologic outcomes of surgery with other treatments for localized prostate cancer. In the absence of this information, patients often base treatment decisions on the side effect profiles of available therapies[7] and rely on their physicians to provide them with accurate information. Presenting only 1- or 2-year outcomes, however, is inadequate and may even be somewhat misleading. Immediate side effects of treatment may continue to evolve or improve, whereas new symptoms may also arise beyond the first 2 years. The normal aging process may also play a confounding role that affects HRQOL over the long term. Knowledge of long-term outcomes thus allows patients to consider treatment side effects in the appropriate context.

The importance of long-term quality of life research is heightened by the changing demographics of prostate cancer in the era of prostate-specific antigen (PSA) testing. Men are now diagnosed with earlier-stage disease and at a younger age. Most patients diagnosed with prostate cancer today can expect to live 10 to 20 years after diagnosis. To limit discussion of the survivorship experience to the first 2 years ignores 80% to 90% of the patient's remaining lifetime. Clearly, we need to appreciate and understand the long-term complications of prostate cancer treatments.

The goal of this chapter is to provide an overview of long-term outcomes following RP. Long-term oncologic outcomes are discussed first, but the focus of the chapter is on long-term HRQOL outcomes, particularly those in the urinary and sexual domains. Comparison of RP with other active treatment modalities, such as external beam radiation therapy, brachytherapy, and androgen-deprivation therapy (ADT), is beyond the scope of this chapter and is not addressed.

LONG-TERM ONCOLOGIC OUTCOMES

Prostate cancer is a heterogeneous disease. Significant percentages of cases have a prolonged natural history. Many men diagnosed with the disease die with rather than of the cancer. As a result, an ongoing debate exists about whether surgery, and in fact any form of active treatment, actually improves overall survival when compared with expectant management (i.e., active surveillance or watchful waiting) among men with early-stage disease. Proponents of surgical treatment cited excellent cancer-free survival rates in several well-known large single-center series as proof that surgical intervention benefits the majority of patients who elect to undergo RP.[8-10] In contrast, opponents quoted large observational studies and meta-analyses that also demonstrated excellent 10-year disease-specific survival rates in men who elected conservative management initially.[11,12] Unfortunately, these supporting data cited by both sides of the argument were flawed by selection bias that limited their generalizability.

A randomized clinical trial from Sweden overcame many of the design flaws of the aforementioned studies and provided the first level I evidence that RP resulted in better overall, disease-specific, and metastasis-free survival rates than did conservative management. This study, initiated before widespread adaptation of PSA screening, randomized 695 men with clinically localized prostate cancer diagnosed between 1989 and 1999 to either surgery or watchful waiting. In 2002, Holmberg and colleagues[13] initially reported that at a median follow-up of 6.2 years, the group randomized to surgical treatment experienced improved metastasis-free and disease-specific survival compared with the group randomized to watchful waiting. However, no difference in overall survival was observed between the two groups.

In 2005, the same group reported updated data at a median follow-up of 8.2 years. These investigators noted that with longer follow-up, improved overall survival rates were observed for men who received surgical treatment, in addition to superior disease-specific and metastasis-free survival rates.[14] Furthermore, the investigators also noted that the magnitude of difference in survival between the two groups appeared to increase over time. It is likely that the relative survival advantage provided by surgical treatment will continue to increase with even longer-term follow-up. The natural history of early, localized disease as demonstrated by men who have undergone conservative management shows that the largest drop-off in cumulative progression-free, metastasis-free, and disease-specific survival rates occurs 15 to 20 years after diagnosis.[15]

Clearly, in selected patients, surgical treatment results in improved survival compared with observation. The real challenge, however, is proper patient selection. To realize a survival advantage, a patient has to have a natural life expectancy of ≥5 to 10 years at the time of surgery. Furthermore, for men with well-differentiated disease, aggressive treatments may not be indicated. Prior large observational studies of men who underwent conservative management indicated that men with well and moderately well differentiated disease have only a small to modest risk of dying of prostate cancer, even with 20-year follow-up.[16] In contrast, men with higher-grade disease have a much higher risk of dying of their disease, and this risk appears to increase or accumulate over time.[15,16] RP provides excellent control of localized prostate cancer, but active surveillance may be appropriate in selected patients (i.e., older patients with less aggressive disease).

Although overall survival and disease-specific survival are the primary clinical end points of interest, recurrence-free survival should also be considered.

Reported 10-year recurrence-free survival rates following RP range from 52% to 75%.[8-10,17] Among patients with recurrent disease, many have isolated biochemical recurrence. Currently, no uniformly accepted definition of a biochemical recurrence following RP exists,[18] and the most conservative definition is a rising PSA >0.4 ng/mL.

Data from Johns Hopkins University in Baltimore showed that at 10 years, 15% of men had an isolated detectable PSA as the only evidence of disease recurrence.[10] A unique characteristic of the Johns Hopkins cohort was the conservative approach used in treating patients with biochemical recurrence. Patients were discouraged from receiving secondary therapy until they become symptomatic, an approach that allowed for the natural history of untreated biochemical recurrence to be observed. The median time from biochemical recurrence to development of metastatic disease was approximately 8 years, and the time from metastatic disease to death was 5 years.[19] A subsequent follow-up study of the same cohort with expanded and updated data demonstrated that most patients who developed PSA recurrence could expect excellent long-term survival. In this cohort, the median time from biochemical recurrence to cancer-specific mortality was not reached even after 16 years of follow-up.[20] PSA doubling time following biochemical recurrence, time to recurrence from surgical treatment, and Gleason score were all found to be significant predictors of prostate cancer–specific mortality following PSA recurrence.[20]

Although many patients who develop biochemical disease recurrence experience an indolent course, even an isolated biochemical recurrence may negatively affect a patient from a quality of life perspective.[21] The reason underpinning the effect of PSA-documented disease recurrence on emotional and psychological well-being is intuitive, but the reason for the effects on other aspects of HRQOL (e.g., in sexual and urinary domains) is less obvious. The likely answer lies in the natural tendency of patients and providers to use secondary therapy on discovery of biochemical disease recurrence. In fact, investigators showed that men who underwent secondary therapy after RP experienced significant, progressive declines in the role-emotional and sexual function HRQOL domains, whereas patients not requiring secondary therapy did not.[22]

Secondary therapy after initial localized treatment is not uncommon. Three important studies examined this issue. The first used the population-based Surveillance, Epidemiology and End Results (SEER)–Medicare data set to assess secondary therapy use after RP.[23] Subjects in this cohort were diagnosed relatively early in the PSA era (1985-1991), and therefore the observed 5-year cumulative secondary therapy incidence of 34.5% did not likely reflect current trends.

Grossfeld and colleagues[24] examined secondary therapy use in the Cancer of the Prostate Strategic Urologic Research Endeavor (CaPSURE) dataset, a large, national, community-based observational registry of men with prostate cancer. In this study, 17% of all patients received secondary therapy within 3 years of treatment. Fifteen percent of patients who received surgical treatment and 24% of those who underwent radiation therapy had received secondary therapy within 3 years of diagnosis.

Finally, researchers from the Urologic Diseases of America Project recapitulated the SEER-Medicare analysis using a more contemporary cohort (1991-1997) with median follow-up of approximately 6 years.[25] These investigators found that 19% of surgical patients and 13% of patients who underwent external beam radiation therapy received secondary treatments. All these studies were published with relatively short follow-up. Therefore, we can expect rates of postoperative secondary therapy to be higher with longer follow-up.

In all these studies, the most common secondary therapy received was ADT.[23-25] Numerous reports have documented the relationship between ADT and certain deleterious clinical side effects, such as hot flashes,[26] gynecomastia,[27] and decreased bone density[28] resulting in increased risk of bone fractures.[29] The concurrent administration of bisphosphonates has been shown reverse the deleterious bony effects of ADT,[30,31] and bisphosphonate use may actually improve functional status and general HRQOL.[32,33] Yet, little is known regarding how widely these agents are used in general practice. In addition to bony complications, ADT may also result in endocrinologic abnormalities,[34] hyperlidemia,[34] and increased risk of fatal myocardial infarctions.[35]

Given that long-term ADT can cause significant additional morbidity, it is not surprising that this therapy negatively affects the HRQOL of patients. Although studies on this topic have often focused on men with metastatic disease, we can extrapolate the results to men who have undergone RP and have experienced an asymptomatic biochemical recurrence for which they are receiving secondary ADT.

Herr and associates[36] compared patients with metastatic disease who were receiving early hormonal therapy with patients who elected to defer treatment until they were symptomatic. These investigators found that the patients who received immediate ADT experienced more fatigue, loss of energy, emotional distress, and a lower overall quality of life. Basaria and associates[37] compared HRQOL outcomes in 20 men receiving ADT with 20 aged-matched controls. In addition to changes in body mass index and bone density, the ADT-treated group had worse sexual function and significant limitations in physical function and perception of physical health.

In a randomized trial of 65 men with nonlocalized prostate cancer who were randomized to receive either immediate or delayed hormonal therapy, Green and colleagues[38] demonstrated that men receiving early therapy reported worse sexual function and decreased role and social functioning. Potosky and colleagues[39] in the Prostate Cancer Outcomes Study (PCOS), studied HRQOL in men who received ADT for localized disease. Compared with men with localized disease who did not receive ADT, men in the ADT group reported worse sexual function and more physical discomfort, a finding once again illustrating the adverse effects of hormone ablation therapy on HRQOL.

In summary, long-term disease-specific survival following RP is excellent. Roughly one third of patients will experience biochemical disease recurrence in the first 10 to 15 postoperative years.[10] The clinical implications of biochemical recurrence vary among patients, but most patients who experience biochemical recurrence can expect prolonged survival. Additional research is sorely needed to refine risk stratification in these patients. When confronted with biochemical recurrence, providers need to consider carefully the purported advantages conferred by early initiation ADT together with its significant side effect profile. The risk of biochemical recurrence and the possibility of secondary therapy should be included in the discussion with patients when initial therapy is chosen. We recommend limiting the use of ADT to patients at greatest risk for prostate cancer–specific mortality.

MEASUREMENT OF HEALTH-RELATED QUALITY OF LIFE OUTCOMES FOLLOWING PROSTATECTOMY

RP is a well-tolerated procedure associated with very low perioperative mortality (<1%) and a rapid postoperative recovery; many men return to unrestricted activity within 30 days.[40] Detailed assessment of HRQOL after the immediate perioperative period provides important insights into how well patients adjust to life after surgical treatment. By convention, discussion of HRQOL typically separates evaluated domains into two distinct types: generic or general and disease-specific. Generic or general HRQOL assesses the overall well-being of the patient. Disease-specific HRQOL, conversely, focuses on specific areas of health affected by the particular disease process and its treatments. Individual components of general HRQOL vary according to the instruments used but can generally be separated into two broad categories: physical well-being and mental or psychological well-being. Ideally, HRQOL should be measured by validated instruments administered directly to patients, with pretreatment assessment, followed by periodic reassessments thereafter.

Many published studies have reported HRQOL outcomes following RP, but most have been single-institution studies and subject to significant selection bias. Furthermore, few studies to date have been able to follow patients longitudinally over the long term, likely secondary to the costs and personnel required. In this context, longitudinal data provided by large-scale, multi-institutional projects are especially valuable.

PCOS is a population-based longitudinal study of men with prostate cancer diagnosed from 1994 to 1995 in three states and three metropolitan areas who were participating in the SEER program. HRQOL and clinical outcomes were assessed at baseline and 6, 12, 24, and 60 months after diagnosis in the PCOS cohort. CaPSURE is longitudinal and observational registry of >13,000 men with biopsy-proven prostate cancer followed at 31 community-based and academic sites across the United States.[41] These two cohorts provide a comprehensive portrait of long-term clinical and quality of life outcomes in the United States. In Europe, the Rotterdam Study, performed within the context of the European Randomized Study of Screening for Prostate Cancer (ERSPC), provides an important non-American perspective on this topic.[42]

Generic Health-related Quality of Life

Available evidence from large cross-sectional studies and a well-known randomized trial indicate that long-term physical well-being and mental or psychological well-being are no different among men with prostate cancer who undergo active treatment or expectant management and age-matched men without prostate cancer. In a study comparing HRQOL among different treatment groups and age-matched controls, Litwin and colleagues[43] noted comparable scores in seven of the eight generic domains of the Short Form-36 (SF-36), a validated and commonly used questionnaire. Patients who underwent watchful waiting reported greater role limitations from emotional problems than did those who underwent active treatment, including RP.[43]

Investigators from the University of Michigan noted similar SF-36 scores on the mental composite summary and the physical composite summary at single time point among patients who underwent surgery, external beam radiation therapy, or brachytherapy a median of 2.6 years after treatment and age-matched controls who did not have prostate cancer.[44] The Scandinavian Prostate Cancer Group Study noted similar physical and psychological functioning between men randomized to RP and watchful waiting at a median of 4 years after diagnosis and randomization.[6]

Does generic HRQOL change over time for patients undergoing active treatment? Longitudinal studies documented the stability of long-term generic HRQOL outcomes. In the University of Michigan cohort, no changes in general HRQOL were noted for any of the active treatment groups after an additional 4-year follow-up.[45] Another study that used the CaPSURE database demonstrated that mental and physical component HRQOL summary scores for those patients who underwent various primary active treatments and watchful waiting changed little from baseline to 4 years after diagnosis.[46]

Investigators from the Rotterdam Study also noted similar stability in generic HRQOL from diagnosis to 5 years after treatment in patients who underwent RP and external radiation.[42]

Thus, published data have consistently indicated that men treated with RP can generally expect excellent general HRQOL outcomes over the long term. However, not all men experience the same outcomes after RP. Patients <65 years old and patients without comorbidities have a higher likelihood of recovering to baseline physical health postoperatively than do older patients and those with comorbidities.[47] Cancer recurrence, as alluded to earlier, also affects generic HRQOL significantly.

In a survey of men who previously underwent RP, lower scores were noted in both physical and mental health domains of the SF-36 among patients who experienced PSA-documented disease recurrence.[21] Tracking the general HRQOL of men who underwent surgical treatment but later required secondary treatment, Arredondo and colleagues[22] noted a large decline in the SF-36 role physical domain (together with smaller but also statistically significant declines in the other domains) beginning approximately 15 months before the onset of secondary treatment. These investigators hypothesized that knowledge of PSA recurrence may account for this otherwise perplexing observation.[22] In conclusion, for men who have undergone RP, generic HRQOL does not appear to be affected negatively by the surgical procedure itself, but generic HRQOL is intimately related to the oncologic outcome resulting from the operation.

Long-term Urinary Outcomes

Anastomotic Stricture

RP can cause postoperative urinary dysfunction through a variety of mechanisms. Stricture at the site of the vesicourethral anastomosis is a well-recognized long-term complication of RP, with a reported incidence ranging between 0.5% and 32%,[48-63] but generally ranging between 5% and 14%. Most cases occur within 1 year of the surgical procedure, and almost all develop within 2 years.[62] In a multi-institutional study by Kao and associates,[64] 21% of patients reported that they had experienced strictures that required dilatation or surgery. When surgical treatment is required, a transurethral incision of the bladder neck is often performed to open the stricture. Although this operation usually treats any obstructive voiding symptoms or urinary retention the patient may be experiencing, it unfortunately carries the risk of increased stress urinary incontinence.

Indirect evidence suggests that anastomotic stricture (AS) formation is at least in part determined by surgical technique. High-volume surgeons as a group seem to have lower rates compared with low-volume surgeons;

but significant variations exist among individual surgeons within each volume strata.[63]

Although no consensus exists on the technical factors that predispose a patient to AS formation, some factors have been repeatedly cited. Excessive tapering during construction of the bladder neck was found in two separate studies to be significantly associated with higher rates of AS formation.[54,60] Excessive bleeding has also been cited as a potential cause, possibly by compromising the quality of the anastomosis because of suboptimal visualization.[49,65] Multiple investigators proposed disruption of the urethral-bladder neck anastomosis as the key event that triggers formation and cited the observed association of postoperative urinary extravasation with higher rates of stricture as evidence.[49,65,66] Delayed bleeding resulting in a pelvic hematoma has also been associated with stricture formation. The authors of this study suggested that the hematoma may cause AS formation through a mechanism other than physical disruption because urinary extravasation on postoperative cystogram was not associated with higher likelihood of AS.[54]

Technical factors aside, patient-related factors may also play a contributory role. Preexisting cardiovascular disease, a history of smoking, a prior history of transurethral resection of the prostate, and a propensity to hypertrophic scar formation have all been cited as potential predisposing factors.[49,51,61] The aggressiveness of the underlying disease, such as indicated by Gleason score and tumor stage, appears to have no relation to AS formation.[51,56,61] Men who develop AS are at greater risk for long-term urinary incontinence.[51,57] In summary, the causes of AS are likely multifactorial. The surgeon should nevertheless always seek to ensure the integrity of the anastomosis and prevent formation of a pelvic hematoma. AS, when it occurs, should initially be addressed conservatively with urethral dilatation because incision increases the risk of long-term stress incontinence.

Urinary Function

Urinary function in the context of prostate cancer generally refers to urinary continence. Stress urinary incontinence is a well-known adverse outcome of RP. The cause of this untoward morbidity is commonly attributed to anatomic changes: a weakened pelvic floor or sphincteric insufficiency resulting from the operation. Reported rates of incontinence after RP vary widely.[60,67,68] This variation may in part result from differences in patient selection, as well as discrepancies in definition of incontinence and reporting methods. We focus our discussion on studies that assessed outcomes with patient-reported data from validated instruments.

Although little dispute exists that surgery can adversely affect urinary continence, the degree to which the surgical procedure itself contributes to urinary dysfunction has been difficult to measure or quantify because answering such a question requires comparison with age-matched controls or with age-matched men with localized prostate cancer who are undergoing expectant management. Data from the University of Michigan cross-sectional study indicated that, compared with age-matched controls without a diagnosis of prostate cancer, men who underwent RP reported lower summary scores in the urinary incontinence domain of a validated questionnaire.[44] This study, however, was limited by the lack of baseline data.

A randomized clinical trial comparing RP with watchful waiting found a higher prevalence of urinary incontinence in men after prostatectomy (49%) than in those managed with watchful waiting (21%).[6] However, not all men who reported incontinence reported severe dysfunction. Specifically, 18% of men randomized to RP reported moderate or severe leakage on follow-up, compared with 2% of men assigned to watchful waiting.[6] This study, although randomized, included only a single assessment of functional outcome with a mean follow-up of 4 years and, more importantly, and did not assess baseline function.

PCOS overcame of some of these common limitations because it provided an assessment of baseline urinary function in addition to long-term longitudinal follow-up. Data from this project indicated that at baseline 1% of men reported total incontinence, 3% reported frequent urinary incontinence, and 10% reported occasional incontinence. In comparison, 5 years postoperatively, 3% of men reported complete urinary incontinence, 11% had frequent incontinence, and 51% had occasional incontinence.[68]

Longitudinal studies indicate that stress urinary incontinence is worst immediately postoperatively, followed by a period of recovery. For example, in the PCOS study cited earlier, 4% of patients reported frequent leakage or no control at baseline; 25% reported this outcome at 6 months after diagnosis, 15.4% reported it at 1 year, 10.4% reported it at 2 years, and 13.9% reported it at 5 years.[68] An understanding of the typical recovery course is of great benefit for patient counseling. From experience, most urologists note that the greatest amount of recovery occurs during the first year. Indeed, such observations have been confirmed by large community-based longitudinal studies.[42,68,69] Long-term follow-up studies report either stability in function or further recovery after year 1. Little additional recovery occurs after year 2, however.[45,46,68] A review of studies that provide longitudinal information on long-term continence outcomes following RP is provided in **Figure 45-1.**

Technical factors aside, the predisposing factors for postoperative urinary incontinence remain undefined. Age, however, appears to play an important role. Rates of postoperative incontinence are significantly lower in younger men.[70] Younger men also have a higher likelihood of recovery to baseline urinary functioning.[47]

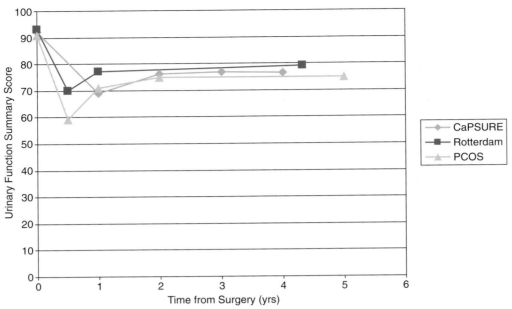

Figure 45-1 Long-term urinary function (incontinence) following radical prostatectomy. Results are from three large datasets.[42,46,68] (Health-related quality of life scores range from 0-100, with higher scores representing better quality of life.) CaPSURE, Cancer of the Prostate Strategic Urologic Research Endeavor; PCOS, Prostate Cancer Outcomes Study.

An often underrecognized effect of RP on urinary function is its positive effect on obstructive voiding symptoms. Unfortunately, most commonly used HRQOL instruments such the University of California Los Angeles Prostate Cancer Index (UCLA PCI) do not capture these outcomes specifically, so neither the PCOS nor the CaPSURE studies (both of which use versions of the UCLA PCI) can inform us of the effect of prostatectomy on obstructive voiding symptoms. However, other studies addressed this issue and documented the positive long-term effect of RP on these outcomes.

The Scandinavian Prostate Cancer Group Study administered the American Urological Association Symptom Score (AUASS) to patients randomized to either surgery or watchful waiting. Patients undergoing RP were significantly less likely to report a weak urinary stream (risk ratio [RR], 0.6; 95% confidence interval, 0.6 to 0.9) and showed a trend toward less involuntary stoppage during urination (RR, 0.6), incomplete emptying (RR, 0.7) and need to urinate every 2 hours (RR, 0.8). The surgical group was significantly less likely to report moderate to severe urinary symptoms (AUASS, 8-35) when compared with the watchful waiting group (35% versus 49%, $P < .05$).[6] Similar findings were reported by Schwartz and Lepor,[71] who noted that RP resulted in significant improvements in all but one question captured by AUASS in men with moderate to severe baseline symptoms. In summary, whereas RP results in increased urinary incontinence, it does appear to have an overall positive effect on lower urinary tract symptoms, likely from relief of previous obstructive symptoms caused by benign prostatic hyperplasia.

Urinary Bother

When one considers urinary function after treatment for localized prostate cancer, it can be difficult to compare therapies because of their differing effects on urinary function. As discussed earlier, surgical treatment can cause long-term stress urinary incontinence, but it can often alleviate lower urinary tract symptoms associated with other prostate conditions or possibly directly resulting from prostate cancer. Radiation therapy usually does not cause stress urinary incontinence, but it can cause irritative symptoms, an increased risk of urethral stricture disease, and urge incontinence.[44] To this end, a more global outcome for assessing the effect of treatment on urination in men with prostate cancer is urinary bother.

Urinary bother measures the distress one experiences from urinary symptoms. This parameter captures distress resulting from irritative and obstructive symptoms in addition to that caused by incontinence. In the Scandinavian Prostate Cancer Group Study, 27% of patients who received surgical treatment reported moderate or great distress from urinary symptoms, compared with 18% in the patients who underwent watchful waiting. Although still significantly different, the magnitude of difference between the surgical and watchful waiting groups was much less pronounced than were the differences noted in urinary incontinence.[6]

The relationship between urinary incontinence and bother should not be discounted, however. Data from PCOS indicated that at 1 year postoperatively, 16% of men who underwent surgery considered urinary incontinence as a moderate or great problem. At 5 years postoperatively, 13% of men remain bothered. The similar percentages of men reporting significant incontinence and significant bother from incontinence suggested a close correlation between the severity of incontinence and the severity of bother. Men who reported daily urinary leakage were much more likely to be bothered compared with those who reported occasional leakage. Similarly, patients who reported continuous incontinence or frequent dribbling were much more likely to be bothered than were those with occasional dribbling or total continence.[43]

Longitudinal data indicate that, similar to the case of urinary function, the greatest degree of recovery in urinary bother occurs in the first postoperative year. Some additional recovery can occur between years 1 and 2, with little change noted after year 2.[42,46,68]

Long-term Sexual Outcomes

Sexual Function

ED or impotence is also a well-recognized adverse sequela of RP. Analogous to the case of postoperative incontinence, reported rates of postoperative ED also vary widely, likely reflecting the culmination of differences in technique, patient selection, and ascertainment. The magnitude of dysfunction caused by the surgical procedure is difficult to assess, but it is likely very significant.

Compared with patients randomized to watchful waiting in the Scandinavian Prostate Cancer Group Study, much higher rates of ED were observed on follow-up among those randomized to RP; ED rates were 45% in the watchful waiting group and 80% in the surgical group.[6] Among 2227 Quebec men who reported be potent preoperatively, only 25% reported postoperative erections adequate for sexual intercourse with long-term follow-up of at least 17 months.[72] In the Rotterdam Study, whereas only 31% of the men undergoing RP reported total ED before treatment, 88% and 88% of this cohort reported total ED at 1 year and 5 years after the surgical procedure, respectively.[42] Reporting on the data from PCOS, Potosky and colleagues[73] observed that 5 years after RP, close to 80% of men were impotent. Abstracting cross-sectional data from men enrolled in a managed care setting, Litwin and colleagues[43] reported that men who underwent surgical treatment had significantly lower sexual function summary scores on the UCLA PCI than did patients who were treated conservatively or age-matched men without prostate cancer.

Longitudinal data indicate that the greatest degree of recovery occurs in the first year postoperatively,[68,74,75]

with continued recovery between year 1 and year 2.[46,68] Penson and associates[68] reported on long-term sexual outcomes following RP in the 1213 men in PCOS with localized disease who underwent this procedure. At baseline, 81% reported erections firm enough for sexual intercourse. This potency rate is probably higher than in the general population and represents either selection bias or recall bias, because healthier, younger men are more likely to undergo surgical treatment and may also overestimate their preoperative erectile function. However, at 6 months after diagnosis, only 9% of men reported erections adequate for intercourse. This number increased to 17% at 1 year, 22% at 2 years, and 28% at 5 years after diagnosis. **Figure 45-2** summarizes results of long-term sexual function outcomes after RP reported by CaPSURE and PCOS.

It was somewhat surprising to see an increase in potency between years 2 and 5 in PCOS. This result may be caused by a true late return of function, but it may also reflect the timing of that particular study. Specifically, year 2 of PCOS was in 1997, whereas year 5 was in 2000. During this interval, sildenafil was approved by the U.S. Food and Drug Administration, and this drug may have positively affected potency rates. These investigators reported a high penetration of sildenafil use in this cohort, with 43% reporting use. However, among those patients who used sildenafil, only 32% reported erections firm enough for sexual intercourse, and only 13% reported that the treatment "helped a lot."[68] It is therefore likely that sildenafil does aid in recovery of sexual function, but only in a minority of men.

The degree of erectile recovery is closely related to preoperative parameters, specifically age and baseline sexual function.[47] Performance of bilateral nerve sparing significantly increases the likelihood of postoperative recovery with regard to unilateral nerve sparing or lack of nerve sparing.[60,68,75] Among men with no baseline sexual dysfunction, postoperative potency rates of 68% were noted for those who underwent bilateral nerve sparing and were 47% for patients who had unilateral nerve sparing.[60]

However, the improved outcomes associated with bilateral nerve sparing were not noted in two earlier studies.[43,76] The reason for the discrepancy remains unclear, but it may be related to the small study size of the two earlier studies or the evolution or learning curve associated with the bilateral nerve-sparing technique. In the PCOS cohort, only 41% of patients who underwent bilateral nerve-sparing surgical treatment reported erections firm enough for sexual intercourse 5 years after diagnosis. However, when stratified by age, 71% of the men >55 years old, 56% of men age 55 to 59 years, and 46% of men age 60 to 64 years who underwent bilateral nerve-sparing surgical treatment reported erections firm enough for intercourse. In contrast, only 18% of the

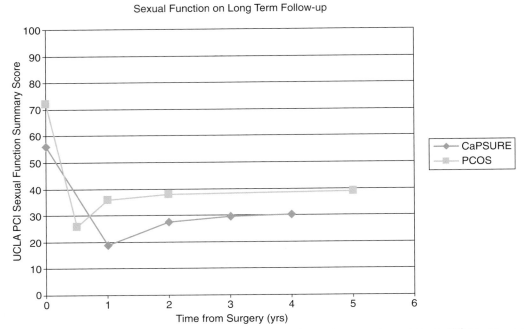

Figure 45-2 Long-term sexual function following radical prostatectomy. Results are from two large datasets.[46,68] (Health-related quality of life scores range from 0-100, with higher scores representing better quality of life.) CaPSURE, Cancer of the Prostate Strategic Urologic Research Endeavor; PCOS, Prostate Cancer Outcomes Study; UCLA PCI; University of California Los Angeles Prostate Cancer Index.

men >65 years old reported erections firm enough for sexual intercourse 5 years after diagnosis.

These findings underscore the close relationship between age and sexual outcomes in prostate cancer. A similar age effect on the effectiveness of sildenafil after bilateral nerve-sparing surgical therapy was seen in the PCOS cohort.[68] Age clearly affects the likelihood of response to treatments for impotence after RP.

Sexual Bother

ED is an important (and arguably the dominant) long-term sexual outcome to consider after RP. It is not the only outcome of interest in the sexual domain, however. All patients have dry ejaculation after RP. In addition to this ejaculatory dysfunction, many patients with prostate cancer experience a decrease in libido, often resulting from the use of adjuvant or secondary hormonal therapy. All these sexual dysfunctions can cause bother for patients, although the degree to which men are bothered by their sexual dysfunction is not as closely related to the degree of their dysfunction as in the urinary domain.[75]

Data from PCOS revealed that at all time points throughout postoperative follow-up, the percentage of patients who reported being moderately or severely bothered by sexual dysfunction was consistently lower than was the percentage of patients who reported impotence. Furthermore, the gap between the two parameters widened over time, a finding suggesting that patients learn to cope with ED. At 1-year follow-up, 61% of men in this cohort reported being moderately or

significantly bothered by their sexual dysfunction, whereas by 5-year follow-up, this percentage had decreased to 46%.[68]

CONCLUSION

RP provides excellent long-term control of clinically localized prostate cancer. Although it negatively affects sexual and urinary function, most men learn to cope with the side effects of surgery, report excellent general HRQOL postoperatively, and are satisfied with their choice. Data from PCOS indicated that 2 years following treatment, 83.1% of men who underwent RP were either mostly satisfied, pleased, or delighted with their treatment,[77] and 90.7% indicated that they would make the same treatment choice again.[77] The degree of satisfaction appears to be maintained with long-term follow-up. In another study examining confidence men had in the treatment they had received 4 to 8 years previously, 77% of men in this cohort who underwent RP were confident that RP provided good cancer control.[78]

In men with localized prostate cancer, the underlying tumor biology may be a primary determinant of cancer outcome, and baseline patient-related characteristics may contribute significantly to post-treatment functional recovery. However, surgical technique also clearly matters for patients who undergo RP. Future investigations should continue to consider measures, both surgical and nonsurgical, to decrease the likelihood of biochemical recurrence, bladder neck contracture, stress incontinence, and sexual dysfunction.

KEY POINTS

1. Although long-term survival following radical prostatectomy is excellent, a considerable number of patients receive secondary therapies. Because secondary therapies, particularly hormonal therapy, have significant negative effects on health-related quality of life, careful consideration must be given as to which patients who experience biochemical recurrence after surgery should be receiving secondary therapy and which should be observed.

2. Although the primary impact of prostatectomy on urinary-specific quality of life domains is stress incontinence, the impact of anastomotic stricture should not be underestimated and surgeons should use techniques to minimize anastomotic strictures.

3. Although urinary incontinence most commonly occurs immediately in the first 3 to 6 months after surgery, studies show that there is often improvement after the initial nadir. However, most patients experience a plateau in return of urinary function by 1 year and do not have additional improvement after this.

4. Erectile dysfunction also occurs most commonly in the first 6 months after surgery, but patients can expect to experience improvement up to 2 years after surgery. After this point, however, it is unlikely there will be any additional natural return of function.

5. Both urinary and sexual dysfunction can cause bother for patients.

REFERENCES

Please see www.expertconsult.com

COMPLICATIONS OF RECONSTRUCTIVE SURGERY

Chapter 46

COMPLICATIONS OF CONDUIT URINARY DIVERSION

Jamie A. Kanofsky MD
Resident in Urology, Department of Urology, New York University Langone Medical Center, New York, New York

Guilherme Godoy MD
Fellow in Urologic Oncology, Bruce and Cynthia Sherman Fellowship in Urologic Oncology, Division of Urologic Oncology, Department of Urology, New York University Langone Medical Center, New York, New York

Samir S. Taneja MD
The James M. Neissa and Janet Riha Neissa Associate Professor of Urologic Oncology; Director, Division of Urologic Oncology, Department of Urology and New York University Cancer Institute, New York University Langone Medical Center, New York, New York

In 1851 Sir John Simon of London attempted open ureterosigmoidostomy in dogs. He reported that the operation was "almost always fatal, and it was plain that the peritoneum would be exposed to much hazard."[1] Although urinary diversion can be dated back to 1851, it was not until 1950 that Bricker[2] reported on the use of ileum for "bladder substitution after pelvic evisceration." Although ileal conduit is the simplest and most popular of diversions, complications are frequent.[3] The surgeon should discuss the options as well as the advantages and disadvantages of conduit and continent diversion with the patient well before the operative day. Critical factors to consider include the patient's age and performance status, manual dexterity, body habitus, motivation and desires, expected long-term functional status, bowel condition, bowel length, prior surgery or radiation, and renal reserve.

Construction of the urinary conduit carries the potential for a great number of unforeseen events. Complications can be divided into two categories, early (≤30 days of the surgical procedure) and late. The rate of early complications has been reported to range from 20% to 56%,[4] and such complications include intestinal obstruction, fistula formation, leakage from the ileal-ileal or ureteroileal anastomosis, wound infection, wound dehiscence, loop necrosis, and pyelonephritis. The incidence of late complications reportedly ranges from 28% to 81%,[4] and these complications include intestinal obstruction, pyelonephritis, renal deterioration, ureteroileal strictures and obstruction, stomal stenosis, parastomal herniation, calculi, metabolic abnormalities, and the development of carcinomas.

In evaluating quality of life issues, Turner and colleagues[5] found that 88% to 95% of patients were satisfied overall, whereas 17% to 19% of patients were bothered by impaired body image. With regard to sexuality, 30% of patients reported decreased libido, whereas 20% felt less sexually attractive.[6] Hart and associates[7] reported frequent difficulty in caring for the collection device in 57% of their patients who had undergone ileal conduit procedures. More recently, Dutta and colleagues[8] found that 85% of patients undergoing ileal conduit would make the same choice of urinary diversion again.

PREOPERATIVE CONSIDERATIONS

Complications related to major intra-abdominal surgery include those secondary to anesthetic, cardiac, pulmonary, and thromboembolic events. Prevention of such complications is discussed elsewhere in the text. Preoperative patient selection and proper evaluation by a cardiologist or pulmonologist may be necessary.

In today's age of managed care, most patients undergo bowel preparation at home. Wolff and colleagues[9] found little difference between aggressive antibiotic preparation and a minimal preparation of enemas, dietary restrictions, and mechanical lavage. This finding suggests that aggressive preparation can be safely avoided, thus reducing the risk of perioperative colitis. We routinely use a 2-day bowel preparation in which patients are started on a clear liquid diet 2 days before the surgical procedure. Magnesium citrate is prescribed for 2 days preoperatively along with two saline laxative

(Fleet) enemas the night before the operation. Alternatively, 1 day postoperatively, patients are asked to drink ≤1 gallon of polyethylene glycol and electrolyte solution (GoLYTELY) until the stool is clear. The classic use of antibiotic preparation is discouraged.

Selection of Bowel Segment

Based on early experience, the use of jejunum in urinary reconstruction has fallen out of favor. Although functional results are not significantly different from those seen with ileum, tremendous metabolic complications arise secondary to water and salt loss. Golimbu and Morales[10,11] used both canine and clinical models to evaluate jejunal conduits. These investigators reported on a series of 30 jejunal conduits used in patients with a history of prior radiation, multiple pelvic surgical procedures, or poor condition of the distal ureters, ileum, or colon. They found that the major complications with use of jejunum were electrolyte abnormality and water loss. However, the resulting hypochloremic, hyponatremic, and hyperkalemic metabolic acidosis, generally accompanied by dehydration, usually responded to increased salt and fluid intake. Despite these findings, jejunum is rarely used today because of the great consequences of fluid shifts, and this method should be considered only when no other option is viable.

The use of ileum and colon has similar functional and metabolic outcomes. In general, those patients with metabolic abnormalities are found to have hyperchloremic metabolic acidosis secondary to luminal bicarbonate loss and active hydrogen ion or ammonium reabsorption.[12] Factors influencing the severity of the metabolic abnormality include the contact time of urine and bowel (conduit length), the drainage of the conduit (adequate stoma), and the underlying renal function of the patient. Other metabolic conditions include encephalopathy from elevated ammonia, weakness from hypocalcemia, neuromuscular dysfunction from hypomagnesemia, and osteomalacia or growth delay in children. Patients with osteomalacia specifically develop bony pain, muscle weakness, decreased phosphate, increased alkaline phosphatase, and excess osteoid in the bone. The physiologic features and management of the metabolic abnormalities accompanying ileal or colon diversion are discussed in detail in Chapter 5. In general, the acidosis is easily treated by one of a variety of medications.[13]

Although functional and metabolic results of colon and ileal conduits are generally similar, Mogg[14] initially described the technique of the colon conduit to be superior to that of ileal conduit because of the thicker musculature, infrequent peristalsis, and the need for less intraperitoneal manipulation. In his review of 48 cases, Mogg found complications in 16 patients: 4 patients developed stones, 2 developed ureteral stenosis, 8 had stomal ulceration, and 2 developed urinary peritonitis.

Morales and Golimbu[15] evaluated 46 colon conduits, of which 39 were constructed using transverse colon. In their study, these investigators observed a 15% mortality rate. Early complications included intestinal obstruction in 3 (6.5%), intestinal anastomotic leak in 2 (4%), and bilateral ureteral obstruction in 1 (2%). Late complications included acute pyelonephritis in 8 (17%) and stomal prolapse in 6 (13%), with 4 (8.5%) of these patients requiring surgical repair. In addition, 6 patients (13%) had ureterointestinal anastomotic obstruction. In evaluating the patients' upper urinary tracts, 32% of normal kidneys showed deterioration postoperatively, 37% of preoperatively abnormal renal units improved, and 25% of preoperatively abnormal renal units deteriorated. The investigators used an intraluminal nipple to achieve an antirefluxing mechanism, and no patient with antirefluxing ureters developed renal damage.

Complication rates with ileal conduit diversion have been similar to those observed with colon conduit. Jahnson and Pedersen[16] reported on 124 patients with ileal conduits followed for ≤20 years. Of the 124 patients, 48% had early complications including urine or intestinal anastomotic leaks, urinary or intestinal obstruction, wound dehiscence, infection, or cardiovascular misadventure. These investigators noted a 6% mortality rate in the perioperative period (4 deaths from septicemia, 2 from myocardial infarction, and 1 from uremia). Jahnson and Pedersen also found an association between preoperative radiation therapy and the rate of wound infection. In addition, the investigators reported a late complication rate of 52%, including 22% of patients with ureteroileal obstruction or stricture.

More recently, Singh and associates[17] evaluated 93 patients undergoing ileal conduit for benign disease and looked at the complication rate after an average of 5 years. These investigators reported a mortality rate of 2.1%. Complications again were related to the stoma (31%); 10% of patients developed a parastomal hernia and 4.3% developed stomal retraction and stenosis. These investigators reported complications of the ureteroileal anastomosis in 7% of the patients. In addition, 34% of patients had upper urinary tract dilatation, 10% with bilateral changes.

In general, it appears that ileal and colon conduit diversions have similar outcomes. Because of the technical ease of ileal diversion, this remains the segment of choice. The decision to use colon is usually based on the condition of the ileum or distal ureters as a result of pelvic irradiation or prior surgical intervention, the length of ureter resected at the time of operation, or the presence of inflammatory bowel disease in the terminal ileum. When the surgeon performs en bloc resection of the colon or rectum, a sigmoid colon conduit may eliminate the need for two bowel anastomoses, or any anastomosis if a colostomy is to be constructed. Finally, if an upper abdominal stoma is required, the transverse colon can be used to reduce technical difficulty associated with bowel mobility. In patients undergoing colon conduit, barium enema should be adequate to rule out the possibility of colonic malignant disease or other abnormalities. In patients undergoing ileal diversion, barium enema is not necessary, but it may be helpful in ruling out potentially obstructive distal abnormalities.

Selecting the Length of Bowel

As mentioned previously, the length of bowel used can be a critical determinant of the severity of metabolic abnormality associated with the pouch. A length of 10 to 12 cm serves as a general guideline. In obese patients with a large amount of abdominal wall to traverse, a longer segment should be isolated. Lengthening and mobilizing the distal conduit can be achieved either through aggressive division of the mesentery (with care taken to preserve the proximal ileocolic branch) or, as a preferred method, resection of a segment of bowel immediately distal to the conduit (**Fig. 46-1**). Another option in the management of a short distal mesentery is the use of a Turnbull loop stoma. In this technique, a "knuckle" of the distal conduit is brought through the fascial opening. The antimesenteric border is incised,

thus allowing circumferential maturation without any tethering from the distal mesentery.

The surgeon should pay careful attention to the anatomic lie of the conduit after maturation of the stoma. The intra-abdominal portion of the conduit should be relatively straight, with no kinking or twisting to impair luminal drainage. A red rubber catheter left in the length of the conduit can allow the conduit to heal in a straight fashion.

In individuals with a thin abdominal wall or small body habitus, as short a segment as possible should be used. Preserving good length of the ureters can allow the ureterointestinal anastomoses to "rise" along the lateral abdominal wall and can thereby minimize the intra-abdominal length of the conduit. Tension on the ureteroileal anastomoses can be avoided by fixation of the proximal segment of the conduit to the sacral promontory or by a lateral retroperitoneal incision.

In patients with impaired renal reserve, as noted by elevated serum creatinine concentration or creatinine clearance <50 mL/minute, the surgeon should make every effort to limit the conduit to as short a length as required by the abdominal wall thickness. Although cutaneous ureterostomy is an option in patients with renal insufficiency, it is generally preferable to interpose at least a short segment of bowel to avoid the stomal

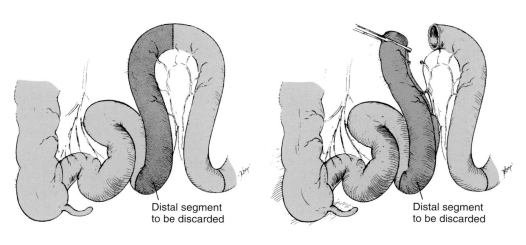

Distal segment to be discarded

Distal segment to be discarded

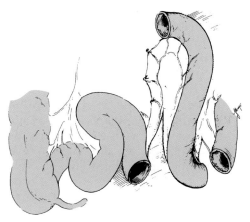

Figure 46-1 Daniel's technique of discarding the distal half of the loop in creating an isolated segment. *(From Ehrlich R. Ileal conduit. J Urol. 1973;109:994.)*

retraction and stenosis seen in cutaneous ureterostomy. Even with significant renal impairment, the patient should have only limited worsening of renal function if the conduit is constructed with the intention of keeping the transit time of urine as short as possible.

Selecting the Site of Stoma

Selection of the stoma site is probably the most important preparatory step for conduit surgery. Ultimately, the stoma predicts the long-term success or failure of the operation. The position of the stoma should be marked preoperatively to ensure adequate fit of the stomal appliance and ease of stomal care on the part of the patient.

Marking of the stomal site should be done with the patient lying down, sitting, and standing, with an attempt to find a flat area on the abdomen. A permanent marking pen or subcutaneous puncture with a needle can be used to mark the planned stoma site preoperatively. Care must be taken to avoid the belt line, abnormal skin creases, and deformities such as scars, bony prominences, valleys, or ridges. Patients should be given the option of wearing a simulation stoma preoperatively, and the surgeon should evaluate the patient carefully to ensure adequate manual dexterity. The stoma should be within the rectus muscle, generally below the umbilicus, on top of the infraumbilical fat mound, and it should be well within the patient's visual field (**Fig. 46-2**).[18]

On rare occasions, a supraumbilical site should be chosen to avoid a protuberant abdomen. This allows the patient to see the stoma clearly and to change the stoma

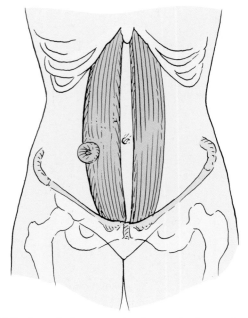

Figure 46-2 Stomal placement. Ample margins from adjacent protuberances and deformities are imperative.

appliance. If such a site is chosen, the conduit is generally brought completely into a retroperitoneal location behind the right colon. The mesentery of the isolated segment can be placed in a retrocolic position or brought through the right mesocolon to place the conduit in the right paracolic gutter. Alternatively, a transverse colon conduit can be used.

Before entering the operating room, the patient must be adequately prepared for the future conduit and its care. The advent of stomal therapists in the 1950s greatly reduced the incidence of stomal complications and permanent defects.[4] When evaluating whether preoperative teaching and marking had any benefit, Bass and colleagues[19] found that those patients who received preoperative teaching had fewer total stomal complications (32.5%) compared with patients who had no preoperative teaching (43.5%). Thus, we strongly encourage that all preoperative teaching and stomal marking be performed by an enterostomal therapist.

COMPLICATIONS

Conduit

Necrosis of the conduit is a rare but disastrous complication. It invariably results from acute ischemia of the conduit, usually secondary to mesenteric injury, twisting, or an inadequately identified blood supply. In the early postoperative period, it is not unusual for the stoma to appear dusky. This discoloration is often caused by venous congestion arising from compression of the segment by local edema above the fascial opening. Within a few days, this phenomenon usually resolves. Drainage is maintained by use of a red rubber catheter inserted beyond the level of the fascia and brought out through the stoma. The red rubber catheter can usually be removed 48 hours postoperatively.

When selecting a bowel segment, the surgeon should identify a clear arterial supply that will be preserved following mesenteric division. This should be separate from the ileocecal artery to maintain blood supply to the bowel anastomosis. The mesentery should be handled carefully, and while the conduit is positioned, no twist or stretch of the mesentery should be present. In closing the mesenteric defect above the conduit, the surgeon should avoid laceration or incorporation of the arteries within the conduit mesentery.

Acute necrosis of the conduit usually manifests with a dusky, oozing stoma and may be accompanied by metabolic acidosis, hyperphosphatemia, or early shock. Alternatively, the patient may not be ill, but the dusky appearance of the stoma may persist for several days postoperatively. In cases of severe acidosis despite a normal-appearing stoma, one should consider a subfascial segmental infarct of the conduit, which can occur on rare occasion. The usual course of action consists of early exploration with resection and replacement of the conduit or diseased segment. Chronic ischemia of the conduit can occur and usually results in a rigid, poorly compliant conduit or stomal stenosis. Chronic ischemia may manifest with upper urinary tract dilatation resulting from poor drainage of the conduit. In this case, surgical intervention with repeat diversion is usually indicated.

Calculi

The incidence of calculi formation in patients with ileal conduits is 5% to 20%.[20-22] These calculi are usually renal in origin, but stones can also form within the conduit itself. The proposed mechanism of stone formation involves a combination of urinary stasis, contact with bowel, and infection. Delayed or incomplete emptying of the conduit allows for longer contact times between urine and the intestinal mucus. This situation results in enhanced and increased chloride and bicarbonate exchange, with subsequent metabolic acidosis. Hypercalciuria develops as the bone buffering mechanisms try to correct the acidosis. When hypercalciuria occurs in the presence of alkaline urine, stone formation is favored. Additionally, infections with urea-splitting organisms release ammonia and may facilitate chloride-bicarbonate exchange and further stone formation.[22,23] Prevention of calculus formation is usually directed at serum alkalinization with bicarbonate (Sholh's solution) or potassium citrate (Urocit-K), prevention of residual urine (catheterization as needed), prevention of infection with urea-splitting organisms (antibiotics), urinary acidification agents (vitamin C), and thiazides to enhance proximal tubular calcium reabsorption.

In addition, stones have been reported to form from retained staples or nonabsorbable sutures. Thus, the surgeon should make an effort to exclude or excise all staples from the bowel lumen during construction of the conduit. The distal staple line of the resected bowel should be completely excised, and the proximal staple line can be excised or excluded from the lumen using Parker-Kerr sutures (a running horizontal mattress stitch) of 2-0 polyglactin 910 (Vicryl). On rare occasions, a staple may erode into the conduit lumen and may cause stone formation.

Upper tract calculi may be treated with extracorporeal shock wave lithotripsy, percutaneous nephrolithotomy, or retrograde techniques, if access is possible. Extracorporeal shock wave lithotripsy may be difficult to perform because these stones are usually infectious, large, and difficult to clear. Cohen and Streem[24] however, reported a 95% success rate with extracorporeal shock wave lithotripsy (occasionally, second therapy was needed). Percutaneous nephrolithotomy has a success rate of 100% and is the method of choice for large renal calculi.

Calculi that develop within the conduit may be treated with endoscopic techniques employing laser lithotripsy. Access can be obtained with a flexible cys-toscope or, in larger conduits, with pediatric endoscopes. The causal factors in conduit stone formation must also be investigated, and any staples should be removed endoscopically if they are identified.

Malignant Disease

Carcinoma within the conduit has been reported since the development of urinary diversions. The first case of ureterosigmoidostomy-associated cancer was reported in 1929, and the incidence of cancer following ureterosigmoidostomy has been reported to range between 6% and 29%.[25] In fact, the risk of developing adenocarcinoma after ureterosigmoidostomy is 400 to 7000 times that of the general population. Husmann and Spence[25] found that 26 years after diversion, 70% of patients had developed adenocarcinoma. However, the rate of carcinoma developing within colon and ileal conduits is <1%.[26] Since 1950, four cases of adenocarcinoma developing in an ileal conduit have been reported.[27,28] The rarity of these cases is likely, in part, the result of the infrequency of primary small bowel tumors.

The origin of adenocarcinoma in bowel conduits is unclear. Gittes[29] found that carcinogenesis of ureterosigmoidostomy depended on the presence of urine, feces, urothelium, and a healing anastomotic suture line. He assumed that the use of bowel segments interposed into the urinary tract would not lead to tumor formation in the absence of feces. This theory has since been challenged. Other hypotheses include chromosomal abnormalities, N-nitrosamines, oxygen free radicals, infection, and chronic inflammation. Malignant transformation in these cases may also be an early event.[26]

Three cases of carcinoid tumor arising in an ileal conduit have also been described in the literature.[30-32] Transitional cell carcinoma developing in the conduit has been reported as early as 9 months postoperatively. Mulholland and coworkers[33] reported finding grade 2 transitional cell carcinoma arising from the bowel mucosa at a site completely separate from the ureter. In any patient undergoing creation of an ileal conduit, the upper urinary tracts must also be followed as well because of the 2% to 9% rate of upper urinary tract transitional cell carcinoma following cystectomy.[34]

Bowel

Bowel complications occurring after conduit surgery are generally related to the ileal resection and anastomosis. When constructing an ileal conduit, the surgeon selects a segment approximately 10 to 15 cm proximal to the ileocecal valve. Despite preservation of the terminal ileum, malabsorptive syndromes can arise, particularly if long segments of bowel are resected. Diarrhea in the early postoperative period is often the result of prolonged antibiotic use and bile salt malabsorption. This complication generally improves spontaneously in ≤4 to 6 weeks. The patient should be encouraged to drink fluids liberally and should avoid the use of motility-suppressing agents. A culture for *Clostridium difficile* should be obtained. In rare cases of severe or persistent diarrhea, oral cholestyramine can be used to form bulk and decrease transit time.

Vitamin B_{12} deficiency can arise from poor absorption following ileal resection. Levels should be monitored periodically starting 6 to 12 months postoperatively. Individuals developing anemia at prolonged intervals following surgery should be evaluated for vitamin B_{12} deficiency.

Anastomotic leak, bowel obstruction, and ileus are common problems following ileal diversion and are discussed in detail in Chapter 22. Early recognition is paramount in avoiding the necessity for bowel resecting or ileostomy.

Stoma

Construction of the stoma is perhaps the most critical aspect of conduit surgery because the stoma is the most likely site of complication. In addition, the stoma greatly influences the patient's quality of life. Preparation of the stoma site, transposition of the bowel segment through the abdominal wall, and maturation of the stoma should be carried out with great caution and meticulous attention to detail. In patients in whom a conduit will undoubtedly be constructed, preparation of the stoma site can be carried out before the midline incision is made. This technique allows the surgeon to align the abdominal musculature in anatomic position with the skin opening, to use the preoperatively marked stoma site without confusion, and to be fresh and alert at the time of site preparation.

Regardless of surgical technique, the essential points of stomal preparation include an abdominal wall opening that can accommodate the conduit without ischemia but is snug enough to provide support, passage through the rectus sheath to avoid herniation next to the stomal opening, and adequate protuberance and maturation of the stoma to ensure good fit of the appliance (**Fig. 46-3**). Although a comprehensive discussion of technique is beyond the scope of this chapter, those points critical in preventing complication are discussed.

Early complications relevant to the stoma are generally related to poor vascularity, as discussed earlier. Delayed or late complications of the stoma are common, and these include parastomal hernia and prolapse, stomal retraction, local dermatitis, and stomal stenosis. As a result, stomal complication is the most common cause of reoperation after conduit surgery. In Bricker's[35,36] evaluation of the complications of 543 ileal

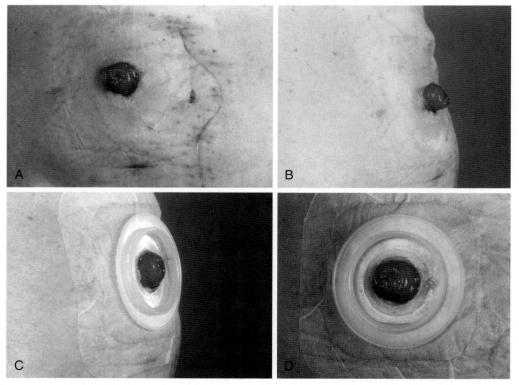

Figure 46-3   **A,** Properly constructed ileal stoma placed directly superolateral to the umbilicus at the edge of the rectus sheath. **B,** The stoma protrudes approximately 1.5 cm from the abdominal wall. No indentation or lateral crease is present in the stoma. **C,** On placement of the appliance, the stoma protrudes into the bag, which provides good drainage and thereby protects the local skin. **D,** Proper fit of the stomal appliance. Less than 1/8 inch of skin is exposed circumferentially. The stoma protrudes into the appliance.

conduits, stomal complications were responsible for reoperation 26% of the time. Cass and associates[37] found that 57% of all reoperations were for stomal problems. Klein and colleagues[38] from the Cleveland (Ohio) Clinic reported their results and noted a 5% overall stomal revision rate. These investigators also found no difference in the complication rates when they compared end stomas with loop stomas.

Cheung[39] analyzed 322 stomas, of which 123 were ileal conduits. The overall complication rate from the stoma alone was >60%, and transverse colostomy had the highest rate of complications at 73%. The overall rate of stomal complications with ileal conduits was 62.6%. With an average 6 years of follow-up, Cheung identified stenosis in 7.3%, parastomal hernia in 27.6%, prolapse in 4.1%, and excoriation in 20.3% of his patients. The average time to stenosis was 128 months, whereas the average time to herniation was 22 months; 23% of all stomal hernias occurred within the first year.[39]

Parastomal Hernia or Prolapse

The reported incidence of parastomal hernia ranges from 4.5% to 6.5% for ileal conduit surgery. Potential contributing factors include obesity, wound infection, chronic cough, steroids, malnutrition, and abdominal distention. Most patients are asymptomatic, but 10% to 20% may have symptoms, including pain, poor-fitting appliances, poor cosmesis, and potential bowel strangulation.[40]

Parastomal hernias arise when a gap exists between the intestinal segment forming the stoma and the surrounding tissue.[41] The fascial defect may be created by tangential forces working on the circumference of the opening that can stretch the fascia.[40] Most commonly, incorrect placement of the stomal opening lateral to the rectus fascia results in gradual opening of the surrounding fascia. Sjodahl and colleagues[41] evaluated 130 patients with intestinal stomas and found the incidence of parastomal hernia to be 2.8% in patients with stomas brought through the rectus muscles compared with 21.6% in patients whose stomas were placed lateral to the rectus muscles. In the operating room, the surgeon should note that the entire fascial opening is within the body of the rectus sheath. Creating the fascial opening before making the midline incision can assure the surgeon that all fascial layers are aligned.

Repair of parastomal hernias can be difficult and should be attempted only if the patient is symptomatic. Conservative options include support belts or appliances to keep the hernia reduced, appliances that eliminate the need to repair the hernia operatively. Surgical options can become complicated and include relocating the stoma to a new site or repairing the fascial defect, either primarily or with the use of synthetic material. The surgeon should realize, however, that untreated parastomal hernias usually worsen, and earlier repair may be technically easier.

Rubin and associates[42] reported on 94 parastomal hernias repaired surgically. These investigators found a 76% incidence of recurrence after fascial repair compared with a 33% incidence after stomal relocation. For patients with recurrent parastomal hernias, fascial repair with synthetic material had the lowest recurrence rates (33%). Overall, 72% of patients developed additional abdominal hernias at the old stoma site, recurrent parastomal hernias, or herniation at the laparotomy incision site. The morbidity associated with surgery was also high; 63% of patients had at least one postoperative complication. These investigators concluded that parastomal hernia is rarely life-threatening, and repair should be avoided if possible because of poor success rates and high rates of morbidity and recurrence.

In another approach to repairing parastomal hernias, reported by Kaufman,[43] the stoma is relocated without a laparotomy incision. The stoma is dissected off the skin and is dissected to its base. Any adhesions are freed. A cruciate incision is made on the patient's contralateral side, and the stoma is delivered to this new site with the use of long sponge forceps and dissection from the herniated side. Such an approach is somewhat blind, and the surgeon should exercise caution in selecting patients with minimal intra-abdominal reaction or adhesion.

A technique described by Leslie[44,45] uses a suprafascial synthetic wrap to close the hernia defect. A skin flap is elevated from medially to laterally, to expose the underlying fascia for 10 to 15 cm circumferentially around the stoma. The stomal skin is left intact. The fascial defect is exposed, the peritoneum is opened, and the conduit and fascial edge are freed from all intraperitoneal contents. The fascial defect is then closed directly or with interposed absorbable mesh. Once the fascia is closed, nonabsorbable mesh is wrapped around the bowel segment and is tacked only to the fascia, approximately 8 to 10 cm away from the conduit. Slight overlap of the edges allows the protuberance of the stoma to be retained by gathering up the bowel centrally. The synthetic material used should be chosen carefully and should not be tacked to the bowel because it has the potential to erode into the conduit over time. Gore-Tex appears to be the material of choice.

Stomal Stenosis

Stomal stenosis has a reported incidence of 2.8% to 19%. Frazier and associates[46] reported on 675 cases performed at Duke University (in North Carolina) in the 1970s and 1980s. These investigators found a 2.8% incidence of stomal stenosis. Factors contributing to the development of stomal stenosis include fascial or muscular constriction, ischemia of the stoma, shape and retraction of the stoma, alkaline urine, hyperkeratosis, and local skin changes.

The most common pathophysiologic features of stomal stenosis usually start soon after the surgical procedure. Poorly fitting appliances, often the result of stomal retraction, can cause skin ulceration and irritation that can eventually lead to hyperkeratosis of the local skin. This complication ultimately results in stenosis (**Fig. 46-4**). Alternatively, stenosis can occur at the level of the fascia in response to an inadequate opening, which over time may result in kinking of the conduit. Abdominal wall muscular spasm in patients with neurologic disease can cause a similar situation. This complication usually responds to antispasmodic medications. When stomal stenosis exists, it can start a cascade of events leading to obstruction, dilatation with reflux, urinary tract infection, sepsis, and renal damage.

When fashioning the stoma, the surgeon must assess for adequate blood supply and adequate mucosal nipple above the skin to guarantee proper fitting of the appliance. The matured stoma should extend 1 to 2 inches above the skin edge for proper appliance fit. If the stoma is too long, this can impair drainage within the bag. Appliances should be no more than 1/16 to 1/8 inch larger than the stoma to minimize urine contact with the skin. Proper maturation of the stoma and selection of the appropriate site for stomal placement are the most critical factors in determining the success of the stoma.

The presence of a bulky mesentery can prevent proper maturation of the stoma. Placement of maturing sutures in positions directly next to the mesenteric edge can allow the distal bowel edge to fold over the mesentery. Ligation of ≤5 cm of the distal mesentery to prevent bowing of the stoma has been advocated by some investigators, but it does have the increased risk of stomal devascularization and associated problems and is not usually necessary. *Defatting,* or removal of excess lateral fat from the edge of the mesentery, can be performed by gently teasing away the fat along the bowel wall.

Care must be taken to avoid laceration of the mesenteric vessels that lie centrally within the mesenteric fat. The tendency to tuck excess mesentery beneath the skin edge should be avoided because it creates a large mound next to the stoma and causes difficulty with the fit of the appliance.

Anchoring the conduit to the rectus fascia to prevent stomal retraction is controversial. In general, if no tension is present on the intra-abdominal portion of the conduit, no retraction should occur. Obesity and postoperative distention can obviously affect this situation. We place two to three sutures from the edge of the anterior rectus fascia opening to the seromuscular layer of the conduit as it passes through the fascia. Additional sutures can also be placed in the posterior rectus sheath. These stitches should not be under traction or they may risk bowel wall ischemia.

We reported a modified technique of stomal maturation before abdominal wall transposition of the conduit or stoma.[47] We observed that this modification allows more symmetric eversion, tension-free anastomosis, and less likelihood of stomal retraction. The technique is begun by defatting the distal 4 cm of mesentery to allow circumferential eversion of the stoma using four seromuscular sutures (**Figs. 46-5** and **46-6**). The bowel intussusception is locked in place with through-and-through sutures from the lumen to the external stomal surface, and the mesentery is then tucked under the everted bowel edge to ensure that no retraction of the stoma occurs along the axis of the mesentery (**Fig. 46-7**).

Hyperkeratosis is characterized by thickening and hardening of the skin and proliferation of the epithelium. This complication can be treated with catheter drainage to avoid urinary contact with the skin, in combination with the application of a heat lamp 12 inches

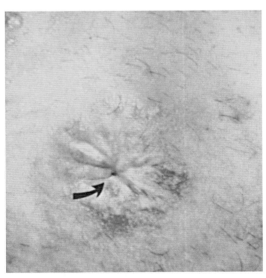

Figure 46-4 Terminal stomal stenosis (*arrow*).

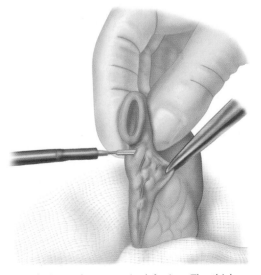

Figure 46-5 Technique of mesenteric defatting. The thickness of the mesentery is reduced by excising excess fat, but the central vascular arcades are preserved.

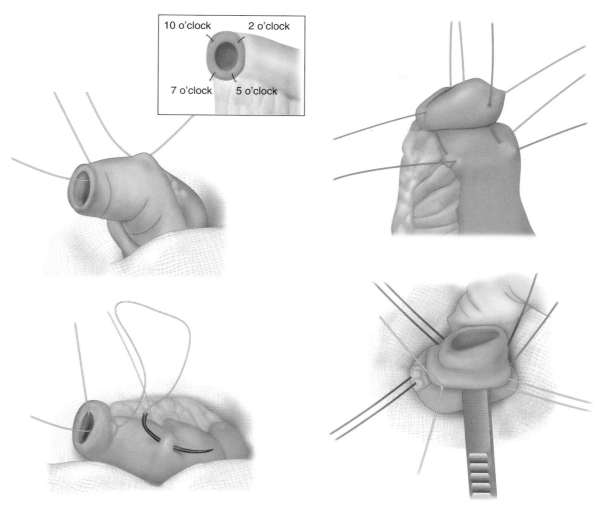

Figure 46-6 Creation of stoma by mucosal eversion and distal bowel intussusception. Sutures are place from the cut bowel edge to the seromuscular layer approximately 4 cm proximal to the edge. If one considers the mesenteric position at 6 o'clock, the everting sutures are placed at 2, 5, 7, and 10 o'clock to maximize eversion to the mesenteric edge and to avoid the necessity for suture placement in the mesentery.

from the skin twice daily. External beam radiation therapy has also been reported to be beneficial in severe cases of hyperkeratosis.[48] Bacterial and fungal infections can initiate stomal deterioration. Continued exposure to alkaline urine can cause stomal encrustation, stomal epithelialization, and eventual stomal stenosis.[18,49] Treatment options include 500 mg of vitamin C four times a day or 0.25% acetic acid washes twice a day. Early local skin care accompanied by urinary acidification is essential to prevent progression of the problem and can often reverse it. If combined with significant stomal retraction, early revision with excision of the hyperkeratotic skin may be advisable.

The techniques for surgical revision of a stenotic or retracted stoma are many. In general, repair can be performed locally through a circumscribing incision at the stoma site (**Fig. 46-8**). The conduit wall is identified in the subdermal tissues, and the conduit is then freed completely to the level of the fascia. Great care should be exercised in avoiding the mesentery of the bowel.

The fascia is freed from the conduit wall, and the bowel is then mobilized intraperitoneally. Extensive conduit length can be achieved in this fashion. The distal stenotic segment of the stoma is then excised along with hyperkeratotic local skin, and rematuration of the stoma is performed (see Fig. 46-8). To facilitate intraperitoneal mobilization, the fascial opening can be extended, but careful closure must then be performed to avoid subsequent herniation.

Alternative techniques of dealing with an incomplete stenosis involve incision of the stenotic ring with either direct reanastomosis to the skin or rotation of a secondary skin flap into the defect (**Figs. 46-9** and **46-10**). The shortcoming of these techniques is that they do not address the problem of stomal retraction. On rare occasions, full laparotomy is required to achieve adequate conduit length for stomal maturation. A preoperative loopogram can provide critical information in determining the intraperitoneal availability of redundant conduit.

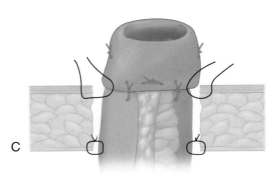

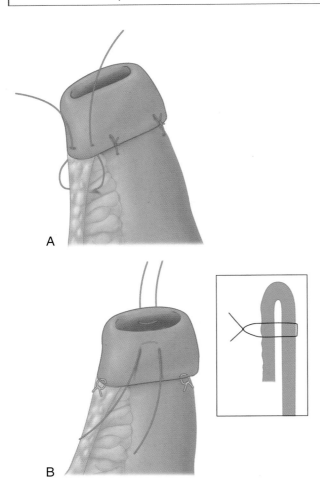

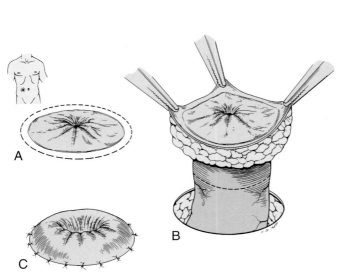

Figure 46-7 **A** and **B**, Eversion over the mesentery is performed by suturing to the mesenteric edge with a U-stitch (*inset* in **B**). The stomal intussusception is held in place with through-and-through sutures from the lumen to the exterior surface. **C**, On abdominal wall translocation, the stomal edge is anastomosed to the skin and fascial sutures are place approximately 3 cm proximal to the everted stomal edge.

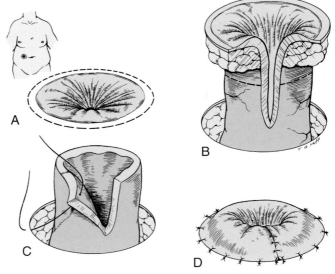

Figure 46-8 Reconstruction with distal amputation. **A**, Circumferential incision is made around the stoma. **B**, Mobilization of stoma and distal conduit and amputation of distal segment are performed. **C**, New stoma is fashioned.

Figure 46-9 Reconstruction of a retracted stoma. **A**, Skin incision is made. **B**, The distal segment is amputated. **C**, Spatulation for a split-cuff stoma is made. **D**, Final stoma.

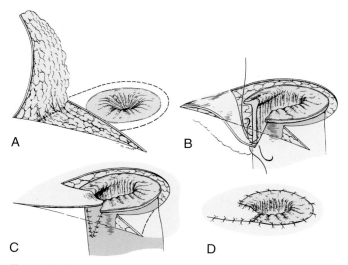

Figure 46-10   Skin inlay reconstruction. **A,** The old stoma and skin flap are mobilized. **B,** The stoma is spatulated. **C,** The skin flap is inlaid. **D,** The skin edges are reapproximated.

Ureterointestinal Anastomosis

During mobilization of the ureter, preservation of the periureteral adventitia is essential to ensure adequate blood supply to the ureter. Before creating the anastomosis, the surgeon must ascertain adequate length from each ureter. In addition, when placing the stoma on the right, the surgeon must pass the left ureter beneath the sigmoid mesocolon with gentle angulation and must be careful to avoid kinking the ureter. These are the basic tenets of constructing the ureterointestinal anastomosis.

Numerous anastomotic techniques exist, and to a large extent, the segment of bowel used, the dilatation of the ureters, and the preference of the surgeon are the deciding factors. Bricker's[2] initial description of the ureteroileal anastomosis employed an end-to-side (ureter-to-bowel) approach with wide spatulation of the ureter. Wallace[50] subsequently reported an end-to-end anastomosis in which the two ureters were converted to a single lumen and were anastomosed to the proximal end of the bowel. Creation of an adequately sized well-vascularized lumen, mucosa-to-mucosa apposition with watertight closure, and sufficient mobilization of the ureter to reduce tension on the anastomosis are necessary. Ultimately, the comfort of the surgeon with an individual technique is likely the greatest predictor of success.

Various techniques for ureterocolonic anastomosis have been described. The technique most commonly used for conduit diversion, however, is antirefluxing tenial anastomosis. As discussed later, the necessity for antirefluxing anastomoses remains to be validated in this setting. The use of a stent in the ureteroileal anastomosis is a subject of great controversy. We routinely use a stent for the following reasons:

1. It ensures the patency of the anastomosis, specifically in the immediate postoperative period when edema is present at the site.
2. It provides access to the kidney and collecting system if retrograde studies are needed.
3. It enhances stomal drainage when long, externally draining stents are used.

Numerous urinary diversion stents can be used, including a single-J stent or a double-J stent with external extension. We prefer the double-J variety because it ensures some urine in the conduit and thus prevents a completely dry anastomosis in the early postoperative period.

Regan and Barrett[51] compared the incidence of stricture and leakage in stented and unstented anastomoses. Those patients who were stented had lower rates of stricture and leakage compared with patients who did not have stents. This was a small study with relatively short follow-up, and the influence of technical factors and selection bias cannot be excluded. Individuals with stents in place may be at a high risk of ascending pyelonephritis and urosepsis in the postoperative period. For this reason, these patients should be administered antibiotic prophylaxis for the duration of stenting, and the stents should generally be removed by postoperative day 5 to 7. Although it is not clear that ureteral stenting is required for ureterointestinal anastomoses, it appears that the potential benefits far outweigh the potential harm.

Ureteroileal Anastomotic Leak

Ureteroileal anastomotic leak (extravasation) is reported to occur in 1.9% to 5.5% of conduits but alarmingly has an associated mortality rate of ≤48%.[52] The factors contributing to the occurrence of leakage include poor surgical technique, prior radiation therapy, recurrent cancer, stomal edema or obstruction, extraluminal hematoma or seroma, and pelvic abscess. During the normal postoperative course, a small amount of leakage from the anastomosis may occur, but this often resolves without any sequelae. Intraoperatively, the surgeon should make every effort to create a watertight anastomosis prevent a perianastomotic urinoma, which may become secondarily infected.

We routinely use a Bricker-type anastomosis in our conduit diversion procedures. During spatulation of the ureter, three directly juxtaposed 4-0 chromic anchoring sutures are placed at the apex, or corner, of the spatulation. Generally, this is the most dependent portion of the anastomosis and thus is the most likely to leak. Interrupted sutures are then placed circumferentially 3 to 4 mm apart. An indwelling stent is always used.

Significant urinary leakage should be suspected in the presence of increased drain output with decreased output from the stoma. Other signs and symptoms may include proximal hydronephrosis or flank pain if no stent is used, sepsis, ileus, bowel obstruction, urinary drainage from the wound, elevated serum ammonia, or elevated blood urea nitrogen (BUN) without a concomitant elevation of the serum creatinine concentration. This last sign is the result of absorption of urine in the peritoneal cavity. Additionally, the creatinine level in the drainage fluid can also be measured. When the drainage fluid is urine, the creatinine level is generally markedly higher than is the serum creatinine. In a study of 1120 ileal conduits, Hensle and colleagues[53] found elevated BUN to be the most reliable indicator of a urine leak (20 of 21 patients).

Once concern of a leak exists, localization of the leak with a loopogram, intravenous pyelogram (IVP), computed tomography (CT) scan, cine loopogram with real time fluoroscopy, or injection of contrast material into the ureteral stent can be helpful. CT loopogram may also help to localize the extent of leakage. The leakage commonly originates from the ureterointestinal anastomosis but can also originate from the middle or back of the loop. In our opinion, loopogram with real time fluoroscopy is most helpful in defining the nature and severity of the leak. In the study by Hensle and colleagues,[53] left ureteral anastomosis was the most common site of leakage. One must also examine the stoma because edema may cause stomal obstruction with increased intraluminal pressure, increased back pressure, and eventual leakage.

When the diagnosis has been established, a conservative approach should be used initially. This approach includes ensuring of adequate drainage with a catheter in the stoma (on low suction if needed), drainage of the collecting system with either percutaneous nephrostomy tubes or ureteral stents, nutritional support, and antibiotic prophylaxis. Early leaks in the stented ureter can be observed initially, provided the patient has no signs of sepsis. Cross-sectional imaging should be used to rule out the presence of an undrained urine collection, which can compress or stretch the anastomosis and thus prevent its ultimate closure. High-output leaks in the presence of a stent should be managed initially by percutaneous drainage of the kidney to minimize urinary extravasation. In the absence of a ureteral stent, it is unlikely a major leak will seal without percutaneous drainage of the kidney and urinoma. Antegrade stenting is an option, but the surgeon should exercise extreme caution to avoid further disruption of the anastomosis.

Delayed leaks occurring >7 to 10 days postoperatively are often the result of ischemic ureteral necrosis. Early attempts at conservative therapy are still worthwhile, and percutaneous nephrostomy is an important adjunct to such therapy. If the leak continues as a high-output fistula despite proximal drainage, it may require early exploration because this finding suggests major ureteral necrosis. If proximal drainage reduces or abrogates fistula output, surgical repair is still likely necessary.

However, waiting for 6 to 10 weeks to allow inflammation to subside is wise.

If the patient does not respond to conservative therapy, early surgical exploration and repair must be attempted. Hensle and colleagues[53] suggested repair after 72 hours if no improvement is noted, whereas Coleman and Libertino[54] suggested waiting ≤3 weeks. In the study by Coleman and Libertino, leaks in 7 of 10 patients resolved after 3 weeks, whereas 3 of 10 patients required open revision. The decision to wait must be based on the patient's condition, the size of the leakage, the output volume, the presence of persistent infection, and the presence of signs of improvement.

In repairing an early leak, surgical exploration usually includes creating a new anastomosis. Simple placement of additional sutures in a preexisting anastomosis is rarely successful and is ill advised. Stent placement in the new anastomosis is strongly advised. The previous opening in the ileum should be identified and closed. To facilitate intraoperative dissection and mobilization, a Foley catheter with 3 to 5 mL in the balloon can be placed in the conduit. Antegrade stenting of the ureters is also helpful in localizing, mobilizing, and repairing the anastomosis.[54] The surgeon should anticipate very friable tissues, and the repair should focus on identification of a viable, minimally inflamed ureteral edge, mucosal apposition, and tension-free anastomosis. Watertight closure is often not possible because of the condition of the tissues. Eyre and associates[52] recommended sending the distal ureter for frozen section during repair, to assess tissue necrosis or small vessel occlusion. However, this condition may be difficult to assess in the presence of acute inflammation.

Patients with a delayed urine leak (10-14 days) usually have ischemic necrosis. This complication can involve a variable length of ureter and, in severe cases, can extend all the way to the renal pelvis. The technique of repair should be based on the length of the defect. Complete resection of the devitalized ureter must be performed with creation of an ileal interposition, transureteroureterostomy, or renal autotransplantation. Minimal to moderate gaps can be closed by mobilization of the proximal conduit itself. In patients with significant ureteral necrosis, critical illness or sepsis, or multiple comorbidities, the surgeon should give strong consideration to nephrectomy if the contralateral kidney is adequately functioning. Before surgical exploration, a renal scan may be performed to assess bilateral function, if necessary. Bowel preparation should be performed, if possible, based on the patient's overall condition.

Anastomotic Strictures

The incidence of ureteroileal strictures ranges from 1.5% to 18.4%.[20] For example, Bricker[35] found a 3.75% incidence of reoperation for ureteroileal obstruction in his initial 54 cases. In addition, Cass and colleagues,[37] and Frazier and associates[46] reported stricture rates of 6.5% and 7%, respectively. More recently, Madersbacher and colleagues[55] noted upper urinary tract obstruction in 13 of 131 (10%) patients as a result of stenosis at the ureteroileal anastomosis, and Gburek and associates[56] reported a 5% rate of stricture in 66 patients, their most common late complication of ileal conduit creation. The possible causes of stricture formation include tension at the anastomosis, devascularization and ischemia of the ureter, prior radiation therapy, prior leakage, and infection. In the setting of prior leakage, dense reaction surrounding the ureteroileal reimplantation results in extrinsic scarring of the anastomosis. Stricture at the anastomosis should be considered in any patient with decreased renal function (increased serum BUN and creatinine levels), hydronephrosis, flank pain, decreased urine output, fever, or sepsis.

The diagnosis of ureteroileal anastomotic stricture can be made with ultrasound, CT scan, IVP, and loopogram. IVP and loopogram can localize and define the length of the stricture. Newer techniques, including three-dimensional reconstructed spiral CT scan, CT urogram, and magnetic resonance imaging urogram, may also be used if available. In patients with poorly functioning or nonfunctioning kidneys, antegrade pyelography is often necessary to define the stricture. Hudson and colleagues[57] reported a rate of correlation between loopogram and IVP of 81%. Although reflux on a loopogram can rule out stenosis, the absence of reflux does not confirm obstruction. In a study by Hudson and colleagues,[57] 84% of obstructed kidneys were on the left, likely the result of extensive left ureteral mobilization and angulation or tension of the left ureter as it crosses behind the sigmoid mesentery. One must also be concerned with recurrent cancer as a cause of stenosis because carcinomas tend to develop at the ureterointestinal anastomosis.[58]

Initially, the conduit should be examined endoscopically to rule out recurrent malignant disease. In patients with established percutaneous access, antegrade endoscopy can further aid in defining the nature and extent of the stricture. The surgeon is then faced with choosing between endoscopic and open treatment. Endoscopic management by antegrade or retrograde methods is discussed in detail elsewhere in the text. Although endoscopic management is increasingly popular, high failure rates are noted unless the stricture is short and uncomplicated.

In the setting of an uncomplicated, short (<1 cm) stricture, most patients should be managed initially with an attempt at endoscopic treatment. The lumen of the stricture should be identified endoscopically. For endoscopic repair, we favor an antegrade approach because the patient is left with a nephrostomy tube as a safety mechanism. If endoluminal ultrasound technology is available, this technique is generally useful. Blind cutting procedures should be avoided because the

anastomosis is often directly next to bowel or vascular structures. The ureter should be stented for 6 weeks following stricture incision. If the stricture is >1 cm long, it may be wise to consider open repair initially.

During open reimplantation of a strictured ureteroileal anastomosis, it is best to place an antegrade stent to the level of stricture. The distal ureter is often encased in fibrotic reaction, particularly in the setting of previous leak or infection, and placement of antegrade stents can allow the surgeon to identify the ureters in an otherwise nondiscernible surgical plane. A catheter is placed in the conduit for similar reasons. The distal ureter must be mobilized, but extreme caution should be taken to avoid devascularization of the healthier proximal ureter. In cases of severe periureteral scarring, it is often preferable to excise the stricture, limit mobilization of the proximal ureter, maximally mobilize the conduit, and bring the conduit to the more fixed segment of viable ureter. We also recommend sending the distal ureteral margin for frozen section pathologic evaluation. If malignant disease is identified, a larger segment of ureter should be resected to achieve a cancer-free ureteral margin. For long stricture defects, numerous surgical options exist, including ileal interposition, transureteroureterostomy, renal autotransplantation, and, on rare occasion, nephrectomy.

When the ureteroileal stricture is identified late and the residual renal unit is nonfunctioning, nephroureterectomy is the treatment of choice. This is particularly true in the setting of underlying urothelial malignant disease because a nonfunctioning obstructed upper tract moiety is difficult to follow up for recurrent malignant disease.

Fate of the Kidney

During the preoperative evaluation, the status of the patient's renal function should be evaluated by sending blood for BUN and creatinine. One of the primary goals of conduit surgery is the preservation of renal function. In patients with a serum creatinine level >2.5 ng/mL or significant renal disease on radiographic studies, a short conduit should be created to help decrease stasis and to minimize electrolyte abnormality.

Pyelonephritis and Renal Damage

The rate of early pyelonephritis ranges from 1.8% to 3.1%, whereas the rate of late pyelonephritis ranges from 3.1% to 13%.[20,46] A reduction in the incidence of pyelonephritis has been reported in contemporary series, perhaps owing to improved technique and better perioperative antibiotics. In early series, Bricker[35,36] observed that ≤33% of his patients suffered from early pyelonephritis. More recently, Madersbacher and colleagues[55] noted that 23% of their patients who had ileal conduits had symptomatic urinary tract infections severe enough to lead to hospital admission. These investigators observed acute or recurrent pyelonephritis in 15 of 131 (11%) patients; this complication was associated with postrenal obstruction caused by anastomotic strictures, stomal stenosis, or urolithiasis in 13 of these patients. Recurrent urinary tract infections without clinically overt pyelonephritis were seen in 10 of 131 (7%) patients, and urosepsis occurred in 5 (4%) patients, associated with upper tract dilatation in 4 of these patients. Gburek and associates[56] observed pyelonephritis as an early complication in 6% of their patients and as a late complication in 2% of their patients.

Refluxing Versus Nonrefluxing Anastomoses

The question whether a nonrefluxing ureterointestinal anastomosis has any added benefit in conduit surgery has been the topic of much debate. Although early experiments suggested renal compromise in the setting of a refluxing moiety,[59] little clinical evidence exists to support this view. Kristjansson and associates[60,61] found no difference in glomerular filtration rate or stricture between refluxing and nonrefluxing anastomoses. A 15% rate of ureterointestinal stricture was noted in each group. Both bacteriuria and renal scarring were more common among refluxing anastomoses. Several investigators demonstrated improvement in hydronephrosis in the majority of patients when nonrefluxing anastomoses were used.[62,63] Stein and associates[64] reported on 105 children who were followed up for 16.3 years after construction of a nonrefluxing colon conduit. These investigators noted a 65.3% incidence of pyelonephritic changes, a rate comparable to that found in other studies, which reported a rate of change in children of ≤68%.

In adults, a conduit with freely refluxing ureters is preferable, mainly for ease of follow-up. Studies show no significant difference in renal damage and, most importantly, no difference in long-term glomerular filtration rates when comparing nonrefluxing and refluxing conduits. In patients with refluxing conduits who have persistent pyelonephritis with renal damage, the physician may consider revision to a nonrefluxing colon conduit.

Bacteriology of the Ileal Conduit

Guinan and colleagues[65] reported on the bacterial milieu of the ileal conduit. The native ileum before creation of a conduit was sterile in 9 of 10 patients, and 1 of 10 grew fungus. Postoperatively, 74% of conduits had urine cultures demonstrating bacterial growth. The most common infectious organism was *Proteus* followed by *Pseudomonas* and *Escherichia coli*. These investigators found IVP changes in 67% of infected conduits but no significant correlation between urinalysis and culture results. The changes seen were most pronounced in the presence of *Proteus* or *Pseudomonas* infection.

We recommend treating patients with significant asymptomatic bacteriuria (>10^5 organisms) in the setting of *Proteus* and *Pseudomonas* infections. Obviously, aggressive treatment is indicated in individuals with pyelonephritis or systemic signs of illness such as fever or leukocytosis. The surgeon must ensure that the conduit is adequately draining, to minimize reflux and the potential for pyelonephritis in the patient with asymptomatic bacteriuria.

Other Potential Complications

The incidence of duplex ureters found on autopsy is 0.3% to 2.5%.[66,67] The presence of this condition, if unknown preoperatively, can greatly compromise the outcome of conduit surgery. Careful examination of preoperative imaging studies is essential for the recognition and management of the duplicated ureter. When this condition is recognized, the ureters can be implanted separately or together with a Wallace-type anastomosis. Another unfortunate but uncommon complication is conduit-enteric fistula. The finding of decreased output, severe watery diarrhea, and fecaluria can lead to the diagnosis of a fistula.[68]

Stomal varices are another rare and problematic complication. Varices are usually seen in patients with cirrhotic or metastatic liver disease. These patients usually present with gross hematuria coming from the mucocutaneous junction and can usually be treated by correcting the underlying coagulopathy.

Occasionally, the use of coagulation or techniques to oversew the varices may be necessary. Transjugular intrahepatic portosystemic shunts have been used to correct the underlying portal hypertension and to stop the bleeding in these patients.[69]

KEY POINTS

1. In performing radical cystectomy, the urinary diversion is the most common source of morbidity.
2. Careful selection of the bowel segment based upon mesenteric arcades is essential in avoiding bowel ischemia or bowel anastomotic leak.
3. In preparing the bowel, the distal mesenteric incision will provide greatest length to the stoma in reaching the skin.
4. Stomal preparation prior to abdominal wall transposition may avoid stomal retraction.
5. Care of the stoma, stomal hygiene, and periodic inspection by an enterostomal therapist may help the patient avoid eventual stomal stenosis.
6. Both Bricker and Wallace style uretero-intestinal anastomotic techniques can be associated with low morbidity, but a tension-free anastomosis with careful attention to ureteral vascularity is essential for success.

REFERENCES

Please see www.expertconsult.com

Chapter 47

COMPLICATIONS OF CONTINENT CUTANEOUS DIVERSION

Eila C. Skinner MD
Professor of Clinical Urology, Department of Urology, Keck School of Medicine, University of Southern California, Los Angeles, California

Matthew D. Dunn MD
Assistant Professor of Urology, Department of Urology, Keck School of Medicine, University of Southern California, Los Angeles, California

Complications related to radical cystectomy and urinary diversion are very common, occurring in ≤35% to 40% of all patients.[1,2] Many of these complications such as bleeding, infection, ileus, bowel obstruction, thromboembolic events, nonurologic infections, and cardiovascular complications are related to the surgical procedure overall, and prevention and management of these complications are covered in Chapter 41. Approximately half of the early complications and three fourths of late complications are related to the diversion itself.[3] This chapter focuses on the management of both early and late complications related to continent cutaneous urinary diversion.

Continent diversion should be considered as a possible alternative to ileal conduit unless the patient has significant renal insufficiency, lack of a suitable bowel segment, or inability to take responsibility for adequate self-care.[4] Many different techniques are available for constructing a continent form of urinary diversion, including orthotopic neobladders as well as continent cutaneous diversions. Continent cutaneous diversion is specifically indicated for male and female patients undergoing cystectomy who are candidates for continent diversion but in whom an orthotopic neobladder is either contraindicated or not desirable. These indications include the following:

1. The patient prefers continent cutaneous diversion.
2. The external urethral sphincter is incompetent.
3. Severe urethral stricture disease is present.
4. The patient is unwilling or unable to catheterize through the urethra.
5. The patient has chronic bladder or urethral pain or severe interstitial cystitis.
6. The patient has known prostatic stroma invasion with urothelial cancer (relative contraindication to orthotopic diversion).

7. Patients who have had previous radical prostatectomy or high-dose radiation therapy to the area of the bladder neck are at higher risk of both incontinence and neobladder-urethral strictures (relative contraindication for orthotopic diversion depending on the severity of the scarring encountered during the surgical procedure).
8. Results of frozen section biopsy of the female urethra or prostatic apex are positive for urothelial cancer.

Many complications are common to all types of diversion (e.g., early urinary leak and ureteral obstruction), but others are unique to continent cutaneous diversion. These diversions are constructed from isolated colon or ileum with a large variety of continence mechanisms. A discussion of the pros and cons of the various techniques is beyond the scope of this chapter. The following discussion focuses on the most common forms of continent cutaneous diversion, including the Indiana pouch and its variations, the right colon pouch with appendix or tubularized ileal stoma, and the cutaneous T-pouch. We also discuss the complications associated with the cutaneous Kock pouch, although that type of diversion is now rarely performed in the United States. Metabolic complications associated with the use of bowel in the urinary tract are covered elsewhere (see Chapter 5).

PREVENTION OF COMPLICATIONS

Careful surgical technique is the key to minimizing complications related to the continent diversion. The choice of bowel segment must allow for adequate pouch volume. In general this requires approximately 44 linear cm of small bowel or 26 to 30 cm of colon for the reservoir portion. If the available colon length is <26 cm, an additional patch of ileum should be used to enlarge the reservoir.

The segment chosen for the reservoir must be isolated from the remaining bowel, with care taken not to compromise the vascular supply of either the reservoir or the remaining bowel. This maneuver is most difficult in patients who have had previous bowel resection. In these patients, it is crucial to take down the previous bowel anastomosis rather than choosing a new site. When a new site is chosen, the risk of vascular compromise of the segment between the old bowel anastomosis and the new one is high. If appendix is to be used it is examined for adequate length and girth, and the tip is amputated to ensure that the lumen is patient (sometimes the lumen is obliterated in older patients). Care must be taken not to damage the main blood supply during mobilization.[5]

The segment chosen for the reservoir must be opened along its entire length to allow for a low-pressure reservoir (**Fig. 47-1**).[5,6] In general the segment should be folded and closed to construct a reservoir that is as spherical as possible, to provide the maximum volume for the surface area used, and that minimizes the reservoir pressure.[7] It is critical to use only absorbable suture (or absorbable staples) to close the reservoir because any permanent suture or staples may become a nidus for stone formation. Closure of the pouch in one or two layers should be watertight, and this should be tested intraoperatively.

An antireflux mechanism is generally believed to be important in cutaneous continent diversion because of the very high rate of bacterial colonization.[4] Some of the commonly used antireflux mechanisms include tunneled ureteral anastomoses, the ileocecal valve, the

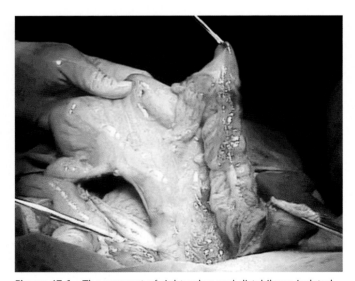

Figure 47-1 The segment of right colon and distal ileum isolated for a right colon pouch with appendix stoma. The entire right colon segment should be incised along one tinea to detubularize the bowel completely. The distal ileum is left intact for implantation of the ureters; the ileocecal valve acts as the antireflux mechanism.

Kock intussuscepted nipple valve, or an extraserosal tunnel (T-pouch).[8,9] Some authors have also reported good results with a refluxing anastomosis.[10]

The choice of technique for the ureteral anastomosis depends on the bowel segment used. We use a stay suture for manipulating the ureter during the anastomosis and avoid grasping it at all with forceps. The ureteral anastomosis with the lowest early and late stenosis rate is the end-to-side ureteroileal anastomosis, with <3% long-term stenosis.[11] This has been our standard anastomosis in the Kock pouch, the Studer and T-pouch ileal neobladders, and the right colon pouch with appendix stoma (using the distal ileum as the afferent limb). A similar direct nontunneled anastomosis to the colon carries a 6% to 7% stenosis rate.[10] The LeDuc method appears to have the lowest stenosis rate for antirefluxing techniques, although results have varied.[12,13] Tunneled anastomoses into the tinea of the colon carry a rate of stenosis of ≥10% to 12%.[11]

Previous ureteral surgery and radiation therapy increase the risk of subsequent stenosis. In patients who have undergone previous pelvic radiation, it is wise to take the ureters well above the field of radiation and to attempt to use a nonirradiated segment of bowel for the implantation.

Construction of the catheterizable efferent limb and stoma requires careful attention. Regardless of the continence mechanism used, the length of the efferent limb has no impact on continence. Therefore, it should be as short and straight as possible, to avoid any redundancy above or below the fascia that can contribute only to difficulty in catheterizing. At each step in construction of the efferent limb the surgeon should pass a catheter to ensure that it is smooth and without obstruction.

Stomal stenosis can be minimized by making a V-shaped flap when opening the skin and dropping the skin flap into the spatulated antimesenteric side of the efferent limb when it is matured to the skin.[14,15] This maneuver is performed whether the stoma is in the right lower quadrant or at the umbilicus. Figure 47-5 (see later) shows such a stoma once it has matured. With an umbilical stoma it is helpful to excise the majority of the umbilical scar to reduce the risk of later stenosis.

Finally, thoughtful placement of catheters, stents, and drains can minimize problems related to urinary leakage in the early postoperative period. All bowel segments excrete a large amount of mucus early on, and this needs to be managed so that catheters continue to drain. We routinely use a 24-Fr stiff two-way hematuria catheter to drain the reservoir placed percutaneously several centimeters away from the stoma, and only a small 12- to 14-Fr red Robinson catheter is placed through the stoma as a placeholder. Pediatric feeding tubes (8 Fr) are used for ureteral stents and can be tied to the hematuria catheter so they are removed together once the pouch has healed.

Alternatively, feeding tubes or stents can be passed up to the kidney and then brought into the pouch and out through the pouch wall and skin to drain externally. We prefer using a soft Penrose plastic drain placed behind the pouch to drain the pelvis passively rather than using a suction drain. A suction drain tends to draw urine out of the pouch and encourages leakage, and it is more difficult to manipulate. We leave the Penrose drain in place until all catheters are out of the pouch and the patient is catheterizing successfully. We also instruct the nurses (and later the patient and family) to irrigate the main catheter regularly to keep it free of mucus.

EARLY COMPLICATIONS

Diversion-related complications account for approximately 40% of the total early complications observed in patients undergoing cystectomy and continent diversion.[1,3] The incidence of early complications is not increased with continent diversion compared with ileal conduit.[16-18]

Urinary Leak

It is very common to have some degree of leakage of urine from one of the suture lines in the pouch in the first few days after the surgical procedure, and this is not a true complication as long as the urine comes out the drain. This leakage may persist for days to weeks but nearly always resolves spontaneously as long as good catheter drainage is maintained. More frequent irrigation of the pouch catheter may hasten resolution of the leak. Sometimes the drain is too close to the pouch and is acting as a wick, so we often will withdraw the drain for a few centimeters to try to resolve this problem.

An undrained leak is potentially serious and may be suspected by the development of abdominal distention or ileus, rising blood urea nitrogen with decreased urine output, or fever. The following measures should be taken in this situation:

1. A gravity cystogram under fluoroscopic guidance to confirm that the catheter is in the proper position. This study may also identify the site of extravasation.
2. Computed tomography (CT) scan to ensure that the patient does not have a large fluid collection in the abdomen or pelvis. If a collection is identified an additional drain should be placed percutaneously under CT guidance. If the CT scan is done with intravenous (IV) contrast in the excretion phase it also may identify the site of leakage.

If leakage is severe and persistent or appears to be arising from one or both ureters or if urine is draining out of the wound or has fistulized to another site (e.g.,

bowel anastomosis or vaginal cuff), then unilateral or bilateral diverting percutaneous nephrostomy tubes should be placed to divert the urine away from the pouch and allow healing. The nephrostomy tubes may be left in place for several weeks if necessary, and antegrade studies can confirm resolution of the leak before the tubes are removed. This method almost always resolves even the most difficult leak.

A basic principle of management of urinary leaks in the early postoperative period is to avoid attempting open surgical repair. Open exploration and primary repair are extremely difficult in this early period as a result of intense inflammatory reaction, and these procedures are rarely successful in achieving a watertight repair. The only situation requiring reoperation is a large, undrained leak that is not amenable to percutaneous drainage. The rare persistent leak that is refractory to all the foregoing steps can be repaired at open exploration 8 to 12 weeks after the initial surgical procedure, once all inflammation has had an opportunity to resolve.

The need for early percutaneous intervention arises infrequently, occurring in 4.7% of 230 patients who underwent cystectomy and neobladder in a prospective study at the University of Southern California in Los Angeles (unpublished data). However, it is crucial that the surgeon performing continent diversion have skilled interventional radiologists available to assist in these situations.

Necrosis of the Efferent Limb of the Pouch

Necrosis of the efferent limb of the pouch should be an extremely rare event if care is taken in mobilizing the pouch and constructing the catheterizable efferent limb. The most distal portion of the efferent limb has the most tenuous blood supply, so slight duskiness at the mucocutaneous border is not uncommon shortly after the surgical procedure. However, if true necrosis is visible, this should be investigated. If complete loss of the limb is suspected, the catheter should be removed and the limb gently inspected with a flexible cystoscope. When healthy mucosa is encountered in the efferent limb, no intervention is necessary. Reoperation with construction of a new efferent limb is required in patients with total necrosis of the limb.[1]

Problems Related to Catheterization

Mucus production is universal in continent diversions made from small or large bowel, and all cutaneous pouches should be regularly irrigated to clear the mucus. Mucus plugging of catheters can usually be managed by aggressive irrigation. Gross hematuria with clots rarely complicates a continent diversion during the initial healing phase. Continuous irrigation, correction of any coagulopathy, and use of products such as aminocaproic acid (Amicar) may be helpful. If a catheter is dislodged or must otherwise be replaced in the early postoperative period, it is advisable to obtain a fluoroscopic cystogram to confirm that the new catheter is in the proper position.

Urinary Infection

Febrile urinary tract infections are relatively common in patients in the early postoperative period, especially while catheters are still in place. Fungal infections and resistant bacterial infections are becoming more common in hospitalized patients and can cause significant morbidity and death, especially if these infections are not recognized early. We routinely add antifungal medications in hospitalized patients who become febrile or have leukocytosis after the first week in the hospital in the absence of other obvious sites of infection, even before the urine culture grows yeast. One must suspect resistant organisms in acutely ill postoperative patients and treat them accordingly.

In a review of 27 perioperative mortalities in cystectomy patients over a 30-year period, 8 cases were caused by overwhelming sepsis.[19] Many of these patients had urine or bowel leak, and all had reoperations during their hospital course.[19] In a more recent series of 230 patients undergoing cystectomy and orthotopic neobladder at our institution, the incidence of early pyelonephritis or urosepsis was <3% (unpublished data) and death resulting from sepsis (not all urinary in origin) was 0.5%.

Bowel Fistula to the Pouch and Other Bowel Complications

A fistula to the pouch is heralded by the presence of fecal material in the urinary drainage bag or drain, possibly associated with fever or pain. It is generally caused by a leak from the bowel anastomosis or a missed bowel injury and should be managed by bowel rest with parenteral nutrition. CT scan is advisable to ensure that an undrained abscess is not contributing to the problem. Again we generally avoid early surgical exploration in favor of delayed repeat exploration and repair if the fistula does not resolve within 4 to 6 weeks of bowel rest.[20]

Other bowel complications include prolonged ileus, partial or total small bowel obstruction, gastrointestinal bleeding (usually resulting from stomach or duodenal ulcers), pseudomembranous enterocolitis caused by *Clostridium difficile* overgrowth, and pelvic abscess caused by a bowel leak. The problems are common to all types of urinary diversion and to most other major abdominal surgical procedures involving bowel resection. Management is conservative whenever feasible, with endoscopic and percutaneous techniques used as needed. Taken together, these types of gastrointestinal complications account for almost one fourth of all early complications in patients undergoing cystectomy and diversion.[3]

General Medical Complications and Complications Unrelated to the Diversion

Many early postoperative complications result from cystectomy itself rather than from the specific type of diversion performed. These complications include hemorrhage, thrombotic events, and medical complications such as cardiac or pulmonary problems. Patients undergoing cystectomy and diversion have an average age of almost 70 years, and increasing percentages of our patients receiving treatment are very elderly (>80 years of age). Previous smoking behavior often contributes to significant cardiac and pulmonary comorbidities in these patients. Other problems that affect surgical healing include diabetes, poor nutrition or obesity, limitations to mobility, and renal insufficiency. General medical problems account for over half of the early complications observed following cystectomy.[3] It is important to optimize the patient's other medical conditions preoperatively whenever possible.

LATE COMPLICATIONS

Infections

Colonization of the urine with bacteria is almost universal in patients with a continent cutaneous reservoir on intermittent catheterization.[17,21] Conversely, late serious infections (pyelonephritis, sepsis) are relatively rare in the absence of upper tract obstruction or stones. *Therefore, it is very important not to subject patients to unnecessary antibiotics for asymptomatic bacterial colonization.* Patients and their primary care physicians need to be instructed in this principle.

Patients with cutaneous diversion who have symptomatic infections should be evaluated for completeness of emptying, hydronephrosis, and the possible presence of stones in the pouch or in the kidney. Occasionally patients with no anatomic abnormality may develop recurrent symptomatic infections that cause pain over the pouch or fevers, often preceded by very foul-smelling urine. This presentation appears to be much more common in patients with a history of interstitial cystitis than in patients with malignant disease. Daily pouch irrigation with saline solution (or even a very dilute bleach solution) should be recommended. A useful approach for patients who suffer recurrent symptomatic infections is to have them take a very short course of antibiotics (e.g., 2-3 days of a sulfonamide or fluoroquinolone) at the first sign of symptoms, no more than once or twice per month. Longer-term antibiotic use serves only to encourage colonization with highly resistant organisms.

Incontinence

Incontinence in a continent cutaneous diversion is virtually always a permanent problem and requires a surgical intervention to resolve.[22] Occasionally what is interpreted as urine leakage is in fact mucus drainage from the efferent limb (which is unavoidable) or failure to pinch the catheter on withdrawal, thus leaving a small amount of urine in the efferent limb. It is always valuable to gather a careful history of the incontinence pattern, including the amount of leakage, and catheterization technique, which should be directly observed. A trial of antibiotics may be worthwhile, but it rarely solves the problem.

Some patients may opt for an external collection device rather than undergoing an extensive workup or open surgical procedure. A pediatric stoma bag is useful if the leakage is of relatively small volume. However, even patients who leak large amounts usually need to continue to catheterize intermittently to empty the pouch completely.

The diagnostic approach depends on the type of urinary diversion that has been constructed, but generally it should include endoscopy of the pouch, a cystogram with drainage views, and possibly urodynamic studies of the pouch (especially if it is constructed from colon).

The following are some considerations for each type of diversion:

1. *Kock pouch to skin.* These procedures are now rarely performed in the United States, but some older patients still have a cutaneous Kock pouch and may require treatment. Incontinence results from incompetence of the intussuscepted nipple valve possibly caused by extussusception of the valve, stones on the nipple valve, or a fistula through the midpoint of the valve (e.g., by traumatic catheterization). Flexible endoscopy allows one to retroflex the scope and see the efferent valve clearly to identify the problem. Detubularized ileal reservoirs generally have reliable low-pressure systems, so urodynamic evaluation is not necessary. Successful repair depends on addressing the problem. Occasionally an extussuscepted nipple valve can be restapled to the back wall of the pouch, or a stone can be removed and the nipple repaired. However, it is often preferable to replace the efferent continence mechanism completely with a new limb (e.g., using a T-limb or other continence mechanism).[22,23]

2. *Indiana pouch and its variations.* Incontinence in this type of right colon pouch is generally the result of incompetence of the reinforced ileocecal valve. It may also be caused by a high-pressure reservoir, especially if the colon was not totally detubularized, so urodynamic studies should be done before the repair is planned. Repair may be accomplished by mobiliz-

ing the pouch and reinforcing the ileocecal valve with additional Lembert silk sutures around the base, with the addition of an ileal patch onto the pouch if high-pressure contractions were seen on urodynamic study.[24] Alternatively, a new efferent limb may be constructed. Temporary improvement may occasionally be achieved with endoscopic subcutaneous injection of collagen around the base of the efferent limb near the ileocecal valve.

3. *Appendix or tapered tunneled ileal segment.* Incontinence in these systems is unusual, but it may result from loss of the reinforced tunnel at the base of the appendix or erosion of the appendix from an indwelling catheter. Again, urodynamic studies and flexible endoscopy are helpful in defining the problem. Urodynamic studies should be performed before surgical repair to identify high-pressure contractions. Repair may be achieved by constructing a new tunnel at the base of the appendix (using the Mitrofanoff principle) or by making a new efferent limb with a tapered ileal segment. Again, injection of collagen in the submucosa at the base of the appendix has occasionally been helpful.

4. *Extraserosal tunnel (T-limb).* Incontinence is usually caused by loss of the extraserosal tunnel, as occurs when the permanent silk backing sutures pull through the serosa, probably because of trauma from daily catheterization.[9] It may be difficult to recognize this situation convincingly on a cystoscopic examination or cystogram because the problem is on the outside of the reservoir. Urodynamic studies should be performed preoperatively if the pouch is made from colon to identify high-pressure contractions. To repair the continence mechanism, the tunnel can be reinforced with a new set of backing sutures or a new efferent limb may be constructed.

Pouch Stones

Stones can develop in any continent diversion, and all patients should be followed with at least yearly plain radiographs, CT scan, or cystogram to discover stones when they are still small enough to manage endoscopically. Stones were very common in Kock pouches because of the metal surgical staples required to maintain the intussuscepted nipple valve.[24] However, they have also been observed in approximately 10% of all types of diversion.[13,25] The risk of stones is related to mucus production, chronic bacterial colonization, and incomplete emptying.

Continent cutaneous diversions have a higher incidence of stones than do neobladders, probably because of a higher rate of bacterial colonization and postvoid residual urine leading to stasis.[26] The incidence appears to increase with longer follow-up, and patients with a history of one pouch stone have a high recurrence rate and should be followed more diligently. These patients should also be encouraged to irrigate their catheters more regularly and may benefit from potassium citrate supplementation to reduce future stone formation.[26,27]

Stones in a pouch may manifest with hematuria, pain, difficulty in catheterizing, urinary incontinence, or recurrent symptomatic infections. The stones are almost always radiopaque and can be identified on cystogram, IV pyelogram (IVP), or CT scan without contrast. However, many radiologists are unfamiliar with the anatomy of this type of reconstruction and may easily miss the presence of stones in the pouch on plain films (**Fig. 47-2**). Therefore it is crucial for the urologist to review these films personally. It is more straightforward to identify even small stones in a pouch on CT scan than on plain films or an IVP (**Fig. 47-3**).

The natural history of pouch stones is that of growth. Not only do they inevitably increase in size with time

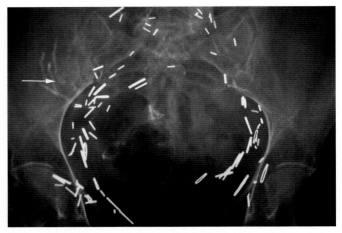

Figure 47-2 Small stones are faintly visible overlying the surgical staples on the efferent intussuscepted Kock ileal nipple valve *(arrow)*. These stones may be missed by an inexperienced radiologist.

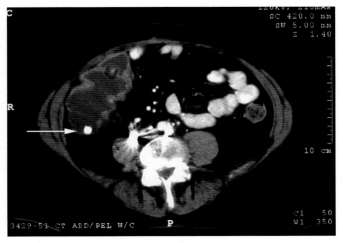

Figure 47-3 CT scan without contrast in the reservoir clearly showing a 1-cm stone *(arrow)* in the pouch.

if they are left untreated, but also they tend to become harder in consistency as more stone deposits in layers. These stones should not be observed but rather treated by complete removal at the time of initial diagnosis.

The goal of treatment is to remove all fragments without damaging the pouch or its continence mechanism. Fortunately, most pouch stones can be removed endoscopically by using techniques similar to those for removal of large bladder or kidney stones. The availability of versatile endoscopes, both rigid and flexible, and of efficient energy sources such as electrohydraulic, ultrasonic, and pneumatic lithotriptors and holmium laser technology has allowed efficient fragmentation and removal of stones even through small stomas. Extracorporeal shock wave lithotripsy is not recommended for pouch stones because of the need to remove all the fragments to prevent recurrence.

Small stones can be easily retrieved with a flexible cystoscope inserted through the stoma. Such scopes have approximately the same caliber size as do the catheters used to empty the pouch. Basket removal or lithotripsy followed by basket removal can safely be performed without too much concern for damaging the continence mechanism. Because these scopes are smaller than their rigid counterparts, however, the smaller working channel makes them less efficient for treating larger stones.

For large stones, a rigid scope, preferably an offset rigid nephroscope or cystoscope, provides a large enough channel to break up and remove the stone fragments efficiently. This technique is preferable to flexible endoscopy whenever possible and a rigid scope can generally be safely inserted through a stoma under direct vision. To protect the continence mechanism from damage during repetitive insertion of instruments during the course of the procedure, an Amplatz sheath can be used. This device definitely dilates the efferent limb and stoma but provides safe access into the pouch without damaging the mucosa of the efferent limb and the continence mechanism. It also allows for continuous flow irrigation, which decreases the pressures within the pouch, allows for efficient irrigation of stone fragments, and improves visibility during the procedure.

Aggressive manipulation of a rigid scope within the efferent limb should be avoided. Fortunately, our patients have not experienced permanent incontinence after endoscopy through a stoma. Some patients may find it difficult to catheterize immediately after endoscopic manipulation because of the presence of edema. This complication is more likely with rigid than flexible endoscopy. It may be helpful to leave a catheter in the efferent limb for 24 hours after the procedure to allow the edema to subside.

In certain situations, rigid endoscopy of the stoma should be avoided. Appendiceal stomas tend to be too narrow for most rigid scopes and the angle entering the pouch limits manipulation. Small stones in such

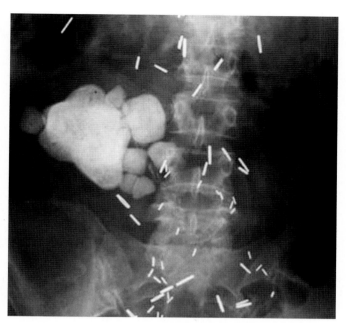

Figure 47-4 Huge stones in a continent cutaneous reservoir. These stones are best removed through a small open incision lateral and inferior to the stoma rather than with endoscopic techniques.

pouches can be removed with a flexible cystoscope, but larger stones or stones in a difficult location within the pouch are better managed percutaneously.[28,29] This procedure can be safely accomplished as long as one is careful to identify a spot where the pouch is up against the abdominal wall without intervening bowel. When a percutaneous catheter had been used perioperatively, use of this old scar is generally safe. If any doubt exists, ultrasound or CT scan can easily identify a safe passage for percutaneous access.

Once access is obtained, the tract can be dilated either by balloon dilation or sequential manual dilators. An Amplatz sheath along the percutaneous tract allows access in and out of the pouch and facilitates irrigation and removal of fragments as well. All stone fragments must be extracted or irrigated out of the pouch at the end of the procedure because they may not pass through the catheter. Retained fragments often stick to the bowel mucosa and become a nidus for additional stones in the future.

Patients who are not followed up with at least annual radiographs may present with huge stones (**Fig. 47-4**). When stones are too large or too numerous, endoscopic management may be difficult and inefficient. In these rare situations, very large stones are more expeditiously extracted through a small open incision lateral or inferior to the stoma.

Kidney Stones

Kidney stones are a known complication of urinary diversions for a variety of reasons. Metal staples from a Kock pouch nipple valve may reflux up into the kidney and form a nidus of stone formation. Metabolic derangements from the interposition of intestinal segments and chronic bacterial colonization with urease-producing bacteria can predispose patients to stone formation as well.[30,31] In patients with cutaneous reservoirs, treatment options for managing kidney stones include extracorporeal shock wave lithotripsy and percutaneous nephrolithotomy. In rare instances, retrograde ureteroscopy can be performed through the stoma but the altered anatomy makes access to the upper collecting system extremely difficult and unreliable.

Treatment options depend on the size and location of the stones. Although no absolute size criteria have been determined for this patient population, smaller stones respond better to extracorporeal shock wave lithotripsy than do larger stones. Overall success rates for extracorporeal shock wave lithotripsy have been variable. More recent reports describe an overall success rate of 81.5%, although 44% of patients may require more than one treatment session.[32] Larger stones, staghorn calculi, and stones within the ureter are more reliably managed percutaneously either through percutaneous nephrolithotomy or antegrade ureteroscopy.

Ureteral Pouch Obstruction

The management of ureteroileal stenosis is covered in detail in Chapter 46. As mentioned earlier, the type of ureteral anastomosis is directly related to the risk of subsequent obstruction. Ureteral obstruction may be discovered incidentally, may occur many years after the diversion, and may be asymptomatic. Therefore, patients with urinary diversion need lifelong follow-up for hydronephrosis, even after the risk of recurrent cancer is past. Obstruction may also manifest with pain, infection or renal insufficiency. The differential diagnosis includes ischemic stenosis and recurrent cancer. These disorders can be differentiated to some extent by their appearance on CT urogram or antegrade nephrostogram and by cytologic study or endoscopic biopsy (**Fig. 47-5**).

Open repair is still considered the gold standard of treatment, with long-term success rates between 76% and 93%.[33-35] However, the morbidity of such repair is not insignificant, and therefore endoscopic techniques are usually the first line of treatment. It can be very difficult and sometimes impossible to access the obstructed ureterobowel anastomosis from the reservoir, so antegrade percutaneous access through the kidney is usually necessary.

Various endoscopic treatment modalities have been described including include balloon dilation, endoureterotomy, and metal stenting. Success rates vary widely and depend on several factors. Wolf and associates[36] reported the importance of renal function on success rates after endoscopic treatment of ureterointestinal strictures. In their series, endoureterotomy failed in all

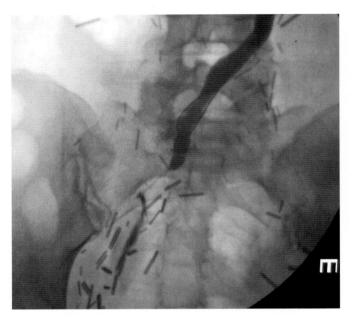

Figure 47-5 Ureteroileal stricture seen on an antegrade nephrostogram. Very little contrast material is seen passing through the stricture. These strictures are most common on the left side and are usually caused by ischemia of the distal ureter. However, cytologic examination and brush biopsy should be performed to rule out recurrent urothelial carcinoma.

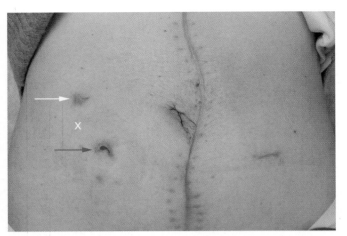

Figure 47-6 Photograph of the abdominal wall of a patient 6 months following cystectomy and nephroureterectomy with a right colon pouch and an appendix stoma. The *red arrow* shows the stoma in the right lower quadrant. The scar from the perioperative percutaneous catheter drain that has been removed is lateral and superior to the stoma (*white arrow*). It is generally safe to drain a pouch percutaneously in the area marked with the *white X* because no intervening bowel should be present in the area between the stoma and the old drain site.

patients with renal unit functioning of <25%. These investigators also observed that repeat endoureterotomy after a failed procedure was considered only when at least a partial radiographic response occurred and when steroid injections were used.[36] Kurzer and Leveillee[37] reviewed the literature on several endoscopic treatment modalities for ureterointestinal strictures after radical cystectomy. These investigators concluded that favorable characteristics for success after endoureterotomy included age <60 years, a right-sided stricture, length <1 cm, mild to moderate dilation, use of a ≥12-Fr stent, and stenting for >6 weeks. In their evaluation, cumulative success rates for various treatment modalities showed that balloon dilation had the worst outcome at 18%, in contrast to endoureterotomy at 63% and metal stenting at 83%. No specific cutting modality (i.e., laser, electrocautery, cold knife) appears to have an advantage over another. These investigators also pointed out that an open repair after multiple endoscopic attempts had a lower success rate and higher morbidity than did an initial primary repair.

These findings clearly emphasize the importance of adequate patient selection for initial treatment. Despite early promising results, metal stents are still not widely accepted because of severe long-term complications such as tissue ingrowth and recurrent obstruction.[37]

Difficulty With Catheterizing

Difficulty with catheterization is one of the most vexing problems for patients with a continent cutaneous diver-

sion and one that causes significant anxiety. This complication usually results from either stenosis at the skin level or tortuosity of the efferent limb in its course from the skin to the pouch. True stenosis of the efferent limb other than at the skin level is rare. Often the source of the problem can be diagnosed by simply catheterizing the patient in the office with the pouch full or observing while patient performs self-catheterization. Occasionally endoscopy is necessary, although that approach often is either impossible or not very helpful.

Complete inability to pass a catheter in spite of multiple attempts is an emergency. A trip to the local emergency room is often not a good solution because most emergency room physicians have little experience with these reservoirs. *The urologist should not delay in becoming involved in trying to solve the problem.* The first attempt should include using a small 14- to 16-Fr Coudé-tip catheter with lots of lubrication. Flexible endoscopy with passage of a wire is occasionally successful if the stoma is open at the skin level.

If these initial attempts fail, one of the most helpful steps is to drain the distended pouch. This maneuver relieves the patient's pain and may straighten out a kink in the efferent limb. This procedure can be done safely percutaneously a few centimeters to the right and inferior to the stoma, given that the right colon and small bowel usually lie medial to the reservoir (**Fig. 47-6**), with a long 18- or 16-gauge angiocatheter such as those used for central line placement. A test pass may be made first with a fine spinal needle, or bedside ultrasound examination may be indicated if the location of the pouch is unclear. Once the tip of the angiocatheter is in the pouch, the needle can be removed and the pouch emptied through the soft plastic catheter. If catheterization through the stoma is still unsuccessful with the pouch less distended, then a wire can be placed through the angiocatheter, the tract can be dilated, and a percutaneous catheter can be placed for temporary drainage until the stoma can be repaired.

Stomal stenosis at the skin level is a fairly common occurrence in appendix stomas and is somewhat less common with other types of cutaneous diversion.[15,38] Stomal stenosis may be more common when the stoma is located at the umbilicus because of the scarring of the umbilical skin. The following sequential steps may be attempted to manage this problem:

1. Office dilation (female urethral sounds work well for this), with a catheter taped in place for a few days to dilate the skin gently further
2. Office incision of the stenotic skin edge or excision of built-up scar tissue
3. Outpatient Y-V plasty of the stoma, by dropping in a new flap of skin
4. Formal revision of the stoma

Formal revision of the stoma, although more involved, is also the most successful in difficult cases. Several months after the original surgical procedure, the efferent limb (appendix or ileum) has usually lengthened significantly and can be mobilized down to the fascia, by excising the old mucocutaneous border and creating a freshly spatulated stoma with an interposed flap of skin.

If the stoma is wide open at the skin but the catheter hangs up inside before entering the pouch, this complication is usually caused by tortuosity of the limb or an outpouching just above the fascia rather than by a true stricture. Changing catheters can often solve the problem. Straight red Robinson catheters are the least expensive and the easiest for patients to find at medical supply shops. However, Coudé-tip catheters or stiffer catheters (e.g., those made by Conveen, Coloplast, Minneapolis) may be more successful for negotiating a tortuous efferent limb or overcoming a lip at the fascia. We often have the patient try several different catheters to see which one works most easily. Sometimes patient position affects the ease of passing the catheter, but because it is not practical for the patient to catheterize only lying down, every effort should be made to find a solution that works with the patient in the seated or standing position.

If changing catheters does not resolve the problem, then open surgical revision is required. In this situation, we usually take down the entire stoma and mobilize the pouch (usually through the old midline incision), resect excess length of the efferent limb, and reconstruct the stoma. This surgical procedure is significant, and one should ensure that all other aspects of the diversion (e.g., continence mechanism, ureteral anastomoses) are

working properly or can be repaired at the same time. The surgeon should be prepared for the possible need to cut a new segment of bowel to construct an entirely new efferent continence mechanism.

Complete reconstruction of the continence mechanism may require several different techniques, and these surgical procedures should be performed by a surgeon with wide experience in continent diversion. Useful techniques include using a tapered ileal segment tunneled into a new tinea of a right colon pouch by a Mitrofanoff technique or construction of an ileal patch with a tapered extraserosal tunnel using the T-pouch technique.[8] Both these mechanisms can be added to a mature right colon reservoir after the old nonfunctioning efferent limb is excised. If the pouch was originally made from ileum then a new T-limb efferent limb may be constructed using a new short segment of ileum.

Conversion From a Continent to a Noncontinent Diversion

Very rarely the patient and surgeon decide that the best management of a problematic continent diversion is to convert it to a continuously draining conduit. Unfortunately, this is not a simple undertaking and sometimes is more complex than fixing the continent diversion. It is unsatisfactory simply to excise the efferent continence mechanism and connect the pouch itself to the skin because this mechanism tends to make a poor stoma, has a high risk of herniation or prolapse, and empties poorly. If an afferent limb is present (e.g., with a Studer pouch or a right colon pouch with the ureters implanted into the distal ileal segment) then the reservoir may be discarded and the afferent limb brought up as an ileal stoma. Care must be taken not to compromise the blood supply to this segment when the rest of the reservoir is excised. In the absence of an afferent limb (e.g., with an Indiana pouch), it is best to discard the pouch and construct a completely new ileal conduit from a new segment of ileum.

Afferent Antireflux Mechanism

The need for an antireflux mechanism in orthotopic neobladders is controversial, but most investigators agree that some sort of antireflux system should be constructed for continent cutaneous diversions.[26] The Kock pouch used an intussuscepted ileal nipple valve that is a very effective antireflux mechanism. Initially, few problems were related to this mechanism other than occasional stones on the surgical staples used to maintain the nipple valve. However, with long-term follow-up, investigators discovered that late stenosis of the nipple valve itself was not uncommon, sometimes occurring 10 years or more after construction of the reservoir.[39] This problem is often silent until the patient has developed significant bilateral hydroureteronephrosis or even renal failure. The diagnosis is made on antegrade study, which shows a dilated afferent limb and delayed emptying into the reservoir.

Endoscopically, these stenotic nipple valves look white and scarred, with only a pinpoint opening that may require IV methylene blue to identify. Treatment involves intubation with an angled catheter and wire and then incision with a hot knife through the stenotic nipple until free drainage of the afferent limb is accomplished. A balloon incision device can also be used under careful direct vision. The main risk of this procedure is bleeding from the cut edge, which can be avoided by careful coagulation. Incision of the valve is usually very effective in resolving the obstruction, although recurrent obstruction can occasionally develop.[40] Most patients who undergo incision of the valve mechanism experience reflux, but that does not usually cause problems, probably because of the high-volume, low-pressure mature reservoir.

The T-pouch extraserosal tunnel mechanism was designed in part to address this risk of late stenosis in the Kock pouch by better maintaining an adequate blood supply to the afferent limb.[41] Stenosis is still occasionally observed, especially in patients who were previously irradiated or in whom the distal afferent limb was tapered during construction. Because of this risk we no longer taper the limb before closing the tunnel over the top of the afferent limb.[42] The absolute risk of late stenosis will not be known until more patients have experienced long-term follow-up. Management is with endoscopic incision, similar to that described earlier for the Kock pouch.

We have also seen occasional afferent limb stenosis that appears to result from fibrosis of the midpoint of the ileal segment itself rather than the nipple valve. These cases closely resemble the late fibrosis and lack of peristalsis seen with very long-term follow-up of ileal conduits.[43,44] An example in a patient with an orthotopic diversion is shown in **Figure 47-7**. As more patients live for many years with these continent diversions, we may find that this problem is more common than currently observed. Management requires replacement of the entire afferent limb with a new segment.

Acute Pouch Rupture

Spontaneous rupture of a cutaneous continent reservoir appears to be quite rare, although the exact incidence is unknown.[45] Mansson and colleagues[46] polled surgeons who performed continent diversion in Scandinavia and reported that 17 patients out of a total of 1070 with cutaneous diversion suffered a spontaneous rupture, for an incidence of 1.6%. The Indiana University group reported rupture in 2 of 69 patients (2.9%).[13] In our experience with the Kock cutaneous ileal reservoir, we have observed very rare spontaneous pouch ruptures. Early rupture can very rarely occur in the first

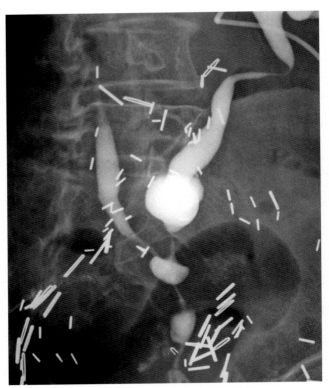

Figure 47-7 Stenosis of the midportion of the afferent limb in a patient with an ileal orthotopic neobladder. The diversion was 11 years old at the time of this diagnosis.

few postoperative weeks in a patient who is noncompliant with catheterization. Late rupture does not always have any obvious inciting event and seems to be more likely in patients who have been previously irradiated.

At presentation, the patient generally has acute severe abdominal pain and distention. Attempts to catheterize the pouch may return little urine. Unfortunately, delay in diagnosis is the rule, and deaths have occurred in this situation as a result of abdominal sepsis. The diagnosis may be made on cystogram, although false-negative cystograms have been reported.[26] A CT cystogram may be more helpful. Rupture should be suspected in any patient with acute abdominal pain and ascites fluid seen on CT scan, even if actual extravasation is not demonstrated. Surgical repair is generally recommended, especially because the urine in these reservoirs is nearly always colonized with bacteria.

Parastomal Hernia

Parastomal hernias have been reported in approximately 4% of patients with continent cutaneous diversions, although the incidence may increase in patients with longer follow-up.[47] These hernias can appear with stomas at any location and are more common in elderly or obese patients and in smokers. These high-risk patients often also have ventral midline hernias from the abdominal incision. The parastomal hernia may lead to difficulty with catheterizing or incontinence. Repair when necessary may be attempted with a semi-circle of permanent mesh placed around the stoma at the fascia level. This procedure is relatively simple for the patient because it does not require full laparotomy or adhesiolysis.

Alternatively, the hernia may be repaired laparoscopically. In either approach, care must be taken to avoid placing the mesh directly against the wall of the efferent limb because that may lead to subsequent erosion of the mesh. Unfortunately, recurrence after these types of repair is not uncommon. The most secure repair involves moving the stoma to a new site, a maneuver that requires open laparotomy and complete mobilization of the pouch. This major undertaking may occasionally require construction of an entirely new efferent limb.

Late Malignant Diseases

The development of late malignant diseases in ureterosigmoidostomy diversions with a mean latency of 25 years was one of the factors leading to the virtual abandonment of this procedure in the United States. However, late malignant diseases have also been reported in nearly every other type of diversion, both ileal conduit and continent diversions using ileum and colon. The risk of such malignancy is unknown, but it appears to be very low.[48] The reason is, partly, that most patients undergoing cystectomy and continent diversion today are elderly, have invasive bladder cancer, and have a limited life expectancy.

Late adenocarcinomas have been reported in patients with continent colonic reservoirs, but with much shorter latency than that seen with ureterosigmoidostomy diversion.[48,49] Because the colon is already predisposed to develop benign and malignant polyps, it seems likely that these tumors may have existed before construction of the diversion. Conversely, Austen and Kalble[50] identified 3 adenomas, 2 carcinoid tumors, and 5 adenocarcinomas reported in ileal conduits 9 to 30 years after construction. In >1500 cases of continent ileal reservoirs spanning 25 years at our institution, we have not yet identified a secondary adenocarcinoma arising from the ileum.

CONCLUSION

Continent cutaneous urinary diversion offers a reasonable alternative to ileal conduit or continent neobladder in properly selected patients. Complications are common after these surgical procedures, and the surgeon undertaking such an operation must be familiar with their diagnosis and management.

KEY POINTS

1. Patient selection is critical to ensure that the type of diversion planned is appropriate for that patient from both a medical and a psychological or social standpoint.
2. Attention to the following technical details during construction of the reservoir can avoid many potential complications:
   - Careful isolation of the segment to be used for the reservoir and complete detubularization of the segment are important.
   - A direct ureteroileal anastomosis carries the lowest risk of subsequent stenosis.
   - The continence (efferent) limb should be short and straight, and the continence mechanism should be tested during construction to ensure complete continence and ease of catheterization.
3. Early urinary leakage should be managed with aggressive catheter irrigation, percutaneous drainage of any urinoma, and diverting nephrostomy tubes as needed. Reoperation should be avoided.
4. Most continent cutaneous reservoirs are chronically colonized with bacteria but symptomatic infections are unusual. Late asymptomatic infections should not be treated.
5. Incontinence from cutaneous continent reservoirs usually requires surgical repair. The exact diagnostic and treatment approach depends on the type of continence mechanism used.
6. Pouch and kidney stones can occur in all types of cutaneous diversions and are usually amenable to endoscopic or percutaneous management.
7. Acute pouch rupture is a rare but potentially fatal complication. Early recognition and surgical exploration are the keys to successful management.
8. Stenosis of an ileal antireflux mechanism may manifest with silent bilateral hydronephrosis and renal insufficiency.
9. Patients with continent cutaneous reservoirs should have annual evaluation to check for pouch and renal stones or upper urinary tract obstruction.

REFERENCES

Please see www.expertconsult.com

Chapter 48

COMPLICATIONS OF ORTHOTOPIC NEOBLADDER

Melissa R. Kaufman MD, PhD
Assistant Professor, Department of Urologic Surgery, Vanderbilt University Medical Center, Nashville, Tennessee

Michael S. Cookson MD
Professor, Department of Urologic Surgery, Vanderbilt University Medical Center, Nashville, Tennessee

Since the 19th century, urologists have used intestinal segments for reconstruction of the urinary tract following extirpative surgical procedures. However, objectives have evolved from a simple diversion of urine with preservation of renal function to the anatomic and functional preservation of volitional voiding without altered body image. In fact, the desire to afford patients with a near-normal state of voiding by preserving the natural continence mechanism while eliminating a cutaneous stoma or absolute requirement for intermittent catheterization led to the development orthotopic urinary diversion. Orthotopic bladder substitution, first pioneered by Lemoine[1] in the early 20th century and popularized by Camey and LeDuc,[2] has been extensively refined[3-6] to a procedure with excellent patient satisfaction and acceptably low morbidity.

Many techniques exist for creation of an orthotopic neobladder.[7-12] Ileum is the bowel segment of choice because of ease of construction, lower storage pressures, less urine absorption, and lower mucus production as compared with large bowel. The most commonly performed ileal reservoirs fall into one of two types: the U-shaped ileal neobladder as described by Studer and associates[13] and the W-shaped reservoir that was initially described by Hautmann and colleagues.[3,10] Basic requirements for an acceptable orthotopic urinary neobladder include a capacious, low-pressure reservoir that provides acceptable continence without compromising cancer control. Both the Studer and Hautmann configurations are easily constructed using an afferent limb or chimney that facilitates the ureteroileal anastomosis.

Multiple large published series and reviews have reported the surgical complications and long-term outcomes of orthotopic neobladders.[14-16] Most potential complications, including the diagnosis and treatment options outlined in this chapter, are generally applicable to all methods of orthotopic neobladder diversion. As discussed in further detail, typical early postoperative complications are similar to those seen with other types of urinary diversion and can include persistent urine leak, pyelonephritis, and bowel complications such as ileus and small bowel obstruction. Late complications can include ureteroenteric and neovesical-urethral anastomotic stricture, urinary fistula, and urolithiasis. Additionally, the issues and complications unique to orthotopic neobladder including patient selection concerns, voiding dysfunction, and incontinence are addressed.

PATIENT SELECTION AND CONTRAINDICATIONS TO ORTHOTOPIC DIVERSION

Fortunately, we practice urology in an era when bladder cancer has become a survivable disease for a substantial percentage of patients and the long-term outlook is a component of the algorithm for the consideration of treatment options. With improvements in anesthesia and surgical technique, radical cystectomy is feasible even in patients of advanced age and with significant comorbid conditions.[17-19] In choosing to perform an orthotopic neobladder, proper patient selection is probably the single most important factor in determining the ultimate success or failure of the procedure. Patients must be cognizant of the medical, physical, and emotional demands of a continent urinary reservoir, must be highly motivated and capable of performing self-catheterization, and must be compliant with the necessary follow-up regimen.[12] Thus, patients with severe mental impairment should not undergo orthotopic diversion.

Preoperative counseling on methods of urinary diversion by a trained wound ostomy continence nurse can aid immensely in both the physical and mental preparations of the patient for the demands of a neobladder and should be obtained for all patients regardless of choice of diversion. The wound ostomy continence nurse should mark the patient for an appropriate stomal

TABLE 48-1	Absolute Contraindications to Orthotopic Neobladder	
Medical	**Oncologic**

Compromised renal function
  Serum creatinine >2.0 mg/dL
  or creatinine clearance
  <60 mL/min
Severe hepatic dysfunction
Compromised intestinal function
  Inflammatory bowel disease
  Radiation enteritis
External sphincter dysfunction
Severe urethral stricture disease
Severe mental impairment
	Bladder neck involvement:
	  female patient
	Prostatic urethral or apical
	  involvement: male
	  patient
	Need for simultaneous
	  urethrectomy
	Failure to achieve negative
	  urethral margin

site on the abdominal wall in the event that intraoperative factors preclude neobladder diversion and noncontinent diversion is performed.

Although some risk factors that were previously considered contraindications to neobladder, including advanced age, have changed with improved technique,[15] absolute contraindications to creation of an orthotopic reservoir still exist (Table 48-1). Sound oncologic principles should always supersede the preference of diversion, most prominently the achievement of negative surgical margins at the site of the neoanastomosis. In women, orthotopic diversion should be reserved for patients whose tumors do not involve the bladder neck or urethra. In men, involvement of the prostatic stroma or apex is an absolute contraindication to neobladder diversion. Investigators have strongly recommended that frozen section analysis of urethral margins be performed intraoperatively before construction of an orthotopic diversion.[20] Orthotopic reconstruction is absolutely contraindicated in patients in whom simultaneous urethrectomy is indicated on the basis of their primary tumor.

Significant benign urethral disease such as profound stricture is also considered an absolute contraindication. Furthermore, patients with external sphincter dysfunction, a damaged rhabdosphincter, or an incompetent urethra should also be excluded from placement of a neobladder. In addition, severe acute or chronic inflammatory bowel disease affecting the chosen bowel segment is a contraindication to construction of a neobladder.[21] In general, continent urinary diversion should not be performed in patients with significant renal or hepatic impairment.[22-24] Isolated case reports have advocated the use of continent urinary diversions in select patients with renal insufficiency.[25,26] However, the prolonged metabolic acidosis associated with neobladder diversion is generally poorly tolerated in patients with any degree of renal compromise.[27] In most adult patients, neobladder diversion should be performed only if the serum creatinine concentration is <2 mg/dL.[28]

Patients considered for continent diversion should have normal liver function because reabsorption of ammonium and chloride can worsen hepatic impairment and can precipitate encephalopathy.[22,29] Some surgeons consider stress urinary incontinence an absolute contraindication for neobladder diversion.[15] However, as discussed later, techniques for management of stress incontinence in patients with neobladders are increasingly acknowledged.

As mentioned earlier, several factors previously considered inadvisable to selection of patients for orthotopic diversion, such as obesity, advanced chronologic age, prior abdominal surgical procedures, or the presence of metastases in pelvic lymph nodes, when taken individually are no longer considered absolute contraindications.[12,30,31] Indeed, management of bladder cancer in the elderly patient is becoming an increasingly important issue as the general population ages. Clark and colleagues[17] demonstrated that radical cystectomy with orthotopic urinary diversion could be performed even in persons of significantly advanced age without escalating operative mortality or diversion-related complications.

Although patients with increased body mass index have been shown to have higher rates of transfusion[32] and of postoperative complications,[33] investigators generally accept that weight per se does not affect cancer-specific survival and is not an absolute contraindication for performing cystectomy with continent diversion.[34] In addition, avoidance of a cutaneous stoma in morbidly obese patients may actually be preferable because of the increased incidence of stomal complications including the development of a parastomal hernia. Multiple studies demonstrated that the incidence of local pelvic recurrence with lymph node–positive disease is approximately 11% and the presence of positive lymph nodes by itself should not preclude placement of an orthotopic diversion.[12,31] In patients who have received prior pelvic irradiation, great care must be taken to select a bowel segment out of the confines of the radiated field. Salvage cystectomy with neobladder diversion is a technically challenging procedure but has been demonstrated to be a viable option in selected cases.[19,35-37] However, patients should be preoperatively counseled on reported incontinence rates approaching 25% following salvage cystectomy with neobladder and the possible need for artificial urinary sphincter placement in the future.[12]

SURGICAL COMPLICATIONS

Proper patient preparation and adherence to meticulous surgical technique are paramount in the prevention of surgical complications. Although controversy exists in the current literature on colorectal surgery,[38] investigators generally accept that urologic patients who have an intestinal procedure on unprepared bowel have an increased incidence of wound infections, intraperitoneal abscess formation, and bowel anastomotic leakage when compared with patients who have preoperative bowel preparation.[28] Accordingly, patients undergoing elective bowel reconstruction should undergo mechanical and antibiotic bowel preparation, which in almost all circumstances can be performed on an outpatient basis.

Various methods are employed for mechanical cleansing of the bowel.[39] Current protocols often administer large volumes of an oral polyethylene glycol solution. Not all patients readily tolerate this treatment because of the large amount of fluid that must be ingested, in addition to the nausea, emesis, and abdominal cramping that are frequent side effects of the bowel preparation. Elderly patients may be unable to complete this regimen as a result of these mentioned side effects in combination with dehydration induced by the profuse diarrhea. Thus, some patients may benefit from preoperative admission specifically for bowel preparation. Alternatively, oral sodium phosphate solutions can produce equivalent mechanical cleansing with the consumption of significantly less volume.[40,41]

Antibiotic bowel preparations are often used in combination with mechanical cleansing and consist of timed doses of neomycin and erythromycin base or metronidazole on the day before the surgical procedure.[42,43] However, articles in the general surgery and colorectal literature have suggested that preoperative bowel preparation with oral antibiotics may be safely omitted in the current era of potent intravenous (IV) antibiotics.[44]

An advisory statement from the National Surgical Infection Prevention Project outlined the use of perioperative antibiotics for prevention of surgical site infections.[45] The work group endorsed infusion of the antimicrobial dose within 60 minutes of incision and suggested that antibiotic prophylaxis be discontinued within 24 hours after the operation. Although the committee did not specifically address urologic surgery, cephalosporins were included in the recommendations for general abdominal, colon, cardiac, orthopedic, gynecologic, and vascular surgical procedures. To decrease wound infection rates in bowel surgery, preoperative IV doses of a second-or third-generation cephalosporin such as cefoxitin, 2 g, should be administered within an hour of incision. For patients with allergies to β-lactam antibiotics, perioperative doses of vancomycin, 1 g IV, in conjunction with clindamycin, 600 to 900 mg IV, should be substituted.

Pulmonary embolism has been recognized in approximately 1% to 3% of patients undergoing radical cystectomy with orthotopic diversion.[46-48] Studies have advocated the use of deep vein thrombosis prophylaxis for major urologic surgical procoedures,[49-51] as under-scored by the knowledge of a higher incidence of deep vein thrombosis in patients with cancer.[52] Low-molecular-weight heparin or alternatively low-dose unfractionated heparin should be administered preoperatively and during the length of hospitalization. Graduated compression stockings and intermittent pneumatic compression may be used in conjunction with systemic anticoagulation. Controversy exists concerning the optimal duration of thromboembolic therapy administered for deep vein thrombosis prophylaxis.[49] Continuation of anticoagulant therapy following hospital discharge is determined at the level of the individual patient with special consideration to the patient's history, age, and mobility.[53]

Intraoperatively, strict adherence to general principles such as preservation of intestinal blood supply, gentle handling of tissue, avoidance of spillage of enteric contents, careful orientation of bowel segments, and realignment of the mesentery is critical in the avoidance of bowel-related complications. Occasionally a patient has such significant bowel adhesions or a tethered mesentery that placement of the neobladder within the pelvis becomes unfeasible. Multiple maneuvers are available for attempts to place the neobladder to the proper anatomic location for urethral anastomosis,[10] but in the event these are unsuccessful, continent cutaneous diversion or incontinent diversion with an ileal conduit should be performed.

Bowel Complications

Early bowel complications are usually related to the bowel resection and subsequent anastomosis. These complications can include anastomotic leak, enteric fistula, bowel obstruction, and prolonged ileus. These entities often manifest in the early postoperative period as wound infections or abdominal abscesses and if undiscovered may progress to sepsis. Fortunately, these complications are relatively uncommon but nonetheless may be a cause of early major morbidity and mortality. This possibility underscores the need for prompt recognition and treatment.

The most common cause of delay in bowel function following intestinal reconstruction is paralytic ileus.[54] The incidence of this complication varies by series, era, and definition but in general approaches 20%. In a series of 304 patients who underwent radical cystectomy, half of whom underwent neobladder diversions, ileus was the most common cause of increased length of hospital stay and was clinically apparent in 18% of patients.[47] Most of these cases resolved with conservative management. Conservative management entails early ambulation, correction of electrolyte abnormalities, and encouraging moderate use of narcotic pain medications. Nasogastric tubes were not used routinely in this cohort and were reserved only for those patients with significant abdominal distention or emesis. Other series also advocated avoidance of nasogastric tubes or their early removal following cystectomy and urinary diversion.[55-57]

Although published evidence is not overwhelming,[58,59] total parenteral nutrition should be considered in patients with prolonged delay in enteral feeding, to avoid subsequent clinical malnutrition and deterioration.[60] More recent series have indicated that early oral or parenteral feeding may not affect the return of bowel function,[61,62] so the use of oral or parenteral nutrition is possibly best reserved for patients with prolonged ileus. Patients who undergo cystectomy should also routinely be treated with a proton pump inhibitor or histamine (H_2) blocker to decrease gastric pH and to facilitate prevention of clinically significant gastric bleeding.[63] Although some surgeons favor the use of metoclopramide as an adjunct to prevent postoperative nausea and vomiting by promoting intestinal motility, no substantial evidence from controlled trials supports this approach.[64]

Bowel obstruction occurs uncommonly in the early postoperative setting, although the historical incidence is between 1% and 15%.[28,54,65] Patients with obstruction may experience any combination of abdominal pain, distention, nausea, emesis, and obstipation. Because mechanical ileus provokes dehydration and electrolyte disturbances, adequate fluid resuscitation, particularly replacement of nasogastric tube output, is critical.

Initial imaging traditionally included flat and upright plain abdominal films to demonstrate distended loops of bowel on the supine view (**Fig. 48-1**), as well as air-fluid levels on the upright view. An unresolving obstruction may merit imaging with computed tomography (CT) including oral contrast or an upper gastrointestinal series with a small bowel follow-through to define the point of mechanical obstruction further. As with paralytic ileus, most partial mechanical bowel obstructions resolve with conservative management, and only a few patients require reoperation.[46,54,66,67] The most common cause of bowel obstruction is adhesions, although fascial and internal hernias can be culpable as well. In addition to careful closure of mesenteric apertures, a novel bioabsorbable membrane of hyaluronate and carboxymethylcellulose (Seprafilm) is available for intraoperative application to diminish the rate of significant bowel adhesions.[68]

Recurrent cancer should always be considered in the differential diagnosis in patients presenting with a late bowel-related complication, even in the absence of demonstrable radiographic findings. When surgical exploration is required, a pathology report should be obtained to rule out recurrent cancer.

Anastomotic bowel leak or breakdown is a potentially devastating complication that has been reported in urologic reconstruction in 1% to 5% of patients.[69] Factors contributing to anastomotic breakdown include

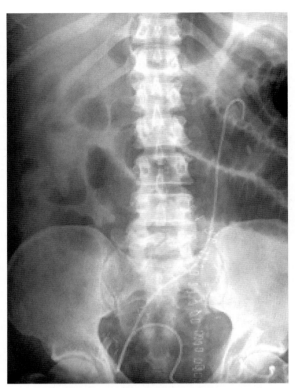

Figure 48-1 Partial small bowel obstruction in an abdominal plain film following cystectomy. Note the substantial dilation of the small bowel and limited air in the distal colon. This patient has a solitary kidney and thus a single ureteral stent emanating from the neobladder.

surgical techniques, bowel ischemia, prior radiation therapy, systemic steroid use, inflammatory bowel disease, and distal bowel obstruction. Attempts to avoid anastomotic breakdown include adequate bowel preparation, irrigation of the bowel segment before manipulation to prevent undue spillage of enteric contents into the peritoneum, use of nonirradiated and well-vascularized bowel, and placement of omentum over the anastomosis.[28,69] Patients with poor nutritional status or chronic pulmonary disease and those who received >2 U red blood cell transfusions also appear to be at higher risk for anastomotic complications.[70]

Unrecognized anastomotic leaks may lead to septic complications including abscess formation, wound dehiscence, and fistula formation. This possibility underscores the importance of early recognition and prompt correction. Fever, leukocytosis, and abdominal pain in the early postoperative period should be aggressively evaluated with abdominal CT scan with oral and IV contrast to delineate the anastomotic leak and any developing abscess. Broad-spectrum antibiotics should be administered early to prevent the development of sepsis, and patients should be kept without oral intake. Although on many occasions the abscess can be percutaneously drained by interventional radiologic means, the surgeon must maintain a high level of vigilance and suspicion for the potential presence of necrotic bowel that would require emergency reoperation.[69]

Resection of >60 cm of ileum for neobladder formation may decrease bile acid reabsorption that cannot be adequately compensated for by hepatic production, with resulting bile salt, lipid, and vitamin B_{12} malabsorption and profound diarrhea.[71] Oxalate levels may additionally become elevated and thus increase the propensity for urinary calculus formation. Cholestyramine has been used to bind excess bile acids and to treat diarrhea, but long-term therapy is poorly tolerated.[72,73] Careful attention to preservation of the ileocecal valve and appropriate use of <60 cm of intestine are the best strategies to prevent sequelae of malabsorption.

Orthotopic diversion allows significant prolonged contact of urine with bowel mucosa. When ileum is used for neobladder construction, ammonium, hydrogen ion, and chloride are reabsorbed with wasting of sodium and bicarbonate into the lumen and resulting hyperchloremic metabolic acidosis, which is reported to occur in ≤10% of patients.[22,74] Early postoperative treatment with sodium bicarbonate (2-6 g/day) may assist in preventing the salt-wasting hypovolemic and acidotic state.[15] Patients are usually weaned from these treatments after the first few months because persistent significant acidosis is rare in patients with normal renal function. However, yearly monitoring of electrolyte status can diagnose and help avert long-term complications of acidosis such as bone demineralization.

Urethral Anastomotic Complications

The ileal neobladder can be complicated by persistent urinary leakage at the neovesical-urethral anastomosis, as manifested by high drain output in the postoperative period. Large series specifically addressing neobladder diversion indicated early urethral anastomotic leak occurrence between 2.1% and 6.6%, with later ileourethral leakage at <1%.[15] Additional series reported rates of urethral anastomotic leak of approximately 3% to 7.7%, with only a minute percentage requiring operative intervention.[46,75,76] Neovesical-urethral anastomotic leaks most often spontaneously close with continued drainage and decompression of the neobladder.

When evaluating anastomotic leak, the surgeon must rule out outlet obstruction as a cause. Urinary retention resulting from mucus obstruction occurs between 1.2% and 4.6% of the time and can contribute to anastomotic leakage as well as the rare but potentially devastating complication of neobladder perforation.[15,77] Regardless of whether a suprapubic tube (which incidentally, we no longer routinely use) is placed in the neobladder in conjunction with the urethral catheter, regular irrigation of the neobladder in the initial postoperative period decreases mucus retention and facilitates emptying to

reduce neobladder-urethral anastomotic leakage and allow optimal healing.

It is also critical to ensure that the Foley catheter is in the proper position and that it has not migrated out of the neobladder into the urethra. We generally use a 20- or 22-Fr Foley catheter with a 10-mL balloon and inflate the balloon to 15 mL to allow a spherical configuration. A larger catheter is necessary to allow for irrigation of mucus or blood clots in the early postoperative period. Occasionally it may be useful to manipulate the placement of the drain lying on the anastomotic suture line to ensure that the drain itself is not perpetuating the leak.[77] A cystogram may be performed before drain or catheter removal to ensure complete closure at the urethral anastomosis. For prolonged urine leakage or in patients who develop metabolic derangements from urinary extravasation, bilateral percutaneous nephrostomy tubes can be placed for temporary diversion along with a Foley catheter and pelvic drain. Prevention of urethral anastomotic leaks may be aided by meticulous mucosa-to-mucosa approximation of a tension-free suture line and avoidance of overdistention of the neobladder resulting from catheter malfunction or mucus plugging.

A later complication of the neovesical-urethral anastomosis is stricture, which often manifests as difficulty with neobladder emptying. The reported incidence of this complication is approximately 2.4% to 9%.[15,46,48,76,78,79] Failure to empty after orthotopic urinary diversion necessitates cystoscopic and radiographic examination to differentiate between dysfunctional voiding and neovesicourethral obstruction. Dysfunctional voiding commonly results from an unsuitable size or shape of the neobladder, from the position, length, or angulation of the neobladder neck, or from a denervated proximal urethra. In contrast, neovesicourethral obstruction is caused by stricture, distal urethral obstruction, local tumor recurrence, cystolithiasis, or obstructive mucosal valves.[78]

Cystoscopy is the primary diagnostic tool allowing direct visualization of the bladder neck and quantitative assessment of the anastomotic stricture. Other diagnostic modalities such as transrectal ultrasound of the vesicourethral anastomosis, ultrasound of postvoid residual, cystography, and CT or magnetic resonance imaging of the pelvis can further assist in differentiating dysfunctional voiding from anastomotic stricture.

Treatment options for anastomotic strictures vary from conservative management with continuous intermittent catheterization or dilation at the level of the bladder neck to transurethral resection or transurethral incision with cold knife, electrocautery, or holmium laser. Although many of these strictures can be managed with transurethral incision or resection, it is paramount to sample tissue and exclude recurrent cancer as a cause. In addition, vigilant follow-up is required to identify early recurrent strictures and to ensure proper emptying. Patients whose neobladder becomes overdistended as a result of outlet obstruction should be instructed to perform intermittent catheterization to ensure proper emptying because the tonicity of the neobladder may not return to baseline. This approach may also serve to check that the stricture has not recurred and that the anastomosis is widely patent.

Ureterointestinal Anastomotic Complications

One of the most difficult complications of urinary diversion is breakdown or stricture of the ureterointestinal anastomosis. Once again, basic surgical tenets are paramount in reducing or preventing anastomotic complications. During mobilization of the ureters, great care must be taken not to devascularize the distal end, and adequate length must be achieved to avoid tension on the anastomosis. Care must be taken to avoid kinking of the left ureter as it is passes beneath the mesentery of the sigmoid colon. Additionally, every effort should be made to create a watertight anastomosis with absorbable suture material.

The incidence of ureteroenteric anastomotic leak decreased significantly with the routine use of soft Silastic stents placed across ureteroenteric anastomosis at the time of diversion.[12,80] This technique is now used almost universally and has a reported rate of urinary leakage of approximately 3%.[46] Studies have investigated placement of self-retaining ureteral stents following neobladder diversion with a similar incidence of complications.[81] Of course, stents alone do not eliminate complications of ureteroenteric anastomosis and can lead to additional complications when they are improperly positioned or are inadvertently sutured to the ureter. Indeed, obstruction or infectious complications including urosepsis may result from occluded ureteral stents.

Ureteral stents are routinely removed before the removal of the pelvic drain. Anastomotic urinary leakage is suspected when drain output is increased or when urinary drainage from the wound is noted, particularly in the setting of decreased urine output. Suspicion of urinary leakage should trigger prompt assessment. Evaluation of the suspected fluid for creatinine content is usually the first step. If the creatinine concentration in the fluid is higher than that of the serum, further testing should include imaging such as a CT scan or IV pyelogram (IVP) to identify the site of urinary extravasation. Most often, initial management is conservative, involving adequate drainage and placement of a percutaneous nephrostomy tube along with continued closed-suction drainage and close monitoring. If leakage persists, usually antegrade stent placement through the nephrostomy will be attempted. Rarely is surgical intervention necessary in the early postoperative period for this complication.

Urinary leakage at the ureteroenteric anastomotic site can lead to periureteral fibrosis and predispose to stricture formation. Other causes of stricture include tension at the anastomosis, ischemia of the ureter, infection, and recurrence of cancer. The incidence of ureteroenteric stricture is between 2% and 7%.[15,28,46,65,76] Ureteral strictures can also occur away from the anastomosis where the left ureter crosses beneath the inferior mesenteric artery.

An exhaustive review of specific ureteroenteric anastomotic techniques is beyond the scope of this chapter, but considerable debate remains about whether a nonrefluxing or refluxing anastomosis is most desirable for orthotopic urinary diversion.[12,77,82] Arguments for provision of an antireflux mechanism include the potential harmful effects on renal function secondary to recurrent pyelonephritis from reflux of colonized urine.[8] Primary opinions supporting a refluxing anastomosis describe a higher incidence of obstruction with the antirefluxing mechanism; these proponents also argue that the neobladder is a low-pressure reservoir and that urine is assumed to be sterile. Studies addressing renal function indicate no detrimental effect on renal function in patients who have neobladders without an antireflux mechanism at an average follow-up of 50 months.[83] However, upper urinary tract deterioration may need to be measured over decades, not months.[12]

Other series additionally indicate a higher level of upper urinary tract deterioration with antirefluxing techniques as a result of stricture formation and obstruction.[84,85] A large cohort with >350 patients who received a Hautmann neobladder with a LeDuc antirefluxing anastomosis had a ureteroenteric stricture rate of 9.3% at average follow-up of 54 months.[86] Abol-Enein and Ghoneim[87] reviewed >300 patients who received a Hautmann neobladder with an antirefluxing serous-lined extramural tunnel technique and reported a 3.8% rate of stricture with unspecified follow-up.

In a series of 166 Kock ileal neobladders in which the ureteroenteric anastomosis was performed with a refluxing end-to-end Wallace technique, the stricture rate was only 0.6% with follow-up of 2.7 years.[88] In a cohort of 32 patients with refluxing ureteroileal anastomosis into a Studer limb, <1% of renal units developed a stricture with 2-year follow-up.[89] Another study examining 130 patients who received either a Studer or a Hautmann neobladder with a refluxing end-to-side Bricker anastomosis found only 3 ureteroenteric strictures at a mean follow-up of 20 months.[90] Thus the rate of ureteroenteric stricture has varied greatly among the large neobladder series that have incorporated both refluxing and nonrefluxing anastomosis, although the general trend reveals lower stricture rates with nonrefluxing anastomoses.

To date, studies evaluating the different anastomotic techniques that are well designed, prospective, and

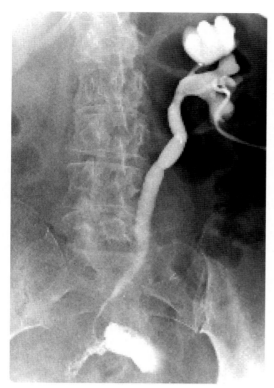

Figure 48-2 Ureterointestinal stricture. Note the dilation of the proximal collecting system above the stricture at the distal ureter in this nephrostogram. Some contrast material still passes through the stricture into the neobladder.

randomized, with appropriate numbers and long-term follow-up, have not been performed. We believe that a simple end-to-side, freely refluxing anastomosis to an afferent limb of a low-pressure neobladder is sufficient and has an acceptably low rate of anastomotic stricture.

Regardless of the technique used for ureterointestinal anastomosis, prompt diagnosis and treatment of anastomotic strictures are paramount to preserve renal function. Although many patients are asymptomatic and the diagnosis is made by the presence of hydronephrosis on routine surveillance imaging, patients with ureteroneobladder strictures may present with flank pain, pyelonephritis, or renal insufficiency.

Ureteroenteric stricture can be diagnosed with IVP, CT scan, or antegrade nephrostogram if obstruction is of high grade and percutaneous intervention with nephrostomy placement is indicated (**Fig. 48-2**). It is imperative that tumor recurrence be excluded in these patients before a specific treatment is initiated. This goal is usually accomplished through a combination of radiographic, endoscopic, and cytologic evaluations. In addition, the function of the involved renal unit should be determined, and in patients with poorly functioning units (<15%), strong consideration should be given to the performance of simple nephrectomy.

Several techniques have been used to treat ureteroenteric strictures including balloon dilation, endoscopic incision with both antegrade and retrograde approaches, and open revision.[77,91] In addition to the potential presence of malignant disease, factors considered in determining the optimal operative strategy must account for the length of the stricture and the history of prior irradiation to the area. Endourologic procedures using balloon dilation have been reported, although success rates are generally no better than 29% with long-term follow-up.[91] Endoscopic incision of strictures has been employed with short-term success rates of approximately 70%.[92] Longer follow-up was not as favorable in this series, which had only a 32% patency rate after endourologic treatment of ureteroenteric strictures at 3 years.

The best results have been seen with short (<2 cm) distal strictures treated when the patient's renal function remains good. Leaving a stent of ≥12 Fr for ≥4 weeks also may increase success rates. Data also suggest improved outcome with local injection of steroids (triamcinolone) into the stricture bed following surgical incision. Success was universally poor for endoscopic treatment in renal units with <25% function.

Open surgical correction with excision of the stenotic segment and revision of the anastomosis yields the highest rate of success but with the tradeoff of a technically challenging and potentially morbid procedure. Anastomotic revision is assisted by placement of an antegrade stent abutting or even through the anastomotic stricture to assist in intraoperative identification of the ureter. This technique is particularly useful in the setting of dense adhesions and fibrosis in which initial identification of the ureter may be difficult. Similarly, a catheter is placed in the neobladder to allow for intraoperative identification. It may also be necessary to revise the contralateral ureteral anastomosis in the event that it is in close proximity to the area of repair.

After recognition and excision of the ureteral stricture, the ureter is spatulated and reanastomosed to the orthotopic diversion. In general, the neobladder enjoys more redundancy than does the ureter, which is often encased in a fibrotic reaction. It is important to evaluate the excised segment of strictured ureter by frozen section pathologic analysis to rule out malignant disease. In the case of large ureteral defects, ileal interposition, transureteroureterostomy, or even nephrectomy may be necessary. These patients should undergo full mechanical and antibiotic bowel preparation to minimize complications and to maximize intraoperative surgical options.

The success rate of open revision of ureterointestinal strictures approaches 90%.[77,93] Not surprisingly, left ureteroenteric strictures are often more difficult because of the longer course and pathway under the sigmoid mesentery. Right ureteroenteric strictures may in certain circumstances be approached from a completely extra-peritoneal approach.

Urolithiasis

Urolithiasis in neobladders can be caused by a variety of factors including metabolic derangements, retained mucus, urinary stasis, and chronic infection.[94] Current opinion is that neobladders are less often colonized compared with continent cutaneous diversions unless long-term catheterization is needed.[95] Reservoirs created with exposed metallic staples have a significantly higher incidence of urolithiasis. Series with the orthotopic Kock neobladder in which exposed permanent staples were used to create the intussuscepted nipple valve reported urolithiasis in the range of 30% at 3-year follow-up.[88] The use of absorbable staples for the afferent nipple valve construction in the Kock neobladder reduced the rate of stones to 4%.[96]

More recent series that did not use staples in neobladder construction reported much lower rates of urolithiasis in the range of 0.5% to 3%.[87,97] As mentioned previously, resection of large portions of ileum may result in increased oxalate absorption and thus raise the risk of urinary calculus formation. For patients with limited stone burden within the neobladder, transurethral techniques may be used, although some investigators favor a percutaneous or open approach to avoid compromising the continence mechanism of the neobladder.[94]

Upper tract calculi are also common complications of urinary diversion. Urinary stasis resulting from chronic dilation is likely a major culprit in stone formation. Most upper urinary tract calculi appear on the left side, a finding suggesting causality with mobilization and transposition of the left ureter.[98] Contemporary treatments include all modalities of management from shock wave lithotripsy to percutaneous nephrolithotomy.[98-101] Planning an operative strategy naturally depends on the stone burden, location, likely composition, and anatomic considerations, as well as the surgeon's comfort with procedures. Retrograde endoscopic management is particularly difficult in orthotopic neobladder diversions even with nonrefluxing anastomoses, and a combination of alternative modalities is often used. Accordingly, almost all ureteral and renal pelvic stones requiring endoscopic intervention are approached by an antegrade percutaneous approach.

Urinary Tract Colonization and Pyelonephritis

Bacterial colonization of the neobladder diversion occurs in 40% to 80% of patients.[102-104] Colonization is strongly associated with both residual urine[105] and the need to perform self-catheterization.[106] Treatment of the neobladder bacteriuria remains a controversial topic in that approximately half of these patients remain asymptomatic from the infection.

In a prospective evaluation of 66 patients with neobladders who were evaluated with urinalysis and culture 2 months to 4 years postoperatively,[103] 55 patients voided normally and 11 performed intermittent catheterization at least once daily as a result of high postvoid residual urine. Of the patients who voided normally, 78% had at least 1 positive urinalysis, and of these bacteria was identified on culture in 50%. Overall, 26 (39%) and 8 (12%) patients had urinary tract infection and urosepsis, respectively. The estimated 5-year probabilities of urinary tract infection and urosepsis in patients who voided independently were 58% and 18%, respectively. Urine culture with >100,000 colony-forming units and female gender were the only factors predictive of urinary tract infection on multivariate analysis. Recurrent urinary tract infection was the only predictor for urosepsis. These investigators recommended prophylactic antibiotics only for patients with recurring urinary tract infections but did not advocate treating patients with a positive urinary culture in the absence of symptoms. However, it is recommended that treatment be pursued in patients with urea-splitting organisms because of the high risk of stone formation.[95]

Approximately 6% of patients with neobladders progress to overt pyelonephritis at some point following urinary diversion.[15] In the absence of obstruction, upper urinary tract infections can be managed with administration of culture-specific antibiotics.

Fistulas

When indications for orthotopic diversion were initially extended to female patients, surgeons were appropriately concern about the rate of neobladder-to-vagina fistula.[107,108] Fortunately, neobladder-vaginal fistula formation was reported at <5% in multiple series.[87,109,110] Surgical refinements that decreased fistula formation include the avoidance of overlapping suture lines and the interposition of omentum when the anterior vaginal wall has been incised or partially excised. When oncologic control is not compromised, the ideal technique includes avoidance of entry into the vagina and preservation of the anterior vaginal wall.[110,111] Most fistulas that develop in the setting of a female neobladder require surgical intervention, and they often are not amenable to repair without complete mobilization and subsequent interposition of omentum or a vascularized pedicle flap (**Fig. 48-3**).

A dreaded complication of neobladder diversion is the development of enterocutaneous or neobladder-enteric fistulas. Mortality is pronounced with these abnormal communications, so diagnosis and treatment must be prompt. As addressed earlier, poor nutritional status, anastomotic leak, devascularization of tissue during the surgical procedure, steroid use, multiple

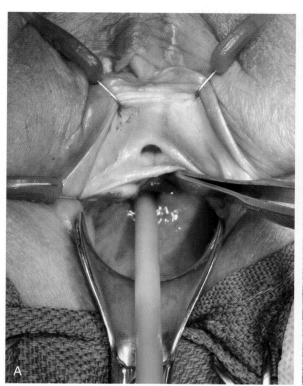
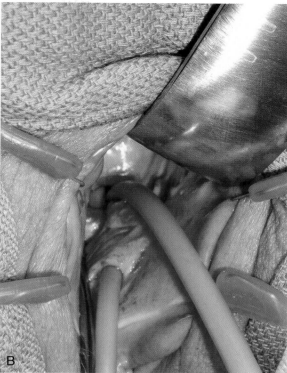

Figure 48-3 Neobladder-vaginal fistula visualized in (**A**) lithotomy and (**B**) prone positions. A catheter is placed into the neobladder through the fistula tract. The urethra is additionally shown catheterized in the prone position.

medical comorbidities, and unprepared bowel all contribute to fistula formation.[54] Enterocutaneous fistulas often manifest between 4 and 7 days postoperatively but of course may become apparent at any time during the follow-up. Patients generally present with fever, leukocytosis, metabolic derangements, and signs of cellulitis that progress to frank spillage of enteric contents onto skin.

Broad-spectrum antibiotics should be briskly administered to ward off sepsis, and CT scan of the abdomen should be obtained to rule out intra-abdominal abscess. Following supportive treatment and stabilization, a fistulogram may assist in localizing the tract and in determining whether further conservative management is merited. In cases of obvious peritonitis, exploration with or without bowel diversion is necessary. In the absence of infection, in patients with sufficient bowel rest and supplementation of nutritional status with either a low-residue diet or total parenteral nutrition, 60% to 80% of enterocutaneous fistulas spontaneously close. For the remainder of patients, operative management is preferable ≤6 weeks of the initial diagnosis.

Fistulas between small or large bowel and neobladder may be more insidious in onset and may manifest with pneumaturia, fecaluria, diarrhea, and general abdominal symptoms. The diagnosis is often confirmed by a traditional or CT cystogram (**Figs. 48-4 and 48-5**). In the absence of gas-producing organisms, the finding of air in the anterior portion of a noninstrumented patient

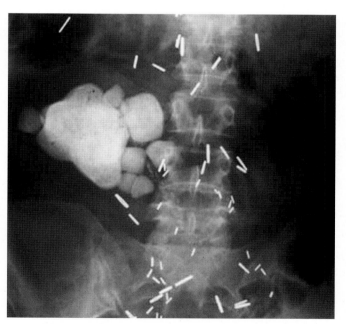

Figure 48-4 Neobladder-enteric fistula on cystogram. Note the extravasation of contrast material into bowel in this postvoid film. Also of interest in this image is ureteral reflux.

on CT scan should arouse strong suspicion of this fistula. Again, conservative measures, which in this case include neobladder catheter drainage, may allow healing of small fistulas,[112,113] but definitive operative management often becomes necessary.[114] At the time of surgical cor-

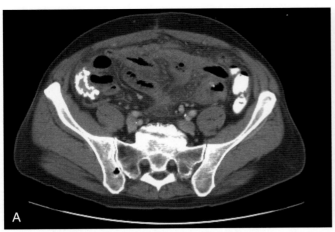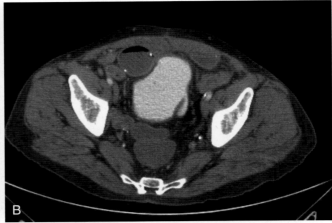

Figure 48-5 Neobladder-enteric fistula on CT cystogram. **A,** Note the presence of gas in the fluid collection anterior to the neobladder that is suggestive of fistula. **B,** Cystogram reveals the fistula tract on the left lateral aspect of the neobladder.

rection, the surgeon should obtain a biopsy sample of the fistula site to exclude recurrent malignant disease as the underlying cause. Rare cases of vascular fistulas with orthotopic diversion have been reported and successfully treated with endovascular repair.[115]

Voiding Dysfunction

The perceived improved quality of life of the orthotopic neobladder as compared with incontinent diversion may be significantly reduced or eliminated in patients with severe voiding dysfunction.[116] Daytime incontinence may range from mild stress incontinence to total incontinence in a small percentage of patients, but complete daytime continence is achieved in close to 90% of patients with neobladders.[15] As many as 50% of patients experience some degree of nighttime incontinence. Alternatively, approximately 8% of patients may develop hypercontinence or high postvoid residuals requiring self-catheterization.[77,117] This situation is particularly common following an episode of urinary retention in which the bladder may become silently overdistended and may fail to recover its natural tonicity.

A comparison of the severity and incidence of voiding dysfunction among various surgical series is confounded by the variability in definitions, end points, surgical technique, and length of follow-up. Additionally, symptoms have rarely been assessed using validated instruments. With these limitations noted, a review of >2000 patients with orthotopic neobladders did provide a clear characterization of associated voiding dysfunction. This meta-analysis showed that 4% to 25% of patients with orthotopic neobladders performed intermittent self-catheterization for incomplete emptying. Daytime incontinence was present in approximately 13% of patients.[116]

As with the fashioning of other types of urinary diversion, general surgical principles must be main-

tained to maximize chances of optimal functional outcomes and to reduce complications. The neobladder must be constructed such that it can accommodate a sufficient volume under low pressure with limited absorption of urine.[12] Intrinsic to the spheroid shape of the reservoir are mathematical principles that dictate the optimal length of bowel to achieve the desired capacity.[73] Ideally, a segment of bowel 50 to 55 cm in length is selected. If the segment is too small, the capacity will be low and will risk unnecessary and avoidable incontinence and urinary frequency.[118] Similarly, if too generous a segment of bowel is selected, poor emptying and urinary retention will ensue. Poor emptying can precipitate not only the need for lifelong self-catheterization but also distention and the rare but devastating complication of neobladder perforation.[119,120]

A report of a large series of neobladder emptying failures in men demonstrated an 8% incidence of mechanical dysfunction and a 3.5% incidence of dysfunctional voiding.[78] The investigators indicated that vigilant reservoir emptying to prevent excessive neobladder distention had a more profound impact on voiding function than did the length of bowel used and the corresponding size of the initial pouch.

During cystectomy, particular attention should be directed toward preserving the rhabdosphincter to protect the continence mechanism.[12,121] In men, the apical prostate dissection should be performed in a manner similar to that of radical prostatectomy. In women, the urethra and uninvolved bladder neck are preserved. In addition, a plane of dissection can be carried posterior to bladder and just above the anterior vaginal wall to preserve urethral innervation. It is also important to handle and preserve vaginal tissues, the levator muscle, and pelvic floor fascia gently. Finally, positioning the neobladder neck in the most dependent portion of the pelvis ensures proper funneling of the bladder outlet on voiding.

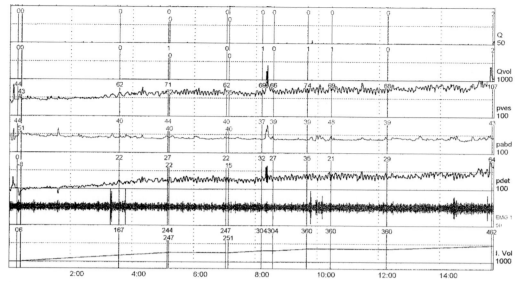

Figure 48-6 Urodynamic tracing of neobladder cystometry in a patient with voiding dysfunction. Note the hyperactivity of the neobladder in the detrusor pressure (pdet) tracing, which reveals neobladder overactivity. EMG, electromyogram; pabd, abdominal pressure; pves, total bladder pressure; Qvol, voided volume.

Urodynamic study is now frequently used to determine causes of dysfunctional voiding in the patient with a neobladder. Indeed, despite bowel detubularization,[122] uninhibited contractions resulting in incontinence may occur in almost half of reservoirs (**Fig. 48-6**).[123,124] These patients often benefit from pharmacologic intervention with anticholinergic agents to decrease neobladder overactivity. Women with de novo stress urinary incontinence following neobladder placement may be candidates for placement of a pubovaginal sling in a modified fashion so the areas of previous surgical intervention are avoided.[125]

In addition to aiding continence, careful neurovascular preservation appears to assist with preservation of sexual function in both male and female patients.[126-128] However, some analyses suggest that sexual function–preserving cystectomy may compromise oncologic control.[129]

Urethral and Pelvic Tumor Recurrence

The historical incidence of urethral recurrence following cystectomy is 10%,[130] but urethral recurrence with ileal neobladder in both male and female patients has been reported in the range of 0.5% to 5%.[48,131-134] This discrepancy is likely the result of both patient selection bias and careful intraoperative evaluation of the urethral margin with frozen section analysis before construction of an orthotopic reservoir.[135,136] Although surveillance cystoscopy or urethral washing for cytologic examination is generally advocated for screening following orthotopic diversion, large series demonstrated that the majority of patients with urethral recurrence actually developed symptoms that led to the diagnosis (discharge, pain, palpable mass) and the pres-

ence of positive cytologic findings did not affect stage or survival.[137,138] Additionally, the sensitivity of urethral wash cytology is extremely low.[139]

Most recurrences are detected within 5 years of cystectomy,[140] but lifelong screening is required because urethral tumors have been found ≤15 years after initial surgical treatment.[141] Whether these tumors actually represent recurrences of the original tumor or are a consequence of the field changes known to occur with urothelial cell cancers is unclear. However, once urethral recurrence is diagnosed, treatment depends on the type of recurrence. For invasive urothelial carcinoma, urethrectomy and conversion of the orthotopic diversion to an incontinent diversion are the therapeutic procedures of choice. Patients with carcinoma in situ have been successfully treated with bacille Calmette-Guérin (BCG) with an 83% response rate.[142] Superficial recurrences have also been managed with endoscopic resection.[131,143]

Pelvic recurrences occur in approximately 7% of patients who have undergone cystectomy,[144] but large-scale analyses indicated that local recurrence with functional impingement on the neobladder that requires resection is rare.[15] In one series, Freeman and colleagues[145] found an overall local recurrence rate of 11% in a study of predominantly male patients with orthotopic neobladders. A similar rate of pelvic recurrence (14%) was reported in another series examining patients with unfavorable histologic features.[146] In these series, one half to two thirds of patients with pelvic disease recurrence retained adequate neobladder function despite death from the disease. In another study, the type of urinary diversion did not change the risk of complications, the response to salvage treatment, or overall survival in patients with pelvic recurrences.[147] In rare circumstances, an ileal conduit or palliative diversion is necessary because of local tumor invasion of the neobladder.

Among women, the rate of pelvic disease recurrence after anterior exenteration was <5% in two separate studies, but in both series the recurrences were in patients without transitional cell carcinoma.[108,148] In a study of patients with squamous cell carcinoma, the pelvic recurrence rate was 12%.[149] Thus, female patients with squamous cell carcinoma and those with nonurothelial histologic features may be at higher risk for local recurrence and may not be appropriate candidates for vaginal sparing. When the anterior vaginal wall was preserved during cystectomy and neobladder formation among women with transitional cell carcinoma, the local recurrence rate was 5%.[110]

Neobladder Rupture

Spontaneous rupture of an orthotopic neobladder has been reported to occur in 1.5% to 4.3% of patients.[119,150] This complication is most commonly the result of acute or chronic overdistention of the neobladder. However, other causes include instrumentation, catheter trauma, mucus retention, and altered sensorium from drug or alcohol effects. Patients prone to overdistention or excess mucus production must be instructed to be vigilant in continuous intermittent catheterization every 4 hours to avoid this uncommon but occasionally life-threatening complication. Patients with orthotopic diversions should be instructed to wear medical alert bracelets to inform medical personnel in the event of an emergency.

The presentation of spontaneous orthotopic neobladder rupture is generally that of acute abdominal pain accompanied by abdominal distention and decreased urine output. In the setting of infection, the patient may present with peritonitis or sepsis. An initial attempt should be made to place a Foley catheter in the neobladder. A cystogram can then be performed to evaluate for extravasation. In addition to a standard CT scan of the abdomen and pelvis, a CT cystogram may be revealing. A high index of suspicion should be maintained if a large amount of free fluid likely representing urine is demonstrated on the CT scan even in the absence of extravasation on cystogram.

The presentation and overall clinical features in part dictate the magnitude of treatment for neobladder rupture. Patients without signs of overt peritonitis or sepsis may be managed initially with conservative measures including catheter drainage, broad-spectrum antibiotics, and careful monitoring of vital signs and urine output.[151] However, patients with altered mental status, intractable pain, hemodynamic instability, or frank peritonitis should undergo emergency surgical exploration. Exploratory laparotomy with drainage of peritoneal urinary ascites and repair of neobladder rupture should be performed. A large-caliber intraperitoneal drain and large-caliber Foley catheter should be placed for postoperative management. Generally, the Foley catheter is removed after 3 weeks, any underlying cause of the complication is corrected, and the patient is monitored closely to ensure that neobladder compromise does not recur.

KEY POINTS

1. Proper patient selection is probably the single most important factor in determining the ultimate success or failure of orthotopic neobladder diversion.

2. Absolute contraindications to orthotopic neobladder include significant renal disease, severe hepatic dysfunction, inflammatory bowel disease, radiation enteritis, sphincter dysfunction, severe urethral stricture disease, inability to manage neobladder care, and any compromise of oncologic control.

3. Most neovesical-urethral anastomotic leaks will spontaneously close with conservative management; however, it is critical to evaluate for outlet obstruction due to mucus retention to prevent neobladder perforation.

4. Ureterointestinal strictures are less prevalent with a refluxing anastomosis. Such strictures are optimally approached in an antegrade fashion for initial endoscopic management.

5. Patient counseling about potential neobladder voiding dysfunction including nighttime incontinence, stress incontinence, and hypercontinence must be thoroughly addressed preoperatively so that outcomes are aligned with expectations.

REFERENCES

Please see www.expertconsult.com

Chapter 49

COMPLICATIONS OF BLADDER AUGMENTATION

Polina Reyblat MD
Urology Resident, Department of Urology, Keck School of Medicine, University of Southern California, Los Angeles, California

David A. Ginsberg MD
Associate Professor of Urology, Department of Urology, Keck School of Medicine, University of Southern California, Los Angeles; Chief of Urology, Rancho Los Amigos National Rehabilitation Center, Downey, California

Augmentation of the bladder with the use of an intestinal segment was first described in 1989 by von Mikulicz. It was not until the 1950s, however, that this procedure became more widely used after a report by Couvelaire described augmentation of small, contracted tuberculous bladders. Bladder augmentation is now a widely accepted technique used to increase bladder capacity. Today, patients are more likely to require bladder augmentation secondary to neurogenic bladder (NGB); other potential indications for cystoplasty include idiopathic overactive bladder, radiation or chemotherapy cystitis, schistosomiasis, and interstitial cystitis. Although ileum is most commonly used, intestinal segments from the stomach to the colon have been chosen for bladder augmentation.

The goal of this chapter is to discuss the presentation and incidence of the various complications seen with bladder augmentation, techniques to avoid these complications during the initial surgical procedure, and therapies and procedures available to treat the complications. Two distinct populations undergo bladder augmentation. Patients with NGB tend to be younger. Although certain complications noted in this chapter may be specific to patients with neurologic disease, these patients are also less likely to encounter some of the complications that may be more common in older, more debilitated patients who do not have NGB.

SHORT-TERM COMPLICATIONS

Relatively few early complications are specifically related to bladder augmentation surgery. As seen with any intra-abdominal procedure, patients undergoing bladder augmentation are at risk for cardiovascular, pulmonary, gastrointestinal, and thromboembolic perioperative events. A mortality rate as high as 2.7% was reported in older literature. The higher mortality rates were also associated with additional surgical procedures. A review by Greenwell and colleagues in 2001[1] noted no deaths in 267 patients undergoing bladder augmentation who were followed up for ≥5 years. Other commonly noted early surgical complications include a 1.9% to 5.7% risk of bowel obstruction requiring intervention and a risk of a significant wound infection of ≤6.4%.[1] Bleeding requiring blood transfusion is seen in ≤3% or less of patients undergoing cystoplasty.[1]

The incidence of early bladder anastomotic leak (**Fig. 49-1**) after augmentation is extremely low.[2] Early leaks are prevented by optimal bladder drainage, which can be achieved with use of both a urethral and a suprapubic catheter. The perivesical space should be well drained. The augmented bladder should be regularly irrigated to evacuate mucus and to minimize the risk of a mucus plug. Mucus plugs can clog a catheter and lead to poor urinary drainage of the newly constructed augment with possible leak at the anastomosis. Small anastomotic leaks that are adequately drained should heal on their own with time. When a trial of conservative therapy fails to heal clinically significant anastomotic leaks, percutaneous drainage of both kidneys and drainage of urinoma, if one is present, are required. Rarely, anastomotic leak can be caused by an ischemic bowel segment, and in these cases conservative management is not successful. Laparotomy with resection of the nonviable segment and repeat anastomosis are necessary.

Infection of a ventriculoperitoneal shunt is an unusual issue that should be specifically watched for in

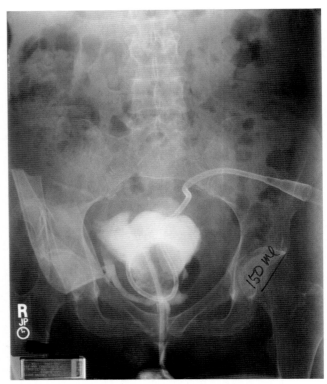

Figure 49-1 Cystogram demonstrating an early leak after augmentation ileocystoplasty.

certain patients undergoing bladder augmentation procedures. Most patients with myelomeningocele have a ventriculoperitoneal shunt and thus are at risk for shunt infection. Appropriate perioperative antibiotics should be given and any risk of intestinal spillage into the abdominal cavity should be minimized. One technique to guard against this complication is the use of the extraperitoneal augment, which allows a significant portion of the operation to be performed extraperitoneally and thus minimizes exposure of the shunt to potential infection. Symptoms of an infected ventriculoperitoneal shunt include fever, headaches, lethargy, change in vision and mental status, and seizures. In addition to significant morbidity, shunt infections are linked to higher risks of future shunt infection and malfunction, intellectual impairment, and even death.[3] If shunt infection is suspected, broad-spectrum antibiotics (vancomycin, frequently in combination with rifampin) should be instituted and neurosurgical consultation initiated.[4]

Intraoperatively, surgeons should also be able to recognize the signs and symptoms of a latex allergy reaction. This allergy is most commonly seen in patients with myelomeningocele and often manifests as a precipitous drop in blood pressure related to the reaction to the latex in the surgical gloves that are in contact with the intra-abdominal contents. Because of the known risk of this potentially life-threatening complica-

tion in this patient population, most centers now require surgeons operating on patients with spina bifida to wear nonlatex surgical gloves and to use latex-free catheters and latex-free surgical drains. If a reaction does occur intraoperatively, recommendations include instant interruption of contact with possible antigens (change gloves, surgical drains, and possibly contaminated instruments), copious irrigation of the field, expeditious completion or termination of the surgical procedure, volume expansion, and appropriate resuscitation and management of anaphylaxis by the anesthesia team.

LONG-TERM COMPLICATIONS

Late complications of bladder augmentation surgery include bacteriuria and urinary tract infections (UTIs), metabolic disturbances, formation of stones, perforation of the augmented bladder, the need to perform intermittent catheterization (IC), and the potential risk of tumor formation. Finally, the outcome of bladder augmentation in pregnancy and obstetric issues in patients with previous bladder augmentation are discussed.

Urinary Tract Infection and Bacteriuria

Asymptomatic bacteriuria is a common finding in patients with bladder augmentation. Most studies have estimated the incidence to be somewhere between 65% and 100% of patients. The need for IC certainly helps predispose these patients to bacteriuria. Because urinary retention and the need for IC are the goals of cystoplasty in patients with NGB, the finding of bacteriuria is as much an expectation as it is a complication in these patients. Patients undergoing bladder augmentation for non-neurogenic reasons are more likely to be able to void on their own and therefore have one less risk factor for bacteriuria. Other risk factors for bacteriuria in patients after bladder augmentation include large residual urine volume and the presence of mucus, which can harbor bacteria.

Symptomatic UTI is not as common as is asymptomatic bacteriuria; most have cited an incidence between 4% and 49%.[5,6] One reason for such a broad range could be the various definitions of symptomatic UTI in these patients. For example, patients with NGB may be insensate; therefore, one cannot reply on the typical symptoms of UTI such as frequency, urgency, and dysuria. Patients with NGB may have vague symptoms such as an increase in spasticity, malodorous or cloudy urine, or symptoms of concomitant autonomic dysreflexia.

Because of the lack of clear-cut symptoms, at times it is not always easy to determine when antibiotics should be instituted for certain patients. In the absence of classic symptoms of UTI, the clinician must rely on clinical judgment. In addition, bacteriuria should be treated if urea-splitting organisms are identified because these organisms may lead to stone formation. Patients often do have a clear idea when their vague symptoms are a sign of true infection. The presence of significant pyuria can also be an indication of more than asymptomatic bacteriuria.

Recurrent UTI can be a significant issue for many patients with NGB at baseline before bladder augmentation. It is not always clear whether a postoperative infection in these patients is a continuation of their preoperative bladder disease or whether the infection is the result of the bladder augmentation procedure itself. Despite the need for IC in patients undergoing bladder augmentation for NGB, these patients have fewer instances of postoperative UTI compared with the preoperative state.[7] This finding may be related to secretion of immunoglobulin A by the bowel that is thought to prevent bacterial adherence to epithelial cells.[8] Several therapeutic options are available for patients with recurrent UTI. Initially, imaging of the upper and lower urinary tract should be performed to rule out potential sources of infection. If results of the radiographic studies are negative, patients can be encouraged to irrigate the bladder regularly during IC. This maneuver may help to remove mucus, which can be a potential source of bacteria. In addition, patients may benefit from changing IC technique by evolving from clean IC and reusing the catheter to sterile IC with one-time use catheter kits. Evidence also indicates that hydrophilic catheters may be helpful in decreasing the risk of recurrent UTI in patients who regularly perform IC.[9]

Stones

The incidence of stone disease in patients with bladder augmentation ranges from 10% to 50%.[10,11] A higher incidence of stones is noted in patients with continent urinary stomas.[12] In fact, compared with findings in patients who have undergone bladder augmentation and who are able to void spontaneously, stones are 5 times more common in patients requiring IC through the native urethra and 10 times more common if IC is performed through a Mitrofanoff urinary stoma.[13] The reason is thought to be related to incomplete urinary emptying and urinary stasis that may be seen with this type of reconstruction as well as a higher incidence of bacteriuria in patients who perform IC. Recurrent UTI and concomitant bladder neck surgery also are significant risk factors for stone formation in patients with an augmented bladder.[14,15] A lower incidence of stone formation has been reported in patients with gastrocystoplasty; potential reasons for this finding include lower urinary pH, less mucus production, and a lower incidence of bacteriuria.[16]

Common symptoms of stones include hematuria, recurrent UTI, and deterioration of urinary continence. However, most patients are more likely to be diagnosed

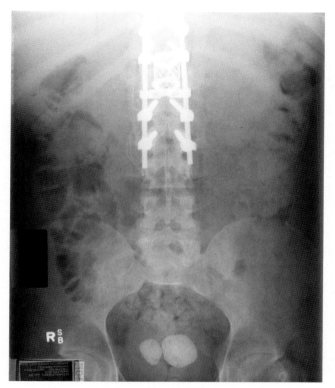

Figure 49-2 Radiographic study of the kidneys, ureters, and bladder. This 45-year-old patient with a T6 spinal cord injury had bladder augmentation 6 years earlier and now has large bladder calculi.

during routine radiographic follow-up of their lower urinary tract reconstruction with either a radiographic study of the kidneys, ureters, and bladder or an ultrasound scan (**Fig. 49-2**). Foreign bodies such as exposed staples, usually associated with a continent stoma, can also serve as a nidus of stone formation.

Therapy is directed at stone removal and can usually be done endoscopically. For large stones, an open procedure can be performed. Percutaneous cystolithotomy should be considered in pediatric patients with urethras too small to accommodate standard endoscopic equipment. This consideration is also important in patients who have undergone a prior Mitrofanoff procedure, which does not allow passage of an endoscope large enough to treat a bladder stone adequately. An Amplatz set can be used to dilate a suprapubic tube tract in preparation for appropriate fragmentation (if needed) with laser or electrohydraulic lithotripsy and removal.[17] It is important to remove all the stone material because any remaining fragments of stone can serve as a nidus of recurrent stone formation. During any type of endoscopic procedure to remove stones, the potential risk exists of unidentified perforation through the much thinner bowel used to perform bladder augmentation; therefore, a temporary catheter should be left in place postoperatively.

One potential therapy to avoid stone formation focuses on removal of mucus. Khoury and colleagues[18] evaluated the mucus of 8 patients who formed stones and of 10 patients who did not and found significantly higher calcium-to-phosphate ($P < .05$) ratios in the mucus of the patients who formed stones. This finding suggests that mucus could conceivably be a nidus of stone formation and removal of mucus could minimize future stone formation. Hensle and colleagues[19] investigated a pediatric population after bladder augmentation (with and without stomas) and found a statistically significant reduction (43% versus 7%; $P < .001$) in the incidence of stone formation in patients receiving a prophylactic irrigation protocol consisting of 240 mL saline solution twice a week and 120 to 240 mL gentamicin sulfate solution (240-480 mg gentamicin/1 L saline).[19]

Perforation

Perforation of an augmented bladder is a rare but potentially fatal complication that was identified in 6% to 9% of patients undergoing cystoplasty in two series[20,21] and in ≤13% of patients in another.[22] The excessive morbidity and mortality associated with a perforation are related to the issue that many patients undergoing bladder augmentation have NGB. The neurogenic cause of their bladder disease often alters and diminishes many of the sensory pathways in these patients. This neurologic deficit can lead to the development of peritonitis and the formation of intra-abdominal abscess with minimal initial symptoms.

The most common presenting symptom is acute abdominal pain; other commonly seen symptoms are nausea, vomiting, oliguria, and fever, as well as shoulder pain secondary to diaphragmatic irritation. Examination should reveal a distended abdomen with peritoneal signs. Cystogram may show extravasation; however, ≤24% of patients may have normal study results.[22] Because of the lack of initial symptoms in certain neuropathic patients combined with the potential that a cystogram not reveal a contrast leak, a high degree of suspicion for this injury should be maintained in patients with bladder augmentation who become acutely ill. A computed tomography urogram may be superior to a cystogram in identifying a perforated augmented bladder.[23]

Factors that appear to place patients at risk for perforation of cystoplasty include a competent bladder outlet that does not allow for a "pop-off" of urine, recurrent UTI, the need to empty the bladder with IC, and chronic overdistention, which is often seen in patients who do not maintain an appropriate IC schedule.[23] In addition, in a review of 500 patients who underwent bladder augmentation, the use of ileum decreased the risk of perforation.[21]

Once the diagnosis of bladder perforation is made, patients should be aggressively intravenously hydrated, they should receive broad-spectrum antibiotics, and they should undergo abdominal exploration to repair the injury. The most common site of perforation is either the junction between the bowel and the bladder wall or the augment segment.

Several causes of perforations of the augmented bladder have been evaluated. Investigators have theorized that bowel ischemia secondary to chronic overdistention and subsequent vascular compromise can lead to rupture.[24] The detubularization of the bowel segment has been investigated as a potential source of bowel necrosis and underlying cause of perforation of the ischemic and necrotic bowel segment.[20] High pressures generated from uninhibited bladder contractions occurring in the augmented bladder also could be the underlying cause of perforation.[24] However, most patients who undergo properly performed bladder augmentation should be able to demonstrate a significant and sustained decrease of their detrusor pressures to acceptable levels and thus should not be at risk of perforation if an appropriate IC regimen is maintained.[25]

Limited reports have described the conservative management of a perforated augmented bladder with catheter drainage of the bladder and percutaneous drainage of any intra-abdominal fluid collections. However, because diagnosis of perforation is often delayed in this patient population, conservative management should be reserved for patients who are hemodynamically stable and do not show signs of progression or worsening of their symptoms.[26]

Carcinoma

A clear association exists between bladder augmentation and malignant disease. However, the actual risk of cancer in patients who have undergone bladder augmentation is not clear. Rates of cancer in patients with an augmented bladder range from as high as 1.2% in 260 patients followed for 10 years[27] to as low as 0% in 267 patients followed for an average of 15 years.[1] Older studies tend to show higher rates of malignancy. This finding may reflect a changing patient population because many of the patients with tumor formation in earlier reports had a diagnosis of tuberculosis or chronic cystitis as the indication for bladder augmentation. The lead time from original augmentation to tumor diagnosis appears to be long. Most tumors are diagnosed >10 years after the original surgical procedure, and approximately 30% of patients die.

Potential risk factors for tumor formation in bladder augmentation include chronic inflammation of the augment patch, recurrent UTI, and urinary stasis.[28-30] The association of recurrent UTI may be related to the impact of bowel and infection on urinary nitrates that are ultimately converted to nitrosamines. Nitrosamines have been implicated in tumors associated with urinary conduits and ureterosigmoidostomies.[31] Adenocarcinoma is the most commonly identified tumor in augmented bladders and is typically found in the region of the anastomosis of the bowel and bladder.[27]

Because no specific symptoms are related to tumors in patients who have undergone bladder augmentation, a high degree of suspicion must be maintained to make the diagnosis. When hematuria develops, an appropriate workup leads to cystoscopy, which enables the clinician to make the diagnosis. However, patients with an augmented bladder perform regular IC and often have microscopic hematuria of benign origin. It is not clear how often and for what degree of hematuria these patients should have a workup for this finding. Although no official guidelines for cystoscopic evaluation and surveillance of these patients exist, a regimen of annual cystoscopy starting after 5 years[32] or 10 years following the augmentation has been proposed.[27] The idea of obtaining regular cytologic studies in these patients to screen for abnormalities suggesting a possible tumor has been proposed; however, cytologic examination is often unreliable in patients who have undergone bladder augmentation, secondary to a chronically infected state.[33] Once a tumor is diagnosed, treatment requires radical cystectomy, removal of the augment segment, and reconstruction. In addition, based on tumor type and stage, chemotherapy may be warranted.

Metabolic Disorders

Hyperchloremic metabolic acidosis is the most commonly noted metabolic abnormality in patients who have undergone bladder augmentation with either an ileal or a colonic segment. This complication is secondary to reabsorption of ammonia and ammonium chloride and secretion of bicarbonate by the bowel segment. Symptomatic acidosis requiring oral therapy with bicarbonate is rare in most series; Greenwell, Venn, and Mundy[1] noted the need for oral bicarbonate in 16% of their patients. An association appears to exist between renal insufficiency and an inability to handle excess acid load that leads to symptomatic acidosis in patients undergoing complete urinary reconstruction. Therefore, patients with a serum creatinine concentration >150 to 200 mmol/L[34] who require complete lower urinary tract reconstruction should undergo conduit formation to minimize the contact time of the urine to the bowel. It is not known whether these values apply to patients undergoing cystoplasty because the native bladder remains in place and thus decreases the total area of bowel in contact with urine.

One potential concern with chronic acidosis is buffering of the acid load by bone, with resulting bone demineralization. Bone disease can be a significant issue

in children undergoing bladder augmentation and can potentially affect bone growth. In fact, Mundy and Nurse[35] noted a halving of growth rate in 20% of children undergoing colocystoplasty. A negative impact on linear growth has not been noted in patients undergoing ileocystoplasty.[35,36] The reason for this finding may be that ileum, as opposed to colon, is able to reabsorb calcium. Boylu and colleagues[37] used bone mineral density to evaluate patients with and without neurogenic disorders before and after ileocystoplasty. These investigators concluded that any changes in bone mineral density were related to the underlying neurologic disease and its locomotor consequences. The decrease in bone mineral density was not thought to be secondary to metabolic changes related to the bladder augmentation.[37] Certainly, no harm exists in following up patients with long-standing bladder augmentation for changes in bone composition, especially in higher-risk patients such as pediatric neurologic patients and postmenopausal women who are already at higher risk for osteoporosis.

Stomach is less commonly used to augment the bladder, and this technique is primarily seen in the pediatric population. Gastrocystoplasty is preferred in patients with underlying renal insufficiency because no additional acid load is generated with augmentation using stomach segment. One issue especially seen with reconstruction using the stomach is the *hematuria-dysuria syndrome*. Symptoms include bladder spasms, hematuria, dysuria, and suprapubic or penile pain. This complication has been noted in ≤26% to 37% of patients undergoing gastrocystoplasty and is related to irritation of the bladder mucosa from acid produced by the stomach segment used for augmentation. This syndrome can usually be managed with histamine (H_2) blockers.[38,39]

Bowel Dysfunction

Postoperative bowel dysfunction can be an especially troubling issue for patients undergoing bladder augmentation. Many of these patients are undergoing cystoplasty for NGB and thus already may have neurogenic bowel dysfunction as well. Possible causes of bowel dysfunction after bladder augmentation include colonization of the distal ileum with colonic bacteria after resection of the ileocecal valve and resection of the terminal ileum that causes bile acid malabsorption. This situation can lead to an increased water and electrolyte load delivered to the colon that cannot be adequately reabsorbed, with resulting diarrhea. In addition, the increased bile acid load can compound the problem by increasing gut motility. Fewer patients with bladder augmentation using sigmoid resection note postoperative bowel dysfunction compared with patients whose bladder augmentation used ileal or ileocecal segments; this finding appears to strengthen the association of ileal resection with postoperative bowel disturbances.[40]

The prevalence of bowel dysfunction after bladder augmentation is not entirely clear from a review of the literature. In a review of 113 patients with ≥3-year follow-up after cystoplasty, Singh and Thomas[40] noted a persistence of bowel dysfunction in 30% of patients. Complaints included an increase in stool frequency (38%), looser stool consistency (38%), and an increase in episodes of fecal incontinence (23%).[40] Husmann and Cain[41] reviewed 63 patients after a hemi-Indiana augmentation procedure and noted an improvement in fecal continence in 23% of patients, no change in 74%, and worsening of fecal control in 3%. Herschorn and Hewitt[42] reviewed 59 patients with a median follow-up of 76 months; 18.6% of patients reported bowel dysfunction, although 7 of those 11 patients noted bowel issues preoperatively as well.[42]

Usual therapy for bowel dysfunction after bladder augmentation includes a low-fat diet and standard oral antidiarrhea treatment (loperamide). Anion exchange resin (cholestyramine) can be used in patients with refractory cases. Despite active treatment, bowel dysfunction persists in a significant portion of these patients. Careful counseling and evaluation of bowel function before surgical intervention may decrease the impact on patients' satisfaction postoperatively.

Incontinence

Persistent urinary incontinence after augmentation cystoplasty can result from several issues. Leakage that only occurs at night is often of multifactorial origin. Potential reasons include decreased urethral resting pressure, increased urinary output at night, and failure of the sphincter to increase its resting tone in response to bladder contractions. Failure to diagnose an incompetent outlet preoperatively can lead to symptoms of stress urinary incontinence. For patients with NGB who use a wheelchair, this complication is often noted with complaints of leakage of urine during transfers or pressure release. Patients may also leak secondary to inadequate bladder augmentation. This complication could result from the use of an inadequately small piece of intestine, an impaired blood supply to the augment segment that leads to decreased capacity or compliance, or the presence of bowel mass contractions.

Evaluation of persistent urinary incontinence after bladder augmentation includes use of a voiding diary and urodynamic study. Voiding diaries can be very helpful in identifying potential reversible causes such as excessive fluid intake and patients who perform IC too infrequently. If the voiding diary is unremarkable, urodynamic studies allow for evaluation of the bladder and the outlet to ascertain the cause of the urinary leakage. Therapy can then be directed accordingly. Potential therapies for an inadequate sphincter include pubovaginal sling, bladder neck reconstruction, bladder neck closure, and artificial urinary sphincter. If the bladder was not adequately augmented with the initial procedure, anticholinergics can be considered. Botulinum toxin has also been used with considerable success in patients with high-pressure NGB, although the use of this agent in patients with treatment failure after bladder augmentation has not been described.[43] If this approach does not resolve the problem, repeat bladder augmentation with ileum was reported to be successful in five patients in whom prior bladder augmentation with either stomach or colon failed.[44]

Pregnancy

A potential issue in young women undergoing bladder augmentation is future pregnancy, including management of the delivery. Possible areas of concern for any woman with lower urinary tract reconstruction and pregnancy include UTI or pyelonephritis, renal deterioration, ureteral obstruction, and premature labor.[45] In a review of 15 patients with bladder augmentation, Hill and Kramer[46] reported development of pyelonephritis in 60% and premature labor in 25% of patients. The most common complication of pregnancy after bladder augmentation is UTI or pyelonephritis. Therefore, frequent urinalysis needs to be performed and infections need to be treated early and aggressively.

No consensus exists on whether delivery should be done by a vaginal or cesarean approach in patients with an augmented bladder. Hill and Kramer[46] recommended proceeding with standard vaginal delivery in patients who had undergone enterocystoplasty alone. In patients who had undergone a concomitant procedure for the outlet, the investigators recommended proceeding with cesarean section to minimize potential disruption to the continence mechanism. However, other investigators did not find this to be an issue and reported vaginal delivery to be safe for all patients who had prior bladder augmentation, even those with prior bladder neck reconstruction.[47,48] If cesarean section is considered, the obstetrician must understand the anatomy of the reconstruction. Cesarean section though a classic upper segment approach should minimize any potential risk to the reconstruction. It may also be helpful to have a urologist available if the obstetrician is unsure of the anatomic features.

KEY POINTS

1. Bladder augmentation is safe, well-tolerated, and effective surgery in appropriately selected patients.
2. Prolonged postoperative anastomotic leak, although rare, is a known early complication of bladder augmentation. It can be prevented and ultimately corrected by continuous bladder drainage and regular irrigation with mucus evacuation. Leaks that initially fail conservative therapy may require percutaneous diversion of the upper tract.
3. Stones may be identified in augmented bladders. Prevention of stone formation can be achieved by regularly removing mucus and appropriately treating urea-splitting organisms in the urine.
4. Perforation of an augmented bladder is a rare but potentially fatal complication. A high degree of suspicion should be maintained for patients with bladder augmentation who become acutely ill. CT cystogram is the optimal study to identify a perforated bladder augment, which requires surgical repair.
5. There is an unclear association between prior bladder augmentation and bladder cancer. Although no official guidelines exist for carcinoma surveillance for these patients, annual cystoscopy starting 5 to 10 years after augmentation is recommended. Gross hematuria needs to be worked up appropriately in augmented patients, as well.

REFERENCES

Please see www.expertconsult.com

Chapter 50

COMPLICATIONS OF FEMALE INCONTINENCE SURGERY

Eric S. Rovner MD

Professor of Urology, Department of Urology, Medical University of South Carolina, Charleston, South Carolina

Urinary incontinence (UI) is defined as the complaint of involuntary leakage of urine.[1] This common condition is an underreported health problem that can significantly affect quality of life.[2,3] Patients with UI may have numerous related problems including depression as a result of the perceived lack of self-control, loss of independence, and lack of self-esteem, and they often curtail their activities for fear of an "accident."[4,5] UI and related overactive bladder may also have serious medical and economic ramifications for untreated or undertreated patients, including perineal dermatitis, worsening of pressure ulcers, urinary tract infections (UTIs), and falls.[6] For these reasons, many individuals suffering from this condition seek treatment. Although surgery is rarely the first choice of treatment,[7] it plays a major role in the therapy of some types of UI. Surgical procedures for UI are some of the most commonly performed operations in the United States by urologists. Thus understanding how to avoid, and when necessary how to treat, complications related to these surgical procedures is important.

TYPES OF INCONTINENCE

Clearly, defining the type of UI before initiating irreversible, expensive, and potentially morbid therapy such as surgery is critical in deciding on the appropriate intervention. A careful preoperative evaluation including history, physical examination, urodynamic study, and cystoscopy, when appropriate, can be essential in understanding the type of UI. The details of this evaluation are beyond the scope of this chapter. However, an incorrect diagnosis not only leads to the wrong surgical procedure but also may result in considerable worsening of symptoms postoperatively.

Simply stated, UI may result from abnormalities of the urethra (including the bladder outlet and urinary sphincter) or the bladder or may be caused by a combination of abnormalities of both structures (Table 50-1).[8]

Abnormalities may result in underactivity or overactivity of the urethra or bladder with the subsequent development of UI.

Urethral underactivity results in stress UI (SUI). *Urodynamic SUI* is the involuntary leakage of urine associated with an increase in intra-abdominal pressure in the absence of a detrusor contraction.[1] Adult female SUI is generally attributed to the following:

1. A failure of the normal transmission of increases in intra-abdominal pressures to the bladder neck and proximal urethra as a result of poor anatomic support of this region (urethral hypermobility or anatomic incontinence)
2. Malfunction, damage, or injury to the intrinsic urethral sphincteric unit (intrinsic sphincter deficiency)
3. A combination of these factors[9]

Surgical correction of female SUI is directed toward either of the following: (1) repositioning the urethra or creating a backboard of support or otherwise stabilizing the urethra and bladder neck in a well-supported retropubic ("intra-abdominal") position that is receptive to changes in intra-abdominal pressure, or (2) creating coaptation or compression or otherwise augmenting the urethral closure forces provided by the intrinsic sphincteric unit—with (i.e., sling) or without (i.e., periurethral injectables)—that affect urethral and bladder neck support.

Urge UI is the involuntary leakage of urine associated with urgency.[1] This disorder is generally although certainly not invariably attributed to detrusor overactivity, as shown by urodynamic assessment. Both phasic bladder overactivity (involuntary bladder contractions) and tonic overactivity (decreased compliance) can contribute to UI. Careful urodynamic evaluation may be necessary in these patients to ascertain lower urinary tract physiology, to assess the risk of deterioration to

TABLE 50-1	Functional Classification of Urinary Incontinence
Abnormality	**Type of Clinical Incontinence**
Bladder overactivity	Urge
Bladder underactivity	Overflow
Urethra overactivity	Overflow
Urethra underactivity	Stress

TABLE 50-2	Goals of Surgical Options for Stress Urinary Incontinence
Surgical Option	**Goal**
Anterior repair	Repositioned urethra or "plicated" sphincter
Retropubic approach Marchetti-Krantz vesicourethropexy Burch colposuspension	Repositioned or stabilized urethra or creation of a "backboard" of support for urethral compression during increased intra-abdominal pressure
Vaginal approach Pereyra Stamey Gittes Raz	Same as retropubic approach with avoidance of a large abdominal incision and associated morbidity
Sling Autologous, cadaveric, synthetic, vaginal wall, etc.	Same as retropubic approach with or without direct urethral coaptation or compression
Tension-free vaginal tape and other polypropylene midurethral slings	Dynamic midurethral support
Artificial urinary sphincter	Intermittent, dynamic urethral coaptation and compression
Bulk agents (injectables)	Improved urethral coaptation

the upper urinary tract, and to search for coexisting urethral or sphincteric UI.

Most of these patients are treated with a combination of behavioral modification, pelvic floor physical therapy, and oral pharmacologic agents. However, for patients with refractory conditions, the goal of surgical intervention is either to reduce or abolish bladder overactivity and the sensation of urgency or to provide a reservoir of adequate size for the low-pressure storage of adequate volumes of urine.

TYPES OF INCONTINENCE OPERATIONS

Except in unusual circumstances, the surgical repair of UI is elective. The decision to treat *symptomatic* UI surgically should be based primarily on the premise that the degree of bother or lifestyle compromise to the patient is sufficient to warrant an *elective* operation and that nonoperative therapy is either undesired or has been ineffective. Therefore, it is particularly troublesome to both the surgeon and the patient when complications arise during or after performance of these elective procedures. In some instances, these complications may be life-threatening or may considerably worsen symptoms or quality of life. Thus, the surgeon must clearly describe and counsel patients regarding potential complications preoperatively. Fortunately however, complications of the surgical treatment of UI are uncommon and when they occur are often amenable to treatment.

Stress Incontinence Operations

The goal of surgical treatment of SUI is to augment urethral closure forces to prevent the egress of urine from the urethra during periods of increased abdominal pressure while at the same time preserving voluntary, low-pressure, and complete bladder emptying. This treatment may involve the use of retropubic or transvaginal suburethral support or compression (slings), periurethral injection (e.g., collagen), or, in male patients, circumferential compression (artificial genitourinary sphincter) (Table 50-2). The precise manner in which each operative procedure improves urethral closure forces and thereby restores urinary continence is not well understood. Nonetheless, >100 different operations have been designed to treat female SUI. Of

these operations, midurethral sling procedures have become, by far, the most widely used for this indication.

The transabdominal approach to vesicourethropexy includes procedures such as the Marshall-Marchetti-Krantz (MMK) vesicourethropexy and the Burch colposuspension. Following development of the retropubic space, these operations elevate or, in some cases, simply prevent rotational descent of the urethra and bladder neck by securing the paraurethral fascia (MMK) or paravesical fascia to a fixed retropubic structure such as the posterior periosteum of the symphysis pubis (MMK) or Cooper's ligament (Burch). In addition to positioning the bladder neck and proximal urethra into a well-supported retropubic location, these procedures may also provide a stable "backboard" on which the urethra and bladder neck are compressed during increases in intra-abdominal pressure.

The advantages to this approach are as follows:

1. The familiarity of retropubic anatomy to most urologists
2. Excellent operative exposure and access to the key anatomic elements for the surgical procedure
3. Long-term data suggesting durability
4. The opportunity to repair coexistent abdominal disease through the same incision or a slightly extended incision

Disadvantages include the following:

1. A large incision
2. Prolonged hospital stay and recovery period
3. The inability to access and repair coexistent vaginal disease through the same incision

The transvaginal or "needle" suspension procedures are alternatives to the retropubic operations for urethral UI resulting from vesicourethral hypermobility. These techniques evolved as minimally invasive alternatives to the retropubic procedures. These two categories of operation have certain features in common: the anterior abdominal wall fascia is not incised and the suspending sutures are passed through the retropubic space from the vagina to the anterior abdominal wall with a specialized long ligature (suture) passer.

Advantages to the transvaginal approach include the following:

1. Avoidance of a large, transfascial abdominal incision and its attendant morbidity, especially in the obese patient
2. Shorter operative times
3. Less postoperative discomfort
4. Shorter hospital stay
5. The ability to repair coexisting vaginal disease (i.e., prolapse) through the same incision or a slightly extended incision

Disadvantages include the following:

1. A potentially lower long-term "cure" rate
2. Poor intraoperative visualization
3. Risk of injury to the bladder and urethra during blind passage of the needles through the retropubic space
4. Risk of significant bleeding in the retropubic space with poor operative access from the vaginal incisions
5. Infection or erosion of a foreign body if suture buttresses are used (i.e., the Stamey operation)

Transvaginal needle suspensions and anterior repairs have fallen out of favor especially following a comprehensive meta-analysis published in 1997 suggesting that these procedures were less durable in the long term as compared with slings and retropubic suspensions.[10]

Originally described more than 100 years ago, slings of various types have had a tremendous resurgence in popularity. This renewed interest may be attributed to several factors including a change in surgical philosophy regarding the pathophysiology of urethral UI in female patients and a perceived if not actual decrease in morbidity associated with sling surgery in the modern era. Fascial slings use either autologous tissue harvested from the patient intraoperatively (e.g., anterior rectus sheath, fascia lata) or cadaveric (allograft) fascia. The

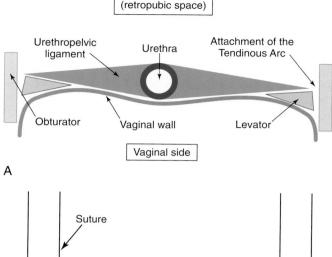

Figure 50-1 Diagrams of the vaginal anatomy in a coronal plane before (**A**) and after (**B**) placement of a fascial sling.

fascia may be full length (extending from the abdominal wall through the retropubic space, under the urethra, and back up to the abdominal wall) or rectangular (extending into the retropubic space on either side but secured to the anterior abdominal wall with nonabsorbable sutures attached to either end of the sling) (**Fig. 50-1**).

Fascial slings are generally placed at the level of the bladder neck and proximal third of the urethra; however, the midurethral polypropylene sling has become the most common type of sling procedure performed in the United States. This popularity is likely the result of the low morbidity, technical ease, and speed of the procedure; its long-term durability and safety; and the rapid recovery and convalescence. These slings, of which many proprietary types are available, are similar in the completely tension-free, minimally invasive technique in which they are placed under the midurethra. Depending on the choice of device, these slings may be placed through a transvaginal, suprapubic, or transobturator approach with no definite advantage to any technique. The actual polypropylene mesh sling material differs from other products.

Bone-anchoring techniques emerged as an alternative method of suture fixation for both transvaginal needle suspensions and some types of slings. Numerous propriety fixation systems have been developed including transvaginal and suprapubic delivery systems, all of which deliver a suture secured to a metallic screw into the cortical bone of the pubic rami on either side of the midline. The initial enthusiasm for these adjunctive procedures was somewhat dampened by the lack of a demonstrable long-term durable benefit over other techniques as well as the cost and potential associated morbidity, including osteomyelitis and osteitis pubis.[11-13]

Periurethral injectable agents have been used for the treatment of SUI in women for decades. Most periurethral agents are injected in a retrograde fashion under direct cystoscopic guidance as an office-based procedure. The exact means by which periurethral injectable agents exert their favorable effects on continence has not been well defined, although an obstructive mechanism or an improved "seal" effect has been suggested.[14] Furthermore, the eventual mechanism of failure for most of these agents is not well understood, although it is believed that biologic reabsorption (e.g., glutaraldehyde cross-linked [GAX] collagen), particle migration, and ongoing degeneration of the sphincteric apparatus may be contributing factors. Generally these agents are safe and have good initial efficacy but lack long-term durability.

The artificial urinary sphincter is used in some centers as primary therapy for female SUI. However in the United States, this device is only very infrequently used in female patients.

Urge Incontinence Operations

Sacral neuromodulation, augmentation enterocystoplasty, and most recently intradetrusor injection of botulinum toxin (BT) have been used for individuals undergoing surgical treatment of detrusor-related UI. Sacral neuromodulation has been used since the 1980s as a therapy for urinary frequency, urgency, bladder overactivity, and UI but has been approved by the U.S. Food and Drug Administration (FDA) for use in the United States only since 1997. A staged implantation technique is most commonly used in which a test stimulation procedure is first performed. In this procedure, a neurostimulator electrode is placed percutaneously in the S3 foramen under fluoroscopic guidance and then is tunneled subcutaneously and externalized. The electrode is attached to an external pulse generator and the patient is evaluated clinically over the ensuing days to weeks. Low-frequency stimulation of the S3 nerve root results in modulation of neural activity in the lower urinary tract and pelvic floor. The exact mechanism by which sacral neuromodulation exerts its therapeutic effects remains unclear. If a suitable clinical response is noted, the patient is taken back to the operating room for placement of a permanent, subcutaneous implantable pulse generator.

Bladder overactivity can be successfully treated by augmentation enterocystoplasty. Principles of urinary reconstruction with intestinal segments include detubularization of the bowel segment, wide opening of the bladder, and anastomosis of the bowel segment to the opened bladder to recreate a shape as nearly spherical as possible. Further discussion and complications related to the use of intestine in the urinary tract are reviewed elsewhere in this textbook and are not considered further here (see Chapter 48).

Finally, intradetrusor injection of BT A has been used in some centers to treat both neurogenic and nonneurogenic detrusor overactivity. BT is produced by the bacterium *Clostridium botulinum* and is the most potent biologic neurotoxin known. This agent been adapted into a useful agent for the treatment of a variety of urologic and nonurologic conditions. Approximately 100 to 300 U of the toxin are injected through the cystoscope with a long, fine needle in a series of 10 to 30 injections. This treatment is most commonly performed using local anesthesia and as an office-based procedure. This therapy is not currently approved by the FDA for use in the urinary tract for any indication, although multiple trials are ongoing. BT produces its motor paralytic effects by inhibiting acetylcholine release at the presynaptic cholinergic neuromuscular junction.

The mechanism of action of BT may also involve some aspects of the afferent limb of the micturition reflex. BT blocks the binding and fusion of the synaptic vesicles to the presynaptic membrane terminal and prevents release of acetylcholine as well as a variety of other neurotransmitters and neuropeptides into the synapse. Clinically this results in muscle weakness, diminished contractility, and muscle atrophy at affected sites. The effect is reversible in 3 to 6 months. The mechanism by which smooth muscle regains contractility over time is not well understood and is not fully explained by axonal sprouting.

PREVENTION OF COMPLICATIONS

Although most complications related to the surgical treatment of female UI are treatable and generally reversible, the optimal situation is to prevent or minimize the potential for an adverse outcome. This process begins in the preoperative period and is initiated during the diagnostic evaluation and workup. Many factors should be considered in determining the optimal surgical therapy for the patient with UI. These include the origin and type of UI, bladder capacity, renal function, sexual function, medical comorbidities, severity of the leakage, the presence of associated conditions such as vaginal prolapse or concurrent abdominal or pelvic disease requiring surgical correction, prior abdominal and pelvic surgical procedures, and finally the patient's suitability for and willingness to accept the risks of surgery. All these factors may affect both the choice of surgical treatment and the risk of surgical complications.

The proper choice of candidate for an anti-UI operation cannot be overemphasized. The diagnosis of SUI must be firmly established to propose outlet-enhancing surgery for the treatment of SUI. Other diagnoses that may mimic SUI should be definitively eliminated including fistula, ureteral ectopy, bladder calculi, urethral diverticula, and overflow UI. Overflow UI in particular, secondary to a neurogenic or myogenic disorder, can be mistaken for SUI and this misdiagnosis can lead to inappropriate intervention and surgical treatment failure. Surgical procedures for SUI should not be performed without the objective demonstration of SUI preoperatively by physical examination (Marshall-Bonney or cough stress test), cystography, or urodynamic evaluation. The patient's history should be consistent with and confirmed by findings on physical examination, and when appropriate, radiographic or urodynamic testing. Apparently conflicting results on preoperative evaluation should be carefully investigated and resolved. Surgical treatment of SUI in the patient with only bladder-related SUI (overactivity or poor compliance) is not indicated and will be unsuccessful.

Reversible factors should be addressed. For patients with postmenopausal, hypoestrogenic vaginal atrophy, topical estrogen replacement may reduce the incidence of postoperative vaginal wound dehiscence or extrusion of sling material. UTI and genital tract infection (e.g., candidiasis) should also be treated before surgical intervention. Nutritional disorders should be assessed and corrected preoperatively before elective surgical treatment is performed. Finally, treatment of any medical comorbidities (e.g., diabetic control, hypertension) should be optimized.

Why do complications occur? Petri and colleagues[15] investigated a series of 328 repeat interventions following midurethral slings at four tertiary care urogynecology centers in Europe. The indications for reoperation were varied and included obstruction and dysuria, among many others. Nonetheless, the most common reason cited for failure of the previous operation was poor surgical technique, and the next most common reason was the wrong surgical indication. Both these factors certainly can be addressed and minimized preoperatively. In fact, another preoperative factor, operative experience with a given procedure, has been cited as an important factor contributing to the risk of operative complications. Kuuva and Nilsson[16] reviewed a nationwide database (Finland) on midurethral slings and noted that operative complications varied inversely with surgical experience. As surgeons performed more procedures, the incidence of complications declined dramatically. This finding supports the notion that sur-

geons who are relative novices at a given procedure are at risk of more complications than are their veteran colleagues.

COMPLICATIONS

The field of SUI surgery has advanced rapidly. As noted previously, the types of procedures performed has evolved from transvaginal needle suspensions and retropubic suspensions to various types of slings, most commonly the midurethral polypropylene slings. This shift has implications for the types of complications seen in contemporary practice as compared with complications seen even a few short years ago. Therefore, the majority of the discussion that follows concerns the midurethral slings.

Choice of Approach

The relative risks of each complication among various types of surgical procedure, especially within a single category such as midurethral slings, regardless of approach (e.g., the risk of bleeding in a transobturator versus suprapubic versus transvaginal approach), are impossible to determine because of the lack of randomized controlled trials comparing procedures and approaches. Currently, small numbers of patients and underpowered clinical trials do not provide sufficient evidence to recommend one procedure or approach absolutely over another based only on complications.

In one of the few well-done randomized controlled trials, Ward and colleagues[17] compared Burch colposuspension with tension-free vaginal tape (TVT). These investigators found that the risk of intraoperative complications such as bladder perforation was higher in the TVT-treated group, whereas the risk of postoperative complications such as delayed voiding was greater in the Burch-treated group.[17] Certainly, some qualitative inferences can be made from the literature and these are discussed later, as appropriate. However, caution must be maintained regarding unsubstantiated marketing claims made by manufacturers regarding the safety and risk of complications related to their proprietary product or approach. Much of what exists is conjecture, theoretical, and anecdotal. Until large, prospective, well-done, multicenter, randomized trials address these issues, with a few notable exceptions discussed later, it is not scientifically valid to claim superiority of one procedure or approach over another with regard to safety.

Risk Factors

Identifying preoperative risk factors such as age, obesity, prior surgical treatment, and impaired contractility that consistently predict for intraoperative and postoperative complications has also been difficult. Much of the existing literature is conflicting.[18] For example, some investigators have found that prior surgical treatment is a predictor of intraoperative bladder injury,[19,20] whereas others have not.[21] This variability may reflect the type of prior SUI surgical treatment: prior retropubic procedures such as Burch or MMK may lead to retropubic scarring and a risk of bladder injury,[22] whereas a prior transvaginal operation such as a Kelly plication wherein the retropubic space is not violated may not. Advanced age is not a contraindication to anti-UI surgery. However, surgical treatment in extremely elderly patients (>80 years old) may be associated with some increased morbidity as compared with younger elderly patients (65-80 years old).[23] Again, well-done, well-powered, randomized trials with adequate numbers of patients are required to address this issue.

Incidence

The overall incidence of intraoperative and postoperative complications is difficult to ascertain. Much of the available literature is from a single center experience and suffers from considerable methodologic limitations. Nevertheless, depending on the definition, the incidence of complications in some series of UI surgery may approach 50%.[19,24] In a review of midurethral sling procedures, Boustead[25] noted that the complication rate in published series ranged from 1% to 40%. Taub and colleagues[26] used the Nationwide Inpatient Sample (a U.S. national database) of >147,000 patients who underwent surgical treatment of SUI from 1988 to 2000 and found an overall complication rate of 13%. Waetjen and colleagues[27] estimated a complication rate of 18% from the 1998 National Hospital Discharge Survey and the 1998 National Census including data on >135,000 patients undergoing surgical intervention. These studies are likely somewhat dated given the shift in types of SUI procedures now performed as compared with the procedures that were popular when these data were compiled.

The actual incidence of any single given complication in the general population cannot be calculated because the total number of procedures performed for UI, especially SUI is, at best, an estimate. These data can be partially captured using government databases as noted earlier or manufacturer's sales figures for proprietary products, but this type of analysis excludes large numbers of patients such as privately insured and uninsured patients who cannot be counted using this methodology. In addition, patients undergoing surgical treatment without the use of a commercially available proprietary product (i.e., until recently, most surgical procedures performed in the United States) cannot be accounted for using this analysis.

Nevertheless, the overall complication rate of all procedures is likely underreported. Deng and colleagues[28] reported on complications in patients referred for repair to a single tertiary care institution over a 4-year period and noted that despite the devastating nature of some of these complications, the reported rate in the literature was much lower than expected based on their experience. Mandatory reporting of operative complications in the United States is not required, nor does a mandatory central database or repository exist for any given procedure. In the United States, for example, surgical complications related to device malfunction can be reported to the FDA Manufacturer and User Facility Device Experience (MAUDE) database.[29] This reporting is completely voluntary, and it possible that the time and effort required in reporting on this site are disincentives to reporting complications. The threat of malpractice litigation also likely contributes to underreporting of surgical complications.

Furthermore, it is difficult to extrapolate the risk of a given complication occurring in the community setting, where most surgical procedures are done. Almost all the literature is published from tertiary care academic centers that may be biased toward reoperative surgery and may be influenced by ongoing resident training. In one prospective Dutch study of TVT, there was an increased risk of complications in teaching hospitals as compared with non-teaching hospitals.[30]

Finally, and perhaps most importantly, the definition of a *complication* is unclear. This lack of standardization permits considerable variability in the reporting of complications. For example, some bleeding is commonly encountered in the performance of transvaginal anti-UI procedures. However, how much bleeding must occur for it to be considered a complication? A surgeon may choose not to report bleeding at all as a complication if it happens quite commonly in his or her experience. Other surgeons may report bleeding as a complication only if it results in the development of postoperative hypotension, the requirement for transfusion, or even hemorrhagic shock and death.

Complications Related to Stress Urinary Incontinence Surgery

Intraoperative Complications

Bleeding The risk of bleeding during surgical treatment of SUI can be minimized but not entirely eliminated by good operative technique. Multiple blood vessels traverse the deep pelvis including large venous channels in the retropubic space. Named vessels in the obturator fossa, along the pelvic sidewall including the iliac vessels, and within the vascular pedicle of the bladder are at risk for injury especially during vaginal surgical treatment of UI because of the lack of direct visualization of these structures during passage of trocars or needles. Major vascular injury can quickly lead to life-threatening hemorrhage if it is not recognized intraoperatively and may result in large retropubic hematomas postoperatively.[31,32]

In a series of >5000 midurethral slings reported by the Austrian Working Group for Urogynecology, bleeding problems were reported in 2.7% of cases.[33] Only 0.8% of patients required intervention for bleeding, and most cases were managed conservatively without operative intervention; <1% of patients required transfusions. No deaths were reported in this series as a result of bleeding. Kuuva and colleagues[16] reported a 1.9% incidence of bleeding >200 mL in >1400 patients who underwent TVT treatment.

Bleeding during retropubic bladder neck suspension is usually easily visualized and controlled with a combination of cautery, suture ligature, and if necessary direct compression. Occasionally, sponge sticks and readjustment of the retractors may be needed to visualize the bleeding vessels optimally. The retropubic anatomy is very familiar to most urologic surgeons, and bleeding during these procedures is rarely problematic.

In contrast to bleeding during retropubic surgical procedures, bleeding during transvaginal operations can be more problematic at times and more difficult to control. The initial dissection of the vaginal wall from the underlying fascia should be associated with minimal bleeding. Bleeding encountered during this early dissection may indicate an excessively deep and incorrect surgical plane within the wall of the bladder or urethra. In this circumstance, immediate recognition and reevaluation are necessary to avoid inadvertent entry into the urinary tract and to minimize bleeding. Following identification of this situation, dissection should then proceed in the proper surgical plane, which, in reoperative surgical procedures, may be difficult to identify.

Another common site of bleeding during transvaginal anti-UI surgical procedures occurs when the endopelvic fascia is traversed. Entry into the retropubic space from the transvaginal side or placement of the suprapubic needles or trocars from the abdominal side may be associated with copious bleeding as the endopelvic fascia is perforated. Again, knowledge of the anatomic features, careful attention to technique, maintenance of countertraction, and proper positioning of the perforating scissors (with the tips curved away from the bladder) or trocar in three planes minimize most bleeding (**Fig. 50-2**). An initial gush of venous bleeding is not unusual during this maneuver, and although it may be unsettling to the operating surgeon, the bleeding dissipates quickly without further manipulation.

If the bleeding continues and is brisk, the vagina can be packed. It can be very helpful to elevate the anterior vaginal wall manually and compress it anteriorly directly against the posterior symphysis pubis for several minutes using the surgeon's hand, a sponge stick, or a retractor. These maneuvers effectively tamponade bleeding in the retropubic space. It is not advisable to "chase" this bleeding using a transvaginal approach. Only very rarely

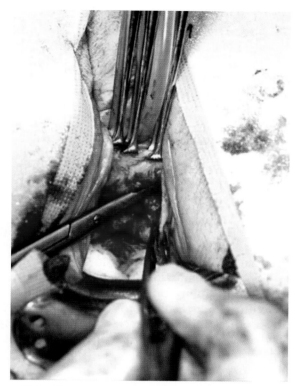

Figure 50-2 The proper plane of dissection. The scissors are directed toward the patient's ipsilateral shoulder. Countertraction is applied to the vaginal wall.

is the exact bleeding point identified and controlled in this manner.

Transvaginal exploration for bleeding results in ongoing blood loss as the surgeon struggles with relatively poor exposure and visualization. Packing and compression lead to adequate control in most cases, and if not, the surgeon should expeditiously complete the procedure, close the incisions, and pack the vagina.[34] Occasionally, in addition to vaginal packing, a Foley catheter inserted through the urethra with the balloon overinflated and then placed on traction adds additional security. Brisk bleeding that does not respond to manual compression for an extended period may suggest a major vessel injury and mandates retropubic exploration.

Urinary Tract Injury   During surgical procedures for SUI, the urethra, bladder, or much more rarely the ureters may be injured. Key to the management of each of these injuries are immediate recognition and repair. Long-term sequelae resulting from unrecognized urinary tract injury can be devastating to the patient and can have potentially substantial medicolegal implications for the physician.

Urethral Injury   From the transvaginal side, injury to the urethra may occur during initial dissection of the vaginal wall off the underlying fascia. As noted earlier, excessively deep dissection, especially in reoperative surgical procedures, risks urethral injury. This injury is usually although not invariably heralded by an unexpected amount of bleeding. Placement of a urethral catheter before incision will help to identify the urethra intraoperatively and in the case of urethral injury will allow immediate recognition as the catheter becomes visible in the operative field.

If a urethral injury is suspected, urethroscopy may be performed. The urethra should be repaired immediately and primarily in two layers by using absorbable sutures in a watertight fashion. The urethra can be repaired over a ≥14-Fr catheter. It is not necessary to leave a drain other than the urethral catheter. The integrity of the repair can be tested by injecting saline through a syringe attached to an angiocatheter (intravenous [IV]) sheath into the urethral meatus adjacent to the catheter with the balloon snugged up against the bladder neck. Failure to recognize the injury or failure to repair it properly risks urethrovaginal fistula, erosion of sling material into the urethral lumen postoperatively (especially synthetic sling material), infection, and a multitude of other potential problems.

The urethra may also be injured during trocar placement in midurethral sling procedures, needle placement for transvaginal suspensions, or cystocele repair. Countertraction during the initial dissection, maintenance of adequate exposure and a working knowledge of the anatomy are helpful in avoiding urethral injury.

In the event of a planned synthetic sling in the setting of a concomitant urethral injury, it is probably advisable to repair the urethra and abort the sling procedure until the urethra is completely healed. An autologous sling may be considered a safer alternative than a synthetic sling as an anti-UI procedure at the time of a urethral injury, but few data support this notion. The urethra is rarely injured during retropubic surgical procedures because the middle and distal thirds are protected by the symphysis pubis.

Bladder Injury Intraoperative bladder injury may occur during transabdominal and transvaginal anti-UI surgical procedures. The potential for urinary tract injury varies considerably with the experience of the surgeon,[35] as well as with the operative approach. Investigators generally believe that the risk of bladder injury is higher with a retropubic approach as compared with a transobturator approach during midurethral sling operations. However, multiple reports of bladder injury during transobturator midurethral sling procedures have been published.[29,36]

The relative risk of urinary tract perforation with a transvaginal versus suprapubic approach to midurethral slings is unclear. Although one study noted an extremely high bladder perforation rate with a suprapubic approach (29% versus 4%, suprapubic versus transvaginal, respectively),[37] others did not.[38] In one small randomized prospective trial comparing transobturator with retropubic midurethral slings, bladder perforation was noted only in the patients who underwent retropubic procedures (4 of 42, 9.5%) whereas vaginal injury was noted only in the patients who underwent transobturator procedures (5 of 46, 10.9%).[39] It is possible that the difference in complication rates results from surgical factors other than approach.

Kuuva and colleagues[16] reported that the risk of bladder perforation during a transvaginal midurethral sling varied with the experience of the operating surgeon. Surgeons performing >80 procedures had almost 50% fewer perforations than did surgeons who had performed <20 procedures.[16] McLennan and colleagues[35] reported that the risk of bladder perforation in a resident training program varied inversely with the number of procedures performed by the trainee. Repeat surgical procedures are almost certainly associated with a higher risk of urinary tract injury in patients undergoing midurethral sling operations. Jeffry and colleagues[20] reported a bladder perforation rate during TVT of 71.4% versus 7.6% in patients with prior surgical treatment versus those without such a history. Similarly, in patients undergoing SPARC (American Medical Systems, Minnetonka, Minn) sling treatment, Deval and colleagues[19] reported a 36.6% versus 7.5% urinary tract injury rate in patients with versus those without a history of prior surgical intervention. Hodroff and colleagues[40] reported an overall bladder perforation rate of 6.7% in 445 patients undergoing retropubic midurethral sling procedures.

Injury to the bladder during midurethral sling procedures is diagnosed intraoperatively by careful endoscopic examination of the bladder and bladder neck with a 70-degree lens following passage of the trocars. The bladder should be filled and then examined to ensure that a small injury does not go unrecognized in a fold of the bladder wall. To avoid injury during trocar needle passage, the urethra should be clearly palpated, the bladder drained, and the pelvic anatomy well delineated. If a bladder injury is noted intraoperatively, the trocar should be removed and reinserted. Bladder injury from a trocar usually does not require primary closure. Postoperative drainage of the bladder with a Foley catheter for several days is, however, desirable to avoid urinoma, fistula formation, and pelvic abscess.

During a transvaginal pubovaginal sling procedure, or during performance of urethrolysis, it is common to perforate the endopelvic fascia intentionally to gain entry into the retropubic space. This perforation maneuver is often done sharply with curved scissors. The surgeon must be aware of lower urinary tract anatomy during this maneuver to avoid injury. Countertraction on the pelvic fascia away from the side of interest as the scissor perforates into the retropubic space will help to avoid injury. If injury occurs, lower urinary tract perforation in this setting is often larger than that seen with the passage of the trocars during a midurethral sling. The injury should be isolated and closed in two layers. A suprapubic drain can be placed and the lower urinary tract drained for several days to ensure healing.

In addition, ureteral patency should be assessed in this setting because the injury can track proximally on the trigone. Injury to the bladder during retropubic operations is usually confined to the anterior bladder wall. This complication is usually easily recognized and repaired. Postoperative Foley catheter drainage is mandatory. During a Burch or MMK procedure, a stitch may be inadvertently placed transmurally into the bladder or urethral lumen. Intraoperative cystoscopic examination identifies these injuries and permits removal and replacement of the suture.[41]

Ureteral Injury Ureteral injury during surgical treatment of UI is uncommon. With the advent of midurethral slings, these injuries are becoming rarer given the expected location of the sling at the level of the midurethra. However, the ureter may be kinked or obstructed during Burch or MMK procedures or during vaginal prolapse repair. Virtually all these injuries can be identified by intraoperative cystoscopy. The administration of IV vital dyes such as indigo carmine permits obvious visualization of ureteral efflux that confirms ureteral patency. Suspected ureteral injuries are confirmed by retrograde pyeloureterography. Most of these injuries are related to suture placement. When found, ureteral injuries may be treated by removal of the offending suture and placement of a temporary indwelling ureteral stent. Ureteral transection requires ureteroneocystostomy.

Intraoperative Cystoscopy Given the low rate of urinary tract injury especially in uncomplicated pelvic surgical procedures, is intraoperative cystoscopy justified in every case? This issue is somewhat controversial.[42-44] Cystoscopy is a low-morbidity procedure that requires little additional time, effort, or resources. However, some additional expense is incurred in performing cystoscopy, and the practitioner requires advanced training in endoscopic examination of the lower urinary tract. Nevertheless, careful cystoscopic examination of the lower urinary tract following anti-UI surgical procedures enables the surgeon to evaluate the patient for almost all lower urinary tract injuries. If IV vital dye is given, ureteral injury can also be excluded by visualizing efflux from the ureters. The bladder must be examined when it is full, and careful attention should be paid at the 10- and 2-o'clock positions at the bladder neck and just inside the bladder neck because these are the locations of the majority of lower urinary tract injuries during UI surgical procedures.

Inexperience with cystoscopy leads to a high rate of missed intraoperative perforations.[35] If perforations are recognized intraoperatively, the lower urinary tract can

be quickly repaired and drained if necessary. Unrecognized urinary tract injuries can lead to infection, sepsis, fistula, stones, and other complications. Despite manufacturers' claims to the contrary, transobturator slings can be associated with injury to the lower urinary tract,[29,36] and thus intraoperative cystoscopy probably cannot be entirely eliminated in these cases.

Bowel Injury Multiple reports of bowel injury during surgical procedures for UI have been reported.[29,40,45] Fortunately this complication is rare. Bowel injury may occur during retropubic dissection for a Burch or MMK procedure, on entry into the retropubic space during an autologous pubovaginal sling or urethrolysis, or during passage of needle passers or trocars during midurethral sling procedures. These injuries can be devastating complications leading to sepsis, abscess, and even death.[29] Unfortunately, most of these injuries are not recognized until the postoperative period, when they lead to considerable morbidity. Initial signs and symptoms heralding a bowel injury may be subtle, including low-grade fever, abdominal pain, and ileus. If bowel injury is suspected, a diagnostic evaluation including plain and upright abdominal radiographs to ascertain the presence of intra-abdominal free air and cross-sectional imaging should be pursued expeditiously. Laparotomy, repair of the bowel injury, and possibly bowel resection are necessary for definitive treatment. In some cases, temporary proximal bowel diversion may be necessary.

Postoperative Complications

Voiding Dysfunction and Urinary Retention Bladder outlet obstruction (BOO) may occur following SUI surgical procedures. This complication manifests as prolonged complete urinary retention, persistently elevated postvoid residual urine volume, or as variably bothersome and poorly categorized lower urinary tract symptoms including combinations of obstructive symptoms and urinary urgency or UI. These last two groups are difficult to identify and are often not recognized as having BOO by many investigators. The incidence of postoperative voiding problems across various procedures is variable and is difficult to compare. Historically the incidence of postoperative voiding difficulties lasting >4 weeks occurred in 3% to 7% of patients undergoing Burch procedures, in 4% to 8% of those undergoing transvaginal needle suspensions, and in 3% to 11% of patients undergoing sling procedures.[10] The incidence of voiding dysfunction, including urinary retention and de novo urgency and urge UI, following midurethral sling procedures ranges from approximately 2% to 25%.[16,19,20,22,40,46-53]

Surgical intervention for voiding dysfunction and urinary retention has been reported in 0% to 5% of patients undergoing midurethral slings.[22,40,46-48,52] As noted previously, short-term voiding difficulties following Burch procedures appear more likely than following TVT.[17] This situation may also be true for pubovaginal slings as compared with TVT.[54] In one multicenter but limited retrospective study, transobturator slings had fewer "obstructive" complications than did retropubic midurethral slings.[55] The minimally invasive midurethral sling procedures are mechanistically tension free, and as such it is not surprising that they likely result in an overall lower incidence of postoperative voiding dysfunction than seen with other types of open SUI procedures.

The finding of absolute prolonged urinary retention makes the diagnosis of obstruction fairly straightforward if the patient had relatively normal voiding dynamics preoperatively. One potential exception is the patient who voids primarily by pelvic floor relaxation. Female patients may void without a perceptible increase in intravesical pressure and in these individuals, even a modest increase in outlet closure forces, such as that caused by a sling, may result in urinary retention. In many other patients, the diagnosis of BOO is extremely difficult. Urodynamic studies, especially videourodynamic studies, are often pursued diagnostically but may not be helpful in many cases because the classic "high pressure–low flow" pattern may not be present. No pressure-flow urodynamic criteria accurately predict successful voiding following urethrolysis.

Various nomograms have been developed for the diagnosis of female BOO but none are absolutely accepted as the gold standard. For patients not in frank urinary retention, the diagnosis of BOO is strongly suggested by the postoperative onset of irritative voiding symptoms, recurrent UTIs, and a poor urine stream. Physical examination may be completely normal or suggest an oversuspended midvaginal segment or the lack of mobility of the urethra following insertion of a metal sound. De novo prolapse should be excluded as a cause of postoperative BOO. An unrecognized and thus unrepaired cystocele may result in BOO following SUI surgical procedures.

Before surgical intervention for postoperative urinary retention is considered, many transient causes should be considered. These are potentially unrelated to iatrogenic BOO and the mechanical effects of the procedure. In the immediate postoperative period, pain is a common reason for delayed micturition. Postoperative pain at the surgical site or catheterization trauma may suppress the micturition reflex.[56] Similarly, postoperative pain relief from narcotic analgesics may suppress micturition as well. These effects are temporary and a period of catheterization for several days postoperatively allows resumption of normal voiding in most cases. Other potential causes of temporary postoperative urinary retention include patient immobility, edema at the operative site, and retropubic hematomas.

Management options for prolonged voiding difficulties include repeated voiding trials, initiation of intermittent urethral catheterization, and incision of the sling or urethrolysis. Some investigators recommended conservative therapy for postoperative voiding dysfunction for ≤3 months before surgical revision is attempted.[57] Most patients resume normal voiding following midurethral slings within 1 to 2 days of the procedure. However, some patients may be delayed for 1 to 2 weeks and those with a history of prior SUI surgical procedures or those undergoing concomitant prolapse repair may be further delayed.[58] However, a prolonged time to intervention for BOO may be associated with long-term, potentially irreversible bladder dysfunction even following successful urethrolysis.[59]

As compared with obstructive symptoms such as hesitancy, straining, and poor force of urine stream, overactive bladder symptoms resulting from iatrogenically induced BOO following an anti-UI surgical procedure are less likely to improve despite a technically successful operation. In one series, voiding symptoms resolved in 82% of obstructed patients following urethrolysis, whereas overactive bladder (storage) symptoms resolved in only 35%.[60] In this series, increased time to intervention was not correlated with persistent detrusor dysfunction.

Once the diagnosis of BOO is considered or established, options include long-term intermittent urethral catheterization, transvaginal or retropubic urethrolysis, or, if applicable, transvaginal incision of the sling. Transvaginal incision of autologous pubovaginal slings is often highly successful in improving voiding dynamics.[61,62] With the advent of midurethral slings, transvaginal incision of the sling is also often attempted as an initial step in these cases.[63] This procedure can be performed as soon as 1 week from the surgical procedure, although investigators vary with respect to the optimal timing of intervention. The incision can be made using local anesthesia in some cases.

Care must be taken to avoid urethral injury while performing a sling incision because the urethral wall may be draped over the taut sling and may be inadvertently pinched and perforated during dissection and isolation of the sling for incision. Generally, the longer the time from sling surgery to sling incision, the more difficult it can be to find the sling during repeat exploration. Following isolation and division of the sling, the edges of the cut sling often separate by 1 to 2 cm, a finding indicating a satisfactory result. Iatrogenic obstruction resulting from autologous fascial slings is often treated in this manner as well.[62] However, historically, some investigators waited ≤3 months before consideration of sling incision for obstructing fascial slings (**Fig. 50-3**).

For patients in whom transvaginal incision fails, or in patients who underwent a nonsling procedure as the

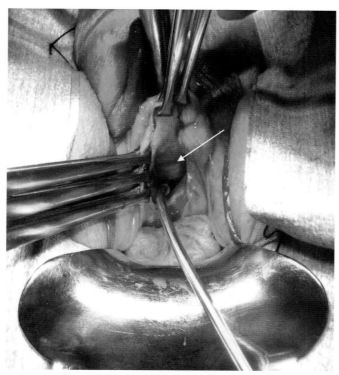

Figure 50-3 Transvaginal incision of a fascial sling. The sling in this case is seen between the tip of the sucker and the *white arrow* as a shiny band of tissue.

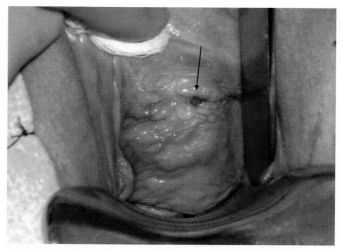

Figure 50-4 A small area of beefy granulation tissue (*black arrow*) is seen along the anterior vaginal wall in this patient, a finding suggesting vaginal extrusion.

cause of their BOO, urethrolysis may be performed.[64,65] Through a transvaginal or retropubic approach,[64,66,67] the retropubic space is entered and the urethra is sharply dissected off the posterior surface of the symphysis pubis and is freed from the surrounding scar. The limbs of the sling or other retropubic attachments are isolated and divided in the retropubic space. Lateral attachments to the pelvic sidewall are incised as needed for patients who previously underwent a Burch or paravaginal repair. A transvaginal, suprameatal approach to urethrolysis has also been described and may be particularly applicable to those patients who previously underwent an MMK procedure.[67]

Recurrence of SUI symptoms following urethrolysis or sling incision may occur in 15% to 20% of patients.[62,68] Patients should be counseled regarding this possibility preoperatively because some may wish to continue performing intermittent catheterization rather than risk recurrent SUI.

Vaginal Extrusion and Urinary Tract Erosion *Vaginal extrusion* refers to the finding of exposed sling material in the vaginal canal postoperatively, whereas *erosion* implies the finding of material within the lumen of the urinary tract at some time interval postoperatively that was clearly documented as not being within the urinary tract intraoperatively.

Extrusion of material may be related to surgical technique, infection, or the physical properties of the implanted material. The extruded material may be located in the midline at the incision line or at the anterolateral vaginal wall. Midline extrusions imply wound dehiscence. Lateral extrusions may result from an unrecognized vaginal wall perforation or injury at the time of sling placement.

Patients are usually symptomatic and have complaints suggesting an extrusion, including a malodorous vaginal discharge, vaginal spotting, vaginal pain, and dyspareunia. Patients may present several days to months postoperatively. On physical examination, the extruded material is often visible, but physical findings may also be quite subtle (**Fig. 50-4**).[69] Granulation tissue suggests the presence of an extrusion. Extruded synthetic mesh is often palpable within the vagina, although the patient's discomfort may preclude a complete examination.

Factors responsible for extrusion include the physical nature of the implanted material, the quality of the vaginal tissues of the host, sling tension, wound healing, and infection.[70] It appears that multifilament materials are at greater risk for extrusion than monofilaments.[71] In addition, a pore size that is large enough to permit fibroblast and macrophage infiltration and subsequent tissue ingrowth is an important factor in preventing extrusion.[72] Some risk factors are not well defined and are specific to the material; as a result, some products were removed from the market.[73,74] Synthetic material placed years earlier may eventually become infected and create a draining sinus or may become a nidus of pelvic infection or recurrent UTIs.[75] These materials will require exploration and explantation.

Small extrusions may heal with conservative management including the application of topical estrogen

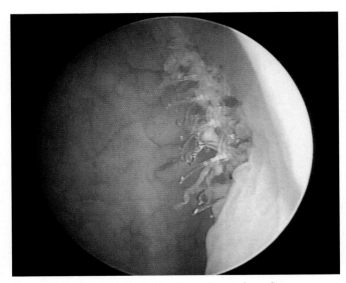

Figure 50-5 Intravesical erosion of a polypropylene sling.

creams. Larger extrusions can be managed with copious irrigation and secondary closure in the operating room. Some patients with large extrusions may benefit from excision and removal of the extruded segment of the sling.

In the immediate postoperative period, avoiding vaginal intercourse or vaginal tampon use should be strongly encouraged for the first 4 to 6 weeks following vaginal surgery to avoid disruption of the vaginal incision and subsequent extrusion of the sling material.

Urinary tract erosion may occur with synthetic, biologic, or autologous materials.[76] This is a devastating complication that unlike extrusion is almost always managed operatively. Whether urinary tract erosion results from a missed intraoperative urinary viscus perforation or from migration of the material into the urinary tract sometime following the surgical procedure is unclear. Patients may complain of irritative lower urinary tract symptoms, recurrent UTIs, hematuria, dysuria, and pelvic pain. The definitive diagnosis is usually made endoscopically (**Fig. 50-5**).

For intravesical erosions, endoscopic scissor or laser transection of the intravesical portion of the eroded sling may permit the remaining sling material to retract outside the urinary tract. If this procedure fails or is technically not feasible, then open operative exploration, removal of the eroded material, closure of the urinary tract, and postoperative drainage will be necessary.

Nerve Injury Several nerves traverse the deep pelvis as well as superficially within the lower abdominal soft tissues. These nerves are at risk for injury during UI surgical procedures in female patients. Stretch or compression injury to the femoral nerve can result from positioning. Femoral nerve compression may occur at the level of the inguinal ligament in response to flexion of the hip joint.[77] This complication results in sensory

changes to the anterior thigh or in more severe cases weakness of hip flexion. Severe abduction and external rotation of the thigh should be minimized during positioning to avoid this complication.

The peroneal nerve can be injured by direct compression while the patient is in the lithotomy position. Lateral direct pressure on the peroneal nerve between the stirrup at the lateral aspect of the knee joint and the fibular head for a prolonged period may result in peroneal nerve palsy and foot drop.[77] This injury may also occur with compression of the fibular head against the stirrup holder, especially when candy cane stirrups are used because the leg rotates externally after placement in the holders. The ilioinguinal and iliohypogastric nerves may be injured by suprapubic trocar placement or dissection resulting in pain in the suprapubic region.[78]

Bone Anchor–related Complications Although the use of bone anchors (BAs) was originally suggested as an alternative and perhaps even superior method of suture fixation during surgical procedures for SUI such as pubovaginal slings and needle bladder neck suspensions, the evidence to date supporting the use of BAs is weak. BAs have been at times touted as effective and minimally invasive; however, since their introduction, a convincing argument for the use of BAs has not evolved clinically or in the literature.[13] With the advent of minimally invasive midurethral slings, the use of BAs has declined.

The complications associated with BAs can be devastating, including osteitis pubis and osteomyelitis of the symphysis pubis. Numerous reports exist of BA-related complications associated with female UI surgical procedures in the urologic, gynecologic, and orthopedic scientific literature.[79-83] Graham and Dmochowski[83] reported on nine patients with pubic osteomyelitis following BA placement elsewhere who were referred for definitive therapy. The BAs were removed successfully from all patients, although residual problems included UI (five of nine patients), and chronic pain (three of nine patients). In a thorough review of the literature, Rackley and colleagues[81] estimated the prevalence of BA-related infections in female pelvic reconstructive procedures to be approximately 0.6%.

Once diagnosed, osteomyelitis related to BAs requires operative exploration and removal of the BA. The BAs are often seated below the cortical bone, a site that mandates partial resection of the overlying bone, usually with fluoroscopic guidance, to locate and remove the BA.

Sexual Dysfunction Historically, female sexual dysfunction following surgery for UI has only infrequently been reported. Whether this finding is the result of a generalized lack of understanding of the condition, a lack of interest in reporting or investigating its occurrence, or an actual low incidence is unclear. Only more recently has the trend been to query female patients regarding sexual dysfunction, and to date few instruments exist.[84]

Female sexual dysfunction is a complex and poorly understood phenomenon,[85-87] and a full discussion is beyond the scope of this chapter. Coital incontinence can be improved following successful sling operations,[88,89] and sexual function scores are similarly improved.[90] However, new-onset sexual dysfunction following sling procedures that is unrelated to vaginal sling erosion has been reported in ≤20% of patients in some series.[91,92] Shah and colleagues[93] reported no difference in female sexual function following distal urethral sling procedures.

Dyspareunia is only one form of sexual dysfunction, but it may occur following anti-UI surgical procedures. Vaginal anatomy is altered by the surgical treatment of SUI. The vaginal axis can be shifted, thus changing the angulation of the vaginal canal. Circumferential narrowing of the vagina may result from excessive trimming of vaginal wall during prolapse repair or simply as a result of aberrant scarring. Dissection along the anterior vaginal wall may cause nerve injury and neuroma formation. Other ill-defined and poorly understood factors contributing to postoperative sexual dysfunction may exist. For example, in some series, 4% to 5% of patients following TVT or intravaginal slingplasty experienced decreased libido.[89,91] The reason for this decreased libido is unclear.

Postoperative dyspareunia should be assessed by a thorough physical examination. When vaginal scarring or narrowing and especially sling extrusion have been excluded, other causes of new-onset sexual dysfunction should be explored and treated.[94]

Other Postoperative Complications Urinary fistula following anti-UI surgical procedures is quite rare. Nevertheless, an unrecognized and unrepaired intraoperative injury to the ureter, bladder, or urethra may result in ureterovaginal, vesicovaginal, or urethrovaginal fistula. Intraoperative recognition of the injury is critical to prevent fistula formation, and thus the importance of a careful intraoperative endoscopic examination and confirmation of urinary tract patency cannot be overemphasized.

De novo vaginal prolapse including cystocele and enterocele may also occur following anti-UI surgical procedures. Alteration of the vaginal axis especially with open retropubic procedures such as the Burch or MMK may result in anatomic changes that predispose patients to postoperative vaginal prolapse. Predicting which patients will develop postoperative vaginal prolapse is exceedingly difficult.

Periurethral Bulking Agents
In general, the morbidity associated with periurethral injectable agents is low. UTI, short-term voiding dys-

function[95] including urinary retention, and hematuria are seen with all the periurethral injectable agents. Minor complications have been reported in ≤20% of patients receiving GAX collagen, although most of these complications are self-limited. Stothers and colleagues[96] reviewed complications related to intraurethral collagen injection in a large series of patients. Of 337 patients injected with intraurethral collagen, approximately 20% had ≥1 minor complication. The most common reported complication was de novo urge UI in 12.6%, followed by hematuria in 5% and urinary retention in 1.9%. Three patients developed a delayed hypersensitivity reaction at the skin test site, 2 of whom patients had significant arthralgias. Although the nature of the complications attributed to intraurethral collagen in this study was somewhat benign and self-limited, even this relatively conservative therapy for the treatment of SUI is not without adverse effects.

Transient dysuria is not uncommon following intraurethral injections. This symptom is generally self-limited. For those individuals with persistent symptoms, UTI should be excluded. Tegress (ethylene vinyl alcohol), which was removed from the commercial marketplace, was associated with persistent dysuria, sometimes on exposure of the material in the urethral lumen following injection. In a series of 17 male patients injected with Tegress for the treatment of SUI, symptomatic urethral erosion of the material was noted in 41%.[97] Distal and systemic migration of periurethral injectable agents including Teflon and carbon-coated beads has been reported. The long-term ramifications of these synthetic materials in the lymph nodes, lungs, and other organs are unknown.[98]

Complications Related to Urge Incontinence Surgery

Botulinum Toxin A
Although BT is potentially quite toxic, few complications have been reported with its use. Local and self-limited complications such as hematuria, dysuria, pain, and infection are infrequently reported. The most worrisome potential complication, respiratory suppression, has not been reported with urinary tract injection of BT. Urinary retention following intradetrusor injection in non-neurogenic detrusor overactivity is uncommon but has been reported in 5% to 16% of patients.[99] Because the pharmacologic effects of BT are not manifest for 7 to 10 days following injection, immediate urinary retention following BT injection is likely related not to the agent itself but rather to other factors including instrumentation. Urinary retention or voiding dysfunction resulting from BT usually occurs 1 to 2 weeks following injection.

Scattered reports of systemic adverse effects have been noted with the use of the Dysport formulation of BT available in Europe. The FDA approved Dysport for

TABLE 50-3	Adverse Events Related to Sacral Neuromodulation (InterStim Implantation) in 219 Patients	
Adverse Event	**Percentage (%)**
Pain at the stimulator site	15.3
New pain	9.0
Lead migration	8.4
Infection	6.1
Transient electric shock	5.5
Pain at the lead site	5.4
Changes in bowel function	3.0

Adapted from Seigel SW, Catanzano F, Dijkema H, et al. Long-term results of a multicenter study on sacral nerve stimulation for treatment of urinary urge incontinence, urgency-frequency and retention. *Urology.* 2000;56(suppl 6):87-91.

use in the United States in April 2009. These reactions have included generalized muscle weakness and hyposthenia in ≤6% of individuals and appear to be dose related because they have not been reported with the use of lower doses of the material.[99] One case of mild arm weakness has been reported with the use of the BOTOX formulation of BT that is available for certain nonurologic applications in the United States.

Sacral Neuromodulation

Several complications related to sacral neuromodulation have been well documented. Overall, the reported surgical revision or removal rate has been reported to be ≤16% to 32%.[100,101] Seigel and colleagues[102] reported adverse events in 219 patients (Table 50-3); in these patients, pain at the stimulator site was the most common event. Pain at the stimulator site is the most frequently reported complication in many series.[101,103] Generally relocation of the device into another buttock or lower abdominal site improves the pain.

KEY POINTS

1. The popularity of midurethral polypropylene slings has changed the types of complications seen in surgical treatment of SUI.
2. New voiding symptoms including overactive bladder symptoms or recurrent UTIs following anti-UI surgical procedures may indicate iatrogenic BOO, which is a very difficult and subtle diagnosis in many patients.
3. Intraoperative trocar injury to the bladder during midurethral sling placement is common, and completion of procedure can be accomplished with minimal morbidity.
4. Currently, few or no data on complications support one approach to midurethral slings over another (i.e., retropubic versus transvaginal versus transobturator) as causing less morbidity.
5. Attention to technique, experience of the surgeon, and careful endoscopic examination of the urinary tract following anti-UI surgical procedures are important factors in reducing operative and postoperative complications.

REFERENCES

Please see www.expertconsult.com

Chapter 51

COMPLICATIONS OF SURGERY FOR MALE INCONTINENCE

Katie N. Ballert MD
Fellow, Department of Urology, New York University School of Medicine, New York, New York

Victor W. Nitti MD
Professor and Vice Chairman, Department of Urology, New York University School of Medicine, New York, New York

Urinary incontinence is a potential complication following surgical treatment of benign prostatic hyperplasia or prostate cancer and has a significant impact on quality of life.[1,2] Most cases of incontinence following radical prostatectomy and some cases of incontinence caused by treatments for benign prostatic hyperplasia result from sphincteric insufficiency.[3,4] The artificial urinary sphincter (AUS) is the current gold standard for the treatment of male stress urinary incontinence. Other treatment options such as male sling (MS) procedures and inflatable balloon compression devices have been described for patients with less severe incontinence and those not desiring a mechanical device.

Three distinct types of sling procedures have been described:

1. The so-called bulbourethral slings compress the urethra and extend from suprapubically to suburethrally.[5,6]
2. The bone-anchored perineal slings compress the urethra from a perineal approach only and are the most commonly used MSs.[7,8] Intermediate-term success rates comparable to those seen with the AUS in appropriately selected patients have been reported with the bone-anchored sling.[9]
3. More recently, the transobturator sling was developed as an additional treatment option for male stress incontinence. The theory is that this sling restores continence not by urethral compression but rather by repositioning the proximal urethra. Tensioning causes proximal movement of the dorsal portion of the proximal bulb that, in turn, affects closure of the urethral lumen and advances the membranous urethra cranial and posteriorly.[10] Outcome data available on transobturator slings are limited.

Each of these procedures has its own set of complications of which physicians and patients should be aware.

In this chapter, we first discuss preoperative evaluation, which can influence potential complications. We then briefly describe the surgical procedures most commonly performed for male urinary incontinence (in order for the reader to appreciate when and why certain complications occur), and finally we discuss the potential complications encountered during the procedures with respect to their temporal occurrence (Table 51-1).

PREOPERATIVE CONSIDERATIONS

Traditionally most urologists agreed that patients should be followed for approximately 12 months before surgical management of postprostatectomy incontinence is pursued. More recently, earlier intervention (e.g., at 6 months) has been recommended in severe cases of incontinence with no temporal improvement. The evaluation of a patient with postprostatectomy incontinence should include a thorough history and physical examination. Important aspects of the history include precipitating factors, associated symptoms (frequency, urgency, nocturia, weak urine stream), severity of incontinence, and impact on quality of life. The history should also address the patient's voiding symptoms before prostate surgery as well as a history of neurologic disease or symptoms, radiation therapy, additional procedures, and earlier attempts at treating the incontinence. During the physical examination, the patient should be instructed to cough or perform a Valsalva maneuver to demonstrate the presence of stress incontinence. In addition, a focused neurologic examination should be performed.

We perform a 24-hour pad test to assess the severity of incontinence objectively as well as to help guide our discussion with the patient regarding surgical options and outcome expectations. In a study by Fisher and colleagues,[11] the only preoperative factor predictive of success following a perineal MS procedure was 24-hour

TABLE 51-1	Complications of Male Incontinence Surgery		
	Intraoperative	**Early**	**Late**
Artificial urinary sphincter	Corporeal injury Urethral injury Device injury Bleeding	Hematoma Retention Infection Erosion	Infection Erosion Urethral atrophy Mechanical Retention
Male sling	Bleeding Urethral injury Obturator nerve injury	Hematoma Retention Infection Pain Paresthesia	Infection Erosion De novo urgency Obstruction Prolonged pain Prolonged paresthesia

pad weight. Patients with high-grade incontinence and those with very low-grade incontinence do not do as well with an MS.[11] The reason for the lower rate of satisfaction among patients with very low-grade incontinence was thought to be related to extremely high expectations in that group.

We also perform urodynamic studies in all patients before surgical treatment of postprostatectomy incontinence. Urodynamic testing allows for determination of the cause and guides the treatment of male urinary incontinence.[12] The main goals of the urodynamic evaluation are to determine the presence of sphincteric insufficiency or bladder dysfunction, to evaluate for obstruction, and to assess detrusor contractility. It is crucial that the study reproduce the patient's symptoms, which in this case would be incontinence. We follow the urodynamic protocol described by Huckabay and colleagues[13] that includes evaluation both with and without a urethral catheter. This urodynamic protocol addresses the subset of men with postprostatectomy stress urinary incontinence who have no leakage with the catheter in place[4,14] and allows for documentation of sphincteric insufficiency in these men. In addition, a flow rate without the catheter allows corroboration of free maximal flow (free Qmax) and Qmax in those patients who have suspected obstruction based on pressure-flow analysis.

PROCEDURES FOR MALE INCONTINENCE

Artificial Urinary Sphincter

Various techniques exist for implantation of the AUS (AMS 800, American Medical Systems, Minnetonka, Minnesota). The classic approach consists of a perineal incision and a lower abdominal incision (either transverse or midline). Other investigators have described placement through a single penoscrotal incision.[15] Traditionally, after placement of a Foley catheter, a midline perineal incision is made and the bulbospongiosus muscle is exposed. The bulbospongiosus muscle can be split or preserved, although we and most other surgeons choose to split it. The urethra is then dissected circumferentially with special attention given to mobilization of the urethra from the intracrural septum. An approximately 2-cm window is made between the corpora cavernosa and the urethra. The urethra is inspected for injury by withdrawing the Foley catheter into the distal urethra and instilling saline solution. The urethra is then measured, and the appropriately sized cuff is placed.

We typically use a transverse lower abdominal incision for placement of the reservoir; however, a midline incision is also an option. The reservoir can be placed preperitoneally, intraperitoneally, or in the retropubic space. We retract the rectus muscle medially, open the transversalis fascia, and place the reservoir in the retropubic space. Typically, a reservoir with 61 to 70 cm H_2O pressure is used and is filled with 23 mL of saline solution. The tubing from the cuff is passed over the pubic bone into the suprapubic incision. Finally, a plane is developed between the suprapubic incision and the ipsilateral hemiscrotum, and a pocket is created in a dependent position for the pump. The components are then connected, and the device is cycled and deactivated.

Male Slings

Bone-Anchored Sling

The most commonly used bone-anchored sling is the InVance sling (American Medical Systems, Minnetonka, Minnesota). We prefer regional anesthesia so that a cough test can be performed during the procedure. A Foley catheter is placed, and a midline perineal incision is made. The bulbospongiosus muscle is identified and the bilateral pubic rami are exposed. Three bone anchors with attached polypropylene suture are placed bilaterally with the use of a drill. The first anchor is placed at the junction of the pubic symphysis and the pubic ramus, the second is placed approximately 3 cm below the first, and the last splits the distance between the two. A 4 × 7 cm silicone-coated polyester mesh sling is secured unilaterally with the polypropylene sutures. Initial tension is determined by performing a cough test

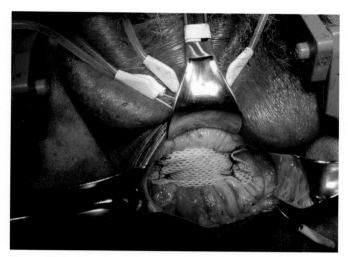

Figure 51-1 Bone-anchored male sling secured into position.

with 250 mL in the bladder. The contralateral side of the sling is secured with a single throw in the sutures, and a retrograde leak point pressure (RLPP) is determined. Tension is readjusted if the RLPP is not ≥60 cm H$_2$O. The sling is completely secured into position (**Fig. 51-1**), and both the cough test and the RLPP are repeated to ensure appropriate tension. The excess mesh is then excised.

Bulbourethral Slings

A percutaneous suprapubic tube and a Foley catheter are placed. A transverse suprapubic incision is made and is taken down to the rectus fascia. A midline perineal incision is made and Colles' fascia is incised laterally to the bulbocavernosus muscle. Finger dissection medial to the ischial arch and lateral to the bulbocavernosus muscle is performed. A modified Stamey needle is passed from the suprapubic incision, lateral to the vesical neck and urethra, and out through the perineal membrane anteriorly between the bulbocavernous muscle and the ischial bone. The sutures on one end of three previously prepared bolsters are passed through the needle, and the needle is withdrawn into the suprapubic incision. The procedure is then repeated on the contralateral side. The bolsters are placed in parallel formation over the urethra to form a sling, and the most posterior bolster is sutured to the bulbocavernous muscle to prevent migration. Tension is placed on the sutures and, using pressure measurements as a guide, they are tied across midline. Cystoscopy can either be performed during or following needle passage to exclude urethral injury.[5] Romano and colleagues[6] described modifications to the procedure that allow placement of an adjustable bulbourethral sling (Argus, Promedon SA, Cordoba, Argentina). The modifications include omitting the suprapubic tube and passing the needle from the perineum to the abdomen in an attempt to decrease urethral injuries.[6]

Transobturator Male Sling

The most commonly used transobturator MS is the Advance (American Medical Systems, Minnetonka, Minnesota). A Foley catheter is placed, and a midline perineal incision is made. The bulbospongiosus muscle is identified, split in the midline, and dissected off the urethra. The urethra is dissected to the level of the perineal body and genitourinary diaphragm. A mark is made on the skin approximately 2 cm below and 1.5 cm lateral to the insertion of the adductor longus. A spinal needle may be used to ensure that the obturator fossa lies at the level of the mark, and a small skin incision is made. A helical passer is then passed through the skin incision, the obturator fossa, the obturator externus muscle, and the obturator membrane. The triangle formed by the urethra, the bulbospongiosus muscle, and the bulbocavernosus muscle is palpated and the trocar is guided onto the surgeon's index finger. A similar procedure is performed on the contralateral side. Cystoscopy is performed to ensure that no injury to the bladder or urethra has occurred. The sling is then attached and is brought out through the skin. The sling is secured proximally and distally in the midline with suture, and tension is placed to provide elevation of the urethra. Cystoscopy is repeated to evaluate urethral coaptation.[10]

Inflatable Balloon Compression

Prostate adjustable continence therapy (ProACT, Uromedica, Plymouth, Minnesota) has been introduced as a minimally invasive treatment for postprostatectomy incontinence. At the time of this writing, ProACT is not available in the United States, although it is used commonly in other countries around the world. The patient is placed in the lithotomy position and cystoscopy is performed. Instillation into the bladder of 50 to 100 mL of contrast material is performed and the cystoscope sheath with its obturator is left in place. A perineal incision is made, and previously a Kelly clamp was used to perforate the pelvic floor.[16,17] More recently, a tissue expansion device has been used to facilitate development of the periurethral space.[18] Following creation of the tract using a special trocar in a U-shaped cannula, the tissue expansion device is inserted. The balloon is then placed in an area beneath the bladder neck and dorsolateral to the urethra. The balloon is filled with 1 to 5 mL of contrast medium and sterile water. A balloon is placed on the contralateral side in a similar fashion. Cystoscopy is performed to confirm balloon position and to exclude urethral injury. Blunt dissection is then performed toward the scrotum, and the balloon ports are placed bilaterally just beneath dartos fascia in the scrotum. This technique allows for percutaneous needle access for future inflation or deflation of the balloons.[16,17]

INTRAOPERATIVE COMPLICATIONS

Artificial Urinary Sphincter

Most intraoperative complications are inconsequential if they are recognized and treated at the time of the surgical procedure. The exception is urethral injury, which requires aborting the procedure in most cases.

Corporeal Injury

In AUS placement procedures, urethral or corporeal injury can occur during mobilization of the urethra from the intracrural septum. Corporeal injury may result in significant bleeding that can impair visualization. Adequate exposure is the key to identifying the injury. Once the injury is identified it can be repaired with absorbable suture.

Urethral Injury

Urethral injury is another potential intraoperative complication and one that should not go unrecognized. Urethral injury typically occurs dorsally, where the spongiosum is thinnest. To detect an unrecognized urethral injury, saline or dilute indigo carmine can be instilled along side the Foley catheter or through the Foley catheter while moving it in a retrograde fashion. If a urethral injury is identified, it should be repaired in multiple layers with absorbable suture, if possible. Most surgeons would abort AUS placement and a leave a Foley catheter for an appropriate period of time. In rare cases if the injury is small and away from the intended site of implantation, the cuff can be placed, although this must be done with extreme caution.

If any question exists regarding the repair or if the cuff cannot be placed away from the site of injury, then the procedure should be aborted. Injury to the corpus spongiosum but not involving the urethra is usually inconsequential especially when it occurs ventrally where the spongy tissue is thick. Such injuries can simply be oversewn to control bleeding. Dorsally, where the sponge this thin, concomitant urethral injury is common.

Device Injury

Care must also be taken to avoid any injury to the device. Damage to the device can result in leakage of fluid from the device and mechanical failure. The tubing should be handled with rubber-shod clamps and care should be taken not to injure the device with sharp instruments or needles. If a device injury is noted, the "injured" component should be replaced. Unrecognized injury results in malfunction of the device as fluid leaks out of the system.

Bleeding

Most significant bleeding with AUS placement results from corpora cavernosa or spongiosum injury (see earlier). Bleeding can also occur with placement of the reservoir from epigastric or retroperitoneal vessels.

Male Sling

Intraoperative complications with sling placement are unusual, and the most common with a bone-anchored sling is bleeding. Minimal literature is available on the newer transobturator placement of an MS. Based on the technique, obturator nerve injury would certainly seem to be a possibility, but it has not yet been reported.

Bleeding

We are unaware of any reported cases of significant intraoperative bleeding following MS procedures, and none of the major series have reported transfusions.[9,11,19-21] However, corporeal injury and bleeding can occur during dissection or during placement of the bone anchors. This bleeding usually occurs when the corporeal bodies are dissected off the pubic ramus to facilitate placement of bone anchors. Bleeding can also occur when a bone anchor is placed through the corpora.

Bleeding from a main or accessory obturator vessel would certainly be possible with transobturator sling placement. When a transobturator sling is placed, it is not unusual to encounter bleeding as the urethra is dissected to the perineal body. This bleeding usually results from small injuries to the spongiosum that can be oversewn with fine absorbable suture (e.g., 4-0 polyglycolic acid). During the same procedure, bleeding can be caused by injury to small vessels along the route of needle passage through the obturator fossa. When this occurs, bleeding can usually can be controlled by tensioning the sling. Certainly, injury to a major obturator vessel is possible, but we are unaware of any reported cases of major vascular injury.

Urethral Injury

Urethral injury with the bone-anchored sling is not reported in the literature but is certainly possible and should be treated as described earlier for the AUS.

Romano and colleagues[6] reported a potential urethral perforation rate of 6% with the Argus adjustable bulbo-urethral sling. This situation was addressed intraoperatively by repositioning the needle and resulted in no further complications.[6] With transobturator sling placement, urethral injury is possible from needle perforation, usually near the bladder neck. Thus cystoscopy after sling placement is essential. If such an injury is seen, the needle or sling should be removed. The injury is usually not in a position that can easily be repaired, so treatment is with catheter drainage for ≤7 days depending on the size of the injury. The sling may be replaced in the same setting at the surgeon's discretion depending on the site and size of the injury.

Inflatable Balloon Compression

No major bleeding complications have been reported during placement of ProACT. Hübner and Schlarp[18] reported an 8% rate of urethral perforation, a 4% rate of immediate balloon rupture, and a 4% rate of intraoperative balloon migration in their initial 50 patients. In the most recent 50 cases, no urethral perforations, balloon ruptures, or migrations have occurred intraoperatively.[18]

Bladder Perforation

Bladder perforation rates of 8% to 18% have been reported. In the majority of cases, this complication resulted in delayed implantation on the affected side with an indwelling Foley catheter for 3 days.[16,17] However, more recently, Hübner and Schlarp[18] reported placing the balloon more distally in cases of "minor" perforation.

EARLY POSTOPERATIVE COMPLICATIONS

Artificial Urinary Sphincter

Hematoma

Scrotal hematoma is a common minor postoperative complication associated with AUS implantation. Hematomas typically resolve spontaneously without intervention; evacuation is rarely indicated.

Urinary Retention

Another early complication is urinary retention as a result of postoperative edema. We typically leave a 14-Fr Foley catheter in place overnight in an attempt to avoid this problem. Bladder neck dilation (for anastomotic stricture) is a risk factor for urinary retention beyond 24 hours. If retention occurs following removal of the Foley catheter, the first step should be examination of the device to ensure deactivation with the cuff in an open position. If catheterization is required, it should be performed carefully with a small 10- to 14-Fr Foley catheter and catheterization time should be kept to a minimum (preferably <48 hours).[22] In addition, if one has even the slightest difficulty in replacing a catheter, this procedure should be performed under endoscopic guidance or a suprapubic tube should be placed. If the patient is unable to void after 48 hours, suprapubic catheter placement may be considered.[23]

Early Infection

Early infection can occur and may manifest with erythema, induration or edema around the pump, purulent drainage, fever, or pain in the scrotum, groin, or perineum. Early infection is most typically the result of bacterial contamination at the time of implantation.

The most common organism in early infection is *Staphylococcus epidermidis*.[24] Another potential cause of early infection is unrecognized urethral injury. Urethroscopy should be performed when the device is removed. Infection requires removal of the entire device and reimplantation after ≥3 months. In selected cases, one may consider device replacement at the time of removal after aggressive wound irrigation with antibiotics, as described by Bryan and colleagues[25] (see later).

Early Erosion

Early erosion can also occur with or without infection. It is likely the result of unrecognized iatrogenic urethral injury, urethral thinning, or early postoperative replacement of a Foley catheter. Erosion may manifest with pain or swelling in the scrotum or perineum, pain referred to the tip of the penis, recurrent incontinence, dysuria, hematuria, or bloody discharge. If erosion occurs without infection, the tubing can be capped at the time of cuff removal. If it is associated with infection, the entire device should be removed. The urethra is repaired with absorbable suture, if possible, and a Foley catheter is left indwelling. A voiding cysto-urethrogram is performed to ensure that the urethra has healed before the catheter is removed, and at the time of reimplantation a different site is selected for the cuff.

Male Perineal Sling

Hematoma

Fassi-Fehri and colleagues[20] reported postoperative hematoma in 4% (2 of 50) of patients undergoing placement of an MS. All cases resolved spontaneously.[20]

Acute Urinary Retention

Fassi-Fehri and colleagues[20] reported transitory acute urinary retention in 12% of patients on initial removal of the catheter following bone-anchored sling procedures. All cases resolved after 48 to 72 hours of catheterization.[20] Rajpurkar and colleagues[21] reported no acute postoperative urinary retention in their series, but two (4.3%) of their patients had high postvoid residual (>100 mL) that resolved within 48 hours. We currently leave a Foley catheter indwelling for 48 to 72 hours after placement of bone-anchored perineal slings to avoid acute postoperative urinary retention. We found a relatively high rate of failure to void when the catheter was removed after 24 hours. Postoperative pain may contribute to early urinary retention. After 48 hours, the risk of urinary retention is <10%. In truth, acute retention can be expected in a certain number of cases and is more of an unfavorable early outcome than it is a true complication.

Romano and colleagues[6] reported a 15% rate of acute urinary retention with the Argus bulbourethral sling. All but one case of urinary retention resolved with short-term Foley catheter placement. One patient required loosening of the sling 15 days postoperatively.[6]

Pain and Paresthesia

Postoperative pain and paresthesia have been reported in all types of MS and have been the most disappointing aspects of bone-anchored MS procedures in our experience. Castle and colleagues[19] reported that immediately following placement of a bone-anchored sling, the majority of their patients experienced significant perineal pain that completely resolved within 3 to 4 months. Rajpurkar and colleagues[21] reported "short lasting" perineal/buttock pain in 4.3% of their patients, whereas Comiter[9] reported that 16% of patients complained of "bothersome" scrotal numbness or pain that resolved in ≤3 months.

Following placement of the Argus sling, Romano and colleagues[6] reported a 21% rate of dysuria associated with perineal discomfort or moderate pain that resolved or became very mild after 1 to 2 months of analgesics and nonsteroidal anti-inflammatory drugs. During the first two cases performed, these investigators used an RLPP of 100 cm H_2O for intraoperative adjustment of the sling. They found that these patients had severe perineal pain that was relieved only by cutting the suprapubic suture at 7 and 25 days postoperatively. Subsequently, the adjustment pressure was decreased to 45 cm H_2O.[6]

Pain without evidence of infection can be managed conservatively with anti-inflammatory medications or analgesics as necessary. Persistent pain should be evaluated. We obtain a computed tomography (CT) scan or bone scan in appropriate cases. In patients with severe or persistent pain, consideration should be given to sling removal.

Infection

Early postoperative infection is possible with MS. As with the AUS, it is probably the result of bacterial contamination at the time of implantation. In approximately 90 cases, we have seen this complication once. The presentation was with erythema, swelling, and spontaneous drainage from the perineal incision.

Inflatable Balloon Compression

Acute urinary retention was reported in 4% to 6% of patients after ProACT placement. Treatment consisted of withdrawing a small amount of solution from the balloons through the injection ports. Infection, erosion, and balloon migration and rupture were also reported, but the time to occurrence was not specified.[16-18] These complications are discussed in the following section on delayed complications.

DELAYED AND LONG-TERM COMPLICATIONS

Artificial Urinary Sphincter

Infection and Erosion

Rates of infection reported in large contemporary series range from 0% to 14%.[26-31] Some investigators have reported higher infection rates in patients after pelvic radiation,[22,32,33] whereas others have reported similar infection rates.[26,30] In contrast to early infections, in which the most common cultured pathogens are skin flora, late infections (>4 months after implantation) are thought to be the result of hematogenous seeding secondary to bacteremia from another source.[23,24] Late infections most commonly present with scrotal pain, but they may also manifest with erythema, edema or induration around the pump, or fever. Infection is most commonly managed by removing all components of the device; however, Bryan, Mulcahy, and Simmons[25] reported management of patients with a salvage technique similar to that used for salvage of penile prostheses. Cystoscopy is performed to rule out urethral erosion. All prosthetic parts are removed, wounds are copiously irrigated according to a seven solution protocol, and a new device is implanted.[25]

In several large series, erosion rates ranging from 2.2% to 6.6% were reported.[26-31,34] Common causes of erosion included prolonged catheterization, catheterization without cuff deactivation, and repeated endoscopic manipulation of the urethra. In a study by Raj and colleagues,[35] patients with hypertension, coronary artery disease, prior radiation, and prior AUS revision (especially for erosion) were found to have a higher likelihood of erosion. These investigators also found that patients undergoing revision for erosion had worse postoperative continence rates than did those undergoing revision for other reasons.[35]

Other investigators also found a higher rate of erosion in irradiated patients. In a series of men with post-prostatectomy incontinence, Walsh and colleagues[32] reported that erosions were more common in patients that had received radiation therapy (23%) than those that had not (1%). On the contrary, Lai and colleagues[26] found no statistical difference in erosion rates among nonirradiated patients, irradiated patients, patients with neurogenic disease, or patients who underwent secondary implantation. In patients who experienced erosion, these investigators found a median time to erosion of 19.8 months.[26]

Potential manifestations of urethral erosion include pain or swelling in the perineum or scrotum, pain referred to the tip of the penis, recurrent incontinence, dysuria, hematuria, or bloody discharge. Erosion is typically into the urethra, but erosion of tubing to the skin can also occur. Urethral erosion typically occurs on the dorsal side of the urethra where the sponge is thinnest, but it can occur anywhere, especially if is associated

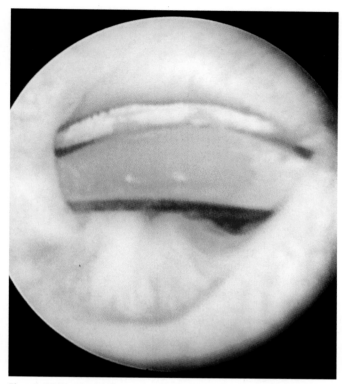

Figure 51-2 Urethral erosion of an artificial urinary sphincter, cystoscopic view. The color indicates that this is likely a long-standing erosion.

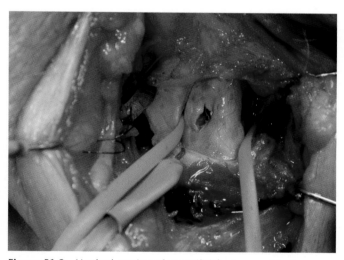

Figure 51-3 Urethral erosion of an artificial urinary sphincter, gross view.

with trauma (**Figs. 51-2 and Fig 51-3**). When urethral erosion occurs, at a minimum the cuff must be removed. If one suspects an associated infection, the entire device should be removed. The site of erosion may be repaired with absorbable suture if it can be easily accessed. However, dorsal erosions are the most common and are often left unrepaired and simply allowed to heal with a

period of catheterization. In either case, a Foley catheter is left indwelling until closure is evidenced by voiding cystourethrogram, usually in 1 to 2 weeks. Reimplantation is performed 3 to 6 months later. Before reimplantation, cystourethroscopy is performed to ensure adequate healing and to rule out formation of a stricture at the site of previous erosion. The new cuff is positioned away from the erosion site.

Guralnick and colleagues[36] described a transcorporeal technique to address patients who require a distal cuff location secondary to previous erosion or urethral atrophy. This technique involves vertical corporotomies with creation of a tunnel leaving a cuff of tunica albuginea on the dorsal surface of the urethra.[36]

Recurrent Incontinence

Recurrent incontinence can result from bladder or sphincteric dysfunction. When it is caused by sphincteric insufficiency, it is likely related to urethral atrophy or mechanical malfunction of the device, as discussed later. Recurrent incontinence can also be a manifestation of infection or erosion, as previously discussed. If it is not clear whether the incontinence is the result of bladder or sphincteric dysfunction, urodynamic evaluation can be helpful. When performing urodynamic studies in a patient who has an AUS, the device should be deactivated with the cuff deflated before the catheter is inserted. Once the catheter is in place, the AUS should be reactivated for filling and stress testing.

Urethral Atrophy

The introduction of the narrow-backed cuff has improved urethral pressure transmission; however, urethral atrophy still accounts for a significant portion of nonmechanical AUS revisions.[28,37] Rates of urethral atrophy have been reported to range from 0% to 14%.[26-31] Obviously, these rates vary depending on length of follow-up.

Urethral atrophy manifests as new-onset incontinence. Examination demonstrates a normally functioning pump. Cystourethroscopy may reveal incomplete coaptation of the urethra, and the urethra may appear thin and pale. Multiple management options have been proposed for urethral atrophy including downsizing the cuff,[38] placing the cuff in a more proximal location,[39] placing tandem cuffs,[40] increasing reservoir pressure, or placing the cuff transcorporeally.[36] In addition, one report demonstrated that in patients who deactivated their cuff at night, recurrent incontinence secondary to urethral atrophy was decreased from 21% to 10%.[37] We prefer to downsize the cuff if possible as the first-line treatment for urethral atrophy. Our second choice is to move the cuff to another position, usually proximally. Placing a transcorporeal cuff is also a viable option when adequate urethral circumference cannot be obtained. Rahman and colleagues[41] also described wrapping the urethra with a biologic material to increase bulk.

Mechanical Malfunction

Mechanical malfunctions can include leakage from one of the components, kinking of the tubing, pump malfunction, and connector separation. Reported rates of mechanical malfunction in several large series ranged from 6% to 25.3%.[26-31] A >50% decrease in mechanical failure rates has been attributed to improvements in the material used to make the AUS and the introduction of the narrow-back cuff.[28,42] Mechanical malfunction typically manifests with recurrent incontinence, but it can also manifest with urinary retention. Physical examination often reveals a pump that is difficult to compress, one that is partially decompressed, or one that takes too long to refill. Intraoperative methods of evaluating component leakage including Ohm testing and volumetric pressure measurements are available. If a component-specific malfunction is identified, the component can be replaced. If the problematic site (e.g., point of leakage) cannot be found or the device is >3 years old, all components should be removed and replaced.

Urinary Retention

Urinary retention that manifests as a late postoperative complication requires endoscopic examination to evaluate the AUS and the bladder neck for contracture or urethral stricture. Contracture and urethral stricture usually result from prostate surgery and not from the AUS per se but nevertheless must be checked. Difficultly with voiding or urinary retention can also be a sign of AUS erosion or late infection. Urinary retention may also be the result of mechanical malfunction.

Male Sling

Infection and Erosion

Reported rates of infection and erosion following a bone-anchored MS are 2.1% to 7.9% and 0% to 2.6%, respectively (**Figs. 51-4 and 51-5**).[9,19-21] All cases of reported erosion occurred with associated infection. There is very little information available regarding the time to infection or erosion. In our experience, patients more commonly present at 6 to 9 months postoperatively. However, Fassi-Fehri and colleagues reported that two of the infections they observed occurred within the first postoperative month and one occurred at 3 months postoperatively.[20] Little information exists regarding the clinical manifestations of infection or erosion. We have noted that patients with infection often present with chronic, low-grade symptoms including mild perineal pain or swelling, or a sinus tract that intermittently drains small amounts of fluid (**Fig. 51-6**) as opposed to acute or systemic symptoms. Removal of the sling is the typical treatment of infection or erosion. However, we

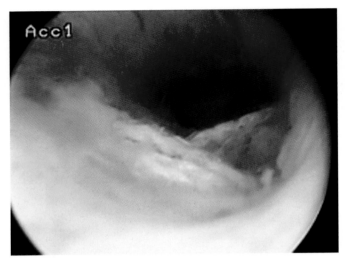

Figure 51-4 Eroded male sling, cystoscopic view.

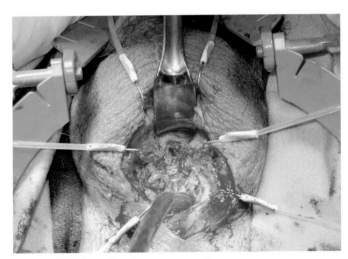

Figure 51-5 Eroded male sling, gross view.

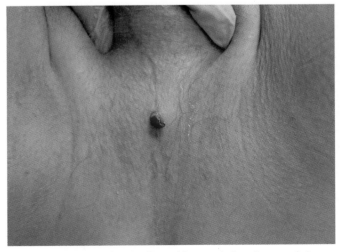

Figure 51-6 Infected male sling with granulation tissue and sinus tract.

have found that despite infection some patients are very reluctant to undergo sling removal secondary to improvement in their continence. We attempted salvage of the sling in two of these patients using the irrigation protocol previously described for salvage of the AUS.[25] This was unsuccessful and both slings subsequently required removal. In addition, we have one patient who has been managed with intermittent antibiotics and fulguration of a chronic sinus tract for >1 year because of his reluctance to have the sling removed.

At 4-year follow-up after bulbourethral sling placement, Stern and colleagues[43] reported an 8% (5 of 62) bolster removal rate in patients who had not received prior radiation therapy and a 22% (2 of 9) bolster removal rate in those who had received radiation therapy. Among patients who had not received radiation therapy, four had bolsters removed secondary to infection or erosion and one had bolsters removed secondary to nonfunction. In patients who had received prior radiation therapy, one required bolster removal secondary to infection and the other underwent removal because of nonfunction.[43] Romano and colleagues[6] reported a 6% (3 of 48) rate of infection and a 4% (2 of 48) rate of erosion following placement of the Argus adjustable sling. All five slings were removed.[6] To date, no known reports exist of infection or erosion with the Advance transobturator sling, but certainly both complications are possible.

De Novo Urgency

To our knowledge, de novo urgency is a previously unreported complication. However, in our series, one patient (1.6%) developed de novo urge incontinence 6½ months postoperatively that was confirmed with urodynamic studies.[11] De novo urgency requires urodynamic evaluation to rule out possible obstruction. If no evidence of obstruction is present, a trial of anticholinergic agents is recommended.

Obstruction

Iatrogenic obstruction following placement of an MS is rare but not impossible. In addition, it was previously reported that the fixed urethral resistance provided by the MS would not result in bladder outlet obstruction.[44] In our experience, however, three patients (4.8%) developed prolonged obstructive symptoms postoperatively.[11] The sling caused the obstruction in two of the patients who experienced urinary retention requiring intermittent catheterization. The other patient had impaired detrusor contractility and the sling did not result in urodynamic obstruction, but it may have increased voiding symptoms. All three patients underwent sling revision. To address obstruction and maintain some improvement in continence, the sling can be loosened. The sling can be isolated in the midline and partially cut (**Fig. 51-7**). Alternatively, or if this does not help, the sling can be completely transected.

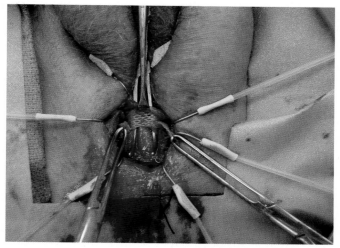

Figure 51-7 A right angle was placed between the intact sling and the urethra and the sling was cut until tension was relieved.

Other options for sling revision include removal and replacement of the sling or release of one side of the sling and replacement of sutures more laterally on the sling. In our experience, the second option has not been possible because the excess sling has typically been excised at the time of sling placement. With regard to the bulbourethral sling, Schaeffer and colleagues[5] reported that one patient (1.6%) had persistent urinary retention requiring clean intermittent catheterization.

Prolonged Pain and Paresthesia

Most patients have perineal pain after placement of a bone-anchored sling; however, most published series have reported resolution of the pain 3 to 4 months postoperatively.[9,19] We found that 8.1% of patients experienced prolonged (>3 months) paresthesia or perineal pain.[11] In addition, Fassi-Fehri and colleagues[20] reported a 12% incidence of prolonged pain requiring analgesic management. In our experience, patients with prolonged paresthesia following bone-anchored sling procedures typically located the symptoms to the scrotum, and those who had prolonged pain experienced it in the perineum. Most of our patients were managed effectively with watchful waiting and anti-inflammatory medications.

In patients with severe, persistent pain, however, we obtain a bone scan and a CT scan to evaluate for osseus or infectious complications. Pain can be a manifestation of sling infection. One patient in our series had persistent pain severe enough to require removal of the sling. Despite unremarkable imaging, the sling was infected at the time of removal.

Clemens and colleagues[45] found that, 9 months after a bulbourethral sling procedure, only 47.5% of patients reported no perineal numbness or pain and 26% reported moderate or severe pain. At 4-year follow-up, however, these investigators found that 82% of patients reported no perineal numbness or pain and only 12% reported moderate or severe pain.[43]

Osseus Complications

A potential risk for osseus complications exist because screws are placed into the bone. To our knowledge, however, no osseus complication, osteomyelitis, or osteitis pubis has been reported following placement of an MS.

Recurrent Incontinence

Following a bone-anchored sling procedure, recurrent incontinence should be evaluated with urodynamic studies. In patients with recurrent stress incontinence, a pelvic radiograph should be obtained to evaluate for bone anchor dislodgment. Comiter[9] reported bone anchor dislodgment in 4.2% (2 of 48) of patients. In this series, patients presented with recurrent incontinence, screw dislodgment was confirmed with pelvic radiograph, and successful sling revision was performed.[9] When bone anchor dislodgement is not the cause of recurrent stress incontinence, other treatment options include bulking agents, repeat MS (if it is thought that compression is not adequate), and placement of an AUS.

Recurrent incontinence following a bulbourethral sling operation is managed with a retightening procedure. Stern and colleagues[43] reported that 14.5% (9 of 62) of patients who did not have prior radiation required a retightening procedure, and three of these patients required a second retightening procedure. Of the patients who had prior radiation therapy, 66.7% (6 of 9) required a retightening procedure, and two of these required a second procedure.[43]

Inflatable Balloon Compression

Balloon Rupture or Deflation

In their first 50 patients, Hübner and Schlarp[18] reported 15 balloon ruptures in 13 patients. Conversely, only 2 ruptures occurred in 2 patients in their most recent 50 patients.[18] The balloons were reengineered to strengthen their attachment to the tubing after several leakages were discovered in the first 50 patients.[16] Trigo-Rocha and colleagues[17] reported a 4% (1 of 25) rate of balloon deflation. These patients were managed with revision to replace the deflated balloons.

Balloon Dislocation

Hübner and Schlarp[18] found a balloon dislocation rate of 18% in their initial 50 patients and a rate of 6% in their most recent 50 patients. These patients were managed with operative repositioning of the balloons.[18]

Erosion

Hübner and Schlarp[18] reported 5 erosions in their first 50 cases and 4 in their most recent 50 cases. However, these investigators did not specify how many patients experienced erosions, and two balloons were placed in each patient. In addition, they did not differentiate between urethral and bladder erosions. Erosions were managed with removal of the devices and reimplantation 6 weeks later.[18] Trigo-Rocha and colleagues[17] reported a single patient (4%) with erosion of one injection port through the scrotal skin. This erosion was managed by removal of both devices. These investigators did not report any urethral or bladder erosions.[17]

Infection

Hübner and Schlarp[18] reported a wound infection rate of 4% in their first 50 patients and no infections in their most recent 50 patients. Infections were managed by removing the balloon on the infected side. These investigators did not mention when or whether the balloons were reimplanted.[18]

CONCLUSION

The AUS, MS, and ProACT balloon compression (not currently available in the United States) are the current surgical treatment options for sphincteric insufficiency following prostate surgery. Each has acceptable complication rates that can be minimized with attention to detail and meticulous surgical and aseptic technique. Patients obviously should be informed of the potential complications associated with the procedures. Along with more minor complications, the AUS, the MS, and the ProACT balloon compression device are associated with a risk of infection and erosion that can result in the need for explantation. In addition, the AUS is a mechanical device that inherently carries a risk of mechanical malfunction and the need for device revision or replacement. Although pain or paresthesia is typically not severe, patients undergoing MS should also be made aware of the possibility of this complication. Patients who understand their treatment options and who are well informed regarding potential risks and complications are more likely to be satisfied postoperatively.

KEY POINTS

1. Most intraoperative complications are inconsequential if they are recognized and treated at the time of the surgical procedure. Conversely, urethral injury typically requires aborting the procedure.

2. To facilitate detection of an unrecognized urethral injury, saline solution or dilute indigo carmine can be instilled next to the Foley catheter or through the Foley catheter while moving it in a retrograde fashion.

3. AUS tubing should be handled with rubber-shod clamps and care should be taken not to injure the device with sharp instruments or needles. Damage to the device can result in leakage of fluid from the device and mechanical failure.

4. Early infection of the AUS, and most likely the MS, is typically the result of bacterial contamination at the time of implantation.

5. Erosion of an AUS is commonly caused by prolonged catheterization, catheterization without

cuff deactivation, or repeated endoscopic manipulation of the urethra.

6. Urinary retention that manifests as a late complication following AUS or MS requires endoscopic evaluation for infection or erosion and evaluation of the urethra and bladder neck for stricture or contracture.

7. De novo urgency following MS procedures requires urodynamic evaluation to rule out obstruction or recurrent stress incontinence.

8. Iatrogenic obstruction following placement of an MS rare but not impossible.

9. Patients with an infected MS may present with chronic low-grade symptoms such as mild perineal pain or swelling or an intermittently draining sinus tract.

10. The AUS is a mechanical device that inherently carries a risk of mechanical malfunction as well as the need for device revision or replacement.

REFERENCES

Please see www.expertconsult.com

Chapter 52

COMPLICATIONS OF URETHRAL RECONSTRUCTION

Joel Gelman MD

Associate Clinical Professor, Department of Urology, University of California, Irvine School of Medicine, Irvine, California

Patients diagnosed with urethral strictures can be managed with observation, endoscopic treatment with dilation or incision, urethral stent placement, or formal open reconstruction with excisional or tissue transfer repair. This chapter reviews the complications that can be associated with the disease itself, the diagnostic testing, and the endoscopic and open surgical treatment of urethral strictures.

COMPLICATIONS OF URETHRAL STRICTURE DISEASE

Observation is always a treatment option, and the potential complications of observation must be discussed when patients are counseled and giving informed consent. Patients often present with obstructive voiding symptoms, and it would be a mistake for a patient to conclude that having to live with obstructive voiding symptoms would be the only potential drawback of observation.

Distal obstruction is associated with high-pressure voiding. The bladder compensates by thickening with the development of trabeculation, and the urethra proximal to the obstruction can become distended (**Fig. 52-1**). High-pressure voiding through the prostatic urethra can be associated with extravasation of urine in retrograde fashion into the prostatic ducts. In a physiologically normal patient, extravasation of contrast material into the prostatic ducts is not seen during retrograde urethrography, but this finding is not uncommon in patients with strictures. Eventually, diverticular formation or bladder decompensation can develop with an increased capacity and residual or urinary retention. Secondary reflux with or without associated recurrent pyelonephritis can also occur. Ultimately, although not common, acute or chronic renal failure can develop as a complication of untreated stricture disease.

In patients with *balanitis xerotica obliterans* (BXO), a disease of the penile skin, glans penis, and urethra (**Fig.** 52-2), stricture progression is common. The obstruction is generally initially within the distal urethra. Often, extravasation into the periurethral glands of Littre is seen during urethral imaging studies in patients with BXO (**Fig. 52-3**), and it is thought that the extravasation of urine into the periurethral glands may be associated with proximal stricture progression. It is not at all unusual for patients with BXO who are conservatively managed to undergo their first retrograde urethrogram and be diagnosed with a >20-cm panurethral stricture (**Fig. 52-4**). Patients who are clinically diagnosed with BXO on physical examination and who have stricture disease limited to the distal urethral stricture disease are best managed with open staged urethral reconstruction or extended meatotomy.[1,2] In summary, the complications of treatment with observation include but are not limited to prostatitis, bladder decompensation, urinary retention, secondary vesicoureteral reflux, pyelonephritis, renal deterioration, and stricture progression in addition to obstructive symptoms.

COMPLICATIONS OF DIAGNOSTIC PROCEDURES

Diagnostic testing procedures for known or suspected urethral strictures include urethral calibration with bougie à boule, urethroscopy, retrograde urethrography (RUG), and voiding cystourethrography (VCUG). Bougie calibration, properly performed to assess the caliber of the urethral meatus and fossa navicularis, does not dilate the urethra and therefore is generally not associated with complications. When urethroscopy is performed, the most common complication is urethral trauma. This trauma can be intentional when scope dilation is performed in an effort to visualize the stricture in its entirety and enter the bladder. This situation represents treatment with dilation before the extent of the stricture is first assessed and the patient is informed of all treatment options. Should the patient be a candidate for open repair, the operation must be delayed for

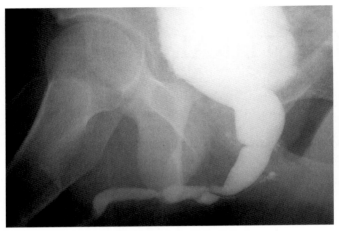

Figure 52-1   Markedly dilated posterior urethra proximal to a narrow-caliber bulbar stricture seen on voiding cystourethrography.

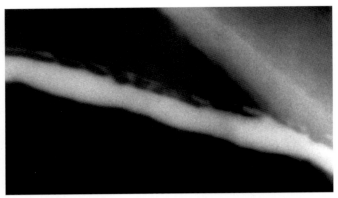

Figure 52-3   Retrograde urethrography with extravasation into the periurethral glands of Littre.

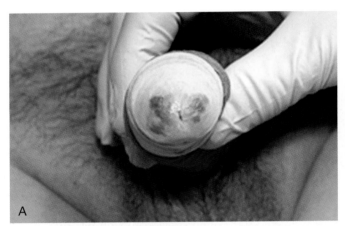

A

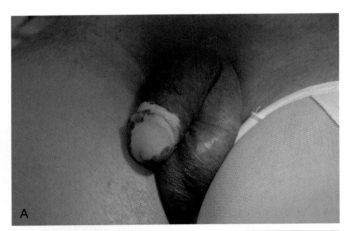

A

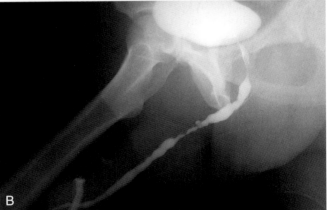

B

Figure 52-4   Appearance of the penis (**A**) and retrograde urethrography of the same patient (**B**) with balanitis xerotica obliterans.

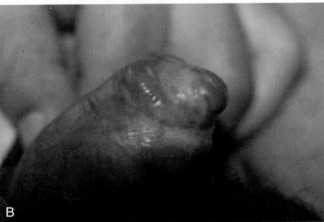

B

Figure 52-2   Balanitis xerotica obliterans can manifest with whitish skin color changes and meatal stenosis (**A**) or with a more severe deformity including a total loss of the coronal sulcus and loss of penile length and girth (**B**).

several months following scope or other dilation because open reconstruction is best performed when the stricture is mature and stable. Urethral contrast imaging is necessary to assess the length and exact location of the stricture because urethroscopy usually identifies only the distal extent of the disease.

Complications of urethral imaging include urinary tract infection with or without sepsis and extravasation. Improperly performed studies can be associated with a higher complication rate. At our institution, diagnostic testing is performed with flat plate imaging, and this includes both RUG and VCUG. The patient is placed in the oblique position. After a scout film is obtained, gauze is wrapped around the coronal sulcus and the penis is placed on stretch. A 60-mL syringe connected

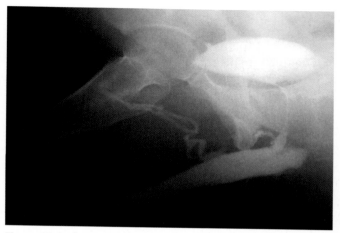

Figure 52-5 Extravasation into the corpus spongiosum and venous system during retrograde urethrography injection.

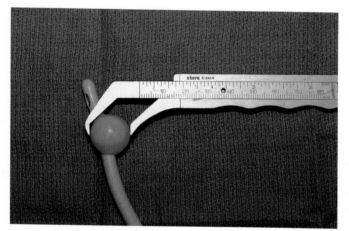

Figure 52-6 Foley catheter after balloon inflation with 2 mL of water. The caliber is >50 Fr (1.7 cm diameter).

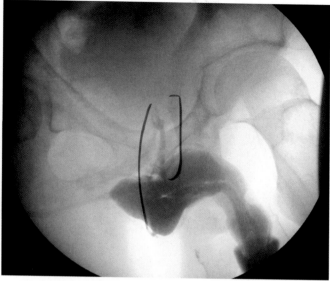

Figure 52-7 Outside retrograde urethrography obtained during a forceful attempt to advance the catheter for the injection procedure.

to a cone-shaped adaptor is placed into the urethral meatus to form a seal, and RUG is performed during the injection of contrast material. The bladder is then slowly filled in retrograde fashion similarly until the patient has the urge to void. VCUG is performed while the patient is voiding.

Extravasation into the corpus spongiosum or venous system is rare when contrast material is instilled gently. However, this complication can occur (**Fig. 52-5**). Sepsis is a concern with extravasation, and when extravasation occurs, prophylactic antibiotics are given. When imaging is performed with alternative techniques at radiology imaging centers, we have observed a high complication rate related to poor technique.

The injections are usually performed with catheter insertion into the urethra and inflation of a balloon within the urethra and subsequent contrast injection through the catheter. We measured the caliber of the balloons of 12- to 16-Fr catheters after inflation with 1 to 3 mL of water. With only 2 mL of inflation, the caliber of the balloon was >50 Fr (**Fig. 52-6**). The caliber of the

penile urethra is approximately 30 Fr, except for the glans and fossa navicularis, which are generally <25 Fr in caliber, and this painful RUG technique often dilates and traumatizes normal urethra. Forceful attempts to insert a catheter through a stricture will both compromise the diagnostic value of the study and damage the urethra (**Fig. 52-7**).

In addition, errors in technique are associated with an incorrect diagnosis of the length and location of the strictures, and this misdiagnosis can compromise subsequent treatment. For example, if the films are taken when the patient is not in the oblique position, the length of the stricture can be significantly underestimated (**Fig. 52-8**). Furthermore, if the penis is not on stretch, the length of the stricture will likely be underestimated. Moreover, if a voiding film is not obtained, the membranous and prostatic urethra and bladder neck cannot be assessed.

When RUG is performed, the normal posterior urethra is coapted and narrowing in this area is a normal finding. Stricture disease cannot be diagnosed or excluded from the injection film. During voiding, however, the bladder neck and posterior urethra are normally widely patent and are often hydrodistended, as shown in Figure 52-1. Wide patency of the posterior urethra confirms the absence of bladder neck and membranous urethral stenosis. Patients with anterior strictures in the absence of pelvic fracture trauma or prior prostate surgical or radiation therapy rarely have disease proximal to departure of the bulbar urethra. However, patients with bulbar strictures can also have membranous strictures. When VCUG is not performed, one possible consequence of incomplete imaging is an error in diagnosis that can be compromise subsequent treatment.

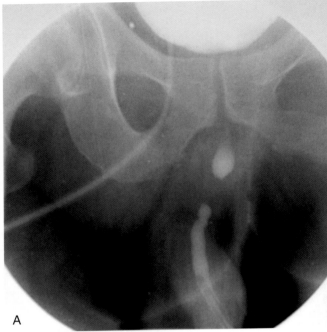

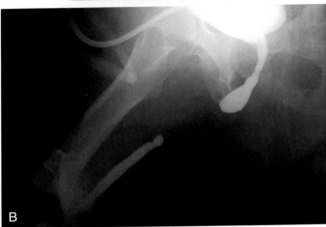

Figure 52-8 **A,** Contrast imaging with the patient in the supine position suggests a 2-cm obliteration. **B,** Repeat study with the same patient appropriately placed in the oblique position confirms that the obliteration is actually 8 cm in length.

COMPLICATIONS OF URETHRAL DILATION

Urethral dilation is commonly used to manage urethral strictures. Dilation techniques include the use of metal sounds, filiforms and followers, catheters, and high-pressure balloons. Ideally, dilation should be performed in the absence of urinary tract infection or colonization. Immediate complications include the creation of a false passage, bleeding, urethral perforation, rectal injury, and failure to achieve the intended increase in urethral caliber. Early complications include sepsis and urinary retention.

Urethral perforation, generally associated with significant bleeding, can be managed with gentle attempts at insertion of an indwelling catheter. The use of a flexible cystoscope to insert a flexible guidewire may facilitate

the placement of a Councill-tipped catheter. Suprapubic tube placement is a very reasonable option when a catheter cannot be placed without further trauma.

The most frequent complication of urethral dilation is stricture recurrence, and recurrent strictures after multiple dilations may be longer and denser. Dilation represents a potentially curative treatment only for very discreet strictures with minimal associated spongiofibrosis. Urethral squamous cell cancer is rare. However, chronic irritation from frequent dilations and self-catheterization is associated with an increased risk of developing this malignant disease. In patients with a history of chronic irritation who develop a fistula to the scrotum, priapism, or a very unusual appearance of the urethral mucosa seen on urethroscopy or contrast imaging, squamous cancer should be suspected.

COMPLICATIONS OF INTERNAL URETHROTOMY

The Otis urethrotome was routinely used to incise urethral strictures blindly before the development of endoscopic equipment that permitted direct vision internal urethrotomy (DVIU) with the use of a cold knife or a laser fiber. Incision of the scar into the corpus spongiosum increases the caliber of the urethra, and generally a catheter is subsequently placed. As with dilation, immediate complications can include bleeding that is generally managed with catheterization and is usually self-limited and damage to the urethra that prevents subsequent catheter placement. Suprapubic tube placement is then indicated. Extravasation of blood or irrigation fluid into the scrotum or penis can occur and generally resolves with conservative management. However, extravasation into the periurethral tissues can significantly complicate dissection and mobilization of the urethra if subsequent open repair is required. Early complications include urinary tract infection and sepsis.

The most common complication is stricture recurrence. Along the circumference of the urethra, epithelium is present except where the urethra was incised. As healing occurs, the outcome is favorable when epithelialization results and leads to a stable increase in the caliber of the urethra. However, more commonly, wound contracture dominates, and the stricture recurs.

The actual recurrence rate after DVIU is not clearly defined in the literature because the multiple reports published on the subject do not include long-term objective follow-up. However, it is known and clearly established that long-term cure with urethrotomy is a reasonable expectation only for strictures that are not recurrent, are <1 to 1.5 cm long, and have minimal associated spongiofibrosis. The recurrence rate with repeated urethrotomies is extremely high, and the standard of care for the initial management of longer strictures or of strictures that recur after incision is open reconstruction.[3,4] Investigators have reported that in patients who require open reconstruction after multiple failed DVIUs, the success rate is lower than when open surgical procedures are performed for initial management.[5,6]

Other complications of DVIU include erectile dysfunction that may be veno-occlusive because a deep dorsal urethral incision can extend into the corpus cavernosum and create a vascular shunt. This complication was reported to be successfully treated with open urethral mobilization and fat pad interposition.[7] High-flow priapism following DVIU has also been reported and can be successfully treated with embolization.[8] Multiple incisions other than at the 12-o'clock position may reduce the incidence of this complication. Incontinence is generally not a complication of urethrotomy unless incisions involve the membranous urethra when the bladder neck is already compromised (e.g., after radical prostatectomy) or when the bladder neck is incised in patients whose membranous urethra is not fully intact.

COMPLICATIONS OF ENDOSCOPIC TREATMENT OF POSTERIOR URETHRAL INJURIES

In men who suffer pelvic fracture trauma and associated membranous posterior urethral disruption, immediate treatment options include a gentle attempt at catheter placement when a partial tear is diagnosed on RUG and suprapubic tube placement with delayed reconstruction. Immediate open urethral reconstruction is not indicated except when the injury is at the level of the bladder neck.[9]

Early primary realignment is a procedure that can be performed immediately in a stable patient or within the first week after the injury when the patient is stabilized. The technique involves endoscopic antegrade and retrograde urethral instrumentation in an effort to place a urethral catheter. As the pelvic hematoma is reabsorbed and healing occurs, the hope is that the catheter will guide the urethra back together in proper alignment, and the patient can then avoid the need for subsequent urethral reconstruction. If a stricture develops after catheter removal, the goals are for the realignment to reduce the length of the stricture or any malalignment and thus to facilitate subsequent repair. The success rate of primary realignment is not clearly established, although this technique is reported to be of possible benefit.[10-12] At this time, it is considered very reasonable to manage posterior urethral disruptions acutely with primary realignment or suprapubic tube placement and delayed reconstruction.

The most common complication of primary realignment is the development of a urethral stricture or total obliteration of the urethra after urethral catheter removal. One significant drawback of primary realignment is that recurrent strictures are then often managed with DVIUs and self-catheterization in an effort to avoid open reconstruction. When a recurrent stricture develops subsequent to urethral catheter removal, delayed open posterior urethral reconstruction is the standard of care and is generally performed approximately 3 months after urethral catheter removal.

In the past, an endoscopic alternative to delayed open reconstruction for obliterative distraction defects was a "cut-to-the-light" procedure. This technique involved simultaneous antegrade and retrograde cystoscopy with "core through" incisions into the obliteration toward the light of the other scope until continuity was established. The failure rate was very high, and this technique fell out of favor and is not recommended.

COMPLICATIONS OF URETHRAL STENTS

The commercially available UroLume (American Medical Systems, Minnetonka, Minnesota) endoprosthesis was developed to provide a simple treatment option for recurrent bulbar urethral stricture disease.[13] The UroLume stent is a self-expanding superalloy braided wire mesh cylinder that is placed endoscopically. Initial reports suggested that the UroLume stent offered an efficacious and durable treatment option for recurrent bulbar strictures and traumatic membranous strictures.[14] However, more recent reports with long-term follow-up described multiple complications with high frequency including pain, infection, incontinence, and recurrent strictures within the stent or proximal or distal to the stent.[15] A long-term study of men who underwent stent placement revealed that only 45% of the patients were free of recurrence and complications and 45% suffered multiple complications. The investigators concluded that UroLume stents should be used only in patients who refuse or are unfit for urethroplasty.[16]

Hypospadias is an absolute contraindication to urethral stent placement because panurethral stricture disease is a potential complication.[17] In patients with hypospadias, the normal continuity of the corpus spongiosum along the distal penile shaft and the glans penis is not present, and the one major blood supply to the anterior urethra is through the bulbar arteries. If this dependent antegrade bulbar arterial supply is compromised by stent compression of the proximal corpus spongiosum, ischemic panurethral stricture formation may occur. Therefore, stent placement should be avoided in patients with hypospadias.

Recurrent strictures that develop after stent placement can be successfully managed with open stent removal with excision and primary anastomosis for relatively short proximal strictures or with tissue transfer reconstruction for longer strictures. Individualized open reconstruction can generally be performed in one stage and has a high long-term success rate.[18]

COMPLICATIONS OF OPEN SURGICAL PROCEDURES

Open surgical procedures for urethral reconstruction include excision and primary anastomosis and tissue transfer reconstruction with skin flaps or grafts. The remainder of this chapter is a discussion of complications associated with patient positioning, excisional repair for posterior and anterior bulbar strictures, graft harvest, and tissue transfer reconstruction.

Patient Positioning

Distal strictures involving the urethral meatus, fossa navicularis, and penile urethra are often repaired with the patient in the supine position. If care is taken to prevent pressure points, positioning complications generally do not occur. In contrast, more proximal strictures are repaired by a perineal approach that requires placement of the patient in the lithotomy position, often an exaggerated lithotomy position (**Fig. 52-9**). This position is associated with many complications including neurapraxia (peroneal nerve in particular) that is often temporary but can be permanent, back pain, compartment syndrome, and rhabdomyolysis.[19-21]

Proper positioning can reduce the incidence of these serious complications. A modified Skytron table (developed by Gerald Jordan, MD) provides pelvic tilt, and modified stirrups allow additional extension of the lower extremities to prevent extreme hip or knee flexion with associated nerve stretch. Proper adjustment of the boots of the stirrups prevents pressure on the calves and reduces the risk of compartment syndrome, a condition that when diagnosed is generally managed with emer-

gency fasciotomies. Investigators have shown that the time spent in the lithotomy position is related to the risk of the development of neurapraxia and rhabdomyolysis. Therefore, when possible, any portion of the surgical procedure (e.g., buccal graft harvesting when indicated) that can be done without the patient's being in the exaggerated lithotomy position should be done with the patient supine.

When neurapraxia develops, it is usually a temporary sensory impairment along the lower leg and the dorsum of the foot in particular. Normal sensation usually returns without treatment in 2 to 3 days. However, more significant and long-term disability can occur along with motor deficits including but not limited to impaired dorsiflexion of the foot.

Rhabdomyolysis is a potentially serious complication of prolonged lithotomy positioning with associated painful muscle damage. The serum creatine kinase level is markedly elevated and myoglobin may be detected in the dark brown urine. Acute renal failure with oliguria and elevation of the serum creatinine may occur. Aggressive treatment is indicated to prevent renal damage, and appropriate management includes hydration and urine alkalinization. Temporary dialysis is required in severe cases. In addition, deep vein thrombosis and pulmonary embolism have been reported as possible complications of high lithotomy positioning.

Excision and Primary Anastomosis for Posterior Disruptions

The most common complication of posterior urethral reconstruction with excision and primary anastomosis is recurrence of the stricture or obliteration. Technical success is defined as durable wide patency of the entire urethra without the need for any subsequent or other intervention. At referral centers for urethral surgery, the success rate of posterior urethral reconstruction (including both initial treatment and revision) is 90% to 98%.[22,23] Factors that increase the probability of a technically successful outcome include the administration of culture-specific antibiotics perioperatively, complete scar excision so the proximal and distal segments of the urethra are widely spatulated to >30 Fr with healthy mucosa circumferentially, and a tension-free repair.[24]

Maneuvers that promote a tension-free repair include midline separation of the corporal bodies along the triangular ligament and, when indicated, infrapubectomy. In rare cases, corporal rerouting has been reported to reduce tension. Investigators have stressed in the literature that posterior reconstructions and urethral reconstructions in general are best performed by urologists with expertise and specialization in urethral stricture surgery because a poor outcome increases the complexity and difficulty of subsequent surgical treatment.

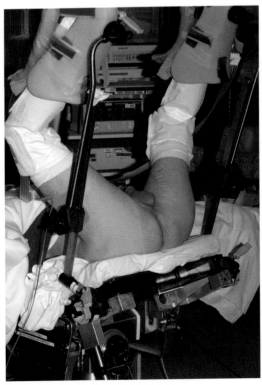

Figure 52-9   Exaggerated lithotomy position.

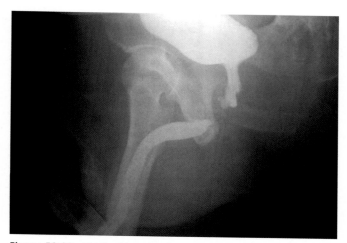

Figure 52-10 Urethral imaging in a patient who previously underwent a technically unsuccessful posterior urethral reconstruction.

Long recurrent total obliterations that develop as early complications of failed surgical procedures (**Fig. 52-10**) are likely caused by inadequate proximal exposure and scar excision. Fortunately, these patients can usually undergo corrective treatment with a very high success rate with repeat excisional repair.[25] The finding that revision surgery was highly successful with the same operation that previously failed before referral suggests that the experience of the surgeon may be significantly related to the success of the operation. Discrete nonobliterative anastomotic recurrences can be successfully managed with urethrotomy. In contrast to the low success rate of DVIU for the initial treatment of strictures, this technique has a high success rate when it is used to treat anastomotic strictures, presumably because these discrete recurrent strictures are not associated with any significant spongiofibrosis.[26]

A potential complication of posterior urethral reconstruction is ischemic stenosis of the anterior urethra.[27] The anterior urethra has a dual blood supply. The bulbar arteries provide antegrade supply to the anterior urethral within the corpus spongiosum. In addition, the dorsal arteries supply the glans penis and the anterior urethra in retrograde fashion. Posterior urethral reconstruction cannot be performed without compromising the bulbar arteries at the time of urethral transection. Therefore, the anterior urethra is subsequently supplied predominantly by the dorsal arteries. If this blood supply is bilaterally compromised by arterial injury, ischemic stenosis can develop as a complication of posterior urethral reconstruction.

Vascular evaluation enables the surgeon to identify patients who may be at risk of developing this complication. Patients with normal erectile function invariably have adequate urethral vascularity. A penile duplex study with pharmacologic erection in patients with postinjury erectile dysfunction identifies patients with bilateral arterial inflow compromise. Patients with severe inflow impairment should then undergo a pudendal arteriogram, and when bilateral dorsal artery compromise is evident, penile revascularization (generally inferior epigastric to dorsal artery) should be performed before urethral reconstruction.

In men who sustain pelvic fracture trauma and associated urethral disruption, erectile dysfunction from nerve or vascular injury is not uncommon.[27] Although erectile dysfunction is a possible complication of posterior urethral reconstruction, impotence is usually secondary to the initial injury. Given that urethral reconstruction generally cures the urethral stricture but does not address the associated erectile dysfunction caused by the initial injury, the most common long-term urologic problem is erectile dysfunction.

Incontinence is also a possible complication of urethral reconstruction. However, when this complication occurs, it is generally at least in part related to the initial injury. The typical location of the urethral injury following pelvic fracture trauma is the membranous urethra. Surgical reconstruction of the urethra does not involve dissection proximal to the apex of the prostate and the dissection is definitely distal to the bladder neck. When the membranous urethra is damaged but the bladder neck is intact, the ability to stop voiding voluntarily is affected, but continence is generally preserved. Incontinence after posterior urethral reconstruction, when present, is therefore related to associated bladder, nerve, or bladder neck damage and not the reconstructive surgical procedure, on the assumption that the anastomosis is made at the most distal area of the patent proximal segment distal to the verumontanum of the prostate. Urodynamic evaluation is indicated if incontinence occurs after urethral reconstruction.

Other potential complications include bleeding, although transfusion should be very rarely indicated. Wound infection is always a potential complication of open urethral surgical procedures. Superficial wound infections should be promptly recognized and managed with incision and drainage if fluctuance is noted. Antibiotics are effective treatment for cellulitis.

Excision and Primary Anastomosis for Proximal Anterior Strictures

Stricture excision and primary anastomosis have long been the open procedures of choice for relatively short strictures of the bulbar urethra. When the surgical procedures are properly performed at a referral center for urethral reconstruction, the success rate is approximately 95%.[28] Strictures 1 to 2 cm long are highly amenable to excisional repair. However, longer bulbar strictures can be managed with primary repair without the development of chordee in selected patients with adequate elasticity of the corpus spongiosum located within the proximal bulbar area.[29]

Suprapubic tubes are routinely placed percutaneously at the time of anterior urethral reconstruction at some centers. Potential benefits include the ability to use a smaller stenting urethral catheter yet maintain adequate bladder drainage postoperatively and the establishment of a secondary source of bladder drainage should one tube become plugged. Potential complications include bleeding and posterior bladder injury. The most serious complication of percutaneous suprapubic tube placement is bowel injury. During suprapubic tube placement, it is important that the bladder be distended, and this can be achieved through slow retrograde filling with saline solution though a flexible cystoscope with the tip of the scope distal to the stricture. The tube should be inserted no more than 2 to 3 cm cephalad to the midline pubic symphysis, and open tube placement or ultrasound guidance should be considered in patients who have a history of prior intraperitoneal abdominal surgical treatment.

Anterior urethroplasty with excisional repair shares many of the complications noted with posterior repair including recurrence, positioning complications, bleeding and infection, and chordee. Fistula and diverticula formation are not at all commonly seen with excisional repair because the corpus spongiosum is present circumferentially to provide support and to prevent diverticular change, and the perineal skin is separated from the urethral lumen by subcutaneous fat, the bulbospongiosus muscle (especially along the midproximal bulbar urethra), and the corpus spongiosum, which is most prominent along the ventral aspect of the urethra.

Graft Harvest

When tissue transfer with grafting is required for urethral reconstruction, the most commonly used graft material currently is buccal mucosa. Grafts are usually harvested from the lateral cheeks, although the lower lip can be used, and occasionally, the upper lip can be a source of additional graft material. Deformity and tightness are greater concerns grafts are harvested from the lower and especially the upper lip, and most grafts are taken from the lateral cheeks. When a lateral buccal graft is harvested, Stensen's duct is identified adjacent to the second upper molar, and the area for graft harvest is then incised inferior to the opening of the duct (**Fig. 52-11**).

Injury to Stensen's duct is a possible complication of buccal graft harvesting, but it can usually be avoided by proper identification of the duct. The morbidity associated with buccal mucosa graft harvest was reported.[30] In this report, most patients experienced significant postoperative pain that was worse than expected. Postoperative side effects included periorbital numbness that persisted for >6 months in 9% of the patients, initial difficulty with mouth opening, and changes in salivation. One patient developed a mucus retention cyst that

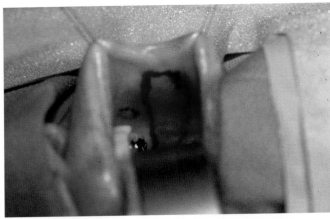

Figure 52-11 Buccal mucosa is marked for harvest, and Stensen's duct is identified.

required excision. Some surgeons close the donor site and others leave the harvest site open. Both options are considered acceptable. However, in this study, the mean pain score for patients with donor site closure was significantly higher than for patients without donor site closure.

In addition to buccal grafts, other autologous graft materials used in urethral reconstruction are split-thickness skin grafts (STSG) often harvested from the thigh, temporalis fascia, and recently, the under surface of the tongue.[31] The harvest of any graft can be associated with bleeding, scarring, contracture (generally not with split-thickness grafts), and infection. However, these grafts can generally be harvested with low morbidity.

Tissue Transfer Reconstruction

All tissue transfer reconstructions, and stricture repairs in general, can be complicated by stricture recurrence, bleeding, urinary tract infection with or without sepsis, wound infection, and breakdown of the repair. However, specific complications are generally associated with flap and graft reconstructions.

Skin flaps by definition retain their blood supply because they are mobilized on a vascular pedicle and are relocated to augment the caliber of the urethra. The most commonly used flap is a penile skin flap. The penile skin is supplied by branches of the superficial external pudendal arteries. These vessels course along the tissue deep to the skin and superficial to Buck's fascia. The supply is axial as opposed to random and is defined. During the elevation of a penile skin flap, under optical magnification, a tissue plane is developed between the superficial and deep plexus of the fascia. Careful attention to technical detail is required so blood supply is maintained both to the skin flap and to the remaining penile skin.

Potential complications of flap elevation include ischemic changes to the penile skin, especially along the distal aspect, and flap ischemia.[32] Distal penile skin ischemia and necrosis are generally managed with débridement of devitalized tissue and wound care. In general, the skin is adequately redundant so that the loss of a small amount of penile skin is not disabling. In patients who previously underwent flap repair and who develop a recurrent stricture, a penile flap may be elevated again by some surgeons. However, once a flap is used, the blood supply of the penile skin is not axial and well defined, but rather random in distribution. Therefore, repeated use of skin flaps can be associated with a higher rate of ischemic flap failure and recurrent stricture formation.

Although currently not commonly used as a urethral replacement, scrotal skin can be used for urethral reconstruction. When scrotal skin is rotated as a flap, it must be nonhirsute. In addition, the skin must be marked on stretch to avoid redundancy that can be associated with diverticula formation (**Fig. 52-12**). Penile skin flaps must also be nonhirsute. In general, the foreskin and distal penile shaft skin are not hair bearing. However, before shaving and draping, when skin flaps are to be used, the skin should be evaluated under optical magnification to ensure that only nonhirsute skin is selected. When hair-bearing skin is used to repair the urethra, hair will then grow within the lumen of the reconstructed urethra (**Fig. 52-13**) and may be a source of infection, stone formation, or recurrent obstruction.

Grafts are detached from their blood supply at the donor site and are transferred to a recipient bed. Grafts obtain blood supply through a process of graft take. Initially, the graft receives nutrients by passive diffusion, a process called *imbibition*. Then, neovascularization occurs. This is called *inosculation*. One possible complication is failure of the graft to take. Proper surgical technique significantly reduces the likelihood of graft take failure. The graft must be firmly approximated to the recipient bed. This is facilitated by creating small slits within the graft to allow blood to escape that may elevate the graft from the recipient bed and prevent neovascularization. In addition, grafts are now often quilted to the recipient bed by using multiple fine absorbable sutures to provide further fixation because graft movement during the process of imbibition and inosculation is deleterious to graft take.

Buccal grafts can be used for one-stage reconstructions as a dorsal, ventral, or lateral onlay or for staged repairs. STSGs are generally used for staged repairs. Buccal mucosa is a better graft material than is STSG because success rates are higher with buccal grafts than with skin grafts, and chordee is less, given that skin is

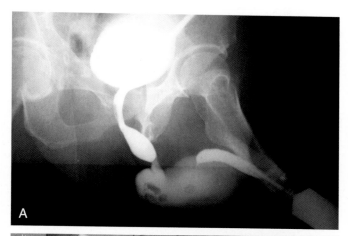

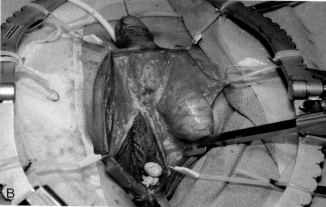

Figure 52-12 **A,** Retrograde urethrography demonstrates a markedly dilated proximal penile and distal bulbar urethral diverticulum that contains filling defects in a patient who previously underwent a one-stage tubed tissue transfer repair with scrotal skin. **B,** At the time of surgery, the massive diverticulum contained multiple stones.

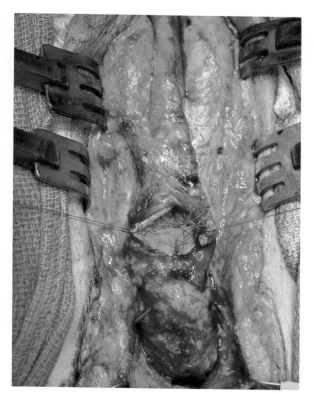

Figure 52-13 Hair developed within the lumen of the urethra after reconstruction using hair-bearing genital skin.

much less elastic than is buccal mucosa.[33] However, the supply of buccal mucosa is limited.

Stricture recurrence is the main complication of urethral reconstruction. In addition to attention to surgical detail, procedure selection is a factor that influences the success rate. In general, the success rate is higher when transferred tissues are used for onlay repair than for tubed reconstruction.[34] In comparison with STSGs and penile skin flaps, buccal grafts appear to have a higher success rate, and the results with onlay buccal mucosa grafts are excellent regardless of whether the graft is placed dorsally and is quilted to the corporal bodies, as originally described by Barbagli and associates,[35] or is placed ventrally or laterally.[36]

Urethral stricture disease associated with BXO was previously commonly managed with penile skin flap repair. However, investigators showed that although short-term success rates with flap procedures were high, the long-term failure rate 10 years postoperatively was extremely high.[37] As a result, the shift in management has been toward staged repairs using extragenital tissues.[38] BXO is a frustrating disease that can recur and lead to stricture recurrence even after technically successful staged repairs. Extended meatotomy or proximal urethrostomy has been proposed for complex cases as the most appropriate surgical treatment.[2]

Diverticula formation and the development of urethrocutaneous fistulas are rarely seen when buccal mucosa is used for urethral reconstruction in patients without hypospadias because the urethra is circumferentially well supported and the penile skin is separated from the urethral lumen by the corpus spongiosum. However, when staged repairs and skin flaps are performed, particularly in patients with *hypospadias,* which is a condition associated with a poorly developed distal corpus spongiosum, urethrocutaneous fistula is a more common complication.[39] These fistulas, when persistent, can be closed primarily but may then recur. Recurrent fistulas may require more complex closure with the interposition of a tunica vaginalis flap.

Incontinence of urine in the bladder is generally not a complication of anterior urethral reconstruction because the surgical procedure is performed distal to both the bladder neck and the external urethral sphincter. However, after tissue transfer reconstruction in particular, the urethra does not coapt normally, and pooled urine present within the reconstructed segment of the urethra after voiding can dribble out after urination.[40] Patients who report this complication should be instructed to "milk" their urethra with their hand from behind the scrotum toward the urethral meatus after urination.

Sexual dysfunction can occur after anterior urethral reconstruction, but one study revealed that the incidence of erectile dysfunction was no higher after urethroplasty than after circumcision.[41] However, another study reported that patient satisfaction with the

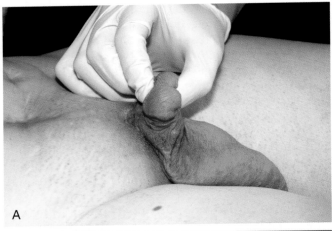

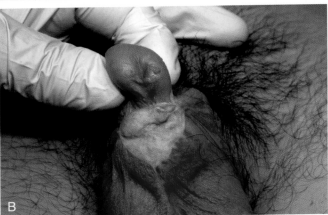

Figure 52-14 **A** and **B,** These two patients previously underwent multiple failed hypospadias repair procedures. The stretched penile length, as shown, is <2 inches.

outcome of urethroplasty was related not only to relief of obstructive symptoms but also to an absence of chordee or tethering.[33] When penile skin is repeatedly used to repair recurrent strictures after failed hypospadias repair, and subsequent salvage procedures fail, patients are at risk for significant compromise of sexual function (**Fig. 52-14**). It is important not to compromise the stretched and erect penile length significantly during repeat urethral reconstruction and not to proceed with tubularization during a staged repair if any chordee has not been fully addressed.

CONCLUSION

Urethral reconstruction, when properly performed using modern techniques, is generally associated with a high long-term success rate and a low complication rate. For all repairs, recurrence is the most common complication. Many published reports include follow-up with urethroscopy or contrast imaging 3 to 12 months after treatment to assess the short-term outcome. This testing is less frequently done after urethrotomy or dilation but is certainly not less indicated given the higher stricture recurrence rate with endoscopic treatment than with open treatment. A low early recurrence rate suggests technical success. However, long-term follow-up reveals that even when short-term success is objectively confirmed, a stricture may recur 5 to 10 or more years after the surgical procedure. This is especially true in patients with BXO and after substitution urethroplasty.[42] Therefore, indefinite periodic follow-up is recommended because the previously mentioned complications of stricture observation are also the possible complications of unrecognized and untreated recurrence.

KEY POINTS

1. The evaluation of urethral stricture disease, prior to treatment, generally includes urethroscopy, a retrograde urethrogram, a voiding cystourethrogram, and Bougie calibration for distal disease. Treatment with dilation using a cystoscope or other instruments should not be performed before a complete evaluation and a discussion of all options with the patient.

2. Stricture recurrence is the most common complication of a DVIU. Because the recurrence rate is high after repeated DVIUs, the standard of care is generally open reconstruction after a failed DVIU.

3. Factors that favor the successful outcome of a urethral reconstruction with excisional repair include spatulation of the proximal and distal ends to 30 Fr after scar excision and a tension-free anastomosis.

4. Factors that are associated with complications of tissue transfer urethral reconstruction include the use of hirsute skin, mobilization of flaps with compromise to the blood supply, and/or inadequate fixation of a graft to the recipient bed.

5. Balanitis xerotica obliterans should not be managed "conservatively" with distal dilations because without relief of the distal obstruction, there can be progression from distal to pan-urethral stricture disease.

REFERENCES

Please see www.expertconsult.com

Chapter 53

COMPLICATIONS OF SURGERY FOR ERECTILE DYSFUNCTION AND PEYRONIE'S DISEASE

Nelson E. Bennett MD
Director, Sexual Medicine and Surgery, Institute of Urology, Lahey Clinic Medical Center, Burlington; Assistant Professor of Urology, Department of Urology, Tufts School of Medicine, Boston, Massachusetts

John P. Mulhall MD
Director, Male Sexual and Reproductive Medicine Program, Urology Service, Department of Surgery, Memorial Sloan-Kettering Cancer Center, New York, New York

Penile prostheses are generally of two types: malleable (semirigid, noninflatable, nonhydraulic) and inflatable (hydraulic) devices. The malleable devices have an outer shell with a central core of metal or plastic. These prostheses are paired solid devices implanted in the corpora cavernosa that produce constant penile rigidity. The primary advantage of these devices is their ease of implantation, whereas the disadvantages include a constantly rigid penis that resembles neither normal erection nor flaccidity, difficulty with concealment, and an increased risk for device erosion.

Inflatable devices are of two varieties: two-piece and three-piece devices. Since its introduction in 1973, the inflatable penile prosthesis has undergone multiple changes in design and manufacturing. American Medical Systems (AMS, Minnetonka, Minnesota) produces both types of inflatable devices (**Fig. 53-1**). Mentor-Coloplast (Santa Barbara, California) produces only three-piece devices (**Fig. 53-2**). Numerous modifications have been made to improve function and survival of the devices. Such modifications include but are not limited to a reservoir or pump lockout valve to prevent autoinflation, antibiotic or antiadherence coating to reduce infection, Parylene (a polyxylylene polymer) coating for the AMS three-piece devices to improve cylinder longevity, and modifications of the scrotal pump to improve ease of use for the patient.

The AMS two-piece device (Ambicor) consists of two cylinders with the distal 2 cm made of solid silicone (**Fig. 53-3**). The cylinders are preconnected to a ball-shaped pump, which is seated within the scrotum. Compression of the pump results in transfer of fluid from the basal part of the cylinders into the middle portion, with subsequent rigidity. The deflation mechanism involves simply bending of the cylinders in midshaft to return the fluid to the basal section. Three-piece inflatable implants have paired cylinders, a small scrotal pump, and a large-volume fluid reservoir. These devices have a greater flaccidity profile that leads to a more natural-type erection.

The ideal penile prosthesis will permit a man to control when he has an erection and will allow penile flaccidity and erection that approximate their natural counterparts as closely as possible. To achieve these goals, fluid must be transferred into expandable cylinders for erection and must back out of the cylinders for flaccidity. A device with a fluid reservoir is required, thus necessitating placement of the reservoir in the retropubic space, although it may be placed in the peritoneal cavity when such an extraperitoneal space does not exist.

It is our practice to place a three-piece device where possible. We routinely use the Mentor device; however, other centers use the AMS three-piece device with excellent results. In certain populations we consider implanting the Ambicor two-piece device. Other authorities use three-piece devices in some of these populations with both excellent safety and satisfaction. These populations include the following:

1. Patients who have undergone renal transplantation or who are about to receive such a transplant
2. Certain patients who have undergone radical prostatectomy. In our experience, approximately 5% to 10% of such patients present great difficulty in placement of the reservoir without an inguinal counterin-

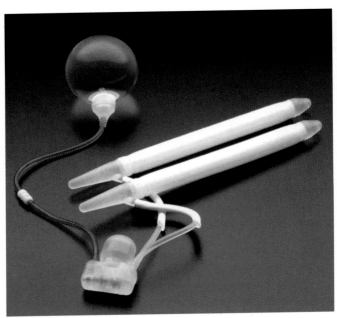

Figure 53-1 AMS 700 series three-piece inflatable implant.

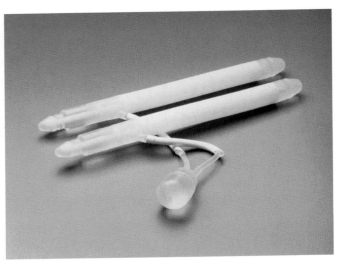

Figure 53-3 AMS Ambicor two-piece penile implant.

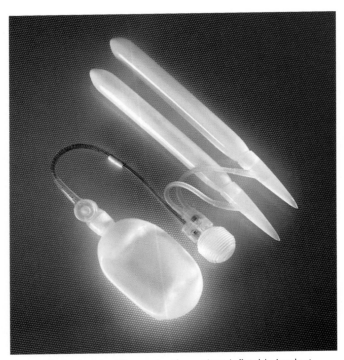

Figure 53-2 Mentor Titan series three-piece inflatable implant.

5. Those older patients whose manual dexterity makes using the three-piece deflation mechanism easier to use

In men who have a fibrotic penis and who are undergoing secondary (repeat) prosthesis implantation, it is our practice to implant a narrow three-piece device, usually in conjunction with the use of a Cavernotome (UROAN 21, Baleares, Spain) or sharp corporal tissue excision. Surgeons in centers that use AMS devices suggest that in men who have had previous cylinder erosion or crossover, CX/CXM (UROAN 21, Baleares, Spain) rather than Ultrex (AMS, Minnetonka, Minnesota) cylinders should be used because avoidance of length expansion (as can occur with the Ultrex device) in these situations is preferable.

The advantages of two-piece over three-piece devices are explained to the patient to enable him to make a more informed choice. We insist that all patients read the device-related literature, view videos of the device, and speak to a patient who has undergone implant surgery. Our patients also have a routine lengthy counseling session with the implant surgeon before they commit to the procedure. Ensuring that the patient has realistic expectations before implant surgery is undertaken is essential to ensuring high postoperative satisfaction profiles. Specifically, we discuss infection rates, rates of reoperation, and the lack of penile length increase with penile prosthesis surgery.

INFECTION

Infection associated with prosthetic surgery is a significant problem. The reported incidence of initial penile prosthetic surgical infections is between 1% and 8%.[1,2] Investigators have reported an increase in this rate with second and third reoperative procedures.[3] Additionally, the risk of prosthetic infection is also increased in

cision; failure to develop an adequate space for the reservoir in these patients significantly increases the chances of autoinflation.
3. Patients who have had bilateral inguinal herniorrhaphy (especially with mesh)
4. Patients with spinal cord injury who desire penile implant surgery for erectile dysfunction as well as for the application of a condom catheter. The solid silicone nature of the most distal 2 cm of the cylinders aids in supporting the condom catheter.

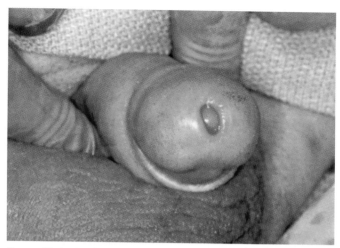

Figure 53-4 Eroding implant cylinder through urethral meatus.

patients with poorly controlled diabetes mellitus (gly-cosylated hemoglobin >11.5%), spinal cord injuries, or a history of urinary tract infection.[4-9]

Skin-dwelling bacteria are usually responsible for operative wound contamination. The most common bacterium associated with penile implant infection is *Staphylococcus epidermidis*. Highly virulent organisms such as methicillin-resistant *Staphylococcus aureus* (MRSA), *Pseudomonas aeruginosa*, *Enterococcus* species, *Prevotella* species (*Bacteroides* subspecies), and fungi have been associated with penile implant infections. Patients with infected penile implants usually present between 1 and 8 weeks postoperatively with fever, pain, and swelling overlying the prosthesis often (but not always) accompanied by purulent wound drainage. Other signs and symptoms of a developing infection are persistent pain over parts of the implant on palpation, elevated white blood cell count, elevated erythrocyte sedimentation rate, cellulitis, fever, chills, erosion (**Fig. 53-4**), or fixation of parts of the prosthesis (tubing or pump) to the scrotal wall. Although it is uncommon, infection may manifest after 8 weeks within the first year after the surgical procedure. Such an infection is usually caused by *S. epidermidis* and manifests in an indolent fashion.

Anecdotally, reports have noted implant infection occurring years after implantation. This phenomenon is believed to result from hematogenously disseminated bacteria leaked into the bloodstream after a surgical or dental procedure. Carson and Robertson[1] described a series of delayed prosthetic infections presumably caused by hematogenous bacterial spread from a remote focus. All six patients underwent uncomplicated prosthesis implantations and had an extended problem-free period of use before the inset of infection.[1] All the devices in this series were explanted.

If the penile prosthesis is infected, it must be removed. Systemic administration of antimicrobial agents alone

is ineffective in destroying all offending bacteria. On an ultrastructural level, biofilm produced by bacteria surrounds the implanted device and thereby radically reduces the ability of antimicrobial agents to penetrate the area where the bacteria are located.[10] Additionally, the human body produces a fibrotic capsule that surrounds the prosthesis. This fibrotic capsule has minimal blood supply, a feature that also reduces the efficiency of antibiotic penetration.

Once the prosthesis is removed, the surgeon must decide whether to reimplant another prosthesis several months later or to perform a salvage procedure. Traditionally, following removal of the prosthesis, the area is copiously irrigated with antibiotic solution. Some experts leave drains in place, and the incision is closed, whereas others do not leave drains. This appears to be a matter of choice because no evidence-based medicine has addressed this issue. Based on intraoperative wound and blood cultures, the patient is treated with appropriate systemic antimicrobial agents. If placed, drains may be irrigated two to three times per day with antibiotic solution for several days. Two to 6 months later, a new penile prosthesis may be reinserted.

An alternative approach is to reimplant a new prosthesis immediately, during the same operative session as the explantation. Procedurally, all parts of the infected prosthesis are removed, the wound is copiously irrigated with a series of antibiotic or antimicrobial solutions, the patient is prepared and draped again, and the new prosthesis is inserted.[11] The benefit is that this approach allows for easier cylinder insertion and abrogates the penile shortening that occurs secondary to corporal fibrosis if the cylinders are removed and are not immediately replaced.[11,12] Mulcahy reported long-term success in 45 of 55 (82%) men who underwent salvage of their penile prostheses in the setting of infection.[12]

Occasionally, the surgeon may determine that only the prosthesis cylinder or pump is infected, not the reservoir. In this instance, although it is controversial, we have on occasion attempted and succeeded in salvaging only the cylinders (acting as stents to prevent penile shortening) and returned later for pump and reservoir placement. Exclusion criteria proposed for salvage include any degree of immunocompromise, sepsis, tissue necrosis, and copious amounts of pus within the corporal bodies.[11] Other relative indications are erosion of the cylinders and the presence of uncontrolled diabetes.

In 2001, Montague and colleagues[13] conducted a retrospective reviewed of 491 patients who received a three-piece inflatable penile prosthesis. These investigators reported infection rates and risk factors in these recipients. Of the 491 total patients, 10 infections (2.0%) occurred. Seven of the infections were in first-time prosthesis recipients and 3 were in recipients of secondary inflatable penile prostheses. The presence of diabetes played a minor role in the development of inflatable penile prosthesis infection because 3 of the total 10 infections were in the 137 men with diabetes mellitus. The remainder of infections occurred in patients who did not have diabetes. Surprisingly, this study[13] did not find statistically significant differences in infection rates between first-time and secondary prosthesis recipients or between diabetic and nondiabetic recipients, findings dissimilar to the conclusions published in studies by Jarow[2] and by Lynch and colleagues.[14]

Jarow[2] reported a higher infection rate in patients undergoing a secondary procedure for corporal reconstruction versus prosthesis revision versus first-time insertion of an inflatable penile prosthesis (21.7% versus 13.3% versus 1.8%). This finding is in contrast to the results of the study by Montague and associates.[13] Jarow[2] found convincing evidence not only that reoperation is associated with higher rates of device-related infections but also that complex corporal reconstruction further increases the chance of postoperative infection of inflatable penile prostheses.

Diabetes mellitus, a reported risk factor for the development of implant infections, has been the subject of articles by luminaries in the field of sexual medicine. One of the first reports in the modern era noted a 22% incidence of infection in patients with diabetes but a 6.7% infection rate in patients who did not have diabetes.[14] Subsequent reports by Wilson and colleagues[15,16] failed to link diabetes (regardless of mean glycosylated hemoglobin levels) to a higher risk of prosthesis infection.

Antibiotic-impregnated Prostheses

In an effort to decrease the rate of prosthetic-associated infection, specially modified implants have been developed. AMS introduced InhibiZone prostheses (which are coated with rifampin and minocycline) and Mentor-Coloplast marketed a device with a low-friction, antibiotic-absorbing coating on their Titan prostheses. In nonrandomized studies, both these coatings were shown to decrease the incidence of implant-related infections.

Carson[17] in 2004 retrospectively reviewed the difference in infection rates between patients who received AMS penile implants impregnated with a combination of rifampin and minocycline and those who received untreated prostheses. He reported that the infection rate was initially 1.59% in the noncoated implant and it decreased to 0.2% at 12 months in the coated implant.[17] These data are based on the use of patient information forms completed at the time of the surgical procedure by the surgeon. Thus, these data are not generated from a randomized study, nor is the surgeon blinded to the device type.

In 2006, Abouassaly and colleagues[18] assessed the impact of prosthesis replacement for mechanical failure in infection rates with an AMS antibiotic-coated prosthesis (coated with rifampin and minocycline). Although the investigators excluded salvage procedures for clinically infected prostheses, 1 of 55 patients experienced postoperative device infection in the 32-month follow-up period. The investigators concluded that insertion of an antibiotic-coated inflatable penile prosthesis may result in lower infection rates in this cohort of men.[18]

In 2007, Wilson and associates[19] reported that "InhibiZone-coated inflatable penile prostheses showed a statistically significant reduction in infection in virgin nondiabetic, virgin diabetic, and revision with washout implants. No reduction in the infection rate occurred among revision patients without washout." Specifically, in 467 patients receiving InhibiZone-coated implants, no infections developed among the 223 first-time implants in nondiabetic patients, 1 of 83 diabetic patients developed an infection, 4 infections were found in 39 patients who underwent implant revisions, and infections developed in 4 of 123 men when a salvage operation was combined with antibiotic washout.[19]

Rajpurkar and colleagues[20] demonstrated the ability of the antiadherence coating on the surface of polyurethane strips cultured with and without antibiotics to decrease bacterial colony counts in rats. After the strips were dipped in a vancomycin-gentamicin solution or saline, they were implanted subcutaneously along with a bacterial solution containing *S. epidermidis*. After 7 days, the strips were explanted, sonicated, and incubated. The antibiotic treatment of coated Bioflex caused a significant reduction in the bacterial colony-forming units compared with uncoated Bioflex, thus representing a 55% reduction in the bacterial count.[20] Hellstrom and associates[21] found similar results when they used antibiotic, hydrophilic-coated, Bioflex disks in rabbits.[21]

MECHANICAL MALFUNCTION

Although infection may be the most serious penile prosthetic complication, mechanical malfunction remains the most frequent reason for reoperation (Table 53-1).[22] Common reasons for malfunction are cylinder aneurysm, tubing leakage, reservoir leakage, cylinder leakage, and connector fracture. Failure rates have been reported to be 15% at 5 years and 30% at 10 years.[23] In the event of malfunction, we believe that replacement of the entire device is prudent if initial insertion occurred >2 years previously because this approach will increase the likelihood of longevity of the device. Frequent updates and revisions of the penile implant devices make it difficult to ascertain their true mechanical longevity scientifically.

Levine and colleagues[24] retrospectively reviewed reliability, complication, and patient satisfaction rates in 131 men with the two-piece AMS Ambicor penile prosthesis. Ten patients had complications, 6 of which resulted from mechanical failure. The Ambicor penile

TABLE 53-1	Mechanical Reliability of Penile Prostheses			
Author	**Year**	**No. Patients**	**Type of Prosthesis**	**Mechanical Failure (%)**
Young	2001	273	AMS CXM700	7.3
Levine	2001	131	Ambicor	4.6
Montorsi	2000	200	AMS CXM700	4
Wilson	1999	410	Original Mentor Alpha I	5.6
		971	Enhanced Mentor Alpha I	1.3
Lewis	1995	56	Mentor Alpha I	1.8
Wilson	1993	64	Mentor 3 piece	18.8
Lewis	1993	275	AMS-700CX	4.7
Quesada	1993	214	AMS-700CX	1.9
Goldstein	1993	112	Mentor Alpha I	3.6
Fein	1992	80	Mentor Mark II	0
Sternkohl	1991	46	Mentor 3 piece	28
	1991	43	AMS-700CX	5
Knoll	1990	94	AMS-700CX	6.4
Wilson	1988	29	AMS-700	14
Furlow	1988	120	AMS-700	8.3
Merill	1988	301	Mentor 3 piece	6
Hackler	1986	46	Mentor 3 piece	0
Fishman	1984	113	AMS-700	1.8

prosthesis historically has had high satisfaction rates coupled with reliable function.

A review by Carson and associates[23] of the reliability of and satisfaction with the AMS 700CX three-piece penile prosthesis encompassed a median follow-up of 47.7 months and had two phases.[23] Phase 1 reviewed the medical record of 372 patients and phase 2 was a telephone interview of 207 patients. Medical record review found that the devices were functionally reliable 92.1% of the time after 3 years and 86.2% after 5 years. Seventy-nine percent of the patients with a device used it at least twice monthly and 88.2% would recommend an implant to a relative or friend. The investigators concluded that the AMS 700CX penile implant was reliable, provided excellent patient and partner satisfaction, and had a low postoperative morbidity profile.[23]

Ferguson and Cespedes[25] prospectively evaluated the long-term reliability of and patient satisfaction with the AMS Dura-II malleable penile prosthesis. In this study, the 94 patients who underwent implantation with the Dura-II device were prospectively examined and asked to complete standardized questionnaires regarding sexual activity, prosthesis function, intercourse satisfaction, and overall quality of life. During the follow-up period of nearly 6 years, 76% and 87% of patients reported satisfactory rigidity and ease of concealing the device, respectively. Quality of life was enhanced by the implant in 87% of men and 88% would recommend this prosthesis to a friend. Malleable penile prostheses appear to be as effective and satisfactory as are fluid-filled models. Patient selection and recipient expectations undoubtedly play large roles in determining the likelihood of a satisfactory outcome.

Wilson and associates[26] published a large, long-term, historical prospective study of 2384 patients to estimate mechanical and overall revision-free survival of 4 different inflatable penile prostheses (Mentor Alpha 1, Mentor Alpha NB, AMS 700 CX, and AMS 700 Ultrex). At 10 and 15 years, mechanical reliability was 79.4% and 71.2%, respectively. More recent Mentor Alpha models improved 10-year survival to ≤88.6%. The newer iterations of the ASM CX devices had a reported 97.9% freedom from mechanical breakdown at 3 years. This large study conducted in 2007 further lends credence to the excellent mechanical durability of modern inflatable penile prostheses.

In an effort to elucidate the chronology of patient satisfaction after implantation of a penile prosthesis, we prospectively evaluated men with the International Index of Erectile Function (IIEF) questionnaire preoperatively as well as 3, 6, and 12 months postoperatively. The investigators also administered the Erectile Dysfunction Inventory of Treatment Satisfaction (EDITS) questionnaire postoperatively at 3, 6, and 12 months.

The study of 96 men found that 6- and 12-month scores were higher than baseline, but satisfaction was statistically higher at 12 months as measured by the IIEF satisfaction domain. This first of its kind study elucidated that satisfaction with penile implant further increases after 6 months, but more importantly it provided physicians with additional information to impart to patients.

EROSION

Erosion of a component of the prosthesis is not rare. The device can erode through skin (cylinder or reservoir) or erode through tunica (cylinder), such that it lies subcutaneously. When erosion through skin occurs, the device is inherently infected and probably eroded in the first place because of a low-grade infection. Our approach to this complication depends on the nature of the erosion.

Erosion of the corporal cylinders extracorporally through the distal portions of the corporal bodies may occur iatrogenically from overenthusiastic corporal dilation or oversizing of the cylinders.[27] Patients with decreased distal sensation such as those with spinal cord injury or diabetes mellitus may have an increased incidence of distal erosion.[28] In addition, we have seen this complication in patients who have received previous pelvic irradiation.

Techniques of distal corporal erosion repair include creation of a new pocket for the tip of the cylinder through a hemicircumferential incision for established or impending distal erosion. In cases of lateral extrusion of corporal cylinders, Mulcahy[29] described the creation of a new corporal cavity to reseat the prosthetic device. In this situation, a hemicircumcising incision is made and the cylinder tip is exposed. Next, a 3-inch lateral longitudinal corporotomy is made proximally over the cylinder. The back wall of the fibrotic sheath is then incised transversely and a new plane of dissection is developed. Finally, the cylinder is inserted into this new cavity.

CRURAL PERFORATION

Proximal (crural) perforation is not uncommon, although no data exist in the literature. This complication usually results from overly vigorous or misdirected proximal dilation such that the dilating instrument perforates the tunica and lies in the perineum. If perforation is noted intraoperatively, no long-term concern exists, but failure to identify this complication at the time of implantation may result in proximal migration of the cylinders out of the glans and into the perineum.

Certain surgical approaches are aimed at preventing proximal slippage of the cylinder without direct repair of the crural tunica. Historically, this goal has been accomplished by wrapping the proximal end of the

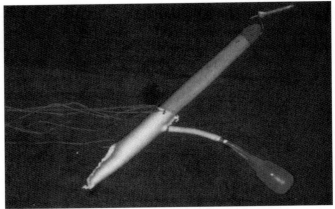

Figure 53-5 Fashioning a windsock around the rear end of the cylinder to prevent proximal migration in the setting of crural perforation. The windsock if used, contemporarily uses an off-the-shelf material such as cadaveric pericardium or intestinal submucosa.

cylinder in a "windsock" made of either synthetic or available natural material such as cadaveric pericardium or intestinal submucosa (**Fig. 53-5**). This windsock is then sutured to the tunica to prevent proximal migration of the cylinder. A second method is to suture the rear-tip extender (if used) to the corporal tunica with nonabsorbable monofilament suture. The cylinder of the prosthesis is then securely seated into the rear-tip extender. A newer approach to this problem is the simple use of a suture hammock around the exit tubing at the proximal end of the cylinder. A simple U-type suture in this setting prevents proximal cylinder migration.

SST DEFORMITY

The *SST deformity* is the name given to the glans of the penis when it appears to bend or hang most commonly downward (but also occasionally upward) limply from the erect penile shaft. This condition may lead to difficulty with penetration or irritation of tissue overlying the ends of the corporal body. The deformity may be the result of inappropriately sized implant cylinders, inadequate distal corporal dilation, or a constitutionally hypermobile glans. This issue may be remedied through a subcoronal incision and dissociation of the glans penis from the distal ends of the corporal bodies. With care taken to avoid neurovascular bundle injury, the glans is then repositioned more proximally on the corporal bodies and is fixed using two nonabsorbable sutures (No. 1 polyester, Ticron, Tyco Healthcare, Waltham, Massachusetts) placed on either side of the midline in a horizontal mattress fashion. These sutures are ideally placed through the tunica albuginea on the corporal body and through the fascial layer on the undersurface of the glans penis.[30,31]

PENILE NECROSIS

The most devastating complication following penile prosthesis insertion is penile necrosis. This rare complication is most often precipitated by local infection; however, pressure dressing or the prolonged presence of a urethral catheter may contribute to the development of necrosis.[32] Adherence to the following basic principles may help avoid this issue:

1. Rigorous sterility of the operative field
2. Limited use of an indwelling catheter
3. Avoidance of circumferential penile compression bandages
4. Proper sizing of penile corporal cylinders
5. Avoidance of prolonged cylinder inflation

Although we have no way to predict who will develop this problem, aggressive treatment may be lifesaving. The prosthesis should be removed, the corporal bodies irrigated, and necrotic tissue débrided. Care must be taken to preserve as much viable tissue (and to avoid amputation) as possible for future penile reconstruction. In the setting of superficial penile gangrene, avoidance of prosthesis removal may be possible but not recommended.[33] Perfusion and healing may be enhanced with hyperbaric oxygen, warm compresses, or vasodilators, although no data exist in the medical literature on these strategies and thus they are purely empirical.

COMPLICATIONS OF PENILE VASCULAR SURGERY

Vascular surgery encompasses penile revascularization and crural ligation surgery for venous leak. Vascular surgery is the only treatment modality that has the potential to allow the permanent return of spontaneous erections without the need for pharmacologic or device support. Specifically, the goal of the surgical procedure is to increase the cavernosal arterial perfusion pressure and inflow in patients with erectile dysfunction resulting from pure arterial insufficiency. The ideal patient is a young man with pure arteriogenic erectile dysfunction who has no other vascular risk factors.

Penile revascularization has undergone many refinements since its first description by Vaclav Michal and associates in 1973.[34] Many variations have been described by Michal and associates,[35] Virag,[36] Hauri, Crespo and colleagues,[37] and Hatzichristou and Goldstein.[38] No further revolutionary changes have occurred in the realm of penile revascularization surgery, nor does consensus exist among experts with regard to the definitive technique.

Complications of penile revascularization occur in approximately 25% of patients.[39-41] Postoperative arterial hemorrhage with hematoma formation may result from disruption of the microvascular anastomosis. This is the culmination of the repetitive stretching and tearing of the vascular anastomosis during coitus or masturbation. In our practice, we recommend abstention from sexual activities involving an erect penis for at least 6 weeks postoperatively.

Another rare complication is glans hyperemia, which occurs when the dorsal vein has been arterialized (inferior epigastric artery or dorsal artery to deep dorsal vein anastomosis).[39,41] The treatment is to ligate the deep dorsal vein distally. Diminished penile sensation may result from dorsal nerve injury but is uncommon because an operating microscope is used for dorsal vessel dissection.[42]

Crural ligation for venous leak has seen a resurgence in use at major referral centers. In an effort to correct isolated venous leak from crural veins, this procedure entails ligation (or exclusion) of the proximal corpora with umbilical tape.[43,44] Two of the more influential studies of this procedure are by John Mulhall and Tom Lue and their associates. Mulhall and colleagues[43] described success using a transscrotal approach, whereas Lue and colleagues[44] favored a 3-inch inguinoscrotal approach. The most common complications in these studies were scrotal hematoma, infection, and continued erectile dysfunction. We had a single case of infection of the umbilical tape, which was removed. We now treat all patients with preoperative, perioperative, and postoperative oral antibiotics.

PEYRONIE'S DISEASE SURGERY COMPLICATIONS

Peyronie's disease is a fibrotic disorder of the tunica albuginea that results in penile deformity, penile pain, and in some patients erectile dysfunction.[45] The etiology and pathophysiology of this disorder have not been completely elucidated.[46-48] Prevalence estimates range from 1% to 8.9%.[49,50] The natural history of Peyronie's disease was initially described by Williams and Thomas in 1970.[51] In this small study, the investigators reported a spontaneous resolution rate of 50%.[51] As a result of this study, many patients with Peyronie's disease are prescribed conservative treatment. In a later report, Gelbard and colleagues[52] described resolution of penile curvature in 13% of patients with nonsurgical treatment.

In 2006, we[53] reported an analysis of the natural history of Peyronie's disease in 246 untreated patients. Mean follow-up was 18 months, at which time 12% of men had an improved curvature, 40% remained stable, and 48% worsened. The most important information from this report is that the average improvement in curvature was 15 degrees, but in patients who experienced worsening of curvature, the mean change was 22 degrees.[53] These and other articles suggest that spontaneous resolution of penile curvature from Peyronie's disease is uncommon.

Peyronie's disease has two phases: acute (inflammatory) and chronic. It is best to correct the penile deformity surgically after the acute phase has passed. Typically, this is 12 to 18 months after the onset of the condition. In the chronic phase, the penile curvature has stabilized and although penile plaque may be prominent and calcified, it is not associated with penile pain. This is the optimal time for surgical intervention.

Indications and Procedures

Tornehl and Carson[54,55] published criteria for the surgical intervention of Peyronie's disease. In our practice, we communicate to patients that no absolute indications exist for curvature correction. However, if the patient can answer any the following questions in the affirmative, if he is ≥12 months from the initial onset of symptoms, and if he has had a stable deformity for ≥3 months, he is then considered to be a candidate for surgical correction of the penile deformity:

1. Does the patient hate the appearance of his penis?
2. Is the patient unable to have penetrative sexual relations?
3. If the patient is able to have penetrative sexual relations, is the experience cumbersome or unsatisfactory?

Once the decision to proceed with operative intervention has been made, the surgeon must choose the most appropriate method of curvature correction based on physical examination (nature and magnitude of deformity) during maximal rigidity erection, baseline erectile function, and penile dimensions. Surgical procedures for correcting curvature resulting from Peyronie's disease fall into three major categories. For a full review of these categories, the reader is referred to the article by Tornehl and Carson[55] in *Urologic Clinics of North America*:

1. Plication: Nesbit, 16-dot, corporoplication, Kelami's corporoplasty, or incisional corporoplasty, Yacchia procedure
2. Plaque manipulation: removal or incision of the plaque with subsequent coverage of the corporal defect with synthetic or nonsynthetic graft material
3. Penile prosthesis insertion

Selecting the correct surgical approach for the individual patient is critical to optimizing results. Patients with complex deformities or those who have at baseline a foreshortened penis are not good candidates for penile plication surgery. Patients with preexisting erectile dysfunction or low-degree simple curvatures are not excellent candidates for plaque incision and grafting surgery. Patients with normal erectile function should probably not undergo penile implant surgery unless they have a complex deformity or a significant hour-glass deformity.

Plication-type procedures are best used in the patient with congenital penile curvature. This approach has a short surgical time, is relatively simple, and has little impact on existing erectile capacity. Plaque manipulation techniques are used in patients with complex deformities, hourglass deformities, normal erectile function, or preexisting penile shortening. Unfortunately, the disadvantages of this method are degeneration of erectile function or dysfunction and dorsal nerve entrapment or damage leading to penile neurosensory alterations. The use of a penile prosthesis in Peyronie's disease is reserved for men with preexisting moderate to severe erectile dysfunction who have unsuccessfully tried oral and injectable agents.

Penile Plication Complications

Complications of plication procedures include hematoma formation, decreased penile sensation (anesthesia, dysesthesia), erectile dysfunction, and bother from suture material palpable after the operation. We perform all dorsal plication procedures after neurovascular bundle elevation.[56,57] This approach minimizes the risk of decreased penile sensation in the postoperative setting. We recommend incising Buck's fascia and using loupe magnification to visualize the dorsal penile nerve bundles. We also use braided nonabsorbable suture (No. 1 polyester [Ticron]) when performing plications because this material is less palpable and may reduce the incidence of patient bother from suture knots.

In 1998, Pryor[58] reported data from 359 patients dating from 1977 to 1992 who had penile plication performed using the Nesbit technique. The investigators convincingly argued that this technique translates into a high patient satisfaction rate (≤90%) while minimizing postoperative complications. These investigators found that Nesbit-related penile shortening was not a significant problem in this patient population; only 6 men were unable to have penetrative sexual relations because of this issue.[58]

A more contemporary series of 68 patients from Spain confirmed the findings of other reports.[59] At 36 months of mean follow-up, 20% of patients had penile shortening of >1.5 cm, but 85% of the men were satisfied with the cosmetic result of Nesbit technique. Complications of the surgical procedure were minimal; 2 men developed phimosis and 2 needed a second procedure for recurrent curvature.[59] Pertinent results of these and other studies are contained in Table 53-2.

Plaque Manipulation Surgery

The risk of complications from plaque-based surgery is low. Initial complications include hematoma (supragraft and subgraft) formation and rarely infection. Hematoma formation may be limited by the use of watertight suture lines, small-diameter suture needles,

TABLE 53-2	Outcomes of Penile Plication Surgery					
Author	Year	No. Patients	Mean Follow-up (mo)	Shortening (%)	Recurrence (%)	Satisfaction (%)
Sulaiman	1994	78	50	?	4	18
Ralph	1995	185	180	?	3	90
Savoca	2000	157	72	14	?	88
Syed	2003	42	84	76	10	50
Savoca	2004	218	89	17	?	83.5
Bokarica	2005	40	81	100	?	?
Moyano	2006	68	36	20	2.9	85

and narrow-gauge needles when erectogenic drugs are administered to generate an artificial erection. Intermediate and late complications are penile skin necrosis, penile length loss, and recurvature. Loss of penile skin, although rare, is caused by the circumferential skin incision. Because the skin of the penile shaft and the skin of the glans have a separate but anastomotic blood supply, we advocate the use of a single circumcising incision. If needed, a transverse scrotal incision can be made in addition to provide access to the proximal corpora.

The recurrence of curvature within a short period postoperatively is the result of either suture failure (we use 4-0 polydioxanone [PDS]) or an inadequately sized graft. Nonabsorbable or delayed-absorption suture must be used in grafting because the tunical forces developed during an erection far exceed the tensile strength of partially absorbed polyglactin (Vicryl, Ethicon, Somerville, NJ) or synthetic polyester (Biosyn, Syneture/US Surgical, Norwalk, Connecticut).

The choice of the best grafting material has been the subject of quiet debate. Synthetic materials (e.g., Gore-Tex) are of historical significance because autologous and cadaveric (processed, prepackaged) grafts are readily available and provide fewer complications. Autologous material (e.g., buccal, dermal, tunical, vein), although available, incites minimal host reaction and infection risk and requires an auxiliary procedure to harvest.

An Italian group led by Montorsi[60] assessed the long-term outcome of vein grafting in 50 patients with Peyronie's disease. After a mean follow-up of 32 months, complete resolution of penile curvature in 40 men (80%), minor residual curvature of ≤30 degrees in 7 men (14%), and recurrence of curvature in 3 men (6%) were reported. The procedure was complicated by penile hypoesthesia, penile hematoma, wound infection, and glandular ischemia. Plaque incision with vein grafting is able to achieve satisfactory clinical results a majority of men.[60] Conversely, processed or prepackaged material (pericardium, dura mater, intestinal submucosa) offers the ability to tailor the graft specifically to the appropriate size, minimizes the host inflammatory response, and abrogates the need for harvesting tissue.

Levine and Estrada[61] published their experience with human cadaveric pericardium. Over a 4-year period, 40 men underwent penile curvature correction with pericardium. Postoperatively, 98% of these men had a straight penis and 95% were able to have penetrative sexual relations; 12 (30%) patients required pharmacologic assistance to achieve a penetration-quality erection. Most interesting is that no major complications occurred in this cohort of men.[61]

Breyer and Lue and their colleagues[62] retrospectively reviewed outcomes with and complications of using intestinal submucosa in the correction of penile curvature in Peyronie's disease. Nineteen patients were treated with tunical incision or excision and grafting with small intestine submucosa. Of these patients, 37% (7 of 19) had significant recurrent penile curvature, whereas 5 of 19 (26%) had recurrent Peyronie's disease plaque. The investigators reported a 37% complication rate, including graft site hematoma and graft infection, as well as reoperation for Peyronie's disease recurrence in a single patient.[62] Despite the ease of use of small intestine submucosa, the high complication rate makes the use of this material less desirable. The results of these and other studies are presented in Table 53-3.

Penile Prosthesis Surgery

Implant surgery for Peyronie's disease is indicated when the patient has both Peyronie's disease and erectile dysfunction that is not responsive to erectogenic pharmacotherapy. General complications of penile prosthesis insertion are listed elsewhere, but penile modeling deserves special comment. Modeling or molding entails powerfully bending the penis in an effort to break or crack the Peyronie's plaque when residual curvature remains after inflation of the device intraoperatively. This method was embraced by Wilson and Delk[63] in 1994 and showed an initial 86% success rate.

TABLE 53-3 Outcomes of Plaque Incision and Grafting

Author	Year	No. Patients	Graft	Length Loss (%)	Correction Rate (%)
Kadioglu	1999	20	Vein	?	75
Montorsi	2000	50	Vein	40	80
Knoll	2001	12	Intestine	0	100
Egydio	2002	33	Pericardium	?	88
Levine	2003	40	Pericardium	?	98
Lue	2007	19	Intestine	63	63

TABLE 53-4 Outcomes of Penile Implant Surgery for Peyronie's Disease

Author	Year	No. Patients	Manual Modeling (%)	Successful Correction (%)	Device
Levine	2000	46	54	100	Two- and three-piece
Wilson	2001	104	100	—	Alpha 1, 700CX
Usta	2003	42	74	26	—
Akin-Olugbade	2005	18	20	100	60%

The specific technique is begun with the device partially inflated and the tubing cross-clamped with rubber shod hemostats. The penis is forcibly bent in a direction opposite to the curvature in a maneuver similar to breaking a twig in both hands for 90 seconds. The procedure is repeated for another 90 seconds. The device is deflated and then reinflated to reseat the cylinders within the corporal bodies.[64] Certain devices are ill advised when penile modeling may be required. The AMS Ultrex, with its girth- and length-expanding capabilities, may cause an increased risk of aneurysm formation when forcibly deformed. Furthermore, the Ultrex device lacks the axial rigidity to straighten a penile curvature.[65] Follow-up studies by Wilson and associates[64] confirmed that implantation and modeling appeared to provide permanent straightening without an increase in revisions as compared with implantation alone.

The major complication of corporal modeling is urethral laceration, which occurs in approximately 4% of cases.[64] This ulceration is usually visible and is repaired using fine absorbable sutures (Table 53-4).

KEY POINTS

1. Infection remains a significant concern, with rates between 1% and 8%.
2. In the setting of infection, device removal is highly recommended. Immediate reinsertion of the prosthesis is associated with long-term success in 45 of 55 patients in one study.
3. Despite the potential complications of the penile prosthesis, satisfaction rates remain high.
4. Peyronie's disease surgery should be undertaken in the properly selected patient with realistic expectations of the potential outcome.
5. Complications of Peyronie's procedures include hematoma formation, decreased penile sensation (anesthesia, dysesthesia), erectile dysfunction, and bother from palpable suture material, penile skin necrosis, penile length loss, and recurvature.

REFERENCES

Please see www.expertconsult.com

Chapter 54

COMPLICATIONS OF SURGERY OF THE TESTICLE, VAS, EPIDIDYMIS, AND SCROTUM

David Fenig MD

Associate Director, Male Fertility and Sexuality, Chesapeake Urology Associates, Baltimore, Maryland

Philip Werthman MD

Director, Center for Male Reproductive Medicine, Los Angeles, California

Since the last publication of this book, the performance of almost all surgical procedures involving the scrotum has transitioned from the hospital operating theater to outpatient surgical centers and physicians' office procedure rooms. Although these procedures are considered minor, they can be fraught with morbidity and can result in significant amounts of pain, anxiety, and lost wages for those patients experiencing complications. In fact, scrotal surgical procedures generate significant amounts of litigation directed toward urologists. Finesse and forethought are necessary requisites for a surgeon to attain a level of proficiency with scrotal procedures.

The subspecialty of male reproductive medicine has experienced significant growth paralleling that of reproductive endocrinology and has required general urologists to expand their knowledge base and skill in this area. Fertility-related procedures encompass a significant portion of scrotal surgery. Many procedures are best performed using an operating microscope and thus necessitate some degree of microsurgical training on the part of the surgeon. The goals of this chapter are to outline the basic principles of surgery of the scrotum and its contents, to describe the potential complications that may arise from each of the individual procedures, and to discuss the treatments of these complications. Most importantly, we hope to convey to the reader some of the pitfalls and situations that may lead to complications and the means to avoid these complications from the outset.

PRINCIPLES OF SCROTAL SURGERY

As with any surgical procedure, patient selection is a key factor to a successful outcome and the avoidance of complications. Indications for surgery on the scrotum or its contents include suspicion of cancer, relief of pain, improvement of fertility, contraception, and cosmesis. Regardless of the reasons for surgical treatment, certain issues must be similarly addressed before, during, and after the procedures, as discussed in this section.

Preparing the patient for surgery must include obtaining informed consent. The surgeon should discuss in detail the procedure, the indications for performing the procedure, all the alternative treatments for the patient's condition, the chances for successful outcome of each of the alternatives, and their advantages and drawbacks. It is important to discuss the recovery process in terms of the patient's occupation and lifestyle. Expectations regarding the procedure and recovery should be realistic. Patients need to be made aware that even very minor procedures can have significant untoward ramifications. A discussion of all the potential risks and complications of a given procedure should be documented in the patient's medical record. For the majority of scrotal procedures the risks include pain, bleeding, swelling, infection, failure of the procedure, testicular atrophy or loss, and potential undesired effects on the patient's fertility or hormone production capacity. Other procedure-specific complications include hydrocele formation and groin or scrotal numbness. Patients should be informed of the small potential for development of chronic testicular or epididymal pain, especially after vasectomy.

Patients should be instructed to discontinue aspirin and nonsteroidal anti-inflammatory medications 7 days before the date of the procedure. Even baby aspirin and some herbal supplements can result in platelet dysfunction that can lead to postsurgical bleeding. The scrotal skin should be shaved in the operating room immediately before the procedure to reduce the risk of infection. The patient should not shave the surgical area at home the day before the procedure. Investigators have shown that small nicks in the skin can become infected and lead to a postoperative wound infection.

Several choices of anesthesia induction are appropriate for these types of cases and include general anesthesia, local anesthesia with or without intravenous sedation, and spermatic cord block. Epidural or spinal anesthesia is hardly ever used in the outpatient setting. A newer needle-less technique using an air gun injector has been described to induce spermatic cord block for vasectomy. The most important considerations in anesthetic choice should include the patient's comfort and anxiety level, safety, the ability to immobilize the patient especially for microsurgical procedures, the risks of the anesthetic technique on the patient's health, and the recovery from the anesthetic.

Some patients may have a high tolerance to local anesthesia such that it is difficult to induce or maintain a pain-free state. Patients who are candidates for local anesthesia should be asked whether they have had any anesthetic issues during dental procedures to identify whether they are resistant to the effects of local anesthetics or require significantly higher doses. Some patients report that local anesthesia wears off quickly. Performing a procedure using only a local anesthetic in the aforementioned groups should be avoided.

The cornerstone of good scrotal anesthesia is the spermatic cord block. The ideal regimen is a 10-mL equal parts mixture of 0.5% bupivacaine with 1% or 2% lidocaine without epinephrine, infiltrated using a 25-gauge needle. The vas deferens is first isolated with the thumb and forefinger and 4 mL is injected around, but not into, the vas. Another 4 mL is then injected into the internal spermatic fascia. The needle is slowly advanced without the use of a back-and-forth motion because this maneuver can lead to hematoma formation. The area of the incision should be infiltrated with 1 or 2 mL to raise a skin wheel. On rare occasions a patient will require an additional injection. Before closing, 5 mL of anesthetic is instilled within the intratunical space and another 5 mL is instilled into the space between the dartos and tunica vaginalis layers. Reinfiltration of the skin incision is then performed before the closing sutures are placed. This regimen should keep the patient pain free for at least several hours and should allow him to leave the facility and return home in little discomfort.

From a surgical standpoint, the scrotum can be an unforgiving area in that a small bleeding vessel can result in a very large expanding hematoma. The many layers of tissue within the scrotum can easy conceal a retracted vessel and can make hemostasis difficult to achieve. To ensure meticulous hemostasis, electrocautery should be used to incise each layer and veil of tissue. On occasion, bleeding can ensue from a spermatic cord block if the needle pierces a vein or more rarely a spermatic artery branch. This situation is more likely to occur in men with large varicoceles, and caution should be taken when inserting the needle into the internal spermatic bundle. The hematoma is usually discovered on entering the tunica vaginalis filled with blood. Persistent low-level bleeding can be stopped with several minutes of manual compression of the upper scrotum and spermatic cord. Brisk bleeding that does not abate with compression necessitates delivery of the testicle and exploration of the spermatic cord with cauterization or ligation of the breeched vessel. Care should be taken to avoid arterial injury while achieving hemostasis.

On closure of the surgical site, all tissue layers should be individually reapproximated at their cut edges with a running suture technique. Minor bleeding at the skin edges can also be controlled in this manner or by placing a Babcock clamp over a gauze pad on the wound for several minutes. The resulting compression of the skin edges usually stops the bleeding.

Use of surgical drains is generally not required for scrotal procedures unless the indication for surgery is to evacuate a hematoma or an infection of a closed space or to repair a large hydrocele. It is wise to consider leaving a drain in place after a procedure in which hemostasis has been less than optimal or when increased inflammation is encountered. Drain placement is easily accomplished by using a hemostat to puncture a hole through the tunica vaginalis, dartos, and skin layers at the base of the scrotum. A ¼-inch Penrose drain is pulled through the drain site and is laid on the posterior surface of the tunica vaginalis under the testicle in a dependant position. Caution must be taken not to incorporate the drain in the wound closure accidentally. A silk or nylon suture is used to secure the drain to the scrotal skin. Patients can be instructed to remove the drain at home on the first or second postoperative day.

Scrotal incisions may be dressed with a small adhesive bandage followed by fluffed gauze and a scrotal support. Athletic supporters tend to be much more comfortable for the patient than do typical surgical supporters. These supporters also can accommodate an ice pack and hold it in place more readily. Turban dressings maintain excellent scrotal compression following bilateral orchiectomy. When increased amounts of postoperative swelling are anticipated, the scrotum can be sutured to the abdominal wall or upper thigh over a gauze roll. This type of dressing is not very practical for outpatient surgical procedures.

Patients should be instructed to continue to use an athletic supporter and ice pack after undergoing any procedure on the scrotum. A variable period of 1 to 5 days of bed rest or light activity should be observed depending on the specific procedure. Postoperative pain can usually be controlled with acetaminophen or a mild narcotic. Ibuprofen and aspirin should be avoided because of their effect on platelet function. Patients should be able to shower on the day after the surgical procedure.

VASECTOMY

Vasectomy is a safe and effective method of permanent male contraception performed on >500,000 men annually in the United States.[1] In the hands of an experienced practitioner, it is a quick, relatively pain-free, and low-risk procedure.[2]

An initial prevasectomy consultation consists of a thorough history and physical examination and a discussion of the procedure, treatment alternatives, and reversibility. Patients should be given a period of time to consider sterilization fully and it is therefore recommended that a vasectomy not be performed at the initial visit or in haste. Exaggerated emotional reactions associated with sterility may lead to an angry and litigious patient should complications arise. A Danish study found that 7.4% of men who underwent vasectomy regretted their decision and 39% of these men were <30 years of age.[3] Approximately 2% to 6% of men will undergo vasectomy reversal. Men contemplating vasectomy should be aware of the costs and success of vasectomy reversal and assisted reproductive technologies should they change their mind and desire children in the future. All patients regardless of age should be given the opportunity to cryopreserve sperm if they so desire. Consideration should be given to whether vasectomy is an appropriate procedure for men who initially inquire about preserving future fertility or in young men who have not fathered a child.

The vasectomy procedure is performed in either the office or outpatient facility and usually with the use of local anesthetic (Box 54-1). After scrotal block as described, the surgeon isolates the vas from the rest of the spermatic cord by using the thumb and forefinger. The skin is anesthetized and then the needle is slowly advanced into and around the perivasal sheath to anesthetize the vas and surrounding tissue. No more than 5 mL need be injected to obtain an adequate block. It often takes several minutes for the block to take effect. It is important not to overinfiltrate the area so the vas can continue to be palpated if necessary. The anesthetic can be massaged into the vas and skin to take effect more rapidly. This facilitates the ability to isolate the vas against the skin completely before the no-scalpel ring clamp is placed on the vas.

BOX 54-1 **Surgical Pearls: Vasectomy**

1. Provide adequate spermatic cord block.
2. Control the vas at all times.
3. Dissect the vas out of its sheath before ligation.
4. Avoid excessive cauterization of the vasal wall; just cauterize the mucosa.
5. Avoid removing very large segments of the vas.
6. Maintain hemostasis.

Vasectomy may be performed either with an incision or with the no-scalpel technique. The traditional vasectomy is performed by incising the skin of the median raphe or over each vas. A site at the midscrotum should be chosen such that a reasonable length of the testicular vasal end is left to accommodate any potential for back-pressure buildup or to allow reversal to be a future option. The dartos muscle is incised with electrocautery and the vas is isolated. The perivasal sheath is incised and the vas is dissected out of its sheath with care to preserve the deferential vessels and nerves. Ligation of the vas is performed, small segment is removed, and the vasal edges and lumen are then cauterized. A segment >1 cm need not be excised because this may lead to increased bleeding, swelling, and recovery time. A fascial segment may be interposed after the vas ends are sutured back on themselves or are buried in the dartos layer. Hemostasis is meticulously achieved and the incisions are closed.

The no-scalpel technique was developed in China in 1974 and has been demonstrated to decrease operative and recovery time as well as complications, including hematoma and postoperative pain.[4-6] Anesthesia is induced as described earlier. After delivering the vas to the skin surface, it is grasped and transfixed in place to the skin with a no-scalpel vasectomy ring clamp. A sharp curved mosquito hemostat is used to pierce the skin, the dartos layer, and the vasal sheath. The vas is delivered out of the sheath and is incised. Ligation of the abdominal and testicular ends of the vas is performed with surgical hemoclips. It is not as important to interpose a segment of fascia or dartos between the cut ends of the vas particularly if surgical clips are used.

Open-ended vasectomy, a procedure in which the testicular end of the vas segment is left untied, has been advocated by some surgeons in an attempt to decrease secondary epididymal obstruction, epididymitis, and pain,[7,8] although it may actually lead to higher failure rates and sperm granuloma formation. Evidence suggests that fascial interposition and cauterization of the vasal ends reduce postoperative failure versus suture-ligation and excision of a segment of vas alone.[4,9]

It is important to maintain constant control of the vas so it does not retract into the scrotum during the procedure. One technique is to have an extra ring clamp available to keep around the testicular end of the vas until the procedure is completed. Care should be taken to dissect the vas out of the vasal sheath and ligate only the vas itself. Incorporating the sheath into the ligature may result in chronic scrotal pain. It is advisable to leave a small hemostat on the vas after completion of the first side so that the same vas cannot be grasped and cut twice, a maneuver that would lead to vasectomy failure.

With the no-scalpel vasectomy, skin closure is usually not necessary although the small hole in the dartos and skin may be cauterized to help achieve hemostasis and reduce its size. A small adhesive bandage is placed over the breach in the skin. Scrotal ice packs and a scrotal supporter are used for ≥24 hours postoperatively, and strenuous activity and sexual activity are avoided for 1 week. Patients are instructed to ejaculate a minimum of 20 times to clear the reproductive tract of sperm. Follow-up semen analyses are mandatory and should begin at 6 weeks after vasectomy. Patients are counseled to use contraception until azoospermia is documented on two consecutive semen analyses.

According to a policy statement of the American Urological Association (AUA), it is not necessary to store or send a segment of the removed vas for pathology examination. It is also important to not overcauterize the testicular end of the vas because that can cause necrosis at the surgical clip site and can result in leakage of sperm with subsequent granuloma formation. Postoperative success is ultimately determined by a negative semen analysis; pathologic confirmation of the vas does not guarantee success. In fact, recanalization may be responsible for failures regardless of the technique performed. Smith and colleagues[10] reported a 1 in 2000 risk of paternity after vasectomy despite postoperative azoospermia.

Specific Complications and Their Treatment

Postoperative hematoma occurs in ≤2% of patients but the rate is slightly higher when fascial interposition is used. This is typically a self-limiting process and a conservative approach is recommended. Initial treatment is with bed rest, ice packs, and a scrotal supporter. Resolution of hematoma occurs over several weeks to months, and patients often require significant reassurance that no permanent sequelae will occur. If the hematoma is expanding, surgical exploration is warranted. After evacuation of hematoma and achievement of hemostasis, a ¼-inch Penrose drain may be placed for 24 to 48 hours. Many times the source of active bleeding is not found. An appropriate cephalosporin is administered.

Wound infection is an infrequent event, occurring in <1% of cases. Immunocompromised patients or patients with diabetes are at an increased risk. Perioperative antibiotics do not appear to confer significant improvement in infection rates, although these drugs may be advantageous in certain patient populations. Treatment of infections must be aggressive to reduce the risk of spread or the development of Fournier's gangrene.

Early or late vasectomy failures may occur as demonstrated by the presence of motile sperm on postvasectomy semen analysis. Identification of nonmotile sperm in the semen on follow-up may result from persistence of sperm in the distal ejaculatory duct or seminal vesicle. Serial semen analyses at 4- to 6-week intervals should be obtained to document azoospermia. An AUA policy statement declared the persistence of sperm in semen to represent a surgical failure. Early failures may be a

result of failure to cut the vas on one side or recanalization. If motile sperm persist at 6-month follow-up, vasectomy should be repeated. Early recanalization may occur in ≤13% of men but this complication appears to be most infrequent when the ends of the vas have been cauterized.[5] Late recanalization is evidenced by the 1 in 2000 risk of paternity after postoperative azoospermia.[10-12]

Sperm granulomas are an inflammatory response caused by the leakage of sperm at the testicular end of the vas. This complication can occur after closed or open-ended vasectomy. Silber[8] found decreased pain and decreased rates of secondary epididymal obstruction in patients with sperm granuloma after open-ended vasectomy with fascial interposition. For some patients, a sperm granuloma may actually cause temporary or long-term scrotal pain and discomfort. A painful granuloma should be treated conservatively with anti-inflammatory medication. Most often the pain is self-limited and resolves within several months of the vasectomy. Patients with intractable pain should consider granuloma excision with or without microsurgical vasectomy reversal.

Chronic scrotal pain, also known as the *postvasectomy pain syndrome*, has been attributed to congestive epididymitis or chronic orchialgia. Subjectively measured, occurrence rates vary, although conservative measures rarely fail. One questionnaire-based study found 18.7% of respondents with complaints of postvasectomy scrotal pain; however, this pain adversely affected quality of life in only 2.2%.[13] In most patients with postvasectomy pain, the pain appears to be a somatic phenomenon rather than psychological in origin. The cause of pain is not necessarily the same for all patients and may be multifactorial. Pain may also be caused by a sperm granuloma, nerve ligation, or neuroma formation.[13] Successful resolution of postvasectomy pain syndrome has been achieved with vasectomy reversal, open-ended vasectomy, excision of sperm granuloma, and total epididymectomy.[7,14] It appears that vasectomy reversal with excision of the vasectomy site and any scar tissue around the vas offers the best chance of cure, with complete resolution in approximately 80% of patients.

Our own experience with converting a closed-ended vasectomy to an open-ended procedure for the treatment of pain was unsuccessful. Several patients developed large granulomas that made subsequent vasectomy reversal more difficult. Epididymectomy should not be performed on these patients because it often does not relieve the pain and makes future reversal impossible. A subset of patients after epididymectomy must undergo subsequent orchiectomy to become pain free. Microsurgical denervation of the spermatic cord may be offered to patients with failed epididymectomies but should not be suggested as first-line surgical treatment of postvasectomy pain.

VARICOCELECTOMY

Approximately 15% of the physiologically normal male population and ≤40% of infertile men have a clinically apparent varicocele.[15,16] Varicoceles are associated with decreased testicular function and may cause testicular atrophy. These lesions are thought to be progressive and may cause deterioration in semen parameters and hormone function over time.[17,18] Indications for varicocele repair include testicular pain, male infertility, hypogonadism, and progressive testicular atrophy. In the adolescent population, varicocelectomy is performed when testicular size discrepancy is evident. Size discrepancy >2 mL or 20% of testicular volume is considered abnormal[19] and usually reverses following corrective surgical procedures.[20,21] Varicocele has been demonstrated to increase sperm DNA fragmentation and correction has been shown to improve the damage. It is important to rule out other causes of infertility in men with severe oligospermia and concomitant varicocele. Patients with bilateral varicoceles have a greater improvement in seminal parameters if they undergo bilateral repair as opposed to unilateral repair.

The treatment options for patients with a clinically significant varicocele include surgical ligation and percutaneous embolization (Box 54-2). Surgical correction may be performed through a retroperitoneal, inguinal, subinguinal, or transperitoneal laparoscopic approach. The goal of varicocele surgery should be to ligate all veins including small branches to prevent recurrence while preserving the arterial supply and lymphatic drainage to optimize testicular function and decrease risk of hydrocele formation. Use of a small incision without cutting the muscle or entering the peritoneum or retroperitoneum decreases pain and recovery time as well as the risks of serious morbidity.

When one evaluates the different techniques in terms of outcomes, recurrence rates and risks, microsurgical inguinal repair appears to be superior to all others. The use of an operating microscopic during the procedure has demonstrated benefit in reducing both recurrences and complications.[22,23] In an attempt to reduce varicocele recurrence through collateral vessels further, delivery of the testis with ligation of the gubernacular and external spermatic veins has been advocated.[24]

Although laparoscopic varicocelectomy is associated with recurrence rates of <2%, it carries the additional morbidity of an intraperitoneal operation and higher cost. No indication exists to perform a surgical procedure that has even a small chance of mortality when more successful alternatives do not expose patients to such risk.

A retroperitoneal repair, as described by Palomo, is performed through a transverse muscle-splitting incision made medial to the anterior superior iliac spine.[25] The peritoneum is swept medially to expose the internal spermatic vessels in the retroperitoneal space. In this technique, the spermatic cord, the internal spermatic artery, and the lymphatic channels are ligated. The drawbacks to this approach are longer recovery time, risk of retroperitoneal bleeding, and high rate of hydrocele formation. The effect of ligating the internal spermatic artery on testicular function is unclear. An artery-sparing approach has been described but has a higher recurrence rate.

An inguinal repair is performed through a small incision just above the external inguinal ring. The aponeurosis of the external oblique is opened, the ilioinguinal nerve is identified and preserved, and the spermatic cord is isolated. Identification of the testicular artery is improved with the use of a Doppler microprobe and operating microscope. The artery is teased away from the surrounding veins. All veins are ligated. Lymphatic branches are spared to reduce postoperative hydrocele formation.

A subinguinal repair is performed through a slightly lower incision over the external inguinal ring. The spermatic cord is dissected without opening the aponeurosis, and a similar procedure is performed as described earlier.

The anatomic basis for varicocele persistence or recurrence is important to understand because it explains the benefits and pitfalls of different surgical approaches. Recurrence after artery-sparing high retroperitoneal repair may result from persistence of small venous collateral vessels associated with the testicular artery. The gubernacular veins have also been implicated as a potential cause. Kass and Marcol[26] found persistent varicoceles in 11% of patients who underwent artery-sparing retroperitoneal repair as opposed to no recurrences in patients who had mass ligation of testicular vessels. Although rates of testicular atrophy are low with laparoscopic or open mass ligation, artery-sparing procedures should be considered in patients with prior inguinal or scrotal surgery because of the possibility of inadequate arterial collateral vessels through the vasal artery.

BOX 54-2 Surgical Pearls: Varicocelectomy

1. Rule out other causes of infertility or pain before varicocele repair.
2. Identify the ilioinguinal nerve in the inguinal canal during inguinal repair.
3. Identify the internal spermatic artery, its branches, and the vas deferens before proceeding with vein ligation.
4. Ligate all internal and external spermatic veins; varicose veins around the vas deferens must be ligated as well.
5. Spare the lymphatic channels.
6. Use of an operating microscope and a Doppler microprobe will decrease recurrence and complications.

In the subinguinal region, the arterial and venous anatomy is more variable. Greater numbers of internal spermatic arteries and veins are present and can make the procedure more tedious and time-consuming.[27] The testicular arterial branches are more intimately associated with and adherent to enlarged veins. Concomitant varicocelectomy and vasovasostomy should not be performed because of the increased risk of arterial injury and testicular atrophy.

Specific Complications and Their Treatment

Minor complications include wound infection, hematoma, and seroma (Table 54-1). These occur in rare instances. Appropriate perioperative antibiotic prophylaxis and meticulous hemostasis mitigate these problems.

The most worrisome complications of testicular devascularization and atrophy are rare.[26,28] Preservation of the vasal artery is necessary for adequate collateral blood flow in the instance of prior internal spermatic artery ligation or injury. Arteries should be carefully spared in all patients but this is critical in patients who have undergone prior inguinal or testicular surgery.

Hydrocele is the most common complication of varicocelectomy, with rates ≤20% following the retroperitoneal approach. Postoperative asymptomatic hydroceles are managed conservatively; however, 10% to 15% of patients may require hydrocelectomy.[28,29] Evidence suggests that hydrocele formation has a negative effect on spermatogenesis secondary to an insulation effect on the testicle. Use of microsurgical lymphatic-sparing techniques has virtually eliminated this complication.

Minimizing varicocele recurrence depends on ligation of all potential venous collateral vessels. Recurrence is rare using microsurgical techniques but increases with nonmicrosurgical inguinal and retroperitoneal approaches.[22,26,29-31] A Doppler ultrasound scan is performed if recurrence is suspected to confirm venous flow in persistent vessels as opposed to previously ligated veins left in situ. Recurrences should be approached using the microsurgical approach because great care must be taken to identify and preserve all arteries in patients undergoing reoperation for persistent varicocele. It is important to ligate the gubernacular veins during surgical procedures for failed varicocele. Consideration should be given to percutaneous embolization of persistent collateral vessels after failed microsurgical varicocelectomy.

Some patients experience anesthesia or paresthesia of the upper thigh or scrotum after inguinal varicocele repair. This complication is secondary to trauma to the ilioinguinal nerve and almost always resolves spontaneously, although it may take many months. Entrapment of a nerve may cause debilitating pain that requires reexploration of the inguinal canal and neurolysis.

Injury or ligation of the vas deferens is fortunately a rare complication. It may be difficult to identify the vas deferens in patients with large varicoceles because a large clotted varix may be indistinguishable from the vas by palpation alone. Immediate microsurgical vasovasostomy must be performed if the injury is recognized.

HYDROCELECTOMY

Hydroceles are serous fluid collections in the space between the visceral and parietal layers of the tunica vaginalis. Hydroceles in the adult population are most often noncommunicating, localized around the testis or confined to the spermatic cord. They occasionally may be septated. These lesions can be idiopathic or the result of trauma, infection, malignancy, or inflammatory disease. Iatrogenic hydroceles may result from varicocele or hernia repair, and the incidence depends on the technique used for varicocele repair.

Patients with a hydrocele typically present with an enlarging scrotum and may complain of pain, a dull heaviness, or discomfort with exercise. Treatments include simple drainage or drainage with sclerotherapy but surgical repair is considered definitive therapy.

In the pediatric population, hydroceles commonly communicate with the peritoneum, a result of failure of the tunica vaginalis to obliterate after testicular descent. Pediatric hydroceles are by definition associated with a congenital indirect inguinal hernia and should be corrected surgically. Children may present with pain or more commonly an enlarged scrotum. Abdominoperineal hydroceles are a rare variant in which an enlarging abdominal component exerts a mass effect on adjacent structures.

Evaluation of a hydrocele includes obtaining a medical and surgical history, physical examination, and scrotal ultrasound. Transillumination may help distinguish a hydrocele from a solid mass. Most hydroceles are the result of benign processes but they can also form secondary to malignant disease. Any testicle that is not completely palpable or irregular in shape warrants ultrasound examination.

Patients should be informed preoperatively that postoperative scrotal edema is common and may take several

TABLE 54-1	Varicocelectomy Recurrence and Complication Rates		
Technique	**Hydrocele (%)**	**Atrophy (%)**	**Recurrence (%)**
Retroperitoneal			
Mass ligation	6-7	<1	2
Artery sparing	<6	<1	11
Open inguinal	3-7.3	<1	6-15
Microscopic inguinal or subinguinal	<2	<1	<2

months to resolve and for the scrotum to return to normal size. It is common for the testicle to feel firm on palpation after hydrocele repair because a layer of scar forms among the dartos, the tunica albuginea, and the imbricated tunica vaginalis.

When results of ultrasonographic examination of the testis are normal, a transscrotal approach to hydrocele repair is most often employed. The incision can be made in either a transverse or a vertical fashion. The hydrocele sac is carefully dissected from under the dartos layer and is delivered intact into the surgical field. The hydrocele sac is opened longitudinally directly over the anterior surface of the testicle and the fluid is drained. Great effort must be made to identify all cord structures, specifically the vas, spermatic vessels, and epididymis. Tunica vaginalis is often thickened or chronically inflamed, thus making visualization of important structures difficult.

The three different surgical methods of hydrocele repair are the Lord procedure, the bottleneck procedure, and a window operation (Box 54-3). The Lord procedure may be used for smaller hydroceles with a thin tunical layer. The hydrocele sac is opened anteriorly using electrocautery and the peritoneal edge of the tunica is plicated using interrupted absorbable suture.[32] For large hydroceles, a bottleneck procedure, as described by Jaboulay, is performed by excising excess tunica vaginalis and then inverting the edges and sewing them closed posterior to the spermatic cord and epididymis.[33] It is critical to leave enough tunica vaginalis to avoid constriction of the spermatic cord. It is also critical to ensure that the epididymis or vas is not incidentally incorporated into the suture line. Imbrication of the tunica above the caput of the epididymis is not necessary. Window operations may adequately treat smaller hydroceles. During this procedure a window of tissue from the tunica vaginalis is excised and the edges are oversewn.[34]

Drain placement should be considered for larger hydroceles or when the surgical field is less than per-

fectly hemostatic. The wound is closed in layers with absorbable suture and the skin is approximated using an interrupted or subcuticular closure. Care must be taken to avoid entrapping the drain in the closure. Either a scrotal supporter with fluffed gauze or a compression dressing should be applied to help reduce postoperative edema.

Hydrocele aspiration combined with sclerotherapy is an alternative to surgery; however, multiple procedures may be required.[35,36] Complete resolution of the hydrocele is rare, although partial reduction in size can be accomplished.[35] This approach may be considered for patients who are poor surgical candidates. The procedure is accomplished by using a 19-gauge needle to aspirate the hydrocele fluid and then inject the sclerosant. Various sclerosant agents have been employed for this purpose. Theoretically, aspiration attempts may introduce bacteria into the hydrocele sac and may thus contaminate the hydrocele fluid and lead to a more serious problem.

Specific Complications and Their Treatment

Hematoma, the most common complication of hydrocelectomy, occurs in 5% to 20% of cases.[35,37] Higher rates of hematoma have been noted with excisional techniques than with techniques that employ oversewing of the tunical edges. A Penrose drain helps to prevent collection of excess serous fluid and blood around the testicle. A scrotal supporter and ice pack also help to reduce the postoperative edema that occurs in most cases. Wound infection or infected hematoma occurs in approximately 5% to 11% of patients undergoing hydrocele procedures.[35,37,38] Meticulous hemostasis, secure closure, proper sterile technique, and perioperative antibiotics may help to reduce rates of infection. Infection in the scrotal space necessitates antibiotic therapy and surgical drainage.

Epididymal or vasal injury has been reported in 5.6% of hydrocelectomies based on evaluation of pathologic specimens for epididymal or vasal tissue. Use of electrocautery should be minimized around the epididymis and vas to prevent thermal injury to those structures.[39] Patients should be made aware of any such injury because it may affect their future fertility status. No specific treatment is usually necessary if the contralateral testicle and excurrent duct system is intact.

Hydrocele recurrence after successful open repair ranges from 0% to 2%, regardless of operative technique.[37,40] Cure rates of 85% to 96% have been reported using sclerotherapy, although multiple procedures may be required to achieve successful resolution.[35-37,41] Complications of sclerotherapy are rare; however, hematoma or edema has been reported in ≤8% of patients receiving sclerotherapy. Infection is the major potential risk.[35] Scarring induced by sclerosant agents may cause secondary epididymal obstruction and azoospermia.

SIMPLE AND RADICAL ORCHIECTOMY

Bilateral orchiectomy can be performed through a scrotal incision as an outpatient procedure or in an office setting with a high spermatic cord block (Box 54-4). Less commonly, unilateral simple orchiectomy is performed to remove a nonviable testis found on exploration for testicular torsion or chronic infection or as a last-line treatment for intractable and debilitating chronic orchalgia. The cause and pathophysiologic features of testicular pain vary among patients, and chances for successful relief of chronic orchalgia following orchiectomy are cause specific.[42,43] Urologists should exercise caution when they contemplate performing orchiectomy for pain relief and should that ensure the patient's expectations are realistic.

Discovery of a solid testicular mass necessitates performance of radical inguinal orchiectomy. A testis suspected of containing cancer should never be approached through a scrotal incision, to avoid violating tissue planes and potentially contaminating the inguinal lymphatic system. Inguinal lymphatic channels drain the scrotal wall, whereas the testicle is drained by the retroperitoneal lymphatic system. Appropriate tumor markers are obtained before radical orchiectomy for patients suspected of having cancer. Sperm banking should be considered in subfertile patients, in patients who may require future chemotherapy, or in those undergoing bilateral orchiectomy.

Simple orchiectomy may be performed using local anesthesia with a spermatic cord block with or without concomitant placement of a testicular prosthesis. Preserving the epididymis or performing a subcapsular orchiectomy can alleviate the feeling of an empty scrotum, which can be disturbing to many men. Patients may prefer one of these approaches for psychological benefit, and these options should be discussed before orchiectomy. A vertical median raphe incision or bilateral transverse scrotal incisions are made. The testis is delivered within the tunica vaginalis. The spermatic cord is separated into three segments: the external spermatic vessels and cremasteric muscles, the internal spermatic vessels, and the vas deferens and vasal vessels. Each bundle is doubly clamped, transected, and then ligated. It is prudent to suture-ligate each bundle to ensure hemostasis. Massive bleeding can ensue if a ligature slips off a retracted spermatic vessel. Intracapsular

---

BOX 54-4 **Surgical Pearls: Orchiectomy**

1. Approach all suspected tumors through an inguinal incision.
2. Doubly ligate and suture-ligate the bundles of the spermatic cord with nonabsorbable suture, and suture-ligate the vas separately.
3. Achieve meticulous hemostasis in the scrotum.

---

orchiectomy is performed by incising the length of the tunica albuginea, sweeping all testicular contents off the capsule, ligating the hilum of the testis, and then closing the tunica albuginea. The epididymis is also spared to provide scrotal bulk.

Radical orchiectomy is approached through an inguinal incision. The external inguinal ring is identified and the external oblique fascia is incised. The ilioinguinal nerve is identified and preserved. This technique is necessary to prevent loss of sensation to a portion of the scrotal skin and upper medial thigh. The nerve is often adherent to the underside of the fascia of the external oblique and can be gently teased off the spermatic cord and isolated. The spermatic cord is dissected off the floor of the inguinal canal and then is surrounded by a Penrose drain. The spermatic cord is mobilized up to the internal inguinal ring. The testis is drawn upward, the plane between the dartos and tunica vaginalis is bluntly dissected, and the testis is released from the scrotum by ligating and dividing the gubernaculum.

Next, the spermatic cord is divided into three bundles, and each is doubly clamped and suture-ligated with 2-0 silk suture to aid in later identification should retroperitoneal lymph node dissection be indicated. Because the spermatic cord may retract into the retroperitoneum after it is divided, sutures should not be cut until adequate hemostasis is ensured. The testicle and spermatic cord are removed from the field intact. Some surgeons incise the testicle on the back table in an attempt to determine tumor type by gross appearance.

Essential to any cancer operation is prevention of tumor spillage. During radical orchiectomy, sterile towels are replaced around the surgical field after the testicle has been removed and dirty instruments are discarded. The scrotum is inverted and all bleeding points are cauterized. The wound is copiously irrigated and closed in layers and dressed. It is important to make sure that the nerve is not entrapped in the suture line when the external oblique fascia is reapproximated.

Specific Complications and Their Treatment

Scrotal or inguinal hematoma or infection may occur following this procedure in a small number of cases. Retroperitoneal hemorrhage is a rare but potentially lethal complication resulting from inadequate ligation of the spermatic cord. Evidence of an expanding hematoma or a significant drop in hematocrit requires surgical exploration. The inguinal incision is opened to identify the bleeding vessel; however, extension of the incision into the retroperitoneum may be necessary if the stump of the spermatic cord has retracted cephalad through the internal inguinal ring.

When a cancerous lesion was inadvertently approached through a transscrotal incision, additional excision of the scrotal scar or postoperative radiation has been recommended. Increases in local recurrence rates of testis cancer have been reported to be <3% and prognosis does not appear to be adversely affected.[44]

Androgen depletion following bilateral orchiectomy has numerous sequelae including hot flushes, decreased libido, erectile dysfunction, and development of gynecomastia. Metabolic changes including changes in body composition, osteoporosis, anemia, fatigue, and changes in mood and cognition may also occur.[45,46] Hot flushes occur in a majority of patients and can be reduced by 85% with the use of megestrol acetate.[47] Erectile dysfunction is treated by the use of oral phosphodiesterase-5 inhibitors, intracavernosal injections, a vacuum erectile device, or a penile prosthesis. Management of complications of antiandrogen therapy for prostate cancer is covered in Chapter 9.

VASECTOMY REVERSAL

Vasectomy is performed on >500,000 men in the United States annually,[1] and ≤6% of men later change their minds and undergo vasectomy reversal.[48] This change is most commonly the result of remarriage or loss of a child, but on occasion a patient desires vasectomy reversal for personal or religious reasons. Vasectomy reversal is also indicated to treat postvasectomy pain syndrome. In vitro fertilization with intracytoplasmic sperm injection (IVF/ICSI) has increasingly been used to treat couples with postvasectomy infertility despite the greater cost effectiveness of vasectomy reversal and the risks to the female partner inherent in IVF.[49-51]

Preoperative evaluation must include a history of prior paternity, complications from the vasectomy, and prior inguinal surgical procedures. Hernia repair in infancy or adulthood may have caused unrecognized distal vasal injury. Physical examination is performed with attention to testicular size, consistency of the epididymis, and the location of the scarred portion of the vas. A short testicular remnant of the vas or removal of a large segment of the vas may complicate standard vasectomy reversal. Epididymal or vasal induration may indicate an epididymal obstruction.

The female partner should be encouraged to undergo a full gynecologic evaluation to assess her fertility status before vasectomy reversal is performed on her partner. Other means of conception and parenthood should also be discussed during the initial evaluation, including IVF/ICSI, donor sperm insemination, and adoption. Increased age of the female partner and prolonged obstructed interval after vasectomy negatively affect the success of vasectomy reversal.[52,53] However, published success rates of assisted reproductive techniques also indicate declining success with advanced female age. Vasectomy reversal provides rates of subsequent pregnancy and delivery that are at least as high as rates of IVF/ICSI after a prolonged obstructive interval and with advanced maternal age.[53,54]

Patients should be made aware of the need for vaso-epididymostomy in the presence of epididymal obstruction. Secondary epididymal obstruction is associated with increased length of time from vasectomy. In a study by Fuchs and Burt,[53] 62% of men undergoing vasectomy reversal >15 years after vasectomy required unilateral or bilateral vasoepididymostomy. Patients should be given the option of sperm retrieval and cryopreservation in the event that vasectomy reversal is unsuccessful; however, this is not necessary in most cases, given patency rates upward of 80%.[52] Cryopreservation is encouraged in men requiring bilateral vasoepididymostomy.

The vas deferens has an intraluminal diameter of roughly 0.33 mm. Surgical reconstruction of structures this minute is best done with the aid of an operating microscope, microsurgical instrumentation, and microsurgical suture material. A surgeon should have a high degree of proficiency in performing these types of procedures after completing the appropriate microsurgical training and should be able to perform both vasovasostomy and vasoepididymostomy if necessary. The successful outcome of a vasectomy reversal is highly dependent on the skill and technique of the operating surgeon and a couple's chances for conception rest on this surgical expertise (Box 54-5).

During vasectomy reversal, each vas deferens is approached through a small vertical incision made over the scarred portion of the vas. Usually, the surgeon does not need to enter the tunica vaginalis or deliver the testis during routine vasovasostomy. The vasectomy site is identified and isolated, and the scar is transected from the healthy vas tissue with the aid of a nerve cutting guide. This technique ensures a straight cut. Fluid from

---

BOX 54-5 **Surgical Pearls: Vasectomy Reversal**

1. The patient's female partner should undergo gynecologic evaluation to assess fertility status before vasectomy reversal is performed.
2. Discuss alternatives with the patient such as sperm harvesting and in vitro fertilization.
3. Biopsy before vasectomy reversal to assess spermatogenesis is hardly ever indicated.
4. Examine the vasal fluid for the presence of sperm intraoperatively.
5. Perform a vasoepididymostomy when indicated.
6. Use the operating microscope and microsurgical technique for best results.
7. The vas should be cut back until healthy tissue with adequate blood supply is encountered.
8. Do not dilate the vas lumen because this may lead to stricture formation.
9. The anastomosis should be watertight and tension free.
10. Evaluate postoperative semen analyses periodically to identify early scarring of the anastomosis.

TABLE 54-2 Reoperative Vasectomy Reversals					
Reference	No. Procedures	No. Patients (%)	No. Pregnancies (%)	Mean Follow-up (mo)	No. Patients With ≥1 Vasoepididymostomy (%)
Belker et al[52] (1991)	199	150 (75)	52 (43)	NA	65 (33)
Matthews et al[55] (1995)	64	43 (67)	17 (27)	22	36 (56)
Donovan et al[57] (1998)	18	14 (78)	8 (44)	NA	10 (56)
Hernandez and Sabanegh[58] (1999)	41	NA (79)	NA (31)	8	30 (73)
Fox[59] (2000)	22	16 (57)	9 (32)	23	0
Paick et al[60] (2003)	62	57 (92)	24 (57)	52	4 (6.5)

NA, not applicable.

the testicular end of the vas is examined grossly and under a microscope. Vasovasostomy is performed in the presence of clear, watery fluid with or without sperm parts. Thick, pasty fluid that is devoid of sperm indicates epididymal obstruction and necessitates the performance of vasoepididymostomy. The lumen of the abdominal vas is cannulated with a 24-gauge angiocatheter and is irrigated with 5 mL of saline solution to confirm patency. No need exists to skeletonize the vas or to perform extensive dissection because this may compromise blood supply and lead to stricture formation. The lumen of the vas should not be dilated with anything other than a soft angiocatheter, to avoid injuring the delicate mucosa.

A microsurgical two-layer anastomosis using 10-0 nylon suture to reapproximate the mucosa and 9-0 nylon to close the muscularis is the preferred technique for vasovasostomy. This technique appears to allow for the most precise and watertight closure. Good patency rates can be expected from a modified single-layer anastomosis.[52]

When an epididymal obstruction is encountered, vasoepididymostomy must be performed. The abdominal end of the vas is mobilized while preserving its blood supply and this is brought down through the tunica vaginalis. The epididymis is examined under the operating microscope, and an area of dilated tubules is selected for the anastomosis, which is performed using an end-to-side or intussusception technique. Postoperatively, the patient is given a scrotal supporter and ice packs for 24 hours. He is instructed to avoid heavy physical activity and sexual activity for 3 to 4 weeks. Semen analysis is performed at 6 weeks and every 2 to 3 months thereafter until pregnancy occurs or semen parameters normalize.

Specific Complications and Their Treatment

Complications of vasectomy reversal are infrequent. When the procedure is performed by an experienced surgeon, scrotal hematoma, infection, and testicular atrophy are all rarely seen. Perioperative cephalosporins may reduce the chances of infection. Given the length of these operations, the use of sequential compressive devices is recommended to prevent deep vein thrombosis.

With careful preparation and proper microsurgical technique, patency and pregnancy rates of 86% to 98% and >50%, respectively, can be achieved.[52,55] The delayed appearance of sperm may occur ≤15 months after reversal.[56] Late treatment failures, characterized by azoospermia following initial appearance of sperm in the ejaculate postoperatively, can occur in ≤10% of cases.[55] Use of methylprednisolone dose packs can decrease scarring and inflammation at the anastomotic site and may aid in the reappearance of sperm in the ejaculate. Patients must be informed of the small chance of aseptic necrosis of the femoral head, an inherent complication of steroid use.

Repeat vasectomy reversal for failed initial reversal is efficacious and cost effective when compared with IVF/ICSI (Table 54-2).[52,55,57-60] The operative principles are similar to those for the initial vasectomy reversal. The obstructed segment of the vas is isolated and excised after determination of distal vasal patency. In the case of proximal epididymal obstruction, vasoepididymostomy is performed. The vasal fluid is evaluated for consistency and the presence of sperm intraoperatively. In the absence of obvious epididymal obstruction, some investigators recommend vasovasostomy regardless of the detection of sperm in the intravasal fluid.[60]

SPERM HARVESTING PROCEDURES

Major advances in the field of reproductive medicine have revolutionized the treatment of the azoospermic patient. With the advent of advanced reproductive technologies such as IVF/ICSI, most men can achieve genetic paternity. Even patients with extremely atrophic testes and follicle-stimulating hormone (FSH) levels >50 mg/dL may have some degree of spermatogenesis. Several procedures have been developed to procure sperm from men with azoospermia. These techniques can be performed percutaneously or as open minor procedures with or without optical magnification. Open microsurgical procedures are associated with higher costs, but more importantly they provide increased chances of finding sperm in the nonobstructed patient and higher yields of sperm from the obstructed patient. Those patients with obstruction have normal spermatogenesis and should have viable sperm present in either the epididymis or the testis. Patients with nonobstructive azoospermia have no sperm in the epididymis.

Therapeutic testis biopsy or testicular sperm extraction (TESE) is appropriate for patients with nonobstructive or obstructive azoospermia. TESE with microdissection improves the sperm yield from the nonobstructed testis and enables sperm localization in men in whom standard TESE approaches are unsuccessful.[61] Microepididymal sperm aspiration (MESA) is reserved for patients with vasal or epididymal obstruction who desire cryopreservation of sperm. Percutaneous techniques for sperm retrieval include percutaneous epididymal sperm aspiration (PESA) and testicular sperm aspiration (TESA). Although it is quick and cost efficient, PESA confers potential risks of unrecognized vascular injury and may fail to obtain live sperm. PESA is indicated for patients with obstructive azoospermia after vasectomy who do not desire future reversal or in patients with congenital bilateral absence of the vas deferens. TESA is indicated in patients with obstructive or nonobstructive azoospermia, anejaculation, and necrospermia. It can be used for diagnostic purposes to determine the likelihood of sperm retrieval for in vitro fertilization (IVF/ICSI) or to obtain sperm on the day of oocyte retrieval for couples undergoing an IVF cycle.[62,63] In addition, fine needle aspiration of the testis may correlate with testis histopathologic findings from open biopsy.[64,65]

Diagnostic testicular biopsy performed without the ability to offer sperm cryopreservation no longer has a role because it unnecessarily subjects the patient to a repeat procedure and its inherent risks. No guarantee exists that sperm will be found on a repeat procedure for patients with very low levels of spermatogenesis.

The choice of sperm harvesting technique should be determined based on achieving optimal results for the patient in the context of his condition as opposed to the surgeon's ability (Box 54-6). The couple's chances of having a genetic child depend in large part on the ability of the surgeon and the IVF laboratory.

Patients with azoospermia need a full preoperative evaluation by a urologist who has expertise in male reproductive medicine and experience in working with reproductive endocrinologists and IVF clinics. Based on history, physical examination of the scrotal contents, and hormonal profile, it is usually fairly easy to ascertain whether a patient has nonobstructive azoospermia

---

BOX 54-6 **Surgical Pearls: Sperm Harvesting**

1. It is crucial to ascertain whether the patient has obstructive or nonobstructive azoospermia; a normal follicle-stimulating hormone level does not mean normal spermatogenesis.
2. Patients need to have appropriate preoperative evaluation, including genetic testing when indicated, before an in vitro cycle is started.
3. Patients need to be given the opportunity to cryopreserve viable sperm.
4. Patients with nonobstructive azoospermia should be informed of the chances of not finding sperm in their testes and should be counseled about the use of donor sperm.
5. Patients with nonobstructive azoospermia need to wait ≥4 to 6 months between sperm retrieval procedures to allow the testis time to recover.
6. Needle biopsy procedures can result in testicular atrophy and hematoma formation.
7. Avoid removal of large samples of testicular tissue, especially from the lower pole area, because this may compromise the main blood supply to the testicle.

---

or an obstruction. What cannot be ascertained preoperatively is the degree of spermatogenesis in a given patient with nonobstructive azoospermia. The only absolute predictor is the finding at testicular biopsy. The patient's pathologic features and the desire to use fresh sperm for ICSI as opposed to obtaining sperm for cryopreservation and future use should dictate the type of sperm harvesting technique used. Patients undergoing PESA should be aware that insufficient numbers of sperm may be obtained for cryopreservation, and an additional procedure may be necessary. It is important to inform patients with nonobstructive azoospermia of the chances of not finding sperm during a retrieval procedure, and the couple should be given the opportunity to have donor sperm available as a backup plan.

Conventional TESE may be performed using local or general anesthesia. After infiltration of the scrotal skin with 1% lidocaine, a 1- to 2-cm incision is made. The tunica vaginalis is entered using electrocautery. An incision is made in the tunica albuginea horizontally to avoid any blood vessels. Extruded seminiferous tubules are excised with iris scissors. Three to six small tissue samples may be taken. The tunica albuginea is closed with 5-0 polyglactin 910 (Vicryl) suture. In microdissection TESE, the tunica albuginea is opened widely near the midportion of the testis, and a search is made for seminiferous tubules with relatively normal-appearing height among scarred or collapsed tubules. These tubules can be identified only using an operating microscope and are excised and opened in the operating room or IVF laboratory to search for sperm.[61]

During MESA, the epididymis is exposed under the operating microscope. A dilated segment of the epididymal tubule is identified and incised. Epididymal fluid is collected with a 24-gauge angiocatheter connected to a syringe containing culture media. Closure of the epididymal tubule may be performed with 9-0 nylon suture, or alternatively the tubule may be cauterized. TESA, as described by Belker and colleagues,[62] is performed by inserting into the testis a 20-gauge needle attached to a 20-mL syringe. Negative pressure is maintained on the plunger and the needle is moved slowly back and forth within the testicle to obtain tissue for a specimen.[62] Aspiration of more than one site is recommended because of wide deviations in quantitative measurements in different areas of the testis.[66] PESA is performed by inserting a 23-gauge butterfly needle into the dilated caput epididymis and aspirating the fluid as the needle is moved back and forth. To facilitate proper placement, the epididymis is held between the thumb and forefinger as the scrotal skin is overstretched.

Specific Complications and Their Treatment

Clinically significant complication rates for each sperm retrieval methods described are exceedingly low. Scrotal hematoma and infection occur in <3% of cases.[67-69] Testicular atrophy is a rare complication. Transient scrotal ecchymosis is quite common.[68] Of 46 men undergoing conventional TESE, 1 patient had a hematocele and wound infection versus no clinical complications in 100 patients undergoing microdissection TESE.[69]

Significantly greater numbers of men have subcapsular hematomas detected ultrasonographically after sperm retrieval procedures; however, most hematomas regress by 6 months.[69-71] In one study, 51% of men undergoing TESE developed diffuse heterogeneity or a hypoechoic area suggesting hematoma compared with 12% of men undergoing microdissection TESE. Only 7.5% and 2.5%, respectively, of hematomas persisted for 6 months postoperatively.[69] Reported rates of testicular hematoma are 6% to 7% in patients undergoing TESA.[70,71] Postoperative use of ice packs and a scrotal supporter for 48 hours may decrease hematoma formation, and strenuous activity should be limited for 1 to 2 weeks.

SPERMATOCELECTOMY AND EPIDIDYMECTOMY

Spermatoceles are benign, cystic outpouchings of the epididymal tubules. They most commonly occur in the caput of the epididymis and contain sperm. Up to 30% of men undergoing scrotal ultrasonography will have a spermatocele discovered, and this lesion is age dependent. Although spermatoceles may grow to uncomfortably large sizes, they usually do not cause epididymal obstruction. Surgical intervention is reserved for painful or very large spermatoceles. Spermatocelectomy should be avoided in men desiring children because of the risk of iatrogenic epididymal obstruction.

Indications for epididymectomy include recalcitrant chronic infection or abscess of the epididymis, multifocal or large spermatoceles in patients not desiring fertility, paraepididymal masses, and postvasectomy epididymal pain. Persistent epididymitis may develop from typical urinary pathogens or as a result of schistosomal, tuberculous, and cytomegalovirus infections.[72] Chronic epididymalgia after vasectomy may be improved by epididymectomy, although success rates vary from 50% to 95%.[14,73-75] Our experience has been to the contrary; epididymectomy has hardly ever provided relief in these circumstances. Microsurgical vasectomy reversal should be attempted to relieve epididymal obstruction before epididymectomy is contemplated. Patients should be informed that fertility may be impaired by epididymectomy. In addition, chronic pain syndromes may not improve in ≤50% of cases.[76] Once epididymectomy has failed, the patient has few options short of spermatic cord denervation or orchiectomy.

In patients with chronic epididymal pain, a thorough evaluation should be performed to identify the cause, which may include infection, trauma, chronic pain syndromes, psychiatric disorders, or the result of prior surgical procedures (Box 54-7). A scrotal ultrasound scan is obtained. Structural epididymal abnormalities noted on ultrasound examination are favorable prognostic factors for performing epididymectomy in comparison with inflammatory causes.[76] Adequate counseling should be given regarding expected improvement or resolution of pain and discussions should be well documented in the patient's record. In our experience, epididymectomy is infrequently successful in resolving chronic pain completely. Men desiring future paternity should be cautioned against spermatocelectomy and should be offered sperm cryopreservation.

A median raphe or longitudinal hemiscrotal incision may be made. The tunica vaginalis is opened and the spermatocele is then dissected free of the epididymal tubules. Operative loupes or an operating microscope may aid the dissection of the spermatocele and may prevent injury to the epididymal tubules. The spermatocele stalk is then divided and ligated or cauterized.

BOX 54-7 Surgical Pearls: Spermatocelectomy and Epididymectomy

1. Optical magnification enables fine dissection of the spermatocele sac off the epididymis.
2. Bipolar electrocautery should be used sparingly to minimize the risk of injury to the epididymis.
3. Care is necessary when dissecting the tail of the epididymis to avoid compromising the testicular blood supply.
4. Appropriate patient selection is critical.

Total epididymectomy requires mobilization of the vas deferens and ligation at the junction of the convoluted and straight segments. The efferent tubules are dissected, ligated, and divided. Care must be taken during these maneuvers to avoid the spermatic cord vessels entering the testicle medial to the epididymis. The base of the resected epididymis is closed using interrupted 4-0 chromic sutures.

The blood supply to the epididymis is through the testicular and vasal branches. Therefore, ligation of either but not both vessels may be acceptable. Spermatic vessels enter the mediastinum testis medial to the epididymis in the upper third of the testis.

Specific Complications and Their Treatment

Complications of epididymectomy and spermatocelectomy are infrequent. Infection may be seen in ≤10% of cases.[38] More serious complications include testicular atrophy resulting from vascular injury, chronic pain, recurrence of the spermatocele, and vasal or epididymal obstruction. In a study by Zahalsky and associates,[39] a portion of epididymis was identified in 17% of spermatocele specimens, a finding suggesting epididymal injury.[39] Although some studies have reported subjective pain relief in 90% of patients after spermatocelectomy[38,77] and epididymectomy,[75] many others have found poor results, a finding that likely reflects patient selection and methodologic differences.[74,76,78] High rates of persistent pain or dissatisfaction with surgery are reported. Worse outcomes have been noted in patients with poorly localized pain[75] and chronic epididymitis[74,76] compared with patients with localized pain after vasectomy or patients with complex cystic disease. Persistent postoperative pain may be addressed with pain management consultation, microscopic denervation of the spermatic cord, or orchiectomy.

KEY POINTS

1. Detailed discussion and documentation of the risks, benefits, and alternatives of each procedure are necessary to ensure realistic patient expectations of improvement and outcome.
2. Meticulous hemostasis is necessary to prevent scrotal hematomas, which may be unsightly and uncomfortable.
3. All patients undergoing vasectomy should be offered sperm cryopreservation.
4. Epididymectomy and conversion to open-ended vasectomy are generally unsuccessful in relieving the postvasectomy pain syndrome refractory to conservative measures; instead, pain may be relieved by vasectomy reversal or excision of sperm granuloma.
5. Particular attention to preservation of vasal and testicular collateral arterial flow is necessary in repeat inguinoscrotal procedures to prevent testicular atrophy.
6. Preoperative testicular ultrasound examination should be performed in all patients with hydroceles to rule out a mass lesion if the testicle not palpable.
7. Transscrotal excision of testicular mass lesions suspicious for cancer should be avoided.
8. Use of an operating microscope and a Doppler microprobe decreases the rates of recurrence and complications in patients undergoing varicocelectomy.
9. All surgeons performing microsurgical vasovasostomy should be proficient at vasoepididymostomy.
10. Testicular biopsy before vasectomy reversal to assess sperm production is hardly ever indicated unless the patient has testicular atrophy or an elevated FSH.

REFERENCES

Please see www.expertconsult.com

COMPLICATIONS OF PEDIATRIC UROLOGIC SURGERY

Chapter 55

SPECIAL CONSIDERATIONS IN THE PEDIATRIC PATIENT

Jennifer S. Singer MD
Assistant Professor, Pediatric Urology and Renal Transplantation, Department of Urology, David Geffen School of Medicine, University of California–Los Angeles, Los Angeles, California

Andrew L. Freedman MD
Director, Pediatric Urology, Minimally Invasive Urology Institute, Cedars-Sinai Medical Center, Los Angeles, California

Since the mid-20th century, dramatic improvements have been made in the care of the pediatric surgical patient. The evolution of pediatric anesthesia subspecialists and of sophisticated monitoring devices has enabled the safe conduct of even complex pediatric operations. Ambulatory care and dedicated pediatric hospitals provide pediatric patients with more comforting environments and resultant decreases in perioperative anxiety. Surgical subspecialization allows pediatric patients to receive their care in the hands of dedicated pediatric surgeons and pediatric urologists and further maximizes the quality of care received.

Despite this progress, families experience inordinate distress when a child has to undergo a surgical procedure. Surgical risk is an ever-present concern. A child is not simply a smaller version of an adult; care pathways are not interchangeable. To that end, in this chapter, we attempt to address the perioperative care of patients undergoing pediatric urologic surgical procedures. Beyond a general overview, we also specifically address complications of penoscrotal surgery exclusive of hypospadias, as well as complications of pediatric pyeloplasty. The goal of this chapter is to outline optimal care considerations that minimize the risk of perioperative complications.

PREOPERATIVE PREPARATION

Psychosocial Preparation

Possibly the most demanding component of preoperative surgical preparation for children is the need to address the anxiety of both the patient and the parent or parents. The behavior of children undergoing surgical procedures directly reflects the stress and anxiety of the parents.[1] Provider efforts to reduce parental concerns should acknowledge the sources of anxiety and the finding that parental fears are often disproportionate to the nature of the anticipated surgical procedure.

The time spent allaying these fears greatly facilitates the outcome. Introducing patients and their families to other members of the perioperative team, including anesthesia, nursing staff, and even residents involved in pediatric patient care, orients family members to the multidisciplinary nature of surgical care and may ease preoperative fears.

The level of psychological preparation required, although important for all children, depends greatly on the age and developmental state of the patient.[1] In young infants <6 months of age, this preparation hinges on addressing the emotional state of the parents. For children 6 months to 5 years of age, managing separation anxiety is paramount. Children in this age group are at the highest risk of developing profound anxiety; they comprehend the threat of separation but lack the abstract perspective to recognize its transience.[2] Many pediatric hospitals provide presurgical visits to introduce children in this age group to the surgical suite and to orient them to the procedures performed.

Preadolescents remain concerned about separation and are at the difficult age of knowing enough to fear the risks of surgery but not enough to prevent irrational fears of loss of bodily integrity. The addition of a child life specialist to the care team was shown to demonstrate significant reductions in anxiety for patients aged 5 to 11 years randomized to the intervention.[3]

Teenagers suffer adjustment problems and the difficult transition from child to adult. Surgical discussions should involve teenagers directly as though addressing adult patients. Beyond developmental stages, children at highest risk for preoperative extreme anxiety include those with inhibited temperaments and those with prior negative encounters with health care providers.[2,4]

Surgical education begins with the parent or parents. Allaying a parent's fears begins with a comprehensive understanding of the nature, risks, and benefits of the surgical procedure. Reduced anxiety among parents diminishes the patients' anxiety. Depending on the age of the patient, the physician should offer patients the opportunity to speak privately, away from their parents. Physicians often underestimate a child's capacity for comprehension. Discussions without the parents enable us to address concerns that the patient may feel but is embarrassed to discuss in front of the parents. Age-appropriate reading materials can ease the transition from the preoperative care unit to the surgical suite and can diminish the patient's concerns preoperatively and in the postoperative recovery period.[4] A simple measure such as a Band-Aid on a stuffed animal at the incision site may help younger children to process the surgical experience.

Children experience the highest level of stress at the moment of anesthetic induction. Parental presence at induction significantly reduces patient and parental stress. In fact, the effect of parental presence at induction has been shown to be stronger than that of preoperative administration of an anxiolytic.[5] The parental role is an important component of patient relaxation because the uninformed, critical, or excessively reassuring parent can exacerbate the child's anxiety.[2] Preanesthesia appointments that educate the family about the surgical environment and the parental role in the induction of anesthesia can prevent these adverse outcomes. An increased emphasis on family-centered care in medicine has helped facilitate parental presence at anesthetic induction, now prevalent at more than half of pediatric specialty hospitals.[6]

Other interventions proven effective include preoperative music therapy, minimizing of the number of individuals interacting with the patient, distraction therapy with video games, and deferring of venous access and other invasive procedures until the child is unconscious.[7,8] We encourage children to bring blankets or stuffed animals with them on the day of the operation. Having separate preoperative and postoperative care areas for children and allowing parents access to the recovery room further cater to the needs of the pediatric patient undergoing a surgical procedure. These efforts to ameliorate the patient's anxiety increase parental satisfaction with perioperative care and promote psychological and clinical convalescence.[2]

Medical Evaluation

Most patients undergoing elective pediatric operations are healthy and are undergoing minor procedures. Thus, preoperative medical evaluation serves to identify those patients with serious cardiopulmonary risk factors who require further evaluation.

The patient's primary pediatrician typically evaluates the patient the week before the surgical procedure. Abnormalities in the cardiovascular and pulmonary systems are of primary concern because these conditions are the most likely to lead to adverse anesthesia-related events. Most anomalies are known from the patient's history. Any preoperative examination should include auscultation for heart murmurs to rule out structural cardiac defects further. Children are particularly susceptible to respiratory infections, and the preoperative examination should further exclude the presence of an active infection.

In the setting of an active lower respiratory infection, the procedure must be postponed. For most elective operations in healthy children, an active upper respiratory infection (URI) should likewise prompt postponement. Lower respiratory tract dysfunction can persist for ≤1 month following an acute URI. Symptoms cannot be used to predict outcome because adverse events do not correlate with the symptoms of the URI.[9] Further, event risk is higher if the surgical procedure is performed ≤4 weeks of the onset of URI symptoms.[9] Complications vary from minor events such as transient hypoxemia to major events including airway obstruction, croup, laryngospasm, and bronchospasm. Anesthetic risks are greatest in infants, whose smaller reserve predisposes them to rapid desaturation.[10] Older children with a mild or resolving URI are probably suitable candidates for anesthesia.[11]

Laboratory Evaluation

Most children undergoing elective minor surgical procedures require no laboratory evaluation. However, we often check the hemoglobin in infants scheduled for elective minor procedures. Infants with anemia, common among those with a history of prematurity, have a higher relative risk of complications related to general anesthesia.[12] Oxygen delivery is most efficient at a hemoglobin level of 10 g/dL.[13] Lower levels increase the intraoperative risks of hypotension and cardiac arrest. Thus, although unnecessary for most older children, a simple hemoglobin measurement is critical to the preoperative evaluation of infants undergoing anything more than minor surgical procedures.

The complexity of the surgical procedure may mandate more involved laboratory analysis as part of the preoperative examination. Surgical procedures with significant risk of hemorrhage or extensive reconstruction mandate determinations of the blood count and electrolyte panels. Children undergoing major urinary tract reconstruction or with a history of urinary obstruction often have an underlying history of chronic kidney disease or renal insufficiency.

In addition to ensuring that values of critical electrolytes such as potassium are normal, attention to proper timing of dialysis in these children should facilitate normalization of the electrolyte panel before induction of general anesthesia. Because these children often receive heparin boluses with dialysis, efforts are needed to minimize heparin administration preoperatively. We check prothrombin and partial thromboplastin times for all dialysis-dependent patients preoperatively and on the morning of the operation. All children listed for renal transplantation at our institution are further assessed with extensive coagulation profiles because undiagnosed coagulopathies are prevalent in this population.

According to guidelines, preoperative urinalysis is not a mandatory component of the laboratory evaluation for patients undergoing urinary tract surgery.[14] However, many of these patients receive reconstructions directed at structural defects implicated in the pathogenesis of urinary tract infections (UTIs). For this reason, and because of the low cost and noninvasiveness of a urinalysis, we perform preoperative urinalysis and culture for all patients scheduled for urinary tract surgery. Although suprapubic aspirate remains the gold standard for urine collection, voided specimens are typically adequate. In infants and younger children, bagged specimens often suffice, although positive results may indicate contamination and must be followed with a catheterized specimen.

Important Medical Conditions

Prematurity increases the risk among infants of postoperative apnea, a potentially lethal complication. Risk factors include anemia and a prior history of apnea.[15] A systematic review attempted to formulate guidelines for former preterm infants undergoing elective surgical procedures, with inguinal herniorrhaphy used as the example.[15] These investigators failed to reach a consensus on a threshold postconceptional age that mandates closer monitoring for postoperative apnea. Infants with postconceptional age of <48 weeks have a ≥5% risk of postoperative apnea and should be monitored overnight. The risk of apnea decreases with increasing age. Similarly, a history of anemia or of apneic episodes in the recovery room, regardless of age, mandates monitoring. In children with a postconceptional age of >60 weeks without history of anemia or recovery room apneic episodes, the risk of postoperative apnea is low enough that monitoring is not necessary. The use of spinal versus general anesthesia does not reduce the risk of postoperative apnea, although desaturation and bradycardia episodes are less common with regional anesthesia.[16]

Asthma is highly prevalent in our pediatric population. Risk stratification divides asthmatic patients into those receiving no medications who have never been hospitalized, those receiving daily medications with occasional exacerbations, and those with frequent exacerbations and hospitalizations. The first category represents a low-risk cohort of patients undergoing surgical procedures. Conversely, the third category represents a population that mandates thorough preoperative evaluation to optimize the child medically as much as possible given the level of urgency of the surgical procedure.

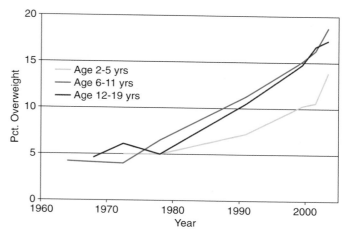

Figure 55-1 Trends in being overweight among U.S. children stratified by age group. *(From Ogden CL, Carroll MD, Curtin LR, McDowell MA, Tabak CJ, Flegal KM. Prevalence of overweight and obesity in the United States, 1999-2004. JAMA. 2006;295: 1549-1555.)*

Standard mask anesthesia, laryngeal mask airway, or regional anesthesia is preferred to endotracheal intubation in these patients. We ask these patients to continue all medications, including leukotriene inhibitors, the morning of the surgical procedure. Depending on the timing and dosage taken, patients may require perioperative steroid supplementation with stress doses at induction of anesthesia. Judicious use of β-agonist inhalers intraoperatively may be necessary, especially in patients requiring endotracheal intubation.

The obesity epidemic has affected the pediatric population as extensively as it has the adult (**Fig. 55-1**), with requisite implications for the delivery of surgical care. Severely obese patients carry a litany of comorbid conditions, among them cardiac disease, asthma and obstructive sleep apnea, fatty liver, endocrinopathies, and comorbid psychiatric illnesses, predominantly depression.[17] Preoperative evaluation should elucidate the nature of comorbid illnesses. Increasing the scope of the preoperative diagnostic evaluation is required compared with nonobese patients. Routine preoperative procedures such as venous access may be complicated, and larger doses of premedication can promote respiratory compromise.[18]

Intraoperative anesthesia monitoring is more difficult. Results of pulse oximetry, crucial in this population at risk for intraoperative desaturation, are less reliable given the extra tissue thickness. That same tissue thickness often compromises surgical positioning and exposure. Postoperatively, wound and pulmonary complication rates are higher in obese patients. The increased comorbidity, functional operative limitations, and higher risk of adverse postoperative events associated with obesity promise to be ongoing obstacles for pediatric urologists. Diligent perioperative care may minimize complications in this population.

Other conditions known to affect surgical care include sickle cell anemia, Down's syndrome, and congenital myopathies such as Duchenne's muscular dystrophy. Sickle cell anemia causes sludging of red blood cells and sickle cell crises during anesthesia. Transfusions to dilute the hemoglobin S fraction to <30% are recommended for patients undergoing major surgical procedures.[19] Children with Down's syndrome have a high incidence of atlantoaxial instability, which complicates head positioning and increases the risk of cervical subluxation or dislocation during intubation.[20] This defect is easily diagnosed with plain film radiographs. Duchenne's muscular dystrophy and associated myopathies confer an increased risk of malignant hyperthermia on administration of inhalational anesthetics. Integration of a medical specialist into the perioperative care of patients with these complicated medical conditions aids in their management.

Bowel Preparation

A complete and thorough bowel preparation is an integral component of the preoperative care of many pediatric urologic patients, especially in light of the increasing use of laparoscopy in these children. Inadequate bowel decompression may limit working space and exposure during laparoscopic surgery and may increase the risk of inadvertent injuries and enteric anastomotic complications, with often disastrous consequences. A survey of pediatric surgeons nationwide demonstrated significant variability in the practice of mechanical bowel preparation among children undergoing elective colorectal surgical procedures.[21]

Typically, laparoscopic procedures require a light mechanical bowel preparation with clear liquids for ≥24 hours preoperatively and a weight-adjusted dose of magnesium citrate (0.5 mL/kg, usually not >200 mL in total dose). More aggressive regimens, including GoLYTELY solution and possible oral antibiotics, are indicated for more involved procedures such as reconstruction with bowel or in patients with extensive surgical histories in whom aggressive adhesions are likely to be encountered. Caution must be exercised when preparing children with chronic kidney disease for bowel reconstruction. Magnesium citrate can cause hypermagnesemia with possible cardiovascular compromise and neurologic complications. Severe hyperphosphatemia and hypocalcemia can result from phosphosoda-based bowel regimens.[22] GoLYTELY was the first bowel regimen without contraindications in patients with renal failure; however, the ingested volume required to produce effective bowel cleansing can be a limitation in that population.

Specific populations requiring bowel cleansing in preparation for pediatric urologic surgery require special mention. For patients with chronic kidney disease who require mechanical bowel preparation preoperatively,

TABLE 55-1	Guidelines for the Recommended Preoperative Fasting Duration for Healthy Children Undergoing Elective Surgical Procedures
Diet	**Hours of Fast**
Clear liquids, chewing gum	2
Breast milk	3
Infant formula	4
Nonhuman milk	6
Light meals	6

From Warner MA, Warner ME, Warner DO, Warner LO, Warner EJ. Perioperative pulmonary aspiration in infants and children. *Anesthesiology.* 1999;90:66-71.

we often conduct the bowel regimen on an inpatient basis, which allows for electrolyte monitoring and ready hemodialysis. Patients with neurogenic bladders, many of whom require enterocystoplasty for low-capacity, high-pressure bladders, often have concomitant neuropathic bowel. Standard bowel regimens must be adjusted in these patients. We often prolong the period of clear liquid restriction to ≥2 days and begin the GoLYTELY 2 days before the surgical procedure to ensure adequacy of bowel preparation. Some patients require hospital admission and nasogastric tube placement for GoLYTELY administration, although one report cited reduced costs without compromising the quality of the bowel preparation using a home health nurse.[23]

Preoperative Fasting

Fasting is designed to minimize the risk of aspiration of gastric contents at anesthetic induction and postoperatively. In children, the requisite fasting time must balance the risk of aspiration with the risk of dehydration, especially in small infants. Most significant aspiration events occur in younger children undergoing urgent or emergency procedures for ileus or bowel obstruction.[24] Mild aspiration events rarely have significant clinical sequelae, important in our predominantly ambulatory patient population.[24] Conversely, dehydration complicates intraoperative venous access and alters hemodynamics on anesthetic induction. Table 55-1 presents current guidelines for the recommended fasting duration depending on the child's diet. Patients admitted preoperatively can be supplemented with intravenous (IV) fluids to prevent dehydration.

INTRAOPERATIVE CONSIDERATIONS

Latex Precautions

Latex allergy is both an occupational health concern and a patient safety concern. Ubiquitous both in society and in the hospital environment, latex can cause type I immediate anaphylactic-type reactions as well as type IV delayed-type hypersensitivity reactions in sensitized patients. Within the pediatric population, those at greatest risk are children with repeated contact with latex-based products. Among pediatric urology patients, those with myelomeningocele are at highest risk, with a prevalence of latex allergy as high as 28% to 67%.[25] These children undergo multiple surgical procedures and frequently manage bladder emptying with clean intermittent catheterization. Multiple urologic and orthopedic procedures and the need for a ventriculoperitoneal shunt confer a higher risk of latex sensitization, although these variables are likely proxies for repeated latex exposure.[26] Other at-risk populations in pediatric urologic practice include patients with prune-belly syndrome, posterior urethral valves, and other forms of neurogenic bladder.

Among health care workers, rates of latex allergy range from 2% to 17%.[25] Latex gloves are preferable to nonlatex gloves because of their elasticity, low cost, and impermeability to viruses.[27] Recurrent use of latex gloves increases the risk of sensitization. For surgeons, a type IV reaction can produce a debilitating dermatitis that prohibits the performance of surgical procedures until the dermatitis resolves. The risks have prompted many surgeons to use latex-free sterile gloves. The technology has improved such that the elasticity and comfort of latex-free gloves rival those of latex gloves.

As with most complications, prevention is critical. For the majority of elective pediatric urologic surgical procedures, latex precautions are unnecessary. For high-risk patients, however, maintenance of latex-free environments is crucial, even among children with no history of latex sensitization. Prophylactic therapy with antihistamines and steroids is not recommended. Although a simple skin test for latex allergy demonstrates good performance characteristics, negative screen results do not preclude a future reaction.[28] Up to 30% of patients with myelomeningocele manifest their initial latex reaction with anaphylaxis.[27] Many children's hospitals are entirely latex free and suitable alternatives are available for most products that are predominantly latex based.

Anesthesia

Beyond fears of disfigurement or surgical complications, the fear most often expressed by parents relates to the risk of anesthesia.[2] In this regard, the value of preoperative visits to the anesthesia provider and the surgical suite cannot be overemphasized. In most centers, the pediatric urology and pediatric surgery teams work closely with pediatric anesthesiologists to provide optimal care, and highlighting this specialty training can help alleviate parental concerns.

Modern anesthetics risks pale in comparison with the risks in earlier eras. The improvement in anesthetic care parallels improvements in neonatal care and the dissemination of neonatal intensive care units, which have facilitated the survival of premature infants at shorter and shorter gestations. Many of these infants require high-risk operations in the neonatal period that confound our understanding of anesthetic risk in the general pediatric population.

A single-institution series reported anesthetic outcomes over a 30-month period in a pediatric teaching hospital.[29] Major intraoperative complications related to anesthesia were more common among infants than among older patients. Respiratory and cardiac events occurred in infants at twice the rate seen in toddlers and older children. Other correlates of major complications included the need for endotracheal intubation, a surrogate for the complexity of the surgical procedure, operations involving the airway, and a higher American Society of Anesthesiologists (ASA) score (3-5 versus 1-2). Among older children, vomiting was the most common complication. Of 24,165 anesthetic regimens, only 8 cardiac arrests occurred, an event rate of 3.3 per 10,000 anesthetics delivered.

The Pediatric Perioperative Cardiac Arrest (POCA) Registry, formed in 1994, catalogues cardiac events in the perioperative period as a quality assurance and quality improvement initiative.[30] This registry received reports on 150 events corresponding to the delivery of anesthesia for an event rate of 1.4 per 10,000 anesthetics. Infants and patients with significant comorbidity were at highest risk. Among healthier patients, oversedation leading to respiratory depression was the most common cause of cardiopulmonary arrest, a finding corroborated in a an analysis of sentinel events.[31] Early detection of respiratory compromise averts adverse outcomes related to these events and highlights the progress made in the instrumentation used in pediatric anesthesia.

Among healthy children, anesthesia is incredibly safe. In the previously cited series, only 1 death occurred in 24,165 anesthetic regimen, and no deaths occurred among patients with an ASA score of 1 to 2.[29] Independent of ASA score, however, age <1 year remained strongly predictive of adverse events, and thus regardless of case complexity, surgical procedures in infants should involve a specialist anesthesia provider.

Hypothermia

Inadvertent hypothermia during anesthesia is associated with platelet dysfunction and coagulopathy, disordered drug metabolism, increased wound infection rates, and cardiac arrhythmias.[32] Pediatric patients, and especially infants, have more surface area over central zones where heat loss is highest, including the head and trunk. Thus, the risk of inadvertent hypothermia is highest among infants. Primary determinants of infant core body temperature are the operating room ambient temperature and the type of surgical procedure performed.[32] Major operations carried a higher risk of postoperative hypothermia, and neonates are more susceptible than infants. Intuitively, exposure of the viscera would increase the risk of hypothermia; however, an analysis of the core temperature of patients undergoing laparoscopic and open surgical procedures showed no difference, with length of the procedure the primary determinant of hypothermia.[33]

To prevent hypothermia, investigators have recommended that the room temperature should be maintained at 80°F for premature and small neonates, 78°F for infants <6 months of age, and 76°F for children ≤2 years of age.[34] As much of the child as possible should be covered, with special attention to the head and trunk, primary sources of heat loss. Air blankets, warming lamps, and warmed IV fluids further help to maintain core body temperature.

Complications of Circumcision

Complications occur in 0% to 2% to 3% of circumcisions.[35] Bleeding is the most common complication. Careful attention to bleeding vessels during the dissection minimizes this complication, and some investigators believe in using cutting current electrocautery for the skin incision to reduce skin edge bleeding.[36] Despite strict attention to bleeding vessels, delayed bleeding may occur. Probably, the culprit vessels were in vasospasm during the procedure. Delayed bleeding usually responds to direct manual pressure or the application of a hemostatic such as silver nitrate in the case of skin edge bleeding. Development of a large hematoma or persistent bleeding despite pressure mandates repeat exploration.

Other complications vary in severity, but they may be classified by the need for further reconstructive surgical procedures. Minor complications that require simple alterations in care or delay until full recovery include surgical site infections and suture granulomas or sinus tracts. Despite the nonhygienic surroundings of the penis, wound infections are relatively rare, likely a function of the excellent blood supply to the penile skin. Suture granulomas are similarly rare, especially in an era of high-quality monofilament absorbable sutures. Most of these granulomas may simply be observed; however, suture site granulomas and sinus tracts that persist may require excision. Although we do not routinely prescribe prophylactic antibiotics postoperatively, we do prescribe antibiotic ointment to be applied to the wound with diaper changes. We believe that this approach maintains wound hygiene and ensures that the parents retract the shaft skin proximal to the wound to prevent glandular adhesions.

Glanular adhesions exemplify a family of minor complications that on occasion require a second procedure or operation. Adhesions occur when the incision heals to the coronal rim of the glans penis. With age, the adhesions thicken and epithelialize. Small, thin adhesions that can be retracted manually in the clinic may not need further intervention. Some unretractable adhesions may be simply excised in clinic with a topical anesthetic such as EMLA (eutectic mixture of local anesthetics) cream. Thicker adhesions or more severe circumferential adhesions require an anesthetic and more formal reconstruction to attempt to recover a good cosmetic outcome.

Postoperative management must include application of a lubricating ointment as the incisions heal to prevent recurrence of the adhesions. Immediately following circumcision, the meatus often appears erythematous and inflamed. Meatal stenosis may occur when this acute meatitis becomes a chronic irritation. This stenosis often responds well to topical steroids, but in the setting of UTIs or a deflected urinary stream it may require secondary meatotomy. Urethrocutaneous fistula is a very rare complication that hardly ever occurs during non-neonatal circumcisions. Invariably the urethra sustained injury during the procedure, usually in the area of the frenulum. Repair is similar to that of fistulas that occur following hypospadias repair with excision of the fistulous tract and a two-layer closure with nonoverlapping suture lines.

Inappropriate excision of the shaft skin typically causes no functional sequelae but leaves the penis covered mostly with inner preputial skin. As children grow, they will have a normal-appearing penis, and reassurance is the best management. In severe cases, one may consider techniques to mobilize scrotal skin to the shaft, despite imperfect cosmetic results.

Following circumcision, development of a concealed or trapped penis results when the penis becomes buried in a large suprapubic fat pad and either is submerged in the fat pad or scars in place. Concealed penis usually occurs in boys with a large suprapubic fat pad, whereas trapped penis results from overzealous removal of shaft skin that produces an accordion-like effect that causes the penis to retract. The repair is similar regardless of the mechanism. Bands of tissue holding the penis in a retracted position must be removed, the penis must be fixed in an unretracted position, and suprapubic dermatolipectomy and penoscrotal tacking often improve the cosmetic result. This operation usually requires placement of an anchoring nonabsorbable or very slowly absorbable suture to fix the dorsum of the penis to the pubic fascia and the ventrum to the scrotal subcutaneous tissue. This technique recreates the penoscrotal angle and elevates the penis from the suprapubic fat pad. Finding skin coverage can be difficult, but preputial skin is usually available. More severe cases require reconstruction with liposuction of the fat pad and Z-plasty techniques to provide coverage. These techniques are reserved for only the most severe cases and most patients are effectively managed with penoscrotal tacking sutures.

Certain anatomic variants have been shown to confer a higher risk for reoperation following circumcision including a prominent suprapubic fat pad, penoscrotal webbing, and a history of prematurity.[37] Many of these risks represent relative contraindications to neonatal circumcision and should prompt referral to a specialist for a decision regarding the timing of the procedure. Often, deferring the procedure until the child is older obviates these outcomes.

Necrosis and amputation of the glans penis are devastating complications that, fortunately, represent a very small proportion of circumcision-related errors. Necrosis typically results from delayed ischemia related to the use of electrocautery. Other reports have implicated the use of a laser for the skin incision.[36] We prefer to obtain hemostasis during non-neonatal circumcision with bipolar electrocautery. Electrocautery should never be used with the Gomco clamp during neonatal circumcision. Inappropriately sized Plastibell clamps have also been implicated. The risk of necrosis emphasizes the need to avoid epinephrine when performing a penile block. Amputation is almost always attributable to neonatal circumcision with a Mogen clamp. When this occurs, the provider should be instructed to place the excised glans in saline-soaked gauze on ice. The hypervascular glans usually survives and the reattachment usually takes without the need for microvascular repair.

Complications of Inguinal Surgery

Orchiopexy

The complications of orchiopexy must be subdivided into those associated with the surgical procedure and those associated with the pathologic features of cryptorchidism. Surgical complications are mostly minor. Postoperative bleeding and hematoma formation are rare. The ilioinguinal nerve can be injured as it courses immediately posterior to the external oblique fascia. Deficits incurred usually involve only sensory neuropathy. Although ilioinguinal nerve injury typically produces numbness in the groin, the deficit may also involve the anterior thigh. The ilioinguinal and genitofemoral branches may also suffer damage during laparoscopic orchiopexy, varicocelectomy, or hernia repair. The ilioinguinal nerve pierces the transverses abdominus lateral to the internal ring just medial to the anterior superior iliac spine of the iliac crest and is less susceptible to injury during laparoscopic procedures than during open inguinal surgery. The genitofemoral nerve and its branches are more prone to injury. The genital branch passes through the internal ring and travels with the spermatic cord to innervate the cremasteric muscle and skin of the inner thigh.

In one study, 4.8% of pediatric patients undergoing laparoscopic varicocelectomy suffered variably transient numbness of the anterior thigh postoperatively.[38] A similar or higher risk of injury must affect patients undergoing laparoscopic orchiopexy. These injuries are usually transient, although long-term sequelae are more common among older patients.

Testicular retraction may also occur, usually as a result of inadequate mobilization of the testis. Opening the floor of the inguinal canal, ligating the inferior epigastric vessels (the Prentiss maneuver), and rerouting the cord structures to a medial course through the inguinal canal may assist in obtaining adequate cord length in proximal cryptorchid testes. High ligation of the patent processus vaginalis further facilitates mobilization. These mobilization techniques are often more easily accomplished laparoscopically in testes located at the internal ring. Placement of a suture to narrow the neck of the dartos pouch may also help prevent retraction.[39] Potential injury to the vas deferens and resultant infertility are discussed later. Careful dissection with frequent identification of the vas helps prevent this occurrence.

Postoperative testicular torsion is a more disastrous complication and likely results from inadequate fixation of the testis to the scrotal wall. The fundamental principles of scrotal positioning include creation of a subdartos pouch and tension-free fixation. Some investigators describe fixation with multiple sutures. We place a single absorbable monofilament suture in the tunica albuginea anteriorly and cephalad on the testis in a watershed area of testicular blood supply. These sutures are then passed through the base of the dartos pouch and are externalized and tied in place. Postoperative fibroblast infiltration then fixes the testis in place as the absorbable suture dissolves.

Testicular atrophy is a rare but frustrating and devastating outcome. Most techniques of standard orchiopexy minimize skeletonization and devascularization of the cord structures. Careful preservation of the main blood supply to the testis consisting of the testicular artery, the artery to the vas deferens, and the Fowler-Stephens membrane minimizes the potential for postoperative atrophy. Monopolar cautery has been implicated as a potential contributory factor in testicular atrophy following orchiopexy.[40] Similar to the risk of testicular retraction, adequate mobilization of the cord reduces tension on the spermatic vessels that may induce ischemia and ischemic atrophy. Performing a Fowler-Stephens orchiopexy significantly increases the risk of postoperative testicular atrophy, whether the procedure is open or laparoscopic. If ligation of the spermatic vessels does not appear to permit tension-free manipulation of the testis into the scrotum, we relegate the operation to a two-stage procedure.

Long-term complications related to the pathologic features of cryptorchidism include an increased risk of testicular cancer and infertility. It was formerly believed that earlier orchiopexy increased the chance of normal fertility.[40] More recent evidence refuted that notion and it now appears that infertility risk is independent of the age at orchiopexy in prepubertal boys.[41] Patients with bilateral undescended testes are at higher risk for infertility than are those with unilateral cryptorchidism. Among postpubertal boys, the risk of infertility is much higher; in those with unilateral cryptorchidism, 83.5% were oligospermic or azoospermic in one study.[42] In these boys, the elevated risk of testicular cancer and the reduced benefit of orchiopexy in fertility outcome should prompt consideration of orchiectomy instead of orchiopexy. Paternity, a more relevant outcome than fertility, is more severely affected in patients with bilateral than unilateral undescended testes.[40] Patients with unilateral cryptorchidism have paternity rates close to those of the general population independent of age at treatment. Current recommendations are to perform orchiopexy when the patient is between 6 and 12 months of age.

The association between cryptorchidism and testicular cancer is well established. The relative risk for the development of testicular cancer for cryptorchid patients compared with the general population was formerly thought to be between 10-fold and 40-fold higher.[40] More recent population-based data estimated the relative risk of cancer to be increased approximately 4-fold.[43] Unlike with fertility outcomes, the risk of testicular cancer does demonstrate some correlation with age at treatment; younger age may be protective. The risk of cancer also correlates with the severity of position. Abdominal testes carry a 6-fold higher risk for the development of cancer than do inguinal testes. Seminoma remains the most commonly encountered histologic subtype in formerly cryptorchid testes. Patients must be counseled about this elevated risk, and patients and their family members must be instructed on testicular self-examination beginning at the onset of puberty.

Herniorrhaphy and Hydrocelectomy

The surgical complications of herniorrhaphy and hydrocelectomy in the pediatric patient mirror the operative risks of orchiopexy. We group hydrocelectomy with hernia repair in the pediatric patient because of their shared physiology and technique of repair. The risks of scrotal hydrocelectomy are quite different and are dominated by postoperative concerns of bleeding and infection. Bleeding and infection are rare following repair of a patent processus vaginalis. Ilioinguinal and genitofemoral nerve injuries related to exposure are similar to those seen in orchiopexies. Dissection of the processus vaginalis from the spermatic cord may incur risks of testicular atrophy and vasal injury. Recurrence is a more prevalent complication than injury to the cord structures during hernia repair or hydrocelectomy.

Complications of Pyeloplasty

The purpose of this section is to review the perioperative management and complications of laparoscopic and open pyeloplasty. Details of endoscopic treatments for ureteropelvic junction (UPJ) obstruction are not discussed. In patients with an indication for surgical intervention, preoperative management should follow the principles discussed earlier. In addition, results of the urine culture should be negative before the surgical procedure. Selection of the surgical technique depends on the age of the patient, the severity of the UPJ obstruction, and the experience of the provider. In younger children and in infants, the dorsal lumbotomy exposure provides excellent access to the UPJ and is associated with rapid convalescence. Older children may benefit from laparoscopic and retroperitoneoscopic techniques, but this choice often is subordinate to the experience of the provider. Traditional open dismembered pyeloplasty through a flank incision remains an optimal exposure, especially in children with pronounced dilatation of the renal pelvis.

Intraoperatively, the fundamental tenets of a successful pyeloplasty include careful preservation of the ureteral blood supply and construction of a widely patent, but watertight, anastomosis. Although myriad techniques are available, most UPJ reconstructions today follow the Anderson-Hynes method of dismembered pyeloplasty. We place an antegrade double-J ureteral stent sized to the patient. To confirm distal placement of the stent and to prevent the unsavory complication of an inaccessible stent, we instill dilute methylene blue into the bladder on placement of the Foley catheter. Following the formula for pediatric bladder capacity (capacity $\approx$ [age + 2] $\times$ 30 mL), we instill a volume of dilute methylene blue of approximately 50% to 75% of the predicted bladder capacity and clamp the catheter at the beginning of the procedure. Blue fluid refluxes up the stent and is seen in the operative field, thus confirming its location. Bladder instillation can also be accomplished with a Y connector to the Foley catheter.

The most common complications of open pyeloplasty are UTI and urine leak. Urine leak occurs in 2% to 4% of patients.[44] Typically, this leakage resolves with drainage through an internalized stent or nephrostomy tube. A nephrostomy tube placed in lieu of a stent obviates the need for a second anesthetic for stent removal. We place an externalized Penrose drain around the area of the anastomosis. On postoperative day 1, if the drain dressing is minimally saturated, the Foley catheter is removed. Most commonly, the following morning, if the drain output remains minimal, the child's pain is controlled, and the child is tolerating a regular diet, we remove the drain and discharge the child. Even in the setting of minimal drainage, some surgeons send the patient home with a drain in place to be removed in clinic 5 to 7 days postoperatively. If the drain output increases following Foley catheter removal, the bladder catheter is replaced. If high volume urine drainage persists for >48 hours, we order an abdominal imaging study to examine for urinoma.

In the absence of a drain, the threshold for imaging the patient is much lower. We generally leave indwelling ureteral stents; however, if no stent was left and the patient has a persistent urine leak, an attempt should be made to pass a ureteral stent across the anastomosis in retrograde fashion. Occasionally, patients require nephrostomy tube placement in this circumstance. If a large urinoma is identified, a percutaneous drain should be placed under computed tomography (CT) or ultrasound guidance. Most urine leaks resolve with prolonged catheter and stent drainage without additional intervention.

UPJ recurrence or pyeloplasty failure occurs in 1% to 2% of patients.[44] Risk factors include prolonged postoperative urinary extravasation, missed crossing vessels, and kinking of the UPJ from a nondependent anastomosis. Investigators have hypothesized that prolonged stenting may predispose patients to treatment failure, although this may be a proxy for a history of urine leak. Retroperitoneoscopic approaches carry a higher likelihood of missed anterior crossing vessels, identified in ≥10% of patients in most series of UPJ obstructions. Directed imaging for crossing vessels, a practice we do not routinely undertake, may be warranted in patients undergoing a posterior approach. In cases of treatment failure, we obtain a contrast-enhanced CT scan to examine for missed crossing vessels. Identification of missed crossing vessels influences the selection of surgical approach.

No discrete algorithm selects the best method of repair for recurrent UPJ obstructions. However, success rates as high as 90% have been reported for endopyelotomy after failed open pyeloplasty. More recent follow-up studies of endopyelotomy demonstrated less satisfactory success rates, and salvage pyeloplasty by open or laparoscopic techniques may offer better success rates than endoscopic treatments.[45]

Laparoscopic pyeloplasty, first described in 1993, has demonstrated success rates equivalent to open pyeloplasty in both children and adults.[46] Operative time is often longer, but the laparoscopic approach may confer decreased incisional pain, quicker convalescence, and potentially better cosmesis. A review of the extensive laparoscopic experience at Johns Hopkins University in Baltimore demonstrated a 13.3% complication rate for adult laparoscopic pyeloplasty.[47] Most complications were minor. Urine leak, the predominant perioperative complication, occurred in 2.3% of patients, and postoperative bleeding or requirement for transfusion occurred in 1.3%. Major complications were rare and consisted of vascular injury in 1% of subjects, likely related to access. Any perioperative complication doubled the length of stay from a median of 2 to 4 postoperative days.

Indwelling stents placed during the surgical procedure are removed 3 to 6 weeks postoperatively. At that time, we usually do not perform retrograde pyelography because the edema from the stent can give a false-positive pyelographic result for persistent obstruction that prompts unnecessary intervention. When nephrostomy tubes are placed, we typically cap the tube before discharge and remove the tube approximately 2 weeks later in the absence of symptoms. No postoperative algorithm has optimally defined necessary follow-up imaging. We obtain an ultrasound scan at 1 month and a diuretic nuclear renogram at 3 months postoperatively. If the ultrasound scan demonstrates stable or improved hydronephrosis and the renogram shows no obstruction, we follow-up the patient with yearly ultrasound scans for 5 years. Data suggest that patients with normal study results immediately postoperatively may be discharged from surveillance after 2 years.[48] Pain or recurrent UTI mandates urgent evaluation with an ultrasound scan, nuclear renogram, or both. We continue antibiotic prophylaxis until the 3-month evaluation. If the 3-month study results are normal, antibiotics are discontinued.

POSTOPERATIVE CONSIDERATIONS

Airway Obstruction

Risk factors for airway obstruction in pediatric patients undergoing general anesthesia include younger age, longer anesthesia time, repeated intubation attempts, and recent respiratory tract infection.[49] Anatomic issues predispose infants to obstruction; infants have disproportionately large tongues and heads relative to their short, hypermobile necks. In all children, however, the trauma of intubation can cause croup, airway narrowing related to postintubation mucosal edema. To prevent croup, anesthesiologists typically avoid using a cuff during general anesthesia with endotracheal intubation for children <8 years of age.[50] The incidence of croup correlates with the absence of an air leak following intubation.

Appropriate management includes humidified oxygen and racemic epinephrine. Patients undergoing minor surgical procedures who experience croup after extubation should be monitored as inpatients to ensure against further adverse events. Laryngospasm, a potentially life-threatening complication of general anesthesia, is more common in younger children. This finding emphasizes the increased risk of anesthesia in younger children with URIs relative to older children. Positive-pressure mask ventilation and vigorous suctioning resolve most episodes, but patients may require reintubation.

Nausea and Vomiting

Postoperative nausea and vomiting commonly complicate recovery from pediatric surgical procedures. Vomiting in the recovery room occurs in 6% of pediatric patients.[29] Use of opiates, early feeding, and a history of vomiting are predisposing factors. Vomiting is of particular concern for patients in ambulatory settings because vomiting may prevent discharge home. For urologic patients, postoperative nausea and vomiting are common after bowel surgery and occasionally after inguinal or scrotal operations. Older children are more susceptible to postoperative nausea and vomiting than are younger children and infants.[29]

Of the prophylactic antiemetics used, the serotonin receptor blockers such as ondansetron and dolasetron reduce postoperative vomiting episodes. A single dose administered near the end of anesthesia effectively protects against vomiting episodes for 4 to 8 hours, enough time to permit postoperative recovery and transportation home for a majority of pediatric patients.[51] Waiting until a child requests fluids postoperatively can further minimize the risk of postoperative vomiting.

Prevention of Wound Infections

Fear of infectious complications often promotes implementation of prophylactic strategies for antibiotic administration that violate recommendations of evidence-based guidelines. The efficacy of antibiotics in preventing surgical site infections is long proven; however, guidelines restrict the use of IV antibiotics beyond 24 hours postoperatively. Initiatives from the Centers for Disease Control and Prevention include adherence to antibiotic prophylaxis measures as a process measure to quantify the quality of care of an individual institution.

For most pediatric urologic procedures, first-generation cephalosporins such as cefazolin provide adequate coverage for the organisms most commonly implicated in surgical site infections.[52] For operations involving the distal intestinal tract such as bladder augmentation or creation of a stoma for administration of a continence enema, the need for anaerobic coverage mandates use of a second-generation cephalosporin such as cefoxitin. Duration of therapy should not exceed 24 hours with transition to oral prophylactic doses when indicated, including patients with residual indwelling tubes and patients previously receiving outpatient antibiotic prophylaxis. Adherence to these guidelines maximizes coverage for surgical site infections while minimizing overuse of antibiotics with unintended risks of bacterial resistance, antibiotic-associated diarrhea, and increased costs of care.

Other measures that reduce the incidence of wound infections include maintenance of normothermia intraoperatively, maintenance of euglycemia especially among children with diabetes, and the preferential use of clippers as opposed to shaving the surgical site. Attention to these processes of care was shown to reduce wound infection rates by 27% in the National Surgical Infection Prevention Project.[53]

Fluid and Electrolyte Management

IV fluids serve multiple purposes in the perioperative patient: they replace fluid losses, maintain tissue perfusion, and cover maintenance fluid requirements.[54] Patients enter the surgical suite with fluid deficits from preoperative fasting and renal or gastrointestinal losses, more significant if a bowel preparation was administered. In patients undergoing ambulatory surgical procedures whose major fluid loss is from preoperative dehydration, maintenance fluid requirements should provide adequate hydration, and the child can resume oral rehydration once fully awake from anesthesia. Patients undergoing major abdominal surgical procedures, especially in the setting of bowel preparation, may present with significant dehydration. Working with the anesthesiologist to ensure adequate hydration overcomes the deficits incurred by general anesthesia and possibly third-space losses and losses from hemorrhage.

Postoperatively, standards for maintenance IV therapy are derived from studies examining weight-dependent metabolic rates among children. The most commonly used regimens are listed in Table 55-2. Additional fluids may be required to replace losses from diarrhea or nasogastric suction. Simply increasing the fluid rate may inadequately cover electrolyte losses specific to the fluid composition of gastric fluid and diarrhea. Gastric fluid is high in chloride content and low in potassium; diarrhea is high in potassium content and low in sodium and chloride concentration. Attention to these particular fluid losses may require an adjustment in the composition of the IV fluids.

Evidence suggests that the maintenance rate and electrolyte compositions shown may predispose patients to hyponatremia, hyperglycemia, and loss of core body

TABLE 55-2	Maintenance Intravenous Fluids for Pediatric Patients Undergoing Surgical Procedures	
Patient Age Group	**Initial 12 Hours**	**Maintenance Thereafter**
Infants (<6 mo)	D5 ¼ NS at 1.5 (MR)	D5 ¼ NS at MR
Children (>6 mo)	D5 LR at 1.5 (MR)	D5 ½ NS + 10 mEq KCl/L at MR
Adolescents	D5 LR at 1.5 (MR)	D5 ½ NS + 20 mEq KCl/L at MR
Renal Failure	Avoid potassium	

D5, 5% dextrose; KCl, potassium chloride; LR, lactated Ringer's solution; MR, maintenance rate; NS, normal saline.
MR: for 0-10 kg give 4 mL/kg/hr
    for 10-20 kg give 40 mL/hr + 2 mL/kg/hr
    for 20-40 kg give 60 mL/hr + 1 mL/kg/hr

temperature. The calculations listed in Table 55-2 overestimate the fluid requirements of the child and can potentially exacerbate hypotonic fluid-induced hyponatremia. This situation can be compounded by the postoperative syndrome of inappropriate antidiuretic hormone with an inability to concentrate urine. Although this condition is more common in cardiac surgery and neurosurgery, it can occur in patients undergoing urologic surgical procedures. Similarly, findings from randomized controlled trials suggest that physicians overdose glucose in maintenance fluids. Use of fluids with dextrose concentrations as low as 1% prevents hypoglycemia with reduced rates of the hyperglycemia associated with 5% solutions. Although no consensus has defined optimal maintenance IV fluids, recommendations for changes in standard regimens include the use of 2.5% concentrations of dextrose or lower and close follow-up of serum sodium concentrations in patients receiving maintenance IV fluids for an extended period of time.

Pain Management

Adequate postoperative pain management in the pediatric patient requires a multimodal approach. Formerly controversial, an infant or child's capacity to feel pain is no longer debated. Inadequate pain management can have behavioral consequences that complicate postoperative convalescence. A combination of opioids, regional anesthetics, and nonsteroidal anti-inflammatory drugs (NSAIDs) successfully addresses pain control for most hospitalized patients. Management should begin in the operating room, to ensure that postoperative regimens serve to maintain pain control rather than reestablish it after the onset of severe discomfort.[55]

Patient-controlled analgesia effectively controls moderate to severe pain in children ≥5 years old and is associated with high satisfaction rates for patients, their families, and nursing staff. A nurse or trained parent may act as a proxy to operate the patient-controlled analgesia apparatus. The use of a proxy has proven safe and effective for younger patients or those with cognitive impairments. Basal rate infusions are rarely indicated and may induce oversedation. Morphine is administered at 25 µg/kg/dose with a lockout at 8 to 10 minutes. Hydromorphone, another drug commonly used in patient-controlled analgesia, is administered at 4 µg/kg/dose with a similar lockout. When narcotic requirements are lower, analgesia regimens typically incorporate intermittent dosing of morphine, hydromorphone, or fentanyl. With morphine and hydromorphone, titration of the dosage facilitates pain control and ease of reversal prevents adverse events, to which infants are particularly susceptible.

Regional anesthesia techniques have become increasingly accepted as a standard of care for pain management in pediatric patients.[56] Caudal blockade is the most commonly used regional anesthetic in pediatric postsurgical pain management. For pediatric urology patients, caudal block provides excellent anesthesia of the perineal and inguinal regions; higher doses may provide effective anesthesia in children undergoing upper abdominal, flank, or dorsal lumbotomy incisions.

Risks of regional anesthesia include ineffective placement and erroneous placement. Erroneous placement may include the following: dural puncture, which is more common in neonates; total spinal anesthetic, which typically wears off in ≤1 to 2 hours; and, rarely, penetration of the sacrum, which may cause injury to pelvic viscera. Sacral penetration is extraordinarily rare, as is urinary retention. Some motor weakness may occur and is tolerated less in older children. Use of a caudal anesthesia block is typically restricted to younger children and infants and may be readministered at the end of the procedure. A catheter placed in the epidural space can provide durable pain relief in children hospitalized following major surgical procedures such as those undergoing lower urinary tract reconstruction. Complications associated with placement are similar to the complications of caudal blockade. Postoperatively, itching, headaches, and hypotensive episodes may necessitate conversion to parenteral or oral forms of analgesia. Patient-controlled epidural analgesia may be appropriate for older patients.

Peripheral nerve blockades are particularly effective in ambulatory patients. Ilioinguinal and iliohypogastric nerve blockade provides skin analgesia for 2 to 8 hours and is best administered to patients undergoing inguinal herniorrhaphy or orchiopexy. Approximately one fingerbreadth medial and superior to the anterior superior iliac spine, a needle is advanced until the fascia is penetrated. On withdrawal of the needle, the local anesthetic, usually bupivacaine, is injected to target the nerves underlying the aponeurosis of the external oblique muscle. In younger children, this blockade overlaps with the skin incision and provides no benefit beyond skin infiltration.

For patients undergoing penile procedures such as circumcision and hypospadias repair, dorsal penile blockade reduces oral narcotic and NSAID requirements. At the caudal extent of the pubic symphysis midway toward the base of the penis, a needle passed on either side of midline is used to inject bupivacaine just under the skin. Additional injections at the base of the penis at the 10-o'clock and 2-o'clock positions immediately under Buck's fascia may provide additional benefit. One should never add epinephrine to the local anesthetic because the penis is an end organ susceptible to ischemia.

Ketorolac, a parenteral NSAID, provides excellent pain relief and reduces narcotic requirements. Ketorolac may also alleviate discomfort from bladder spasms following ureteroneocystostomy. An initial dose of

1 mg/kg should be given intraoperatively 20 minutes before closing. For those hospitalized, follow-up interval doses of 0.5 mg/kg every 6 hours can be given for ≤72 hours, although limiting administration to 48 hours reduces the risk of bleeding, gastrointestinal injury, and acute renal failure. As part of a standard pain control regimen, ketorolac is typically combined with oral or parenteral opioids for inpatients following pediatric urologic surgery. Acetaminophen serves patients as both an analgesic and an antipyretic and can be given orally or per rectum. The standard recommended dose is 10 mg/kg, although this dose may achieve insufficient blood levels for analgesic effect and studies have demonstrated the safety and efficacy of using a loading dose of 30 mg/kg followed by interval doses of 15 mg/kg no more than every 6 hours. Rectal administration necessitates higher doses.

Successful pain management relies on the ability to assess a patient's pain level accurately. As a clinician, we usually rely on self-report: patients verbalize a level of pain and medications are administered appropriately. These estimates are less reliable in young children and in patients who are cognitively impaired. Adaptations of visual analog scales using diagrams of facial expressions or color scales enable clinicians to assess pain levels successfully in younger children. In infants, careful observation of physiologic measures and of facial expressions directs administration of pain medications.

ETHICS

Tackling the ethics of pediatric urologic interventions mandates entry into a veritable quagmire. Many procedures in pediatric urology involve clear risk-to-benefit ratios. For these procedures, decision analyses are less controversial. However, procedures that are largely cosmetic or that appeal to cultural divisions represent the majority of ethical dilemmas in pediatric urology. In this regard, circumcision dominates ethical discussions in pediatric urology.

Bioethics operates on the principles of beneficence (advocate for the patient), nonmaleficence (do no harm), autonomy (concept of informed consent), and justice (equity of access to care). With regard to elective circumcision, parents and physicians represent the patient's advocates, and in the absence of parental consensus, the procedure should not be performed. The principle most often expounded in discussions of the ethics of circumcision is the lack of the patient's involvement in the consent process. Clearly, an infant under-going elective neonatal circumcision lacks autonomy. Legal briefs have used this factor as parcel of an argument that parental consent should be subordinate to a child's right to "body integrity."[57] Children of reasonable age should participate in the decision-making and consent processes.

Ethics also intersects with pediatric urology in the field of fetal medicine. High-risk deliveries, including high spinal level myelomeningoceles and fetuses with bilateral hydroureteronephrosis, megacystis, and oligohydramnios, integrate medical and ethical concerns into the decision-making process. The physician-parent relationship is crucial to this quandary. Guiding the parents through the medical and legal information and incorporating parents' religious preferences should be the product of a multidisciplinary team approach. In most cases, expert panels have decreed that in the modern medical environment, in which long-term healthy survival is possible even for high-risk fetuses, aggressive intervention is recommended when possible.[58,59]

Intersex conditions require delicate attention to the psychologic state of the parents and certain ethical concerns. Most ethicists believe that procedures involving genitoplasty, unless absolutely necessary, should be deferred to the point at which the patient may participate in the discussion. The additional time allows the patient to form and verbalize gender identity that may guide the decision-making process regarding reconstruction.[60] In some instances, phenotypic abnormalities associated with severe intersex anomalies or cases of cloacal exstrophy challenged by insufficient phallic structures, early discussions regarding gender assignment must be tackled. In these cases, a multidisciplinary approach including parents, pediatricians, neonatologists, child psychiatrists and psychologists, pediatric urologists, and ethicists remains critical to a satisfactory outcome. In such cases, parental understanding and acceptance of realistic functional outcomes are crucial to a child's healthy psychosocial development.

CONCLUSION

The safe and effective delivery of pediatric care requires special attention to preoperative, intraoperative, and postoperative management concerns. Ensuring that patients and their families are prepared for a surgical procedure eases their perioperative care. Attention to these processes makes surgery safe and comfortable for the patient and his or her family and an extremely rewarding experience for the physician.

KEY POINTS

1. In pediatric patients undergoing surgical procedures, psychosocial preparation of the patient and parents is as important to the outcome as is the medical evaluation. Efforts to alleviate anxiety include thorough explanations of the surgical procedure, possibly using visual tools, distraction therapies, and involvement by the parents in the anesthetic induction.

2. The preoperative medical evaluation should rule out complicating cardiopulmonary disease and active infections, especially respiratory tract infections that may exacerbate anesthetic risks. Infants carry the highest risk of adverse events.

3. The most common complication of circumcision is bleeding, which is usually successfully managed with manual pressure. Devastating complications of glans amputation and necrosis are rare and require the immediate attention of a specialist.

4. Surgical complications of orchiopexy are typically minor. Long-term effects of cryptorchidism can have more severe consequences, with at least a fourfold increased risk for testicular cancer and significant detriment in fertility outcomes.

5. The most common complication of pyeloplasty, whether open or laparoscopic, is urinary extravasation. Conservative management with prolonged bladder and upper tract drainage resolves nearly all leaks. Recurrent obstruction is rare but may be managed with excisional repairs as opposed to endoscopic interventions.

6. Standard maintenance IV fluid regimens in pediatric patients may predispose those with longer admissions to electrolyte abnormalities. Consideration should be given to lower dextrose concentrations, and sodium levels should be followed regardless of the tonicity of the solution.

7. Multimodal treatment is integral to successful pain management in pediatric patients. Regimens commonly combine regional and local anesthesia, NSAIDs such as ketorolac, and opioids.

REFERENCES

Please see www.expertconsult.com

Chapter 56

COMPLICATIONS OF PEDIATRIC LAPAROSCOPY

Yagil Barazani MD
Resident, Department of Urology, Beth Israel Medical Center, New York, New York

Steven E. Lerman MD
Associate Professor of Urology, Department of Urology, David Geffen School of Medicine, University of California–Los Angeles, Los Angeles, California

Despite the rapidly expanding application of laparoscopy in adult urology, the emergence of general usage of advanced laparoscopic techniques in pediatric urology has been slow by comparison. The main reasons are lack of laparoscopic training and the smaller number of indications in children than in adults.

Because much of pediatric urology is reconstructive rather then extirpative, relatively few procedures such as nephrectomy are performed that facilitate learning of laparoscopic skills. With a limited number of renal operations as an experience base, it is difficult for surgeons to move to other more technically advanced procedures. It is also difficult for any one practitioner to develop experience with a given operation, such as may occur in an adult urology practice in which a single procedure may be performed almost exclusively. Even at larger academic centers, pediatric urologists perform >20 different procedures, only few of which may be adaptable to laparoscopic approaches.[1,2]

Moreover, it is difficult to improve on the results of open pediatric surgery, which offers an expected postoperative result and a course similar to that of laparoscopy.[3] In particular, infants and young children experience less postoperative morbidity than adults; therefore, the incentive and demand for minimally invasive approaches are reduced.[4] The wide range in age and size of pediatric patients also contributes to the difficulty in demonstrating that laparoscopy is superior to open approaches.[2] Together, these barriers have caused pediatric urologic laparoscopy to lag behind adult urology.

In spite of the aforementioned obstacles, laparoscopic techniques in pediatric urology are evolving at an increasing pace. The original application for determining the presence and location of the nonpalpable testis (NPT) has become nearly the standard of practice,[2] and with the burgeoning development of instrumentation and techniques for laparoscopic surgery, increasing numbers of centers are performing more advanced laparoscopic procedures in infants and children. Indications have evolved from diagnostic to ablative and, more recently, to reconstructive procedures.[1,3,5] The advent of robotic assistance offers an exciting new horizon that may popularize challenging procedures such as ureterovesical reimplant and dismembered pyeloplasty, which are still limited to a few high-volume centers.[1,2] This chapter is a review of the current indications, techniques, complications, and results of various laparoscopic procedures in pediatric urology.

GENERAL LAPAROSCOPY IN CHILDREN

Advantages and Disadvantages

Laparoscopic surgery provides many advantages over standard open techniques, including improved intraoperative visualization and magnification, reduced postoperative morbidity, faster recovery, less postoperative pain and consequently a lower analgesic requirement, and improved cosmesis. Commonly cited disadvantages include technical difficulty, increased operative time, and conversion of retroperitoneal open surgery to transperitoneal surgery. However, the techniques that were developed in adults have been refined for the pediatric population, and as surgeons continue to gain experience in these techniques, the procedures become less technically challenging and operative times decrease.[6]

Laparoscopic Approach: Transperitoneal Versus Retroperitoneal

A major consideration in pediatric laparoscopic urology is the choice of the most suitable way to reach the urinary tract. Until a few years ago, the transperitoneal route was the only route to the kidney and the urinary tract. This approach was initially preferred because it is technically easier and allows the surgeon to work in the wider and more familiar peritoneal chamber. Usually, three to four trocars are necessary, and after the colon is reflected medially, the kidney and upper urinary tract are easily identifiable. The lower urinary tract, testis, and spermatic vessels are also accessible using this approach.[5]

As some surgeons gained more experience in pediatric laparoscopy, they began to prefer retroperitoneoscopy for cases of urologic disease.[5] This approach offers a limited working space that makes suturing more difficult and can increase operative time. However, retroperitoneal access requires less dissection to reach the kidney and avoids the peritoneal cavity, thereby decreasing the risk of abdominal organ injury. The retroperitoneal approach also ensures that urine leaks and bleeding will be confined to the retroperitoneal space.[7] Despite the difficulties associated with the smaller operating chamber, retroperitoneoscopy is therefore suitable for reaching the upper urinary tract,[5] and this approach seems to be gaining momentum as more and more cases are reported.

Laparoscopic Access

Laparoscopic access in the pediatric patient can be achieved by placing trocars with either an open or a closed technique. The approach first described by Hasson using open trocar placement under direct visualization is favored over blind insertion of the Veress needle and primary trocar because the open approach minimizes the risk of visceral or vascular injury.

Complications of access range from insufflation of the abdominal wall or falciform ligament to more serious complications including damage to solid organs and intestinal and vascular injuries. Injury to the inferior epigastric vessels can occur, leading to profuse bleeding or hematoma formation that may not be evident until removal of the trocars. This complication can be averted by visualizing the inferior epigastric vessels before placing the trocar and can be controlled using sutures or clips or with a coagulation instrument. Evisceration may occur, although this injury is easily repaired and may be avoided by closing all trocar sites in small children. Finally, although minor vascular injuries, enterotomies, and solid organ injuries can be managed laparoscopically, major vascular injuries warrant rapid conversion to open surgery.[8]

Anesthesia

Laparoscopy is generally well tolerated by children; however, several anatomic and physiologic differences are worth mentioning. The major differences are in neonates and infants and the relevant features include rate-dependent cardiac output resulting from reduced ventricular compliance, a short trachea, primarily diaphragmatic respiration (which may make splinting of the diaphragm a serious problem), pleuroperitoneal membranes that may be patent, the possibility of right-to-left cardiac shunts, and a tendency to bradycardia in response to visceral stimulation, hypoxia, or hypovolemia.[9]

Although few studies have described the physiologic changes associated with laparoscopy in infants and children, some of the potential problems have been highlighted by data collected in a retrospective audit of members of the French Association of Paediatric Anaesthetists. These data show that in children and infants >4 months old, cardiorespiratory changes are similar to those in adults as long as the intra-abdominal pressure is <15 mm Hg. In neonates and children <4 months of age, an intra-abdominal pressure >15 mm Hg may seriously impair cardiac output because of a decrease in contractility and compliance of the left ventricle. An intra-abdominal pressure ≤6 mm Hg has therefore been recommended in this age group, in whom the high peripheral vascular resistance can lead to right-to-left flow through cardiac shunts.[9]

Halachmi and colleagues[10] retrospectively reviewed 62 patients undergoing laparoscopic procedures and reported that intraperitoneal and extraperitoneal insufflation resulted in only minor changes in heart rate and oxygen saturation. Although the effect of pneumoperitoneum on cardiovascular function is negligible in a child with normal cardiac parameters, the physiologic effect of carbon dioxide (CO_2) insufflation on children with comorbid cardiopulmonary compromise is an important consideration.[4] To this end, studies of high-risk cohorts of children with end-stage renal disease or ventriculoperitoneal shunts demonstrated the safety and feasibility of pneumoperitoneum even in these patients.[11,12]

Laparoscopic procedures in neonates and infants have some limitations as a result of the cardiac and pulmonary disturbances produced by pneumoperitoneum. The main effect of pneumoperitoneum on the heart relates to mechanical compression of the inferior vena cava, with subsequent reductions in preload, cardiac output, and potentially blood pressure. Moreover, the CO_2 used for insufflation has a direct cardiovascular depressant effect. Pulmonary effects are both mechanical and metabolic. Pneumoperitoneum pushes on the diaphragm and transmits pressure to the thoracic cavity. This pressure results in a restrictive syndrome, with decreased lung compliance, increased peak expiratory airway pressure, increased end-tidal CO_2 concentration, and reduced functional residual capacity.[13] In addition, the trachea deviates superiorly during pneumoperitoneum, and this change can result in right bronchial intubation particularly in infants.

The metabolic effects consist of increased amounts of CO_2 that must be eliminated by ventilation intraopera-

TABLE 56-1	Physiologic Effects of Laparoscopy in Neonates and Children <4 Months of Age	
System	**Effect of Pneumoperitoneum/Intra-abdominal Pressure >15 mm Hg**	**Potential Complications**
Cardiovascular	Increased systemic vascular resistance	Impaired cardiac output Right-to-left flow through cardiac shunts

Pulmonary	Restrictive syndrome
	    Decreased lung compliance
	    Increased peak airway pressures
	    Increased end-tidal carbon dioxide concentration
		Oxygen desaturation

tively to avoid a decrease in blood pH. Additionally, the increase in airway pressures, coupled with an overall reduced respiratory compliance, may lead to oxygen desaturation.[4]

Given these cardiac and pulmonary effects of pneumoperitoneum, emergency procedures are not eligible for the laparoscopic approach in neonates and infants. Furthermore, patients with a history of severe respiratory distress syndrome (e.g., hyalin membrane disease, bronchodysplasia, pneumothorax) or some congenital cardiac malformations should be denied laparoscopic treatment. Insufflation pressures must not exceed 6 to 8 mm Hg, and complete exsufflation of the pneumoperitoneum in the strictly horizontal plane should be guaranteed at the end of the procedure (Table 56-1).[13]

TOTAL NEPHRECTOMY

Laparoscopic nephrectomy in adults was initially reported in 1991 by Clayman and colleagues and has since become the standard of care in the adult population with nonfunctional kidneys and renal cancer.[2,14] In 1993, Koyle and associates[15] performed the first pediatric laparoscopic nephrectomy, and subsequently others have documented successful results of laparoscopic nephrectomy and nephroureterectomy in the pediatric population.[14] These reports have demonstrated the efficacy of laparoscopic nephrectomy, partial nephrectomy, heminephrectomy, and nephroureterectomy in children for a variety of disorders.[4]

The most common indication for laparoscopic nephrectomy in the pediatric population is nonfunctional kidneys secondary to multicystic dysplastic kidney disease, obstructive uropathy, vesicoureteral reflux (VUR), ectopic ureteral implantation, or dysplastic or hypoplastic kidneys. Other less commonly reported indications include nephrectomy for xanthogranulomatous pyelonephritis, hypertensive nephropathy, severe nephrotic syndrome, and severe hemolytic uremic syndrome, as well as before transplantation.[1,4,14,16-18]

The laparoscopic approach is excellent for most of these cases and has been shown to shorten the hospital stay significantly without increasing operative duration when compared with open nephrectomy.[19] However, indications for nephrectomy in children remain infre-

quent and should not be modified because of laparoscopy. Specifically, malignant renal diseases are not believed to be suitable for laparoscopic nephrectomy in children, and not all multicystic kidneys should be removed from patients.[4,14,16]

Although the treatment approach initially described by Koyle and colleagues[15] was transperitoneal, use of the retroperitoneal approach in children is progressively gaining popularity among different centers.[1] Retroperitoneal access obviates the need to transgress the peritoneal cavity and mobilize the colon and has therefore been purported to decrease the incidence of complications such as adhesion formation, collateral injury to intra-abdominal viscera with bacterial contamination of the peritoneal cavity, omental or visceral herniation through port sites or specimen incisions, and postoperative ileus, although some studies do not support this assertion.[4,18,20-22]

Laparoscopic nephrectomy, both retroperitoneal and transperitoneal, is technically feasible at any age with minimal intraoperative complications, robust recovery for most patients, and a low incidence of conversion to an open surgical procedure.[14,17,18,23] El-Ghoneimi and associates[14] described their initial experience with pediatric laparoscopic renal surgery through a retroperitoneal approach in 1998. Of the 31 patients undergoing laparoscopic nephrectomy in this study, no patients required conversion to an open procedure; mean operative time was 104 minutes and average hospital stay was 2.4 days.[14] A retrospective review of 100 pediatric laparoscopic nephrectomies by Gundeti and colleagues[17] demonstrated a 2% conversion rate to open operation. Shanberg and colleagues[18] similarly reported a single conversion to an open procedure in 37 patients (2.7%) undergoing nephrectomy or nephroureterectomy, with minimal blood loss in all but 1 patient and a hospital stay of <24 hours in all but 5 patients.

Few reports in the literature have compared laparoscopic with open procedures in pediatric patients. Hamilton and colleagues[24] retrospectively compared children who had undergone open (10 patients) or laparoscopic (10 patients) nephrectomy for benign disease and reported that hospital stay was 46% shorter for patients who underwent laparoscopic compared with open nephrectomy (22.5 versus 41.3 hours, respectively), with no major perioperative complications and minimal

TABLE 56-2 Pediatric Laparoscopic Nephrectomy Studies

Reference	No. Procedures	Approach	Mean Operative Time (min)	Mean Hospital Stay	No. Converted to Open Surgery	No. Complications
El-Ghoneimi et al[14] (1998)	31	RP	104	2.4 days	0	1 (postoperative bacteremia)
Gundeti et al[17] (2007)	100	RP + TP	112 (TP) 96 (RP)	2 days (TP) 1 day (RP)	2 (for bleeding)	6 (1 intraperitoneal abscess, 1 chest infection, 1 pleural effusion, 1 urinoma, 2 port site wound infections)
Shanberg et al[18] (2001)	37	RP		<1 day in all but 5 patients	1 (for bleeding)	0
Hamilton et al[24] (2000)	10	RP + TP	176	22.5 hr	0	0 major complications

RP, retroperitoneal; TP, transperitoneal.

blood loss in either group. Although pediatric laparoscopic nephrectomy is now generally accepted as safe, a prospective randomized study comparing the open and laparoscopic approaches has not yet been conducted (Table 56-2).

PARTIAL NEPHRECTOMY

The primary indication for a partial nephrectomy or heminephrectomy in a child is to remove a nonfunctioning upper or lower pole resulting from complicated duplex anomalies of the kidney. This indication differs from those in adults, in whom partial nephrectomies are typically carried out because of malignant disease.[1,4,14,25] In contrast to adults, who have no anatomic plane to follow for partial nephrectomy, pediatric patients with duplication anomalies present with a clear vascular and anatomic plane to be followed between the upper and lower poles. This feature makes the laparoscopic approach for partial nephrectomy in children more straightforward than in the adult population and decreases the risk of damage to the vascular supply of the remnant pole.[2] Moreover, laparoscopic techniques are well suited to partial nephrectomy by allowing perfect global exposure to the anatomy of the full kidney and its vessels without the need to mobilize the remaining part of the kidney.[1] However, laparoscopic partial nephrectomy is technically more demanding than is total nephrectomy and requires more laparoscopic experience, as shown by higher rates of conversion to an open procedure (0%-15%), and of renal or extrarenal complications (7%-58%).[14,19,25]

In a prospective nonrandomized study, Robinson and colleagues[26] compared outcomes of laparoscopic partial nephrectomy with open surgical procedures in children. These investigators found that whereas patients undergoing laparoscopic partial nephrectomy experienced decreased hospital stays, lower analgesic requirements, and improved cosmesis, the costs and

operating time were increased for this group.[26] However, another series comparing laparoscopic retroperitoneal partial nephroureterectomy with conventional open surgical procedures found that patients in the laparoscopy group experienced shorter hospital stays (1.4 days versus 3.9 days) with similar operative duration (152 minutes versus 146 minutes).[19]

These results were duplicated by Lee and colleagues[27] in a retrospective, case-controlled study comparing an age-matched cohort of 28 pediatric patients undergoing open partial nephrectomy with patients undergoing laparoscopic partial nephrectomy. The laparoscopic cohort had a mean operative time comparable to that of the open surgical group (194 minutes versus 193 minutes, respectively), but decreased mean hospital stays (1.7 days versus 4.7 days, respectively) and lower postoperative narcotic requirements, without significant complications or the need for conversion to an open procedure.[27] These series, in contrast to that of Robinson and colleagues,[26] demonstrate that laparoscopic operative times can be equivalent to open surgical times as experience develops.[2]

Initially described by the transperitoneal approach by Jordan and Winslow,[28] laparoscopic partial nephrectomy is currently performed in children by either a transperitoneal or a retroperitoneal approach. Both approaches have been shown to be efficacious and safe, with low postoperative morbidity, even in young children, and with operative times similar to those of open procedures.[4,25]

Although the transperitoneal approach offers excellent exposure of the kidney and its vasculature because of a larger working space and makes it possible to perform complete ureterectomy when needed, the main difficulties of this procedure lie in identifying and dissecting the polar vessels without traumatizing the main renal vessels. Conversely, the retroperitoneal approach provides a technique comparable to that of conventional renal surgery. The main advantage is the rapid and easy exposure of the renal pedicle that minimizes injury to the other polar vessels. Because the peritoneal cavity is not entered, the risk of postoperative adhesions and of injury to peritoneal organs is reduced. Postoperative urinoma or hematoma collections are confined to the retroperitoneum. The main disadvantage of the retroperitoneal approach is the minimal working space in smaller children.

Both the transperitoneal and retroperitoneal approaches to laparoscopic nephrectomy are associated with minimal morbidity, although the indications for each differ. In a series comparing transperitoneal and retroperitoneal heminephrectomy, Castellan and colleagues[29] found that complication rates depended on the age of the patient rather than on the surgical approach; patients <1 year of age were at greatest risk. These investigators found no significant differences between transperitoneal and retroperitoneal laparoscopic heminephrectomy techniques with regard to operative time, complication rates, or hospitalization time. Castellan and colleagues[29] recommended the transperitoneal approach in patients <12 months old, those in whom total ureterectomy is necessary, and those with large kidneys. The retroperitoneal approach is preferred in patients >12 months old who need an upper or lower pole heminephrectomy with partial ureterectomy.[29]

Retroperitoneal access can be achieved either posteriorly with the patient in the prone position or with the patient in a lateral decubitus position.[1,4,14,19] Borzi[30] compared the two retroperitoneal approaches and found that the lateral approach created more inferomedial space, gave better access to ectopic kidneys, and permitted complete ureterectomy in all cases. The posterior retroperitoneal approach was noted to give easy and quick access to the renal pedicle, thus making it preferable for isolated renal or polar excision without extended ureterectomy. This approach also allowed for nearly complete ureterectomy in children <5 years of age.[30]

MANAGEMENT OF NONPALPABLE TESTIS

Diagnostic Laparoscopy

The incidence of cryptorchidism is approximately 1% in the male population, and approximately 20% of these patients will have an NPT.[4,31] The historical approach to the NPT was first to identify the location of the testicle using radiographic studies,[31] despite the limited sensitivity and specificity of both ultrasound and magnetic resonance imaging in the diagnosis of NPT.[32] Subsequent to either identification or lack of visualization of testis, groin exploration would be performed. If a viable testicle was encountered, standard orchiopexy was performed. If a testicular remnant with associated testicular vessels and vas deferens was found, it was removed.[31] However, if cord vessels were not

visualized during inguinal exploration, laparotomy was the standard procedure to search for the testis or for blind-ending vessels.[4]

This approach to NPTs proved frustrating for surgeons and parents alike because the operation was performed without a preoperative diagnosis or a predefined treatment plan. Moreover, the morbidity of an abdominal exploration in the era of laparoscopy was seen as unacceptable by many urologists with regard to recovery and cosmetic outcome.[31]

The stable incidence of undescended NPT has led to the frequent use of laparoscopy in diagnosis and treatment.[31] Diagnostic laparoscopy was first used for NPT by Cortesi and colleagues in 1976,[33] and since that time the laparoscopic technique has become the gold standard for detection of intra-abdominal testes.[4]

Multiple studies demonstrated the efficacy and accuracy of laparoscopy in identifying and characterizing testicular morphology and location, and from these reports laparoscopy is estimated to be 97% accurate in identifying and locating testicles when they are present.[31,34] Cisek and colleagues[35] reported that diagnostic laparoscopy was highly consistent and specific as a technique. It precluded unnecessary abdominal exploration in 13.2% of cases and optimized the surgical approach for open inguinal exploration in 66% of cases based on testicular location.[35] Given these and other similar findings, pediatric surgeons and urologists have pushed to give laparoscopy more of a primary role in diagnosing and locating NPT.[31]

Laparoscopy is by far the most sensitive and specific procedure for localizing an NPT,[1] but the real diagnostic superiority of laparoscopy for NPTs is the ability to characterize the location and quality of the testicle, testicular vessels, and vas deferens accurately.[31] Reports have characterized testicular location in various ways, including at the pelvic brim, in the iliac fossa, in the retroperitoneum, high, low, and at the internal ring (peeping), as well as by documenting the testicle's distance from the internal ring.[31]

Findings during diagnostic laparoscopy for NPT generally point to one of the following three clinical situations:

1. If blind-ending intra-abdominal vessels and vas deferens are present proximal to the internal ring, a vanishing testis is diagnosed and no further action is taken.
2. If the vessels and vas deferens are seen and appear to enter the internal ring, then inguinal or scrotal exploration is warranted.
3. If an intra-abdominal testis is visualized with normal vas deferens and vessels, its location and quality are assessed.[4]

High testicular position implies that primary orchiopexy is not feasible and that a Fowler-Stephens orchiopexy should be performed, whereas a low-positioned testicle near the internal ring is amenable to primary orchiopexy with or without laparoscopic mobilization of the testicular vessels.[31]

The likelihood of finding the NPT in the location described by each of the aforementioned situations is remarkably consistent as reported by several investigators. One study reported blind-ending cord structures or an intra-abdominal testis during 31% to 83% of laparoscopic evaluations for NPT.[4] Blind-ending vas deferens and vessels are seen in 20% to 25% of patients, normal vas deferens and vessels entering the internal ring are seen in 40% to 50%, a low-lying intra-abdominal testicle is seen in 20% to 30%, and a high-lying intra-abdominal testicle is seen in 10% to 15% of cases. The ability to identify the location and quality of the testicle is a valuable asset that laparoscopy brings to the diagnosis of the NPT. Once the NPT is identified, the surgeon can determine the optimal therapeutic plan based on laparoscopic findings, including treatment by the laparoscopic approach.[31]

Laparoscopic Orchiopexy

The adaptation of novel laparoscopic materials to pediatrics has encouraged surgeons to apply laparoscopy as a therapeutic modality in patients with NPT. When an NPT is detected during diagnostic laparoscopy, it is evaluated for size and location. If a testicular remnant or atrophied testicle is visualized, orchiectomy is warranted. If the testicle seems relatively normal in appearance and is deemed viable, laparoscopic orchiopexy may be performed. Currently, all the open surgical procedures described for orchiopexy are performed by laparoscopy.[1] First, the ability to mobilize the testicle to the scrotum is assessed by measuring its distance from the internal inguinal ring. If the decision is made to proceed, the next step includes the dissection and mobilization of the spermatic cord and testis. If vessel length prevents the testis from reaching the scrotum, either a one-stage or a two-stage Fowler-Stephens procedure can be performed laparoscopically.[2,36]

Initial laparoscopic orchiopexy series reported high success rates in the treatment of NPT,[36-41] but these series were criticized for originating from high-volume centers with greater laparoscopic experience.[4] In a large multi-institutional analysis of laparoscopic orchiopexy with data gathered from 10 centers in the United States, Baker and colleagues[38] reported success rates higher than those historically ascribed to open orchiopexy, with no significant differences in success or complication rates between series from centers with large laparoscopic experience and smaller series from centers with less experience. This large retrospective study demonstrated that when compared with open orchiopexy, laparoscopic orchiopexy is an acceptable and successful approach to the management of NPT.

Deciding whether to perform orchiopexy with the vessels intact as opposed to dividing the testicular pedicle as part of a one-stage or two-stage Fowler-Stephens procedure is challenging because no specific criteria have been determined.[4] This decision is largely based on intraoperative measurement of the distance between the testis and the internal ring, observation of the spermatic cord anatomy, the presence of a normal contralateral testicle, and the capacity of the intra-abdominal testicle to reach the opposite inguinal ring after dissection.[4] Baker and colleagues[38] reported that atrophy occurred in 2.2% of testes after primary laparoscopic orchiopexy, in 22.2% of testes after a one-stage Fowler-Stephens orchiopexy, and in 10.3% of testes after a two-stage Fowler-Stephens orchiopexy (with 3-6 months between surgical procedures), for an overall success rate of 92.8%.

Esposito and colleagues[42] reported comparable results in a series of laparoscopic orchiopexy procedures performed without dividing the spermatic vessels. However, lower atrophy rates were reported by Lindgren and colleagues[36] in a review of patients treated with the laparoscopic Fowler-Stephens orchiopexy in one or two stages. In this study, all patients without previous surgical intervention were free of atrophy at follow-up, whereas two testes on which previous surgical procedures had been performed atrophied postoperatively. These success rates of 89% overall and 100% in patients without prior testicular surgical procedures exceed those of open orchiopexy in patients with abdominal testes.[31,36] Similar results were published by El-Anany and colleagues,[43] who found that only 4.3% of testes atrophied following laparoscopically staged Fowler-Stephens orchiopexy.

These studies demonstrate that laparoscopic transection of the testicular vessels is safe in boys with high abdominal testes that do not reach the scrotum after high retroperitoneal dissection. Moreover, although the one-stage Fowler-Stephens procedure avoids a second anesthetic regimen and the extensive dissection occasionally required during reoperation,[36] laparoscopically staged Fowler-Stephens orchiopexy is the procedure of choice for high intra-abdominal testis not amenable to the one-stage approach (Table 56-3).[43]

PYELOPLASTY

Since the first description of dismembered pyeloplasty by Anderson and Hynes in 1949,[44] open pyeloplasty has been the gold standard for treatment of ureteropelvic junction (UPJ) obstruction in adults as well as in children, with success rates >90%.[45,46] Laparoscopic pyeloplasty, introduced in 1993 by Schuessler and colleagues,[47] became the first minimally invasive option to match the long-term success rates of open pyeloplasty. The advantages of laparoscopic pyeloplasty are reduced morbidity and postoperative incisional discomfort,

TABLE 56-3	Results of Studies Comparing Different Laparoscopic Orchiopexy Techniques			
Reference	No. Procedures	Mean Operative Time (min)	Testicular Atrophy (%)	Complications (%)
Baker et al[38] (2001)	178 testes (primary orchiopexy) 27 testes (one-stage FS orchiopexy) 58 testes (two-stage FS orchiopexy)	142 (unilateral primary) 206 (unilateral primary) 133 (unilateral one-stage FS) 50 (bilateral first-stage FS = clipping) 118 (unilateral second-stage FS = mobilization) 150 (unilateral first stage FS + contralateral second stage)	2.2 (primary orchiopexy) 22.2 (one-stage FS orchiopexy) 10.3 (two-stage FS orchiopexy)	4.8
Esposito et al[42] (2002)	24 (primary orchiopexy)	60 (median)	4	4 (rupture of the spermatic vessels)
Lindgren et al[37] (1998)	44 (primary orchiopexy, one-stage FS orchiopexy, and two-stage FS orchiopexy)	135	0	5.4 (persistent communicating hydrocele, ileus)
El-Anany et al[43] (2007)	117 (primary orchiopexy, two-stage FS orchiopexy)	15 (laparoscopic diagnosis), 50 (primary orchiopexy), 20 (first-stage FS orchiopexy), 70 (second-stage FS orchiopexy)	0 (primary orchiopexy) 4.3 (two-stage FS orchiopexy)	0

FS, Fowler-Stephens.

shorter hospital stays, and improved cosmetic outcomes.[4] In 1995, Peters and coworkers[48] reported the first case of transperitoneal pediatric laparoscopic pyeloplasty, in a 7-year-old boy. Several years later, Tan[49] reported the first pediatric series of transperitoneal laparoscopic dismembered pyeloplasty in 18 children aged 3 months to 15 years. The mean operative time was 89 minutes; no conversions to open surgical procedures were necessary, and 2 patients required repeat laparoscopic pyeloplasty for persistent obstruction.[49]

Other series since demonstrated that transperitoneal pyeloplasty has efficacy and success rates comparable to those of open surgical procedures.[50-52] In a retrospective review of 27 consecutive children who underwent transperitoneal laparoscopic dismembered pyeloplasty, Braga and colleagues[52] reported that all patients experienced a reduction in the degree of hydronephrosis. No conversions to an open approach were required; however, 2 patients subsequently underwent retrograde endopyelotomy secondary to persistent obstruction. Mean operative time was 221 minutes.[52]

Ravish and colleagues[50] yielded similar results in a prospective study comparing laparoscopic and open pyeloplasty in 29 children with UPJ obstruction. In this study, a single treatment failure occurred in the laparoscopy group (6.7%) that required retrograde endopyelotomy, compared with no failures in the group undergoing open surgical procedures. The mean operative time was significantly shorter in the open surgical group (159 versus 214 minutes). However, patients in the laparoscopic group experienced less postoperative pain, shorter hospital stays, and earlier return to normal activity.[50]

Although experience has shown that laparoscopic pyeloplasty in adolescents is akin to the same procedure in adults, with a similar learning curve and postoperative outcomes, other studies have focused on younger pediatric patients. In one such study, Cascio and colleagues[51] retrospectively reviewed the results of transperitoneal laparoscopic dismembered pyeloplasty in 11 children <2 years of age. In this study, mean operative time was 100 minutes, and only 2 patients required repeat pyeloplasty, findings suggesting that laparoscopic pyeloplasty can also be performed in young children with good results.[51]

Laparoscopic pyeloplasty in children has followed the same evolution as nephrectomy, with the transperitoneal approach paving the way for the retroperitoneal approach.[1] Yeung and colleagues[53] reported the first series of retroperitoneal laparoscopic pyeloplasties in 13 infants and children. Mean operative duration was 143 minutes (103-235 minutes), and only 1 patient (7.7%) required conversion to an open surgical approach (Anderson-Hynes). However, a report of 22 retroperitoneal laparoscopic pyeloplasties by El-Ghoneimi and colleagues[54] found that 4 procedures (18.2%) were converted to open operations secondary to difficulty in completing the anastomosis. In this series, the mean operative duration was 228 minutes (170-300 minutes), and the mean hospital stay was 2.5 days (2-4 days). The investigators commented that the long operative duration and high conversion rate could be reduced with experience.

In a retrospective comparison between laparoscopic and open pyeloplasty for UPJ obstruction, Bonnard and colleagues[7] compared the results of 22 children who underwent laparoscopic dismembered pyeloplasty through the retroperitoneal approach with those of 17 children who underwent similar procedures by an open surgical approach. The investigators found that mean operative time was significantly shorter in the open surgical group than in the laparoscopic group (96 versus 219 minutes, respectively). However, mean postoperative use of acetaminophen was less and mean hospital stay was shorter in the laparoscopic group than in the open surgical group (2.4 versus 5.0 days, respectively).[7]

Controversy still exists regarding which laparoscopic pyeloplasty approach to chose: transperitoneal or retroperitoneal. Arguments for one approach over the other are more theoretical than based on objective criteria,[50] although some real differences may be taken into consideration during planning of the procedure. Although the retroperitoneal approach makes for an easier dissection and duplicates the principles of the standard open approach, working space is limited. This limitation makes suturing more difficult, particularly in smaller children and infants, and may lead to increased operative time. Some question also exists about whether crossing vessels are more easily missed. However, the transperitoneal approach transgresses the peritoneal cavity and requires more dissection to reach the kidney, thus theoretically increasing the risk of injury to peritoneal viscera. Moreover, urine leakage and bleeding would be more poorly tolerated in the intraperitoneal cavity as compared with the retroperitoneal space.[1,4,7] In the first study to compare retroperitoneoscopic and laparoscopic repair of UPJ obstruction in children at a single institution, Canon and colleagues[13] reported that these two approaches should be considered equal with regard to the successful correction of UPJ obstruction.

Robotic Pyeloplasty

The evolution of laparoscopic surgery in pediatric urology has been limited by the challenge of laparoscopic suturing. Robotic technology may offer the means to overcome this major impediment of laparoscopic surgery by allowing three-dimensional visualization, 6 degrees of wrist movement, and tremor filtering to make suturing and fine motor movements more intuitive. The advent of clinically useful robotic systems to facilitate reconstructive laparoscopic surgery in pediatric urology opens new doors to minimally invasive procedures.[55,56] Laparoscopic pyeloplasty seems a natural choice as a robotic procedure, given the delicate intra-corporal suturing required to complete the ureteropelvic anastomosis in smaller children and infants.[1,4,57,58]

Few studies have examined the application of robotic technology to the field of laparoscopic surgery in pediatric patients. In the first series of computer-assisted retroperitoneoscopic pyeloplasty in children using the da Vinci Surgical System (Intuitive Surgical, Inc, Sunnyvale, California), Olsen and colleagues[58] reported their outcomes of 15 retroperitoneal pyeloplasties with respect to operation time and complications. The procedures were performed without open conversion in any patient, with a median operative time of 173 minutes and a median postoperative hospital stay of 2 days. Two patients had postoperative complications related to the double-J catheter; however, all patients had satisfying outcomes during the preliminary follow-up period of 1 to 7 months.[58]

In the first study to compare the outcomes of laparoscopic versus robotic pyeloplasty primarily in the pediatric population, Franco and colleagues[57] studied 29 patients who underwent pyeloplasty, including a robot-assisted procedure in 15 patients and a laparoscopic procedure in 12. All surgical procedures except 1 were deemed successful. Mean intraoperative time for robot-assisted pyeloplasty was 223.1 minutes, compared with a mean time of 236.5 minutes in the laparoscopic group. Based on these results, the investigators concluded that robot-assisted laparoscopic anastomoses produced similar outcomes in pediatric patients who underwent pyeloplasty, with similar operative times. Thus, there appeared to be no quantifiable benefits between the two procedures.[57] Other initial studies in the pediatric urology literature demonstrated that robot-assisted laparoscopic pyeloplasty is safe and offers results comparable to those of open pyeloplasty but with similar or longer operating times.[59-61]

Although robot-assisted laparoscopic pyeloplasty offers no clear advantage in terms of postoperative morbidity compared with standard laparoscopic pyeloplasty, this modality comes at a significantly greater cost.[56] Early results with robot-assisted laparoscopy are encouraging, however, and the technique continues to be investigated in both the pediatric and adult populations. As robotic technology improves, this method of repair may become the minimally invasive treatment of choice for pyeloplasty and may popularize this challenging procedure in additional centers with less laparoscopic experience.

TREATMENT OF VESICOURETERAL REFLUX

VUR is one of the most common uropathies in children (0.4%-1.8% in the pediatric population), yet optimal management of this condition remains controversial. Laparoscopic surgery for the treatment of VUR has not been widely used, because early series demonstrated that the technical demands and longer mean operative times of the laparoscopic approach outweighed its benefits.[4,62,63] However, in more recent series, excellent results comparable to those of established open procedures were achieved with laparoscopic ureteral reimplantation, with a significant reduction in postoperative discomfort and a shorter recovery.

In one of the largest series to date of laparoscopic extravesical reimplantation, Lakshmanan and colleagues[64] modified the Lich-Gregoir laparoscopic extravesical approach and reported a 100% success rate with 71 refluxing ureters, with no persistent VUR or obstruction in any of their patients. These investigators reported that patients had markedly decreased postoperative morbidity and generally returned to normal physical activity in approximately 7 days.[64]

Riquelme and colleagues[65] presented similar results in a study of 15 children (19 ureters total) who underwent laparoscopic extravesical transperitoneal reimplantation by the Lich-Gregoir technique. All procedures were successfully completed laparoscopically and VUR was corrected in all but a single patient, whose grade III VUR changed to grade I. The mean surgical times for unilateral and bilateral VUR repair were 110 and 180 minutes, respectively, and the longest hospital stay was 72 hours.[65]

In a smaller series of six postpubertal female patients who underwent laparoscopic extravesical ureteral reimplantation, Shu and colleagues[66] reported that all patients had resolution of VUR. The average length of hospital stay was 36 hours, the mean time to resumption of full activity was 8 days, and the mean operative times for the unilateral and bilateral procedures were 1.75 and 3.75 hours, respectively.[66]

These studies demonstrate that laparoscopic ureteral reimplantation provides patients with the advantages of quicker recovery, shorter hospitalization, and improved cosmesis while maintaining the same safety and efficacy as established open procedures. The only major drawback of the laparoscopic operation is its longer operative time compared with the open reimplant procedure, which can be performed in approximately 90 and 180 minutes in unilateral and bilateral cases, respectively.[64] However, when laparoscopic ureteral reimplantation is performed by pediatric urologists competent in advanced laparoscopic techniques, operative times approach those of the open surgical procedure, and the laparoscopic approach thus offers an attractive minimally invasive alternative in carefully selected patients.[64] Such patients include those with bilateral simultaneous and duplex ureters,[65] although ureters with ureteroceles and megaureters needing a taper are unsuitable. Moreover, the working space in the pelvis of children <4 years old may be inadequate for efficient use of laparoscopic instruments.[64] Although laparoscopic surgery is not yet commonly suggested in patients with VUR, these studies suggest that in the future, laparoscopic ureteral reimplantation may be offered routinely to properly selected patients.

LAPAROSCOPIC VARICOCELECTOMY

Varicocele is a disorder that can lead to progressive dysfunction of the testicle and epididymis in children and may result in subsequent testicular atrophy and infertility. The incidence among men is 15%. However varicocele is less common in children, with a reported incidence of approximately 5%. Although this lesion is rare before puberty (<1%), the incidence of varicocele in postpubertal children approaches that in adulthood (15%-16%). Indications for treatment include severe dilatation of testicular vessels (grade II and III varicocele), symptoms (discomfort, chronic pain, or dragging sensation), testicular atrophy, and bilateral varicocele.[67] Predicting which varicoceles will lead to impaired fertility is impossible, therefore, the main indication for varicocele repair is ipsilateral testicular hypotrophy.[4] After successful repair, catch-up growth of the smaller testis has been reported in ≤80% of patients.[68]

Varicoceles are most commonly treated surgically by one of several techniques, including the Palomo technique (high retroperitoneal mass ligation of all enlarged vessels above the internal inguinal ring), the Ivanissevitch technique (inguinal ligation of enlarged testicular vessels), internal spermatic artery–sparing techniques, the lymphatic-sparing technique, and plication of the spermatic fascia over the enlarged vessels.[67] Postoperative complications including hydrocele, testicular atrophy, and varicocele recurrence or persistence are fairly common, and the likelihood of these complications is predictable based on the surgical method used.[67] Traditionally, the most popular treatment of varicoceles in pediatric patients was open high retroperitoneal ligation of the internal spermatic vein and artery according to the Palomo technique. However, laparoscopic varicocelectomy (the laparoscopic Palomo procedure) has gained popularity and offers results comparable to those of the open technique.[4,67]

Several studies compared outcomes between open and laparoscopic therapies for pediatric varicoceles. Riccabona and colleagues[69] compared four techniques of varicocele ligation in boys and young adolescents: laparoscopic, the inguinal testicular artery–sparing, the standard Palomo (high mass retroperitoneal ligation), and the modified Palomo. The modified Palomo approach involved suprainguinal and retroperitoneal ligation of the veins and artery and microsurgical sparing of the blue-stained lymphatic pathway of the testis. The investigators reported the following rates of postoperative varicocele and hydrocele: 11% and 5%, respectively, in the laparoscopy group; 14% and 0%, respectively, in the inguinal testicular artery sparing group; 0% and 12%, respectively, in the standard Palomo group; 2% and 0% in the modified Palomo group. In the group undergoing laparoscopic varicocelectomy, testis volume increased in 84% of patients.[69] These results demonstrate that outcomes of laparoscopic varicocelectomy are comparable to those of other techniques, with the exception of the modified Palomo group, which has the best overall results.

Other studies assessed the safety and effectiveness of laparoscopic Palomo varicocelectomy, with encouraging results. Pini Prato and colleagues[67] described a series of 41 pediatric patients operated on by this approach. The investigators reported that 90% of symptomatic patients improved significantly postoperatively, and 62% of patients with preoperative testicular atrophy showed postoperative catch-up growth of the involved testis. However, 1 patient (2.4%) showed varicocele recurrence and 12.2% of patients experienced persistent postoperative hydrocele requiring further surgical intervention.[67]

In another multicenter study on the laparoscopic treatment of pediatric varicoceles, Esposito and colleagues[70] reported an average operating time of 30 minutes, with a postoperative hydrocele formation rate of 5.6% and an overall varicocele recurrence rate of 2.5%. These results are comparable to those of other published series,[71,72] and they demonstrate that the laparoscopic Palomo procedure is safe and effective for the treatment of pediatric varicoceles, although it carries a fairly high risk of postoperative hydrocele in the absence of lymphatic-sparing techniques.[67]

Hydrocele is thought to result from disruption of gonadal lymphatics, and lymphatic-sparing techniques have been shown to decrease the incidence of this otherwise common postoperative complication. Hydrocele formation rates have been reduced to 0% to 2% in some series that incorporate a microsurgical approach into the treatment of varicoceles in children.[73,74]

Golebiewski and colleagues[73] randomly assigned boys affected by varicocele grade III to undergo laparoscopic varicocelectomy, either by a lymphatic-nonsparing approach (26 patients) or a lymphatic-sparing approach (26 patients). Before the surgical procedure in the lymphatic-sparing group, blue dye was injected under the tunica dartos. No recurrent varicocele or testicular volume reduction was detected. Four patients in the lymphatic-nonsparing group (15.4%) developed a hydrocele, and it required operation in 1 patient (3.8%). No patient from the lymphatic-sparing group developed a hydrocele, a finding suggesting that staining gonadal lymph vessels is an effective method of visualizing lymphatic drainage from the testis and minimizes hydrocele development.[73]

Podkamenev and colleagues[75] compared laparoscopic lymphatic-sparing versus open lymphatic-sparing treatment of pediatric varicoceles. In this study, 434 patients underwent laparoscopic varicocelectomy and 220 patients underwent open varicocelectomy. In both groups, the operations were performed by a modified Palomo technique with preservation of lymphatics and mass ligation of the artery and veins in the retroperito-

neum above the internal inguinal ring. The investigators reported that the clinical efficacy of the laparoscopic approach was superior to that of traditional open varicocelectomy because the laparoscopic group experienced similar rates of varicocele relapse (1.8% versus 1.4%), but lower rates of postoperative hydrocele (0.2% versus 1.8%), wound complication (0.2% versus 7.7%), and testicular or scrotal edema (3.9% versus 13.1%), as well as shorter hospital stays and operating times.[75]

With advances in operative technology, laparoscopic varicocele repairs are being performed faster and with lower complication rates, as well as with reduced hospital costs that approach those of traditional open repair.[4] Some studies demonstrated that laparoscopic varicocele ligation is a feasible procedure and can be performed safely without much experience in laparoscopic surgery. When laparoscopy is chosen, however, the Palomo modified varicocelectomy with lymphatic preservation is the optimal surgical procedure to treat varicocele in adolescents because this approach reduces the incidence of postoperative hydrocele (Table 56-4).[1]

COMPLICATIONS OF PEDIATRIC LAPAROSCOPY

Although children experience the same complications as those reported in adults, few reports on the incidence and nature of complications related to pediatric laparoscopy have been published.[2,4] As in adults, laparoscopic complications include subcutaneous emphysema and preperitoneal insufflation as well as great vessel laceration, abdominal wall herniation, and bowel or bladder injury.[4,19] Such abdominal injuries are often related to surgical access, with complications generally occurring during placement of the first trocar. The pediatric abdomen requires less force to enter, so penetration injuries to abdominal viscera occur more easily. Moreover, the smaller working space in pediatric patients increases the risk of injury to visceral and vascular structures from the laparoscopic working elements.[4]

Bowel and retroperitoneal vascular injuries comprise the majority of initial access injuries and although rare, these injuries have serious consequences with a mortality rate of ≤13%. The most common vascular injury caused by trocar or Veress needle insertion is damage to the inferior epigastric artery. More severe and life-threatening injuries can occur with puncture of retroperitoneal vessels. These usually result from blind insertion of the initial trocar access. Signs of major vascular injury include blood on initial visualization, blood aspirated through the insufflation needle, and retroperitoneal staining with expansion. These rare injuries can result in significant morbidity and mortality and in most cases necessitate immediate laparotomy to achieve control. Tamponade should always be employed promptly unless immediate conversion to an open procedure is elected.

TABLE 56-4	Pediatric Varicocelectomy Studies			
Reference	No. Procedures	Mean Operative Time (min)	Varicocele Recurrence Rate (%)	Postoperative Hydrocele Rate (%)
Lymphatic Nonsparing				
Riccabona et al[69] (2003)	19 (laparoscopic varicocelectomy)		11.0	5.0
Pini Prato et al[67] (2006)	41 (laparoscopic varicocelectomy)		2.4	12.2
Esposito et al[70] (2000)	161 (laparoscopic varicocelectomy)	30	2.5	5.6
Lymphatic Sparing				
Golebiewski et al[73] (2007)	26 (lymphatic-nonsparing laparoscopic varicocelectomy) 26 (lymphatic-sparing laparoscopic varicocelectomy)		0	15.4 (lymphatic-nonsparing group) 0 (lymphatic-sparing group)
Podkamenev et al[75] (2002)	434 (lymphatic-sparing laparoscopic varicocelectomy)	15	1.8	0.2

Visceral organ damage can also occur during insertion of the Veress needle and trocar. Injury to the intestine, stomach, or bladder is not as easily detected as is injury to a blood vessel. Many abdominal perforations therefore can go undetected, with resulting postoperative ileus and peritonitis. If detected intraoperatively, the injury should be repaired with intracorporeal suturing or stapling. When bowel or bladder punctures are made with the trocar, it may be necessary to repair the tear by open laparotomy or exteriorization of the injured bowel segment. Bladder drainage is part of the management of any bladder injury.

Other less common complications include gas embolism and subcutaneous emphysema. Gas embolism is a rare but potentially fatal complication. The most common reported cause is direct insufflation of a vessel. Sudden decreases in end-tidal CO_2 and blood pressure are hallmarks and warrant immediate evaluation for gas embolism, particularly in the context of initial Veress access or an open vein in the field. Subcutaneous emphysema with crepitus under the skin usually results from insufflation outside the peritoneum with initial access or leak at trocar sites. This complication is concerning in patients with impaired gas exchange, who may require postoperative hyperventilation to "blow off" the excess gas.

In an attempt to assess the incidence and nature of laparoscopic complications in pediatric urologic procedures, Peters[5] reported the results of >5400 laparoscopic surgical procedures performed by 153 pediatric urologists. In this study, complications were reported in 5.4% of cases. Excluding preperitoneal insufflation or subcutaneous emphysema, the complication rate was 1.2%. Complications requiring surgical repair occurred in 0.4% of cases, including bowel, bladder, and great vessel injury. The clearest predictor of complication rate was laparoscopic experience. The technique used to obtain pneumoperitoneum was also important, because the

Veress needle technique was associated with a 2.6% significant complication rate compared with 1.2% for the open technique.[5]

In a similar study, Esposito and colleagues[76] evaluated the results and complications of 701 laparoscopic urologic procedures performed at 8 Italian centers of pediatric surgery. Most procedures were in patients with cryptorchidism or varicoceles, but a few were complex renal procedures. The investigators identified no deaths and 19 complications (2.7%) in their series, one third of which required conversion to open operations. Some of the complications were of relatively little significance, such as peritoneal perforation during retroperitoneal surgery and instrument problems, but more serious complications were also noted, including vascular, bowel, and bladder injury.[76] Together, these studies demonstrate that complication rates for pediatric laparoscopy are comparable to the rate of 4% reported in most adult series,[21] and these events can be minimized by experience of the surgeon and team.

CONCLUSION

Indications for laparoscopy in pediatric urology are expanding as more centers gain proficiency in the various minimally invasive urologic procedures. Although early experience with laparoscopy was hindered by bulky equipment and limited tools, technologic advances enable laparoscopy to be used not only as a diagnostic tool but also as a method for intricate reconstructive intervention.

The benefits of minimally invasive surgery have been clearly demonstrated in adults, with reduced postoperative morbidity and shorter convalescence. Although these advantages are less obvious in the pediatric population, the cosmetic advantages of minimally invasive surgery are more important in children and in some cases may even be an indication for use of the laparoscopic approach.[77] Moreover, the disadvantages commonly attributed to pediatric laparoscopy, including technical difficulty and longer operative time, are gradually being overcome as increasing numbers of surgeons continue to gain experience in performing advanced laparoscopic procedures.

The spectrum of pediatric laparoscopic urologic surgery continues to expand, although it lags behind laparoscopic urologic surgery in adults.[4] Currently, a few indications have already been confirmed and are widely accepted as alternatives to open surgery, if not the gold standard. These include laparoscopic exploration for undescended testicles, laparoscopic orchiopexy, and laparoscopic nephrectomy. More technically demanding procedures such as laparoscopic pyeloplasty, laparoscopic ureteral reimplantation, and laparoscopic modified Palomo varicocelectomy with lymphatic preservation have been introduced and are still limited to selected centers, with excellent results.[1,4,77]

Although numerous publications have described the results of laparoscopic procedures in pediatric urology, efforts are still needed to validate the benefits of laparoscopic procedures over open operations. Moreover, the emergence of robot-assisted laparoscopic surgery has the potential to popularize challenging reconstructive procedures such as pyeloplasty and ureterovesical reimplantation,[1] although further studies are needed to evaluate the efficacy of the robotic approach. As more outcomes data become available and surgical experience with these procedures increases, it is likely that pediatric urologic laparoscopy will be incorporated into the standard repertoire and thus will make minimally invasive approaches to urologic conditions more widely available to children in the future.[4,77]

KEY POINTS

1. Indications for laparoscopy in pediatric urology are expanding, as laparoscopy has progressed from a diagnostic tool to a reconstructive modality.

2. Laparoscopic approaches to exploration for undescended testicles, orchiopexy, and nephrectomy are now widely accepted.

3. Laparoscopic pyeloplasty, ureteral reimplantation, and modified Palomo varicocelectomy have been performed at selected centers with promising results.

4. Robotic approaches to reconstructive procedures such as pyeloplasty and ureterovesical reimplantation continue to be investigated and may one day offer a minimally invasive alternative to these open procedures.

REFERENCES

Please see www.expertconsult.com

Chapter 57

COMPLICATIONS OF SURGERY FOR POSTERIOR URETHRAL VALVES

Ellen Shapiro MD
Professor of Urology, Director of Pediatric Urology, Department of Urology, New York University School of Medicine, New York, New York

Jack S. Elder MD
Clinical Professor of Urology, Case Western Reserve University School of Medicine, Cleveland, Ohio; Chief, Department of Urology, Henry Ford Hospital; Associate Director, Vattikuti Urology Institute, Detroit, Michigan

The management of posterior urethral valves (PUVs) has evolved since the late 1990s. With prenatal diagnosis and in utero intervention, the spectrum of the problems associated with this anomaly poses new challenges to the neonatologist, pediatric urologist, pediatric nephrologist, and transplant surgeon. Despite these advances, children continue to present in childhood or adolescence with subtle findings often overlooked during routine pediatric care. This chapter addresses complications of in utero intervention, valve ablation, ureteral tailoring and reimplantation, and delayed presentation. The evaluation and treatment of bladder dysfunction are also reviewed because this condition directly affects the success of ureteral surgery and kidney transplantation and dictates the need for augmentation cystoplasty.

IN UTERO INTERVENTION

Since the mid-1980s, surgeons have been cautiously optimistic about the role of antenatal bladder decompression for obstructive uropathy and oligohydramnios.[1] The purpose of this intervention is to restore the amniotic fluid to a more normal volume and thereby prevent pulmonary hypoplasia, which is the pulmonary complication of oligohydramnios. Techniques used include vesicoamniotic shunt placement and cutaneous vesicostomy through hysterotomy.

Moderate enthusiasm for this new technology was generated following a report by Manning and associates[2] of the International Fetal Surgery Registry that suggested that fetal intervention resulted in survival of ≤44% of cases with oligohydramnios. However, a careful review of all reported cases of fetal intervention for suspected obstructive uropathy yielded only two documented cases in which antenatal bladder drainage could

have improved the outcome.[3] More recently, refinements in the technology and better criteria for intervention have allowed the diagnosis and appropriate selection of candidates who may benefit from in utero therapy.[4,5]

Fetal sonographic techniques have improved. In some cases, however, upper urinary tract changes that result from PUVs are not apparent before 24 weeks of gestation.

Fetuses with PUVs and normal-appearing anatomic features at 20 weeks of gestation tend to have more normal renal function, and consequently prenatal therapy probably would not be beneficial in this group with a better prognosis.[6] A structural ultrasound scan performed at 20 weeks permits systematic evaluation of the urinary tract. The kidneys appear echodense in most cases. Large kidneys with mild parenchymal changes are seen in early obstruction, whereas small kidneys suggest significant parenchymal damage. Discrete focal cysts are a common sonographic manifestation of renal dysplasia.[5,7-13]

The ureters are assessed for dilation. Abnormal patency and dilatation of the ureterovesical junction (UVJ) suggest advanced urinary tract changes with poor prognosis. Bladder distention is almost always noted and the classic "keyhole" sign is observed at times (**Fig. 57-1**). Bladder wall thickening is also important to characterize. Symmetric thickening suggests PUVs, whereas asymmetric thickening of the lower half of the bladder relative to the dome region suggests the prune-belly syndrome.[5,10-13]

Because oligohydramnios can be present on the initial examination, amnionic infusion with warm lactated Ringer's solution restores the amnionic fluid volume for in utero sonographic surveillance.[5] The incidence of chorioamnionitis has been reduced by the

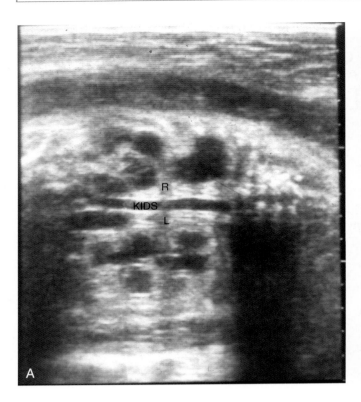

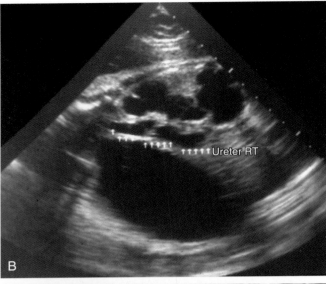

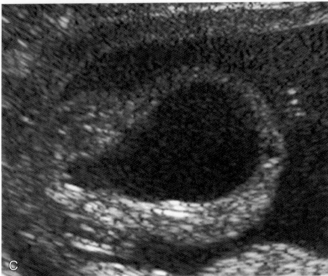

Figure 57-1 Fetal ultrasound scan shows bilateral hydronephrosis (**A**), right (R) hydroureteronephrosis and a distended bladder (**B**), and a distended bladder with a "keyhole" sign (**C**). KIDS, kidneys; L, left; Ureter RT, right ureter.

routine administration of parental antibiotic therapy at the time of the infusion followed by 10 days of oral antibiotics. Fetal karyotyping is performed with chorionic villous sampling or cordocentesis to rule out aneuploidy and to confirm the fetal sex. Knowledge of the sex of the fetus is important because shunting of dilated urinary systems in patients who were later found to be female with cloacal malformations provides no benefit in this setting.[5]

The most recent addition to our diagnostic selection criterion is electrolyte determination on serial vesicocentesis performed at 48- to 72-hour intervals.[4,13-15] Normally, fetal urine is hypotonic, whereas urine in renal dysplasia is more likely to be isotonic.[13] Normal fetal urine has a sodium concentration <100 mEq/L, a chloride concentration <90 mEq/L, and osmolality <210 mOsm/L. Analysis of fetal urine aspirated from the bladder allows analysis of fetal renal function; urine with normal electrolyte values suggests that fetal renal function will be adequate following bladder decompression.

The other important parameter to measure is β_2-microglobulin; levels >10 are highly suggestive of irreversible renal dysplasia.[16] However, an elevated level noted after a single bladder aspiration may be misleading because this value may represent stale urine.[17] Instead, sequential aspiration is more reliable. If the fetal urine parameters improve, this finding is an indication that fetal renal function may be acceptable. Using serial vesicocentesis, Evans and associates[4] and Freedman and colleagues[18] reported a 60% survival and a 33% incidence of renal failure in high-risk fetuses identified in the first trimester with severe bilateral hydroureteronephrosis, bladder distention, and oligohydramnios.

Although percutaneous vesicoamniotic shunts have been used for >2 decades, these shunts continue to have significant limitations.[2,3] Vesicoamniotic shunts become obstructed or displaced in 25% of cases, a situation necessitating additional procedures that can cause increased morbidity to the mother and to the fetus, with a 5% procedure-related fetal loss rate.[5] The shunt provides only palliative therapy and does not treat the anomaly or the pulmonary hypoplasia and renal dysplasia that are responsible for up to half the deaths in patients with PUVs. In addition, vesicoamniotic shunting does not alter long-term renal function significantly in most cases.[11-13]

Despite the advances of the Rodeck shunt, which places the proximal and distal pigtails at 90-degree angles, shunt displacement continues to occur in 25% to 30% of cases.[5,19,20] The site of shunt placement is important. The shunt must avoid the dome and be positioned in the midline just above the pubic symphysis. Even when no problems with shunt placement and function are noted in the appropriate candidate, unusual and unexpected outcomes can occur.[5] Johnson and Evans[5] shunted three fetuses with sonographic resolution of the urinary tract dilation within 6 to 8 weeks. These fetuses developed oligohydramnios that ultimately led to fetal demise. Autopsy revealed small kidneys with significant fibrocystic dysplastic changes suggesting progressive degeneration despite successful intervention.[5]

The first reports of percutaneous fetal cystoscopy at 19 weeks and subsequent endoscopic fulguration of the valves were published in 1995.[1,21] At the time of the first vesicocentesis, a 0.7-mm fiberoptic endoscope was threaded through the lumen of an 18-gauge thin-walled needle, similar to the technique used to performed transabdominal embryofetoscopy. At 22 weeks of gestation, a 10-gauge trocar was inserted through the maternal abdomen and into the fetal bladder. A 2.5-mm steerable endoscope with a 1.3-mm operating channel was passed through the trocar. A soft-tip 0.025-inch guidewire was used and the endoscope was advanced along the wire. The valves were electrocauterized with a 2-Fr ball-tip monopolar flexible electrode with 25 W of coagulating current. Following the 2-hour procedure, improvement in the urinary tract dilation with restoration of the amniotic fluid was seen on the post-treatment ultrasound scan. Delivery occurred at 31 weeks as a result of preterm labor, and the infant weighed 2000 g, with an Apgar score of 5[1] and 7.[5] A 10-mm abdominal wall defect with minor omental herniation was present at the site of the trocar. The infant died of pulmonary hypoplasia on day 4 of life.

Outcomes

Holmes and colleagues[22] reviewed the University of California San Francisco experience with fetal intervention for obstructive uropathy over 2 decades since 1981.

These investigators evaluated 40 patients, and 36 of these fetuses underwent surgical intervention. Only 39% (14 of 36) of the fetuses had a postnatal diagnosis of PUVs. The remaining patients had prune-belly syndrome or were females with urethral atresia or urogenital sinus anomalies. All fetuses underwent karyotyping and serial vesicocentesis for electrolytes and those with PUVs had favorable electrolyte values.

Intervention was performed at a mean gestational age of 22.5 weeks. Only two patients were noted to have renal cortical cysts, and one also had increased parenchymal echogenicity. The fetuses underwent various in utero surgical procedures including cutaneous ureterostomies (1), fetal bladder marsupialization (2), in utero valve ablation (2), and placement of a vesicoamniotic catheter (9). One patient who underwent valve ablation subsequently required a vesicoamniotic shunt for significant ascites. Another patient required multiple shunt placements as a result of malfunction or migration of the shunt. Before delivery, fetal demise occurred in 43% (6 of 14). One pregnancy was electively terminated because of significant pulmonary hypoplasia and the remaining deaths were resulted from prematurity and respiratory failure.

Long-term follow-up (mean, 11.6 years) in five of eight living patients revealed that 63% had chronic renal insufficiency (mean serum creatinine, 2.5 mg/dL after 1 year of age). Two patients required renal transplantation. Five of the eight living patients underwent urinary diversion (vesicostomy or cutaneous ureterostomy) or augmentation cystoplasty. This study underscores the finding that intervention does not alter the outcome of renal failure, despite "favorable" fetal renal function and suggests that intervention may primarily assist in keeping the fetus viable to term.

Biard and colleagues[23] reported their long-term outcomes in 7 of 18 children treated by vesicoamniotic shunting and who had PUVs. Other diagnoses included urethral atresia (4) and prune-belly syndrome (7). These investigators followed their algorithm for prenatal evaluation including fetal karyotyping and serial vesicocentesis for electrolytes and management.[23] Parents requested shunting in 3 cases with poor predicted prognoses. Most cases (13 of 18) had good prognostic findings. The mean gestational age at first vesicocentesis was 19.8 weeks (range, 15-28 weeks) and at vesicoamniotic shunting was 21.9 weeks (range, 15-29 weeks). Eight complications were associated with vesicoamniotic shunting including shunt displacement in 5 requiring replacement in 4, abdominal omental herniation in 2, and premature rupture of membranes 4 days following shunt placement in 1. Mean gestational age at delivery was 34.6 weeks. In boys with PUV, long-term renal function was acceptable (creatinine clearance >70 mL/minute) in 3 of 7. Mild renal insufficiency was defined as creatinine clearance <70 mL/minute not requiring renal replacement therapy and was found in 3 of 7.

Only 1 of 7 required renal transplantation at 10 years of age. Five patients voided spontaneously, 1 required catheterization, and 1 voided spontaneously and was also catheterized. In the overall group of children who underwent shunting, normal physical and cognitive development was noted in 78%.

INITIAL MANAGEMENT OF PATIENTS WITH POSTERIOR URETHRAL VALVES

The newborn with PUVs may have an abdominal mass (49%), failure to thrive (10%), urosepsis (8%), or urinary ascites (7%).[24] In many cases antenatal sonography has demonstrated bilateral hydroureteronephrosis and a distended bladder (**Fig. 57-2**). When the bladder is empty, one often feels or palpates a walnut-size, firm mass in the pelvis that corresponds to the trabeculated bladder muscle. In addition, dyspnea associated with pneumothorax or pneumomediastinum may be the initial sign of severe urethral obstruction.[25,26] A normal urinary stream is an infrequent finding.[24]

A voiding cystourethrogram (VCUG) should be obtained promptly to establish the correct diagnosis. (see Fig. 57-2C) Alternatively, suprapubic or perineal ultrasound imaging has been used to make the diagnosis because a dilated prostatic urethra may be apparent.[27] Sonography usually shows significant hydronephrosis bilaterally. Demonstration of the corticomedullary junction is a favorable prognostic sign for renal function. Conversely, echogenic kidneys, subcortical cysts, and failure to demonstrate the corticomedullary junction on the initial and follow-up ultrasound studies are unfavorable signs.[10,12,24]

Prenatal urinomas are thought to serve as a protective mechanism to reduce pressure-related impairment of renal function (**Fig. 57-3**). Patil and colleagues[28] studied two groups of patients with PUVs. Group 1 had ascites with and without urinoma and no vesicoureteral reflux (VUR) and group 2 had urinoma formation alone (unilateral or bilateral) and bilateral VUR. Moderate renal failure was seen in the three boys with ascites alone and mild renal failure was present in the three boys with urinoma and ascites. The investigators speculated that ascites without urinoma suggests bladder rupture and more severe renal damage. The three boys in group 2 with bilateral urinomas had normal glomerular filtration rates (GFRs), whereas the nine boys with unilateral urinomas showed impaired renal function on the side of the urinoma.

The foregoing findings suggest that bilateral urinomas and bilateral VUR have a protective effect, whereas renal function is impaired on the side of the urinoma and most patients have impaired global renal function. A treatment algorithm recommends aspiration in patients with deteriorating clinical features including increasing urinoma, rising plasma creatinine concentration, infection, hypertension, and parenchymal com-

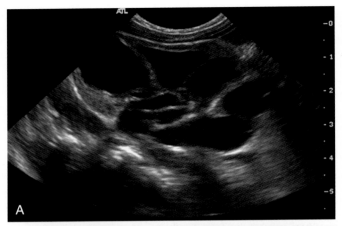

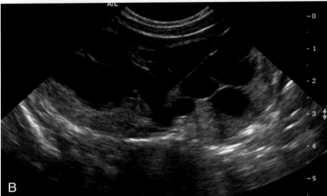

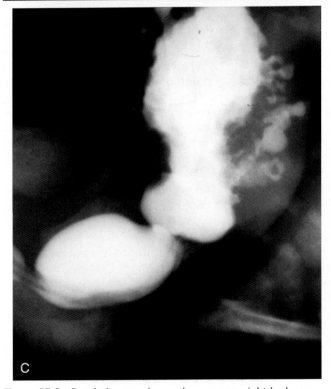

Figure 57-2 Renal ultrasound scan shows severe right hydronephrosis and hydroureter (**A**), severe left hydronephrosis (**B**), and voiding cystourethrogram demonstrating typical findings of type I posterior urethral valves (**C**).

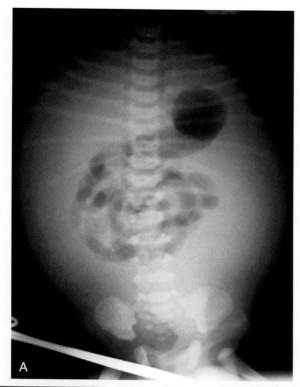

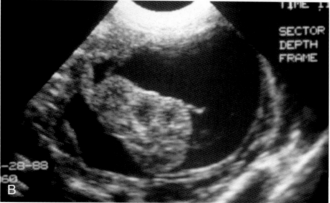

Figure 57-3 Newborn with an abdominal mass. **A,** Abdominal plain film shows the ground-glass appearance of abdominal ascites. **B,** Renal ultrasound scan demonstrates an extracapsular urinoma and complete decompression of the collecting system. (Courtesy of Dr. Anthony Caldemone.)

association between renal function and urinoma formation.[29]

The initial treatment for neonates suspected of having PUVs is directed at decompressing the urinary tract with a 5-Fr feeding tube passed transurethrally. Attention must be given to pulmonary function and fluid and electrolyte management. We recommend passing the catheter at the time of the first ultrasound scan immediately following birth. The catheter can be difficult to pass because of the dilation of the posterior urethra and the hypertrophy of the bladder neck. Sonography confirms the placement of the catheter within the bladder because a catheter that is coiled in the posterior urethra will cause the majority of urine to drain around the catheter. Similarly, if too much of the catheter is coiled in the bladder, the tip may extend distally through the external sphincter and provide some drainage of the bladder with continuous leakage around the catheter. Foley catheter use is discouraged because the balloon can obstruct the ureteral orifices when the thick-walled bladder is decompressed, or it can cause severe bladder spasm that can obstruct the intramural ureters. Although anuria can result from the noncompliant, hypertonic bladder wall and can lead to relative obstruction of the UVJ, mechanical occlusion can also be the source of anuria in some cases.[30]

Antibiotic prophylaxis is commonly prescribed. In the absence of suspected sepsis, ampicillin or cephalexin is administered at the time of catheter placement.[24] Judicious use of aminoglycosides or other nephrotoxic antimicrobial agents is warranted. It is best to avoid nephrotoxic agents that may cause further tubular dysfunction. Finally, neonatal circumcision should be recommended in these boys because it also helps reduce the risk of urinary tract infection (UTI).

Primary Valve Ablation

Infant urethral sounds should be passed to calibrate the urethra. The term newborn male urethra generally accepts an 8-Fr endoscope. Dilation of the urethra to pass a larger instrument may lead to urethral trauma and stricture formation. Vigorous dilation may result in iatrogenic hypospadias due to splitting of the glans to the subcoronal level. Vesicostomy remains the treatment alternative for the infant whose urethra is too small to accept the currently available endoscopes.[24]

Smith and colleagues[31] reported valve ablation using the 6.9-Fr cystoscope and the 3-Fr Bugbee electrode in premature infants as small as 2500 g. The coagulating current was used to ablate the valves. In older patients, the 11- or 13-Fr Storz resectoscope can be used with the cutting current and the right-angle loop. In addition, the neodymium:yttrium-aluminum-garnet (Nd:YAG) laser may be used.[32] In the series by Bhatnagar and associates,[32] this modality was successful in 16 of 20 patients, and 4 patients underwent repeat valve ablation.

pression. In the study by Patil and colleagues,[28] intervention was necessary in all boys in group 1, whereas six of nine boys in group 2 underwent aspiration of the urinoma. If is no improvement or stabilization occurs, percutaneous nephrostomy, ureteral stenting, or ureterostomy is recommended.

Patil and colleagues[28] hypothesized that if renal extravasation is extracapsular, it could have a protective effect on renal function, whereas if the extravasation is subcapsular, the renal parenchyma is compressed, thus possibly leading to the deleterious effects of a urinoma. If the type of urinoma cannot be determined, this may explain the results of other studies that showed no

Varying methods are used to ablate PUVs. The valves should be incised at the 12-o'clock position and the lateral leaflets should be cut at the 5- and 7-o'clock positions.[33] Passing a cystoscope or resectoscope that is too large may result in urethral stricture.[34] In the past, alternative methods of valve ablation in neonates and small premature infants included the Whitaker diathermy hook and the venous valvutome; these techniques are rarely used now, and the Whitaker hook is no longer made.[35,36] Chertin and colleagues[37] reported a series of 35 cases of valve ablation under fluoroscopic guidance using a 4-Fr Fogarty balloon catheter filled with 0.5 mL of saline. A postoperative VCUG revealed no residual valve in 34 of 35 patients (97%). Other methods include creation of a temporary perineal urethrostomy into which the cystoscope or resectoscope is passed or performance of the procedure in an antegrade fashion through a percutaneous cystostomy.[38]

A small feeding tube is left indwelling for 1 to 2 days, and a VCUG may be obtained at the time of catheter removal. Although it is likely that the posterior urethra will be dilated on this early study, no valve remnant should be visualized. Performing the VCUG at the time of catheter removal alleviates the concern about residual valve leaflets as the cause of increasing hydronephrosis or a rising creatinine concentration when catheter drainage is discontinued. If the VCUG is not obtained before discharge from the hospital, it should be obtained 2 to 4 weeks postoperatively to confirm satisfactory valve ablation. In addition, a renal sonogram confirms satisfactory bladder emptying.

Another method to assess adequacy of valve ablation is the preoperative and postoperative urethral ratio.[39] This ratio is determined by measuring the diameter of the posterior urethra transversely at a point halfway between the bladder neck and the distal end of the membranous urethra and the diameter of the anterior urethra at the transverse diameter at the point of the maximum distention in the bulbar urethra. Measurements are most accurate on voiding films in which the catheter has been removed (**Fig. 57-4**). In one study,[39] the median urethral ratio before ablation was 8.6 (range, 4-14.7) and that of normal age-matched controls was 2.6 (range, 1.3-5.5). The postoperative urethral ratio was 3.1 (range, 1.9-4). A second group of patients with a postoperative urethral ratio of 8 (range, 5-15.5) after the first ablation underwent a second ablation with a final urethral ratio of 3.1 (range, 2.9-6.4).[39] Valve ablation is successful in >90% of patients. Long-term stricture formation is uncommon.[34]

Alternatives to Valve Ablation: Cutaneous Vesicostomy and Upper Tract Diversion

An alternative to primary valve ablation is the creation of a temporary cutaneous vesicostomy.[40,41] A small transverse incision is made midway between the umbi-

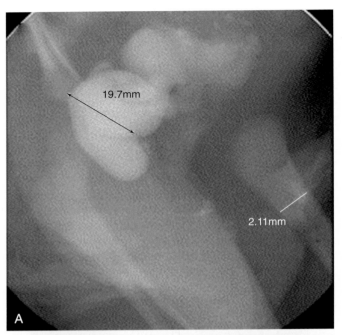

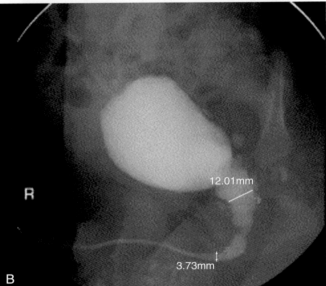

Figure 57-4 Posterior urethral measurements to determine the urethral ratio on a preoperative (**A**) and postoperative (**B**) voiding cystourethrogram. *(From Bani Hani O, Prelog K, Smith GHH. A method to assess posterior urethral valve ablation.* J Urol. 2006;176: 303-305.)*

licus and the pubic symphysis, and the dome of the bladder is brought to the skin. If the anterior bladder wall rather than the dome is exteriorized, prolapse may occur. The vesicostomy should calibrate to 24 to 26 Fr to avoid stenosis. In addition, daily dilation of the stoma with a plastic medicine dropper helps minimize contraction of the stoma. The vesicostomy drains into the diaper and no urinary collection device is necessary.

Cutaneous vesicostomy has been shown to be as effective as valve ablation for initial therapy.[42] This form of management allows the bladder to cycle with voiding at low pressure through the stoma and does not reduce bladder capacity. A cutaneous vesicostomy should not be performed in the presence of active UTI because contraction of the bladder may occur. These babies should be maintained on antibiotic prophylaxis. In some cases breakthrough febrile UTIs occur and vesicostomy closure is necessary.

In the past, proximal high diversion with cutaneous pyelostomy or cutaneous ureterostomy was advocated for neonates and infants with severe hydronephrosis and a persistently elevated creatinine concentration following catheter drainage.[24,43] In addition, high diversion provides the opportunity to sample the kidneys for biopsy and may allow the urologist to predict the child's ultimate renal outcome. One would think that proximal diversion could provide better renal drainage than vesicostomy, particularly in patients with ureterovesical obstruction, and could thereby optimize the potential for ultimate renal function. Indeed, Krueger and colleagues[44] claimed that high diversion yielded improved renal function and somatic growth. In that series, however, small patient numbers and the absence of statistical significance failed to support their claims.

Furthermore, UVJ obstruction seems to occur only when the bladder is filling and results from an elevation of intravesical pressure, not from obstruction secondary to detrusor hypertrophy. Furthermore, proximal high diversion therapy has not been shown to prevent end-stage renal disease (ESRD) because ≤85% of these patients have renal dysplasia.[45] In addition, by diverting the urine away from the bladder, regular cyclic vesical contraction may not occur and result in a smaller, less compliant bladder compared with vesicostomy.[46] Finally, cutaneous pyelostomies require placement of a diaper across the abdomen and flank, and even then the child's clothes may become wet. Consequently, this form of diversion generally is reserved for rare cases in which valve ablation or vesicostomy have failed to show improvement in upper urinary tract drainage or when urosepsis is secondary to pyonephrosis.[24,43]

If cutaneous vesicostomy, ureterostomy, or pyelostomy is chosen as initial therapy, valve ablation should not be performed simultaneously because the urethra will remain dry, and urethral stricture formation is common (**Fig. 57-5**).[47] Another case illustrating the importance of choosing well-planned diversionary procedures and delaying primary valve resection is shown in **Figure 57-6**. Alternatively, the Sober-en-T ureterostomy has been performed at the time of primary valve ablation or soon thereafter because this type of urinary diversion permits rapid decompression of the upper urinary tract while permitting urine to pass into the bladder.[48] **Figure 57-7** shows a modification of the original Sober-en-T ureterostomy.

Another initial approach is to perform total urinary reconstruction, with valve ablation, ureteroneocystos-

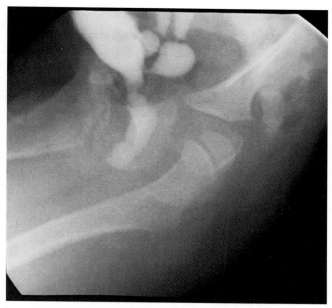

Figure 57-5 A newborn underwent bilateral cutaneous pyelostomies and transurethral ablation of posterior urethral valves. Before upper tract reconstruction at age 4 years, a catheter could not be passed at the time of the voiding cystourethrogram. The cystogram through a cutaneous ureterostomy shows a complete proximal anterior urethral stricture requiring a perineal approach for reconstruction.

tomy, and excision of large bladder diverticula.[49] We think that this approach is rarely necessary because significant improvement in reflux and bladder function may occur after elimination of the obstructing valve leaflets.

Controversies in Initial Management of Posterior Urethral Valves

The initial management of PUVs continues to be controversial. In 1997, Close and colleagues[46] suggested that early valve ablation permitted recovery of the normal bladder appearance and function when the procedure was performed within the first months of life. In their patients, urinary diversion was believed to be deleterious to ultimate bladder function because of the absence of normal bladder cycling. Patients who underwent diversion had worse compliance and less resolution of bladder wall anomalies. Delayed development of daytime urinary continence occurred in 80% of patients who underwent diversion procedures as opposed to 33% of those who underwent primary valve ablation. However, both groups developed similar degrees of renal dysfunction in the long term.[46]

Podesta and colleagues[50] studied a group of patients with PUVs who were undergoing either vesicostomy and delayed valve ablation or primary valve ablation. These investigators demonstrated that approximately 50% of the diverted group had detrusor overactivity, which was rarely observed in the primary ablation

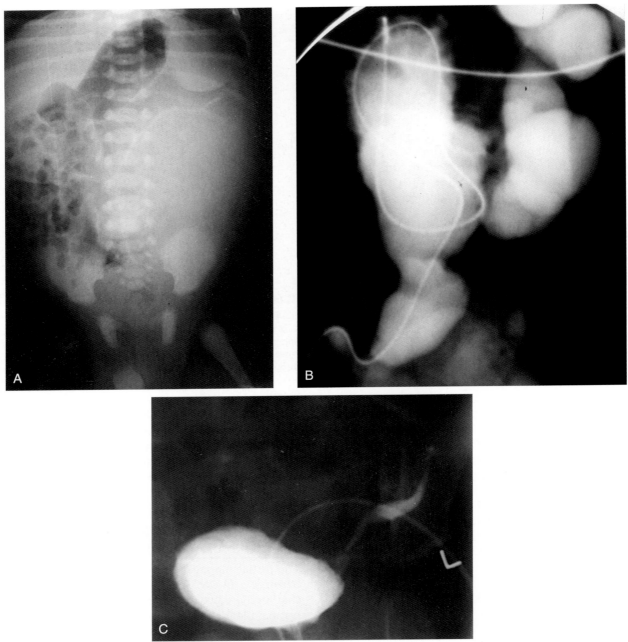

Figure 57-6 A newborn boy was noted prenatally to have left hydronephrosis and a distended bladder. **A,** Abdominal plain film shows a large left urinoma. **B,** Voiding cystourethrogram shows high-grade left vesicoureteral reflux and posterior urethral valves. His creatinine concentration was 0.5 mg/dL after 1 week of catheter drainage. During passage of the resectoscope, the glans split, creating a subcoronal hypospadias. Valve ablation proceeded and a left ureterostomy at the midureteral level was performed. Postoperatively, all his urine is noted from the left ureterostomy. Before urinary diversion at age 3 years, a renal scan demonstrates that the left kidney contributes 20% to the total renal function and a cystogram (**C**) shows reflux into a nondilated left distal ureter, mild trabeculation, and normal capacity for his age (150 mL). Left proximal ureterogram shows no obstruction. Takedown of the left ureterostomy with excision of the left distal ureter and ureteral reimplantation with a psoas hitch are performed. This case demonstrates several points: (1) ureterostomy is not usually indicated for reflux; (2) ureterostomy should not be performed midureter when reimplantation will be required; (3) once the valve is resected, procedures should not be performed that completely divert urine from the bladder; and (4) care should be exercised when instrumenting the infant male urethra.

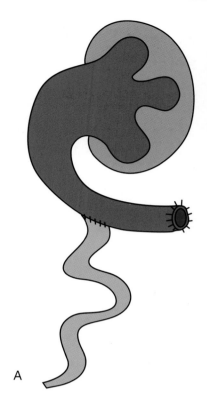

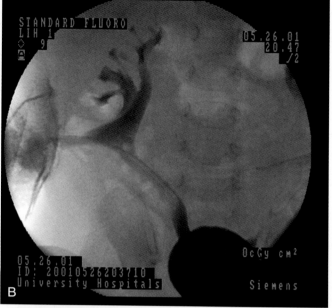

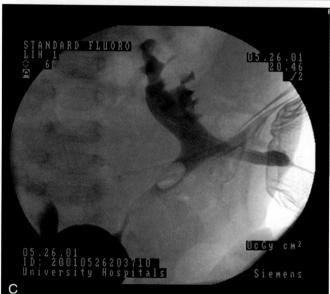

Figure 57-7 **A,** Sober-en-T ureterostomy decompresses the upper urinary tract and permits urine to pass into the bladder. The proximal ureter is divided below the lower pole of the kidney. The upper end is diverted to the skin. The lower end is anastomosed to the proximal ureter just below the renal pelvis, but not to the pelvis as originally described by Sober. Ureterograms showing the right **(B)** and left **(C)** kidneys 1 year after Sober Y-en T ureterostomies. *(A, From Liard A, Seguier-Lipszyc E, Mitrofanoff P. Temporary high diversion for posterior urethral valves. J Urol. 2000;164[1]:145-148.)*

group. The primary ablation group also had a lower detrusor filling pressure at expected bladder capacity for age and improved detrusor compliance.

Although these groups advocated primary valve ablation, their observations on bladder function differed from the 1996 report of Smith and colleagues.[51] Smith and associates examined the long-term outcome of 100 patients treated with primary valve ablation (74%), vesicostomy (13%), or high diversion (90%). Thirteen percent developed ESRD by age 15 years. Treatment choice did not influence the age at which they developed ESRD. The incidence of chronic renal failure was 34% at age 10 years and 51% at age 20 years. Almost all patients had delayed development of daytime urinary

continence; only 19% developed continence by age 5 years and 46% by age 10 years. Although formal urodynamic testing was performed in only 10 patients, only 1 patient was thought to need an augmentation cystoplasty.[51]

Kim and associates[52] compared the urodynamic findings in patients with PUVs who had undergone primary valve ablation, vesicostomy, or proximal diversion with pyelostomy or ureterostomy. When the urodynamic findings of end-filling detrusor pressure and bladder capacity were compared, no statistical difference was found in any of these groups. In fact, the vesical or proximal diversion groups had somewhat better urodynamic findings. The investigators concluded that the initial management of valve ablation or vesical or proximal diversion does not affect ultimate bladder function.

A report of the long-term follow-up of bilateral high Sober-type urinary diversion in 36 patients with PUVs who underwent urodynamic testing not only after diversion but also before and after ureterostomy closure showed well-preserved bladder capacity or compliance in 80% and 69%, respectively, and stable detrusor activity in 89%. An increase in bladder capacity was demonstrated in 33% (13/39).[48]

Narasimhan and colleagues[53] performed a prospective study of boys with PUVs who were undergoing primary ablation or vesicostomy. These investigators analyzed the effect of the modality on renal function and somatic growth and whether the presence of VUR and an abnormal serum creatinine concentration affected somatic growth. At birth, body weight and length and serum creatinine concentrations were similar in the two groups but the valve ablation group lagged behind the vesicostomy group at 3 and 6 months in weight and length measurements. The investigators concluded that treatment modality did not affect the outcome of renal function because at 1 year the serum creatinine concentration decreased to 0.7 ± 0.2 ng/dL in the valve ablation group and to 0.9 ± 0.7 ng/dL in the vesicostomy group. Both groups showed delayed growth when compared with normal age-matched controls. Serum creatinine concentration >1.0 mg/dL and the presence of VUR were significantly associated with somatic growth delay by the end of the second year. Vesicostomy appeared to assist with catchup growth in weight and height by the end of the first 2 years of life. Although all these studies vary in their conclusions, this evaluation lends support to the earlier observations of Krueger that influenced surgical management of patients with PUVs in the 1980s by suggesting that initial treatment with high urinary diversion resulted in better somatic growth.[44]

With improved instrumentation, primary valve ablation is recommended as the initial treatment modality of choice when fulguration can be performed safely and when the patient has had improvement in upper tract dilatation with catheter drainage unless the neonate is ill and small.[54] Antibiotic prophylaxis should be continued until the massive dilation of the upper urinary tract shows significant improvement, a process that may take several years. In addition, if the child has VUR, prophylaxis should be continued until the reflux resolves spontaneously or is corrected surgically. Most patients benefit not only from long-term urologic management but also from nephrologic care initiated at birth.

Common problems include significant polyuria secondary to an inability of the kidneys to concentrate urine, metabolic acidosis (which may complicate somatic growth), renal insufficiency with hypocalcemia and hyperphosphatemia, and hypertension.[55] If the patient remains clinically well with good somatic growth, periodic follow-up with sonography and evalu-

ations of electrolytes, blood urea nitrogen, creatinine, urinalysis, and blood pressure will ensure satisfactory growth and development.

PROGNOSIS FOLLOWING INITIAL THERAPY

The prognosis for satisfactory renal function may be predicted by several factors. A serum creatinine concentration <0.8 mg/dL 1 month following initial treatment or at 1 year of age is associated with favorable ultimate renal function.[54] Other investigators concluded that the most significant prognostic factor for the future development of chronic renal failure is the GFR at 1 year of age, and the development of proteinuria portends a worse prognosis.[56] These investigators found no differences in age at diagnosis, initial management, VUR status, UTI, and hypertension in the development of chronic renal insufficiency, whereas sonographic observations may be useful in identifying patients who will develop renal insufficiency. The presence of the corticomedullary junction on renal sonography has been associated with a favorable outcome.[57] This radiologic finding may not be present on the initial ultrasound study but may become apparent during the first few months of life.

In another study, Duel and colleagues[58] showed that 90% of boys with PUVs who were followed up for a mean of 8.5 years and who ultimately developed poor renal function had echogenic kidneys, whereas 46% of patients with good renal function also had echogenic kidneys. In addition, 60% of the patients with echogenic kidneys developed poor renal function compared with 13% of the patients with normal renal echogenicity. Increased cortical echogenicity and loss of corticomedullary differentiation were relatively insensitive predictors of eventual renal function in patients with PUVs. These investigators found that the serum creatinine concentration following 4 days of catheterization was a more sensitive predictor of outcome in these boys.

Achieving diurnal continence by the age of 5 years also is recognized as a favorable feature.[59] Another favorable prognostic feature is the presence of a pressure pop-off mechanism, such as massive reflux into a nonfunctioning kidney (termed the *VURD syndrome* for valves, unilateral reflux, dysplasia), urinary ascites, or a large bladder diverticulum.[60,61] Although short-term studies suggested that these mechanisms may allow more normal renal development, Cuckow and colleagues[62] reported that at 8 to 10 years of age, only 30% of boys with the VURD syndrome had a normal serum creatinine concentration. The finding that pop-off mechanisms may not always be protective was further supported by Patil and colleagues,[28] who observed that ascites may result from bladder rupture, and GFR in those patients approaches the severe renal failure range.

The detrimental or beneficial effects of reflux on renal function in patients with PUVs remain controversial. Some investigators suggest that reflux contributes to the deterioration of the upper urinary tract and others propose that reflux, especially when associated with the VURD syndrome, protects the upper urinary tract from high intravesical pressures. Hassan and colleagues[63] reported that reflux in their 73 patients did not serve as a significant prognostic factor for renal function. Alternatively, persistent reflux with or without renal deterioration in the absence of UTI may indicate bladder dysfunction and the need for lower urinary tract evaluation.

Other adverse prognostic factors include persistence of the serum creatinine concentration >1.0 mg/dL following initial therapy, identification of small subcapsular cysts beneath the renal capsule (indicative of renal dysplasia), and failure to visualize the corticomedullary junction.[54] Diurnal incontinence in patients >5 years old also is associated with a poorer prognosis. This factor probably is related to detrusor instability and detrusor sphincter dyssynergia, which can result in elevated upper urinary tract pressures and gradual deterioration in renal function.[59,64]

VESICOSTOMY CLOSURE

The decision to close a cutaneous vesicostomy must be made carefully. If the patient has had breakthrough febrile UTIs, vesicostomy closure is important because it will reduce the risk of bacterial contamination. In other patients, this procedure may be necessary as a prerequisite to renal transplantation. In most cases, vesicostomy closure is performed after the upper urinary tract has stabilized and the child is large enough to undergo simultaneous valve ablation, generally between 6 months and 3 years.

Preoperatively, VCUG should be obtained through the vesicostomy to assess the presence of significant reflux and to evaluate the bladder. In selected cases, urodynamic studies are helpful to assess bladder compliance.[65] If reflux is significant and the child is quite young, it is usually safe simply to close the vesicostomy and delay reflux correction until the child is older.

After closure of the vesicostomy, the upper urinary tract should be monitored carefully to ascertain whether hydronephrosis is worsening and ensure that the child is emptying the bladder satisfactorily. In some cases, anticholinergic medication alone or with clean intermittent catheterization may be needed to improve compliance and bladder emptying.[54] α-Blocker therapy may be effective in improving uroflowmetry and bladder emptying in some patients with PUVs.[66]

VESICOURETERAL REFLUX

VUR is present in approximately 50% of boys with PUVs at presentation, with half bilateral and half unilateral. Following valve ablation, ≥20% of patients show spon-

taneous reflux resolution and VUR may resolve as long as 3 years following initial treatment.[64] Antibiotic prophylaxis should be prescribed and assessment with cystography and upper tract imaging should be performed regularly. Hassan and colleagues[63] showed that the rate of reflux resolution was related to the function of the involved kidney, with decreased resolution rates in the more poorly functioning renal units.

VUR should be corrected if breakthrough UTIs occur or if it remains high grade. Although most pediatric urologists are adept at performing ureteral reimplantation surgery, reimplanting thick, dilated ureters into the abnormal valve bladder can be most challenging, and a 15% to 30% complication rate has been reported.[67]

Gearhart and colleagues[68] studied dilated ureters from patients with PUVs and demonstrated an increased ratio of collagen to smooth muscle. This quantitative histologic finding was associated with less distensible ureters, which may predispose to failed ureteral reimplantation. In addition, Freedman and colleagues[69] performed quantitative morphometry of 20-week gestational age bladders with PUVs and demonstrated a significant increase in both the smooth muscle and collagen components. Both these observations show that the ureter and bladder can be suboptimal tissues for reconstruction despite the surgeon's best efforts and experience. For these reasons, endoscopic therapy with dextranomer/hyaluronic acid copolymer is an attractive alternative to open surgical intervention in some cases, but no long-term data in patients with PUVs are available to support the efficacy of this approach.[70]

In boys with the VURD syndrome, nephrectomy should be performed at some point.[50] The ureter should be removed, unless the bladder is small or poorly compliant, in which case ureterocystoplasty should be considered.[71] Following this procedure, the solitary kidney should be followed carefully for the development of hydronephrosis, because the pressure pop-off mechanism has been removed.[72] Narasimhan and colleagues[73] demonstrated that when the contralateral kidney demonstrates evidence of renal scarring, renal function is more likely to be impaired.

BLADDER DYSFUNCTION

Children with PUVs have a spectrum of urodynamic findings. Favorable prognostic signs include pop-off mechanisms such as VURD syndrome (valves, unilateral reflux, unilateral renal dysplasia), bladder diverticulum, patent urachus, and urinoma.[60,61] These pop-off mechanisms protect the bladder and assist in predicting bladder function. Kaefer and associates[61] found that 71% of their patients had at least one pop-off mechanism, and 87% of these patients had favorable urodynamic findings such as satisfactory compliance and bladder capacity. Only 55% of patients without a pop-off mechanism had favorable urodynamic findings. In the group who had no pop-off mechanism and unfavorable urodynamic findings, five of seven patients underwent augmentation cystoplasty.

Urinary incontinence in patients who have a history of PUVs has several causes.[74,75] These include myogenic failure and overflow, uninhibited detrusor contractions, severe polyuria, high-pressure voiding secondary to incomplete valve resection with resultant outlet obstruction, stress urinary incontinence, and valve bladder syndrome (**Fig. 57-8**). The term *valve bladder syndrome* refers to the bladder with poor detrusor compliance resulting from fibrosis secondary to long-standing obstruction. This condition may cause secondary ureteral obstruction with worsening hydronephrosis if bladder pressure is >35 cm H_2O. The full valve bladder syndrome often is complicated by polyuria, which results from an inability of the chronically obstructed kidneys to concentrate urine. Polyuria results from nephrogenic diabetes insipidus caused by impaired medullary development with a paucity of collecting duct formation. This problem is common and may make it necessary for the child to void frequently to avoid upper urinary tract changes. Therefore, continence is difficult to achieve.

Initial therapy probably should consist of double or triple voiding. In addition, these patients usually require anticholinergic therapy and clean intermittent catheterization with or without augmentation cystoplasty.[75] Options include the usual segments of bowel, although these patients may then require bicarbonate supplementation unless stomach or ureter associated with a nonfunctioning kidney is used for augmentation.[71,76]

Koff and associates[77] evaluated the pathophysiology of the valve bladder syndrome. The investigators proposed that the cause of the valve bladder was chronic

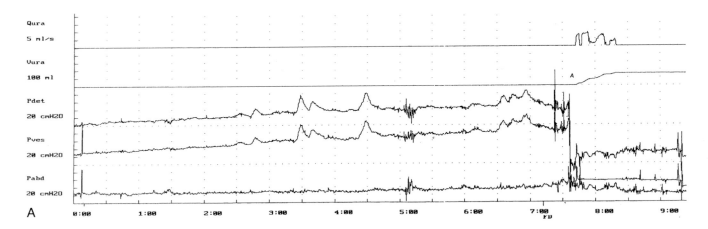

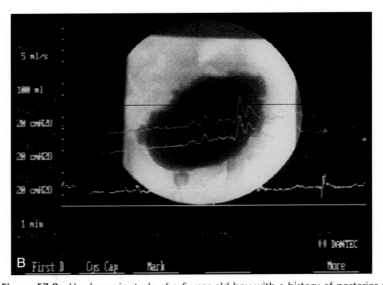

Figure 57-8 Urodynamic study of a 5-year-old boy with a history of posterior urethral valves resected at the age of 4 years. He has day and night incontinence and bilateral hydronephrosis evident on an ultrasound scan. **A,** Urodynamic tracing shows progressive loss of compliance with detrusor instability and no urinary flow with the urethral catheter in place. When the catheter is removed at A, the flow is weak and intermittent. **B,** The video portion of the study shows a trabeculated bladder with multiple diverticula and residual valve. Pabd, abdominal pressure; Pdet, detrusor pressure; Pves, total bladder pressure; Qura, uroflow rate; Vura, voided volume. *(From Horowitz M, Combs AJ, Shapiro E: Urodynamics in pediatric urology. In: Nitti VW, ed. Practical Urodynamics. Philadelphia: WB Saunders; 1998:262.)*

overdistention of the bladder during sleep as a result of polyuria, impaired bladder sensation, and residual urine. Because daytime decompression alone was insufficient, the investigators proposed nocturnal bladder emptying by placement of an indwelling catheter, intermittent nocturnal catheterization, or frequent nocturnal double voiding. Chronic hydronephrosis improved significantly or resolved completely in all patients. Serum creatinine concentrations improved in 6 of 18 patients, 4 of whom deteriorated and 2 of 4 of whom underwent renal transplantation.[77] In boys who resist overnight catheterization through the penis, a Mitrofanoff appendicovesicostomy may be performed.

Several distinguishable urodynamic patterns have been recognized in patients with PUVs and vary depending on age (**Fig. 57-9**). Holmdahl and colleagues[78] showed that the urodynamic pattern in infancy is characterized by hypercontractility and low bladder capacity. During the first 3 years of life, the pattern changes with resolution of the hypercontractility to instability with emptying difficulties. Bladder emptying resulting from some degree of myogenic failure is again seen as a late, postpubertal problem.

Holmdahl and colleagues[79] also studied bladder dysfunction before and after puberty. In prepubertal patients, urodynamic features at presentation were again noted to be uniform with hypercontractility and diminished bladder capacities. The voiding pattern in early childhood was one of small, frequent voids during the day and no voids during sleep. Hypercontractility improved with age. After puberty, the bladders were found to be highly compliant, whereas instability and emptying difficulties remained unchanged. The bladders increased to a normal capacity in the prepubertal boy, but bladder capacities were twice normal size in postpubertal patients. Fifty percent of these dilated, decompensated bladders could not develop a sustained detrusor contraction. In these patients, a Valsalva maneuver was required to empty the bladder. The development of myogenic failure may be associated with polyuria. Because the urodynamic pattern changes during infancy, in early childhood, and before and after puberty, it is important to follow up these patients carefully to identify changes that may ultimately affect upper urinary tract function and drainage.[80]

DELAYED PRESENTATION OF POSTERIOR URETHRAL VALVES

Bomalaski and colleagues[81] described 47 patients ages 5 to 35 years (mean, 8 years) who were investigated for diurnal enuresis (60%), UTI (40%), and voiding pain (13%) and were found to have PUVs. Hydronephrosis was observed in 40% and reflux in 33%. Only 10% presented with a poor urine stream, gross hematuria, and proteinuria. The serum creatinine concentration before valve ablation was elevated in 35%, whereas 10% had

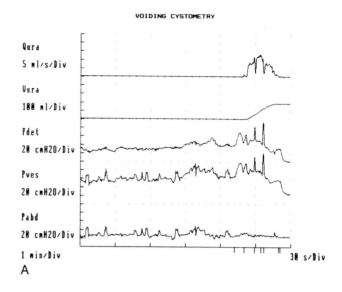

A

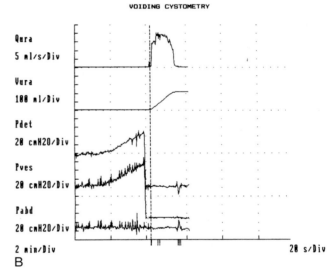

B

Figure 57-9 Urodynamic study of an 8-year-old boy with a history of posterior urethral valves who had a previous valve ablation. The child has persistent incontinence day and night. **A,** Tracing from the terminal portion of the urodynamic study demonstrating instability and impaired compliance (Pdet = 40 cm H_2O) before voiding. During voiding, with a 7-Fr urethral catheter in place, a choppy flow pattern is noted with Qmax = 14.2 mL/second with 192 mL voided and no postvoid residual. A significant component of the voiding pressure came from elevated pressure secondary to impaired compliance. **B,** Repeat study, with a faster fill, demonstrating a similar degree of impaired compliance (Pdet = 40 to 45 cm H_2O at capacity). The catheter was removed, and the patient voided with a Qmax of 20.7 mL/second with a normal shaped flow curve. This study demonstrates the existence of bladder dysfunction; however, it is not secondary to persistent obstruction. Pabd, abdominal pressure; Pdet, detrusor pressure; Pves, total bladder pressure; Qura, uroflow rate; Vura, voided volume. (*From Horowitz M, Combs AJ, Shapiro E: Urodynamics in pediatric urology. In: Nitti VW, ed.* Practical Urodynamics. *Philadelphia: WB Saunders; 1998:263.*)

ESRD at presentation. These investigators noted that if the VCUG had been performed only in patients with an abnormal renal ultrasound scan or UTI, 30% of PUVs would not have been diagnosed. Only 1 of those patients had an elevated creatinine concentration, a finding supporting the notion that severity of signs and symptoms is significantly associated with renal impairment. The investigators recommended performing VCUG in boys >5 years old who have voiding complaints especially associated with diurnal enuresis or UTI.

Schober and colleagues[82] studied a group of 70 boys (mean age, 7.46 years; range, 2-14 years) with delayed presentation of PUVs who were undergoing valve ablation. Dysfunctional voiding was the most common symptom, with nocturnal enuresis in 67% and urinary frequency in 60%. UTI occurred in 17%. Microhematuria was found in 30%, and mild age-corrected hypertension was noted in 17%. Serum creatinine concentrations were normal in all patients. Despite adequate valve resection, 63% of these patients had persistent voiding dysfunction.

Ziylan and colleagues[83] reported on a group of 36 patients with PUVs who were diagnosed at a mean age of 8.8 years (range, 5-14 years). The investigators compared the post-treatment urodynamic findings and renal function in the delayed presentation group ($n = 20$ with a mean age of 10.65 years at urodynamic evaluation) with age-matched controls who were children with PUVs diagnosed and treated at <5 years of age ($n = 19$ with a mean age of 8.52 years). Abnormal urodynamic findings included detrusor overactivity in 3 (15%), significant postvoid residual in 9 (45%), and an enlarged bladder capacity in 9 (45%) patients. No significant difference was noted in bladder capacity, compliance, or postvoid residual in the late presentation versus control group, whereas detrusor overactivity was significantly lower in the late presentation group. After approximately 5 years of follow-up, age-specific creatinine levels were increased in 13 of 27 patients with late presentation, and 7 (25.9%) of these patients developed ESRD. Renal function was significantly impaired in the late presenters compared with controls (48.1% versus 13.7%), with mean serum creatinine levels of 2.17 and 1.03 mg/dL, respectively. Although renal function was significantly impaired in the patients with late presentation, the investigators reported a similar pattern of bladder dysfunctions in this older age group with PUVs.

PROGRESSION TO END-STAGE RENAL DISEASE AND RENAL TRANSPLANTATION

Proteinuria in infancy is related to a worse prognosis.[55] Proteinuria results when the kidney has decreased functional reserve.[56] To keep up with the child's growth, the functioning nephrons undergo hyperfiltration to attempt to maintain normal renal function. Excessive filtration leads to proteinuria and focal segmental glomerulosclerosis and renal failure. In a study of boys with PUVs, proteinuria was present in 79% of patients with chronic renal failure compared with only 17% with normal renal function. One study suggested that angiotensin blockade may effectively control proteinuria and stabilize renal function in children with non-diabetic proteinuric kidney disease.[84]

Chronic renal failure affects puberty by influencing hypothalamic control of the onset and progression of pubertal growth and gonadarche, but puberty also affects chronic renal failure.[85] Pubertal acceleration of kidney dysfunction has been observed in VUR and PUVs, whereas sex steroids alter kidney growth and function. Androgens are known to stimulate the renin-angiotensin II system by producing higher blood pressures in male patients. Androgens also promote normal and abnormal kidney growth and have been shown in animals to promote kidney damage.[85]

Holmdahl and Sillén[86] reported on long-term outcomes in patients with PUVs who were 31 to 44 years old; these investigators focused on renal function, bladder function, and paternity. Of 19 male patients available for follow-up, 32% were uremic, 21% had moderate renal failure, and 47% had had no follow-up since adolescence. All patients were continent, although bladder dysfunction was reported in 40%, all of whom described detrusor weakness including weak urine stream, the need for double voiding, and urinary residual. Only 5 of 19 patients had experienced daytime continence at age 5 years. Infertility was associated with uremia. This study highlights the importance of long-term follow-up because of the risk of late renal impairment in 25% to 50%.[51] These investigators further noted that 50% of their patients who initially had favorable renal function and a low incidence of reflux had no clinical problems related to renal function.[86]

Of all male patients with ESRD, 0.2% have a primary diagnosis of congenital obstructive uropathy.[87] Although early transplant at <5 years of age is thought to result in better somatic growth and neurologic development, bladder compliance and stability at >5 years of age is usually more favorable for transplantation.[43] Specific attention has focused on treating bladder dysfunction because it influences the success of renal transplantation. Graft survival rates, patients' survival rates, and serum creatinine concentrations in boys with a history of PUVs are now similar to those of patients without bladder outlet obstruction who require renal transplantation.[88] Careful urodynamic evaluation and management of lower tract dysfunction with anticholinergic medication with or without intermittent catheterization ensure success in this selected group of patients. Most of these patients do not require bladder augmentation. If augmentation is required, it should be performed before renal transplantation and the start of long-term immunosuppression. If bladder augmentation is needed after the transplant, one should proceed when the immunosuppressive regimen has been tapered.

Salomon and associates[89] reviewed renal transplantation in 66 children with PUVs. The graft survival rates in the PUV and control groups were 69% and 72% at 5 years, and 54% and 50% at 10 years, respectively. A significant increase in serum creatinine was noted at 10 years in children with PUVs. This study suggested that renal transplantation can be successful and that long-term deterioration of graft function in the past was most likely related to lower urinary tract dysfunction.

Ross and colleagues[90] reported a 20-year experience with 16 patients with PUVs. Ten of the patients had supravesical urinary diversion before the development of ESRD. All but one kidney was transplanted to the native bladder. Two- and 5-year growth survival rates were 70% and 58%, respectively. The 15 surviving patients have allografts that were functioning at a mean of 86 months after transplantation, with a mean serum creatinine concentration of 2.0 mg/dL. Significant complications occurred in approximately 20% of transplant recipients.

More recently, DeFoor and colleagues[91] reported their experience between 1990 and 2000 with 10 patients with PUVs, mean age 10 years, who underwent 13 renal transplants. Although the mean follow-up in this report was only 3.9 years, cumulative allograft survival was 85% and 64% at 1 and 5 years, respectively. Nine of 10 patients had functioning living related donor transplants, and 1 patient lost 3 cadaveric transplants through chronic rejection. The mean serum creatinine concentration of patients with functioning grafts was 1.1 mg/dL. No grafts were lost to infection or bladder dysfunction. This study underscores the need for meticulous management of lower urinary tract dysfunction because prompt recognition and treatment of lower tract dysfunction result in successful graft function comparable to that of the general transplant population and obviate the need for augmentation cystoplasty in many cases.

CONCLUSION

The diagnosis and management of PUVs continue to evolve with improved ultrasound technology and new techniques for fetal intervention. Advances in endoscopic instrumentation permit early surgical intervention for most neonates. Improved understanding of bladder dysfunction in these boys has resulted in maximizing preservation of renal function and furthering our knowledge of the underlying pathophysiology of bladder outlet obstruction.

KEY POINTS

1. PUVs can be diagnosed during prenatal sonographic screening, but may patients present in infancy with an abdominal mass, failure to thrive, urosepsis, or urinary ascites.
2. Antenatal intervention is considered for bilateral hydroureteronephrosis and a distended bladder when hypotonic electrolytes are found on serial vesicocenteses.
3. The VCUG remains the gold standard for diagnosing PUVs.
4. Renal function is determined postnatally by following the fall in the maternal creatinine level.
5. Primary valve ablation is the treatment of choice when the urinary tract decompresses with catheter drainage.
6. A serum creatinine concentration <0.8 mg/dL 1 month following initial treatment or at 1 year of age is associated with favorable renal function.
7. Hydronephrosis may be chronic as a result of reflux, incomplete bladder emptying, or poor detrusor compliance.
8. Bladder dysfunction is manifested primarily by detrusor overactivity and incomplete bladder emptying.
9. Pop-off mechanisms including the VURD syndrome, bladder diverticulum, patent urachus, and urinomas are thought to protect the bladder.
10. Delayed presentation of PUVs should be considered in boys >5 years old who present with diurnal enuresis, UTI, voiding pain, and urinary frequency.
11. In boys with a history of PUVs, graft survival and serum creatinine concentrations following renal transplant are now similar to those in patients without bladder outlet obstruction because meticulous attention is paid to the management of lower urinary tract dysfunction.

REFERENCES

Please see www.expertconsult.com

COMPLICATIONS OF URETERAL REIMPLANTATION, ANTIREFLUX SURGERY, AND MEGAURETER REPAIR

Rosalia Misseri MD
Assistant Professor, Pediatric Urology, James Whitcomb Riley Hospital for Children, Indiana University School of Medicine, Indianapolis, Indiana

Richard C. Rink MD
Professor and Chief, Pediatric Urology, James Whitcomb Riley Hospital for Children, Indiana University School of Medicine, Indianapolis, Indiana

The first successful attempt at surgical correction of vesicoureteral reflux (VUR) was reported by Hutch in 1952.[1] Since that time, multiple surgical, endoscopic, and minimally invasive techniques have been described. Surgical correction remains the gold standard, with success rates >98% in most pediatric centers.[2,3] Despite excellent surgical results, most children with reflux are managed medically, and increasing numbers of children are managed with endoscopic techniques. Given multiple treatment options, it remains imperative that the urologist understands the potential risks and complications of each.

NONSURGICAL COMPLICATIONS

Because primary VUR often resolves, the initial management is typically nonsurgical. Although it is impossible predict which child will outgrow VUR, the disorder is most likely to resolve in younger children with lower grades of reflux.[2] The primary goal of the treatment of VUR, whether medical, surgical, or endoscopic, is to prevent pyelonephritis. Pyelonephritis may lead to reflux nephropathy with subsequent hypertension, poor somatic growth, renal insufficiency, and end-stage renal disease.

Antibiotic prophylaxis has proven effective in preventing urinary tract infection (UTI) in children with VUR.[4] Because reflux nephropathy may progress in patients with recurrent UTI, it is imperative to maintain sterile urine with daily antimicrobial prophylaxis.[5] The effectiveness of the use of continuous prophylactic antibiotics in preventing breakthrough UTI and renal scars is well supported in the literature. Rates of breakthrough UTI and renal scarring in patients compliant with antibiotic treatment are reported to be as low as <5% and 0.5%, respectively.[6,7] Certainly, with longer periods of conservative management (5-10 years), the risk of UTI-related morbidity is likely to increase.

Unfortunately, despite aggressive medical and surgical management of VUR, reflux nephropathy accounts for 3% to 25% of cases of end-stage renal disease in children and 10% to 15% of cases of renal failure in adults.[8-11] Reflux-related complications also increase the risk of pregnancy-related morbidity including UTI, pregnancy-related hypertension, and low birth weight.[12]

Risks of Medical Management

Some uncertainty exists regarding the ideal antimicrobial prophylaxis for use in this population. The most commonly used antibiotics include sulfamethoxazole-trimethoprim, trimethoprim alone, nitrofurantoin, and amoxicillin for neonates and young infants, in doses one fourth to one half of treatment doses on a daily basis. Although side effects are lower than with treatment doses, adverse effects are reported.[13] Common side effects of sulfamethoxazole-trimethoprim including allergic skin reactions, nausea, vomiting, and diarrhea are reported in 15% to 22% of patients.[2] Additional adverse effects are neutropenia, thrombocytopenia, and photosensitivity reaction. Stevens-Johnson syndrome, although extremely rare, is the most serious side effect.

Nitrofurantoin suspension may cause gastric upset, nausea, vomiting, rash, and fever. Its foul taste may worsen compliance with treatment. Liver toxicity and interstitial pneumonitis are rare but reported with the use of nitrofurantoin. The use of the macrocrystal preparation eliminates the foul taste, gastric upset, nausea, and vomiting.

Because fructose is used to prepare drug suspensions, children may be at increased risk of dental caries. Sulfa-based drugs and nitrofurantoin are contraindicated in children <2 months old because these drugs are hepatically metabolized. For this reason, amoxicillin and cephalexin are used in the first 2 months of life. To date, no data suggest that the use of low-dose antibiotics for urinary prophylaxis is dangerous.

Patient and family compliance with respect to daily prophylaxis and follow-up certainly affects successful prevention of pyelonephritis and reflux nephropathy. In a public health system model, compliance rates exceeded 90%.[6] However, >34% of patients with reflux in the United States are lost to follow-up.[14]

Current recommendations for patients with unresolved reflux after years of medical management vary, ranging from surgical correction of moderate-grade reflux after 4 years of observation[15] to complete discontinuance of antibiotic prophylaxis and clinical monitoring of patients after 6 or 7 years of age.[16] The recommendations of the American Urological Association (AUA) are to proceed with surgical therapy for children 6 to 10 years old who have moderate- to high-grade VUR with or without scarring. No recommendations for lower grades of reflux are available because of a lack of consensus.[2] Currently, the AUA is updating the consensus report. In female patients, ongoing VUR may increase the risk of pyelonephritis, especially during pregnancy and with sexual activity.[17,18] Therefore, surgical or endoscopic therapy may be warranted in female patients regardless of VUR grade if the disorder does not resolve.

BLADDER DYNAMICS AND VESICOURETERAL REFLUX

Patients with voiding dysfunction often present with wetting, UTI, and VUR. Treatment of the underlying disease with a combination of bladder retraining, treatment of constipation, anticholinergic therapy, and biofeedback frequently eliminates incontinence, UTI, and at times VUR and thus obviates the need for surgical or endoscopic intervention. Normal voiding habits and normal bladder dynamics are essential for successful antireflux surgery. One of the most common problems with failed reimplants is undiagnosed or underestimated bladder disease. This error may have a significant effect on surgical and endoscopic outcomes and also increases the risk of postoperative UTIs. Most cases of persistent postoperative reflux will likely resolve with the treatment of voiding dysfunction.[19]

SURGICAL COMPLICATIONS OF URETERAL REIMPLANTATION IN THE NONDILATED URETER

Technical Considerations

Many different techniques with similar success rates have been described for ureteral reimplantation. The technical aspects of these procedures are discussed else-

where and are not reviewed here.[20-22] To ensure a successful result, several common principles of ureteral reimplantation must be followed. The most critical point is to provide adequate detrusor backing for the ureter in its submucosal tunnel. As advocated by Hendren,[23] an atraumatic no-touch technique should be employed to mobilize the ureter. Submucosal tunnel lengths should be four to five times the ureteral diameter. Other important technical considerations include the following:

1. Preservation of ureteral blood supply
2. Creation of a tension-free anastomosis
3. Adequate proximal and distal ureteral fixation
4. Adequate closure of the muscular hiatus
5. Placement of the hiatus posteriorly and medially, in the immobile portion of the bladder
6. Avoidance of ureteral torsion, kinking, or J-hooking

Postoperative Evaluation and Identification of Complications

Complications of antireflux surgical procedures may be evident in the immediate postoperative period; however, many complications do not become evident until years after an assumed successful repair. Early complications of antireflux surgical procedures are symptomatic and clinically evident, whereas late complications are often asymptomatic. We typically obtain a renal ultrasound scan 4 weeks postoperatively to evaluate for hydronephrosis. Dilation of the upper urinary tract may be seen as a result of edema at the ureterovesical junction (UVJ) if the image is obtained <4 weeks after the procedure. If dilation is noted on the postoperative ultrasound scan, a diuretic renal scan is obtained to rule out significant obstruction.

We no longer routinely obtain postoperative voiding cystourethrograms (VCUGs) after uncomplicated reimplant procedures at our institution. Although this practice is supported by other surgeons,[24,25] the decision to obtain a postoperative VCUG should be based on the surgeon's experience and individual success rates. If a VCUG is obtained, it should be performed 3 to 4 months postoperatively to allow for resolution of edema or inflammation of the submucosal tunnel. Suppressive antibiotics are continued for 3 months postoperatively. Renal ultrasound scans are obtained on a yearly basis for 3 to 4 years to screen for delayed complications of surgical treatment of VUR. Yearly blood pressure measurements and urinalysis are obtained to identify hypertension in children with renal scarring and UTI.

Early Complications

Low Urine Output

Low urine output may be a sign of several different complications of antireflux surgical procedures. The most frequent cause of decreased urine output (<1 mL/kg/hour) after ureteral reimplantation is mild ureteral obstruction secondary to transient edema at the UVJ. Mild dehydration secondary to preoperative fasting and supraphysiologic secretion of antidiuretic hormone in response to surgical stress also contribute to low urine output. This condition generally responds to fluid boluses (10 mL/kg lactated Ringer's solution or 0.9% normal saline solution) and resolves ≤4 to 6 hours after the surgical procedure with no long-term sequelae. Dehydration may be avoided with vigorous intraoperative hydration to compensate for fasting and third-space losses.

Profound oliguria and anuria occur infrequently and most commonly in bilateral cases or after surgical correction of reflux in a solitary kidney. In both unilateral and bilateral obstruction, the patient may complain of worsening abdominal pain, nausea, and vomiting. Oliguria or anuria can be a sign of a technical error leading to ureteral obstruction or of severe ureteral or UVJ edema. It may be worsened by bladder spasm or obstruction of the orifices by the balloon of the urethral catheter. Treatment with anticholinergics and removal of the balloon catheter are useful in differentiating between these factors. Overly aggressive fluid replacement with hypotonic solutions should be avoided because it may lead to hyponatremia. A renal and bladder ultrasound scan is useful if oliguria persists after volume replacement. Hydroureteronephrosis or urinary extravasation may be evident (**Fig. 58-1**). These findings may be confirmed with a diuretic renal scan (**Fig. 58-2**).

Decompression of the upper urinary tract with a temporary percutaneous nephrostomy tube with or without ureteral stenting is recommended in cases of ureteral obstruction. We agree with surgeons who advocate early stent internalization to avoid a "dry reimplant."[22] The ability to place a retrograde stent is limited in the early postoperative period, particularly after a Cohen ureteroneocystostomy. Open retrograde stent placement may become necessary if less invasive techniques fail. Stents are generally left in place for 4 to 6 weeks to allow for resolution of edema at the UVJ. The ultimate outcome is usually that of a successful reimplant. Once the stent is removed, urine output is monitored and serial renal ultrasound scans are obtained. If hydroureteronephrosis persists, a diuretic renal scan is obtained and the patient is treated accordingly (see later). In our practice, ureters that are plicated or tapered and the ureter of a solitary kidney are routinely stented at the time of reimplant.

Postoperative urinary extravasation is an uncommon problem and is usually related to inadequate closure of the detrusorotomy. This complication can be managed conservatively by replacing the urethral catheter for an additional 72 hours. Some surgeons routinely prefer to leave perivesical Penrose drains after reimplantation,

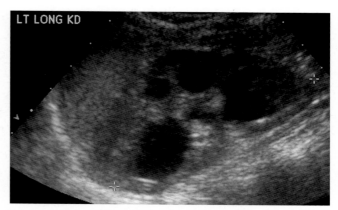

Figure 58-1   Renal ultrasound scan 2 days after routine ureteral reimplantation shows moderate hydronephrosis. LT LONG KD, left longitudinal kidney.

although we have not found this approach to be necessary.

Infections and Voiding Dysfunction

Postoperative febrile UTI and urosepsis may occur after reimplantation. A preoperative urine culture is obtained 5 to 7 days before the surgical procedure. If results of the culture are positive and the patient is asymptomatic, the patient is treated with the appropriate antibiotics. If the patient is asymptomatic, the bladder is inspected cystoscopically to identify signs of inflammation before the incision is made. Inflammation may increase both the difficulty of the surgery and postoperative complications. If the preoperative culture grows unusual or resistant organisms or if a patient is symptomatic, urine culture should be repeated and results should be negative before the surgical procedure is performed. Generally, we postpone the operation to allow the inflammatory response to resolve.

The incidence of recurrent cystitis after successful reimplantation has been reported to be ≤32% to 39%, and ≤8% of patients have clinical pyelonephritis.[26,27] Parents should be forewarned of this complication because it may cause severe anxiety in the postoperative period.

Transient voiding dysfunction is common after intravesical ureteral reimplantation. Daytime urge incontinence, nocturnal enuresis, and urinary retention may continue for several weeks. These symptoms typically resolve as bladder inflammation resolves. Patients with significant bladder spasm or pain on urination may require anticholinergic therapy or phenazopyridine HCl.

Postoperative urinary retention is rare following intravesical reimplantation. However, much concern and controversy exist regarding urinary retention after bilateral extravesical repair. The reported incidence of urinary retention after bilateral extravesical repair varies from 3.2% to >22%.[28-31] In the series reported by Fung

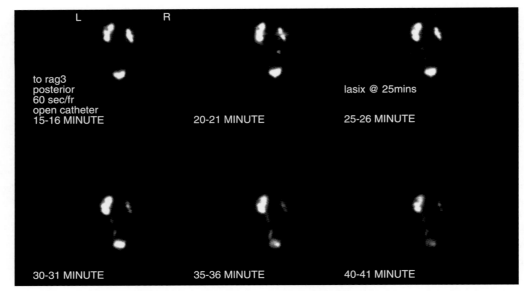

Figure 58-2 Diuretic renal scan confirms obstruction at the ureterovesical junction. This obstruction may be related to edema in the early postoperative period.

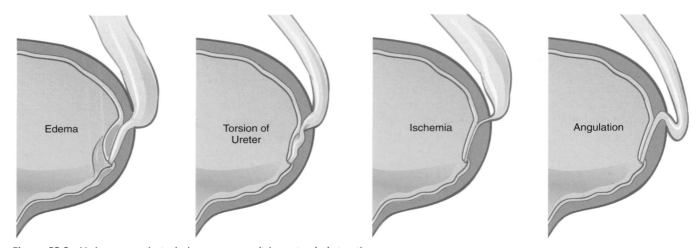

Figure 58-3 Various errors in techniques may result in ureteral obstruction.

and colleagues,[31] urinary retention persisted in 5.2% of their patients at 8 weeks postoperatively, and two patients had prolonged urinary retention and required temporary cutaneous vesicostomy and a catheterizable channel. Nerve-sparing techniques have been described because urinary retention is thought to be the result of neurapraxia related to detrusor nerve manipulation.[32] Using such modifications, the rate of immediate urinary retention was reported to be 2% with no long-term urinary retention or voiding dysfunction.

Following transvesical reimplant, hematuria is expected to persist for several weeks as the detrusor and mucosa heal and as spasms resolve. Meticulous closure of mucosal incisions minimizes this problem. Although rare, retrovesical hematoma may result in ureteral obstruction.[33] To avoid this complication, great care

must be taken when the ureter is dissected, particularly in the retroperitoneum.

Late Complications

Ureteral Obstruction
When prolonged ureteral obstruction occurs postoperatively or when obstruction is identified during routine follow-up, the cause is not typically related to transient edema, as is common in the early postoperative period. Late ureteral obstruction may be associated with abdominal or flank pain, nausea, vomiting, or UTI or it may be completely asymptomatic.

Late ureteral obstruction is most commonly the result of an error in surgical technique (**Fig. 58-3**). The most common causes of obstruction are mechanical obstruction and devascularization of the distal ureter. Ureteral obstruction is rare, occurring in <2% of case.[2,34] Although technical problems may become apparent early in the postoperative period, they are more commonly noted on radiographic examination in an asymptomatic patient. Often these changes are associated with significant loss of renal function.[35,36] It is unlikely that ureteral obstruction diagnosed early in the postoperative period that does not resolve spontaneously or after stent placement or obstruction diagnosed long after the surgical procedure will improve without reoperation.

The diagnosis of obstruction can be made with ultrasound or renal scan. A diuretic renal scan has the additional advantage of estimating the function of the affected kidney. Occasionally, an antegrade nephrostogram or Whitaker study may become necessary to differentiate persistent nonobstructive hydronephrosis from true obstruction (**Fig. 58-4**).

Devascularization of the distal ureteral segment may lead to ischemia and stricture. Devascularization may be avoided by gentle manipulation of the ureter and cautious use of electrocautery when the ureter is dissected from the detrusor hiatus. Torsion of the reimplanted ureter within the submucosal tunnel can also lead to obstruction. Placement of a traction suture at the ureteral meatus allows for gentler manipulation of the ureter. Additionally, this suture serves as a marker for proper orientation after mobilization of the ureter.

The submucosal tunnel should be created with care to ensure adequate width, length, and hemostasis. Bleeding from the submucosal tunnel can cause ureteral compression and early postoperative obstruction. The submucosal tunnel should allow the ureter to sit freely within it without compression. The distal ureter is anchored to the detrusor muscle with a long-lasting absorbable suture to prevent ureteral retraction. An additional suture is used to secure the ureter to the detrusor muscle at the level of the hiatus to provide two-point fixation of the ureter at both ends of the submucosal tunnel. The ureter should be approximated to the bladder mucosa with a fine absorbable suture to prevent the uncommon complication of ureteral meatal obstruction.[37]

If the new ureteral hiatus is placed too far laterally on the mobile portion of the bladder, especially when one uses the Leadbetter-Politano technique or other suprahiatal techniques, intermittent ureteral obstruction caused by "J hooking" and obstruction of the ureter as the bladder fills can result.[38] This diagnosis can be difficult to make because the complication manifests silently and requires upper urinary tract studies with the bladder empty and full. If the obstruction is mild and is identified with only significant bladder filling, these patients can be managed with frequent bladder emptying because the functional obstruction occurs only when the bladder is full.

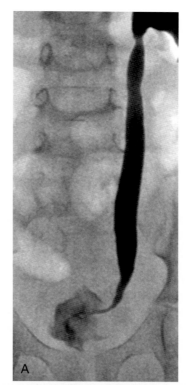

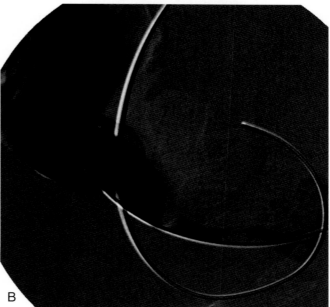

Figure 58-4 A, Antegrade nephrostogram shows narrowing at the ureterovesical junction. This condition was secondary to edema and resolved. **B,** Antegrade nephrostogram demonstrates massive dilation of the proximal ureter. The obstruction resulted from ischemia and required a tapered reimplant with a psoas hitch.

Most patients with J hooking require revisionary surgical procedures. This complication is related to redundancy in the ureter or lateral placement of the hiatus and therefore requires straightening and excision of the redundant ureter or movement of the ureteral hiatus medially onto the fixed portion of the posterior bladder wall.

Ureteral obstruction may also occur with a narrow neohiatus, a hiatal defect that is closed too tightly, or an acute angulation as the ureter enters the submucosal tunnel (commonly the result of a prominent lip of tissue at the detrusor hiatus). Kinking and narrowing may be avoided by incising some detrusor fibers at the inferior portion of the neohiatus to create a trough for the ureter.[22,39]

If the original hiatus is used, the defect must be closed carefully to ensure adequate mobility of the ureter within the detrusor portion of the tunnel. The hiatus should be left wide enough to allow passage of a tonsil clamp or similarly size instrument adjacent to the ureter. In this manner, the hiatus is of sufficient caliber to prevent constriction but is narrow enough to prevent formation of a postoperative diverticulum. The incidence of postoperative diverticulum has been reported to be ≤17% following a Cohen reimplantation. Diverticula have been blamed for both recurrent reflux and postoperative obstruction.[40]

Care must be taken to pass the ureter under direct vision during transvesical procedures that require creation of a neohiatus, to avoid passage of the ureter into and out of the peritoneal cavity. Late ureteral obstruction has been attributed to adhesions within the transperitoneal course of the ureter, placement of the ureter through bowel segments, and placement of the ureter through the broad ligament.[35,41,42] Blunt dissection of the peritoneum off the posterior bladder wall and passage of a right angle through the neohiatus under direct vision should help prevent these complications.

In male patients, care must be taken to avoid injury to the vas deferens during transvesical mobilization of the ureter. Additionally, ureteral obstruction may occur if the hiatus is moved superiorly within the bladder and ureter is not moved anterior to the vas, with resulting acute angulation.

Postoperative Reflux

Ipsilateral Reflux

Following surgical treatment of VUR, reflux may persist in the affected ureter or may occur in the contralateral ureter in approximately 2% and ≤32% of patients, respectively.[2,43] Significant evidence indicates that persistent reflux, identified on postoperative VCUG, may resolve without intervention because it may be caused by a transient voiding dysfunction and inflammation. Persistent postoperative VUR is reported to resolve spontaneously in 24% to 100% of cases.[44-49] Because the rate of postoperative resolution of persistent reflux is so high, our practice is to prescribe long-term prophylactic antibiotics for these patients. A repeat VCUG is delayed for approximately 1 year.

Persistent reflux is most commonly attributed to inadequate tunnel length, but it may also result from persistent inflammation at the submucosal tunnel (**Fig. 58-5**). An infrequent cause of postoperative reflux is the development of a ureterovesical fistula.[50,51] Formation of a ureterovesical fistula is attributed to entrapment and devascularization of the intravesical portion of the ureter with suture used to close the bladder mucosa. This complication can usually be recognized on cystoscopy and requires reoperation with resection of the ureter distal to the fistula with remobilization of the ureter and reimplantation with an appropriate tunnel. Bladder diverticulum at the hiatus may prevent adequate tunnel length and may result in persistent reflux.

Contralateral Reflux

The incidence of contralateral reflux after unilateral reimplantation is 0.6% to 32%.[42,52-54] Spontaneous reso-

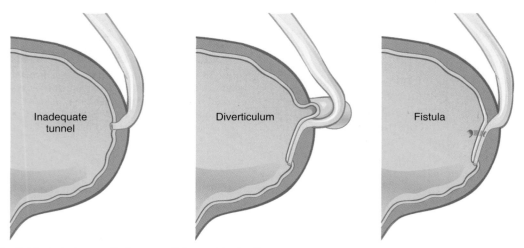

Inadequate tunnel   Diverticulum   Fistula

Figure 58-5 Potential technical errors that can result in persistent reflux.

lution has been reported in 61% to 98% of cases with a minimum of 3 years of follow-up, and most investigators recommend observation while the patient is receiving prophylactic antibiotics as an initial treatment measure.[23,43,52,53,55] Additionally, treatment of voiding dysfunction, if present, with behavioral modification, medical therapy, or both is indicated during this period. In children with breakthrough UTIs, correction of postoperative reflux should be considered. Although most cases of postoperative contralateral reflux resolve spontaneously, this potential risk should be discussed preoperatively.

Several reasons have been proposed for the development of contralateral reflux. An incidence of contralateral VUR of ≤18% was reported by Hoenig and Diamond and their colleagues.[56] Warren and colleagues[43] suggested that patients with an abnormal shape or position of the ureter were at greatest risk. Other theories to explain contralateral VUR include operative trigonal distortion or a pop-off mechanism; however, these theories have been challenged.[56-61] In a review of 107 patients, Noe[62] identified two possible contributors to contralateral VUR: (1) age at initial operation, which correlates with a smaller number of cystograms and fewer opportunities to identify contralateral VUR; and (2) the presence of dysfunctional voiding. Like many other surgeons, we perform bilateral reimplants in any patient with a history of bilateral VUR even after unilateral spontaneous resolution.

Managing the Failed Reimplant

A reoperative surgical procedure after failed (persistent reflux or obstruction) ureteral reimplantation is often difficult and involves longer operative times. Surgical planes are challenging, and the risk of future complications related to devascularization and contralateral ureteral injury is increased. More aggressive extravesical mobilization and the use of a psoas hitch or a Boari flap are more likely to become necessary to prevent reflux successfully in repeat surgical procedures.

Patients whose initial reimplant fails should receive long-term antibiotic prophylaxis. Reevaluation of reflux should include renal and bladder ultrasound scan, VCUG, and diuretic renal scan. Additional studies including a Whitaker test may be necessary in cases of equivocal obstruction. We believe that all children with persistent reflux after reimplantation should undergo urodynamic evaluation.

In a child with postoperative obstruction, reoperation should be delayed for ≥3 to 6 months to allow the distal ureter to reestablish sufficient vascularity. Diversion with a percutaneous nephrostomy tube decompresses the collecting system and permits repeat investigation with a Whitaker test if necessary.

If the decision is made to reoperate on a child with persistent reflux or obstruction, the surgeon must indi-

vidualize the management of each patient and be prepared with a variety of reconstructive options. Preoperative cystoscopy may aid in identifying a short mucosal tunnel, diverticulum, or fistula as the cause of persistent VUR. Retrograde ureteropyelography or intravenous urography can provide useful information about the severity of ischemic changes or angulation of the distal ureter if an antegrade study cannot be performed. Occasionally, the ureteral orifice may be completely obliterated by severe scarring.[35]

Various procedures have been used for reoperative ureteral reimplantation including the Cohen, Leadbetter-Politano, Paquin, and a combined intravesical-extravesical approach, each with good results.[30,63-65] We have usually been able to mobilize the ureter adequately through the Pfannenstiel incision, although a vertical midline incision may also be employed for more exposure. The ureter must be carefully mobilized, to preserve all tissue surrounding the ureter. Sacrificing the gonadal vessels to improve the blood supply to the distal ureter is occasionally necessary and has been suggested by some surgeons. If the ureter is dilated >1 cm, it should be tapered to allow an adequate submucosal tunnel. A psoas hitch may be necessary when the ureter is short or when a longer tunnel for a tapered reimplant is necessary.[64,66] In rare cases, bowel interposition, transureteroureterostomy, or transureteropyelostomy may be necessary.[64,67] Percutaneous balloon dilation of UVJ strictures following reimplantation of the ureter has been described in a limited number of patients with favorable short-term outcomes.[68]

Dextranomer/hyaluronic acid (Dx/HA) has been used as an alternative to reoperation in patients with persistent postoperative VUR.[69,70] In each series, patients identified with postoperative VUR were initially observed. During the period of observation, Jung and colleagues[70] maintained patients on antibiotic prophylaxis and treated voiding dysfunction in those affected. Seventy to 80% of the renal units injected had complete resolution of reflux after one injection. A second injection was successful in two thirds of the patients in the series by Jung and colleagues.[70] No complications resulting from injections were reported.

COMPLICATIONS OF ENDOSCOPIC CORRECTION OF VESICOURETERAL REFLUX

Endoscopic therapy of VUR was first introduced in 1984.[71] This technique has become increasingly popular since the introduction of Dx/HA (Deflux, Q-Med Scandinavia), which was approved for use in the United States in 2001. Dx/HA is indicated for the treatment of grade II to IV VUR. The use of this agent is contraindicated in patients with active voiding dysfunction, UTI, ureters with associated Hutch diverticulum, ureteroceles, and nonfunctioning kidneys.[72] The treatment of duplex systems has not been studied prospectively.

Success rates between 76% and 94% have been reported after a single injection.[73,74] However, these successes vary based on the experience of the endoscopist, the grade of reflux, the underlying bladder disease, and ureteral anomalies such as duplications and ectopia.[75-78] The incidence of contralateral reflux following endoscopic injection with Dx/HA ranges from 4.5% to 12.5%.[74,79,80]

In cases of failed Dx/HA, the material appears to migrate away from the subureteric orifice or migrates to the extravesical space or along the periureteral sheath (**Fig. 58-6**). Although this issue is controversial, volume reduction may occur in time and may lead to failure.[72,81,82] In the meta-analysis by Elder and associates,[83] repeat therapy was successful in 68% of ureters, whereas Elmore and colleagues[82] reported a success rate in 89% of ureters undergoing second injections.

Open ureteral reimplantation after failed injection is more difficult than is a primary open reimplantation procedure and may be related to granuloma formation secondary to injection. In our practice, higher rates of obstruction have been noted after open reimplantation for failed injection therapy.[84] In addition to persistence of reflux and new contralateral reflux, extravesical ureteral obstruction has also been reported (**Fig. 58-7**).[85] Given the relatively recent introduction of injection therapy, it remains difficult to comment on long-term complications.

SURGICAL COMPLICATIONS OF LAPAROSCOPIC/ROBOTIC REIMPLANT

Both extravesical and transvesical laparoscopic and robotic ureteral reimplantation procedures have been performed. Some significant series have been reported. Correction of reflux varied from 47% in one group with follow-up of 30 to 37 months[86] to 99% after modifications in technique in another group.[87] Higher success rates using open procedures, the ease of endoscopic therapy, and limited access to a robot have made minimally invasive techniques a less attractive option for most urologists.

SURGICAL COMPLICATIONS OF MEGAURETER REPAIR

Some controversy exists regarding the timing of megaureter repair. Today, many children with megaureters present as asymptomatic neonates referred for evaluation of antenatal hydroureteronephrosis.[88,89] Surgical treatment of the refluxing megaureter and of the nonrefluxing, nonobstructed megaureter is often unnecessary because improvement in high-grade reflux occurs commonly in the first year life.[2] The megaureter that is neither refluxing nor obstructed often maintains normal function and reverts to normal caliber in time.[90] Obstructed refluxing megaureters often require surgical

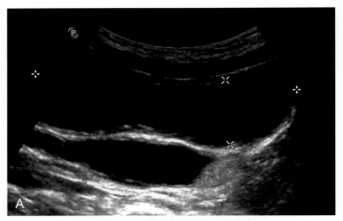

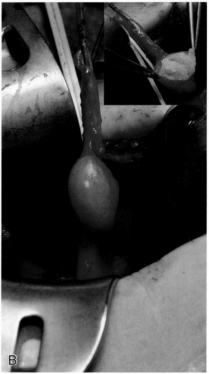

Figure 58-6 Migration of dextranomer/hyaluronic acid used in the treatment of vesicoureteral reflux. **A,** Hyperechoic material at the distal end of the ureter. **B,** Encapsulated migrated material consistent with ultrasound findings. The *inset* shows the granular makeup of dextranomer/hyaluronic acid.

intervention. However, the treatment of obstructed megaureters remains controversial.[85,91,92]

Regardless of the timing or indications for megaureter repair, the procedure is technically challenging and carries a significantly greater risk of postoperative complications than in the case of a nondilated ureter.[87] Reconstruction of the megaureter may be achieved using an excisional technique described by Hendren[93] or by one of the imbricating methods, most commonly those described by Starr[94] and Kalicinski and colleagues.[95]

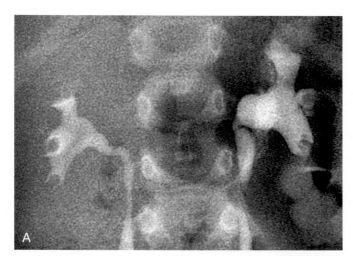

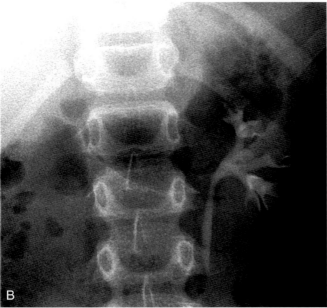

Figure 58-7   A, Preoperative voiding cystourethrograms with bilateral VUR after endoscopic therapy. **B,** Postoperative voiding cystourethrograms with resolution of right VUR and minimal improvement of left VUR. The dextranomer/hyaluronic acid "mound" was not sonographically identified on the left.

Excisional tapering of a megaureter requires careful attention to ureteral blood supply during resection of the redundant ureter and closure of the tapered ureter. Injury to the vascular supply of the ureter may lead to devascularization, obstruction, fistula, and urinary leakage. Inherent ureteral characteristics such as increased collagen and altered smooth muscle of the distal ureter may also contribute to surgical failure.[87,96,97] Reported success rates for excisional tapering range from 74% to 90%.[98-102]

Tapering should be performed when a submucosal tunnel long enough to fulfill the 5:1 rule of tunnel length to ureteral diameter cannot be achieved. Hendren's series[93] remains the largest reported, and the complications are well detailed.[90,98] Of 160 patients with primary and secondary megaureter, 14 had transient obstruction requiring percutaneous nephrostomy tubes, 11 had obstruction requiring reoperation, and 8 had postoperative reflux, for an overall success rate of 88%.

Success rates for imbricated techniques are slightly better and are reported to be 93% to 95%, with lower rates of vascular injury when compared with excisional techniques.[92,95,96,101,103] The slightly better success rates in the imbricated group may be a consequence of selection bias because plication was limited to ureters with smaller diameters in some studies.[96] Persistent reflux, seen in both the Kalicinski and Starr techniques, is most likely the result of failure of reimplantation rather than failure to narrow the ureter. The plicated ureter is bulky, a characteristic that renders creation of a submucosal tunnel more difficult.[104] One of the greatest advantages of folding and plication techniques is that these procedures can be performed on moderately dilated ureters entirely intravesically.

Patients in whom megaureter repair has failed and patients with iatrogenic megaureter secondary to obstruction after ureteral reimplantation must be carefully evaluated for factors contributing to treatment failure such as voiding dysfunction or poor bladder compliance. Patients with new or persistent VUR after megaureter repair should be given prophylactic antibiotics because reflux may resolve with observation.

In cases of obstruction, a percutaneous nephrostomy tube should be placed. Occasionally, the obstruction resolves with diminishing edema. Upper urinary tract drainage with the nephrostomy tube allows for antegrade radiographic examinations, Whitaker tests, and time for healing before a corrective surgical procedure is attempted. Altered ureteral histologic features may limit the ureter's capacity for proper peristalsis. As in any reimplantation procedure, bladder dynamics must be examined. In some cases clean intermittent catheterization, anticholinergics, or frequent bladder emptying may become necessary.

SURGICAL COMPLICATIONS OF URETEROCELE REPAIR

A *ureterocele* is a cystic dilation of the terminal ureter within the bladder, urethra, or both that creates diagnostic and therapeutic dilemmas once it is identified. Management of ureterocele varies and depends on the presence of obstruction, reflux, and incontinence, as well as the function of the affected kidney or renal moiety. Ureteroceles occur most commonly in white patients and are four to six times more frequent in girls than in boys.[105] Ectopic ureteroceles are four times more common than are intravesical ureteroceles.[106]

Today, ureteroceles are more likely to be diagnosed based on prenatal ultrasonography rather than on UTI. Hydronephrosis and dysplasia of the upper pole moiety are commonly associated with a ureterocele.[104] Rarely, ureteroceles may manifest with bladder outlet obstruction because ectopic ureteroceles can prolapse. Ureteroceles found in adults are usually intravesical and are associated with a single collecting system. Adult ureteroceles may be acquired rather than congenital, as in children. Function of the affected kidney is less likely to be impaired in an adult.[107]

The diagnosis of ureterocele may be difficult. A ureterocele may be collapsed and thus not visible on an ultrasound scan if the bladder is overfilled. If the bladder is underfilled, a large ureterocele may fill the entire bladder and give the impression of a partially filled bladder. A VCUG should be obtained to evaluate for VUR in association with the ureterocele. Reflux to the ipsilateral lower pole occurs in approximately 50% of cases, and contralateral reflux occurs in approximately 25%. This complication is likely the result of distortion of the bladder base by the ureterocele.[108] Occasionally, a ureterocele may evert during VCUG and resemble a diverticulum. Nuclear renal scans are useful to evaluate the function of the moiety associated with the ureterocele and that of other moieties. Poorly functioning moieties may not be worth salvaging.

Once the ureterocele has been radiographically evaluated, treatments range from endoscopic decompression to complex reconstruction. Nonoperative management has also been advocated in cases involving nonobstructed duplex systems with relatively good preservation of renal function, associated multicystic dysplastic moieties, or completely nonfunctioning upper pole moieties.[109] Additionally, watchful waiting may have a role in cases of prenatally detected ureteroceles without bladder outlet obstruction, ipsilateral lower moiety obstruction, and ipsilateral lower moiety VUR less than grade IV.[110]

It is beyond the scope of this chapter to discuss each of the different management techniques; however, the complications encountered are directly related to the treatment options selected. Endoscopic incision or puncture is simple and minimally invasive. It typically requires a short anesthetic regimen and usually can be performed as an outpatient procedure. The procedure has been reported to offer definitive therapy in ≤93% of patients with intravesical ureteroceles.[111] No consensus exists on the effectiveness of technique for treating ectopic ureteroceles. Although it may not be curative, incision may relieve obstruction of both the involved and uninvolved moieties and may thus prevent further loss of function and UTI.

If incision does not result in a cure, it allows the delay of definitive treatment until the child has grown. Additionally, the decompressed system may be easier to reconstruct.[112-114] Other investigators have argued that this approach may commit the child to future lower urinary tract reconstruction.[115] Despite controversy, investigators agree that endoscopic puncture of an ectopic ureterocele is indicated for patients with uncon-

trolled sepsis, azotemia, and bladder outlet obstruction. New reflux may be created in 30% to 47% of patients as a consequence of ureterocele incision, and the procedure may fail to decompress the involved moiety in 10% to 25% of cases.[108,111]

The traditional upper urinary tract approach for ureteroceles associated with a duplicated collecting system and minimal function of the upper pole segment is partial nephrectomy with subtotal removal of the upper pole ureter and ureterocele aspiration. Complications of upper pole heminephrectomy include inadvertent ligation of branch vessels to the lower pole resulting in devascularization. Additionally, traction on the lower pole of the kidney may lead to intimal injury and thrombosis of lower pole vessels. Consequently, significant atrophy of the lower pole occurs in 7% to 10% of cases.[116,117] Careful handling and the use of topical papaverine (30 mg/mL) to prevent vasospasm minimize this complication. Additional complications include prolonged urine leak as a result of entrance into the lower pole collecting system, hemorrhage, and new-onset lower pole VUR. Postoperatively, the ureterocele may prolapse and urinary retention may occur in ≤10% of patients.[114]

Complete reconstruction of the ureterocele includes partial nephrectomy, excision of the ureterocele, and reimplantation of the lower pole ureter in patients with a nonfunctioning upper pole or ureterocelectomy and a common sheath reimplant with or without tapering in patients with preservable function in the upper pole. The ureterocele must be excised in its entirety to avoid postoperative urinary retention secondary to an obstructing lip of tissue.

Ureteral reimplantation associated with a ureterocele is more difficult than is uncomplicated reimplantation and is associated with higher failure rates. To increase the chance of success, our recommendation is to create the tunnel for reimplantation above the area of ureterocele excision. This technique allows normal muscle backing for the reimplanted ureter and precludes working in the area of the reconstructed bladder base or marsupialized ureterocele. Success rates for reimplantation of single system ureteroceles approach those of uncomplicated reimplantation procedures.

Other potential complications of ureterocele excision include bladder neck injury, urinary incontinence, bladder diverticulum, vesicovaginal fistula, and urethrocutaneous fistula. These complications may be avoided with careful dissection of the posterior wall of the ureterocele off the bladder neck musculature and reconstruction with approximation of the attenuated bladder neck.

CONCLUSION

Ureteral reimplantation of a normal-caliber ureter into a normal bladder can be accomplished successfully with minimal complications. Newer endoscopic techniques are also successful and have few associated complications. Successful outcomes depend on thorough preoperative evaluation of bladder dynamics and meticulous surgical technique. Careful postoperative evaluation allows early recognition and treatment of the uncommon complications.

KEY POINTS

1. Open surgical correction of VUR remains the gold standard, with success rates >98% in most pediatric centers.

2. The primary goal of the treatment of VUR is to prevent pyelonephritis that may lead to reflux nephropathy with subsequent hypertension, poor somatic growth, renal insufficiency, and end-stage renal disease.

3. Despite aggressive medical and surgical management, reflux nephropathy accounts for 3% to 25% of cases of end-stage renal disease in children and 10% to 15% of cases of renal failure in adults.

4. Undiagnosed or underestimated bladder disease is a common cause of failed ureteral reimplants.

5. Important technical considerations for ureteral reimplantation include the following:
   - Adequate detrusor backing for the ureter in its submucosal tunnel
   - Preservation of the ureteral blood supply
   - Creation of a tension-free anastomosis
   - Adequate proximal and distal ureteral fixation
   - Adequate closure of the muscular hiatus
   - Placement of the hiatus posteriorly and medially, in the immobile portion of the bladder

   - Avoidance of ureteral torsion, kinking, or J-hooking.

6. The most frequent cause of decreased urine output in the early postoperative period is mild ureteral obstruction secondary to transient edema. Additionally, dehydration resulting from preoperative fasting and supraphysiologic secretion of antidiuretic hormone in response to surgical stress may also contribute.

7. Late ureteral obstruction is most commonly the result of an error in surgical technique including mechanical obstruction or devascularization of the distal ureter.

8. Following surgical treatment of VUR, reflux may persist in the affected ureter or may occur in the contralateral ureter in approximately 2% and in ≤32% of patients, respectively.

9. Reported success rates with Dx/HA for the endoscopic treatment of VUR have been between 76% and 94% after a single injection.

10. Excisional tapering of a megaureter requires careful attention to ureteral blood supply during resection of the redundant ureter and closure of the tapered ureter. Injury to the blood supply may lead to devascularization, fistula, and urinary leakage.

REFERENCES

Please see www.expertconsult.com

Chapter 59

COMPLICATIONS OF EXSTROPHY AND EPISPADIAS REPAIR

David J. Hernandez MD
Assistant Professor, Division of Urology, University of South Florida College of Medicine, Tampa, Florida

John P. Gearhart MD
Professor and Chief of Pediatric Urology, Brady Urological Institute, Johns Hopkins Medical Institutions, Baltimore, Maryland

The surgical management of classic bladder exstrophy remains a challenge to the pediatric urologist and pediatric surgeon. Several reconstructive procedures are being used to repair classic bladder exstrophy. The modern staged repair approach to functional closure of bladder exstrophy (MSRE) has provided increasingly successful results.[1-3] This method of treatment consists of bladder closure with posterior urethral, abdominal wall, and pubic closure the day after birth or soon thereafter. Pelvic osteotomies are performed as needed. Concomitant epispadias repair can be performed in very selected cases, but only by experienced exstrophy surgeons. In most cases, the epispadias repair is performed when the patient is 6 months old. This repair precedes bladder neck reconstruction; by adding outlet resistance, it thereby facilitates bladder growth to an adequate capacity for bladder neck reconstruction. Along with an antireflux procedure, bladder neck reconstruction is usually performed at 4 to 5 years of age when the patient has achieved satisfactory bladder capacity, wants to be dry, and will comply with an intense postoperative voiding regimen. This chapter identifies the complications of all current forms of exstrophy and epispadias treatment and highlights methods to avoid many of these problems.

The modern era of exstrophy reconstruction began in the early 1970s when Jeffs and colleagues[4] and Cendron[5] introduced a staged approach to functional closure of bladder exstrophy. Formerly, this treatment regimen consisted of bladder closure, later bladder neck reconstruction, and finally epispadias repair. However, since the middle to late 1980s with MSRE, reconstructive procedures have evolved and have been altered such that exstrophy closure is performed at birth, epispadias repair is performed at 6 months of age, and bladder neck reconstruction is undertaken at 4 to 5 years of age.

The success of the MSRE approach has been quite encouraging. In specialist centers, continence is achieved in ≤80% of children.[6-8] In a series of 67 patients treated at the Johns Hopkins Hospital in Baltimore by a single surgeon and followed up for ≥5 years, 70% achieved continence (daytime and nighttime) and 80% achieved social continence (dry for ≥3-hour intervals).[8]

This review of complications associated with classic bladder exstrophy and epispadias includes the experience of 213 patients who have been seen and treated at the Johns Hopkins Hospital between 1988 and 2004 by Gearhart and colleagues.[8] These patients, as well as those referred either for exstrophy complications or after initial closure for epispadias repair or bladder neck reconstruction, form the substance of this chapter.

To achieve a successful treatment result by way of functional closure, the needs of each child with bladder exstrophy must be carefully considered at birth. Numerous factors determine the surgical success of bladder exstrophy closure, including the newborn's bladder template size and condition, tension-free closure, free egress of urine, secure placement of suprapubic tubes and stents, wound care and avoidance of infection, movement, and prevention of raised intra-abdominal pressure as occurs with straining, coughing, and postoperative ileus.[9-11]

Bladder size and functional capacity of the detrusor muscle are important factors in the ultimate outcome of functional closure. It is imperative not to confuse apparent bladder size with potential bladder capacity; true bladder size can be accurately assessed only while the patient is under anesthesia. Although the bladder may appear small on preliminary examination, an examination while the patient is under anesthesia may reveal a bladder with suitable capacity that indents easily when it is depressed by a gloved finger.

If the initial bladder capacity after successful closure is estimated to be ≥5 mL, one can expect the bladder to develop adequate size and capacity over time. However, repeated irritation or trauma not only produces a bladder that is unsuitable for closure, but also hinders subsequent bladder growth. In addition, a small fibrotic bladder patch without elasticity or contractility may not be appropriate for primary closure. Other conditions that prevent successful primary closure include ectopic bowel, severe upper tract changes, and significant hamartomatous polyps.

In some neonates with small bladder templates, it may be prudent to wait until the child is 4 to 6 months of age, to allow the child and the bladder to grow, and then undertake closure with epispadias repair under testosterone stimulation, rather than risk a failed closure in the newborn period.[12] Conversely, many patients with small bladders do undergo closure, and some obtain a volume that can yield a satisfactory dry interval after bladder neck reconstruction. In addition, a small bladder that is successfully closed can be subsequently used as a template for ureteral reimplantation and bladder augmentation if adequate bladder capacity is not eventually attained.

The main complications of primary bladder exstrophy closure are complete wound dehiscence (**Fig. 59-1**), bladder prolapse (**Fig. 59-2**), and urethral outlet obstruction (**Fig. 59-3**). Other resultant complications of bladder closure include bladder and renal calculi. With the modern treatment of bladder exstrophy, the incidence of all the aforementioned complications has declined significantly. These complications and methods to avoid them are discussed in the following sections on initial bladder closure, epispadias repair, bladder neck reconstruction, and long-term considerations.

INITIAL BLADDER CLOSURE

Overview

The technique for primary bladder closure that has been previously described and diagramed is to close the bladder template, bladder neck, and proximal posterior urethra up onto the shaft of the penis in a secure manner to allow free egress of urine.[3] In very selected cases, this technique can be combined with formal epispadias repair in patients who have a generous bladder template, an adequately sized penis, and a deep urethral groove. However, this complex procedure should only be performed by surgeons experienced in treating bladder exstrophy. Regardless of the chosen method, free egress of urine during healing is essential.

To prepare the newborn infant for later bladder neck repair in an attempt to achieve continence, the bladder, bladder neck, and posterior urethra must be placed well within the pelvis. This placement allows the bladder to drain under a well-closed pubic arch and for the pelvic floor musculature to aid in eventual continence by com-

pressing the urethra to interrupt the urinary stream. In addition, ultimate tailoring of the bladder neck in a "funnel" manner and suspension of the vesicourethral angle are more readily accomplished when the bladder and bladder neck are located deep in the pelvis. These later maneuvers are distinctly more difficult when the bladder is superficial and is covered merely by skin or attenuated fascia and when continued mobility of the tissue between the pubic bones exists.

The distance from the anal verge to the umbilicus is significantly reduced in exstrophy. Therefore, deeper structures are crowded into a smaller space. Positioning these structures into the deep pelvis can be accomplished only by radical mobilization of the urogenital diaphragm and medial aspects of the pubic bone down to the level of the levator hiatus. This maneuver allows the posterior urethra and bladder to be placed deeper into the pelvis and to exit the pelvis more posteriorly. At the same time, sectioning of the suspensory ligament and anterior attachments of the penis helps correct dorsal chordee and allows the penis to gain length and to lie in a more dependent position.

Formerly, paraexstrophy skin flaps were used to lengthen the urethra and to allow the bladder neck to recede into the pelvis. However, with the modern techniques of epispadias repair, including modified Cantwell-Ransley repair, this procedure is performed only rarely. In our practice, paraexstrophy skin flaps are only used if the verumontanum is located distal on the shaft of the penis near the glans; in this situation, the foreshortened urethral plate makes placing the posterior urethra and bladder deep into the pelvis impossible. These flaps are constructed with great care and are monitored carefully for the first several months after closure.

Complications

The previously discussed bladder and posterior urethra closure appears to be easily accomplished when it is performed with a sterile field and with tissues that could be brought into apposition without tension and immobilized during the healing period. Infection, tension, and movement, along with an indwelling urethral catheter, can cause wound separation and exposure of deeper holding sutures that can result in subsequent minor or major degrees of bladder prolapse or even complete dehiscence.

Infection

To limit the potential for infection, the bladder should be closed as soon after birth as possible. From birth until the time of bladder closure, the bladder should be protected with a nonadherent plastic film such as plastic (Saran) wrap to prevent petroleum jelly, gauze, umbilical clamps, or the diaper itself from denuding the mucosa and removing the epithelium and natural surface antibodies. The bladder surface should be irrigated at each

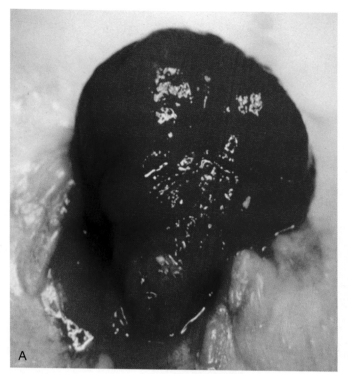

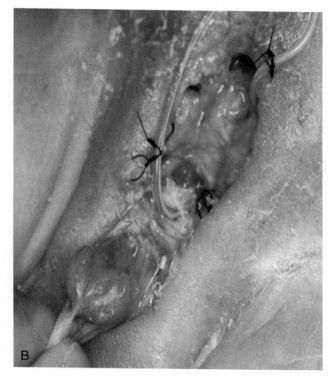

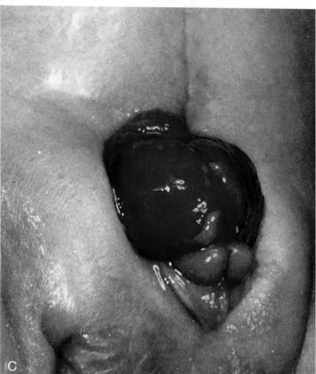

Figure 59-1 **A,** Complete bladder dehiscence in a 2-month-old girl whose primary exstrophy closure was performed at 2 days without osteotomy. **B,** Bladder dehiscence with early granulation tissue following initial exstrophy closure with insufficient mobilization of the vesicourethral unit. **C,** Bladder dehiscence from the lower end of the midline abdominal incision in a boy with loss of penile skin.

diaper change with sterile saline solution at body temperature. All efforts should be made to minimize diaper rash and ammonia burns that occur in this area from contamination with urea-splitting organisms.

At the initial closure, antibiotics (typically ampicillin and gentamicin) are given preoperatively and are con-

tinued for 10 to 14 days postoperatively. Antibiotics remain an essential adjunct to successful bladder closure because exstrophic bladders and the surrounding tissues inevitably become contaminated. The administration of antibiotic therapy is an attempt to convert the contaminated area into a clean surgical wound. In addition, the

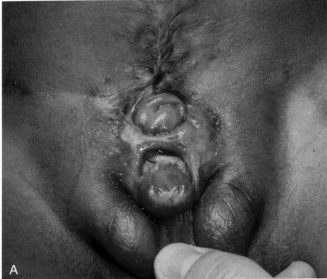

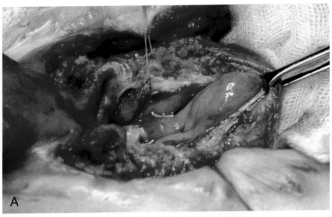

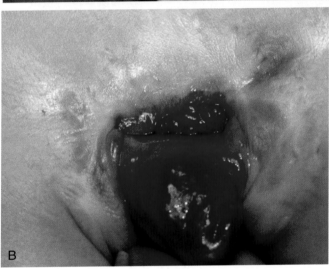

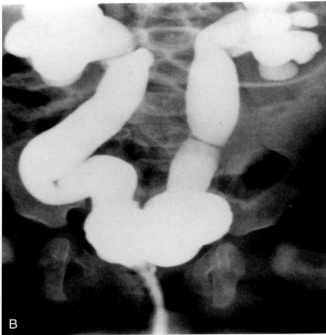

Figure 59-2 **A,** Bladder prolapse 5 weeks after initial exstrophy closure in a newborn boy. **B,** Minor bladder prolapse that developed within 3 months in a 16-month-old boy who underwent exstrophy closure at 3 days without osteotomy. Reclosure was performed with epispadias repair and osteotomy at 18 months.

Figure 59-3 **A,** Dense urethral stricture following initial exstrophy closure using paraexstrophy skin flaps with a thickened bladder and posterior urethra. **B,** Resultant bladder and upper urinary tract decompensation.

local area is thoroughly washed and cleansed with povidone-iodine, and the bladder and its interstices are liberally soaked.

At the initial closure, the patient is prepared from the nipples to the knees anteriorly and from the base of the scapula down to the popliteal fossa posteriorly. The entire area is then draped into the operative field. This method allows access to the posterior body while manipulating the pelvic ring to bring the pubic bones together and to the orthopedic fixating device should an osteotomy be performed. Finally, gauze or an adhesive surgical dressing is inserted into the patient's anus to prevent stool contamination during the procedure.

Wound Tension and Mobility

Wound tension and mobility also contribute to wound dehiscence. These situations are prevented by firm anterior fixation of both sides of the pubis, whether or not an osteotomy is performed. After the induction of anesthesia, the patient is examined to reapproximate the pubic diastasis, and the elasticity of the pubis is noted. As long as the pubic bones can be easily coapted without tension, closure is performed without osteotomy. This situation typically occurs when the pubic diastasis is ≤4 cm, in particular when the newborn undergoes the closure procedure in ≤72 hours. If the diastasis is >4 cm or if any uncertainty exists about the mobility of the pubic bones, an osteotomy is immediately performed.

Those patients with a very large bladder template and a wide pubic diastasis stand to benefit the most from successful closure, and a bilateral osteotomy will help protect the closure and ensure an excellent result. This maneuver reduces tension on the midline wound closure and therefore is most valuable in those patients who do not undergo closure procedures at birth, those in whom an earlier closure procedure has failed, and those with a wide separation of the pelvic ring secondary to a large bladder template.

Our experience with combined anterior innominate and vertical iliac osteotomy in >100 patients led us to adopt this procedure because of decreased blood loss and operating time (**Fig. 59-4**).[13] When the operation is performed using this position, the anterior apposition is achieved without flattening the pelvis and thus without drawing the penis inferiorly under the pubic closure. Therefore, penile length is enhanced rather than decreased by the osteotomy procedure.

Movement during healing often results in excessive moisture, eventual infection, and subsequent dehiscence. Fixation of the wound is vital for initial healing. A three-part plan is recommended to obviate the problem:

1. An attempt is made to coapt the pubic bones with a horizontal mattress suture tied on the outside of the closure. When this is accomplished, another heavy suture can be easily placed in the lower rectus fascia at the junction of the rectus fascia onto the top of the pubic bone, which is now closer to the midline. The pubic stitch must be of very large caliber, usually number 2 nylon, to give the initial strength required for closure. The same caliber suture is also used in an interrupted fashion above the pubic closure in the lower rectus fascia. As shown by biomechanical testing by Sussman and associates,[14] number 2 nylon horizontal mattress suture provides the best load-to-failure ratio among several methods of pubic approx-

imation using various commonly employed suture materials. However, all approaches are weak compared with the intact pelvis.

2. Patients who undergo a closure procedure without pelvic osteotomy are kept in external fixation with modified Bryant's traction for 4 weeks to complete pelvic ring closure and pubic healing. Patients who undergo combined anterior innominate and vertical iliac osteotomies are kept in an external fixating device and modified Buck's traction for 4 weeks in primary closures and 6 weeks in secondary closures (**Fig. 59-5**). Plaster casting, mummy wrapping, and other maneuvers have been used by other surgeons but are not recommended because these methods are less effective and are associated with significant complications (**Fig. 59-6**).[9,15] In a series of 86 failed closures in patients referred to the Johns Hopkins Hospital for definitive treatment, these alternative measures were associated with failure of the closure in a majority of cases because they provided insufficient immobilization.[15]

3. The child's muscular activity, incisional pain, and bladder spasms must be controlled to permit wound fixation. In our unit these goals are achieved mostly through the members of our pediatric anesthesia group who place a tunneled epidural catheter, which is left indwelling for 2 weeks after primary closure. This epidural catheter, along with supplemental intravenous narcotics, diazepam, and anticholinergics, keeps the child still and obviates pain. This treatment necessitates a team approach with physicians, nurses, parents, and members of the pediatric pain service who pamper the child to ensure that pain, frustration, hunger, and muscle and bladder spasms do not produce undue or prolonged activity that defeats attempts to prevent wound mobility.

Mothers are encouraged to nurse and cuddle their babies while these infants are in traction and to assist

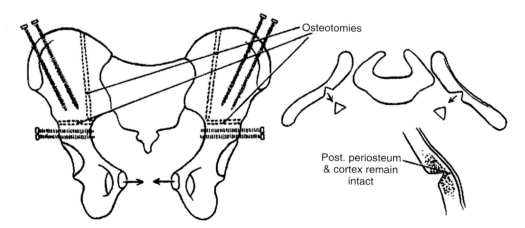

Figure 59-4   Combined anterior innominate and vertical iliac osteotomy and pin placement with preservation of posterior periosteum and cortex.

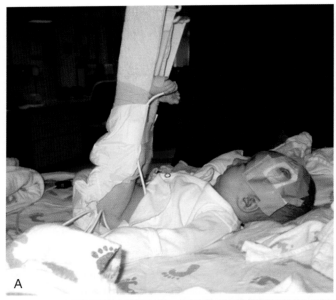

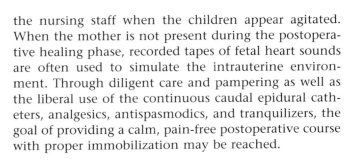

Figure 59-5 Adequate postoperative pelvic and lower extremity immobilization. **A,** No osteotomy: modified Bryant's traction for 4 weeks. **B,** With osteotomy: Buck's traction and external fixator for 4 weeks (6 weeks in secondary closures).

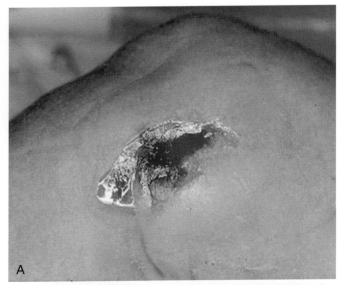

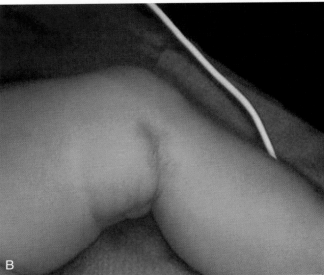

Figure 59-6 Complications of mummy wrap. **A,** Pressure sore on the medial knee after wrap removal. **B,** Persistent scar after 3 months.

the nursing staff when the children appear agitated. When the mother is not present during the postoperative healing phase, recorded tapes of fetal heart sounds are often used to simulate the intrauterine environment. Through diligent care and pampering as well as the liberal use of the continuous caudal epidural catheters, analgesics, antispasmodics, and tranquilizers, the goal of providing a calm, pain-free postoperative course with proper immobilization may be reached.

Osteotomy Complications

We believe in performing pelvic osteotomies as indicated because 90% of children referred to our institution following partial or complete bladder dehiscence do not have an osteotomy or adequate lower extremity

immobilization.[15,16] Controlled fracture of the pelvis allows the pubic rami to be approximated in the midline and thereby permits the bladder to be placed in a more physiologic position. Although various anatomic approaches to osteotomy have been implemented, we favor the combined anterior innominate and vertical iliac technique because of its technical practicality and equivalent or improved outcomes.[17,18]

In series reported by Baird, Sponseller, and Gearhart[13] of 68 patients who underwent combined anterior innominate and vertical iliac osteotomies, no episodes of osteomyelitis and only one external fixator pin site infection occurred. The complete absence of osteomyelitis in this modern series is probably the result of the use of broad-spectrum antibiotic coverage as well as the meticulous pin site care given by the nursing staff at our institution. With careful attention to wound care, even superficial pin site infections are rare.

Another complication of the osteotomy procedure described in some older series is partial femoral nerve palsy.[17] We have since changed our practice such that currently, after fixator placement, we do not tighten the device until ≥7 days after the primary surgical procedure. The external fixating device is then rotated medially to help ensure complete pubic bone apposition. With this modification, we have observed only 2 partial femoral nerve palsies in our last 100 patients, and both completely resolved.[13]

Undue blood loss has not been a problem with pelvic osteotomy, even in very young patients. Nevertheless, osteotomy wounds do ooze fairly frequently until clot formation inside the osteotomy is adequate. In some patients who have undergone failed closure and who need repeat pelvic osteotomy, blood loss can be more extensive and some patients may require transfusion. Nonetheless, the added benefit of closure performed with repeat pelvic osteotomy is worth the slight increase in operative blood loss.[18]

The return of pubic diastasis to a lesser degree than its preoperative width occurs in all patients, but especially in young infants in whom the pelvic bones are not as strong. However, when patients undergo bladder neck reconstruction, the residual diastasis is narrow and a firm intrasymphyseal bar exists. This observation underscores the importance of adequate fixation and solid closure of the pubis to allow a strong intrasymphyseal bar to form. Although it is not sufficient to prevent ultimate recurrence of some degree of pubic diastasis, this union is essential during the immediate postoperative period of wound closure and healing. This point was aptly demonstrated in the report by Gearhart and Baird,[13] who noted that none of the patients with classic bladder exstrophy who underwent a combined osteotomy developed bladder prolapse or wound dehiscence.

Bladder Outlet Obstruction

When paraexstrophy skin flaps are used, urethral stricture can occur where the flaps join in the midline or to the bladder neck. These strictures have generally been treated successfully with dilation alone and only a few have required operative revision. However, several patients referred to our institution developed severe stricture at this location that resulted in massive hydronephrosis and reflux; these patients generally required multiple procedures to correct this problem.

In a review by Gearhart and associates,[19] 31 of 78 patients (40%) who had undergone paraexstrophy skin flap procedures with initial bladder exstrophy closure developed strictures. Various maneuvers were employed to correct these problems including direct vision urethrotomy in 12 cases, urethral dilation in 4 cases, open revision in 3 cases, and full-thickness grafts in 5. The other 7 patients had such complex strictures that they required continent diversion (5), colon diversion (1), or cutaneous ureterostomy (1). The last two patients had undergone vesicostomy for their strictures elsewhere before they were referred to our institution.

The use of paraexstrophy skin flaps has decreased markedly. However, when the urethral plate is very short, skin flaps may still be required to position the bladder in the deep pelvis behind the pubic closure. The use of paraexstrophy skin flaps demands special attention to design, careful placement, and avoidance of urinary drainage catheters through the urethra. Indwelling catheters through the urethra can cause ischemia and the complications mentioned earlier. When paraexstrophy skin flaps are used, careful follow-up, especially in the immediate 4 to 6 postoperative months, is mandatory to avoid complicating strictures and their sequelae.

We have also seen severe urethral strictures after complete repair of bladder exstrophy (CPRE), as described by Grady and Mitchell,[20,21] and after the Kelly repair[22] using radical soft tissue mobilization.[23,24] In many of the patients undergoing these repairs, urethral closures associated with stricture formation occurred. Whether these complications resulted from ischemic damage of the urethral plate or technical error is unclear. However, severe strictures can be seen after both the CPRE repair and the Kelly repair.[23,24]

Another outlet complication of primary closure is erosion of the intrapubic stitch into the posterior urethra during the healing process. This complication can manifest as urinary tract infection a few months after primary closure, increasingly dry diapers in the 2 or 3 months after closure, or high residual urine volumes in the postoperative state after healing has occurred but before removal of the suprapubic tube. Immediate cystoscopy should be performed to rule out any form of obstruction if hydronephrosis is seen on a postoperative ultrasound scan, if a urinary tract infection occurs, if high residuals arise after healing is completed, or if diapers seem dryer.

An intrapubic stitch that has eroded into the posterior urethra >4 months after the operation can easily be removed through a small suprapubic incision. When this complication occurs in the immediate postoperative state, we typically leave the suprapubic tube in place for 2 to 3 months and then remove the stitch through a small suprapubic incision. Although this complication is rare, it led us to use AlloDerm (collagen matrix) as an extra level of soft tissue between the intrapubic stitch and the posterior urethra in our 30 most recent primary exstrophy closures. With this modification, no stitch erosions into the posterior urethra have occurred.

Penile Complications

Most penile complications have been seen in CPRE and the Kelly radical soft tissue mobilization procedure. Loss

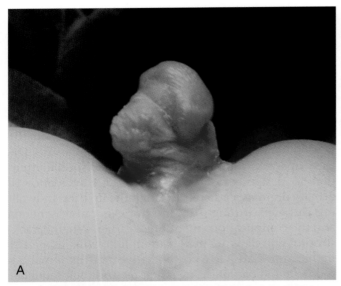

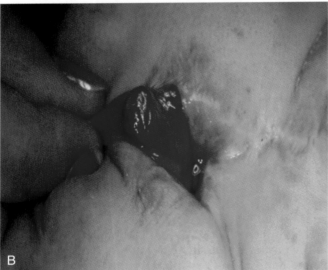

Figure 59-7 **A,** Loss of left hemiglans following complete primary repair of exstrophy. **B,** Loss of right hemiglans and distal corpora.

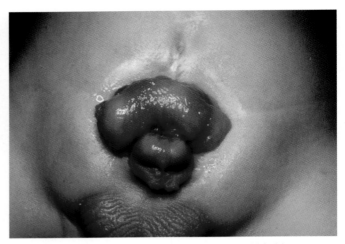

Figure 59-8 Complete dehiscence after closure of bladder exstrophy without osteotomy.

of the glans, loss of one or both corpora, and loss of the entire urethral plate have been reported (**Figs. 59-7** and **59-8**).[23-25] Whether these disastrous complications are the result of damage to the terminal arteries of the penis or injury to the bulbar artery as it exits into the corpus spongiosum from the common penile artery is unclear. In addition, excess venous congestion of these tissues from overzealous pubic closure could be implicated. If congestion occurs after pubic closure, the intrapubic stitch should be removed and replaced more cephalad on the pubic rami. Whatever the cause, this operation carries significant risks and should be performed only by experienced surgeons.

Other Complications

Penile lengthening procedures must not be taken lightly because brisk bleeding can occur during mobilization of

the prostatic plate in the male patient and can lead to damage to the corpus cavernosa or spongiosum. Care must be taken during dissection over the corporal bodies, especially between the lower edge of the urogenital diaphragm and the urethral plate on top of the corpora cavernosa. In some referred patients, corporal damage was so severe that it resulted in the inability to achieve erection in the corpus on one side. If this condition is not corrected, it will permanently interfere with erections and sexual function.

Hypertension remains a major concern in patients undergoing primary closure. This problem can be eliminated by ureteral intubation begun at the time of closure and maintained for 10 to 14 days postoperatively. Bladder drainage is accomplished with a suprapubic Malecot catheter. However, if the ureteral tubes are draining well and the child will be in traction for 4 to 6 weeks, we frequently do not remove the stents until healing is complete.

A commonly seen complication of ureteral intubation is blockage of the small ureteral stents. Normally, these stents are 3.5- to 5-Fr pediatric feeding tubes that have a small perforation at the end. These tubes are easily clogged by debris or small blood clots and we simply incise the end of the tube to make one large hole that is easier for irrigation. These stents are secured to the suprapubic tube at the skin line with Steri-Strips to keep them in position and to prevent inadvertent removal. The stents and the suprapubic tube are irrigated at regular intervals to ensure patency.

Late Postoperative State

To prevent complications after the period of immobilization, external fixation, and healing, the adequacy of the bladder outlet should be tested before discharge. After the ureteral stents are removed, an ultrasound scan is obtained to rule out hydronephrosis. The suprapubic tube is then clamped and residual urine volumes are measured over a few days. If the residual urine volumes are consistently low, the suprapubic tube is removed. A sample for urine culture is always sent from the bladder through the suprapubic tube before its removal to ensure that the bladder urine is sterile. If the residual urine volumes are high, cystoscopy is undertaken to look for a stricture or an erosion of the intrapubic stitch.

Patients are administered long-term suppressive antibiotics postoperatively, and the effectiveness of these drugs is monitored by monthly urine cultures. Renal and bladder ultrasound scans are obtained 6 weeks after discharge and again at 4 months. This monitoring ensures that the upper urinary tract drains appropriately and that obstruction or reflux is not causing any undue change in the upper urinary tract.

Treatment of the newborn with bladder exstrophy is a significant undertaking that requires a high-quality team of neonatologists, pediatricians, pediatric anesthesiologists, nurses, pediatric orthopedists, and surgeons. To protect against and manage complications, a concentrated team effort should be organized so that the child can be adequately prepared for a formal continence procedure at a later date.

Incontinent Interval

Although patients who underwent successful newborn exstrophy closure may appear free of obvious complications, detailed follow-up is required for early detection of impending problems. Normal bladder closure converts a child with exstrophy into one with complete epispadias and incontinence. When epispadias repair is combined with bladder closure in the newborn period, the child remains incontinent and the follow-up is precisely the same. Ultrasound scans are repeated at regular intervals during the 2 to 3 years after closure to detect any upper urinary tract changes that can result from obstruction, reflux, or infection.

Conclusion

The ability of functional closure of bladder exstrophy to yield a 75% to 80% continence rate with preservation of renal function was documented by several series.[2,6-8,10,26] However, the success of initial bladder closure most significantly affects the eventual ability to achieve continence through spontaneous voiding without the use of clean intermittent catheterization. After one failed bladder exstrophy closure, the chance of achieving adequate capacity for bladder neck reconstruction is reduced to 68%, and the chance of attaining ultimate dryness after bladder neck reconstruction is only 30%.[27] After two failed exstrophy closures, only 40% of patients achieve enough bladder capacity for bladder neck reconstruction and only 20% overall

achieve continence; 80% of these patients require intermittent catheterization and bladder augmentation.[9] Thus, after two or more failed exstrophy closures, only 20% of patients are continent and voiding through the urethra. Clearly, an initial bladder exstrophy closure can be expected to be successful when it is performed at an excellent and experienced center and when the procedure includes the use of osteotomies when needed as well as appropriate pelvic fixation and immobilization.

EPISPADIAS REPAIR

Overview

Many surgical techniques have been described for reconstruction of the penis and urethra in patients with classic bladder exstrophy. Four key concerns must be addressed to ensure a functional and cosmetically acceptable penis:

1. Dorsal chordee
2. Urethral reconstruction
3. Glandular reconstruction
4. Penile skin closure

Historically, most epispadias repairs stemmed from Cantwell's original description in 1895.[28] Although these early pioneering steps in penile reconstruction were initially accepted, devascularization of the urethral closure occurred and led to the abandonment of this approach. Young[29] modified Cantwell's technique by leaving the urethral plate attached to one corpus and transposing this plate ventrally.

Although some penile lengthening can be achieved with release of chordee during the initial bladder closure, it is often necessary to perform penile elongation with release of chordee at the time of epispadias repair in patients with bladder exstrophy. All remnants of the suspensory ligaments and residual scar tissue must be excised, and further dissection of the corpus cavernosa from the inferior pubic ramus is often required. Lengthening of the urethral groove is also essential. Regardless of whether paraexstrophy skin flaps were used at the time of bladder closure, further lengthening is needed. The urethral plate must be completely dissected from the corporal bodies both proximally to the bladder and distally toward the glans to achieve maximal penile length. However, the urethral plate is left attached to the distal centimeter of the glans to preserve blood supply.

Furthermore, to release dorsal chordee, one can lengthen the dorsomedial aspect of the corpora by incision and anastomosis of the corpora and by placement of dermal graft to allow lengthening of the distal aspect of the corpora. Ransley and colleagues[30] introduced this concept of releasing dorsal chordee by incision and anastomosis of the dorsomedial aspect of the corpora over the urethra and ventral meatotomy at the distal end of the glans and thus moving the urethra to a more anatomic position. Various authors have reported success with the Cantwell-Ransley repair and modifications thereof.[31-35]

Urethral reconstruction is an important aspect of external genital reconstruction in patients with bladder exstrophy. This procedure can be accomplished by many reported methods. In the late 1980s, we began to use the Cantwell-Ransley repair exclusively for the repair of epispadias in patients with bladder exstrophy or epispadias. We reported on our long-term experience with this procedure.[35] In our variation of the Cantwell-Ransley repair, the urethral plate is mobilized almost completely from the glans penis to a location above the prostate and is transferred to the ventrum of the penis under the separated corpora. Mitchell and Bagli[36] reported a technique of complete disassembly of the corpora from the urethral plate in an attempt to lengthen the penis and to correct dorsal chordee. Unfortunately, 30% to 70% of these patients are left with hypospadiac meatus requiring hypospadias repair.[36-38]

Historically, bladder neck reconstruction was performed before urethral or penile reconstruction. However, the finding of a significant increase in bladder capacity after epispadias repair in those patients with small bladder capacity prompted a change in our management program in the late 1980s. In a review of patients with small bladders after initial closure that were deemed inadequate for satisfactory bladder neck repair, we noted a mean increase of 55 mL after only 22 months following urethroplasty for epispadias.[39] These patients subsequently underwent successful bladder neck reconstruction. At present, construction of a neourethra, penile lengthening, and dorsal chordee release are performed between 6 and 10 months of age. Because most boys with bladder exstrophy have a small, widened penis and a shortage of available skin, all our patients undergo testosterone stimulation before urethroplasty and penile reconstruction.

Complications

The most common complication of epispadias repair is a urethrocutaneous fistula. In a series of 129 Cantwell-Ransley repairs by Baird, Gearhart, and Mathews of the Johns Hopkins Hospital,[35] fistulas developed in the immediate postoperative period in 16% of patients with bladder exstrophy and in 13% of patients with complete epispadias. In 5 of 18 patients, the fistulas closed spontaneously in the first few postoperative months. The other 13 patients underwent a separate procedure to close the fistulas.

Fistulas in this group of patients all uniformly appeared at the base of the penis, where the urethra comes up proximally between the corporal bodies and then goes under the pubic bone. Initially, we thought that this location would be the most common area of fistula formation when paraexstrophy skin flaps were used. However, fistulas occurred more often in patients with an intact urethral plate. In all patients, whether paraexstrophy skin flaps were used or not, fistulas occurred at the base of the penis. Currently, while performing epispadias repair, we harvest and de-epithelialize the inner aspect of the ventral foreskin as a soft tissue flap to cover the urethral repair at the base of the corporal bodies before it dives under the corpora to the level of the prostate. Our hope is that adding this extra layer of soft tissue will further reduce the incidence of fistula.

Although the most common complication of epispadias repair is urethrocutaneous fistula, in a series of 129 Cantwell-Ransley repairs, 9 cases of urethral stricture occurred, all at the proximal anastomosis.[35] One of these strictures responded quite well to direct vision internal urethrotomy. Other techniques included urethral dilation and intermittent catheterization, free full-thickness skin grafts, and buccal grafts. Currently, we use a buccal mucosal graft to replace the urethra instead of a full-thickness skin graft; therefore, the incidence of stricture formation should decrease in time.

Another complication of epispadias repair is loss of penile skin. As mentioned previously, these patients have a preexisting paucity of skin, and testosterone is used to increase the vascularity and availability of local penile skin. In the previously mentioned series by Baird, Gearhart, and Mathews,[35] 15 patients had minimal separation of dorsal skin that granulated without incidence. No instances of substantial skin or glans loss have been observed in our entire experience with the Cantwell-Ransley repair.

Another epispadias repair procedure is complete penile disassembly, as described by Mitchell and Bagli in 1996.[36] The fistula rate reported with this repair was 18% in a small published series.[40] Some of the most worrisome complications of epispadias repair have been observed with this approach. Loss of the glans, loss of the corpora, and loss of the urethral plate were reported in a combined series by Husmann and Gearhart.[25] In addition, data by Purves and Gearhart showed similar risks with the Kelly radical soft tissue mobilization technique.[24] These serious complications point to the risks of this procedure, especially when it is performed by a surgeon who does not routinely operate on delicate, infant tissues, because they can doom the ability of the child to undergo later bladder neck repair and further reconstruction.

Dorsal chordee can persist after epispadias repair. In the review of 129 patients with the Cantwell-Ransley repair, most patients had penises that were straight or deflected downward, but many of these patients were still quite young.[35] Patients >18 years old who engage in satisfactory sexual intercourse state that their penises are quite acceptable, both functionally and cosmetically. Whether simple rotation of the corpora is adequate or whether corporal incision and anastomosis are required is a judgment call at the time of the surgical procedure. Whether these patients require further penile straightening as they achieve sexual maturity is unknown, but they certainly will require prolonged follow-up.

Our experience with older children finds that mobilization of the urethral plate and corporal rotation are inadequate to correct the chordee completely. Incision and anastomosis of the corporal bodies or dermal grafts are required to achieve penile straightness in these older patients. With current methods of epispadias repair, the urethra is straight under the corporal bodies. The urethra obtains a more anatomic and straighter course and is supported dorsally by the more normally placed corporal bodies. This issue has become increasingly important because, should intermittent catheterization be needed in the future, an easily catheterized urethra may obviate the need for a continent urinary stoma. More than 100 patients have undergone cystourethroscopy or urethral catheterization and a smooth urethral tube that is easy to negotiate was present in all patients.

BLADDER NECK RECONSTRUCTION

Overview

Bladder neck reconstruction is usually performed at the age of 4 to 5 years when the child is mature enough to want to be dry and participate in a postoperative voiding training program. Bladder capacity is measured with a gravity cystogram obtained while the child is under anesthesia. If the bladder capacity is ≥85 mL, bladder neck reconstruction can be considered.[10] Because all patients with bladder exstrophy have vesicoureteral reflux, an antireflux procedure is required at the time of bladder neck repair. One common problem that we have seen in multiple patients is bladder neck reconstruction performed when the child is 2 to 3 years of age. At that time, the child has no interest or need to be continent and these operations are doomed to failure.

Some repairs such as the CPRE and the Kelly repair have been purported to decrease the number of operations and to obviate the need for bladder neck reconstruction. In a series by Grady and associates,[41] 72% of female patients and 86% of male patients who underwent CPRE required bladder neck reconstruction, as did 63% of patients in another series by Borer and colleagues.[42] In a series by Gearhart and colleagues,[43] 100% of referred CPRE patients required bladder neck repair to be continent.

At the time of initial bladder neck repair, an attempt is made to obtain continence by creating a long, narrow bladder neck and an elongated posterior urethra in the modified Young-Dees-Leadbetter manner.[44] The reflux is corrected by transtrigonal or cephalotrigonal reimplants, which are also necessary to move the ureters away from the bladder neck repair so that trigonal tissue

can be used to create the bladder neck. In the past, the classic Cohen transtrigonal procedure was used exclusively.[45] However, when the ureters lie low and laterally on the bladder floor, our preference is a more cephalic course for the ureters that involves using the same hiatus but constructing a submucosal tunnel in the cephalad position.[46] This procedure brings the ureteral meatus from each ureter together near the midline of the bladder. This approach works quite well with ureters positioned onto the upper aspect of the trigone and away from the newly reconstructed bladder neck.

Outlet pressure and continence length can be measured by intraoperative urethral pressure profilometry, and resistance of the bladder neck is measured after bladder closure. Our research indicates that urethral closure pressure of 70 to 100 cm H_2O over a length of 2.5 cm is necessary to achieve a successful outcome.[47] Finally, a Marshall-Marchetti-Krantz bladder neck suspension is performed to further increase the continence and urethral closure pressure further.[48] This repair must be allowed to heal for 3 weeks without indwelling urethral stents and with a suprapubic tube to drain the urine before voiding trials begin.

Numerous factors account for a successful outcome after bladder neck repair. Leadbetter[44] considered the length of the bladder neck to be the most significant factor contributing to continence. Therefore, we follow his recommendation and construct the bladder neck approximately 3 cm in length.[44] In addition, bilateral pelvic osteotomies performed at the time of initial closure permit placement of the urethra in the pelvic ring. This maneuver allows for the levator ani and puborectalis muscles to aid in voluntary urinary control. A bladder neck suspension aids in preventing static and stress incontinence. The effectiveness of bladder neck suspension has been demonstrated intraoperatively using urethral pressure profilometry.[47]

The mechanism for achieving urinary continence must not compromise renal function. Both intravenous pyelography and ultrasound studies have been used to evaluate the upper urinary tract in our patients following bladder neck reconstruction. In a series of 189 patients treated by a single surgeon at our institution from primary closure through bladder neck reconstruction, 67 male patients were identified who had a minimum of 5-year follow-up. Of these, only 1 patient developed hydronephrosis after bladder neck reconstruction, and that complication was corrected with reoperative surgical repair.[8]

Complications

Complications of bladder neck reconstruction do occur and include the following:

1. Difficulty with urinating after bladder neck repair
2. Persistent incontinence

3. Development of hydronephrosis
4. Formation of bladder stones

In the previously mentioned series of 67 bladder neck reconstructions with long-term follow-up, difficulty with urination developed in 20% of patients postoperatively.[8] All these patients learned to void except a single patient, who required long-term intermittent catheterization for continence.

Obstruction to the flow of urine occurring at the end of the 3-week healing period may be managed by continued suprapubic drainage, gentle dilation of the urethra with passage of an indwelling urethral catheter, or intermittent self-catheterization. As an initial step, an 8-Fr Foley catheter is placed while the patient is under anesthesia; the surgeon uses a pediatric cystoscope and glidewire during catheterization, and the catheter left in place for 3 to 5 days. After removal of the catheter, voiding usually occurs. If difficulty persists, an extended period of catheter drainage is employed before another voiding trial is attempted.

As indicated from the results of our study, urinary continence with a long-term dry interval does not occur immediately after bladder neck reconstruction and can take ≤2 years to achieve. In our series, the interval between bladder neck reconstruction and urinary continence ranged between 4 and 23 months, with a mean time of 14 months.[8] Nighttime dryness varies but can also take ≤2 years to obtain. Most patients have dry intervals of 3 hours within the first year. During the second year, a few additional patients achieve successful continence. However, if they are still not dry for 3 hours during the day after the second year, bladder neck reconstruction has failed.

The bladder must also adjust to a new environment and new constraints. In addition, and probably more important, the patient must learn for the first time to recognize bladder filling and must be able to initiate voluntary detrusor contractions. With cooperation and time, urinary continence can be achieved in 75% to 80% of patients who have had a successful initial closure operation.[8]

If stress incontinence or dribbling is present 3 to 4 weeks after bladder neck reconstruction, the chance of obtaining adequate control is almost nonexistent. As noted, some patients gain continence with time, usually by increasing their bladder capacity and dry interval rather than by achieving better closure of their outlet. In male patients, growth of the prostate was formerly thought to help produce control of voiding. However, research by Gearhart and colleagues[49] showed that the prostate probably contributes little to the eventual attainment of continence.

Continuous postoperative dribbling typically indicates that further intervention will be required. Although the injection of substances (e.g., bovine collagen and dextranomer/hyaluronic acid [Deflux]) into the bladder neck after modified Young-Dees-Leadbetter bladder neck reconstruction is simple and safe, and although this approach has been used to try to improve continence, the success rate is approximately 45%.[50,51] Unfortunately, this procedure is typically not sufficient to create continence and should be used only as an adjunct to bladder neck reconstruction.

Bladder neck reconstruction can be repeated a second time if it fails. However, bladder capacity must be superb and urodynamic studies must reveal a stable bladder with absence of uninhibited contractions. In a series by Gearhart and colleagues,[52] only 50% of patients with failed prior bladder neck reconstruction were candidates for reoperative surgical procedures. In this highly selected group, continence rates (dry day and night) were approximately 85% after the reoperative bladder neck repair. All these patients had excellent bladder capacity (>100 mL) and stable function demonstrated on urodynamic examination before the reoperation.

Hydronephrosis can persist after bladder neck plasty and reimplantation. Careful follow-up to provide frequent evaluation of the upper urinary tract must be undertaken to prevent this complication. If hydronephrosis occurs and a small bladder capacity persists, bladder augmentation can be performed to protect the urinary tract and to achieve improved continence. In a review by Surer and colleagues,[53] 91 patients whose bladder exstrophy reconstruction failed required either bladder augmentation or continent urinary diversion. Of these patients, 62 had undergone previous bladder neck reconstruction but remained incontinent because of small bladders that did not grow after bladder neck reconstruction. None of these patients had reflux after their failed bladder neck procedures.

Treatment options in this group of patients include the following:

1. Placement of an artificial urinary sphincter and bladder augmentation
2. Reoperative bladder neck repair
3. Bladder augmentation with or without continent abdominal stoma
4. Continent stoma along with bladder augmentation and bladder neck transection or replacement

The prospect of reoperation around the bladder neck after earlier failed surgical procedures makes the artificial sphincter and reoperative bladder neck procedures less attractive. However, in a bladder without reflux, the bladder neck can usually be transected safely and the bladder used as a template for augmentation and continent stoma construction.

In a series of 35 patients with bladder exstrophy who had multiple treatment failures, when the bladder capacity was >50 mL, reimplantation of the ureters into the bladder template and stoma creation were usually possible.[54] In these patients, when the bladder capacity was <50 mL, a continent stoma was implanted in the taenia of the bowel used for reconstruction and the ureters were reimplanted into the bladder template. In some cases, bladder capacity after treatment failure was so small that the entire bladder was replaced and the stoma channel was implanted into the neobladder. No major complications occurred in this group of patients. Therefore, we believe that in patients with failed exstrophy reconstruction, augmentation cystoplasty or continent urinary diversion provides prolonged stability in the upper urinary tract and continence, and this approach has proved a successful alternative to urinary diversion.

Finally, stones can form in the urinary tract after bladder neck repair. In a series of 67 bladder neck repairs, bladder stones developed in 7 patients and renal stones in 1 patient.[8] Most of these patients had difficulty with urinating after bladder neck repair and required prolonged suprapubic drainage. Thus, proper hydration and tube removal as soon as possible may aid in decreasing stone formation after bladder neck repair.

LONG-TERM CONSIDERATIONS

Penile Appearance

Most patients in our series had not reached adulthood and therefore may ultimately develop problems that occur in older patients. Some older patients seen at Johns Hopkins Hospital have problems pertaining to their exstrophy repair. Most of these young adults handle their problems well. However, the most severe problems are encountered in patients who underwent urinary diversion previously.

Certainly, penile shape and size are problems for some of these patients. Although many patients make good and imaginative use of their phallus, others voice concerns about its short and broad appearance. In addition, certain patients complain of residual chordee. Some patients have been counseled and learned to live with their problems and others have undergone surgical treatment, depending on their emotional and penile status.

The penile lengthening procedure, as described by Johnston,[55] can be performed in adulthood to achieve a more dependent penile position, especially in the patient who has undergone previous urinary diversion. Sometimes, these patients can obtain greater length (usually ≈1 inch) by a repeat penile lengthening procedure, which must be carefully performed. Persistent dorsal curvature can also be corrected by dermal grafts used as corporal substitutions, which can be especially helpful in achieving a straight penile length when dis-

proportion exists in size and length of the corporal bodies.

In an article by Mathews and colleagues from our institution,[56] the use of subcutaneously placed tissue expanders was found to be of great benefit in adult and adolescents with a history of bladder exstrophy. Penile skin can be stretched, and a considerable amount of new penile skin can be achieved in this manner. All remaining remnants of the suspensory ligaments and scars are radically excised and the penis is covered again with the newly generated penile skin. This procedure has been especially helpful in patients who have lost skin on one side of the penis or who have an overall paucity of skin secondary to surgical procedures in infancy and childhood.

Penile and Introital Difficulties

Another problem encountered in older patients is ejaculatory dysfunction. Again, many patients who underwent previous urinary diversion may have a seminal fistula located in the mons area at the base of the penis. Ben-Chaim and associates[57] measured seminal volumes in 16 patients who were voiding through the urethra and found that 10 reported an ejaculatory volume of a few millimeters, 3 ejaculated only drops, and 3 had no ejaculations. Overall, patients with a history of bladder exstrophy ejaculate only small amounts compared with their physiologically normal colleagues.

In adolescent female patients, the anterior location of the vaginal introitus can cause difficulty with sexual intercourse. A relaxing incision can often be made to facilitate intromission. Great care must be taken, however, because uterine prolapse has been reported after these procedures. These patients typically have short and wide vaginas, similar to the penises seen in male bladder exstrophy, and the cervix is very near the vaginal introitus. In girls who have not had an osteotomy, when one opens the vaginal introitus to make it suitable for sexual intercourse, the uterus sometimes descends, even in virginal female patients. In this case, we perform abdominal sacral colpopexy using a synthetic sling to allow sexual intercourse and pregnancy.

Many patients present with a bifid clitoris and a less than ideal appearance of the mons and surrounding area. Both uterine prolapse and an unsuitable appearance of the external genitalia appear to be less common in those patients who underwent osteotomy in the newborn period. When the pubic bones have been brought together in proper apposition, a mons-like appearance above the genitalia is created that facilitates subsequent feminizing genitoplasty without tension. Many of these female patients want a more cosmetic appearance to this area at puberty. Skin flaps and tissues expanders have been used in this area with great success.

Fertility and Pregnancy

Reconstruction of the male genitalia and preservation of fertility were not primary objectives in the early surgical management of bladder exstrophy. Many accounts of pregnancy in female patients and impregnation by male patients with bladder exstrophy have been reported. In a review by Shapiro and associates[58] of 2500 patients who had undergone exstrophy and epispadias repair, 38 male patients had fathered children and 131 female patients had given birth. Ejaculatory fertility is rare in patients with a history of bladder exstrophy. However, in our database of >890 patients with bladder exstrophy who we have treated and followed up, we have had 18 patients deliver healthy babies with in vitro technology, and so far none of the newborns has had bladder exstrophy. In an article by Mathews, Gan, and Gearhart,[59] sexual function and pregnancy were normal in a selected group of female patients.

Libido in patients who have undergone bladder exstrophy repair remains high. The erectile mechanism in patients who underwent epispadias repair appeared intact in >90% of patients in our series who had erections following epispadias repair.[60] In a series of adult patients with long-term follow-up, all the women had normal and regular menstrual periods.[57] All these women had serious long-term relationships and were sexually active. Most experienced orgasm.

As mentioned previously, surgical complications include cervical and uterine prolapse. These young women must be informed of the likelihood of uterine and cervical prolapse even after one pregnancy. Birth by cesarean section is mandatory for women who have undergone closure and bladder neck repair or continent urinary diversion, to alleviate stress on the pelvic floor and to avoid trauma to the surgically reconstructed lower genitourinary tract.

Malignant Disease

Most reported malignant diseases have occurred in patients with exstrophies that were left unclosed.[61] The most common tumor is adenocarcinoma, often resembling colonic malignant disease on immunohistochemical staining.[62] Investigators have suggested that rests of ectopic colonic epithelium serve as the origin of these adenocarcinomas.[63,64] Published case reports and other sources found rhabdomyosarcomas in three patients with bladder exstrophy.[65,66]

The inherent malignant potential of the closed exstrophic bladder has not been determined because long-term follow-up of a large cohort of patients with bladder exstrophy without urinary tract infections, obstruction, or chronic irritation has not been published. In an article by Novak and colleagues,[67] polyps associated with bladder exstrophy were evaluated pathologically and were found to be either fibrotic or edematous. Cystitis glandularis was often described, typically in polyps removed from bladders undergoing secondary exstrophy closures. Although no dysplasia was noted, cystitis glandularis is associated with adenocarcinoma of the bladder, and we believe these patients warrant surveillance with routine urine cytologic and cystoscopic examination as they enter adult life. We must be prudent to maintain a high index of suspicion until long-term studies become available.

Adenocarcinoma of the colon adjacent to the ureterointestinal anastomosis in ureterosigmoidostomy as well as in trigonocolonic diversion has been reported.[68,69] Gittes[70] calculated the long-term risk of developing a malignant tumor in the ureterosigmoidostomy at approximately 5%. In a study of patients who had a ureterosigmoidostomy for >15 years, the risk was found to be 11%.[71] In this study the risk of developing malignant tumors at the ureterocolonic anastomosis by 36 years of age was 11%. Although these types of urinary diversions are not commonly performed in North America at this time, we still see one to two patients a year with rectal cancer secondary to ureterosigmoidostomy. Thus, any patient who has a ureterosigmoidostomy should have an annual colonoscopy.

Social Adjustments

Studies have shown that these patients are relatively normal and well adjusted with good psychological integration and a positive attitude toward life.[57,72] However, the exstrophy-epispadias complex may be associated with an increased risk of anxiety disorders.[73] A recurring theme in all these patients is concern about penile length and chordee. The main objective of surgical intervention in bladder exstrophy repair is to enable these patients to achieve normal social interactions with their families and communities. With continuing excellent results of MSRE, it is gratifying that great progress has been made toward the realization of this goal.

CONCLUSION

This review of the complications of all methods of modern treatment of bladder exstrophy emphasizes the complexity of reconstruction of the bladder exstrophy spectrum. In experienced hands, the surgical results of primary bladder closure, epispadias repair, and bladder neck reconstruction are quite acceptable. A review of MSRE by Baird and Gearhart demonstrated that a secure abdominal wall closure, urinary continence, preservation of the upper urinary tract, and a cosmetically acceptable penis can be achieved in patients with a successful primary closure and in a reasonably high percentage of patients with an unsuccessful primary closure.[8] Similarly, in a review by Gearhart and associates,[54] all 35 patients in whom bladder exstrophy reconstruction failed were doing well following bladder augmentation or continent stoma. Therefore, although complications such as dehiscence, deterioration of renal function, and fistula do occur, with careful attention to surgical detail and frequent follow-up, these patients can have a normal childhood and can become contributing members of society.

ACKNOWLEDGMENT

This chapter is dedicated to the memory of Robert Douglas Jeffs, MD, FRCS(Can) (1924–2006), Emeritus Professor of Pediatric Urology at the Johns Hopkins Hospital in Baltimore, a respected teacher, colleague, and friend.

KEY POINTS

1. Continence can be achieved in ≤75% to 80% of children following the MSRE regimen (exstrophy closure at birth, epispadias repair at 6 months, and bladder neck reconstruction as well as an antireflux procedure at 4 to 5 years). Although other repairs (complete primary repair and the Kelly repair) have been offered, long-term outcomes are lacking.

2. The success of bladder exstrophy closure depends on the newborn's bladder template size and condition, a tension-free closure, free egress of urine, secure placement of suprapubic tubes and stents, wound care, and avoidance of infection and movement.

3. The complications of any primary exstrophy closure include infection, wound dehiscence, bladder prolapse, and urethral outlet obstruction.

4. Diligent care and pampering as well as the liberal use of an indwelling epidural catheter, analgesics, antispasmodics, and tranquilizers may provide for a calm, pain-free postoperative course with proper immobilization.

5. Although various anatomic approaches to osteotomy have been implemented, the combined anterior innominate and vertical iliac technique is preferred because of its technical practicality, comparable outcomes, and long-term success.

6. The most common complications of epispadias repair are urethrocutaneous fistulas, urethral strictures, loss of penile skin, and persistent dorsal chordee, but loss of glans or corpora can occur.

7. Modified Young-Dees-Leadbetter bladder neck reconstruction and ureteral reimplantations (transtrigonal or cephalotrigonal) are performed at 4 to 5 years of age when the child wants to be dry, will participate in postoperative voiding training, and has a bladder capacity of ≥85 mL.

8. Complications of bladder neck reconstruction include difficulty with urinating, persistent incontinence, the development of hydronephrosis, and the formation of calculi.

9. Most patients with failed exstrophy reconstruction require augmentation cystoplasty or continent urinary diversion to provide prolonged stability in the upper urinary tract and continence.

10. Long-term considerations include the appearance of the external genitalia, ejaculatory dysfunction, introital difficulties, uterine prolapse, and malignant disease.

REFERENCES

Please see www.expertconsult.com

with reference to commonly used techniques.

PREVENTION OF COMPLICATIONS

To provide insight into the learning curve for hypospadias repair among fellowship-trained pediatric urolo-
and the anesthetic risk to the child. Genital awareness begins at approximately 18 months of age and tends to become significant by age 3 to 5 years. Several investigators reported that patients undergoing earlier repair (usually <12 months of age) experienced less anxiety and had improved psychosexual outcomes when com-

pared with older children undergoing hypospadias repair.[5-7] Patients operated on at a younger age may also experience fewer complications, a finding that reinforces the need for early correction.[8] In medical centers possessing appropriately trained pediatric anesthesia specialists, hypospadias repair can be performed safely in very young children. After 6 months of age, anesthesia outcomes approach those of older children and adults.[9,10] Based on studies such as these, the American Academy of Pediatrics Section on Urology[11] suggested that the optimal time for hypospadias repair is between 6 and 12 months of age.

History and Physical Examination

The initial evaluation of all patients presenting for repair of hypospadias requires a careful history and physical examination. In the patient who has not previously undergone penile surgical procedures, the history is directed toward identification of coexistent anomalies that could affect surgical care. The inquiry should focus on a history of prior urinary tract infections, voiding dysfunction, and associated medical diseases such as asthma or bleeding diatheses.

We refer patients with bleeding diatheses or a family history of bleeding diathesis for hematologic evaluation before the operation because significant bleeding may have a profound impact on wound healing, hematoma formation, and the overall outcome of the hypospadias repair. Patients with a history of other systemic anomalies should be evaluated with a screening ultrasound scan for the presence of upper urinary tract abnormalities.[12] The physical examination focuses on the severity of chordee, the location of the meatus, and the presence or absence of penoscrotal transposition. Finally, patients with unilateral or bilateral undescended testes, perineal hypospadias, or ambiguous genitalia must be carefully assessed because the risk of an intersex disorder is much higher in this group.[13-16]

Surgical planning continues after the induction of anesthesia. Following antiseptic preparation of the genitalia and administration of intravenous antibiotics, the genitalia are carefully examined again. We do not find it necessary to perform routine cystoscopy except in cases of severe proximal hypospadias. Because hypospadias and intersex conditions are associated with prostatic utricles in >10% of patients and occur more frequently in proximal hypospadias, cystoscopic examination may be useful in these particular situations to identify and characterize utricle abnormalities that could interfere with proper catheter placement or may need surgical management later.[17,18]

Operative Technique

The initial step in hypospadias repair is the thorough resection of penile chordee (orthoplasty). The adequacy of resection can be assessed intraoperatively using arti-

ficial erection as described by Gittes and McLaughlin[19] or by pharmacologically induced erection.[20] Some children may achieve erections with induction of anesthesia or with simple corporal occlusion through perineal pressure. During the release of chordee, the meatus often recedes to a position far more proximal than anticipated preoperatively. We recommend use of a urethral catheter or sound for evaluating the hypospadiac meatus because the sound may reveal the overlying ventral skin to be deceptively thin and unusable for urethral coverage. The surgeon must anticipate this possibility and have a wide array of techniques available so as not to be limited in approach.

After the resection of chordee, the surgeon must recreate a functional urethra. The techniques of neourethral construction can be broadly classified as those using flaps of genital skin, those using grafts of preputial or extragenital tissue, and urethral tubularization procedures. Although we prefer to use flaps of local genital skin if possible, in patients undergoing revision hypospadias repair this is not always feasible. Many surgeons have reported their experience using the tubularized incised plate urethroplasty for both primary and revision hypospadias surgical procedures.[21-23] This technique allows dorsal incision of the urethral plate to increase lateral and ventral coverage of the neourethra.[24] In a survey of pediatric urologists, the tubularized incised plate technique was used >90% of the time for distal hypospadias repairs and 80% of the time for midshaft repairs.[25] Numerous techniques are available for the management of proximal or complex hypospadias. The use of hair-bearing skin is discouraged because it renders the neourethra susceptible to stone encrustation and to the development of recurrent urinary tract infections.

Perhaps more important than the choice of tissue for the urethroplasty is the technique with which the tissue is handled. The preservation of blood supply to tissues is crucial to the prevention of complications and is greatly aided by the use of operative magnification. Ischemia results in fibrosis and contraction of tissues, predisposes patients to infection, and potentiates the breakdown of suture lines. Although topically applied dihydrotestosterone gel is not used at our institution, evidence indicates that this agent may improve local tissue vascularization and reduce complications.[26]

Flaps must be mobilized generously to minimize tension on suture lines and to prevent ischemia. Subcuticular neourethral approximation with epithelial inversion has been shown to decrease complications when compared with full-thickness approximation.[27] The delicate nature of the genital tissues demands meticulous atraumatic technique. Tissue trauma can be minimized by the use of fine forceps, skin hooks, and stay sutures. For urethral reconstruction we prefer a fine absorbable monofilament such as polydioxanone (PDS) or polytrimethylene carbonate (Maxon). Next, the use of multiple

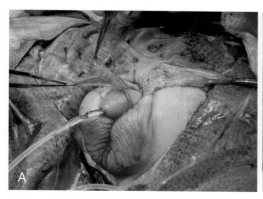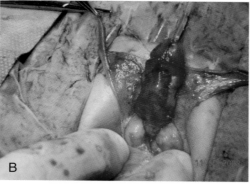

Figure 60-1   Dartos flap for second layer urethral coverage. **A,** Harvesting of the dartos flap from the dorsal preputial skin. **B,** Placement of the flap over the newly tabularized urethra.

tissue layers is vital in the reduction of complications. Savanelli and colleagues[28] and other investigators showed that dartos interposition flaps reduced fistula formation after tubularized incised plate repair (**Fig. 60-1**).

Finally, careful hemostasis should be maintained with the use of pinpoint bipolar cautery and a compressive bio-occlusive dressing (**Fig. 60-2**). This dressing can be formed from an adhesive membrane such as Tegaderm, which is applied circumferentially from the level of the glans to the penoscrotal junction. The glans must be included in the dressing to avoid excessive swelling. Care must be taken to prevent a constricting ring at the proximal extent of the dressing

Postoperative Care

The importance of good postoperative care cannot be overemphasized. This often overlooked aspect of hypospadias management is clearly as important as surgical technique in determining eventual outcome. Catheters must be well secured before the patient leaves the operating room. We use a two-diaper drainage system with the catheter draining into the outside diaper to facilitate keeping the inside diaper and thus the repair dry during the catheterized period (**Fig. 60-3**).

Excellent pain control is crucial and can be achieved with a caudal regional block as well as a circumferential penile block. In our institution, we prefer a caudal block and have not seen any significant complications of this technique. The effect can be improved when preoperative and postoperative blocks are performed for both types of blocks.[29,30] In addition, ketorolac (0.5 mg/kg), given as a single dose 30 minutes before the conclusion of the procedure, is a safe and effective adjunctive pain medication that is associated with less emesis than are opioid analgesics.[31]

Postoperatively, the surgeon must take every precaution to prevent damage from high urethral pressures. Bladder spasm is common after urethroplasty and can result in voiding around stents and catheters. This complication is easily treated with an anticholinergic agent such as oxybutynin, which is started in the postoperative period and continued until 24 hours before removal of the urethral stent. Perioperative antibiotics and pro-

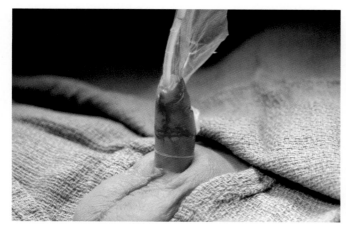

Figure 60-2   Dressing for one-stage hypospadias repair. **A** and **B,** Transparent adherent dressing is applied from glans to level of penoscrotal junction, with care taken to prevent a constricting band at the proximal extent. A 6-Fr silicone urethral stent is sutured to the glans to allow free passage of urine.

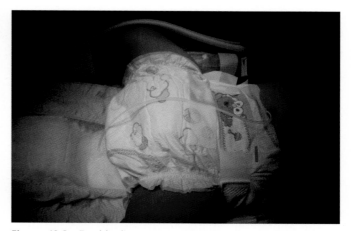

Figure 60-3   Double-diaper urinary drainage system. Placing a second diaper on the child allows the urinary catheter to drain into the second diaper and thus effectively keep the inside diaper and the dressing dry during the postoperative period.

phylactic antibiotics during the postoperative catheterization period have been shown to reduce postoperative complicated urinary tract infection and thus potentially to decrease overall fistula and stenosis rates.[32]

MANAGEMENT OF COMPLICATIONS

Early Postoperative Complications

Ischemia

Tissue ischemia is involved to some degree with most of the acute and chronic complications of hypospadias surgical procedures. Ischemia potentiates edema and infection, delays healing, and promotes fibrosis. Common techniques in urethroplasty employ either the transfer of tissue islands on a delicate blood supply or the use of grafts that must rely on diffusion of nutrients from the recipient tissue bed. These tissues are predisposed to ischemic damage, which can result in the formation of fistula or stricture. Ischemia of flaps used for skin coverage generally leads to marginal necrosis, eschar formation, and wound contraction.

Thoughtful operative technique can usually prevent ischemic complications. Every attempt should be made to minimize postoperative edema or hematoma formation. Flaps must be conceived with adequate blood supply and appropriate dimensions. Ideally, poor perfusion is discovered during the procedure. Tissue edges that blanch when they are sutured are usually under excessive tension and should be modified. Despite meticulous technique, ischemia to the penile skin may not become apparent until after removal of the wound dressing. Treatment is initially conservative. Necrosis of skin flaps is usually partial and results in a small eschar with gradual re-epithelialization of the defect. If a clearly demarcated edge exists, débridement of the eschar is appropriate. Grafting and revision surgical procedures are rarely necessary and are reserved for extensive tissue defects.

Bleeding and Hematoma

The formation of wound hematoma should be relatively uncommon after hypospadias repair if intraoperative hemostasis is adequate and an effective compressive wound dressing is used. In its most severe form, the mass effect of blood may distort tissue planes and interfere with perfusion of tissue flaps or prevent inosculation of blood vessels into a graft. A large hematoma can result in skin separation. A hematoma may serve as a nidus for infection, and resorption of the blood can result in inflammation, scarring, and fibrosis. All these factors increase the potential for late complications such as fistula, stricture, and recurrent chordee.

The appropriate management of this complication depends on the size of the hematoma and the time when it is noted. If a significant hematoma is present at the end of the procedure, the skin should be opened, the clot evacuated, and the source of bleeding identified and controlled. A patient with a large hematoma discovered early in the postoperative period should be returned to the operating room for evacuation of the hematoma and placement of a drain in the subcutaneous tissue. Occasionally, a large hematoma is recognized several days postoperatively. When the surgeon believes that these hematomas may affect flap survival or the success of the operation, the hematoma should be evacuated. Smaller hematoma rarely cause long-term problems and can usually be managed conservatively.

Wound Infection

Because of the excellent blood supply of the genital structures, severe infections rarely occur after genital operations in children. Nevertheless, poorly perfused flaps, skin grafts, and traumatized tissue have a propensity to develop mild localized infections. These infections generally result from gram-positive skin flora and are usually the predominant organism cultured from the perimeatal tissues at the time of the surgical procedure.[33]

Urinary tract infections can also occur in patients with catheter urinary diversion and represent organisms that migrate along indwelling catheters. The most common of these organisms are *Klebsiella* and *Escherichia coli*.[32] Meir and Livne[32] showed that the addition of perioperative antimicrobial therapy and the continuation of prophylaxis during the catheterized period reduced the number of infectious complications and decreased the occurrence of bacteruria. This finding is in line with our practice to administer cephalexin to our patients until all catheters are removed. When infections do occur, aggressive management is important to prevent inflammation, which can delay wound healing and predispose to fistula or stricture formation.

Wound and urine cultures should be obtained in all patients developing skin infectious, and antibiotic coverage should be tailored to treat the offending organism. When possible, devitalized tissue should be gently débrided. Any subcutaneous collection of fluid should be drained immediately. Superficial infections usually respond quickly to these measures and generally have a minimal impact on function or cosmesis. More extensive infections, in particularly those associated with *Pseudomonas,* or leakage of urine may occasionally require admission to the hospital for treatment with intravenous antibiotics.

Wound Separation

The origin of wound separation is multifactorial. Infection, ischemia, and hematoma formation predispose to breakdown of the suture line. Postoperative erections, frayed suture material, and tension on the wound closure may disrupt the wound, as can a variety of patient-related factors such as trauma from manipulation of the genitalia or stents. Management of this complication is straightforward. If the defect is small and not infected, it generally closes by second intention with minimal morbidity. An attempt to place additional sutures is not recommended because this maneuver invariably requires anesthesia and may lead to ongoing infection or inflammation. If wound disruption occurs several days postoperatively and is associated with excessive tissue edema, the surgeon must entertain the possibility of infection or urine extravasation. The management of this complication is discussed earlier.

Late Postoperative Complications

Urethrocutaneous Fistula

Urethrocutaneous fistula is the most commonly reported major complication of hypospadias repair, and the more extensive the urethroplasty, the higher is the frequency of this complication (Table 60-1). The incidence of fistula has been steadily decreasing as the equipment and operative technique have improved. An incidence of <5% for distal hypospadias repair is now to be expected.[34,35]

The development of fistula is a multifactorial phenomenon. Edema-attenuated vascular supply, infection, and hematoma may combine to impair healing of the neourethra. Distal urethral obstruction from meatal crusting or stenosis results in high urethral pressures during voiding and may result in disruption of a proximal suture line. Finally, technical factors such as overlapping of suture lines, inadequate inversion of the epithelium, or use of poorly absorbable suture material have been implicated.[36]

Management of urethral fistula depends on size, location, and interval from the surgical procedure. A urine leak usually becomes apparent in the first few days after initiation of voiding and most are noticed in the first 6 months.[37] In our practice, we have also observed children who present later, when toilet training occurs. It is most likely that the fistula occurred much earlier but came to be noticed at this time because parents are actively observing their child's urinary stream during voiding. Although replacement of a urethral catheter can be attempted, in our experience this maneuver is rarely successful. No attempt should be made to place additional sutures to close the fistula because this approach invariably exacerbates the inflammatory process and worsens the problem.

Small fistulas noted perioperatively, without concomitant inflammation or meatal stenosis, occasionally close. Larger fistulas and those persisting beyond several weeks invariably require operative intervention. This intervention must be delayed until tissues have thoroughly healed from the previous operation. Six months is generally adequate time to allow ingrowth of blood vessels and resolution of inflammation and edema.

TABLE 60-1	Reported Complications of Common One-Stage Hypospadias Repairs				
Reference	No. Patients	Complications (%)	Fistula (%)	Meatal Stenosis (%)	Neourethral Stricture (%)
Tubularized Incised Plate					
el-Kassaby et al[35] (2008)	764	3.4	2	1	—
Stehr et al[82] (2005)	100	22	5	17	—
Baccala et al[83] (2005)	101	5	2	3	—
Elicevik et al[23] (2007) (primary procedure and reoperation)	360	30	11	10	1
El-Sherbiny et al[84] (2004) (primary procedure and reoperation)	133	15	9	5	0.8
Snodgrass and Lorenzo[85] (2002) (proximal)	33	33	21	3	3
Borer et al[86] (2001) (primary procedure and reoperation)	206	7	6.5	0.5	—
Mathieu					
Samuel et al[30] (2002)	211	15.2	12.3	0	—
Minevich et al[87] (1999)	201	1.5	1	—	—
Ghali et al[88] (1999)	205	16	10	0.5	0
Uygur et al[89] (1998)	197	—	21	—	—
Onlay Island Flap					
Sedberry-Ross et al[90] (2007)	421	10.6	8.7	0.9	—
Castanon et al[91] (2000) (proximal)	38	31.5	18.4	2.63	—
Barroso et al[92] (2000)	47	25	17	5	—
MAGPI					
Ghali et al[88] (1999)	92	10	2	0	0
Uygur et al[89] (1998)	91	8	0	0	0

MAGPI, meatal advancement with glanuloplasty incorporated.

Effective management demands a careful evaluation for associated urethral disorders such as chordee, stricture, and diverticula. The surgical approach is dictated by these findings, as well as by the size and location of the fistula. Intraoperatively, it is important to calibrate the urethra distal to the fistula with an 8- to 10-Fr bougie à boule to ensure adequate size (**Fig. 60-4**). The penile shaft must be evaluated for the presence of other unrecognized fistulas. The fistula tract can be cannulated with a lacrimal probe to determine the site of entrance into the urethra. This maneuver is useful in planning the orientation of skin flaps for coverage of the fistula. The lacrimal probe can also be a useful aid for the dissection of the fistula tract. Once the origin of the fistula is appreciated, it can be closed with delicate 7-0 or finer absorbable suture.

Small-caliber fistulas can be closed primarily without compromising the diameter of the urethral lumen. Larger fistulas may require coverage with a trap-door or island flap of penile shaft skin. In general, better results have been achieved when a second layer or flap coverage is possible especially in cases of recurrent urethral fistula.[38-40] Skin coverage can be obtained by several methods to avoid overlap of urethral and skin suture lines (**Fig. 60-5**).

Despite a well-performed repair, 20% or more of fistulas will recur.[3,41,42] This recurrence rate can be decreased by the interposition of a nonepithelialized layer between the urethral closure and the skin. We have been impressed with the use of a scrotally based tunica vaginalis flap as advocated by various investigators.[43-45] Scrotal dartos tissue has been used in a similar fashion.[44,46] De-epithelialized flap repair is another technique that has shown promise.[39] Other surgeons have shown and we agree that no need exists to divert the urine for simple repairs, but for larger repairs we routinely divert the urine for 7 to 10 days with a silicone urethral stent.[39,47] Finally, in cases of severe fistula problems, buccal mucosa grafts have been used with some success.[48] In our experience, repeat hypospadias repair may be the best choice for complex fistula management especially in patients with stricture disease.

Urethral Stricture

Urethral stricture is the second most frequently reported complication of hypospadias repair. These strictures tend to form at anastomotic suture lines such as the meatus, the end of the glans closure, or the proximal anastomotic suture line. Strictures generally become apparent ≤3 months after hypospadias repair with diminished force of urine stream, straining to void, or urinary tract infection. Alternatively, the patient may present with splaying of the urinary stream, urethral fistula, or occasionally urinary retention.

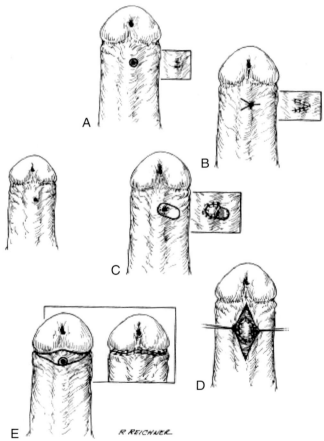

Figure 60-5 Techniques of fistula repair after hypospadias correction. **A,** Excision and primary closure. **B,** Y-V skin advancement after excision and closure of the fistula. **C,** Trap-door flap of penile skin. **D,** Full-thickness patch graft. **E,** A small coronal fistula is excised and penile shaft skin is advanced to cover the defect. *(From Winslow BH, Vorstman B, Devine CJ: Complications of hypospadias repair. In: Marshall FF, ed.* Urologic Complications: Medical and Surgical, Adult and Pediatric. *Chicago: Year Book; 1990.)*

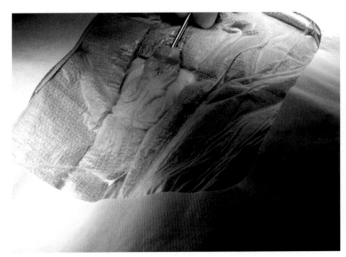

Figure 60-4 Probe in a urethral fistula. This child has a large urethrocutaneous fistula that is being shown with a urethral sound.

Several factors promote the formation of neourethral stricture. Poor design of the neourethra is an important example and includes formation of a conduit of insufficient caliber, tension on suture lines, and poor spatulation of the anastomosis. Tissue ischemia, trauma, or infection can result in inflammation and concentric scarring of the lumen. In tubularized pedicle flaps, a stricture may be functional, secondary to a redundant neourethra kinking at the proximal anastomosis. It is best to characterize the stricture by cystoscopic examination with a 0-degree lens while the patient is under anesthesia and with care taken to obtain an accurate estimation of length and location of the stricture as well as the extent of coexistent urethral disease.

In most cases, initial management is conservative and consists of dilation or endoscopic treatment. Husmann and Rathbun[49] showed success rates with urethrotomy for stricture disease after hypospadias repair of 22% to 24% regardless of whether clean intermittent catheterization was employed. These investigators reported success rates of 72% and 63% for onlay urethroplasty strictures and urethral plate urethroplasty strictures, respectively, findings suggesting that this type of repair may be more amenable to urethrotomy than are other types of tubed grafts or tubed flaps. The outcome tends to be better for short anastomotic strictures and when conservative treatment is initiated ≤3 months after operation.[50,51]

Strictures not responding to initial dilation and those noted to be extensive on the initial evaluation generally require revision urethroplasty. Attempts at repeated dilation or urethrotomy in these patients are usually not successful and should be discouraged because of the possibility of worsening the existing fibrosis.[52]

Urethral Diverticulum

Urethral diverticula generally manifest in ≤6 months after hypospadias repair with weak urinary stream, postvoid dribbling, urinary tract infection, and occasionally hematuria. The patient or caretaker may notice ballooning of the penile shaft during voiding (**Fig. 60-6**) or lateral displacement of the penile shaft or may complain of the need to "milk" residual urine from the penile urethra. In our practice as in others, we have noticed this complication more commonly in patients with onlay flaps and two-stage repairs,[53] most likely as a result of lack of spongiosum combined with a longer urethroplasty.

Diverticula generally occur as diffuse dilations of either the neourethra or the native urethra. These complications have been reported in ≤10% of patients undergoing island flap repairs and probably result from a combination of factors.[53-55] Chief among these is the intrinsic weakness of the neourethra resulting from a lack of supporting spongiosum. The creation of a neourethra of excessive caliber may be a contributing factor. Distal urethral obstruction potentiates the formation of

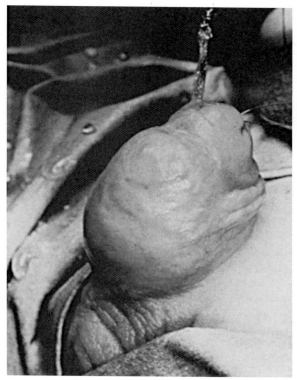

Figure 60-6 Urethral diverticulum in an 18-month-old child, 6 months following double-faced transverse preputial island flap repair. *(From Elder JS, Duckett JW. Urethral reconstruction following an unsuccessful 1-stage hypospadias repair. World J Urol. 1987;5:19.)*

diverticula and may result from a noncompliant or inadequate-caliber distal urethra, meatal stenosis, kinking of the neourethra at the glans, or a marked step-off in diameter at the level of the neourethral anastomosis.

Urethral diverticula are commonly found in association with other forms of urethral disease such as stricture and fistula. Their presence must be appreciated during the surgical procedure so treatment of these complications can be incorporated into the operative plan. The intraoperative approach must include an assessment of the distal urethral caliber with a bougie à boule or lacrimal probe. Cystoscopy should be available to inspect the distal urethra, and the presence of fistulas must be ascertained.

A localized saccular diverticulum can usually be excised and reduced in a longitudinal fashion. The more commonly encountered megaurethra has traditionally been repaired by excision of redundant tissue and multilayered closure.[56] The tissue is usually elastic and well vascularized, thus making it suitable for use in the repair of fistula and distal strictures. Various flap techniques have been employed to reconfigure redundant diverticular tissue for this purpose (**Fig. 60-7**).[57] Interposition of a tunica vaginalis flap between the skin and the repair may decrease the incidence of postoperative fistula.

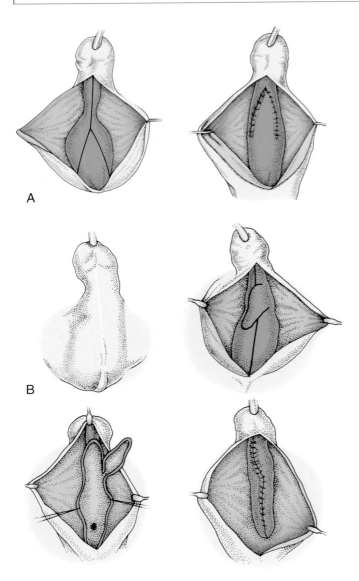

Figure 60-7 Use of diverticular tissue to correct distal stenosis. **A,** Repair of urethral diverticulum with distal stricture using Y-V plasty. **B,** Repair of urethral diverticulum with distal stricture using rotation flap.

Alternatively, a dartos flap or a de-epithelialized flap may be employed.

Heaton and colleagues[58] advocated a urethral plication procedure alone or in combination with distal stricture repair for megaurethra after hypospadias repair. Because the urethra is not opened, this technique has the theoretical advantages of preserving the neourethral blood supply and decreasing the risk of postoperative fistula. After repair of the diverticulum, urine should be diverted for 7 to 10 days.

Meatal Complications

Procedures that rely on tunneling of the neourethra through the glans are at risk of causing *meatal stenosis.* Ischemia or inflammation may exacerbate stenosis in tunneled flaps with marginal perfusion. Intraopera-

tively, it is imperative to excise a small core of the glans during formation of a glans tunnel as opposed relying on incision and forcible dilation. Usually, a stenotic meatus can be managed conservatively with routine meatal dilation with the tip of an ophthalmic ointment tube.[59] Lorenzo and Snodgrass[60] showed, however, that regular dilation after tubularized incised plate repair does not reduce the rate of meatal stenosis complications. When the stenosis is refractory to dilation, various operative interventions have been described, ranging from simple dorsal meatotomy to Y-V glanulomeatoplasty or ventral flap using a tissue onlay.[61,62]

Meatal retrusion is a complication occasionally encountered after the meatal advancement with glanuloplasty incorporated (MAGPI) technique and the Mathieu hypospadias repair in which the glansplasty has broken down. Meatal retrusion likely is caused by selection of the wrong repair for the patient's anatomic features. A urethra that is immobile or a meatus that is noncompliant results in retrusion of the neourethra to its original position. In the Mathieu repair, an inadequate ventral skin flap may lead to premature dissolution of the glansplasty sutures with the same result. The consequences of this complication are predominantly cosmetic rather than functional. However, if significant splaying or deflection of the stream occurs, revision of the meatus may be worthwhile.

Persistent Chordee

Persistent chordee is an unfortunate complication of hypospadias repair that may result in the sacrifice of a functional urethroplasty. Historically, persistent or recurrent penile chordee was common and required the use of multistage repair of hypospadias. With the use of intraoperative erection, all but the most complicated repairs can now be completed in one stage. The occurrence of persistent chordee lies primarily in the misinterpretation of intraoperative erection, although rarely this complication may result from corporeal disproportion or extensive urethral fibrosis.

Residual chordee can be corrected through a systematic approach. Artificial erection is used at each stage of the resection to determine the degree of residual penile curvature. The previous operative site should be exposed through a circumferential coronal incision. The penis is then degloved to the penoscrotal junction. An adequate dissection may require elevation of the neourethra and resection of scar on the ventral aspect of the corporal bodies.[63] If chordee persists after this procedure, elevation of the urethral plate down to the bulbar urethra if necessary has been shown to be another effective treatment (**Fig. 60-8**).[64] Scar tissue exposed by this maneuver is excised.

If after these maneuvers bow-stringing of the urethra remains, one may consider division of the neourethra at the point of maximal curvature. This technique alone rarely straightens the penis, and residual curvature after

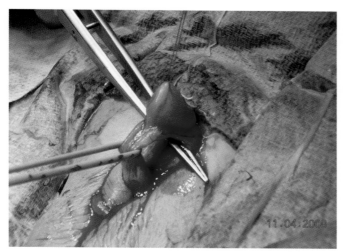

Figure 60-8 Urethral plate elevation for correction of chordee. The urethral plate is elevated to allow for further correction of significant chordee.

division of the neourethra usually requires dorsal plication.[65] Severe residual ventral chordee may require ventral transverse corporal incision with corporal grafting of a piece of dermis harvested from the groin or a piece of porcine small intestine submucosa. However, this is usually encountered in the first hypospadias repair and is uncommon in the management of recurrent chordee because it is usually associated with recurrent scarring or skin tethering.

Other Urethral Problems

If hair-bearing skin is used for the hypospadias repair, the patient may eventually experience complications related to *hair in the urethral lumen*. In the most severe form, hair may protrude from the meatus and resemble a urethral beard. This complication usually occurs after multiple-stage procedures or complex reoperations in which a paucity of non–hair-bearing skin is available. Hair in the urethral lumen occasionally results in stone formation or recurrent urinary tract infections. Laser ablation has shown some initial success.[66,67] Stone debris can be readily removed during urethroscopy in the majority of cases. In severe cases or those associated with recurrent urinary tract infections, the affected neourethra is best excised and repaired with hairless skin by means of a small patch graft or a short island pedicle.

Some patients develop *recurrent urinary tract infections*. A thorough evaluation generally uncovers urethral diverticulum, redundant urethroplasty, or stricture. Occasionally, a voiding cystourethrogram demonstrates an enlarged prostatic utricle as described earlier. The presence of an enlarged prostatic utricle can promote urinary stasis and can provide a chronic reservoir for bacteria. If no other source of infection can be found in these patients, consideration should be given to either excision or fulguration of the utricle.[18]

Psychiatric Consequences

Psychiatric consequences have been identified in both children and adults who have undergone hypospadias repair. In a study of 6- to 10-year-old patients, Sandberg and colleagues[68] identified more behavior problems and poorer school performance in patients with hypospadias when compared with age-matched controls. These factors correlated positively with the extent of the initial hypospadias repair. In a series of adults who underwent hypospadias correction at an average age of 5 years, 38% had limited or no sexual experience (mean age, 27 years).[69] Overall, these patients tended to have fewer sexual partners and were older when they began sexual activity.

In general adult patients with a history of hypospadias repair do not manifest major psychiatric disturbances. However they tend to be less satisfied with penile appearance, have more inhibitions in seeking sexual contacts as a result of embarrassment, and have a more negative genital appraisal. These patients tend to manifest more anxiety, hostility, and lower self-esteem, some of which may be ameliorated by operating at an earlier age.[70,71]

Complex Hypospadias

Although the majority of complications arising from hypospadias repair can be readily managed with one or two interventions, a small subset of patients becomes caught in a cycle of repeated operations, each more difficult than the previous and with a less successful outcome. These patients with complex hypospadias represent a formidable challenge to the pediatric urologist. The penis is often inordinately scarred and lacks supple, well-vascularized tissues for reconstruction. Patients generally have several coexistent problems to be corrected, and the existing deformity is often worse than the original congenital defect.

Devine[72] reasoned that "once complications have occurred in hypospadias repairs, the surgeon has a tendency to attempt small operations, hoping to convert failure with a minimum of effort. This generally makes matters worse. In these cases, extensive resection of scarring, major shifts of tissues and meticulous reconstruction will usually be found necessary to transform a difficult problem into a therapeutic success." We fully agree with this stance. The successful approach to these patients invariably requires radical excision of diseased tissue and aggressive reconstruction of the defect.

Although we prefer to use local skin flaps to grafts in urethral construction, patients with complex hypospadias rarely possess sufficient usable genital skin. This situation necessitates the transfer of tissue from extragenital sites. Several sources for tissue grafts have been proposed. We have been less than enthusiastic about one-stage rolled skin grafts. Although many surgeons have reported initial success, significant late complications such as graft shrinkage and stricture led us to abandon the use of these grafts.[73] Furthermore, the initial enthusiasm for bladder mucosal grafts in these patients has waned. Keating and associates[74] extensively reviewed the results of this technique and reported an overall 40% complication rate. Complications related to the neomeatus have been the major drawback of bladder mucosal grafts. The neomeatus may prolapse in a cauliflower-type deformity in $\leq$38% of patients.[75]

A search for other sources of extragenital tissue led several investigators to favor the use of buccal mucosa in complex urethra reconstruction.[76,77] This tissue is ideally suited to urethral reconstruction. It is well adapted to contact with both fluid and air. The tissue is permissive to the ingrowth of blood vessels and resistant to infection, and it causes little morbidity at the donor site. Because of its elasticity and good tensile strength, buccal mucosa can be used as an onlay graft, an inlay graft, or a tube graft and can generally be used to reconstruct the urethra in a single stage.

Harvesting the buccal graft proceeds as outlined by Eppley and colleagues.[78] Strict attention to removing all nonmucosal tissue is important for future revascularization. Construction of a graft 20% larger than the needed surface area allows for graft contraction. When choosing between labial and buccal grafts, we prefer to use the labial graft because intraoperative access is easier. For longer defects in complex cases or in older children, buccal mucosa can be used because it allows for a larger graft size. Our practice has been to close the defect when harvesting these grafts.

Mohkless and associates[79] described the technique of graft placement well. When the graft is placed as an inlay, the urethral plate is split all the way to the location of our future neomeatus to form a deep groove in the glans for good recession of the graft and for creation of sufficient space to close the glans wings over the neourethra easily. The graft is secured laterally and at multiple sites over the length of the graft. These surgeons described a technique of placing small incisions in the graft to prevent blood accumulation, but we have not found this technique necessary in our practice. When performing a staged operation, we usually allow 6 months before proceeding with tubularization and skin closure.

Bracka[80] popularized a two-stage technique for the repair of hypospadias that is especially applicable to complex hypospadias with limited genital skin. He reported success with initial resection of scarred tissue and correction of chordee, creation of a glans slit, and at the same time grafting of buccal mucosa or preputial skin in the urethral and glandular bed. In a second stage, the vertical strip of grafted tissue is then used to form the neourethra, with adjacent layers of water-proofing coverage provided by local tissue flaps. This method is versatile and can be applied to both primary proximal hypospadias and reoperative hypospadias.[79,81] Although Bracka initially described this technique using a preputial graft, more recent studies reported excellent use with buccal mucosa grafts. Histologic analysis of grafted buccal mucosa showed favorable neovascularity and excellent graft uptake.[79]

CONCLUSION

The surgical repair of hypospadias remains one of the most challenging issues in the field of pediatric urology. Although improvements in technique, instrumentation, and perioperative care have profoundly advanced this surgical endeavor, a successful outcome still places great demands on the physician. By understanding the factors involved in the development of complications and by possessing a rational plan for the management of these complications, urologists are better equipped to provide their patients with optimal care.

KEY POINTS

1. Hypospadias repair requires meticulous attention to detail, especially with regard to tissue handling and creation of local tissue flaps.
2. When faced with complex hypospadias either in primary or reoperative situations, the surgeon must have a variety of techniques available to be able to individualize the operation to the needs of the patient.
3. When necessary, staging of the hypospadias operation may provide adequate time for graft healing and chordee corrections, thus facilitating more effective urethroplasty at a second stage.
4. Use of a barrier layer with local tissue is crucial for reinforcing the urethroplasty and for preventing the formation of fistulas.
5. When evaluating a hypospadias complication, the surgeon should be careful to address all factors that may have contributed to the complication and not just the complication in isolation.
6. In a patient with a complication, the surgeon must be willing to revise the entire repair if other treatments would leave the patient less than satisfied or at high risk of a second, later complication caused by correction of the initial complication.

REFERENCES

Please see www.expertconsult.com

Chapter 61

COMPLICATIONS OF SURGERY FOR DISORDERS OF SEX DEVELOPMENT

Jason M. Wilson MD
Associate Professor, Division of Urology, Department of Surgery, University of New Mexico, Albuquerque, New Mexico

Laurence Baskin MD
Professor and Chief, Pediatric Urology, University of California–San Francisco Children's Hospital, San Francisco, California

Disorders of sex development (DSDs) can be defined by congenital conditions in which development of chromosomal, gonadal, or anatomic sex is atypical. These abnormalities comprise a myriad of disorders as illustrated in Table 61-1.[1] Debate has centered on the timing of genital surgery and on whether surgical treatment should be delayed until such time as the patient can be involved in the surgical decision-making process. Surgical procedures in patients with 46, XX DSD are most commonly encountered and have traditionally been performed early in life to avoid potential psychological stressors involved in rearing the child. The difficulty in the objective assessment of perceived psychological complications associated with genital ambiguity contributes to a lack of culturally adjusted, control-matched data that may help in solidifying the medical consensus in regard to management.

Discussion shall proceed under the assumption that patients in whom surgical treatment is deemed necessary have met and evaluated by an assembled gender assignment team composed of chosen, experienced individuals in the fields of endocrinology, pediatric urology or surgery, psychology, social work, and genetics or dysmorphology. The purpose of such a team is to inform the legal guardians thoroughly of all available options including expectant management and the current state of and expected outcome in each area of reconstruction considered. Particular attention should also be given to discussion of psychosexual outcomes data or lack thereof. In patients who require surgical treatment, the surgeon has the responsibility to outline the surgical sequence and subsequent consequences from infancy to adulthood. Only surgeons with specific expertise in the care of these patients and specific training in the surgical treatment of DSDs should undertake these procedures.

For the purpose of discussion, it is useful to categorize patients in whom surgical treatment is necessary into three general groups:

1. Overvirilization
2. Vaginal agenesis
3. Undervirilization and gonadal abnormalities
   Each category is discussed in turn in this chapter.

OVERVIRILIZATION

The most common cause of overvirilization is congenital adrenal hyperplasia (CAH), and 21-hydroxylase is responsible for 90% of cases. Surgical treatment should be considered only in cases of severe virilization (Prader III, IV, and V) and should be performed in conjunction, when appropriate, with repair of the common urogenital sinus. Parents now appear to be less inclined to choose surgical treatment for children with less severe clitoromegaly.[1] The only known function of the clitoris is in contribution to sexual pleasure.[2-3] Because orgasmic function and erectile sensation may be disturbed by clitoral surgery, the surgical procedure should be anatomically based to preserve erectile function and the innervation of the clitoris. Further delineation of neurovascular anatomy has allowed a more direct and conscious approach when clitoral surgery is necessary, to preserve the neural architecture important in the sensory aspect of sexual pleasure.[4-6]

Nerve density is lacking in the 12-o'clock position in contrast to the densely innervated 11- and 1-o'clock positions in respect to dorsal nerve distribution. In one report, cavernous nerves were noted to perforate the tunica albuginea of the dorsal clitoral bodies near the crus.[6] The nerve distribution suggested by this study seems to correlate with reported areas of sensitivity and ease of orgasm as demonstrated by Schober and associates.[7] Despite evolving understanding of the neurovascular anatomy of the clitoris, it remains difficult to predict what types of surgical procedure will irrevocably alter clitoral sensation and sexual pleasure. Investigators have suggested that any type of clitoral surgery significantly alters sensation. Crouch and colleagues[8] reported

TABLE 61-1	**Classification of Disorders of Sex Development**	
Sex Chromosome DSDs	**46,XY DSDs**	**46,XX DSDs**

A. 45,X (Turner's syndrome and variants)	A. Disorders of gonadal (testicular) development
	  1. Complete gonadal dysgenesis (Swyer's syndrome)
	  2. Partial gonadal dysgenesis
	  3. Gonadal regression
	  4. Ovotesticular DSDs
		A. Disorders of gonadal (ovarian) development
		  1. Ovotesticular DVDs
		  2. Testicular DSDs (e.g., SRY+, dup 5OX9)
		  3. Gonadal dysgenesis

B. 47,XXY (Klinefelter's syndrome and variants)	B. Disorders in androgen synthesis or action
	  1. Androgen biosynthesis defect (e.g., 17-hydroxysteroid dehydrogenase deficiency, 5α-reductase deficiency, StAR mutations)
	  2. Defect in androgen action (e.g., CAIS, PAIS)
	  3. LH receptor defects (e.g., Leydig cell hypoplasia, aplasia)
	  4. Disorders of AMH and AMH receptor (persistent müllerian duct syndrome)
		B. Androgen excess
		  1. Fetal (e.g., 21-hydroxylase deficiency, 11-hydroxylase deficiency)
		  2. Fetoplacental (aromatase deficiency, POR)
		  3. Maternal (e.g., luteoma, exogenous)

C. 45,X/46,XY (mixed gonadal dysgenesis, ovotesticular DSD) D. 46,XX/46,XY (chimeric, ovotesticular DSDs)	C. Other (e.g., severe hypospadias, cloacal exstrophy)	C. Other (e.g., cloacal exstrophy, vaginal atresia, MURCS, other syndromes)

AMH, antimüllerian hormone; CAIS, complete androgen insensitivity syndrome; DSDs, disorders of sex development; LH, luteinizing hormone; MURCS, müllerian, renal, cervicothoracic somite abnormalities; PAIS, partial androgen insensitivity syndrome; POR, cytochrome P-450 oxidoreductase, StAR, steroidogenic acute regulatory protein.

that five of six women who had undergone feminizing genitoplasty had abnormal sensation results in response to temperature and vibration. One of the patients had undergone surgical treatment within 1 year of the study and conceivably had benefited from improved surgical techniques.[8] This finding demonstrates a typical situation in that it is often difficult to determine exactly what type of surgical procedure has been performed and whether newer techniques will impart preserved neurovascularity.

Two case reports in the literature noted that the preservation of dorsal and ventral neurovascular bundles while preserving the glans during reduction clitoroplasty imparted no difficulty in achieving orgasm or perceived decreased clitoral sensation. These surgical techniques were suggested as reproducible operations in children.[9-10] Thus, emphasis is on functional outcome rather than on strictly cosmetic appearance. Clinical trials in which success is judged solely on an acceptable aesthetic result are conspicuously insufficient and ignore the potential loss of psychosexual adjustment. It is also unreasonable to assume that preservation of neurovascular anatomic features will result in "normal" development and a gratifying sexual life. Investigators generally believe that surgical procedures performed for cosmetic reasons in the first year of life relieve parental distress and improve attachment between the child and the parents.[1]

The current recommendation is that surgical treatment, when necessary, be performed between the ages of 6 and 12 months. Evidence on the establishment of functional anatomy is inadequate to abandon the practice of early separation of the vagina and urethra.[1] The rationale for early reconstruction is based on guidelines on the timing of genital surgery from the American Academy of Pediatrics, the beneficial effects of estrogen on tissue in early infancy, anecdotally reported and experienced difficulty in performing feminizing surgery in adolescent and adult patients, and the avoidance of potential complications from the connection between the urinary tract and the peritoneum through the fallopian tubes.[1] It is anticipated that surgical reconstruction in infancy will need to be refined at puberty.[1]

Although it is considered acceptable to undertake surgical correction of the common urogenital sinus at an early age, one must be aware and accepting of the likelihood of further surgical intervention in adolescence. Fourteen girls who had early surgical procedures were reassessed near adolescence and were found to have abundant fibrosis and scarring.[11] Another series reported the need for further surgical procedures in similarly treated young girls with CAH in 43 of 44 patients to correct poor cosmesis or to correct introital stenosis.[12] It is currently unknown whether newer surgical techniques will lessen the need for surgical treatment later in life.

Several studies suggested that urogenital sinus mobilization, when possible, may decrease the risk of vaginal stenosis, especially if this procedure is performed early in life. These findings led to the further application and refinement of partial urogenital mobilization in feminizing surgery for the patient with CAH.[13-16] Encouraging early results based on position and caliber of vaginal introitus require longer follow-up to clarify further whether improved technique and early surgical treatment obviate the need for revisions in pubertal female patients. The current trend toward delayed operative intervention paralleled by the continued refinement of early surgical technique may produce enlightening outcomes data on psychological, physiologic, and anatomic function in these differently managed groups of patients.

VAGINAL AGENESIS AND VAGINOPLASTY

An absent or inadequate vagina (with rare exceptions) requires a vaginoplasty performed in adolescence when the patient is psychologically motivated and a full partner in the procedure. No one technique has been universally successful; self-dilation, skin substitution, and bowel vaginoplasty each has specific advantages and disadvantages.

Considering a low vaginal confluence, the most popularly employed technique of vaginoplasty is skin substitution of the posterior vagina through an omega flap. The omega flap is a modification of the perineal skin flap proposed and developed by Fortunoff, Lattimer, and Edson.[17] Twenty-eight patients with a salt-losing form of CAH underwent posterior flap vaginoplasty between 1997 and 2001. Twenty-six of these patients had a low vaginal confluence. The age of these patients ranged from 5 months to 17 years, and follow-up was between 1 and 4 years. Nine patients had undergone previous surgical procedures but none had had prior vaginoplasty. None of the patients required further surgical treatment of vaginal stenosis or inadequate caliber, although 2 patients were undergoing continued vaginal dilation without reported difficulty.[18]

Jenak and colleagues[19] described the use of a narrow-based (omega) perineal skin flap to create a widened introitus. Four of the six patients had CAH and follow-up ranged from 1 to 9 months. The mean vaginal calibration in four patients was 10.5 Hegar.[19] The initial cosmetic results noted in these two reports were encouraging, but long-term follow-up is needed to determine the functional capacity imparted in early versus late surgical vaginoplasty.

Another technique described, requiring 1.5 to 2 cm of urethral length, combines urogenital sinus mobilization with creation of urogenital sinus flaps. These urogenital sinus flaps can be posteromedially rotated to form a posterior vagina that is mucosa lined and thus obviate the need for a perineal skin flap. The group reported a mean follow-up of 2.5 years without vaginal stenosis or the need for vaginal dilation. The age range was 3 months to 13 years and CAH was present in 7 of the 11 patients. Most of these procedures were accomplished with a perineal approach (8 of 11).[20] A major concern is whether the vagina will undergo stenosis or fibrosis that will increase the possibility of painful or unpleasant penetrative sexual intercourse in the future. Because assessment of successful results should incorporate both the feasibility and the quality of sexual intercourse, continuing methods of evaluating the quality of sexual life must be developed.

High vaginal confluence is generally considered to be >3 cm.[13] From a surgical standpoint, a high vaginal confluence indicates a position near or proximal to the urethral sphincter and the need for a vaginal pull-through procedure.[21-22] The likelihood of encountering this anatomic feature in a patient with CAH is 5%.[23] Vaginal pull-through requires separation of the vagina from the urethra and increases the probability of complications such as urethral stricture, urethrovaginal fistula, and urinary incontinence.

Hendren and Atala[21] reported the results of 16 female patients with high vaginal confluence and CAH who had undergone repair procedures using the described technique for pull-through with superior and inferior U-flaps and partially mobilized labia majora between 1962 and 1993. At the time of the report, 9 of 16 women were adults and 6 of the 9 were sexually active (5 of 6 with heterosexual preference and 1 of 6 with bisexual orientation). One woman had given birth to a child by cesarean section, and at the time this was the first reported birth after a pull-through operation for high vaginal confluence.

In 1994, Donahoe and Gustafson[24] advocated a one-stage repair for patients at an early age and cited a high incidence of vaginal stenosis with the two-staged pull-through procedure. Three older patients aged 2, 3.2, and 9.2 years required the use of posterior buttock flaps. Three younger children aged 8, 8, and 12 months did not require such flaps, and vaginoplasty was undertaken with the use of local tissue and a posterior, perineal skin flap. Follow-up at 6 weeks with endoscopic and anesthetic-aided examination and follow-up at 5 to 17 months indicated no fistulas and an adequate introital caliber. These investigators noted the importance of long-term follow-up to detect delayed vaginal stenosis. They also noted that injury to the urethra was of particular concern.[24]

A posterior approach as described by Pena and colleagues[25] included division of the rectum and creation of a diverting colostomy. Subsequently, Rink and associates[26] described a posterior prone approach in which the rectum was retracted and division avoided. Eight patients aged 6 months to 25 years underwent the procedure. Four had ambiguous genitalia and the other half had a pure urogenital sinus anomaly. Follow-up ranged from 6 months to 5 years and one patient was sexually active. These investigators noted greater mobility of tissue and no increased technical difficulty in the younger patients. One of the older patients required ongoing vaginal dilation for mild vaginal stenosis and a teenaged patient had an asymptomatic urethrovaginal fistula noted during cystoscopic examination.[26]

True vaginal agenesis is a rare condition consisting of primary amenorrhea and an intact hypothalamic-pituitary-gonadal axis in a genotypically and phenotypically normal female patient. Numerous techniques are described, dating as far back as 1817, when Dupuytren described creation of a pouch that could epithelialize without the use of a mold, to create a vagina in place of its absence or in place of a small vaginal dimple.[27] Technique has evolved with a common goal: creation of a functional vaginal vault in concordance with the desire of the patient, who accepts the ongoing need for self-dilation and commits to that regimen.

Nonsurgical dilation was first described by Frank in 1938.[28] Subsequently, the technique was described as successful and easier to perform using the patient's weight instead of digital pressure, especially when patients had no history of earlier surgical procedures and were motivated by an active sexual relationship.[28-32] Vaginal creation has been successful in 43% to 91% of patients by using the technique as described by Frank and further modified by Ingram.[33] In these patients, success is determined by the presence of a vagina that allows satisfactory penetrative sexual intercourse. Ingram's modification and initial report[33] involved 12 women with primary vaginal agenesis, and 62.5% of a total of 24 women (12 of whom had vaginal stenosis) reported comfortable sexual intercourse after 4 to 6 months of progressive dilation.

Surgical management of vaginal agenesis (**Figs. 61-1 and 61-2**) can be broken down into three categories:

1. Creation of space between bladder and rectum and use of mold and covering
2. Vulvovaginoplasty using skin flaps
3. Bowel segment vaginoplasty

The primary advantage at the time of inception of the first-described use of a mold in a created perineal space was avoidance of the peritoneum. Different coverings have been used with variable success, including peritoneum, split-thickness skin grafts (STSG), bladder mucosa, amnion, and peritoneofascial flaps.[34-37]

Thirty-two women aged 17 to 39 years underwent surgical creation of vagina using a mold and STSG harvested from gluteus or thigh.[35] On postoperative day 7, the mold was removed to allow determination of STSG take, and it was then used continuously for 3 months. After time, it was possible to use the mold for 1 hour per week to avoid shrinkage. In judging the success of the procedure, these investigators used several criteria: STSG take, presence and degree of pseudomucinous metaplasia and associated sensitivity, vaginal dimensions and variation over time, and characteristics of sexual relationships. No regrafting was needed, and the

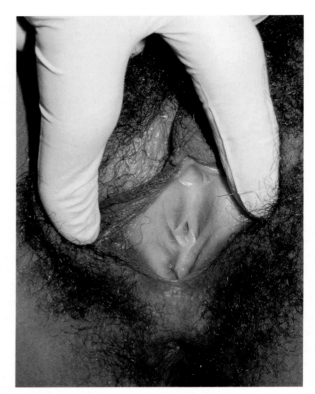

Figure 61-1 Gross photograph of the introitus of a female patient with vaginal agenesis.

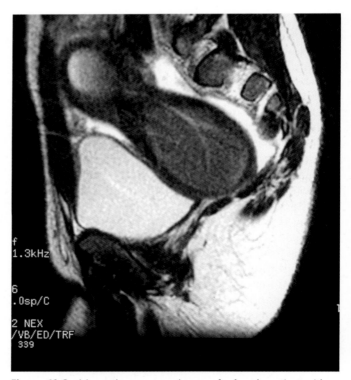

Figure 61-2 Magnetic resonance image of a female patient with complete vaginal agenesis. Note the dilated uterus with retained menstrual fluid.

rate of complete STSG take was 90.6%. Average vaginal dimensions were 10 cm in length and 4 cm in diameter. Twenty-seven of 32 (84.3%) women reported normal sexual activity with good sensitivity and 5 did not engage in sexual intercourse. The rate of complications was 9.3% for partial take of STSG and 6.2% for partial vaginal stricture. One patient had total vaginal stricture. Success in outcome depended on mold management adherence or regular sexual activity.[35]

Long-term outcome in this type of reconstruction is directly related to the patient's motivation and willingness to comply with postoperative management and the desire for or presence of sexual intercourse.[38] An extensive retrospective review of 201 cases was reported in 1996.[39] A modified Abbe-McIndoe procedure was performed in all cases with an average patient age of 20.5 years. In most cases, the impetus for performing reconstruction was the patient's desire to engage in sexual relationships. Follow-up was from 3 to 16 years and the investigators reported low morbidity and high success rates. In this review, 156 women completed a sexual satisfaction questionnaire; 112 (71.8%) reported their sexual life as good or satisfactory, considering the presence of lubrication and the absence of dyspareunia, and some within this group noted insufficient vaginal lubrication. Reported complications were low and included graft site infection (5.5%), graft infection (4%), and rectal perforation (1%). The investigators recommended that surgical reconstruction be delayed until regular sexual intercourse is anticipated or desired by patient.

The use of skin in vulvovaginoplasty has been described by several surgeons, with modern approaches derived from those described by Sheares, Fortunoff, Williams, and Hendren. Use of local skin in creation of a distal vagina in the case of a severely masculinized female patient with whom the decision has been made for reconstruction often requires more than a perineal skin flap. A proximal vaginal confluence increases the concern for incontinence and vaginal stenosis after reconstruction. Hendren and Donahoe[40] described the creation of lateral and anterior walls of the distal vagina by using bilateral, medially rotated buttock flaps. Passerini-Glazel[41] described the use of local skin for creation of distal vagina, advocated this technique for patients with proximal and distal vaginal confluence, and suggested that the procedure could be used at any age.

The use of musculocutaneous flaps is avoided in this patient population secondary to the considerable bulk of such flaps. The use of tissue expansion in the labia minora can create hairless, abundant, elastic, and well-vascularized flaps for creation of the distal vagina.[42] Donahoe and Gustafson[24] noted in 1994 that in patients presenting for vaginal exteriorization as part of a two-staged procedure, the use of bilateral rotated buttock flaps was necessary. In management of infants with a proximal vaginal confluence, no additional skin was needed for a posterior perineal-based flap and an anterior subphallic skin flap.[24] Based on the experience and comparison between the two techniques, the investigators recommended early, one-stage reconstruction and emphasized the mobility of tissue and the use of labia minora and majora flaps for anterior and lateral introitus construction.[24]

Long-term follow-up in patients undergoing Passerini-Glazel feminizing genitoplasty demonstrated a significant difference in incidence of vaginal stenosis between two groups of patients. The first group, who had undergone the surgical procedure at a mean age of 2 years, was noted to have a 45% (10 of 22) incidence of vaginal stenosis. The incidence of vaginal stenosis was 25% (6 of 24) in the group who underwent the procedure at a mean age of 14 years and who had a history of other surgical procedures performed at younger ages. The overall incidence of vaginal stenosis was noted to be 35%.[43]

When multiple approaches and the timing of surgical treatment are taken into consideration, the incidence of vaginal stenosis ranges from 11% to 94%. The decision to perform early reconstructive surgery should include the expectation for minor surgical procedures (i.e., introitoplasty) near the adolescent period.[11,12,21,44,45] Repair of vaginal stenosis should be undertaken at puberty when estrogen levels are high, to facilitate healing and to decrease the likelihood of recurrence.

Bowel segment vaginoplasty was initially described by Baldwin in 1904 and was subsequently avoided because of complications including several deaths.[27] The use of bowel to create a functional vagina has been associated with long-term complications unique to the use of a colonic segment such as the reported occurrence of diversion colitis associated with mucous discharge and bleeding.[46] Other complications or unwanted long-term associations include enteric segment prolapse, stenosis, and the long-term need for daily use of absorbent liners or douching for copious mucoid discharge.

Parsons and associates[47] reviewed 28 patients who had undergone colovaginoplasty and identified the following postoperative complications: introital stenosis (4 of 28), mucosal prolapse (4 of 28), partial small bowel obstruction (2 of 28), perineal hematoma (2 of 28), wound infection (2 of 28), and vaginal prolapse (1 of 28). The complication rate was 50%. The mean follow-up period was 6.2 years, and the patients in the review believed that adolescence was an appropriate time to undergo the procedure. Despite the high complication rate, long-term patency and cosmesis were not affected and 15 of 16 adult patients were sexually active.[47]

Hendren and Atala[48] reported on a large volume of patients who had undergone bowel segment vaginoplasty for various conditions. The most common complication was mucosal prolapse, occurring in 16 of 65 patients. The prolapse was easily repaired with a simple trimming and the investigators believed that technical changes to avoid this minor complication would predispose the patient to more serious complications such as stenosis or bowel segment retraction. Recommendations from this report included early reconstruction to avoid the psychological ramifications of an absent vagina and daily douching with normal saline solution to prevent the accumulation of foul-smelling mucoid concretions.[48]

A published review of sigmoid vaginoplasty performed at a mean patient age of 16.8 years in 14 female patients with congenital vaginal agenesis indicated that the procedure provided a cosmetically suitable, self-lubricating vagina without the need for routine dilation, although daily irrigation and dilation were implemented for 8 weeks postoperatively. The psychosexual status of these patients was reported as acceptable, and no complaints of dyspareunia were reported. The patient population in the study was unique in that they had all presented at the inception of marriage arrangements. This finding indicates that the successful results were associated with older patients motivated, presumably, by the prospect of an active sexual life. Mean follow-up was 4.1 years.[49]

A review of the literature suggests that very few patients with CAH require the use of an enteric segment for construction of a functional vagina. In deciding whether to proceed with early as opposed to delayed reconstruction, one must weigh the potential psychological aspects of an absent vagina throughout childhood and early adolescence against the reported complications of vaginal stenosis and chronic discharge. Once again, evidence-based literature to help in establishing an algorithmic approach to decision making in this type of reconstruction is conspicuously lacking, and it is of utmost importance to consider each patient individually and to incorporate anatomic, physiologic, and psychosexual facets of personal development into the decision-making process. Family counseling and education with a multidisciplinary team approach are crucial.

UNDERVIRILIZATION AND GONADAL ABNORMALITIES

The undervirilized newborn with a DSD should be approached in the same manner as previously described, with a multidisciplinary approach in an experienced medical center. The historically described emergency status of the newborn with ambiguous genitalia has been challenged, and referral to an experienced center is always possible after the workup has ruled out true emergencies such as salt-wasting adrenal hyperplasia. 46,XY DSD is characterized by a spectrum of medical conditions including hypospadias, genetic syndromes, androgen receptor abnormalities, defects in androgen biosynthesis, and gonadal abnormalities. A specific

diagnosis is identified in 50% of children with 46,XY DSD, in contrast to those children with 46,XX DSD.[1] Assuming that each patient has been carefully evaluated with full family participation and education, surgical treatment can proceed appropriately after consideration of factors including fertility, sexual function, degree of in utero exposure to androgens, psychosexuality, and culture.

In the case of a DSD associated with hypospadias, standard techniques for surgical repair such as chordee correction, urethral reconstruction, and the judicious use of testosterone supplementation apply.[1] An animal model of penile growth subsequent to testosterone stimulation indicated that the early use of synthetic androgen to achieve a more normal penis in childhood may ultimately result in the absence of further growth during puberty and result in a significantly smaller phallus.[50] Therefore, caution should be exercised when testosterone supplementation is considered.

The magnitude and complexity of phalloplasty in adulthood should be taken into account during the initial counseling period if successful gender assignment depends on this procedure.[51] At times this may affect the balance of gender assignment. Patients must not be given unrealistic expectations about penile reconstruction, including the use of tissue engineering. No evidence indicates that prophylactic removal of asymptomatic discordant structures, such as an utriculus or müllerian remnants, is required although future symptoms may indicate surgical removal.

In a review including 57 patients over 20 years who were undergoing masculinizing genitoplasty, only 2 patients required excision of an utriculus. In this review, 77% of patients had severe penoscrotal hypospadias and 33% had perineal hypospadias.[52] Technique-specific, long-term outcome data are not sufficient to determine whether refinement in surgical technique will decrease the incidence of long-term complications. One-stage techniques may offer superior cosmetic and functional outcomes without the potential psychological trauma of repeated genital surgery.

Miller and Grant[53] reported on 19 patients in whom staged procedures had been performed for severe hypospadias. Only 7 patients reported satisfactory ejaculation and 15 reported satisfactory erection and orgasm. A questionnaire completed by 22 men aged 18 to 26 years in whom surgical treatment had been performed in childhood for hypospadias (severe, 11) identified penile size as a cause of dissatisfaction.[54] Age-matched controls showed no significant differences in sexual behavior, and a slightly higher rate of dissatisfaction was reported in the surgical group (40.9% versus 34.2%).

Using the described modern surgical techniques involving inner preputial skin, Chertin and colleagues[52] performed masculinizing genitoplasty in 39 patients at a median age of 1.8 years. With a median follow-up of 6 years, 10 patients required further surgical procedures for urethral breakdown (3), urethrocutaneous fistula (5), and excision of utriculus (2).

Lam and associates[55] reported on the outcome in 27 male patients who had undergone two-stage repair of hypospadias in infancy for congenitally located meatus at midshaft or more proximally. Five patients had a DSD and hypospadias. Additional surgical treatment had been necessary in 5 patients for excision of diverticulum, in 3 patients for fistula, and in 4 with minor urethral strictures. Forty percent of patients experienced spraying of the urinary stream but were able to stand and urinate. Nine of 20 patients who were able to ejaculate reported the need to "milk" the ejaculate. All patients reported satisfaction with genitourinary function and 23 of 27 were happy with their penile appearance.[55]

When considering masculinizing genitoplasty for the patient with a DSD, one must be mindful of potential complications of müllerian remnants and dysgenetic gonadal tissue. Utricular manifestations may include chronic urinary dribbling, recurrent urinary tract infection, and multiple failed attempts at hypospadias repair. Desantel and colleagues[56] found a high risk of infertility in patients undergoing surgical treatment for symptomatic utricles. This condition was thought to be either secondary to abnormal anatomic insertion of ejaculatory ducts or vas deferens or caused by operative injury.

The severity of hypospadias or micropenis should not be considered when one determines the sex of rearing in the patient without an androgen receptor defect. Current data do not support the amputation of sexually sensitive and functional but small male phallic structures.[51,57,58] Another review of patients with micropenis noted that either male or female gender assignment was possible, and no patients sought gender reassignment. The investigators noted a higher complication rate in feminizing surgery and a higher rate of dissatisfaction with external genital appearance and concluded that male gender assignment was preferable.[59]

In management of the patient with a DSD, removal of gender-discordant structures is generally directed by symptoms or risk of malignant disease. Specifically, varying degrees of gonadal dysgenesis may be present and may necessitate surveillance or removal of this tissue. This situation is encountered in the patient with a DSD and Y chromosomal material. Several gene mutations that have been identified and documented are associated with DSDs and a propensity toward gonadal malignant disease.[1,60]

Historically, gonadal biopsy and excision were performed using laparotomy. More recent trends support the use of laparoscopy for diagnosis, biopsy, and excision of aberrant or discordant structures.[61-64] Standard laparoscopic techniques apply, and three-port placement is sufficient for surgical procedures in the pelvis. Bladder drainage increases visualization and reduces the chance of injury during laparoscopic pelvic surgical procedures, particularly in the patient weighing <15 kg.

The testes in patients with complete androgen insensitivity syndrome and in those with partial androgen insensitivity syndrome who are raised as girls should be removed to prevent malignant disease in adulthood.[1] The availability of estrogen replacement therapy allows for the option of early removal of testes at the time of diagnosis. This approach also takes care of the associated hernia, psychological problems with the presence of testes, and the malignancy risk. Parental choice allows deferment of treatment until adolescence, because the earliest reported malignancy in complete androgen insensitivity syndrome occurred at 14 years of age.[1]

The streak gonad in a patient with mixed gonadal dysgenesis who is raised as a boy should be removed laparoscopically (or by laparotomy) in early childhood.[1] Bilateral gonadectomy is performed in early childhood in girls (bilateral streak gonads) with gonadal dysgenesis and Y chromosome material. In patients with androgen biosynthetic defects who are raised as girls, gonadectomy should be undertaken before puberty. A scrotal testis in patients with gonadal dysgenesis is at risk for malignant disease.

Current recommendations are testicular biopsy at puberty to seek signs of the premalignant lesion termed *carcinoma in situ* or *undifferentiated intratubular germ cell neoplasia*. If results of the biopsy are positive, the option is sperm banking before treatment with local low-dose radiation therapy, which is curative.[1] Surgical management of DSDs should also consider options that will facilitate the chances of fertility. In patients with a symptomatic utriculus, removal is best undertaken laparoscopically to increase the chance of preserving continuity of the vasa deferentia.

Patients with bilateral ovotestes are potentially fertile from functional ovarian tissue.[1] Separation of ovarian and testicular tissue can be technically difficult and should be undertaken, if possible, in early life. Four fifths of ovotestes will demonstrate tissue that is adjacent and clearly demarcated in an end-to-end fashion.[65]

Growing numbers of specialty trained and experienced physicians, advocacy and support groups, and well-informed patients and families herald a future for the child with a DSD that is free of stigma and abounds with the opportunity for a life of choice. It is quite clear that technical advances have decreased the number of surgical procedures and complications associated with DSDs. The possibility of delaying surgical treatment when it is not immediately necessary will perhaps provide the community with a patient population that is older and more involved in the treatment decision-making process. This would provide the community with a control population to illuminate the areas of neuroanatomic and psychosexual functioning further. For example, we may learn that, regardless of age at surgical reconstruction, the patient with a DSD is more likely to have difficulty in adjusting.

Education and further clinical trials undoubtedly will clarify this issue in the future, particularly with emphasis on all facets of outcome, including an extrapolation of the previously held notion that successful outcome was based on appearance and the ability to engage in conventional sexual intercourse. Expanding models of sexuality will aid in defining a reproducible measure of sexual function and psychological well-being. Critical factors should remain well within the foreground during discussions with family and health care providers: preservation of fertility, preservation of sexually sensitive tissue, measures for determining successful outcome, cultural and societal factors, and the time honored, sage admonition—*primum non nocere.*

KEY POINTS

1. The newborn with a DSD must be evaluated for salt-wasting adrenal hyperplasia.
2. An assembled team of multidisciplinary experts should be assigned the task of educating and treating patients with DSD and their families.
3. Surgical procedures must be undertaken cautiously with knowledge of the accumulated and growing body of data, stressing functional and psychosexual adjustment outcomes.

REFERENCES

Please see www.expertconsult.com

Index

Note: Page numbers followed by b, f, and t indicate boxes, figures, and tables, respectively.